LEDDY & PEPPER'S

PROFESSIONAL NURSING

NINTH EDITION

LEDDY & PEPPER'S

PROFESSIONAL NURSING

NINTH EDITION

Lucy Jane Hood, RN, PhD

Professor and Department Chair, Pre-Licensure
Nursing Education
MidAmerica Nazarene University
Olathe, Kansas

Professor Emeritus
Saint Luke's College of Health Sciences
Kansas City, Missouri

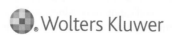

Philadelphia • Baltimore • New York • London
Buenos Aires • Hong Kong • Sydney • Tokyo

Senior Acquisitions Editor: Christina Burns
Associate Product Development Editor: Dan Reilly
Editorial Coordinator: Amberly Hyden
Editorial Assistant: Hilari Bowman
Senior Production Project Manager: Alicia Jackson
Design Coordinator: Holly McLaughlin
Illustration Coordinator: Jennifer Clements
Manufacturing Coordinator: Karin Duffield
Marketing Manager: Sarah Schuessler
Prepress Vendor: Aptara, Inc.

9th edition

9 8 7 6 5 4 3

Printed in China

Library of Congress Cataloging-in-Publication Data

Names: Hood, Lucy J., author.
Title: Leddy & Pepper's professional nursing / Lucy Jane Hood.
Other titles: Leddy & Pepper's conceptual bases of professional nursing |
   Leddy and Pepper's professional nursing | Professional nursing
Description: Ninth edition. | Philadelphia : Wolters Kluwer, [2018] |
   Preceded by Leddy & Pepper's conceptual bases of professional nursing /
   Lucy Jane Hood. Edition 8. 2014. | Includes bibliographical references and
   index.
Identifiers: LCCN 2017020451 | ISBN 9781496351364
Subjects: | MESH: Nursing Theory | Nursing–trends
Classification: LCC RT41 | NLM WY 86 | DDC 610.73–dc23 LC record available at https://lccn.loc.gov/2017020451

CCS0519

To all professional nurses who have a passion for nursing that enables them to share their values, beliefs, and skills to make differences in the lives of others and to shape the nursing profession. To Dr. Susan Leddy and Dr. Mae Pepper, who saw the need for a textbook to meet the needs of registered nurses who were continuing their education. To all the readers of this text who have the courage to take the risk of returning to school or pursuing a professional nursing career. To the following persons whose actions, values, and beliefs enabled me to live out my dream of being a professional nurse: my parents, Bob and Helen Chamberlin; Mary Belle Hickey, RN, my first nurse manager, who always challenged me to be the best possible nurse and gave me the confidence to pursue higher education; my dear mentor, Dr. Susan Leddy, professor of nursing who showed me the essence of nursing scholarship; and my loving husband, Michael, who selflessly gives me the time, support, and humor to live out my dreams.

L.J.H.

In Memory

J. Mae Pepper

January 18, 1936–March 19, 1997

For 20 years, Mae was Susan Leddy's colleague, coauthor, mentor, and friend. In 1977, Mae joined the faculty at Mercy College in Dobbs Ferry, New York. Mae's previous teaching experience at the University of North Carolina-Chapel Hill, New York University, and Bronx Community College, as well as her vision, wisdom, and dedication, was crucial to the development and accreditation of the new baccalaureate program for registered nurses and to the subsequent development of the first master's program at the college.

Mae held the position of Chairperson of the Nursing program from 1981 until her sudden death in March 1997 from a ruptured aortic aneurysm. Although she talked for years about leaving administration in order to do more scholarly work, she continued to serve as Chair out of a sense of duty and responsibility. She was devoted to the students and faculty, and very conscientious in her service to the College and many civic and professional organizations.

Mae found time to read voraciously, listen to music, care for animals, and to enjoy outdoor white-water rafting, camping, and bird watching. She loved her garden, was a careful craftsperson in her furniture refinishing, and liked to go to garage sales and flea markets looking for collectibles. Mae had a good sense of humor and loved a good time. Devoted to her friends and family, she willingly gave time and attention to anyone who asked. She was a great listener, and her counsel was always wise and kind. Mae lived her belief in mutuality, genuineness, and respect for others.

Susan Kun Leddy

February 23, 1939–February 23, 2007

For 14 years, Susan was my mentor and friend. We met in 1993 when I became a doctoral student at Widener University. Susan had a long distinguished career in nursing education. She set high academic standards for herself and also expected her students to attain them. Her favorite question posed to us was "So what?" thereby forcing us to verify the significance of what we said or wrote.

Susan earned a Bachelor of Science nursing degree from Skidmore College in New York in 1960. In 1965, she completed a master of science in nursing degree from Boston University. She completed a doctor of philosophy degree in 1973 at New York University. Never wanting to stop learning, she did postdoctoral work at Harvard University in 1985 and the University of Pennsylvania from 1996 to 1998.

During her first 4 years as a nurse educator, Susan taught in diploma schools and taught in the baccalaureate program at Columbia University before completing her doctoral studies. She and three other faculties founded the RN-BSN program at Pace University. In 1976, she was asked to do a feasibility study and generate a proposal to the state of New York to develop a new RN-to-BSN nursing program at Mercy College. As program chair, Susan and Mae Pepper both opened the program in 1977. The two of them realized the need for a textbook to meet the needs of registered nurses returning to school for baccalaureate education and co-wrote *Conceptual Bases for Nursing Practice* that was first published in 1981. After a trip to Wyoming, Susan became enthralled with the mountains. She moved to the state and became the first dean of the School of Nursing at the University of Wyoming in 1981. In 1984, she was appointed as the

Dean of the reconstituted College of Health Sciences at the University of Wyoming. In 1988, she returned to the East Coast as the Dean of the School of Nursing at Widener University in Chester, Pennsylvania until 1993 when she gave up her administrative position to assume teaching responsibilities mainly in the doctoral program.

Susan was a prolific scholar and has many journal publications. After her retirement and while battling breast cancer, Susan continued to write. In addition to previous editions of this text, she authored *Integrative Health Promotion: Conceptual Bases for Nursing Practice* and *Health Promotion: Mobilizing Strengths to Enhance Health, Wellness & Well-Being*. Both of these books received Book of the Year Awards from the *American Journal of Nursing*.

Susan made time to travel and visited nearly every place in the world. She found her trips exhilarating and stimulating. She incorporated many of the ideas from her travels into her Human Energy Model. Susan also enjoyed quilting, weaving, and dabbling in watercolors. She was very energetic and always had a project to accomplish.

Susan deeply loved her daughters, Deborah and Erin, and made certain that they had what they needed to pursue successful lives. She adored her granddaughter, Katie, who always got her to laugh and smile even through some very rough times.

Susan exemplified the life of a true scholar, superb teacher, and devoted mother. It is my hope to live up to the standards of my beloved mentor and friend. I miss her great words of wisdom and support.

Contributor

Karen D. Wiegman, PhD, MSN, RN
Dean, School of Nursing and Health Science,
    Professor
MidAmerica Nazarene University
    Olathe, Kansas

Reviewers

Elizabeth W. Black, MSN, RN
Assistant Professor
Gwynedd Mercy University
Gwynedd Valley, Pennsylvania

Billie Blake, RN, MSN, BSN, EdD, CNE
(Retired) Associate Dean of Nursing
St. Johns River State College
Orange Park, Florida

Laura Blank, RN, MSN
Associate Clinical Professor
Northern Arizona University
Flagstaff, Arizona

Annie Boucher, RN, MScN
Professor
Cambrian College
Sudbury, Canada

Mary Boylston, EdD, MSN, BSN, AHN-BC
Assistant Professor
Eastern University
St. Davids, Pennsylvania

Beryl K. Broughton, MSN, CRNP, CS, CNE
Nursing Faculty
ARIA Health School of Nursing
Trevose, Pennsylvania

Jennifer Bryer, PhD
Acting Assistant Dean, Chairperson,
    Associate Professor
Farmingdale State College
Farmingdale, New York

Kathy Burlingame, EdD, MSN, RN
Dean of Nursing
Galen College of Nursing
Louisville, Kentucky

Paula Byrne, DNP, RN
Assistant Professor and Chair
The College of St. Scholastica
Duluth, Minnesota

Ruth Chaplen, DNP, MSN, BSN
Associate Professor
Rochester College
Rochester Hills, Michigan

Betty Daniels, PhD, RN
Assistant Professor
Brenau University
Gainesville, Georgia

Karen Davis, DNP, RN, CNE
Clinical Assistant Professor
University of Arkansas for Medical Sciences
Little Rock, Arkansas

Lori A. Edwards, DrPH, MPH, RN, PHCNS-BC
Assistant Professor, Associate Director for Global
    Occupational Health
University of Maryland
Baltimore, Maryland

Marcus M. Gaut, DNP, RN
Assistant Professor
The University of Southern Mississippi
Hattiesburg, Mississippi

Evalyn J. Gossett, MSN, RN
Lecturer
Indiana University Northwest
Gary, Indiana

Debra Kantor, PhD, RN
Associate Professor
Molloy College
Rockville Centre, New York

Coleen Kumar, PhD, RN
Dean of Nursing
SUNY Downtown Medical Centre College of
    Nursing
Brooklyn, New York

**Kathleen M. Lamaute, EdD, MS, FNP-BC,
NEA-BC, CNE**
Associate Professor
Molloy College
Rockville Centre, New York

Debra Lee, PhD, BSN, RN
Assistant Professor, Dean of School of Nursing and
    Health Sciences
Malone University
Canton, Ohio

Rosemary Macy, PhD, RN, CNE, CHSE
Associate Professor
Boise State University
Boise, Idaho

Kari Mardian, MEd, BN, RN
Instructor
Medicine Hat College
Medicine Hat, Canada

Tammie McCoy, BA, BSN, MSN, PhD
Professor/Chair
Mississippi University for Women
Columbus, Mississippi

Valerie O'Dell, DNP, RN, CNE
Associate Professor/MSN Program Director
Youngstown University
Youngstown, Ohio

Teresa O'Neill, PhD, APRN, RNC
Distance Education Coordinator, Professor Emerita
University of Holy Cross
New Orleans, Louisiana

Cheryl Passel, PhD
Assistant Professor
Marian University
Fond du Lac, Wisconsin

JoAnne Pearce, MS RNC, APRN-BC
Assistant Professor
Idaho State University
Pocatello, Idaho

Theresa T. Quell, PhD, RN
Assistant Dean for Academic Programs
Fairfield University
Norwalk, Connecticut

Janet Reagor, RN, PhD
Interim Dean, Assistant Professor
Avila University
Kansas City, Missouri

Debra Simons, PhD, RN, CNE, CHSE, CCM
Associate Dean
College of New Rochelle
New Rochelle, New York

Diane Spoljoric, PhD, RNC, FNP
Associate Professor
Purdue Northwest
Westville, Indiana

Nancy Steffen, MSN
Instructor
Century College
White Bear Lake, Minnesota

Alicia Stone, PhD, MS, RN, FNP
Professor
Molloy College
Rockville Centre, New York

Wendy Wheeler, RN, BScN, MN
Continuous Nursing Faculty
Red Deer College
Red Deer, Canada

Sylvia K. Wood, DNP, APRN, ANP-BC
Assistant Professor
St. Joseph's College
Brooklyn, New York

Ronda Yoder, PhD, ARNP
Faculty
Pensacola Christina College
Pensacola, Florida

Karen Zapko, PhD, CNS, MSN, RN
Assistant Professor
Kent State University at Salem
Salem, Ohio

Tamara Zurakowski, PhD
Clinical Associate Professor
Virginia Commonwealth University
Richmond, Virginia

About the Author

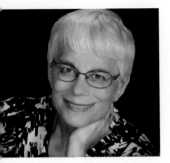

Lucy Hood, PhD, RN is the daughter of an American auto worker. She graduated from St. Luke's Hospital of Kansas City Diploma Nursing School. She returned to school and earned a BSN from Webster College (now Webster University), an MSN from UMKC, and a PhD in Nursing from Widener University, Chester, Pennsylvania. With 14 years of experience in the areas of medical-surgical and neuroscience nursing, she embarked on a career in nursing education. Dr. Hood currently serves as the Department Chair, Pre-Licensure Nursing Education in the School of Nursing and Health Sciences at MidAmerica Nazarene University in Olathe, Kansas. Prior to her current position, she has more than 25 years of teaching experience in traditional undergraduate, RN to BSN, and graduate nursing programs at Saint Luke's College of Health Sciences in Kansas City, Missouri and MidAmerica Nazarene University. She also has taught in the Clinical Pastoral Education Program at St. Luke's Hospital of Kansas City. Professional nursing activities include membership in the ANA, MONA, ONS, NLN, and AANN. She has been a member of the MONA Advocacy Committee which involves political activism. She is a volunteer musician for St. Margaret of Scotland Catholic Church. Currently, she and her husband enjoy antiquing, gardening, and caring for their dachshund, Yoda.

Preface

In the early 1980s, Susan Leddy and Mae Pepper realized the need for a professional development textbook for registered nurses who were returning to school to earn baccalaureate degrees in nursing. This edition builds on the previous contributions that Leddy and Pepper made in earlier editions of *Professional Nursing*. So that the memory of Susan Leddy and May Pepper will continue, their names have appeared as part of the book title since 2003.

I express my sincere appreciation to the following persons for their creativity and attention to detail during the revision process: Christina Burns, Senior Acquisitions Editor; Dan Reilly, Associate Development Editor; Amberly Hyden, Editorial Coordinator; Jennifer Clements, Art Director; Holly McLaughlin, Design Coordinator; and Karan Singh Rana and the Production Team staff. A special note of thanks to Dr. Cheryl Stetler for permission to reproduce the Stetler Model of Evidence-Based Practice.

Organization

The ninth edition is organized into the following sections.

- Section 1, Exploring Professional Nursing
- Section 2, The Changing Health Care Context
- Section 3, Professional Nursing Roles
- Section 4, Envisioning and Creating the Future of Professional Nursing

Content revisions to the ninth edition include the following.

- Chapter 1: The Professional Nurse
  Presentation of key core competencies essential for effective professional practice including the Massachusetts Department of Higher Education's *The Nurse of the Future Nursing Core Competencies©* along with updates related to the Institute of Medicine's recommendations for improving nursing practice and education has been updated.
- Chapter 2: The History Behind the Development of Professional Nursing
  Presentation of changes from the early 21st century that continue to impact today's professional practice.

- Chapter 4: Establishing Helping and Healing Relationships
  Updates from The Agency for Healthcare Research and Quality program TeamSTEPPS® 2.0 has been added to this chapter.
- Chapter 9: Health Care Delivery Systems
  Updated content on the changes made to health care delivery as the revisions to health care delivery in the United States that have occurred during the implementation of the Affordable Care Act.
- Chapter 13: Environmental and Global Health
  Updated information on the state of the global environment has been added and the nurse's role in disaster planning, mitigation, and recovery for natural and human disasters has been placed here.
- Chapter 14: Informatics and Technology in Nursing Practice
  New and updated content presents more specific information about informatics in health care encountered by nurses in daily practice, improvements in technology for patient safety and other recent technologic advances that affect consumer health, professional practice, and health care delivery.
  Recognizing that all baccalaureate nursing programs contain a course in community health nursing, the chapter on Community Health Nursing was omitted.
- Chapter 15: Nursing Approaches to Client Systems
  Expanded content on the concept as community as clients appears in this chapter along with career opportunities for nurses in community health settings.
- Chapter 16: The Professional Nurse's Role in Teaching and Learning
  Updated statistics related to health literacy of Americans is contained within this chapter with implications for nurses to consider when planning and implementing health education.
- Chapter 18: Quality Improvement: Enhancing Patient Safety and Health Care Quality
  This chapter has been co-authored with Karen Wiegman, PhD, RN, CS and provides updated information on Accountable Care Organizations and value-based purchasing.

- Chapter 19: The Professional Nurse's Role in Public Policy

  This chapter contains updated information about current legislative issues, policies, and professional nursing organization initiatives to improve health care safety and advance the nursing profession. In addition, the chapter highlights specific nurses who have contributed and are currently representing professional nursing in the public policy arena.

- Chapter 22: Shaping the Future of Nursing

  Revised information on the future of nursing practice and education based on predictions from the United States Health Resources and Services Administration and from current futurists who analyze current trends to predict the future.

Learning Tools

Continued efforts have been made to make this book more "user-friendly" and to engage students in the learning process and in the application of this material to practice. The book received an updated look to facilitate reading and mastery of concepts essential for effective professional nursing practice. Features from the previous editions have been renamed and revised and new features added. In addition to such textbook standards as **Key Terms and Concepts, Learning Outcomes**, and **References**, each chapter also includes the following.

- **Real-Life Reflections** (formerly *Vignettes*): Case studies are presented at the beginning of each chapter and revisited at chapter's end, highlighting for students the application of the chapter's content to practice and providing questions for thought as they read the chapter.

- **Questions for Reflection** (formerly *Think Time*): Questions posed throughout the text help students think about their own life experiences in the context of their learning.

- **Focus on Research:** Current journal articles are synopsized to relate research to learning and practice.

- **Concepts in Practice:** Hypothetical clinical situations teach professional nurses how they can best incorporate text concepts into real-life practice.

- **From Theory to Practice:** End-of-chapter questions ask students to think about each chapter's content in the context of their own lives.

- **Nurse as Author:** Short writing exercises designed to strengthen critical thinking and writing skills. The nature of the written exercise in each chapter relates to and depends upon the nature of chapter content.

- **Your Digital Classroom:** At the end of each chapter, online resources are brought together to provide students with opportunities for further study and reflection. These include *Online Exploration* (compilation of websites appropriate to each chapter's content); *Expanding Your Understanding* (Internet-based exercises); and *Beyond the Book* (a link to and instructions for accessing the numerous online resources now available with this text).

Text boxes have been categorized to help students identify the purpose of their content.

- **Professional Building Blocks:** Highlight clinical and professional implications.

- **Learning, Knowing, and Growing:** Provides students with information to help them grow both personally and professionally.

- **Professional Prototypes:** Provide examples of documents, concepts, philosophies, and more with suggestions for personal and professional growth.

Students who follow the Beyond the Book link to the www.thePoint.lww.com can access

- Fully searchable eBook
- Learning Objectives
- Literature Assessment Tool (includes current journal articles and questions for students at different experience levels)
- Video interviews with RNs relating chapter concepts to practice
- Spanish–English Audio Glossary
- Web link exercises
- Time Management Strategies
- Nursing Professional Roles and Responsibilities supplemental reading

To facilitate reading, this edition is being printed in full color and photographs have been added to break up large chunks of printed material.

As Mae Pepper and Susan Leddy noted in the preface to the third edition,

> During these changing times, we have been pleased with the utilization of our book in many educational settings, particularly in baccalaureate and graduate programs. Although the first edition of the book was targeted for upper division RN baccalaureate programs, we have become aware of its utilization in generic baccalaureate programs, masters programs, and practice settings.

It is my hope that this ninth edition of *Professional Nursing* will carry on the tradition of previous editions and continue to make a meaningful contribution to the profession.

L.J.H.

Contents

Section 2
The Changing Health Care Context   213

Section 4

Envisioning and Creating the Future of Professional Nursing 529

EXPLORING PROFESSIONAL NURSING

To people outside the nursing profession, being a nurse means taking care of those who are ill or injured, in a variety of complex and sometimes chaotic situations. Nurses make key contributions in the delivery of health care services by providing safe, high-quality care to individuals, families, and groups. Since its beginning, however, nursing has struggled to attain professional status. The therapeutic relationships nurses establish with clients play a significant role in making differences in the lives of the people they serve. Learning the art and science of nursing requires time and perseverance. When nurses provide solid evidence of their impact on client outcomes, the unique contributions they make become apparent to the other members of the health care team and to the public. Professional nurses engage in lifelong learning to remain competent in the areas of clinical practice.

The Professional Nurse

KEY TERMS AND CONCEPTS

Professional nurses
Professional nurse
   contributions model
Core competency
Nurse of the Future
   Nursing Core
   Competencies©
Caregiver
Client advocate
Teacher
Change agent
Coordinator
Counselor
Colleague
Socialization
Resocialization
Role theory

Role
Role conflict
Returning-to-school
   syndrome
Transitions
Professional self-concept
Novice-to-expert model
Characteristics of a
   profession
Associate's Degree in
   Nursing (ADN)
Diploma nursing
   program
Bachelor of Science in
   Nursing (BSN)
Differentiated
   competencies

Graduate nursing
   education
Postgraduate nursing
   education
Critical thinking
Creative thinking
Reflective thinking
Autonomy
State boards of
   nursing
Licensure
Professional
   organizations
General-purpose nursing
   organizations
Specialized nursing
   organizations

National League for
   Nursing (NLN)
American Association
   of Colleges of Nursing
   (AACN)
National Council of State
   Boards of Nursing
   (NCSBN)
American Nurses
   Association (ANA)
International Council of
   Nurses (ICN)
Sigma Theta Tau
   International (STTI)
National Student Nurses'
   Association (NSNA)
Ethical codes

LEARNING OUTCOMES

By the end of this chapter, the learner will be able to:

1. Outline key elements for professional nursing contributions to health care.
2. Identify strategies for thriving in the nursing education environment.
3. Specify a process for socialization into the profession.
4. Discuss methods to facilitate socialization and resocialization into the nursing profession.
5. Outline a process for developing a professional self-concept.
6. Identify the characteristics of a profession.
7. Explain how nursing meets the characteristics of a profession.
8. Discuss additional work that needs to be done to fulfill all characteristics of a profession and attain professional status on a par with that of other professions.

REAL-LIFE REFLECTIONS

Sue graduated from an Associate's Degree in Nursing (ADN) program and has been work-ing as a night charge nurse on a medical-surgical unit. Her nurse manager recently hired a new nurse with a Bachelor of Science in Nursing (BSN) degree. Sue thinks that perhaps she should go back to school and earn a BSN in order to feel secure about her current position. While speaking with a friend, Sue says, "I am a good nurse even though I don't have a BSN.

(continued on page 4)

I don't see how more education will make me more professional or improve my patient care, but I see where it may make my charge nurse position secure."

- *What assumptions has Sue made relative to the importance of education in nursing practice?*
- *How would you respond to her?*
- *What are your thoughts about the BSN and higher education for nurses?*

Professional nurses comprise the largest group of health care workers in the United States. More than 3 million registered nurses (RNs) are living in the United States, about 2.8 million of whom are employed as professional nurses (Kaiser Family Foundation, 2016; U.S. Bureau of Labor Statistics [BLS], 2015a [U.S. Department of Health & Human Services, 2014]). Professional nurses are RNs with a broad scope of practice that is determined by each state.

Some people consider all caregivers as "nurses." This logical confusion stems from the fact that people who tend to the sick, injured, disabled, or elderly commonly have the word "nurse" in their job title, such as nursing assistants or licensed practical/vocational nurses (LPN/LVNs). However, professional nurses offer a specialized service to society. They assume ultimate accountability for client outcomes, and they supervise and educate LPN/LVNs and unlicensed assistive personnel (UAP) as they assist in nursing care delivery. Although they frequently perform tasks that could be done by other health team members, professional nurses bring an ability to improvise while individualizing client care in a variety of settings. **Professional nurses** use science and theories as a basis for professional practice along with art when modifying care approaches. Thus nursing is often considered both an art and a science (see Box 1.1, Professional Prototypes, "Essential Features of Professional Nursing").

CHARACTERISTICS OF PROFESSIONAL NURSING PRACTICE: THE HOOD PROFESSIONAL NURSE CONTRIBUTIONS MODEL

As interdisciplinary health team members, nurses make many unique contributions to health care delivery in clinical settings. The **Professional Nurse Contributions Model** (Fig. 1.1) synthesizes the affective, cognitive, behavioral, and psychomotor domains of professional practice. The model's circular form designates how the interprofessional health care team surrounds health care consumers. A solid outer circle emphasizes the importance of all team members working cohesively for the benefit of care recipients. Each of the concepts in this model is integrally connected to the others to result in a unified whole.

In an ideal world, all health care team members share an altruistic attitude toward the individuals they serve. Many people enter the nursing profession because they genuinely care (caring) about other people and have a desire to help others in time of need (compassion). *Caring, compassion,* and *commitment* are the key affective domains for optimal professional nursing that are intricately linked and comprise the outer circle of the model. The attitudes of caring, compassion, and commitment are key for nurses to view nursing as a profession rather than just a job. Two

1.1 Professional Prototypes

Essential Features of Professional Nursing

Professional nurses assume responsibility to the public for using the best evidence to provide safe, high-quality health-related services for all whom they serve. In *Nursing's Social Policy Statement,* the American Nurses Association (2010) identified the following "key essential features of professional nursing" (p. 9).

1. **Provide** "a caring relationship" that facilitates health and healing.
2. **Attend** "to the range of human experiences and responses to health and illness within the physical and social environments."
3. **Integrate** "assessment data with knowledge gained from an appreciation of the patient or the group."
4. **Apply** "scientific knowledge to the process of diagnosis and treatment" by using "judgment and critical thinking."
5. **Advance** "professional nursing knowledge through scholarly inquiry."
6. **Influence** "social and public policy to promote social justice."
7. **Assure** "safe, quality, and evidence-based practice."

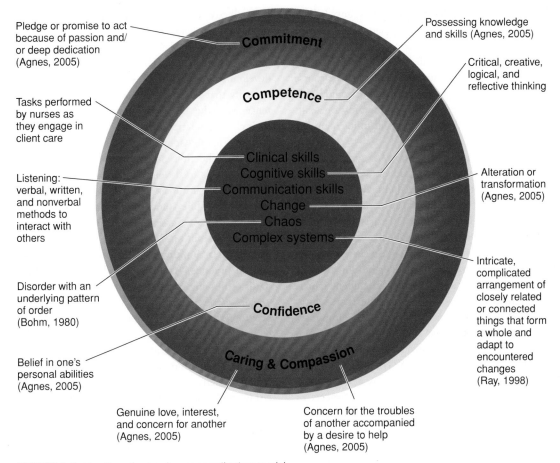

Pledge or promise to act because of passion and/or deep dedication (Agnes, 2005)

Possessing knowledge and skills (Agnes, 2005)

Commitment

Critical, creative, logical, and reflective thinking

Competence

Tasks performed by nurses as they engage in client care

Clinical skills
Cognitive skills
Communication skills
Change
Chaos
Complex systems

Alteration or transformation (Agnes, 2005)

Listening: verbal, written, and nonverbal methods to interact with others

Intricate, complicated arrangement of closely related or connected things that form a whole and adapt to encountered changes (Ray, 1998)

Disorder with an underlying pattern of order (Bohm, 1980)

Confidence

Belief in one's personal abilities (Agnes, 2005)

Caring & Compassion

Genuine love, interest, and concern for another (Agnes, 2005)

Concern for the troubles of another accompanied by a desire to help (Agnes, 2005)

FIGURE 1.1 Hood's professional nurse contributions model.

additional attributes of nurses that are closely linked are competence and confidence. Clients expect *competence* from health care providers. Likewise, health care providers expect competence from each other. To provide safe, effective patient care, nurses must have competence with clinical skills and decision making. Many nursing education programs use simulations with high- or low-fidelity manikins to provide students with the opportunities to learn essential clinical skills and clinical decision making in a safe learning environment (Wilson & Rockstraw, 2012). Current literature emphasize that students gain and retain knowledge, learn clinical skills, and develop confidence in nursing abilities from simulated learning experiences (Alexander et al., 2015; Aqel & Ahmad, 2014; Engum & Jeffries, 2012; Weaver, 2011).

Before competence can be achieved, however, professional nurses must have *confidence* in their ability to execute the clinical, communication, and cognitive skills needed for effective practice. Simulated clinical experiences in nursing education also build

confidence in nursing students (Weaver, 2011). As the nurse's confidence improves, he or she becomes willing to question orders and actions by others that may not appear to be logical or safe. Patients and families feel more at ease when receiving care from a confident nurse. For example, the nurse who knows how to start an IV line and has confidence in his or her ability will attempt to start IVs. As the nurse gains experience in starting IVs, he or she refines his or her technique and eventually possess the ability to start IVs in any patient. The nurse's colleagues identify him or her as the IV starting expert on the unit (confidence booster). The nurse gains more experience starting IVs even when colleagues cannot (increasing competence). Thus, there appears to be a symbiotic relationship between confidence and competence in nursing practice.

The innermost circle in the model depicts the overlapping skills and circumstances with which nurses must work and cope. The roles assumed by nurses require that they have a repertoire of *clinical, cognitive,* and *communication skills.* The nurse must always have sound reasons behind clinical decisions and actions and be able to communicate the reasons well. A broad knowledge base related to all information and strategies available enable the nurse to decide the best course of action to take in any given clinical situation. Highly refined clinical, cognitive, and communication skills delineate professional nurses from all other members of the health care team.

Nurses deliver health care in *complex systems,* so it is important that they understand the nature of these systems and are able to manipulate them. Wiggins (2008) described health care systems as complex adaptive systems in which interdependency exists among individuals and groups. Each individual's actions within complex adaptive systems are based on current knowledge and past experiences. Just like the human body is composed of interacting systems, the client is part of a community, communities form states, states form nations and nations are part of the global community. The earth is part of a solar system which is part of a galaxy which is part of the universe.

Nurses frequently encounter complicated client situations and must adapt to *change* as new scientific evidence emerges, reforms occur in legal aspects of health care delivery, and, most importantly, patient conditions fluctuate. Finally, professional nursing practice has an element of unpredictability and disorder that is conceptualized as *chaos.* Nurses continuously make complex and multiple decisions and may bring order in today's clinical environments. Once order is achieved, something occurs that results in disorder. The pattern of ever-emerging chaos creates constant challenges for nurses. Upon acknowledgment of the deeper underlying, uniform pattern of chaos, nurses understand that they cannot control all clinical practice events. Even though a clinical setting may have a well-defined organization, nurses must adapt to and work in an ever-changing, highly complex, and chaotic environment.

CORE COMPETENCIES FOR PROFESSIONAL NURSES

The concept of **core competency** arose in the 1990s. A core competency can be defined as "a defined level of expertise that is essential or fundamental to a particular job; the primary area of expertise; specialty; the expertise that allows an organization or individual to beat its competitors" (Dictionary.com, n.d.). In professional nursing, core competencies are fundamental knowledge, abilities, and skills that enable nurses to provide

safe, effective care to other persons in health care settings. In many health care settings, professional nurses are expected to display competence in a particular area of practice on an annual basis. Frequently, nursing staff development departments design and deploy activities to verify that nurses possess a certain level of competence with the knowledge and skills appropriate to their clinical practice areas.

In 1973, the American Nurses Association (ANA) published the first *Standards of Nursing Profession.* The goal was to develop a generic list of standards for professional nurses that would apply across practice settings. The standards primarily focused upon nursing process (assessment, diagnosis, planning, implementation, and evaluation) which at the time articulated a thinking model for all nurses to use in clinical practice. As time passed, the original standards of nursing practice have evolved into the *Scope and Standards of Nursing* that outline all key elements of professional nursing practice including nursing process and key competencies (knowledge and skills) for meeting each standard of professional practice. Although the competencies are designated, the execution of each competency may be context dependent. For example, Standard 3 Outcome Identification and Standard 4 Planning specify that the patient, significant others, and other health team members should be involved in determining the desired outcomes and how to achieve them (ANA, 2015c). If the patient is unconscious or has been legally declared mentally incompetent, then the patient is unable to be an active participant in the determination of care goals and planned actions to attain them.

By the 1990s, the ANA recognized the need to develop standards of practice for nursing specialty areas and collaborated with the nursing specialty organization to develop context-based scope and standards or practice including those for school faith community, psychiatric–mental health, transplant, holistic, pediatric, forensic, hospice and palliative care nursing, and nursing administration. The ANA's (2015c) third edition of the *Nursing: Scope and Standards of Practice,* contains 6 standards addressing nursing process (assessment, diagnosis, outcome identification, planning, implementation, and evaluation) and 11 standards related to professional performance (ethics, culturally congruent practice, communication, collaboration, leadership, education, evidence-based practice and research, practice quality, professional practice evaluation, resource utilization, and environmental health) (ANA, 2015a). Disposing used needles and sharp implements (e.g., needles, disposable scissors) into hard, impermeable boxes labeled "biohazard" is an example of a competency related to environmental health. In 1990s, the Institute of Medicine (IOM) published a series of reports outlining safety and quality concerns within the American health care system. The Robert Wood Johnson Foundation provided funding to Linda Cronenwett, PhD as principal investigator and the American Association of Colleges of Nursing (AACN) for the Quality Safety Education for Nursing Initiative to develop strategies for nursing practice and education for continuously improving and enhancing safety in health care delivery. During the first phase of the project, the following six core competencies were identified for professional nursing: "patient-centered care, teamwork and collaboration, evidence-based practice, quality improvement, informatics, and safety" (QSEN Institute, 2014, para 4). Along with identifying the competencies, the initiative developed sets of knowledge, skills, and attitudes for each of them. The project initially addressed pre-licensure nursing education, but eventually was expanded to address graduate nursing education (QSEN Institute, 2014).

In March 2006, the Massachusetts (MA) Department of Higher Education and the MA Organization of Nurse Executives held a workshop *Creativity and Connections: Building the Framework for the Future of Nursing Education and Practice* that was attended by 32 key stakeholders in nursing education and practice. An outcome of the workshop was the formation of a subcommittee to develop a set of core professional nursing competencies to facilitate a seamless continuum for progression in nursing education. Between 2006 and 2009, the committee reviewed the best practices, standards and initiatives education progression to create a list of nursing competencies for each level of nursing education. Results of the review were compiled into a set of 10 core competencies that were then compared to outcomes required for associate degree and baccalaureate degree program accrediting agencies. Funded by the MA Department of Higher Education and the Johnson and Johnson Promise of Nursing for the MA Nursing School Grant Program, the Nurse of the Future Competency Committee identified 10 core competencies that are essential for professional nursing practice known as **The Nurse of the Future Nursing Core Competencies**© (Fig. 1.2). The identified competencies are patient-centered care, professionalism, leadership, systems-based practice, information and technology, communication, teamwork

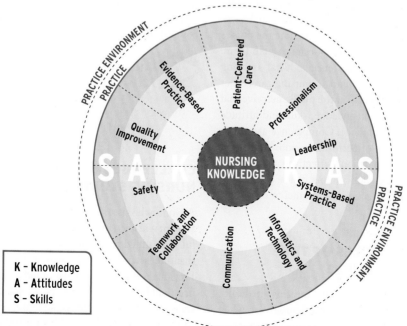

FIGURE 1.2 Massachusetts Nurse of the Future Nursing Core Competencies Graphic.

TABLE 1.1   Hood's Professional Nursing Contributions Model and the Nurse of the Future Nursing Core Competencies© Linkages

Hood's Professional Nursing Contributions Model	Nurse of the Future Nursing Core Competencies©
Caring	Professionalism, patient-centered care
Compassion	Professionalism, patient-centered care
Competence	Professionalism, safety, patient-centered care
Confidence	Professionalism, communication, collaboration and teamwork
Clinical skills	Informatics and technology, safety, patient-centered care
Cognitive skills	Leadership, informatics and technology, quality improvement, patient-centered care
Communication skills	Communication, collaboration and teamwork, leadership, informatics and technology, patient-centered care
Chaos	Leadership, systems-based practice
Complex systems	Systems-based practice, informatics and technology, patient-centered care

and collaboration, safety, quality improvement, and evidence-based practice (Massachusetts Action Coalition, 2014; Massachusetts Dept. of Higher Education, 2010). Similar to QSEN competencies, each one of *The Nurse of the Future Nursing Core Competencies©* contain specific knowledge, skills, and attitudes for nurses to display. The identified competencies include the hallmarks of baccalaureate education: systems-based thinking, evidence-based practice, and nursing leadership (AACN, 2008). Table 1.1 links the Hood Professional Contributions Model with *The Nurse of the Future Nursing Core Competencies©*. Caring, compassion, commitment, and confidence are the key attitudes that provide the affective domain of professional nursing practice. Caring and compassion denote the nurse's genuine concern for others and a desire to help them. When a nurse displays confidence in what is being done as a professional, recipients of nursing care, other health care team members, and the public perceive that the nurse possesses the knowledge, skill, and attitude for effective role performance. Competence ascertains that nurses are capable of performing skills (cognitive, clinical, and communication) effectively to provide safe, optimal care. Complex systems, chaos, and change describe the clinical practice environments of professional nurses.

THE MULTIPLE ROLES OF THE PROFESSIONAL NURSE

Nurses assume multiple roles while meeting the health care needs of clients. They serve as **caregivers** when providing direct client care. Their **client advocate** role emerges when they intervene on behalf of clients to ensure that adequate information and decision-making resources are provided and that client wishes are respected at all times. They assume the role of **teacher** when providing education to UAP, clients, family members, students, each other, and interprofessional colleagues. When working to reform public policy, modify work processes, or transform workplace environments, nurses become **change agents**. They accept the role of **coordinator** when assuming supervisory and managerial responsibilities. Nurses also act as **counselors**, providing emotional and spiritual support to clients. Finally, they assume the role of **colleague** among all health team members. To execute these multiple roles effectively and with genuine compassion, nurses must commit themselves to lifelong learning.

Take Note!

To execute multiple roles effectively and with genuine compassion, nurses must commit themselves to lifelong learning if they are to effectively and compassionately execute their multiple roles.

CHALLENGES OF THE PROFESSIONAL NURSING STUDENT

Anyone who assumes the role of professional nursing student will need to make lifestyle changes to be successful. The added responsibilities of nursing school means that life as previously known will be greatly altered. Previous routines will be disrupted and personal sacrifices will be needed. Money once used for recreation is spent on tuition, student fees, books, and other school supplies. Less time is available to spend with family and friends. Families and friends have different reactions as the nursing student role is assumed. The reactions vary from feeling neglected (which may result in actions to derail the educational process) to intense pride (as they watch their significant other grow). Ongoing communication between the new student, family, and friends enables all involved parties to understand how roles will be altered and what lifestyle changes will need to occur (Dunham, 2008; Quan, 2006).

Meeting job and school responsibilities may be challenging for employed students. Employers may not support educational endeavors. Some coworkers may add to the difficulties by complaining about or refusing work schedule changes; others may express pride in their colleague and help to accommodate the student's schedule.

Part of the toll of returning to school is entering into unfamiliar learning situations. The once-confident honor student or professional nurse may question his or her ability to survive in an intense academic program. The educational process is designed to change people. During times of change, people frequently encounter feelings of discomfort.

REAL-LIFE REFLECTIONS

Remember Sue, from the beginning of the chapter.
- *What obstacles might she encounter at home and in the workplace if she decides to return to school?*
- *Can you suggest strategies Sue can use to defray the potential chaos that returning to school might bring?*

SKILLS FOR EDUCATIONAL SUCCESS

In ideal educational situations, students and faculty interact with each other as colleagues. Faculty design educational experiences and students bear the responsibility for active engagement in learning activities. In traditional education, faculty members serve as authoritarian experts who impart knowledge to students and may create oppressive climates. In educative-caring education, students and faculty members hold equal status and faculty members strive to create effective learning climates based on active and participative learning (Bevis & Watson, 2000; Billings & Halstead, 2005; Young & Paterson, 2007). Such egalitarian interactions with faculty members provide students with experience in collegiality.

When students assume responsibility for learning, they reap maximum benefits from the educational process. To make professional transitions, nurses focus their educational efforts on refining previously learned skills while establishing theoretical foundations for professional practice. Theory-based practice enables professional nurses to understand complex situations and anticipate potential complications in clinical settings. Learners need a variety of skills to be successful in the educational process.

Take Note!
To make the most of the educational process, students must assume responsibility for learning and utilize a variety of skills.

Reading, Listening, and Speaking

Reading constitutes a major component of a successful education experience, but finding time to read remains a challenge for today's busy students—especially as they juggle multiple roles. Effective reading skills streamline the study process. Trying to read and digest each word printed on a page (or screen) is inefficient. When students master the skill of reading for major ideas within a passage, reading becomes more efficient (Dunham, 2008; Osuna, 2014). Strategies to develop reading effectiveness and efficiency include reading for general understanding of ideas, using learning outcomes to identify key concepts, taking notes while reading, highlighting key points, and taking brief reading breaks between major headings within a chapter. During reading breaks, some students find it beneficial to paraphrase what has been read.

In educational settings, effective speaking and listening skills are essential to success. Students listen to faculty members as they share their nursing expertise. Taking time to think before responding to faculty-posed questions enables better organization of thoughts and selection of the best words to convey an answer. Most nursing programs require that students give oral classroom presentations to facilitate refinement of public speaking skills.

Asking questions is essential to avoid making errors in both education and health care settings. Most people (especially clinical nursing faculty and nurses) welcome questions from students. However, fear prevents some students from asking questions. Sometimes, the most difficult task to master is learning what questions need to be asked and having the courage to ask them.

Because nursing relies on teamwork, faculty frequently assign group project. Some students dread group projects because of the difficulty finding time to connect with group members. Osuna (2014) offers the following suggestions to survive group projects:

1. Provide all members of the group with contact information to facilitate the sharing of project information.
2. Appoint a group leader who organizes the project timeline, requests member project sections, pulls the entire project together for a finished product (edits writing for consistent style and finalizes required formatting), serves as a resource person and tackles issues when they arise.
3. Develop a project timeline with the equal input of all group members.
4. Define specific tasks (including the format for each member to submit the section to the leader) required for the project and make group assignments.
5. Hold all members accountable for sections of the project.
6. Communicate openly, timely, and respectfully.

Hopefully, by following the aforementioned suggestions, the project gets completed following instructions outlined in the course syllabus. When problems arise, the group should be able to manage them. However, sometimes faculty involvement may be needed should an irreconcilable issue arise.

Writing

Writing is another critical skill for educational and career success. Professional nurses use writing skills to document client care, develop clinical practice policies, compose email messages and letters, publish articles, develop budgets, and submit change proposals (Fig. 1.3). Writing requires nurses to use critical and reflective thinking (Broussard & Oberleitner, 1997).

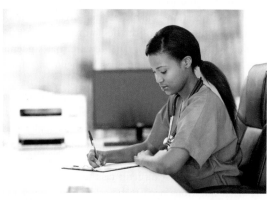

FIGURE 1.3 Writing by hand in the clinical setting enables the professional nurse to have key information readily available for change of shift reports, report key patient information to physicians, and record patient assessments in the event of computer failure.

Written course assignments provide opportunities to polish writing and thinking skills. Success requires understanding the purpose of the writing assignment, setting a timeline for completion by the designated deadline, allowing time for multiple drafts, and having a trusted friend or family member proofread the work before submission.

Perhaps the most difficult aspect of preparing an assignment is narrowing the topic appropriately to fit assignment criteria and enabling a realistic approach for gathering relevant and reputable resources among the vast sources of information. Librarians and faculty welcome the opportunity to help students secure reliable resources such as books, peer-reviewed journal articles (online, in print, or on microfilm), nursing experts, government documents, and online information from academic, nonprofit organizational nurse specialty group and government websites (Dunham, 2008; Stebbins, 2006).

Students should be cautious when considering information from for-profit sources and some special interest organizations. If an assignment requires detailed information about a particular medication, then perhaps the drug manufacturer's website might contain appropriate information. However, some websites serve as a "virtual soapbox" for any person, organization, or company. Health professionals and students must carefully evaluate the validity of information from websites used for personal, professional, and client education (Table 1.2).

Hyperlinks appearing within a website may send viewers to websites of lesser quality. Some website information can disappear without warning, and unless the website has security mechanisms, the information may be susceptible to unauthorized and accidental changes (Alexander & Tate, 1998; Stebbins, 2006; University of Southern Maine, 2012). For example, any person who accesses the online encyclopedia, Wikipedia, has the capability to change posted information. Therefore, this particular site should not be considered a reliable resource.

Writing style for student work varies according to assignment criteria. Nonfiction prose can be developed using description, narration, exposition, and argumentation. Description is used to create a dominant impression. When storytelling is the goal, narration serves as an effective tool. Exposition, which is used to show the how and why of something, can employ one or more of the following tools: (1) exemplification (providing illustrations or examples for a concept); (2) process analysis (giving step-by-step instructions for how to do something); (3) compare and contrast (outlining

TABLE 1.2 Guidelines for Evaluating Online Information

Criteria	Questions to Ask Yourself
Accuracy	■ Is the information error free and consistent? ■ Does the information conflict with known scientific information?
Authority	■ What are the qualifications of the expert or organization providing the information? ■ Are the sources stated? ■ Is there a way to contact author(s)?
Objectivity	■ Does the information seem biased or attempt to sway the reader, such as by selling a product or advocating a specific viewpoint?
Currency	■ Are the initial posting dates and updates presented?
Scope	■ Is the topic covered in-depth?
Site format	■ Is the target user clearly identified? ■ Is the information visually appealing and well organized (especially intrasite links)? ■ Does the site include images that enhance the information? ■ Is it easy to access information from the site?
Cost and accessibility	■ Is the site available to everyone, or do you need to register by providing a username and password? ■ Is there a fee for using part of or the entire site?

Adapted from Alexander, J., & Tate, M. A. (1998). *Web resource evaluation techniques.* Chester, PA: Widener University; University of Southern Maine. (2012). *Checklist for evaluating web resources.* Retrieved from www.usm.maine.edu/library/checklist-evaluating-web-resources. Accessed October 5, 2012.

similarities and differences); (4) analogy (comparing something unknown to something familiar); (5) classification (placing into groups based on common features); (6) definition (explaining the meaning of something); and (7) causal analysis (outlining cause-and-effect relationships). Finally, argumentation can be used to present an objective rationale to support a position (Fondiller, 2007). A casual or informal debate among friends or colleagues involves a presentation of diverse viewpoints based on personal opinions. However, a scholarly debate consists of having some form of evidence (scientific, statistical, research, or ideally information from a peer-reviewed reference) to substantiate the various views being discussed.

Effective writing requires that authors select words to convey messages clearly. Reading serves as a vehicle to expand vocabulary that can be used in writing

(Fondiller, 2007; Martinez, 2000). Dictionaries and thesauri provide a rich source of words for use in writing. Many dictionaries also provide grammatical rules for written language, and word-processing programs offer spelling and grammar check features. Some writers find it useful to read aloud written passages (Dunham, 2008).

Most educational programs have a standard format for written assignments. Students enrolled in these programs should purchase the publication manual for the selected format. Students also may find internet sites that provide assistance with questions about frequently encountered formats such as the American Psychological Association guidelines for manuscript preparation. However, nothing supersedes proofreading by another person to verify that what is written clearly communicates the intended ideas and follows the proper writing guidelines.

In recent years, much attention has been paid to plagiarism. Use of computers and the internet can entice students to cut and paste large pieces of text into assignments and then pass it off as their own work. Plagiarism is best avoided by citing all sources used, avoiding the use of too many citations, paraphrasing and summarizing information carefully, limiting the use of direct quotations, and never purchasing a paper from a friend or paper mill (Stebbins, 2006).

Organizational Skills

Scholastic success requires good organizational skills. Previously learned organizational skills transfer readily in helping to balance personal and professional responsibilities. Work–life–school balance means simply to have a feeling of control, achievement, and enjoyment in daily life (Malloy, 2005; Young & Koopsen, 2011). Key organizational skills for success include managing information, refining test-taking skills, and managing personal time.

Managing Information

The enormous amount of information that one must review, evaluate, and study to remain current in today's professional practice environment challenges all nurses, not just students. Scientific discoveries and changes in health care delivery systems surface quickly. Students and professional nurses spend much time sorting through large volumes of correspondence, publications, advertisements, and professional information. Going through information immediately as it arrives eliminates clutter. Setting priorities for action facilitates meeting professional, personal, and school deadlines. Time spent organizing personal libraries and files saves time by making available resources easier to find (Dunham, 2008; Osuna, 2014; Quan, 2006). To stay abreast of the latest information, some nurses subscribe to online newsletters and service lists (LISTSERV) that offer summaries of new developments in the health care arena.

Refining Test-Taking Skills

Testing serves as a means for assessing learning, yet many students find test taking stressful. Optimal test preparation, which increases the chance of a favorable performance, includes reading all required class assignments, attending class, asking questions during class, taking notes, reviewing learning objectives for each class, reviewing class materials frequently, attending test reviews (if available), and talking with faculty members to clarify content when needed. Some students find they are better prepared if they participate in a peer study group, establish a study schedule, make audiotapes of class sessions (if permitted), outline readings, recopy notes, or create study cards (Dunham, 2008; Osuna, 2014).

Some students become overly anxious during examinations, which may result in poor performance. For some students, a bit of stress may be helpful. Each student perceives stress in a different manner. However, when stress produces anxiety, the following tips might be helpful: arriving 15 minutes early to the test site, practicing relaxation techniques (deep breathing exercises, visualizing success, and guided imagery), skimming notes and textbooks, and talking with classmates. Quan (2006) and Osuna (2014) suggest that study groups offer the opportunity to talk with others about the content covered in courses while also helping to establish new friendships. Complementary health practices such as aromatherapy (e.g., smelling the essential oil of mandarin [citrus reticulate], which evokes feelings of calmness, thereby allaying anxiety) may be also useful (Leddy, 2003).

Managing Personal Time

Time takes on paramount importance for all students enrolled in a nursing program because of role conflicts. Balancing work, professional, student, and family responsibilities is an art. Family members may feel neglected. Scheduling time to tend to the needs of family and friends may provide a welcome study break and facilitate the maintenance of optimal mental and spiritual health (Dunham, 2008; Malloy, 2005; Osuna, 2014).

Success in education requires a team effort. Learning to say no and asking for help without feeling guilty are essential time management techniques. Delegation of household tasks (such as cooking, cleaning, and laundry) to other family members frees time for study while providing other family members with an opportunity to learn or refine life survival skills (Dunham, 2008; Malloy, 2005; Quan, 2006). Finally, networking with one's colleagues can result in time saving ideas, such as sharing quick, easy recipes.

IMAGE AND PHYSICAL APPEARANCE

Physical appearance plays a role in projecting a professional image. Nursing caps became obsolete in the 1970s, and nurses quickly abandoned their white uniforms for colorful scrub suits and dresses. Clean, pressed scrubs and dresses present a professional appearance. However, when nurses wear printed scrubs with cartoon characters, they may fail to project the desired professional image unless they are working with children.

Cleanliness and safety should be priorities when preparing for professional practice. Clean clothing, well-manicured natural nails, and clean shoes decrease the spread of infection. Dangling earrings and necklaces serve as hazards for nurses if they encounter confused or combative clients. Tongue piercing impairs the clarity of a nurse's speech. Visible body piercing and extensive tattooing might create distress for some clients. Clients have more confidence in nurses who display a professional appearance.

SOCIALIZATION AND RESOCIALIZATION INTO THE NURSING PROFESSION

Nurses who assume a different role undergo the processes of **socialization** and resocialization. In simple terms, socialization is the process of preparing someone for a particular societal role. The definition of professional socialization is expanded to include the "formation and internalization of a professional identity congruent with the professional role" (Lynn, McCain, & Boss, 1989, p. 232). **Resocialization** occurs when someone adapts his or her role to a new setting. As they pursue new jobs or educational endeavors throughout their careers, professional nurses have many socialization and resocialization experiences.

Traditionally, the study of socialization emphasizes how external factors, such as family, peers, school, and other institutions, affect a person's development.

Professional socialization addresses the processes by which a person develops a professional identity along with how a profession accepts an individual into its ranks.

Significant environmental changes (e.g., changing a job, moving to a different practice setting, returning to school) stimulate the resocialization process. Thus, resocialization is also a lifelong occurrence. Nurses can reduce the discomfort of resocialization by understanding all aspects of the change processes required for successful professional transitions.

For example, some nursing students select a path of educational mobility as their route to enter the nursing profession. These students start health careers as UAP, then become LPN/LVNs or associate degree nurses before pursuing a baccalaureate or higher nursing degree. Resocialization is needed at each level of education to help the nurse synthesize a changed theoretical foundation for practice, adapt to new professional role expectations, and form a new professional identity. The IOM (2011) advocates this model to advance the nursing profession, and proposed that by 2020, 80% of all nurses should hold a baccalaureate degree and that the number of nurses with a doctorate should be doubled.

Nurses returning to school provide a rich source of information to educational programs. Because of previous client care experiences, they possess a sense of self as a nurse; know how to use current health care technologies; understand governmental and accrediting agency regulations; know how to interact with other health care team members; have encountered human suffering and death; have coped with personal fears, anxiety, concerns, and shortcomings; have worked within complex organizations; have seen others who model lifelong learning; and acknowledge the inevitability of change (Diekelmann & Rather, 1993).

Despite their knowledge and expertise, nurses returning to school still face the process of resocialization. Nurses typically undergo a transformation in the way they practice after earning a new degree. In some cases, however, resocialization may be ineffective and students may finish programs with more knowledge but without changes in their internalized professional self-image.

Take Note!

Throughout their education and careers, nurses will face numerous circumstances in which adaptability—their ability to socialize and resocialize—will be a key to their success.

REAL-LIFE REFLECTIONS

- *Describe the resocialization process that Sue might experience if she decides to return to school.*
- *How might she make the process easier?*
- *What advice would you give to a student just beginning her nursing education to help him or her navigate the socialization process?*

Role Theory

Role theory serves as the basis for socialization. As a concept, roles link persons and society. Linton (1945) proposed that a **role** contains three key pieces: values, attitudes, and behaviors. Professional socialization focuses on preparation for a particular role that offers service to society rather than life in general. Because roles are viewed as separate and discontinuous, it is assumed that stress occurs when a person takes on a new role or new expectations within an existing role (Bradby, 1990). When getting married, for example, a person adopts the new role of spouse, and new expectations might be assumed as part of that role (e.g., homemaker, breadwinner, and child caregiver). Adult nursing students often hold multiple roles that sometimes compete for attention, such as employee, spouse/significant other, and parent. When a new role is assumed (becoming a "student" again), students must adjust how they meet all current life roles. **Role conflict** arises when roles assumed by a person compete with each other for time and attention (Bradby, 1990). The newly acquired student role competes with other roles because of school demands.

Most students enter nursing because they want to help others. In contrast, the professional educational image of the nurse differs somewhat from societal views. These differences include "an increased emphasis on health maintenance and promotion, establishment of analytic and therapeutic nurse–client relationships, strong technical skills along with a broad scientific knowledge base to guide professional interventions, use of critical inquiry processes to creatively individualize nursing care to address client concerns and needs, and the assumption of responsibility and accountability for patient care decisions" (Hinshaw, 1976, p. 5). Clearly, the socialization process involves changes in knowledge, skills, attitudes, and values that may trigger strong negative emotional reactions.

Take Note!
The changes in knowledge, skills, attitudes, and values required by the socialization process may trigger strong negative emotional reactions.

QUESTIONS FOR REFLECTION

1. What potentially competing roles may surface in your life as you begin your nursing education or return to school?
2. Why is it important to identify potentially competing roles?
3. List your roles in order of priority. Why did you list them in this order?

Shane's Returning-to-School Syndrome

Shane (1980) described a **returning-to-school syndrome** encountered by RNs seeking to earn higher nursing degrees. Although the syndrome was described decades ago, it remains relevant today.

The first phase, the honeymoon, is positive. Nurses identify similarities between their previous educational experience and the present experience that reinforce their original role identity as a nurse. The nurse feels energetic about learning new things.

The next stage, conflict, is characterized by turbulent negative emotions. Conflict arises during the first nursing theory or clinical nursing course when faculty challenge nurses to change their ways of thinking and/or practicing. Feelings of professional inadequacy may emerge during this stage and may be expressed by angry outbursts, feelings of helplessness, or depression.

Successful resolution of conflict results in the next stage, the beginning of reintegration. Here, nurses struggle to hold on to cherished beliefs about practice and frequently wonder why they decided to pursue a higher degree. Hostile feelings toward the nursing program and faculty are common during this phase.

Once the nurse works through the first three stages, the final stage of integration emerges. This stage is characterized by the ability to blend the original culture of work with the new culture of school. The integration of the old with the new results in a positive resolution of the returning-to-school syndrome. Nurses recognize that a transformation has occurred. They notice that their clinical practice has forever changed, and they incorporate their newly acquired theoretical knowledge into practice. Using in practice what they have learned in school stimulates these nurses and fosters a new curiosity to learn more.

Moving into a new practice arena or position may mean that despite years of clinical experience and specialized education, an expert nurse becomes a novice again. By recognizing the various stages of socialization and resocialization processes, nurses can identify sources of actual and potential feelings of discomfort and work effectively by steering rather than reacting to the processes of change.

REAL-LIFE REFLECTIONS

- *Thinking back to Sue, what assumptions can you identify that she has made about the benefit of seeking a baccalaureate degree in nursing?*
- *What personal transitions will be required of Sue to successfully work through resocialization using Shane's returning-to-school syndrome?*
- *Why are these transitions important?*

Bridges' Managing Transitions

Bridges (2003) offered an explanation for understanding the psychological impact of returning to school. He proposed that persons undergo **transitions** (psychological adaptations to changes) whenever they are exposed to changes, and developed a three-step process to facilitate transitions that "starts with an ending and finishes with a beginning" (p. 5). People do not move sequentially through the phases; instead, they experience the phases, at times, simultaneously.

The first phase is "letting go" of previous ways and identities. Professional nursing students frequently experience stress as they embark on a new educational program because they realize that what they have done in past practice may not have always been the best practice.

The second phase Bridges called "the neutral zone," which is when the old identity has vanished but the new one is not fully developed. People going through this phase experience an unsettled feeling because they may not know how to act or what questions to ask. They try new ways of looking at and doing things without discarding old ways. When starting a new course or educational program, students sometimes do not know how to begin. In a beginning nursing program (ADN or BSN), students assume a new role of nurse. Nurses returning to college for a bachelor's or advanced nursing degree must assume the role of a student and reconcile with the new role of a professional or an advanced practice nurse (APRN). Feelings of fearful uneasiness surface as the person tries to reconcile the new with the old. If a person leaves the neutral zone before repatterning is solidified, the change will most likely not be successful. Because "the neutral zone is a lonely place" (Bridges, 2003, p. 47), communication is critical. Creative use of the neutral zone involves setting short-term goals, spending time in personal reflection to examine the meaning of change, discovering new ways of doing things, experimenting with the new role, taking time to embrace setbacks and losses, and networking with others in similar transitions. Students enrolled in the same program frequently and effectively support each other while experiencing the neutral zone. After working through the uncertainty and obscurity of the neutral zone, they make an emotional commitment to start anew.

Bridges (2003) called the final phase the new beginning, which is a mental image or experience hallmarked by "a release of new energy in a new direction" (p. 57). A new beginning means a new commitment and identity. Bridges specified that new beginnings require four P's: "the purpose, a picture, the plan, and a part to play" (p. 60). Quick successes such as the accomplishment of small goals facilitate the process of internalizing a new identity. For example,

Professional nursing students who actually use theories derived from best evidence to guide clinical practice may see the positive effects of a theoretically based practice. Take the situation of a nurse caring for a patient who is having difficulty sleeping. A theoretical approach to the problem analyzes and addresses the environmental, psychological, and spiritual factors that may be interfering with the patient's ability to sleep. Instead of immediately administering a sedative, the nurse rubs the patient's back and spends time talking with the patient who expresses concern about the impact of the current illness on his or her family. After sharing the concerns with the nurse and with the muscle relaxation that occurs from the massage, the patient is able to sleep.

DEVELOPING A PROFESSIONAL SELF-CONCEPT

As a person develops patterns of behavior, the self-system becomes organized and strives to actualize itself, although it is continually being repatterned. The self-system interacts symbiotically with the environment, providing the conditions from which a personal view of the self emerges—the self-concept. The self-concept encompasses all beliefs about oneself and personal interpretations about the past, present, and future (Jones, 2004). Because humans develop personal selves first, those personally organized sets of

behaviors form the basis of the selves brought into the profession. Thus, the personal self strongly influences the emerging professional self.

The development of the **professional self-concept** (how a person perceives oneself as a nurse) follows the same path as that of development of the personal self. In every profession, the professional has significant others. During various stages of professional growth and development, nurses have different significant others who help them during times of transitions. For example, beginning nursing students may view faculty members as significant others, while novice nurses may identify experienced nursing colleagues and/or nurse managers as significant others.

The significant others in professional self-development serve as role models or mentors as nurses adjust to changing situations and try to be the kind of person capable of meeting situational demands. Role models provide nurses with examples of how to be, and mentors provide guidance and emotional support. Professional self-concept development also requires that individual nurses engage in episodic self-appraisal along with a willingness to accept the challenges and criticisms of mentors and role models. The personal self-concept cannot be separated from the professional self-concept, although professional significant others are different from personal significant others.

Successful implementation of professional nursing roles and tasks reinforces one's perception of the professional self. Repeated successes in practice solidify the concept of being a competent professional nurse, resulting in increased self-confidence. Because the development of a professional self requires interactions with others in the profession, separating the developmental from the socialization processes may be impossible.

Benner's Novice-to-Expert Model

Benner (1984) devised a model of stages from novice to expert that has relevance for experienced nurses. Benner's **novice-to-expert model** describes stages in the progression of patient care expertise that can result from practicing nursing experience (Table 1.3). This model, based on the work by Dreyfus and Dreyfus (1980), suggests the following three general aspects of skilled performance.

1. Movement from reliance on abstract principles to the use of past concrete experience as paradigms.
2. Change in perception of what is needed in a particular situation from a compilation of equally important bits of information to a more or less complete whole in which only certain parts are relevant.

TABLE 1.3	Benner's Stages From Novice to Expert				
	Stage I	**Stage II**	**Stage III**	**Stage IV**	**Stage V**
Title	Novice	Advanced beginner	Competent	Proficient	Expert
Experience level	Student	New graduate	2–3 yrs in same setting	3–5 yrs in same setting	Extensive time in one or many settings
Characteristics of performance	Is inflexible Exhibits rule-governed behavior	Formulates principles Needs help with priority setting	Plans Has feelings of mastery	Perceives "wholes" Interprets nuances	Has an intuitive grasp

From Benner, P. (1984). *From novice to expert* (pp. 21–34). Menlo Park, CA: Addison-Wesley.

3. Passage from detached observer to involved performer who is engaged in the situation.

Stage I, the novice stage, corresponds to the student experience in nursing school. Because no background understanding exists, the novice depends on context-free rules to guide actions. Although this approach enhances safety, "rule-governed behavior is extremely limited and inflexible" (Benner, 1984, p. 21). When nursing students encounter situations that do not conform to the rules learned, they become highly critical of what happened and cling steadfastly to what they learned in class.

The new nursing graduate demonstrates marginally acceptable performance as an advanced beginner in stage II. The advanced beginner relies on basic theory and principles and believes that "clinical situations have a discernible order" (Benner, Tanner, & Chesla, 1996, p. 54). The advanced beginner can formulate principles for actions, but because all actions are viewed as equally important, help is needed for priority setting. Advanced beginners typically become very uncomfortable when they encounter chaotic clinical situations.

The competent practitioner, who has reached stage III, typically has worked in the same setting for 2 to 3 years. This person has conscious awareness of long-range goals and can engage in deliberate planning based on abstract and analytical contemplation. As a result of this planning activity, the practitioner has a feeling of mastery and the ability to cope with contingencies and feels efficient and organized. Competent practitioners typically must think about what can be done before acting in novel or chaotic situations.

By stage IV, which requires 3 to 5 years of experience, the nurse is a proficient practitioner. The proficient nurse perceives situations as "wholes" rather than as accumulations of aspects, and performance is guided by maxims. Actions do not need to be thought out, and meanings are perceived in relation to long-term goals. In addition, the proficient practitioner can interpret nuances in situations and recognize which aspects of a situation are most significant. Proficient practitioners automatically use creative adaptive strategies when they encounter complex, unfamiliar, or chaotic clinical situations.

The fifth and final stage—expert practitioner—is achieved only after extensive experience. The expert has an intuitive grasp of situations and thus does not have to think through actions analytically. In fact, experts are so skilled at grasping the situation as a whole that they often are unable to think in terms of steps. Expert nurses instinctively act effectively for the client's welfare in any clinical situation.

Professional Nursing Roles

Benner (1984, p. 6) identified that nurses use many competencies as they engage in clinical practice. She organized them into the following seven categories according to the roles and key function that fall within the domain of professional nursing.

1. "The helping role" provides the foundation for the roles of caregiver (provider of direct client care), colleague (helpful team member), and client advocate (person looking out for the client's best interests).
2. "The teaching–coaching function" provides the foundation for the roles of teacher (provider of education and information) and counselor (one who provides emotional support and encouragement).
3. "The diagnostic and patient-monitoring function" provides the foundation for the caregiver and critical thinker (someone who uses complex thought processes) roles.
4. "Effective management of rapidly changing situations" provides the foundation for the caregiver, change agent (person who initiates and guides the change process), and coordinator (person who manages, leads, and verifies that things get done) roles.
5. "Administration and monitoring of therapeutic interventions and regimens" provide the foundation for the caregiver and change agent roles.
6. "Monitoring of and ensuring the quality of health care practices" provide the foundation

for the roles of coordinator, client advocate, and change agent.

7. "Organizational and work-role competencies" provide the foundation for the client advocate, change agent, and coordinator roles.

According to Benner, experience is absolutely necessary for the development of professional expertise.

CHARACTERISTICS OF A PROFESSION

The **characteristics of a profession** (what differentiates a professional from a technician) have been debated for many years. The Flexner Report issued by the Carnegie Foundation in 1910 served as the criteria for determining medicine as a profession. Since the 1950s, the nursing profession has been analyzed using sociologic theories that define a "profession."

Although considered a profession for many years, an assessment of the characteristics of a profession reveals that nursing fails to meet all required criteria and is more accurately classified as an "emerging profession" (Table 1.4). Although nursing does use a specialized knowledge base, has autonomy and control over its work, requires specialized competence, regulates itself,

TABLE 1.4 Professional Status Progress: Nursing Meets All But One Criterion How Nursing Meets Characteristics of a Profession

Professional Characteristics	How Nursing Meets the Criteria or Characteristic
Authority to control its own work	▪ Nurses work for physicians or health care agencies unless engaged in private advanced nursing practice. ▪ State boards of nursing set rules and regulations for practice in nurse practice acts.
Specialized body of knowledge	▪ Nurses pull from a variety of fields to provide holistic nursing care. ▪ Nursing research generates new scientific knowledge for practice.
Specialized plan of formal education	▪ Currently, there are three levels of education for entry into professional nursing practice: associate degree, diploma, and baccalaureate nursing programs.
Specialized competence	▪ Nurses demonstrate assessment skills; possess an understanding of pharmacology, various branches of physical sciences, pathophysiology, diagnostic tests, and surgical procedures; and have skills to manage the technical equipment used in client care. ▪ Many nurses hold certification in specialized areas of nursing practice.
Control over work performance	▪ Nurses make independent judgments based on client situations and area of practice. ▪ Some nurses work in organizations that use shared governance and quality management frameworks.
Service to society	▪ Nursing care focuses on the client system. ▪ Caring for others serves as a major theme in most nursing theories. ▪ Nurses receive middle-income pay for taking care of others.
Self-regulation	▪ Nurses abide by the nurse practice act of the state in which they practice. ▪ Individual state boards of nursing regulate nursing practice.
Credentialing systems to certify competence	▪ Nurses take the National Certification Licensing Examination (NCLEX) developed by nurses, which measures minimum competence for safe nursing practice. ▪ Nurses obtain certification in specialized areas of nursing practice from nurse specialty organizations. ▪ Some states require continuing education for continued licensure.
Legal reinforcement of professional standards	▪ All nurses are held liable for their actions based on what a reasonable and prudent nurse would do in a given client care situation. ▪ Individual state boards of nursing have the power to restrict the practice of nursing within a state.
Ethical practice	▪ The ANA and International Council of Nursing have both published a Code of Ethics for Nurses.
A collegial subculture	▪ Professional nursing organizations offer networking opportunities, shared governance, and clinical practice partnership models, and they enhance collegiality among staff nurses and nursing administration.
Intrinsic rewards	▪ Many nurses derive deep personal satisfaction from making a difference in the lives of clients and families. ▪ Some nurses view the profession as an opportunity to practice religious beliefs on a daily basis.
Societal acceptance	▪ Nursing has been ranked as the most honest and ethical of all the professions for 14 yrs according to polling done by Gallup (2015).

possesses a collegial subculture, and has public acceptance (Freidson, 1994; Miller, Adams & Beck, 1993), nursing fails to have standardized education criteria for entry into the profession.

Take Note!

Although considered a profession for many years, an assessment of the characteristics of a profession reveals that nursing fails to meet all required criteria and is more accurately classified as an "emerging profession."

Currently, three levels of education qualify persons to take the licensing examination for professional nurse registration. The **Associate's Degree in Nursing (ADN)** consists of 2 years of concentrated study focused on clinical skills in the community college setting. The **diploma nursing program** offers 3 years of nursing education focused on learning nursing skills in a hospital-based setting. In diploma nursing programs, students typically receive the most clock hours of clinical instruction. The **Bachelor of Science in Nursing (BSN)**, or baccalaureate, degrees consist of 4 years of nursing education in institutions of higher learning (4-year colleges and universities). Along with education focused on the art and science of nursing, BSN programs also emphasize the importance of a liberal education, nursing research, and community health nursing. The AACN (2015b) reported that 55% of all practicing nurses held BSN or higher degrees in nursing.

Trends in the initial preparation of professional nurses have changed over time. Table 1.5 summarizes key changes. Diploma nursing programs prepared the majority of new nurses until 1971, associate degree nursing programs prepared most of the new nurses by the mid-1970s and continue to be the dominant form of educational preparation for newly licensed professional nurses. However, the number of baccalaureate-prepared nurses appears to be continually rising.

Intellectual Characteristics

Because nurses make decisions that affect clients' lives, they need the intellectual capability to master scientific concepts, understand the impact of self on others, use this information in clinical practice, and understand potential consequences of alternative actions (AACN, 2008). Professional nurses possess the following three intellectual characteristics.

TABLE 1.5 Percentage of Graduates From Baccalaureate, Associate Degree and Diploma Nursing Programs 1960–2015

Year	Baccalaureate (%)	Associate Degree (%)	Diploma (%)
1960–1961	13	3	84
1970–1971	21	31	48
1980–1981	33	50	17
1990–1991	27	65	8
2001	36	60	4
2010	39.3	58	2.7
2015	44.9	53.4	1.7

Note: The National Council of State Boards of Nursing reporting years changed from July 1st to June 30th to a traditional calendar year in 1997.

Hood, L. J., & Leddy, S. K. (2006). *Leddy & Pepper's conceptual base of professional nursing* (6th ed.). Philadelphia, PA: Lippincott Williams & Wilkins; National Council of State Boards of Nursing. (2012). *Revised 2010 nurse licensee volume and NCLEX® examination statistics.* Retrieved from http://www.ncsbn.org/12_REVISED_2010NCLEXExamStats_Vol52.pdf. Accessed October 10, 2012; National Council of State Boards of Nursing. (2016a). *2015 Number of candidates taking NCLEX examination and percent passing by type of candidate.* Retrieved from https://www.ncsbn.org/Table_of_Pass_Rates_2015_(3).pdf. Accessed February 14, 2016.

1. A body of knowledge on which professional practice is based.
2. A specialized education to transmit this body of knowledge to others.
3. The ability to use their knowledge in critical and creative thinking.

Because of the global nature of professional nursing to meet client care needs, nurses frequently use knowledge that originated in other professional disciplines. However, they use the cognitive skills of critical and creative thinking to adapt this knowledge to the realm of professional nursing practice.

Specialized Body of Knowledge

Professional practice is based on a body of knowledge derived from experience (leading to expertise) and research (leading to theoretical foundations for knowledge and practice). Most state boards of nursing (SBN) specify that an ADN serves as the minimum educational qualification for practice as an RN. However, according to the IOM (2011) extensive literature review, patients who receive care received from baccalaureate-prepared nurses had better outcomes than those who received care from associate degree–prepared nurses. Areas of improved outcomes included reduced incidences of hospital-acquired pneumonia, urinary catheter–associated infections, and failure to rescue (recognition of early signs of life-threatening complications and taking action before patients experienced a respiratory or cardiac arrest).

Most states require advanced education and professional certification for nurses who assume advanced practice roles. Professional nurses make clinical judgments based on solid, scientific rationales. They modify plans and actions to meet the demands of specific client situations. ADN programs tend to emphasize technical skills over theoretical concepts. New nurses and nurses who have been education with a skills focus seek out a single "right" answer when delivering patient care. However, seasoned nurses who use theory in practice, anticipate complications before they occur, analyze all aspects that affect health care delivery, and adapt institutional policies and procedures when needed to address complex patient care situations.

Liberal arts education serves as a hallmark of professional education. A liberal arts education provides a knowledge base that enhances a person's ability to practice citizenship, communicate effectively, appreciate advantages of diverse viewpoints, and understand more deeply what it means to be human. Liberal arts courses foster the development of thinking and communication skills, cognizance of historical contributions, understanding of science, exploration of personal values, appreciation of the fine arts, and sensitivity of human diversity (AACN, 2007). Associate degree nursing educational programs require nearly 2 years of liberal education, especially in science and mathematics, and baccalaureate degree programs include courses in the fine arts, statistics, and social sciences that provide baccalaureate degree nurses with a broader perspective of what it means to be human. Knowledge and skills derived from a liberal arts education enhance the nurse's ability to adapt knowledge and skills to novel situations through the use of global rather than narrow thinking.

Whether nursing has a unique body of knowledge or applies knowledge borrowed from the fields of medical, behavioral, or physical science has long been a matter of debate. In the early days of nursing, nurses derived knowledge through intuition, tradition, and experience or by borrowing it from other disciplines (Kalisch & Kalisch, 2004). Today, the nursing profession uses nursing models and frameworks as a foundation for practice. These models and frameworks provide guidance for nurse researchers to substantiate scientifically the unique contributions that nurses make in health care delivery.

Specialized Plan of Formal Education

The NCSBN coordinates efforts to license registered and practical nurses. The National Council Licensure Examination for Registered Nurses (NCLEX-RN) provides computer adaptive testing that measures minimal competence for safe professional nursing practice. Examination content includes health promotion, pharmacotherapeutics, nursing assessment, clinical decision making, nursing interventions, and client care outcome evaluation.

Education for other health care professions (pharmacists, social workers, physical therapists, occupational therapists, chaplains, and physicians) requires postbaccalaureate education. Some nursing leaders have proposed requiring a master's degree (or even a doctorate) as the educational entry level for professional nursing. The IOM (2011) recommends that by 2020, 80% of all RNs hold a bachelor's degree in nursing. The IOM report also recommends interdisciplinary education of all future health team members, including professional nurses. Some collegiate health science programs offer interdisciplinary learning experiences that provide nursing students an opportunity to collaborate with other future interprofessional health team members.

In 1965, the ANA issued a white paper (a detailed proposal) that specified that the entry level into professional nursing should be the BSN degree. The AACN concurs with this position. Efforts during the mid-1980s resulted in **differentiated competencies** for ADN- and BSN-prepared nurses. Professional nursing has two accrediting agencies for nursing education programs; the National League for Nursing (NLN) (all levels of nursing education from practical/vocational nursing through doctoral programs) and the AACN for baccalaureate and higher-degree programs (Kumm et al., 2014). Distinguishing program outcomes and competencies for each level of nursing education has been difficult. In the following Focus on Research section, a group of nurse researcher wanted to determine if there were indeed differences in program outcomes and competencies at the end of associate degree and baccalaureate nursing programs.

FOCUS ON RESEARCH

Baccalaureate Educational Outcomes Being Met by Associate Degree Nursing Programs

The purpose of the study was to determine which baccalaureate nursing program outcomes were being met by 17 associate degree nursing programs that graduated 92% of AD-prepared nurses in a Midwestern state. The authors designed a 114-item structured questionnaire that asked 5 demographic questions and 109 questions pertaining to the AACN Essentials for BSN education programs. Following Institutional Board approval, data were collected from 30 nurse educators who attended a workshop addressing the differences between associate degree and baccalaureate nursing education. The study reveals that 42 of the BSN essentials that were met by ADN programs were found under the domains of information and application of patient care technology, professionalism and professional values, and generalist nursing practice. ADN programs effectively met outcomes for technology centered on electronic health record use and acquiring information for safe, quality patient care. Generalist nursing practice outcomes were centered on providing bedside care to patients and families. ADN programs covered legal issues surrounding professional

practice and what it means to be a member of a profession. Professional outcomes not met by the ADN programs included nursing history, analysis of contemporary nursing issues, lifelong learning, managing ethical dilemmas, comprehensive environmental assessment, genetics and genomics, providing care within a community, supervising other health team members, emergency preparedness, and tolerance for ambiguity. Six areas not included in ADN education are liberal education, organizational and system leadership for patient safety and quality care, evidence-based practice and nursing scholarship, health care policy, financing and regulatory systems, interprofessional communication and collaboration to improve patient outcomes and clinical prevention, and population health. Weaknesses of this study include that data were collected exclusively in one Midwestern state that requires national accreditation of all ADN programs. Information from this study can be used to refine differentiated ADN and BSN competencies/outcomes and be used for nursing faculty to design relevant curricula for RN-to-BSN programs.

Kumm, S., Godfrey, N., Martin, D., Tucci, M., Muenks, M., & Spaeth, T. (2014). Baccalaureate outcomes met by associate degree nursing programs. *Nurse Educator, 39*(5), 216–220. doi: 10.1097/NNE0000000000000053.

However, in 2010, the NLN developed a list of differentiated competencies for professional nurses based upon earned degrees. The NLN model of differentiated competencies fall under the domains of human flourishing, nursing judgment, professional identity, and spirit of inquiry (NLN, 2010). Table 1.6 outlines the different expectations of ADN- and BSN-prepared nurses. All nurses advocate for their patients and act as interprofessional colleagues. ADN competencies tend to center around caregiver, counselor, and educator roles with patients and families, while BSN competencies include working with communities. However, in recent years, ADN nurses are educated to provide nursing care following established evidence-based policies and procedures while using critical thinking skills to make decisions when deviations to policies and procedures are needed. BSN-prepared nurses are educated to engage in independent thinking, analyze current

evidence-based practices, critique new research findings, and spearhead efforts to change practice standards for improved nursing care. ADN and BSN nurses practice in a variety of settings. Because of the independence required and the complexity of community health nursing, BSN preparation has become the minimal education preparation for this specialized area of professional nursing practice.

However, implementation of the different levels of practice has been very difficult because after gaining years of valuable clinical experience, ADN-prepared nurses have effectively assumed leadership and supervisory roles in many health care organizations. However, many health care organizations require at least BSN and sometimes graduate nursing degrees for nursing management positions. Some health care organizations use clinical ladders for promoting staff nurses and many of these require a BSN degree to reach higher levels. Along with organizational

TABLE 1.6 Differentiated Core Competencies for ADN- and BSN-Prepared Nurses

ADN-Prepared Nurses	BSN-Prepared Nurses
Advocate for patients and families when needs arise during the provision of nursing care services	Advocate for patients, families, and communities during the provision of nursing care services AND in the political process to affect health care policy development
Make evidence-based practice judgments to provide safe, high-quality care to promote patient health recognizing the effects of the patient's family and community	Make evidence-based and theoretical-based nursing judgments using nursing and borrowed theories to provide safe, quality care to promote the health of patients, families, and communities
Practice professional nursing with diverse patients and families in a responsible, ethical manner with utmost integrity and develop an ever-changing professional self-identity with a commitment to caring for others using evidence to guide practice and serving as an advocacy role when needed	Practice professional nursing with diverse patients, families, and communities and families in a responsible, ethical manner with utmost integrity and develop an ever-changing professional self-identity with a commitment to caring for others, using evidence to guide practice, serving as an advocacy role when needed providing leadership to others, and assuming leadership in the change process to improve care services
Challenge the status quo of clinical practices, examine evidence underlying assumptions for current practice, and offer suggestions to improve the quality of care for patients and families	Challenge the status quo of clinical practices, identify questions to ask to guide accessing evidence to answer clinical questions, seek out high-quality evidence, critique the available evidence to either substantiate current practice or identify key areas for practice changes, propose nursing innovations when needed and follow established processes for making changes within the context for care delivery to improve the quality of care for patients, families and communities Use concepts and theories from liberal arts studies to guide professional practice and engage with patients, families, health care team members, and communities while understanding, appreciating, and respecting care variation, increased complexity, and increased use of all available resources (organizational private, and public) required for attaining, maintaining, and retaining optimal health for all Develop, design, manage, and coordinate care for patients, families, and communities
Use computer technology effectively for direct patient care to access reliable evidence for practice and obtain relevant and accurate patient and family education materials	Use computer technology effectively for direct patient care to access reliable evidence for practice and obtain relevant and accurate patient, family, and community education materials Effectively conduct computerized database searches for relevant and valid evidence for critique
Use critical thinking and nursing process effectively	Use critical and *creative* thinking and nursing process effectively and *incorporate reflection in action and reflection on action into daily clinical practice*
Follow rules, laws, and regulations when engaging in professional practice	Engage in legal professional practice and participate in political and legislative processes to improve health care policies, regulations and laws
Conducts physical, psychological, and spiritual patient assessments	Conducts holistic patient, family, and community assessments by paying close attention to environmental factors that affect the quality of human life
Use material, financial, and human resources effectively to implement health care services to patients and families	Use and coordinate material, financial, and human resources to maximize access to and implementation of health care services to patients, families, and communities
Identify issues and trends that affect the nursing profession, clinical practice, and health care delivery	Identify and analyze using technology to understand and generate possible solutions for issues and trends affecting the nursing profession, clinical practice, health, quality of life, and health care delivery for patients, families, communities, and society
Apply basic principles of disaster preparedness and contagious disease control and prevention for patients and families.	Use principles and theoretical models of epidemiology for contagious disease and control, evidence-based risk reduction and theoretical models for disaster preparedness, and response and recovery when providing services to patients, families, and communities.

National League for Nursing (2010). *Outcomes & competencies for graduates of practical/vocational, diploma, baccalaureate and masters nursing programs.* New York: NLN.

American Association of Colleges of Nursing. (2008). *The essentials of baccalaureate education for professional nursing practice.* Washington, DC: Author.

Texas Board of Nursing (2011). *Differentiated essential competences (DECs) of graduates of Texas nursing programs evidenced by knowledge, clinical judgment and behaviors.* Austin TX: Texas Board of Nursing.

requirements, multiple research studies have demonstrated that patients have improved outcomes when receiving care from BSN-prepared nurses and nurses who hold certification in a specialized area of clinical practice.

■ QUESTIONS FOR REFLECTION

1. Which of the BSN outcomes/competencies listed in Table 1.6 do you think will be of utmost interest to you as you pursue your degree? Why does this one interest you the most?

2. Which of the BSN outcomes/competencies listed in Table 1.6 do you not find particularly interesting to you? Why do you find this not as interesting?

3. Do you agree with the list of differentiated competencies for ADN- and BSN-prepared nurses found on Table 1.6? Why or why not?

Currently, LPNs provide direct resident care in extended facilities and RNs provide supervision. Many times, the RN supervisor in an extended care facility has been prepared at the associate degree level. The PEW Health Professions Commission (1998) emphasized the importance of strengthening career mobility paths within the nursing profession and proposed a seamless educational path from nursing assistant to RN and RN to nursing doctorate (PEW Health Professions Commission, 1998). Aiken, Clarke, Cheung, Sloane, and Silber (2003) published a landmark study that found that surgical patient outcomes differed based on the educational level of RNs caring for them. The study findings suggest that when clients receive care in an acute care unit staffed with 50% BSN-prepared nurses, mortality is reduced by 5% and substantial reductions are found in incidences of failure to rescue, nosocomial pneumonia, and pulmonary failure. In 2007, the Agency for Healthcare Research and Quality examined the findings of 94 studies using meta-analysis techniques and found that lower client mortality rates were apt to occur when nurses had BSN preparation and had more than 7 years of nursing experience. The study also showed that statistically significant reductions occurred in failure to rescue, patient falls, urinary tract infections, nosocomial pneumonia, and pulmonary failure when nurse to patient ratios fell from 1:5 to 1:4. This and other studies also found that the likelihood of a nurse making a medication or treatment error increased threefold when shift lengths exceeded 12.5 hours. This and other consistently support BSN preparation for all nurses as a means to improve the quality of health care in hospitals.

Graduate nursing education programs offer advanced education for nurses interested in pursuing careers in advanced practice nursing (certified nurse midwifery, nurse practitioners, or clinical nurse specialists), or in nursing education, nursing administration, or nursing informatics. Most graduate nursing education programs offer a master's degree, which can usually be completed within 3 years if a student assumes a full-time plan of study. The majority of programs give students up to 7 years to complete graduate work.

In 2004, the AACN noted several issues with the educational preparation of APRNs at the master's degree level. First, the amount of time spent by nurses engaged in nursing graduate study surpassed the amount of time spent by members of other health care disciplines earning master's degrees (60 vs. 45 credit hours, respectively). Second, some APRNs specified a need for more education to meet the demands of advanced practice. The AACN proposed that all future APRNs would earn a Doctor of Nursing Practice (DNP) degree by 2015. Many other members of the interprofessional health care team, including pharmacists and physical therapists, hold doctorates. The AACN proposed that graduate nursing programs prepare the clinical nurse leader, who would provide "care in all health settings at the point of care, and assumes accountability for client care outcomes by coordinating, delegating, and supervising the care provided by the health care team" (AACN, 2004, p. 10). Currently, there is much debate over the implementation of the DNP requirement for APRN certification and practice.

Postgraduate nursing education leads to a doctorate in nursing. Traditional doctoral nursing programs offer a philosophy degree (PhD) to prepare nurse researchers and collegiate faculty. Nurses engaged in PhD programs have the expectation to generate new nursing knowledge through a rigorous, scientific research study. The practice nursing doctorate (DNP) is a clinically focused degree targeted toward an advanced area of nursing practice. Nurses engaged in DNP programs conduct a final, extensive, evidence-based project that is practice and application oriented. Instead of generating new nursing knowledge, DNP students are expected to translate new scientific advancement to practice situation. Nurses with DNP preparation have the credentials to be clinical faculty in nursing education programs (AACN, 2015). Although less common, some institutions of higher learning still offer clinical doctorates such as Doctor of Nursing (DN), or the Doctor of Nursing Science (DNS or DNSc). Grants and scholarships are available for nurses interested in doctoral work.

Using Knowledge by Critical Thinking

Critical thinking has cognitive and affective characteristics. Critical thinking imposes standards (Paul, 1992) and prevents illogical thinking. Rubenfeld and Scheffer (2015) identify the following habits of the mind associated with critical thinking: "confidence, contextual perspective, creativity, flexibility, inquisitiveness, intellectual integrity, intuition, open-mindedness, perseverance, and reflection" (p. 7). They also identify the cognitive skills of critical thinking as "analyzing, applying standards, discriminating, information seeking, logical reasoning, predicting, and transforming knowledge" (p. 7).

Creative Thinking

As a key component of critical thinking (Rubenfeld & Scheffer, 2015), **creative thinking** generates alternative approaches to clinical situations. Creative thinking requires an ability to think outside of what usually is done and results in novel approaches to client care. If not tempered with critical thinking, however, solutions generated with creative thinking may be hazardous. For example, when using therapeutic touch to relive a client's pain, the nurse notes that the client experiences a substantial fall in blood pressure resulting in hypotension. If the hypotension results in the client fainting when getting out of bed after the therapeutic touch session and sustaining an injury, the nurse is accountable for the adverse outcome. Nurses engage in creative thinking when confronted with clients who have complex integrative health problems that require individually designed plans to attain desired outcomes.

Reflective Thinking

Reflective thinking is engaging in purposeful analysis about what one is currently doing and about what one has done (Schon, 1987). Reflection plays a key role in professional nursing practice (Fig. 1.4). Consider the following clinical situation.

Ms. S has advanced cancer and lives in constant pain. Because the pain is unbearable, Ms. S's physician orders patient-controlled analgesia (PCA) with morphine. Ms. S is fearful that the morphine will not ease her pain, will result in addiction, and will produce a loss of consciousness. Her fear and anxiety cause increased muscle tension. As the nurse initiates

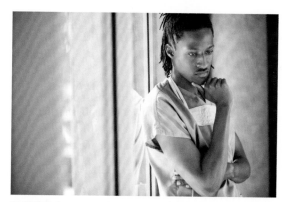

FIGURE 1.4 Reflective thinking enables nurses to analyze and improve their professional performance.

the morphine drip, she remembers the pharmacologic action and potentially adverse effects of the morphine. She educates Ms. S about morphine and how best to use the PCA device for optimal pain control. As the nurse talks with Ms. S, she performs a back massage, knowing the theoretical benefits of human touch and the physiologic response to muscle massage.

When nurses think about theoretical and scientific principles while delivering client care, they engage in reflection in action (Clarke, James, & Kelly, 1996; Kim, 1999; Powell, 1989; Schon, 1983).

Schon (1983, 1987) advocated for reflection on action, another form of professional reflection. Reflection on action occurs when the professional practitioner conducts a retrospective analysis of action taken (Clarke et al., 1996; Schon, 1987). Returning to the example above, the nurse analyzes care given to Ms. S, considering what interventions were implemented and whether they were successful. Reflection on action enables the practitioner to develop a deeper understanding of practice and provides a vehicle to learn from experience (Clarke et al., 1996; Schon, 1987). Journal writing also provides practice with reflection on action.

> **Take Note!**
> Cognitive skills such as critical, creative, and reflective thinking help nurses make sound clinical decisions when providing client care.

Independent Clinical Decision Making

Professional nurses make independent decisions to solve problems in clinical practice. Sometimes, nurses act prematurely because of inadequate information and insufficient time to generate alternative approaches.

Concepts in Practice IDEA → PLAN → ACTION

Visiting Hours

Which of the following actions would you take with a patient whose visitors insist on staying beyond the visiting hours established by hospital policy?

1. *Possible action 1:* Tell the patient and the visitors that the visitors must leave.
2. *Possible action 2:* Allow the visitors to stay for an additional hour.
3. *Possible action 3:* Explore the reasons why the visitors want to stay and the significance of having the visitors spend time with the patient. Base your decision on the result of information generated.

As a nurse, you would use critical thinking to realize that collecting more information surrounding the situation will result in an optimal decision. Perhaps the visitors have arrived from out of town and have no place to stay. Maybe the client has not seen them in a long time or the client may be afraid to be left alone in the hospital the night before a potentially life-threatening procedure.

When nurses use critical thinking and logical reasoning to support the actions taken, they make effective clinical decisions.

Nursing Process

Nurses use the nursing process, a systematic thinking method to process information about specific client care situations. This problem-solving process consists of five interacting steps: assessment, diagnosis, planning, implementation, and evaluation (Fig. 1.5). Assessment consists of collecting subjective (what clients say) and objective (measured or verifiable by another) information about clients. Nurses then categorize data into clusters to determine nursing diagnoses (an actual or potential client response) upon which a care plan is developed. After the care plan is implemented (executed), nurses evaluate the effectiveness of the plan and start the process again with assessment. Effective use of the nursing process requires critical, creative, and reflective thinking.

Service to Society

Ever since nursing began, it has been associated with serving others. However, the intrinsic motivation "to care" is only one way to look at caring. Morse, Bottorff, Neander, and Solberg (1991, p. 122) identified the following five conceptualizations of caring: (1) caring as a human trait; (2) caring as a moral imperative; (3) caring as an affect; (4) caring as an interpersonal interaction; and (5) caring as a therapeutic intervention. Obviously, caring encompasses more than just intuitive concern for others. Several nursing theories use caring as a major concept or central theme.

Professional service to society requires impeccable integrity, individual responsibility for ethical practice, and lifelong commitment. However, some nurses view nursing as a job rather than a profession.

Many nurses leave the profession (permanently or temporarily) to pursue personal interests or to raise a family. Some nurses work to supplement family income, and others work because they are sole or primary income providers for their family. Nurses needing job security avoid confronting less-than-ideal nursing practice situations. Employing agencies sometimes exploit these nurses. Regardless of high client-to-nurse ratios, rotating shifts, and floating, some nurses make do and maintain the status quo. However, other nurses confront poor working conditions and always do what is best for clients.

Service to others involves ethical and legal responsibilities. Nurses must have the integrity to do what is right, especially in situations that cause moral dilemmas. The International Council of Nurses (ICN) has published a Code of Ethics and the ANA (ANA, 2015b) also has published a Code of Ethics and Social Policy Statements for nurses to follow. Fowler (2015b) articulates that the *ANA's Nursing's Social Policy Statement* serves as a reciprocal contract between nurses and society. Society expects nurses to offer caring services with the patient as the primary concern of the nurse when services are offered. Nurses are expected to have the necessary knowledge, skill, and competence to execute their professional duties. Nurses also acknowledge that there are hazards associated with patient care (violent patients, exposure to contagious diseases and placing oneself in peril to negotiate hazardous weather conditions to report for duty). Nurses as individuals and as members of the profession are accountable and responsible for professional practice endeavors. Professional nurses are expected to develop and stay abreast of new scientific knowledge to improve the health for all people. They also must engage in ethical practice as specified by professional nursing codes of ethics. As members of an interprofessional health care team, they are expected to collaborate with other team members and recipients of care to identify care needs, set care outcomes, and plan care. Nurses are also expected to promote the health of

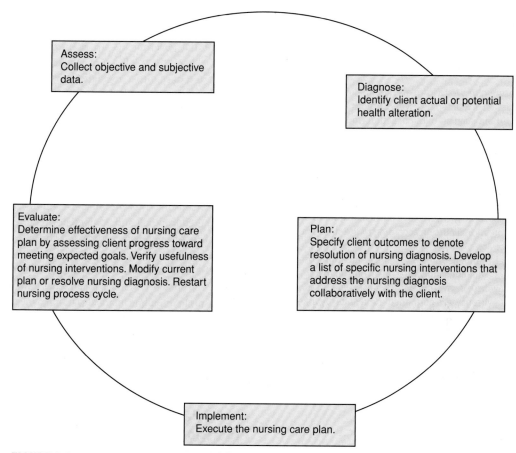

FIGURE 1.5 Nursing process as a continuous cycle.

the public by addressing health disparities and intervene to protect the public via whistleblowing and advocacy efforts. In return, nurses expect society to authorize practice autonomy, extend self-governance, protect the title of RN and scope of practice, receive respect and fair remuneration for services, be free to practice nursing to the full extent of educational preparation, receive support to sustain the nursing profession, and be protected from hazardous service activities.

Service to society requires legal assurances that practitioners are competent. Credentialing systems, such as **licensure**, provide a means to certify minimal competence for safe practice by a person legally permitted to use the title "registered nurse." State nurse practice acts also provide legal reinforcement against incompetence. Upon initial state licensure, the nurse receives a copy of his or her state's nurse practice act. Printed copies of specific nurse practice acts can be obtained from individual SBNs (a fee usually is charged), or copies may be downloaded from SBN websites. When litigation occurs, courts of law hold nurses accountable for what a usual and prudent nurse would do in a particular client care situation.

Autonomy and Self-Regulation

Autonomy means that professionals have control over their practice. Autonomy involves independence, a willingness to take risks, and accountability for one's actions, as well as self-determination and self-regulation. In the United States, each state has a nursing board that governs practice that occurs within its borders. **State Boards of Nursing (SBNs)** regulate professional nursing practice by issuing professional licenses to qualified individuals. Through licensure and the legal system, society protects consumers from unsafe nursing practice by holding nurses responsible for their professional actions. SBNs have legal authority to ensure that all nurses follow the state's nurse practice act. Thus, the nursing profession regulates itself.

Nurse practice acts define various levels of nursing practice, determine rules that guide each level of

1.2 Professional Building Blocks

Licensure Versus Registration

Licensure refers to "a form of credentialing whereby permission is granted by a legal authority to do an act, without such permission, action would be illegal, trespass, a tort, or otherwise not allowable" (Loquist, 1999, p. 105). A professional nursing license is a legal document that certifies that an individual has met minimum standards for qualified practice. As a state function, licensure protects citizens from unsafe or incompetent health care providers. Upon licensure, nurses become registered in a particular state to practice professional nursing according to the state's nurse practice act.

Registration denotes "enrolling or recording the name of a qualified individual on an official roster by an agency of government" (Loquist, 1999, p. 15). Although licensure is permanent (unless it is revoked for illegal or immoral behavior), registration must be renewed periodically (usually every 1 to 2 years) by paying a fee to each state in which current registration is desired.

nursing practice, and provide specific guidelines for continued licensure. The SBN has legal authority and accountability to implement the nurse practice act. Most SBNs are composed of a group of persons typically appointed by the state's governor, with nurses holding most of the positions. Requirements for RN licensure appear in each state's practice act. Most nurse practice acts contain information related to reasons for licensure, nursing definitions, minimum standards for nursing education programs, licensure requirements, licensure exemptions, reasons for license revocation, endorsement provisions for nurses licensed in other states, development of a state board of examiners, nursing board responsibilities, and penalties for practicing nursing without a license or not in accordance with the state nurse practice act (see Box 1.2, Professional Building Blocks, "Licensure Versus Registration"). Each SBN has the responsibility for carrying out activities covered in its nurse practice act.

Recognizing the need for a united approach to nursing licensure and education, the 50 SBNs formed the NCSBN in 1978. This national board has developed licensure examinations for professional and practical nursing, a mutual compact for interstate nursing licensure, and educational materials for new and experienced nurses.

As in the United States, Canadian legislation to regulate nursing practice is passed by the provincial and territorial governments. In all provinces (except Ontario, where the College of Nurses of Ontario assumes responsibility), regulation of professional nurse registration lies with the provincial or territorial professional nursing associations. Canadian nursing regulatory bodies determine educational and practice standards and define the scope of nursing practice. They also specify who may use the title RN and outline mechanisms for professional discipline. Finally, the regulatory bodies also approve educational programs to prepare persons for entry into practice and to establish continuing educational and competency requirements for members of the nursing profession (Brunke, 2003; Ross-Kerr, 2011).

Because the profession of nursing defines nursing practice, sets practice standards, and has established mechanisms to discipline members failing to meet practice standards, nursing fulfills the element of autonomy and self-regulation. In some cases, the regulatory bodies also provide a means for professional nurses to engage in the activities resulting in the creation of a collegial subculture, another hallmark of a profession.

A Collegial Subculture (Accrediting, Professional, and Student Nursing Organizations)

Professions also have a collegial subculture that helps their members to support one another and ensure continuance. Like other professions, nursing has many national and international **professional organizations** that set practice standards, advocate, and provide networking opportunities for members. More than 100 professional specialty nursing associations have been formed to date in the United States (Shinn, 2012), each of which creates its own collegial subculture.

Professional nursing organizations can be divided into two categories: **general-purpose nursing organizations** (which address the issues and concerns of all nurses) and **specialized nursing organizations** (which address specific issues and concerns of nurses practicing within a specific specialized practice arena). Specialty nursing organizations link nurses who practice in a particular area and create subcultures of nurses with common interests within the profession. Each organization specifies its mission, goals, and constituency.

Only about 6% of professional nurses belong to the ANA (2010). Some nurses believe that membership in specialty organizations (e.g., Oncology Nursing Society, American Assembly for Men in Nursing) better fits their professional needs than membership in a general nursing organization. Others (Milstead, 2008; Shinn, 2012) have argued that if all professional nurses would join a single, general-purpose organization, nurses would become more influential in health care delivery and policy formation. In 2001, the Nursing Organization Alliance was formed to bring all nursing organizations together so that a strong, cohesive voice and action plan could address common issues of concern to all professional nurses (Shinn, 2012). The following discussion presents some of the major broad-purpose organizations.

National League for Nursing

The **National League for Nursing (NLN)**, which may be the oldest nursing organization in the United States, was formed in 1893 (Dock & Stewart, 1920; NLN, 2016a). The NLN is committed to advancing the quality of all levels of nursing education, from licensed practical nursing to nursing doctorates. Membership is open to nursing education institutions, nurses and other health care professionals, health care agencies, and anyone interested in improving the quality of nursing education. The NLN has over 40,000 individual members and 1,200 institutional memberships (NLN, 2016a). NLN (2016b) core values are caring, integrity, diversity, and excellence that guide its work and services. Its mission is to promote "excellence in nursing education to build a strong and diverse nursing workforce to advance the health of our nation and the global community" (NLN, 2016c, para 1). The NLN has the four following key goals: (a) to become one of the most renowned leaders in national and international education; (b) build a sustainable, culturally diverse, and member-led organization; (c) serve as the champion for nurse educators by being their voice and forwarding their interests in the academic, political, and professional domains; and (d) advance the science of nursing education by promoting the scholarship of teaching and evidence-based nursing education practice (NLN, 2016c). The NLN Commission for Nursing Accreditation accredits associate's degree, diploma, baccalaureate, and upper-degree nursing programs to foster high quality nursing education.

Along with its accreditation activities, the NLN provides consultation services, continuing education programs, analysis of statistical data related to nursing education and nursing workforce resources, various examination and testing services, information about legislative affairs affecting nursing, journals, continuing education seminars, grants for nurse educators conducting research, nurse educator certification, and a variety of information packages to promote recruitment and the image of professional nursing.

American Association of Colleges of Nursing

The **American Association of Colleges of Nursing (AACN)** acts to guide and increase the quality of baccalaureate and higher-degree programs in nursing. Its mission is to become a key national asset that serves the public by "setting standards, providing resources, and developing the leadership capacity of member schools to advance nursing education, research, and practice" (AACN, 2016b). AACN envisions that, by 2020, nursing will be a highly educated and diverse profession that will assume leadership in health care delivery, quality, and development of new knowledge that will improve health and health care delivery. Membership consists exclusively of deans and directors of higher education nursing programs, but the association offers seven leadership networks for faculty and staff who engage in instruction, research, leadership, faculty practice, business operations, research, graduate student recruitment, and communications/development. To standardize program curricula, AACN publishes essential documents for baccalaureate, graduate, and postgraduate nursing programs that outline competency expectations for graduates (AACN, 2016a).

Along with developing standards for nursing programs, the AACN provides government advocacy, research and data services, conferences and webinars, and special projects such as integrating and certifying clinical nurse leaders, determining best practices for end-of-life nursing care, establishing cultural competency, developing and implementing quality and safety in nursing education competencies, and facilitating the requirement of the DNP as the minimal education level for advanced nursing practice (AACN, 2016b).

The AACN has an autonomous entity, the Commission on Collegiate Nursing Education (CCNE) that accredits baccalaureate and graduate nursing programs. The CCNE specifies the criteria that outline the hallmarks of nursing education programs to prepare effective professional nurses. Through program identification and assessment, the CCNE serves the public by publishing a list of accredited programs. CCNE accreditation means that a program offers effective educational practices (CCNE, 2013).

National Council of State Boards of Nursing

The **National Council of State Boards of Nursing (NCSBN)** and individual SBNs work together on common issues and concerns that might affect public health, safety, and welfare, including setting standards for minimal competence for safe nursing practice (measured by the NCLEX). The NCSBN assumes the responsibility for development and administration of the NCLEX for professional and practical/vocational nurses. Along with licensure examination, the NCSBN keeps records on nursing license suspensions, tracks professional nursing demographics, spearheads the effort toward interstate licensure and conducts research to develop evidence-based regulation for nursing practice. In collaboration with the ANA and other advanced nursing practice groups, the NCSBN and SBNs set guidelines for licensure of APRN at state levels (NCSBN, 2016a). Membership is limited to the boards of nursing from the 50 US states. Associate membership includes five colleges and seven associations of nursing from Canadian provinces, the Bermuda and New Zealand Nursing Councils, Nursing and Midwifery Boards of Ireland and Australia, and the Singapore Nursing Board (NCSBN, 2016c).

American Nurses Association

In 1896, 10 representatives from 10 different alumni association of nursing programs met at the Manhattan Beach Hotel with the aim of starting a national professional nursing organization and named it the Nurses' Associated Alumnae of the United States and Canada. The name was changed to the **American Nurses Association (ANA)** in 1911 and officially established the current organization (Flanagan, 1976). The current mission of the ANA is "Nursing advancing our profession to improve health for all" (ANA, 2015a, p. 1). The vision of ANA is to have nursing become "the unifying force for advancing quality of health for all" (ANA, 2015a, p. 1) Membership criteria require professional nursing licensure. When professional nurses join the national organization, they obtain membership at the state and local district levels. The ANA represents nurses in all 50 states, the District of Columbia, Guam, and the US Virgin Islands. The ANA offers a wide variety of services to members and plays a key role in promoting healthy workplaces for nurses through continuing education programs, certification programs for specialized and advanced practice, nurse workforce data, political activism and public policy analysis, programs to promote the economic and general welfare of nurses, and the development and publication of nursing practice standards, handbooks, journals, newsletters, social policy statements, and an ethical code. Members receive discounts on nurse liability insurance, publications, journal subscriptions, conferences, and online educational programs (ANA, 2016b). In 2016, the ANA launched a campaign "2016 Culture of Safety"

with the slogan "Safety 360, Taking Responsibility Together" aimed at improving the safety of health care delivery for consumers and nurses. The ANA addresses national nursing issues through membership in various national nursing councils that meet regularly to discuss the issues and concerns about nursing practice. The ANA also sponsors activities of the American Academy of Nursing, a group of distinguished nurses who have made major contributions to the nursing profession, and the American Nurses Foundation, a program that provides funding for nursing research and other projects to advance the profession (ANA, 2016a). The American Nurses Credentialing Center (ANCC) is a wholly owned subsidiary of ANA. The ANCC provides certification examinations for nurse practitioners and clinical specialists, programs recognizing health care organizations for positive and safe work environments for nurses and processes for approval of nurse continuing education providers (ANCC, 2016). The ANA is also a member organization of the ICN (ANA, 2016c).

The International Council of Nurses

Founded by nurses in Great Britain, Canada, Germany, Scandinavia, and the United States, and located in Geneva, Switzerland, the **International Council of Nurses (ICN)** unites national nursing organizations from 128 nations in a single confederation. The founders included nurses from nursing organizations in Great Britain, Canada, Germany, Scandinavia, and the United States. Since 1899, the ICN has worked to preserve the professional welfare of nurses, address interests of women, and improve global health. By living the core values of visionary leadership, inclusiveness, flexibility, partnership, and achievement, the ICN strives to bring nurses together globally, advance the profession worldwide, and influence health policies (ICN, 2011). The ICN addresses a wide array of nursing concerns, including nursing regulatory issues, the global standardization and credentialing of nurses, human rights, ethics, socioeconomic welfare of nurses, occupational safety, health policy formation, career development, and position statements on health issues.

The ICN serves as an advocate for more than 13 million nurses and for all the people of the world. Current efforts by the ICN focus on establishing a global definition of professional nursing practice (International Classification for Nursing Practice), addressing the global shortage of nurses, credentialing nursing competence, measuring the value of professional nursing contributions on client outcomes, addressing a variety of global health issues, and furthering advanced nursing practice. The organization has advised the United Nations on global health issues. In addition to its *Code of Ethics for Nurses* (ICN, 2012), the ICN has published position statements that have been presented for consideration to governments when making health care policy decisions (ICN, 2011).

Sigma Theta Tau International

Four nursing students at the University of Indiana formed Sigma Theta Tau in 1922. In 1985, **Sigma Theta Tau International (STTI)** became an international honor society for nurses. The organization has more than 123,000 active members form 90 countries. The society has more than 500 chapters in close to 695 institutions of higher education throughout the world. Chapters are located on every continent except Antarctica. STTI holds membership in the Association of College Honor Societies. The mission of STTI is "advancing world health and celebrating nursing excellence in scholarship, leadership, and service" (STTI, 2016, para 1). The vision for STTI "is to be the global organization of choice for nursing" (STTI, 2016, para 2).

To become a member of STTI, a nurse must demonstrate superior scholastic achievement, professional leadership potential, and/or marked achievement in the nursing field. STTI contributes to the advancement of nursing via research grants, scholarships, monetary awards to nursing, online continuing education programs, conferences, and publications. The organization publishes *The Journal of Nursing Scholarship, Worldview on Evidence-Based Nursing,* scholarly books, *Reflections on Nursing Leadership, Chapter Leader Emphasis,* and *STTIconnect.* STTI also sponsors writers' seminars, offers a media development program, and bestows awards for outstanding contributions to the nursing profession. Local chapters also present educational programs, awards, and scholarships. STTI runs the Virginia Henderson International Nursing Library, a state-of-the-art electronic library and information resource center that holds more than 38,000 abstracts from research studies and nursing conferences. All nurses are invited to submit scholarly papers to the repository. Before they are posted, each paper undergoes a peer-review process (Virginia Henderson Nursing e-Repository, 2016).

National Student Nurses' Association

The **National Student Nurses' Association (NSNA)** is an inclusive association for students from all types of nursing educational programs. Over 60,000 student members finance and run the autonomous organization. Members live in all 50 states, the District of Columbia, Puerto Rico, and the US Virgin Islands. NSNA goals, according to the group's mission statement, are "to mentor the nursing students preparing for initial licensure as RNs and to convey the standards, ethics, and skills that students will need as responsible and accountable leaders and members of the profession" (NSNA, n.d.).

NSNA offers a variety of activities and services to implement its mission. The association participates on committees of NLN, ANA, and ICN. The NSNA Foundation administers a scholarship program and publishes the journal *Imprint,* the newsletter *NSNA News,* and a variety of reports and handbooks. As members of NSNA, students enjoy discounts on health insurance, publications, conference attendance fees, mobile device applications, cell phones, and state board review courses (NSNA, n.d.).

■ QUESTIONS FOR REFLECTION

1. Are you currently a member of a professional nursing organization? Why or why not?
2. If you are a member of an organization, how would you go about recruiting another nurse to join a professional nursing organization?
3. If you are not a member of an organization, what factors prevent you from joining one?
4. Is a nurse more professional if he or she holds membership in a professional organization? Why or why not?

Ethical Practice

Ethical professional practice has been defined by several broad-purpose nursing organizations through published **ethical codes** (statements defining honest, honorable, humane, and fair practice). Ethics permeates all areas of professional practice. Nurses with solid professional identities possess strong individual and professional values that provide the foundation for ethical dimensions of professional practice. Caring emerges as a shared value within the nursing profession. Clients trust nurses with their lives, and professional nurses must never violate this sacred trust.

Sometimes, a nurse's professional duties will be in conflict. Nurses have individual, professional, and societal duties (Bandman & Bandman, 1995; Fowler, 2015a). As science and technology advance and resources dwindle, nurses confront increasingly difficult, complex, and conflicting issues in daily practice. Ethical systems provide nurses with a set of values and behaviors to use when situations without clearly right or wrong answers arise. By studying ethics, nurses identify and examine personal biases and values. A code of ethics assists nurses to make decisions when confronted with ethical dilemmas.

Bandman and Bandman (1995) stated, "Effective nurses function as moral agents" (p. 46). When acting as moral agents, nurses assume responsibility and accountability to do no harm. Nurses assume responsibility for action when they assume blame or credit for their own actions. Accountability encompasses the ability to provide sound reasons, explanations, and defenses for the actions taken (Sullivan & Christopher,

1999). When nurses encounter practice situations with multiple correct actions and answers, they often agonize about which of the imperfect and alternative choices would serve the best interests of the client. Table 1.7 identifies some common ethical dilemmas encountered by nurses in clinical practice.

Nurses use multiple ethical codes depending upon the context in which they practice. Common principles appear in original versions of the *ICN Code of Ethics for Nurses* (ICN, 2012) and the ANA *Code of Ethics for Nurses with Interpretive Statements* (Fowler, 2015a). Nurses can read specific ethical codes online. Although

TABLE 1.7 Ethical Issues Encountered by Professional Nurses in Practice

Ethical Principle	Definition	Practice Dilemmas
Sanctity of human life	Human life is sacred and must be preserved at all costs	■ Quality vs. quantity of life ■ Pro-choice vs. pro-life ■ Capital punishment ■ Withholding life-saving treatments ■ Euthanasia and assisted suicide
Autonomy	Individual freedom to make rational and unconstrained decisions	■ Lack of client knowledge about available treatments ■ Coercive power ■ Paternalism ■ Cognitively impaired individuals ■ Individual decisions that interfere with another person's rights
Veracity	Truth telling	■ Whistle-blowing ■ Concealing a chemical or physical abuse pattern ■ Falsification of legal documents to cover errors ■ Covering up reasons for care errors or poor performance ■ Informed consent
Distributive justice	Allocation of limited resources	■ Managed care ■ Reduced access to care based on inability to pay for services ■ Judicious use of high-tech equipment for prolonging life ■ Deciding who gets resources based on fitness, cost–benefit analysis, equal chance, equal share, or equal consideration
Respect for personal beliefs	Accepting individual beliefs as a basis for decision making	■ Religious preferences not to subject self or family to "impure" acts ■ Conflicts of research evidence on personal health habits
Nonmaleficence	Do no harm	■ Securing court orders for life-saving therapies ■ Withholding therapy ■ Assisted suicide ■ Right to leave clients alone
Beneficence	Do only good	■ Balancing what is morally right with what is legal and practical; highly individualized for each situation and shares actions with many of the principles presented above
Confidentiality	Keeping privileged information private	■ Reporting health problems that interfere with safe driving to state officials ■ Telling families about poor prognoses before informing clients ■ Disclosing alternative lifestyles
Fidelity	Keeping promises	■ Not keeping one's word ■ Failing to followup with what one says one will do
Justice	Treating people fairly	■ Treating clients differently based on their ability to pay or other socio-cultural characteristics ■ Singling out special clients for extra nursing care ■ Denying health care access to anyone

ethical codes are often updated, all ethical codes contain the following common principles.

- Respect for human dignity and uniqueness
- Protection of confidential information
- Actions to safeguard persons receiving nursing care
- Responsibility and accountability for nursing actions
- Maintenance of nursing competence
- Use of informed judgment
- Participation in research and other activities to generate new nursing knowledge
- Participation in activities to improve and implement nursing standards
- Integrity of the nursing profession
- Collaboration with coworkers, other health care professionals and consumers

Ethical codes are morally, not legally, binding.

Societal Acceptance: Legal Reinforcement of Professional Standards

Nurses must know and function within the legal parameters of nursing practice in the state where nursing services are offered. People know what services professional services nurses provide and hold them accountable for providing high-quality, safe and effective nursing care. If nurses have ethical or legal concerns about medical treatment or client situations, they must share their concerns with medical and institutional authorities. Because nurses are responsible for client well-being, they may refuse to execute a treatment, but they must not attempt to circumvent the physician by interfering with treatment without the physician's knowledge. Nurses and physicians must collaborate, not compete, with each other. Members of society trust nurses. For many years, Gallop poll findings reveal that Americans have consistently rated nursing as the most ethical of all the professions (Gallup, 2015; Jones, 2012).

Future Work for the Nursing Profession to Attain Full Professional Status

In nursing, several barriers to fulfilling all criteria for professional stature exist. First, while most professions have a single, specialized plan of study before persons can enter them, professional nursing has multiple levels of education for entry. Many recipients of nursing services do not know the differences in educational preparation. To them, a nurse is a nurse.

Along with an inconsistent educational entry level, many nurses have become specialists in a particular area of practice (e.g., oncology, cardiology, critical care). Frequently, some of these nurses find themselves having to choose between joining a specialty or general-purpose nursing organization because of limited time and monetary resources. Other nurses may not even join a professional organization (Shinn, 2012). By failing to unite, nurses reduce their political effectiveness and collective identity, which may create opportunity for others to exploit them.

In addition, society tends to devalue nurses more than other health care team members. Although nurses hold the lives of other persons in their hands when they practice, some clients view nurses simply as "hired help." In a capitalistic society, the amount of money received for a service is based on the perceived value of the service. Professional nurses tend to receive comparatively less compensation than other interprofessional health team members. According to the (BLS) (2015a), the average salary for full-time employed RNs in 2014 was $69,790 and certified RN anesthetists earned an average annual salary of $158,900 (BLS, 2015b). Nurses with graduate degrees made $30,000 more on average than nurses holding BSN and ADN degrees (BLS, 2015c). In comparison, based on 2015 data from the BLS (2015d), physician generalists earned a mean income of $221,419 (mean salaries for some specialty physicians topped $464,000) (Forbes, 2016). Pharmacists earned a median income of $120,950 (BLS, 2015e), physical therapists earned $82,390 (BLS, 2015f), and dental hygienists earned $71,520 (BLS, 2015g). The disparity in salary could be related to the fact that all of the above health team members (with the exception of dental hygienists) typically hold at least a master's degree in their practice area and some require doctorates for entry into practice.

Professional nurses must work together to showcase the contributions they make to society while developing ways to overcome the barriers to attaining full status as a profession. There are more professional nurses than any of the other members of the interdisciplinary health team. If efforts by the profession were channeled toward cooperation rather than competition, nurses could make substantial contributions toward the betterment of health for all.

REAL-LIFE REFLECTIONS

Recall the situation of Sue, who is considering returning to school. What advice would you give to Sue as she enters a baccalaureate nursing program? Why do you think each piece of advice you will give her is important?

Summary and Significance to Practice

Because nursing fails to meet all criteria for a profession, it is sometimes referred to as an emerging profession. The process of becoming a professional nurse involves change and growth throughout various stages of a career. Over time, being a professional nurse may become embedded into one's personal identity and being. The profession calls on nurses to engage in moral and ethical practice to provide what is best for clients. Through educational and occupational experiences, the nurse develops attitudes, beliefs, and skills as knowledge expands and deepens. A professional nurse should expect to commit to a life of continuous learning, growth, and development. Any change in clinical specialty practice area and formal education results in resocialization. The professional nurse assumes many roles when engaged in clinical practice. Effective implementation of these roles requires deep commitment; authentic caring; genuine compassion; technical competence; self-confidence; cognitive, clinical, and communication skills; and the ability to work in and cope with nonstop change, highly complex systems, and chaos.

From Theory to Practice

1. Has your perception of professional nursing changed since reading this chapter? Why or why not?
2. What do you think is a major barrier to nursing achieving status as a profession? Why do you think this is a major barrier? What steps could the nursing profession take to eliminate this barrier to attaining full status as a profession?

Nurse as Author

Write a 400 to 500 word essay about why you have decided to pursue a BSN in nursing and how this will affect your future nursing career. Remember that an essay has an introductory paragraph, several supporting paragraphs, and a concluding paragraph. If you need a refresher in how to write an essay, here is a link to the Writing Center at the University of Minnesota: **http://writing.umn.edu/sws/assets/pdf/ quicktips/academicessaystructures.pdf**

Be certain to follow instructions found in your course syllabus for this and any other written course assignment.

Your Digital Classroom

Online Exploration

American Association of Colleges of Nursing: **www.aacn.nche.edu**
American Nurses Association: **www.nursingworld.org**
International Council of Nurses: **www.icn.ch**
National Council of State Boards of Nursing: **www.ncsbn.org**
National League for Nursing: **www.nln.org**
Sigma Theta Tau International: **www.nursingsociety.org**

Expanding Your Understanding

1. Visit **www.nursingworld.org,** the official website of the ANA, to analyze the benefits and costs of membership. Would you join the ANA? Why or why not?
2. Search the internet for any specialized area of nursing practice, and see if you can find a professional nursing organization to support nurses practicing in that field of nursing. Analyze the benefits and costs of membership. Compare and contrast two professional nursing organizations.
3. Visit **www.ncsbn.org,** the website for the NCSBN. Identify key issues surrounding safe nursing practice. What states have enacted the multistate compact for professional nursing practice? Visit your SBN website to identify key information about license renewal, announcements, and news.

Beyond the Book

Visit **thePoint® www.thePoint.lww.com** for activities and information to reinforce the concepts and content covered in this chapter.

REFERENCES

Agnes, M. (2005). *Webster's new world college dictionary* (4th ed.). Cleveland, OH: Wiley Publishing.
Aiken, L. H., Clarke, S. P., Cheung, R. B., Sloane, D. M., & Silber, J. H. (2003). Educational levels of hospital nurses and surgical patient mortality. *Journal of the American Medical Association, 290,* 1617–1623.
Alexander, J., & Tate, M. A. (1998). *Web resource evaluation techniques.* Chester, PA: Widener University.
Alexander, M., Durham, C. F., Hooper, J. I., Jeffries, P. R., Goldman, N., Kardong-Edgren, et al. (2015). NCSBN simulation guidelines for prelicensure nursing programs. *Journal of Nursing Regulation, 6*(3), 39–42.
American Association of Colleges of Nursing (AACN). (2004). *AACN position statement on the practice doctorate in nursing, October 2004.* Retrieved from www.aacn.nche.edu/DNP/pdf/DNP.pdf. Accessed October 10, 2012.

AACN. (2008). *The essentials of baccalaureate education for professional nursing practice.* Washington, DC: Author.

AACN. (2015a). *The doctor of nursing practice: current issues and clarifying recommendations. Report from the task force on the implementation of the DNP.* Retrieved from http://www.aacn.nche.edu/aacn-publications/white-papers/DNP-Implementation-TF-Report-8–15.pdf. Accessed August 28, 2016.

AACN. (2015b). *Fact sheet: the impact of education on nursing practice.* Retrieved from http://www.aacn.nche.edu/media-relations/EdImpact.pdf. Accessed March 6, 2016.

AACN. (2016a). *About AACN.* Retrieved from www.aacn.nche.edu/about-aacn. Accessed March 11, 2016.

AACN. (2016b). *Mission and values.* Retrieved from http://www.aacn.nche.edu/about-aacn/mission-values. Accessed March 11, 2016.

American Nurses Association. (2010). *Nursing's social policy statement: The essence of the profession.* Silver Spring, MD: Author.

American Nurses Association (ANA). (2015a). *2014 annual report.* Retrieved from http://nursingworld.org/FunctionalMenu Categories/AboutANA/Annual-Report.pdf. Accessed March 12, 2016.

ANA. (2015b). *Code of ethics for nurses with interpretive statements.* Silver Spring, MD: Author.

ANA. (2015c). *Nursing scope and standards of practice* (3rd ed.). Silver Spring, MD: Nursebooks.org.

ANA. (2016a). *2016 culture of safety.* Retrieved from http://nursingworld.org/MainMenuCategories/ThePracticeofProfessionalNursing/2016-Culture-of-Safety. Accessed March 12, 2016.

ANA. (2016b). *Member benefits.* Retrieved from http://nursingworld.org/MainMenuCategories/ANAMarketplace. Accessed March 12, 2016.

ANA. (2016c). *FAQs.* Retrieved from http://nursingworld.org/FunctionalMenuCategories/FAQs#about. Accessed March 12, 2016.

American Nurses Credentialing Center (ANCC). (2016). *ANCC certification center.* Retrieved from http://www.nursecredentialing.org/Certification Access March 12, 2016.

Aqel, A. A., & Ahmad, M. M. (2014). High fidelity simulation effects on CPR knowledge, skill acquisition, and retention in nursing students. *Worldviews on Evidence-Based Nursing, 11*(6), 394–400.

Bandman, E. L., & Bandman, B. (1995). *Nursing ethics through the life span* (3rd ed.). East Norwalk, CT: Appleton & Lange.

Benner, P. (1984). *From novice to expert: Excellence and power in clinical nursing practice.* Menlo Park, CA: Addison-Wesley.

Benner, P., Tanner, C. A., & Chesla, C. A. (Eds.). (1996). *Expertise in nursing practice: Caring, clinical judgment and ethics.* New York: Springer.

Bevis, E. O., & Watson, J. (2000). *Toward a caring curriculum: A new pedagogy for nursing.* Sudbury, MA: Jones & Bartlett.

Billings, D., & Halstead, J. (2005). *Teaching in nursing: A guide for faculty* (2nd ed.). St. Louis, MO: Elsevier Saunders.

Bohm, D. (1980). *Wholeness and the implicate order.* London: Routledge.

Bradby, M. (1990). Status passage into nursing: another view of the process of socialization. *Journal of Advanced Nursing, 15,* 1220–1225.

Bridges, W. (2003). *Managing transitions, making the most of change.* Cambridge, MA: Perseus.

Broussard, P. C., & Oberleitner, M. G. (1997). Writing and thinking: a process to critical understanding. *Journal of Nursing Education, 36*(7), 334–336.

Brunke, L. (2003). Canadian provincial and territorial professional organizations and colleges. In M. McIntyre, & E. Thomlinson (Eds.), *Realities of Canadian nursing: Professional, practice and power issues.* Philadelphia, PA: Lippincott Williams & Wilkins.

Clarke, B., James, C., & Kelly, J. (1996). Reflective practice: reviewing the issues and refocusing the debate. *International Journal of Nursing Studies, 33,* 171–180.

Commission on Collegiate Nursing Education. (2013). *Standards for Accreditation of Baccalaureate and Graduate Nursing Programs.* Retrieved from www.aacn.nche.edu/ccne-accreditation/Proposed_Standards_Clean_3–2013.pdf. Accessed May 20, 2013.

Dictionary.com. (n.d.). *Dictionary.com's 21st Century Lexicon.* Retrieved from http://dictionary.reference.com/browse/core competency. Accessed February 14, 2016.

Diekelmann, N. L., & Rather, M. L. (Eds.). (1993). *Transforming RN education: Dialogue and debate.* New York: National League for Nursing.

Dock, L., & Stewart, I. (1920). *A short history of nursing.* New York: Putnam.

Dreyfus, S., & Dreyfus, H. (1980). *A five-stage model of the mental activities involved in directed skill acquisition.* Washington, DC: Storming Media. Retrieved from www.dtic.mil/cgi-bin/GetTRDoc?AD=ADA084551&Location=U2&doc=Get TRDoc. Accessed May 20, 2013.

Dunham, K. S. (2008). *How to survive and maybe even love nursing school!* (3rd ed.). Philadelphia, PA: F. A. Davis.

Engum, S. A., & Jeffries, P. R. (2012). Interdisciplinary collisions: bringing healthcare professionals together. *Collegian, 19*(3), 145–151.

Flanagan, L. (1976). *One strong voice.* Kansas City, MO: Lowell Press.

Fondiller, S. H. (2007). *Health professional style manual.* New York: Springer.

Forbes. (2016). *The 10 best paying medical specialties.* Retrieved from http://www.forbes.com/pictures/eekj45fmdl/the-10-best-paying-medical-specialties/ Accessed March 6, 2016.

Fowler, M. D. M. (2015a). *Guide to the code of ethics for nurses with interpretive statements, development, interpretation and application* (2nd ed.) Silver Spring, MD: American Nurses Association.

Fowler, M. D. M. (2015b). *Guide to Nursing's social policy statement: Understanding the profession from social contract to social covenant.* Silver Spring MD: American Nurses Association.

Freidson, E. (1994). *Professionalism reborn: Theory, prophecy and policy.* Chicago: University of Chicago Press.

Gallup. (2015). *Honesty/ethics in professions.* Retrieved from http://www.gallup.com/poll/1654/Honesty-Ethics-Professions.aspx. Accessed February 13, 2016.

Hinshaw, A. S. (1976). *Socialization and resocialization of nurses for professional nursing practice (National League for Nursing Publication No. 15–1659).* New York: National League for Nursing.

Institute of Medicine. (2011). *The future of nursing: Leading change, advancing health.* Washington, DC: National Academies Press.

International Council of Nurses (ICN). (2011). *Our mission.* Retrieved from www.icn.ch/about-icn/icns-mission/. Accessed October 10, 2012.

ICN. (2012). *The ICN code of ethics for nurses.* Revised 2012. Retrieved from http://www.icn.ch/images/stories/documents/about/icncode_english.pdf. Accessed February 13, 2016.

Jones, J. M. (2012). *Nurses top honesty and ethics list for the 11th year.* Retrieved from www.gallup.com/poll/145043/nurses-top-honesty-ethics-list-11-year.aspx. Accessed October 8, 2012.

Jones, R. (2004). The science and meaning of the self. *Journal of Analytical Psychology, 49,* 217–233.

Kaiser Family Foundation. (2016). *Total number of professionally active registered nurses.* Retrieved from http://kff.org/other/state-indicator/total-registered-nurses/. Accessed February 13, 2016.

Kalisch, P., & Kalisch, B. (2004). *The advance of American nursing: A history* (4th ed.). Philadelphia, PA: Lippincott Williams & Wilkins.

Kim, H. S. (1999). Critical reflective inquiry for knowledge development in nursing practice. *Journal of Advanced Nursing, 29*(5), 1205–1212.

Leddy, S. K. (2003). *Integrative health promotion.* Thorofare, NJ: Slack.

Linton, R. (1945). *The cultural background of personality.* New York: Appleton.

Loquist, R. S. (1999). Regulation: parallel and powerful. In J. A. Milstead (Ed.), *Health policy and politics: A nurse's guide.* Gaithersburg, MD: Aspen.

Lynn, M. R., McCain, N. L., & Boss, B. J. (1989). Socialization of RN to BSN. *Image—The Journal of Nursing Scholarship, 21,* 232–237.

Malloy, A. (2005). *Stop living your job, start living your life.* Berkeley, CA: Ulysses.

Martinez, M. E. (2000). *Education as the cultivation of intelligence.* Mahwah, NJ: Lawrence Erlbaum.

Massachusetts Action Coalition. (2014). *The Massachusetts Nursing Core Competencies: A toolkit for implementation in education and practice settings.* Retrieved from http://www.mass.edu/nahi/documents/Toolkit-First%20Edition-May%202014-r1.pdf Accessed February 14, 2016.

Massachusetts Department of Higher Education Nurse of the Future Competency Committee. (2010). *Nurse of the Future Nursing Core Competencies Graphic.* Boston: MA: Department of Higher Education. Retrieved from http://www.mass.edu/nahi/documents/NursingCoreCompetenciesGraphic.pdf Accessed February 14, 2016.

Miller, B. K., Adams, D., & Beck, L. (1993). A behavioral inventory for professionalism in nursing. *Journal of Professional Nursing, 9*(5), 290–295.

Milstead, J. A. (2008). *Health policy and politics: A nurse's guide* (3rd ed.). Sudbury, MA: Jones & Bartlett.

Morse, J. M., Bottorff, J., Neander, W., & Solberg, S. (1991). Comparative analysis of conceptualizations and theories of caring. *Image—The Journal of Nursing Scholarship, 23*(2), 119–126.

National Council of State Boards of Nursing (NCSBN). (2016a). *2015 Number of candidates taking NCLEX examination and percent passing by type of candidate.* Retrieved from https://www.ncsbn.org/Table_of_Pass_Rates_2015_(3).pdf. Accessed February 14, 2016.

NCSBN. (2016b). *About NCSBN.* Retrieved from https://www.ncsbn.org/about.htm. Accessed March 10, 2016.

NCSBN. (2016c). *Member Boards.* Retrieved from https://www.ncsbn.org/member-boards.htm. Accessed March 11, 2016.

National League for Nursing. (2010). *Outcomes and competencies for graduates of practical/vocational, diploma, associate degree, baccalaureate, master's, practice doctorate and research doctorate programs in nursing.* New York: National League for Nursing.

National League for Nursing. (2016a). *About NLN.* Retrieved from http://nln.org/about. Accessed March 6, 2016.

National League for Nursing. (2016b). *Core values.* Retrieved from http://nln.org/about/core-values. Accessed March 6, 2016.

National League for Nursing. (2016c). *Mission and goals* http://nln.org/about/mission-goals. Accessed March 6, 2016.

National Student Nurses Association. (n.d.). *About us.* Retrieved from http://www.nsna.org/about-nasa.html. Accessed June 7, 2017.

Osuna, M. (2014). *Nursing school thrive guide.* Lexington, KY: Author.

Paul, R. (1992). *Critical thinking: What every person needs to survive in a rapidly changing world* (2nd Rev. ed.). Santa Rosa, CA: Foundation for Critical Thinking.

PEW Health Professions Commission. (1998). *Recreating health professional practice for a new century.* San Francisco, CA: University of California, San Francisco Center for the Health Professions.

Powell, J. H. (1989). The reflective practitioner in nursing. *Journal of Advanced Nursing, 14*(10), 824–832.

QSEN Institute. (2014). Project overview. Retrieved from http://qsen.org/about-qsen/project-overview/. Accessed February 14, 2016.

Quan, K. (2006). *The everything new nurse book.* Avon, MA: Adams Media.

Ray, M. (1998). Complexity and nursing science. *Nursing Science Quarterly, 11*(3), 91–93.

Ross-Kerr, J. (2011). Credentialing in nursing. In J. Ross-Kerr, & M. Wood (Eds.), *Canadian nursing issues & perspectives.* Toronto: Elsevier Canada.

Rubenfeld, M. G. & Scheffer, B. K. (2015). *Critical thinking tactics for nurses* (3rd ed.). Burlington MA: Jones & Bartlett Learning.

Schon, D. A. (1983). *The reflective practitioner.* London: Temple Smith.

Schon, D. A. (1987). *Educating the reflective practitioner: Toward a new design for teaching and learning in the professions.* San Francisco, CA: Jossey-Bass.

Shane, D. L. (1980). The returning-to-school syndrome. In S. Mirin (Ed.), *Teaching tomorrow's nurse.* Wakefield, MA: Nursing Resources.

Shinn, L. (2012). Current issues in nursing associations. In D. Mason, J. Leavitt, & M. Chaffee (Eds.), *Policy & politics in nursing and health care* (6th ed.). St. Louis, MO: Elsevier Saunders.

Sigma Theta Tau International. (2016). *STTI Organizational Fact Sheet.* Retrieved from http://www.nursingsociety.org/why-stti/about-stti/sigma-theta-tau-international-organizational-fact-sheet. Accessed March 12, 2016

Stebbins, L. F. (2006). *Student guide to research in the digital age.* Westport, CT: Libraries Unlimited.

Sullivan, M. C., & Christopher, M. M. (1999). Ethical issues. In E. J. Sullivan (Ed.), *Creating nursing's future.* St. Louis, MO: Mosby. https://www.bon.texas.gov/pdfs/publication_pdfs/delc-2010.pdf

United States Bureau of Labor Statistics (USBLS). (2015a). 2.75 million employed in nursing practice. *Occupational Outlook Handbook Dec. 2015.* Retrieved from https://www.bls.gov/ooh/healthcare/registered-nurses.htm. Accessed February 13, 2016.

USBLS. (2015b). *Occupational employment & wages, May 2015, 29–1141 Registered Nurses.* Retrieved from http://www.bls.gov/oes/current/oes291141.htm. Accessed March 6, 2016.

USBLS. (2015c). *Nurse anesthetists, nurse midwives and nurse practitioners.* Retrieved from http://www.bls.gov/ooh/health-care/nurse-anesthetists-nurse-midwives-and-nurse-practitioners.htm. Accessed March 6, 2016.

USBLS. (2015d). *Physicians and surgeons.* Retrieved from http://www.bls.gov/ooh/healthcare/physicians-and-surgeons.htm#tab-5. Accessed March 6, 2016.

USBLS. (2015e). *Pharmacists.* Retrieved from http://www.bls.gov/ooh/healthcare/pharmacists.htm. Accessed March 6, 2016.

USBLS. (2015f). *Physical therapists.* Retrieved from http://www.bls.gov/ooh/healthcare/physical-therapists.htm#tab-1. Accessed March 6, 2016.

USBLS. (2015g). *Dental hygienists.* Retrieved from http://www.bls.gov/ooh/healthcare/dental-hygienists.htm. Accessed March 6, 2016.

USBLS. (2016). *U.S. Department of Labor, Occupational Outlook Handbook, 2016–17 Edition, Registered.* Retrieved from http://www.bls.gov/ooh/healthcare/registered-nurses.htm. Accessed February 14, 2016.

University of Southern Maine. (2012). *Checklist for evaluating web resources.* Retrieved from http://www.usm.maine.edu/library/checklist-evaluating-web-resources. Accessed October 10, 2012.

Virginia Henderson Global Nursing e-Repository. (2016). *About the Henderson repository.* Retrieved from http://www.nursing-library.org/vhl/pages/about.html. Accessed March 12, 2016.

Weaver, A. (2011). High-fidelity patient simulation in nursing education: An integrative review. *Nursing Education Perspectives, 32*(1), 37–40.

Wiggins, M. (2008). The challenge of change. In C. Lindberg, S. Nash, & C. Lindberg (Eds.), *On the edge: Nursing in the age of complexity.* Bordentown, NJ: Plexus Press.

Wilson, L., & Rockstraw, L. (2012). *Human simulation for nursing and health professions.* New York: Springer Publishing.

Young, C., & Koopsen, C. (2011). *Spirituality, health and healing: An integrative approach.* Burlington, MA: Jones & Bartlett.

Young, L., & Paterson, B. (2007). *Teaching nursing: Developing a student-centered learning environment.* Philadelphia, PA: Lippincott Williams & Wilkins.

2

The History Behind the Development of Professional Nursing

LEARNING OUTCOMES

By the end of this chapter, the learner will be able to:

1. Trace the history of nursing from ancient to current times.
2. Outline the key societal trends that affected recruitment and retention of nurses in the workforce.
3. Explain the parallels between past nursing history and current nursing practice.
4. Describe how history could be used to address current and future nursing issues.

REAL-LIFE REFLECTIONS

Marita, Carol, and Joe received an assignment to give a class presentation on nursing history that could be used to prepare the nursing profession for a future challenge. At first, they view this assignment as busywork. However, as they explore the history of nursing, they come to appreciate significant events and persons. They acknowledge that the profession may need to look at history to solve current and future problems.

- *How much do you know about the history of nursing?*
- *Do you think knowing the history of the profession might be helpful as you embark on this phase of your education? Why or why not?*

With advances in technology, the field of health care is increasingly initiating targeted efforts to explain the interrelationships of health, longevity, multiculturalism, socioeconomics, and spirituality. In many ways, nursing has helped forge the path to this holistic view of health care. An examination of nursing history provides professional nurses with an understanding of the profession's unique place within the health care arena and may offer answers for current and future challenges.

Take Note!

An examination of nursing history provides professional nurses with an understanding of the profession's unique place within the health care arena and may offer answers for current and future challenges.

NURSING IN ANCIENT CIVILIZATIONS (BEFORE 1 CE)

Humans learned how to care for one other by observing how animals relied on each other in times of need (Nutting & Dock, 1935a), such as uninjured animals bringing food to injured companions and helpless offspring. By watching animals, humans learned therapies such as licking wounds as a form of an antiseptic cleaning (from canines and felines), applying pressure to control bleeding (from apes), amputating extremities when ensnared in traps (from rats), ingesting salt (from deer, cows, and antelope), wrapping wounds in a spiral fashion (from birds), applying splints (from snipe), traveling great distances to soak in healing water (from deer), and entombing the dead (from bees).

Early cultures believed that a person's soul (or life-giving spirit forces) existed independent of the body. Human tragedy, including illness, was blamed on the spirit world. Early therapies for illnesses and injuries focused on the religious domain and societies believed that some of their members possessed special powers that could ease suffering, enhance healing, and cure diseases by appeasing the spirits. Techniques used by early healers included pummeling (a form of massage), administering herbs, exposing persons to smoke, squeezing, starving, purging, applying roots or balms to the skin, or twisting the body into various positions. Along with touch, medicine magicians frequently applied warm poultices and held healing ceremonies using drumming, smoking, and chanting to drive out evil spirits (Nutting & Dock, 1935a).

Egypt

The oldest written recordings about medicine and nursing come from Egypt and date to 3000 BCE. The Ebers Papyrus outlines over 700 therapies derived from minerals, plants, and animals. Compounded prescriptions were made up in the forms of decoctions, pills, tablets, injections, infusions, lozenges, powders, potions, inhalations, lotions, ointments, and plasters (Kalisch & Kalisch, 2004; Nutting & Dock, 1935a). The art of medicine in ancient Egypt consisted of two branches. The theurgic class devoted themselves to magical cures, while the practitioners used natural cures. Along with disease treatment, the Egyptians practiced public hygiene and sanitation. Although there is no evidence of hospitals or nursing in ancient Egypt, there is mention of temple priestesses without reference to their duties (Nutting & Dock, 1935a).

India

Details of nursing are also recorded in Lesson IX of the *Charaka Samhita*. This ancient Indian record describes the following four qualifications for a nurse: (1) knowledge of drug preparation, (2) cleverness, (3) devotion to patients, and (4) purity of body and mind (Nutting & Dock, 1935a). The ancient Indians were the first to link hygiene to health (Jamieson & Sewall, 1954; Kalisch & Kalisch, 2004; Nutting & Dock, 1935a).

In the third century BCE, King Asoka of India developed community institutes to care for sick travelers. These precursors of hospitals were described as spacious and roomy mansions protected from strong winds, breezes, smoke, sun, dust, and rain. In **ancient nursing practice**, the sick were cared for by male attendants noted for their purity and cleanliness of habits; they were characterized as kind, clever, and skillful in providing service to others. Along with providing good nutrition, ventilation, and a clean environment, the attendants read stories, chanted hymns, played musical instruments, and conversed with the infirm while attending to all their needs. In many ways, these earliest known nursing interventions were the **roots of holistic nursing practice**. At the same time, records from Ceylon wrote about women who provided care for the sick as part of the Buddhist tradition of mercy, compassion, justice, and humane treatment for all living things. Caring for the infirmed in the ancient Far East was done by both men and women (Nutting & Dock, 1935a).

Babylonia

The Babylonians shared some ideas with the Egyptians, but they also believed that numbers possessed magical powers and displayed a great interest in astrology (Jamieson & Sewall, 1954). Like the Egyptians, the Babylonians viewed illness as punishment for displeasing or sinning against the gods and they used methods to banish demons and developed ways to avoid evil spirits. However, the Babylonians also left records outlining surgical procedures, and in 1900 BCE, King Hammurabi developed a code that provided the first sliding scale of fees for goods and services. Hammurabi's law also specified that citizens had to compensate each other equally for transgressions. Therefore, a surgeon could have his hands amputated if he performed unsuccessful surgery (Jamieson & Sewall, 1954; Nutting & Dock, 1935a).

China

The ancient Chinese developed the concept of yin (the passive, negative, feminine energy force) and yang (the active, positive, masculine energy force) and defined health as a balance of these two forces. By 2000 BCE, the Chinese were practicing dissection, performing acupuncture, and prescribing herbal therapies to enhance health and cure illness. They used baths to reduce fever and bloodletting to remove evil spirits from the body. The Chinese were the first to outline detailed principles of physical examination (look, listen, ask, and feel) (Jamieson & Sewall, 1954).

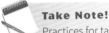

Take Note!
Practices for taking care of the ill date back to the beginning of civilizations.

Persia

A Persian epic dated 642 BCE mentions three kinds of physicians: one healed by the knife, another by exorcism and incantations, and a third by using plants. The Persians excelled at chemistry: they tested bodily fluids, studied drug, and were the first to introduce medications derived from plants. They built beautiful hospitals and cared for patients in specialized wards. Patients were treated with skills and kindness. Although Persian records make no mention of nurses, they describe numerous procedures, many of which fall within the domain of current nursing practice, such as detailed ways to care for wounds, provide hydration, and control discomfort (Nutting & Dock, 1935a).

Palestine

The Hebrew culture adopted sanitary measures from Egypt during the period of enslavement around 1200 BCE. The ancient Hebrews adopted natural cures but rejected magical therapies. The Old Testament outlines food inspection, vital statistics records, and infectious disease quarantine followed by fumigation. Hebrew law also placed an obligation on people to show sympathy, cheer, and aid to the sick. One of the seven acts of charity mentioned in rabbinical literature is visiting the sick. The Hebrews developed sick houses that were connected to rest houses for travelers and the destitute (Nutting & Dock, 1935a).

Greece

Like Egypt, Greece traced medical arts to divine myths. The Greeks also divided the healing arts into two branches, with one retaining priestly powers and the other having medical functions.

In *The Iliad*, Homer identifies Asklepios, the father of Machaon and Podalirius, as the "blameless physician." Temples of Asklepios were reported to exist as early as 1134 BCE.

Hospitality was a sacred obligation in Greek culture. In large Greek cities, the "xenodochium" served as a municipal inn for strangers, the poor, and the sick (Nutting & Dock, 1935a). In addition to the public xenodochium, the Greeks established "iotrions" (temples for healing services) where surgery was performed and dispensaries were located. Only persons who could be cured were admitted to the iotrions. Temples had a place devoted to the sick called the "abaton." Ruins reveal that the abaton contained a large room with an altar surrounded by smaller rooms that could accommodate a single person. The abaton was staffed with priests and a variety of others, including physicians, bath attendants, slaves, and priestesses. The Greeks believed that birth and death caused permanent pollution where they occurred. Therefore, the terminally ill were left on the street to die (Nutting & Dock, 1935a).

The great physician Hippocrates outlined the role of physicians as assisting nature to bring about a cure. Hippocrates set standards for bathing, bandaging, and other cures. Although he provided no treatise on nursing, his work specified that he used assistants (Kalisch & Kalisch, 2004; Nutting & Dock, 1935a).

Rome

The Greeks introduced the Romans to medicine sometime in the third century BCE. Before then, Romans believed that lost health could only be restored by the gods. The Romans constructed drains, aqueducts, good roads, sewage systems, and proper cemeteries, as well as an organized system of medicine that enhanced public health. Nero organized a Roman medical service and appointed a superintendent of court physicians. Slaves of rich families cultivated knowledge of practical medicine. Many slaves earned freedom by curing owners with their skills. The Romans reserved the best medical and nursing care for their soldiers (Kalisch & Kalisch, 2004; Nutting & Dock, 1935a).

Northern Europe

Civilization in northern Europe at the time of the Roman Empire was less organized. The ancient Teutons, Norsemen, and Druids revered their wise women. These women, usually elders, gathered herbs that they knew had medicinal and remedial qualities.

As time progressed, various superstitions followed both wise women and medicine men. According to Finnish mythology, the ancient healers practiced **white magic** or healing magic, which was primarily medicinal in nature. However, society grew to believe that these persons with special healing powers also had connections to evil spirits and could use "black magic," which caused natural catastrophes or human illness and injury (Nutting & Dock, 1935a). The healing women may have been seen as early prototypes of witches.

Germany

Like the northern Europeans in the last millennium before the Christian era, the Gauls and Germans held certain women in high regard. They believed that these women could communicate readily with the gods. Many women also possessed great knowledge and skill in medicine and surgery. German women established expertise in treating wounds from war, providing obstetrical care, and treating animals (Nutting & Dock, 1935a).

■ QUESTIONS FOR REFLECTION

1. Are any ancient nursing interventions used today to tend to the ill and infirmed?
2. Why do you think that some ancient nursing interventions and medical therapies had to be "rediscovered"?

NURSING IN THE EARLY CHRISTIAN ERA (1–500 CE)

Roman Matrons

As early as the second century CE, Roman converts to Christianity transformed their homes into places to care for the sick and poor. Women from well-established Roman families enjoyed dignified and respected positions in the society. Wives in such families were considered equal to their husbands. These **Roman matrons** organized and delivered care to persons in need.

The earliest female workers in the Catholic Church who were concerned with nursing were the deaconesses and widows. Early converts to Christianity, especially affluent women, viewed comforting the afflicted as a sacred duty. Deaconesses were married women who were commissioned to serve in a church-related agency such as a hospital or social outreach program, although men also performed nursing duties. In 60 CE, Phoebe became the first parish worker, friendly visitor, and district nurse and is credited as the mother of visiting nursing (Nutting & Dock, 1935a).

Early church deacons and deaconesses sought out those in need, established a system of visiting nurses, and sometimes brought the ill into their homes. As home hospitals were organized, the deaconate became associated with the work of nursing. Eventually, the bishops followed the deaconate example and opened their homes to tend to the sick. As congregations grew and more poor people joined them, the church established the Christian xenodochium, or home for strangers. The xenodochium contained one section for ordinary travelers and another section for the poor and infirm. Nursing the sick was seen as proper penance for past sins and solace for unhappy lives (Nutting & Dock, 1935a).

Between 249 CE and 263 CE, an extensive epidemic hit Rome, resulting in many deaths among the deaconate. In 350 CE, another epidemic hit the city of Edessa, where desperate wealthy inhabitants freely gave money to Ephrem to provide care for the ill. Ephrem, who was later canonized as a saint, used the donations to build the first hospital. Along with the matrons, widows, old men, and the disenfranchised provided nursing care in the hospital established by Ephrem.

In the fifth century CE, Emperor Justinian granted the bishops authority over hospitals. With great zeal, the bishops built shelters, hospices, foundling asylums, and nosocomials (nursing hospitals) within the confines of monasteries. Nursing religious orders were formed and flourished. Men and women joined the religious orders. Because arranged marriages were common in this era, women could join a religious order and embark on a life of caring for the ill within these establishments resulting in living a life that was intellectually stimulating and personally satisfying (Jamieson & Sewall, 1954; Nutting & Dock, 1935a).

Advances in Greece

Although **early Christian nurses** were instrumental in the development of modern nursing, other groups played a key role in the advancement of nursing practice. In 100 CE, Aretaeus emphasized the necessity for strict cleanliness of bedclothes, the use of powders on moist skin, and mouthwashes for patients who were not allowed to drink. He directed that, for fevers, rooms should be light and airy and patients should be lightly covered and receive only liquids for nourishment. Excitable patients should be kept in small, undecorated rooms, with constant temperature. Aretaeus outlined strategies for pain control that included hot baths, fomentations, hot water bladders, light massage, plasters, and salves. Music was also used to soothe and lull persons in distress.

In 138 CE, the Greeks established a maternity hospital and a home for the dying (Nutting & Dock, 1935a).

NURSING IN THE MIDDLE AGES (500–1500)

The first mention of a nursing uniform surfaced in 1190, when a Bavarian monk insisted that religious women wear distinctive dress to be recognized when out in public performing charitable acts. As monasteries flourished as centers of learning, nuns became distinguished for work in academia and service. By the 13th century CE, monks and nuns were said to have more medical knowledge than the rest of the society (Nutting & Dock, 1935a).

Because of the societal power of the monks and nuns possessed from their medical knowledge, the Lateran Council in 1123 forbade monks and priests from the practice of medicine. The Benedictine sisters, however, covertly and actively continued to expand the knowledge of medicine and practiced medicine and nursing without the support of the church. Monks secretly joined the nuns and they conjointly cared for the sick: the monks cared for men and the nuns cared for women. The nuns took charge of the hospital while the monks served as priests (Nutting & Dock, 1935a).

Hildegarde, a nun, perhaps heralded the beginning of female dominance in nursing. She possessed extraordinary intellectual powers and amassed great knowledge of medicine through her nursing experiences. Between 1151 and 1159, she wrote volumes devoted to medical works that include accurate physiology related to reproduction, circulation, and the nervous system (Nutting & Dock, 1935a).

The Crusades and Nursing Knights

During the Crusades, hospitals were built on the routes to and in Jerusalem where men delivered care to travelers and battle-scarred warriors. The Knights Hospitallers of St. John of Jerusalem started as an exclusive nursing order. The Teutonic Knights had both nursing and military duties. The Knights of St. Lazarus was a nursing order from the great hospital in Jerusalem built by Basil in AD 329. Along with the Knights of St. Lazarus, the Sisters of St. Lazarus, an order of nuns, provided care.

In England, the Order of St. John consisted of men devoted to charitable work, including the formation of cottage hospitals, convalescent homes, and nurse training for the poor (Kalisch & Kalisch, 2004; Nutting & Dock, 1935a).

In the 11th century, two hospitals were built in England: one to care for lepers and another to care for other persons. Religious brothers attended to the sick men and nuns attended to the sick women. The hospital for lepers (St. Giles) was run by an order of nuns known as the Poor Clares. Ladies of noble birth added attending to the sick as a social duty (Nutting & Dock, 1935a).

Religious Orders of Nursing for Women

In the 12th century France, nursing became part of the manual labor performed by several orders of Roman Catholic sisters. Secular orders of nuns also engaged in nursing. One French hospital staffed itself with laywomen who were either widowed or repenting from sins of impurity (Nutting & Dock, 1935a). **Nurses from religious orders** provided a structured approach to the care of the ill and infirm, whereas other women haphazardly cared for them. In Paris, the Augustinian order of nuns provided nursing care in hospitals. Those in the Augustinian order shared with one another information on how to care for the sick. In 1212, the Catholic Church passed statutes to regulate the nursing orders to exercise control over them. To join, both men and women took permanent vows of poverty, chastity, and obedience. Within 150 years, the various orders became corrupt and many leaders skimmed off donated resources for personal gain. The men and women actually caring for the sick became demoralized because they had no respite from the unrelenting toil. Religious orders, especially the nuns, accumulated much money and many possessions and focused their efforts to manage them. When an epidemic of syphilis spread, hospitals became centers of infection. During this time, many persons left monasteries and convents taking whatever they could carry, further depleting resources for the care of the infirmed (Nutting & Dock, 1935a).

THE ESTABLISHMENT OF NURSING IN EUROPE, ENGLAND, AND THE NEW WORLD (1500–1819)

France

In 1505, France's King Louis XII decreed that jurisdiction of the hospitals be temporarily removed from the Catholic Church and governed by secular directors. In 1526, the rectors of a hospital located in Lyons directed staff members to wear a white uniform to denote purity of character. In 1562, the dress changed from white to black, with a white linen apron and an unstarched white cap. The apron was worn when directly caring for the sick. By the middle of the 16th century, the secular rectors introduced stringent regulations and required nursing service members to become part of a religious order. Male nurses were required to wear blue robes and silver crosses. Female nurses could only leave nursing to marry or to care for aging parents. Nursing service members worked in hospitals, visited the sick at home, and distributed herbal medications (Nutting & Dock, 1935a).

England

In England, the control of hospitals moved from the church to become the responsibility of the cities. Philanthropy and state aid became the major funding sources. Members of religious orders were replaced by ordinary lay servants and attendants hired by civic authorities who had little knowledge about caring for the infirm. The matron, who had the status of an untrained housekeeper, usually had some knowledge of how to run a hospital, supervised all attendants, and was responsible for finding staff. Frequently, the matron found care attendants from jails and debtor prisons. The title "sister" was bestowed on the head nurse of a ward. A "sister" had no formal nursing education, but assumed responsibility for the staff that cared for patients and the work performed on a ward. Because of their social status, an ordinance passed in 1699 denoted that only wives of free men could hold the position of sister. Patients received care from heartless attendants and under nurses (female servants who were hired by the matron, but learned how to care for patients from a sister), who were required to work 12 to 48 hours without a break. In some cases, patients nursed each other as the servant nurses slept (Nutting & Dock, 1935a).

The late 1700s marked the earliest beginning of the worldwide hospital reform movement. John Howard's work on reforming hospitals evolved from his crusade to reform prisons (Jamieson & Sewall, 1954). In his 1789 notes on the state of hospitals throughout Europe and England, Howard wrote that hospitals staffed by members from religious orders tended to be quiet, neat, and clean, with careful attention to patient hygiene and infection prevention. When describing secular hospitals, he wrote that patients were dirty, pest infested, and without bed linens (Nutting & Dock, 1935b).

Nursing in the New World

As the New World was settled, French and Spanish religious orders opened hospitals. In what is now Canada, the Jesuits opened a hospital for settlers and native people. The native people shared remedies for scurvy with the French. Likewise, the Jesuits shared their knowledge of medicines with the native populations. The nuns assumed most of the patient care in hospitals. As hospital labors for nuns grew heavier, the native women also quickly began providing patient care (Nutting & Dock, 1935b).

Sometime before 1524, Cortez built the Hospital of the Immaculate Conception in the location of what is now Mexico City. Nursing staff consisted primarily of a religious order of men. In 1531, the second oldest hospital of the New World was founded in what is now Santa Fe, New Mexico, where a community of over 30,000 members of the Pueblo tribe practiced hospitality and charitable works (Nutting & Dock, 1935b).

In the English colonies, the growth of hospitals was slow. Often, a ship's captain assumed the role of religious deacon, and frequently his wife assumed midwife responsibilities. Early treatment for illness in the English colonies consisted of prayer and superstitious practices. Early American hospitals admitted the poor and destitute along with the sick. Care was provided from uneducated persons from public workhouses and houses of correction. When hospitals opened in New York in 1751 and Philadelphia in 1771, they admitted only ill persons. Although the New York and Philadelphia hospitals relied solely on private donations for support, administrators exercised care in selecting the person who provides patient care services. The hospitals offered basic training in patient care. Dr. Valentine Seaman of the New York Hospital was the first physician known to have lectured American nurses in the areas of anatomy, physiology, maternal nursing, and care of children (Jamieson & Sewall, 1954; Kalisch & Kalisch, 2004).

> **Take Note!**
> As the New World was colonized, members of religious orders established the earliest health care systems.

During the American Revolutionary War, Catholic nuns were the only organized group of nurses. Women followed husbands to the battlegrounds and provided nursing care to the wounded and infirmed soldiers. Many homes and barns became hospitals. In 1786, the Quakers established the Philadelphia Dispensary, where physicians practiced disease prevention. In New York, a residential insane asylum was founded in 1798. In Canada, the Augustinian nuns from France established hospitals, visiting nurse programs, schools, and orphanages (Jamieson & Sewall, 1954; Nutting & Dock, 1935b).

THE MOVEMENT OF NURSING TO A RESPECTABLE PROFESSION (1820–1917)

Although efforts to educate nurses did not become formalized until the early 19th century, at the end of the 18th century, nursing manuals began to appear. Some contained commonsense information, while others were scientifically based. Dr. J. D. Phahler's manual gave specific instructions on how to arrange and maintain a sick room, procedures for various treatments, instructions for use of equipment, and maintenance of written records. Along with procedures, Phahler's manual emphasized the importance of attending to patients' psychological needs. Dr. Franz May's nursing manual provided more general approaches to patient care and also emphasized the importance of maintaining the health of caregivers. In 1836, Pastor Gossner, who assumed responsibility for a German evangelical hospital, favored the word "Pflegerin" (nurse) to title care attendants in Prussia (Nutting & Dock, 1935b).

In 1821, Pastor Theodor Fliedner arrived in Kaiserworth, Germany, to find himself the pastor of a financially depressed congregation. Fliedner founded a hospital there for two purposes: to care for the sick and to provide a field for deaconess instruction. In 1836, Gertrud Reichardt, a physician's daughter who helped with her father's practice, became the first probationer of the hospital. A probationer was a young woman who expressed an interest in becoming a nurse, but was uncertain if she had the stamina, fortitude, and determination to learn how and to provide patient care services. Under the leadership of Pastor Fliedner's wife Fredrike, the hospital tended the sick and probationers received clinical and theoretical instruction on the art of nursing. Upon completion of their education, the newly ordained deaconesses provided services to the poor, imprisoned, and infirmed (Jamieson & Sewall, 1954; Nutting & Dock, 1935b). The deaconesses from **Kaiserworth** established an honorable reputation of nursing that spread worldwide. In 1850, Fliedner took several deaconesses to Pittsburgh, Pennsylvania, where they staffed a hospital. The movement progressed to Milwaukee, Wisconsin, where the Deaconess Home and Hospital was founded (Jamieson & Sewall, 1954; Nutting & Dock, 1935b).

In 1811, Stephen Grellet (a French American) became appalled at the living conditions of the children who had been born in prison. He consulted Elizabeth Fry, an English friend, to help. Fry had developed a program for the women prisoners to make and sell goods. Revenue generated from the sale of the goods provided funds to feed, clothe, and care for the children. As she traveled throughout Europe setting up similar programs, Fry became acquainted with Kaiserworth, a German training program for nurses. Fry referred **Florence Nightingale** to Kaiserworth upon learning of Nightingale's interest in nursing (Jamieson & Sewall, 1954; Nutting & Dock, 1935b).

In 1831, a group of Irish women under the leadership of Catherine McAuley formed the Religious Sisters of Mercy and provided nursing services throughout Ireland and the world. The Irish sisters devised a system of **careful nursing** that comprised "physical care and emotional consolation provided from a spiritual perspective" (Meehan, 2003, p. 99). In the realm of careful nursing, each client was cared for with great tenderness, gentleness, kindness, and patience. Patients received highly skilled care from nurses who practiced with spiritual love, sought to create an environment of calmness, created restorative environments, strove for perfection in keeping patients safe and comfortable, provided health education, collaborated with physicians and other health care providers, and took care of themselves. During the Asian cholera epidemic of 1832, there was a substantially lower mortality rate among recipients of nursing services from McAuley and her colleagues (Meehan, 2003).

The Nursing Society of Philadelphia was founded in 1836 and primarily provided home maternity services. This group selected its nurses from the applicants who displayed stable character. In 1850, the Nursing Society opened a home and school where systematic instruction was given on cooking and obstetrics. Students received clinical instruction in client homes (Jamieson & Sewall, 1954).

Florence Nightingale and the Birth of Nursing as a Profession

The beginnings of nursing reform evolved from efforts to reform prisons and hospitals. Florence Nightingale (Fig. 2.1) led the efforts to reform patient care and established nursing as a profession.

Nightingale was born into an affluent English family. Her father delighted in teaching her Latin, Greek, and other languages, as well as mathematics, science, and reading. According to her diary entries, Nightingale identified nursing as her life passion from her experiences accompanying her mother on hospital visits. Although the elder Nightingale expressed concern about her daughter keeping company with drunken, immoral nurses and tending to the needs of people with unhealthy bodies in prison-like, dirty, smelly hospitals,

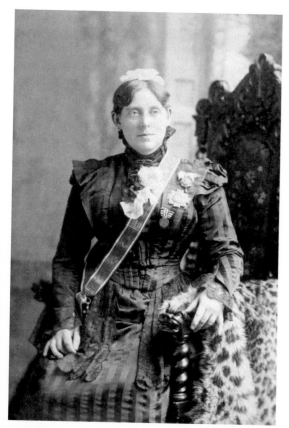

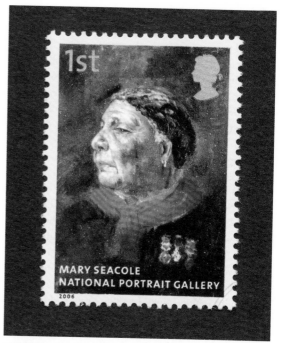

FIGURE 2.2 A postage stamp printed in the United Kingdom circa 2006, bearing the portrait of Mary Seacole (1805–1881), highlights how the profession of nursing has been shaped by nurses from diverse cultural backgrounds.

FIGURE 2.1 Florence Nightingale (1820–1910) photograph, circa 1880.

when Nightingale turned 25, her parents allowed her to attend a British hospital–based nurse's training program. Nightingale did not practice nursing full time after her training, but continued to travel with her parents.

After visiting with nuns in Rome, Nightingale explored the option of starting a community of trained nurses. A friend of the Nightingale family informed Nightingale about Kaiserworth. Nightingale attended Kaiserworth in 1850 and 1851, where she was instructed in the art of nursing (Jamieson & Sewall, 1954; Kalisch & Kalisch, 2004; Nutting & Dock, 1935b). At age 34, Nightingale became the superintendent of a small London institution that provided shelter to homeless women and nursing services to sick governesses.

When the British became involved with the Crimean War, they discovered that they had no sisters to assist with injured and infirmed troops. In 1854, the British government appointed Nightingale as the superintendent of the nursing staff because of her demonstrated ability to obtain and organize resources for the homeless and her ability to provide effective nursing services care. She and 38 other women

(including Joanna Bridgeman, a colleague of Catherine McAuley) went to Scutari, Turkey, where they found two hospitals in deplorable condition. Nightingale obtained funding and supplies from friends and transformed the hospitals into clean, well-ventilated buildings that provided nutritious meals for the patients. The hospitals' mortality rate of 40% declined to 2% after the implementation of Nightingale's reforms (Jamieson & Sewall, 1954; Kalisch & Kalisch, 2004; Meehan, 2003). Nightingale also considered the physical and psychosocial needs of the ill and injured. She wrote letters for soldiers, employed wives who had accompanied spouses to the battlefield, and made night rounds in the wards with a lamp.

Power, admiration, and fame came to Nightingale. Before long, army nursing under Nightingale evolved into a health service valued by the British government.

During the Crimean War, Nightingale met **Mary Seacole** (Fig. 2.2), a Jamaican nurse volunteer who also nursed the soldiers. Seacole saw the need for holistic outreach nursing services for civilians who had been injured or displaced. She set up a hotel where she provided shelter, relaxation, and excellent food. When guests became ill, she prescribed medicines. After the war, Seacole dedicated her life to elevating nursing to a respectable profession (Wheeler, 1999).

In 1855, prominent British citizens established the "Nightingale fund" to enable Nightingale to establish a school to train women in the art of nursing. Nightingale expected graduates of her school to teach nursing to the entire world. Besides establishing a formalized program of nursing education, Nightingale continued her efforts at reforming hospitals, public health, and nursing (Jamieson & Sewall, 1954; Nutting & Dock, 1935b).

Along with Nightingale, several American women influenced the reform of health care and nursing. In 1893, Lillian Wald and Mary Brewster opened a Nurses' Settlement House in New York City. They used the term "**public health nurse**" to describe the trained nurses who responded to nursing needs outside the hospital. These nurses responded to calls from individuals as well as physicians to provide home nursing services. The program provided services regardless of the ability of recipients to pay. In 1895, Wald and Brewster moved to larger accommodations that became known as the Henry Street Settlement House. By 1900, 20 district nursing organizations employed 200 trained nurses across the United States (Roberts, 1954).

▌ QUESTIONS FOR REFLECTION

1. Did you know about the contributions of others to professional nursing in the 19th century?
2. Why do you suppose these contributions were overlooked?

THE BIRTH OF FORMAL NURSING EDUCATION

In the Victorian era (1837–1901), upper- and middle-class women led circumscribed lives: They were deemed the property of their fathers or husbands, had no independent rights, and were considered incapable of intellectual development. Some in Victorian society even thought that education would damage women's reproductive organs. Women from lower classes, for whom work was a necessity, found socially acceptable employment as retail clerks, factory workers, governesses, or domestic servants. Nursing, however, was considered an unacceptable profession and reserved for female paupers from workhouses or those who served prison time for drunkenness, vagrancy, or prostitution.

Nightingale's service in the Crimean War elevated the nursing profession. The society began thinking of nursing as an art that "must be raised to the status of a trained profession" (Kjervik & Martinson, 1979, p. 22),

and efforts to standardize the training were made. Although Nightingale established a theoretical model for nursing practice, she proposed that nurses should follow protocol rather than use independent thinking. She emphasized that nurses should be taught how to carry out physicians' orders. To maintain discipline, Nightingale delineated a strict nursing service hierarchy. Good character superseded intellectual ability when the Nightingale nursing school selected students. Education in Nightingale's school focused on teaching nurses what to do and how to do it, following physicians' orders, knowing why, training a nurse's senses, and linking these things with reflection to decide what should be done (Kalisch & Kalisch, 2004).

Civil War Nursing

As nursing became more acceptable, women volunteered during the Civil War to be nurses. American women transformed the ballrooms of their homes into wards for injured and infirmed soldiers, resulting in the birth of **Civil War nursing**. Dorothea Dix, who was appointed as the superintendent of female nurses in the Union Army, founded the first American Army Nursing Corps, and was given full power to organize human and material resources to care for sick and injured soldiers.

Along with the Army Nursing Corps, female volunteers and family members also provided nursing services to Civil War casualties. Author Louisa May Alcott served as a nurse during the war and wrote about her tragic experiences caring for soldiers. Mary Ann "Mother" Bickerdyke diligently searched to find living soldiers who had been wounded in battle but had been mistakenly placed among the dead. Clara Barton (Fig. 2.3), a former school teacher from New England, independently organized a large relief effort to provide supplies to care for those injured or displaced on both sides of the battle, and occasionally provided nursing care. In 1881, Barton persuaded the United States government to ratify the Geneva treaty of the Red Cross and is credited with starting the American Red Cross.

Jane Stuart Woolsey, a Union hospital nurse kept detailed records of her observations. She and her sister served as supervisors of the nursing and cooking department for a Union hospital located on a Virginian hillside. Woolsey had the opportunity to visit various types of hospitals during the Civil War and noted that the hospitals run by nuns seemed to have a system for patient care along with discipline and order, in contrast to the haphazard care provided by most military and public hospitals (Kalisch & Kalisch, 2004). Along

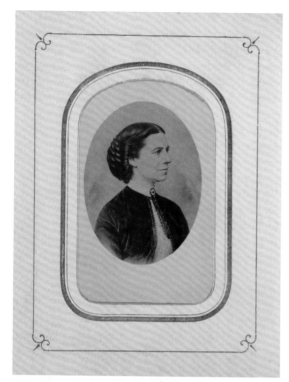

FIGURE 2.3 Clara Barton (1821–1912) at the end of the Civil War during which she lead nursing efforts for wounded Union troops, circa 1865.

Women and Children in Boston" (Kalisch & Kalisch, 2004, p. 361). Nursing programs were opened for black nursing students in the 1880s (Kalisch & Kalisch, 2004). By 1880, 15 programs existed. Within a decade, the number of programs had grown to 432 and had graduated 3,465 nurses (Burgess, 1928).

The early hospital training schools had some autonomy in determining the nursing program of study, but rapidly became dependent on hospitals for financial support, eventually becoming nursing service departments within the affiliated hospitals. Students worked 7 days a week, 50 weeks per year, for 1 to 2 years in exchange for on-the-job training, a few lectures, and a small allowance. Only unmarried women (single or widowed) were accepted as students. Students followed strict rules and schools tolerated no misconduct. Staffing the hospitals with students and faculty proved financially advantageous, and hospitals without training programs quickly established them. Hospitals quickly discovered that they could care for more patients and reap large profits when they provided nursing education. Between 1880 and 1926, the number of hospital-based nursing programs increased from 15 to 2,155 (Burgess, 1928).

The United States was not the only nation to provide formal nursing education in hospitals; Australia and Great Britain also educated nurses within the confines of hospitals. Hospital training programs became the dominant form of nursing education in the early part of the 20th century. However, untrained nurses continued to practice nursing, especially in rural areas (Kalisch & Kalisch, 2004; Madsen, 2005) where they filled a need and held the respect of their communities. Unlike their trained counterparts, untrained nurses willingly provided housekeeping services along with patient care. They also filled the need for caregivers in long-term care institutions (Madsen, 2005).

Nursing program graduates found themselves in hospital supervisory positions or in homes as private duty nurses. Hospitals with nursing students used the students as staff or contracted their services with families and pocketed the money for the services rendered. Typical private duty nursing cases required the nurse to live with families and to be available 24 hours a day. The average wage earned was $120 per month. The nurse remained idle if not on a private case. As nurses aged, they lacked the stamina required for all-night vigils, and the hard work required for safe, effective patient care (Goldmark, 1923).

Because of perceived lack of social prestige, many African American women steered away from entering the nursing profession. In 1930, there were 5,728

with female volunteers, Young Men's Christian Association (YMCA) members volunteered to serve as nurses (Jamieson & Sewall, 1954).

In Confederate states, most of the nursing care was delivered by Southern "matrons" who volunteered their services. Efforts made by these women focused on cooking, making bandages, and sewing. Slaves and plantation mistresses and daughters worked together at times to provide care for wounded and sick soldiers (Kalisch & Kalisch, 2004).

American Hospital Training Programs and Diploma Schools

In the United States, nursing training programs started simultaneously when the society accepted and provided opportunities for college education for upper-class women. As medical education moved into the postgraduate university, nursing education became established as apprenticeship training under the control of physicians and hospitals. The first nursing training programs were established in 1872 and 1873 in Boston, New Haven, and New York City. In 1879, Mary E. P. Mahoney earned a diploma in nursing "from the School of Nursing of the New England Hospital for registered black nurses for a total black population of 11,891,143 black Americans. Most of these nurses worked in hospitals (63%) or in the area of public health (28%). There were more untrained black midwives than there were professional nurses at this time.

QUESTIONS FOR REFLECTION

1. Do you think that today's nursing students and professional nurses are exploited by their employers? Why or why not?
2. How do you think that today's employers exploit professional nurses?
3. What safeguards are in place to prevent exploitation of nurses by employers? Why are these important?

Proliferation of Nursing Education Programs

The proliferation of nursing programs between 1880 and 1900 resulted in widespread variance in nursing education quality. Linda Richards, a graduate of a Canadian nursing program and the first trained American nurse, led reforms in major American nursing programs (Jamieson & Sewall, 1954). Isabel Hampton Robb questioned the qualifications of nursing faculty and spearheaded the first educational program for nursing faculty at Teacher's College in New York in 1901 (Dock, 1912). Widespread public concern arose regarding the safety of nursing and medical care. Reforms in nursing education followed reforms in medical education. In 1910, the Flexner Report broadcasted problems with the quality of medical education, resulting in drastic reforms (Flexner, 1910). Nursing leaders of the time hoped the Flexner Report would also result in nursing education reform. The Goldmark Report (1923) and other studies and surveys conducted at the time indicated that the root of most of the difficulties related to nursing training stemmed from the nursing schools' dual purpose of providing education and nursing service. Unfortunately, these studies resulted in limited reform. Table 2.1 highlights the development of modern nursing education programs.

Baccalaureate Programs

In 1893, the School of Medicine at Howard University (Washington, DC) established the first nursing diploma program within a university setting. The program, designed for African American students, lasted only 1 year before being assumed by Freedmen's Hospital. The University of Texas recognized nursing in the early 1890s and gave an endowed professorial chair to Hanna Kindborn, who lectured to both nursing and medical students (Dock, 1912). In 1909, the University of Minnesota established a 3-year diploma nursing program within its College of Medicine. In subsequent years, colleges adopted the pattern of combining academic and professional courses that led to both a diploma and a Bachelor of Science in Nursing (BSN) degree. Students attended academic courses at the university and received professional nursing courses using the apprenticeship model at the hospital (Dock, 1912; Jamieson & Sewall, 1954). In 1909, Dr. Richard Olding Beard instituted a plan to make nursing a college major at the University of Minnesota (Jamieson & Sewall, 1954).

In 1923, Yale University established a nursing program that had its own dean and endowed funds. Other universities that established baccalaureate nursing programs included Case Western Reserve University (in 1923), the University of Chicago (in 1925), and Vanderbilt University (in 1930). As nursing education moved to the collegiate setting, physicians voiced opposition because they thought that higher education and theoretical knowledge might lead nurses to question their authority (Kalisch & Kalisch, 2004).

Associate's Degree Programs

The Brown Report (Brown, 1948) and the Ginzberg Report (Ginzberg, 1949), two privately commissioned reports, specified that professional nursing education should be removed from hospitals and transferred to the collegiate setting. In her 1951 doctoral dissertation, Mildred Montag suggested that education for the technical nurse should occur in community college settings. She proposed that technical nurse education would result in a terminal degree and that technical nursing would attain a unique and semiprofessional identity (Montag, 1951). Upon graduation, the technical nurse would be completely prepared for hospital or nursing home employment. Community college nursing programs flourished. Graduates of Associate's Degree in Nursing (ADN) programs were given the same professional nursing licensure examination as graduates from diploma and baccalaureate nursing programs.

QUESTIONS FOR REFLECTION

1. How did the associate degree nursing program affect the nursing profession?
2. What differences do you see between nurses educated at the associate degree, diploma, and baccalaureate degree levels?

TABLE 2.1 **The Development of Modern Nursing Education Programs**

Event	Year
First school for training practical nurses opens	1897
Daughters of the American Revolution serve as the examining board for military nurses	1898
North Carolina becomes the first state to require registration of nurses	1903
1,006 hospital-based nursing training programs and 90 mental health institution–based nursing programs exist	1911
The Goldmark Report proposes that additional education beyond the basic diploma is needed for practice in public health, nursing education, and supervision	1923
University of Minnesota starts a baccalaureate degree nursing program	1909
Apprenticeship approach dominates nursing educations	1920s
25 nursing programs grant Bachelor of Arts (BA) or a Bachelor of Science degree in Nursing (BSN), with Yale opening the first separate university nursing department in 1924	1926
11 practical nursing programs operate in the United States	1930
1,472 hospital-based education programs, 70 collegiate nursing education programs, and 36 practical nursing programs exist	1936
Crash programs are developed to train nursing aides to alleviate the nursing shortage of World War II	1941
The Brown Report ranks nurses as important to the society as teachers and ranks collegiate nursing education as equal to other professional education programs	1948
Accreditation programs are created for practical and professional nursing schools	1952
296 practical nursing programs are in existence	1954
Birth of ADN programs in community colleges	1958
Toward Quality in Nursing Needs and Goals. A Report of the Surgeon General's Consultant Group in Nursing is released by the U.S. Public Health Service	1963
The Nursing Training Act is enacted	1964
The ANA releases its *Position Paper on Education for Nursing*	1965
797 hospital-based, 218 ADN, and 210 BSN programs exist	1966
288 hospital-based, 742 ADN, and 402 BSN programs exist	1982
60 hospital-based, 890 ADN, and 661 BSN programs exist	2003

From Kalisch, P. A., & Kalisch, B. J. (2004). *The advance of American nursing* (4th ed.). Philadelphia, PA: Lippincott Williams & Wilkins.

THE AMERICAN PUBLIC HEALTH MOVEMENT

As the field of public health nursing grew, basic principles specific to the specialty emerged. Reform efforts indicated a need to provide nursing services to all who were sick, without considering the ability to pay, religious affiliation, or ethnic background. District nurses identified the need to keep formal client records to facilitate consistency in service. To avoid duplication of services and prevent gaps in fulfilling client needs, nurses learned the importance of cooperation with other groups providing community care. During the rise of the public health movement, the family became the basic care unit (Spradley, 1990). Some public health nurses acknowledged the limitations of their hospital-based education and sought additional education in institutions of higher learning to develop a global approach for community nursing.

Public health nursing prospered from 1900 until the outbreak of World War I. The patient home served as the major location for nursing practice, as hospitals had become places to receive charity, contract infection, and die.

Other Social Reform Movements

Other social reform movements in the early 1900s impacted the nursing profession. William Booth founded the Salvation Army to protect the poor, the ex-prisoners, the old, the young, and any who were miserable and had been perceived by the society as having fallen from the grace of God. Jane Addams established Hull House in Chicago, which provided day care, kindergarten, and library services to immigrant women and children. Christian associations of young men and women were formed to build character and provide community services. The associations were the forerunners of today's Young Men and Young Women Christian Associations (YMCA & YWCA). Medicine experienced reforms that emphasized science and invention over superstitious practices. The spread of the telegraph and telephone also helped spread the word of these movements across the United States and throughout the world (Jamieson & Sewall, 1954; Kalisch & Kalisch, 2004).

NURSING DURING THE EARLY 20TH CENTURY, THE WORLD WARS, AND THE POST-WORLD WAR II ERA (1890–1960)

North Carolina led the efforts to **state registration** of nurses in 1903 by establishing guidelines for professional registration. Requirements included graduation from an established diploma nursing school. New Jersey and New York quickly followed. By 1912, 29 states and the District of Columbia had registration requirements for nurses. To renew initial registration, nurses were given a 3-year grace period to practice, then were required to take a licensing examination that emphasized dietetics, patient comfort, skilled handling of patients, and general management (Dock, 1912).

Registration as a professional nurse was not limited to females. The few male nurses suffered discrimination in professional practice. According to Kalisch and Kalisch (2004), male nurses were described in a 1914 hospital administration manual as being a composite of genius and drunkenness, but seemed more easy-going than their female colleagues. They were accused of taking sips of whisky while on duty to cope with the daily stresses of clinical practice. During World War I, trained male nurses were assigned to National Guard units and gained expertise in psychiatric-mental health nursing (Kalisch & Kalisch, 2004).

As the United States entered World War I in 1917, unmarried trained nurses entered the Army and Navy Nurse Corps. Volunteers from well-to-do families served as nurses' aides at their own expense. The government launched a publicity campaign to recruit women into nursing. Advertisements glamorizing nursing appeared in newspapers and magazines. However, on the battlefields, the nurses encountered the horrors of battlefield injuries. At times, the ratio of nurse-to-patient rose to as high as 1:60. Nurses were required to perform surgery to save lives. The flu epidemic of 1918 to 1919 only compounded the need for more nurses (Kalisch & Kalisch, 2004).

Nursing sustained an image problem in the 1920s. Movies portrayed nursing in unrealistic and unflattering ways. Reduced prestige for the profession resulted from several factors: (1) 95% of nurses were women, (2) most nursing leaders were unmarried, (3) societal expectations were that the woman's place was in the home as a devoted wife and mother, and (4) nursing was portrayed as an altruistic, self-sacrificing profession in a time that focused on frivolity and self-indulgence.

By the 1920s, most trained nurses were employed as private duty nurses. However, technologic advances in patient care and improvements in hospital facilities led to more patients being hospitalized for treatment and surgery. Public acceptance of going to the hospital for acute and serious illnesses reduced the demand for private duty nurses working in home settings (Kalisch & Kalisch, 2004). The hospitals relied on student nurses for patient care, leaving program graduates unemployed. In 1939, the National League for Nursing (NLN) reported that the typical hospital connected with a school of nursing. By the 1920s, most trained nurses were employed as private duty nurses. However, technologic advances in patient care and improvements in hospital facilities led to more patients being hospitalized for treatment and surgery. Public acceptance of going to the hospital for acute and serious illnesses reduced the demand for private duty nurses working in home settings (Kalisch & Kalisch, 2004). The hospitals relied on student nurses for patient care, leaving program graduates unemployed. In 1939, the NLN reported that the typical hospital connected with a school of nursing during 1938 employed only an average of 10 graduate nurses for general duty (National League for Nursing, 1939).

During the Great Depression, trained nursing graduates willingly worked for room and board. As the economic state improved, hospitals kept these trained nurses on staff while paying them an hourly wage. Medical advances increased the demand for educated registered nurses (RNs). A few nurses found employment with the new aviation industry as nurse-stewardesses. Other nurses participated in the Civil Works Administration (CWA) and Works Progress Administration (WPA) programs and became employed in public hospitals, clinics, and public health agencies.

Efforts to find best practices for nursing procedures started during this era. Even though nursing research was not a formalized process, nursing all over the world disseminated information through publications such as *The American Journal of Nursing*, *The Canadian Nurses* and *Kai Tiaki* (New Zealand). A description of nurses during

FOCUS ON RESEARCH

Standardized Nursing Practice: Striving for Best Practice

In the 1930s, nurses identified the need to standardize nursing procedures to improve patient care and to strengthen nursing education. In New Zealand, the head of the National Nursing Association, Mary Lambie, had responsibility for all nursing matters in the country. She formed a Nursing Education Committee (NEC) with members of nurses from a variety of practice areas. The NEC goal was to develop best practices for nursing procedures. The committee sent surveys about two to three nursing procedures to nurse administrators of all training hospitals. They combined the survey responses and constructed a model method for each nursing procedure. These results were published in *Kai Tiaki*. The journal was then circulated to all nurse training schools by the Department of Health.

Starting in the 1940s, the model procedures consisted of a series of recommended steps, but also contained rationale for underlying key principles for nurse consideration. Nurses then could vary the procedure steps and supplies according to local conditions, but would pay close attention as to not violate the key principles. The model procedures were reviewed by a medical committee of physicians and many times they specified that more study was required.

Some of the standardized procedures developed by the NEC included the following: nurse hand hygiene, cleanliness of nursing uniforms, isolation procedures, sterile dressings, bedsore prevention, bedpan use, oral care, temperature taking, ursine testing, and all routes of medication administration. Before finalizing each procedure, the NEC submitted them to a medical advisory committee who agreed with, but did not approve them. The goal was to have the training hospitals develop film strips

and guidelines for test questions, but World War II derailed the project.

Formalized nursing research studies can be traced back to the early 1930s when research studies were performed in the United States and Canada for establishing the effectiveness of intramuscular injections of camphor oil to ease postpartum breast engorgement, comparing ways to optimally disinfect thermometers, and to determine the effectiveness of cod liver oil use to treat wounds and burns. In New Zealand, a nurse compared two treatments of scales, two treatments for impetigo, and four treatments for pediculosis and compared costs, number of required treatments, and days of treatment needed to obtain a cure.

At the 1927 International Council of Nurses conference, the ICN cautioned against the use of standardized practice because it might interfere with the best interest of the patient or the well-being of the nurse. However, the group also concluded that identification of standardized practices could be applied to develop scientific nursing practice. The search for the one way to perform nursing procedures became the search for the best way.

Results of this reveal the importance of having key underlying scientific principles to guide professional nursing practice in order to provide optimal nursing care. The perception of standardized practice as becoming monotonous routine practice without being able to individualize patient care to best meet patient needs persists today. Like the search for standardized procedures, evidence-based practice protocols will continually be challenged as ways of health care delivery change.

Wood, P., & Nelson, K. (2013). Striving for best practice: standardizing New Zealand nursing procedures, 1930–1960. *Journal of Clinical Nursing, 22*, 3217–3224. doi: 10.1111/jocn.12456

---

this era is explained in the following research box that examines artifacts from the times to specify the process for determining best practices for nursing procedures.

Although most nurses were women in 1940, there were five nursing schools that exclusively educated male nurses. Of these four were accredited by the NLN and enrolled 212 men. There were also 63 coeducational programs with a combined enrollment of 710 men and 3,798 women.

Hospital administrators noted improvement in the care of male patients especially in the areas of psychiatric and genitourinary nursing (Kalisch & Kalisch, 2004).

In 1941, President Franklin Roosevelt issued an executive order that declared that all Americans were encouraged to fully participate in national defense programs. He proclaimed that the nation could only be defended with success if all Americans could work together. In addition, Roosevelt extended steps toward equality in America by appointing the Fair Employment Practices Committee. The efforts of the committee opened up new employment opportunities for all Americans because of the need for increased production of war-related products. Between 1940 and 1944, black employment in manufacturing rose by close to 700,000 persons and the number of blacks employed in governmental service more than tripled (Kalisch & Kalisch, 2004).

By World War II, graduate nurses and RNs had become accepted members of hospital staffs. When hospitals discovered that hiring RNs could cut costs, many nursing schools closed. However, as news of war loomed in Europe, the government took steps to promote the entry of young women into nursing. Recruitment methods included advertisements in printed media and the Nurse Cadet program (Fig. 2.4). The Nurse Cadet program was designed to provide nurses for essential and military nursing for the duration of World War II. The Nursing Cadet program was open to all young women who wanted to become nurses. Two thousand young black women entered the program with 20 all-black nursing schools enrolling 1,600 of them (Kalisch & Kalisch, 2004). As RNs joined the military, a civilian nurse shortage resulted. Hospitals employed civilian workers who held certificates from the Red Cross and hired the volunteers who had been helping nurses with nonprofessional duties.

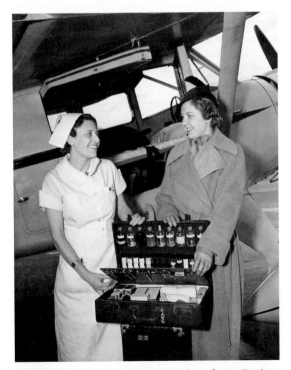

FIGURE 2.4 Cadet nurse thanking a donor for medications for use during the war effort.

In addition, black nurses were permitted to join the American Nurses Association (ANA), but only if they secured membership in a state nurses association that specified no restrictions for race as a condition for membership (Kalisch & Kalisch, 2004). Previously, these nurses could join the National Association of Colored Graduate Nurses (NACGN) that was founded by Martha Minerva Franklin. Like the ANA, the NACGN worked toward advancing the welfare of its members. In addition, the NACGN fought to win integration of African American RNs into all nursing employment opportunities, nursing education programs, and nursing organizations (African American Registry, 2013). By 1951, the NACGN merged with the ANA.

After World War II, the United States experienced a time of great economic growth. Companies offered health insurance as a fringe benefit for workers and a concession for not increasing wages. Workplace reforms led to an 8-hour day and a 40-hour workweek.

Insurance reimbursement of hospital care resulted in an increase in the number of hospital beds. Hospitals also became profitable and provided a central location for advancements in medical technology. However, the nursing shortage worsened as more hospital beds became available. Many nurses left practice to pursue marriage, better-paying jobs outside the profession, and more autonomous positions in industry or public health.

Segregation became outlawed in the United States in 1954 with the Supreme Court Ruling in the *Brown v. Board of Education in Topeka* case. This decision overturned the long-held doctrine of "separate, but equal" and espoused that all students (regardless of race) are offered "equal protection of the law." This landmark case created opportunities for all Americans to pursue educational endeavors that had previously been unavailable to them. Before the ruling, the National League for Nursing had issued a position that nursing education should be open to all persons. Prior to World War II, only 42 American nursing schools would admit black students. The number rose to 710 programs following a 1953 position statement of the need to open nursing program enrollment to all students by the NLN in 1953 (Kalisch & Kalisch, 2004).

NURSING IN THE MODERN ERA (1960–1999)

The 1960s

The 1960s ushered in a time of great change in American culture. The Civil Rights Movement to end racial segregation, begun more than a decade earlier, accelerated; and civil rights marches and acts of civil disobedience increased awareness among all Americans about the inequalities that were evident in everyday life. In 1965, Congress enacted President Johnson's "Great Society" legislation to create a society in which all citizens would have equal access to employment, education, and health care. Many of today's current social programs, such as Medicare and government grants for education, grew out of the Civil Rights movement and the "Great Society." Equal rights meant equal rights for all, including all women. In the early 1960s, the health care system consisted primarily of independent, not-for-profit hospitals; small, independent physician offices; and neighborhood pharmacies and medical supply stores. Persons unable to afford care sought health care services in local government-managed hospitals and clinics. By working independently or in small practices, physicians enjoyed autonomy and control over patient care. Hospitals recruited physicians to join medical staffs. Private insurance companies or patients reimbursed physicians based on fee-for-service payment systems. In the health care system of the 1960s, nurses were viewed as subservient to physicians.

Although the NLN, in the 1960s, denied accreditation to hospital diploma schools that used students to staff hospitals, hospital-based diploma schools remained the dominant educational pattern for registered nursing until the early 1970s. Educational reforms instituted in the 1960s resulted in increased expenditures for hospitals that sponsored diploma programs. Some hospitals offered solid nursing education, but at a marked financial deficit. The federal government offered hospitals with diploma programs, direct reimbursement for the number of student practice days to defray education-induced costs. In response to a predicted need for 680,000 additional professional nurses by 1970, the federal government increased funding for nursing education through a series of initiatives, including Professional Nurse Traineeships, The Nurse Training Act of 1964, and the Health Professions Educational Act of 1963 (Kalisch & Kalisch, 2004).

In 1965, the American Nurses Association (ANA, 1965) published the *ANA Position Paper on Education for Nursing,* which specified that the minimum educational level for beginning professional nursing practice should be the BSN, the minimum educational preparation for technical nursing practice should be the ADN, and all unlicensed care assistants should receive education in vocational education centers instead of on-the-job training. The proposal assumed that hospital diploma nursing schools would collaborate with either baccalaureate degree-granting institutions or community colleges to develop either professional or technical nursing programs. However, instead of collegial collaboration among hospitals and other educational institutions, the result was a deep division among members of the nursing profession (Flanagan, 1976; Kalisch & Kalisch, 2004).

Growth of the Professional Nurse Workforce

In addition to societal upheavals, the 1960s was also a time of biomedical advancements leading to expensive, life-saving technologies. Complex surgical procedures, new pharmaceuticals, and new technologies increased not only the cost of health care delivery but also the need for highly skilled and educated nurses. By this time, employers offered health care insurance as a standard benefit to workers. In 1965, the federal government introduced Medicare and Medicaid to provide health care coverage to the elderly and the poor. Improved insurance coverage meant improved access to health care services for the employed and the elderly citizens. Demand for hospital care and physician services increased. Hospital admissions rose and along with that came the need for highly educated, clinically competent professional nurses for patient care.

ADN programs were viewed as a means to provide a quick way to increase the number of nurses capable of hospital practice. Many hospitals that provided nursing diploma programs found themselves struggling to maintain their nursing programs because of the financial costs. The U.S. Public Health Service (1963) issued a report, *Toward Quality in Nursing: Needs and Goals,* that outlined the following concerns: severe deficiencies in the current nursing education, not enough young people entering the nursing profession, high turnover within the nursing profession, the need for collegiate and university-based nursing programs, the persistent low socioeconomic status of nurses, the ineffective use of available nursing personnel, and not enough research being conducted to advance the practice of professional nursing. The report served as evidence for the Nurse Training Act of 1964, which provided federal funding for diploma nursing schools to defray nursing education costs. The act also provided federal monetary support for ADN programs in community colleges and BSN programs in 4-year colleges and universities (Kalisch & Kalisch, 2004).

During the days of the early Vietnam conflict, the Army Student Nurse Program (instituted in 1956), enabled diploma nursing students to receive a free nursing education in return for 2 years of service in the

Army Nurse Corp. However, because of the unpopularity of the Vietnam war (1955–1975), the number of nurses willing to serve in the military declined. In 1966, a bill was passed authorizing male nurses to serve as regular forces in the Air Force, Army, and Navy Nurse Corps. By 1967, 22% of the Army Nurse Corp consisted of male professional nurses (Kalisch & Kalisch, 2004). Some military reservists and soldiers who had served in the military opted to use GI education benefits toward acquisition of a professional nursing education.

The 1970s

The 1970s saw an increase in inflation and unemployment. Consumers revolted against tax increases. To decrease the economic burden of supplying health care, the government employed mechanisms to monitor health care delivery to Medicare and Medicaid recipients. Although ineffective, these mechanisms, such as utilization review to reduce lengths of hospital stays and physician peer review programs, have become common practice. Hospitals and physicians are still required to participate in these programs or lose Medicare and Medicaid reimbursement.

Insurance providers also carried increased risks as consumers and employers exerted pressure on them to keep premiums from rising. In 1974, the Employment Retirement Security Act added incentives to businesses to self-insure their employees. A few for-profit investor hospitals were established, but medical and hospital care proceeded as usual. Self-insurance enabled employers to negotiate with health care organizations to become preferred providers for an employer-based health insurance program in attempts to curb health care costs. Some professional nurses found differences in working conditions between for-profit and not-for-profit hospitals, with higher workloads in the for-profit hospitals.

During this era, community colleges prospered as the society placed emphasis on equal opportunity for all American citizens to education. ADN-prepared nurses successfully passed the professional nursing licensure examination and soon filled vacant nursing positions, where they provided effective nursing care services. Costs for hospital-based nursing education programs continued to rise.

Graduate nursing education programs proliferated in the 1970s, offering advanced study in clinical specialty areas, nursing education, and nursing administration. Nurse practitioner programs were started to improve health care delivery while reducing costs.

Nursing research became a hallmark of advanced nursing education and practice.

In 1971, the National Institutes of Health (NIH) noted the importance of nursing research and established the National Center for Nursing Research. Compared to medical research, nursing research has been hampered by inadequate financial support. Between 1971 and 1981, the government awarded $40 million to the National Center for Nursing Research. During the same period, the NIH received $1.7 billion for general biomedical research.

The 1970s also ushered in the women's movement, called women's liberation, the modern feminist movement, or second-wave feminism (Malka, 2007). Equality for all oppressed persons became a dominant societal theme during this decade. The perception of nursing as a vocation became outdated. For many persons, the selection of a professional career focused upon high salary and status rather than pursuing a career as a religious calling (Bradshaw, 2010) (see Focus on Research, "Nursing as a 'Vocation'"). Women strove to discover their authentic selves, find personal meaning in their existence, and enjoy social equality. Women found they could pursue other careers besides nursing and teaching, and no longer did the nursing profession attract the best and brightest young women. The ability of women to select other careers seems to have contributed to the current nursing shortage (Malka, 2007).

FOCUS ON RESEARCH

Nursing as a "Vocation"

The 1972 Briggs Report resulted in a new model of nursing and nursing education for the United Kingdom. The purpose of Bradshaw's historical research study was to review the concept of "vocation" in the nursing literature of the 1960s and 1970s and to compare these findings with those of the Briggs Report. The investigator examined literature published between 1937 and 1975, including nursing textbooks, journal articles, nursing research studies, and primary and secondary works on nursing history. Analysis of the resources verified the reliability, coherence, consistence, and transparent interconnection of the historical data.

The study revealed that nursing as a vocation was addressed in the publications of the era. Many nurses who entered the profession in the 1960s and 1970s did so for altruistic reasons and because they expressed feelings of being "called" to the profession. The concept of vocation was seen as a hindrance to the development of the nursing profession.

This study exemplifies the influence of feminism on the development of the nursing profession. From 1960 to 1970, nursing literature fostered the use of science and empowerment rather than subservience and exploitation. However, as nurses look for meaning in their careers, they cannot overlook the spiritual elements embedded into the reasons for joining and remaining employed in the profession. More research is needed to explicate the meaning of professional vocation in nursing as well as the attitudes, values, and motivations of nurses and how these affect the quality of patient care.

Bradshaw, A. (2010). An historical perspective on the treatment of vocation in the Briggs Report (1972). *Journal of Clinical Nursing, 19*, 3459–3467. doi: 10.1111/j.1365–2702.2010.03359.x

A shift also occurred in women's behavior and attitude from that of pleasing men toward an opportunity for self-expression and fulfillment. Medicine, a male-dominated profession, dictated how health care was delivered, resulting in further oppression of some nurses. However, other nurses saw the feminist movement as a means to assert themselves and use female empowerment to transform the role of nurses from dutiful servants to competent professionals with an obligation to question physician orders when needed to protect patients. Many nurses asserted their rights as persons and professionals. Changes abounded in practice settings: nurses no longer stood when physicians entered nursing units, gathered charts for rounds, or got coffee for them. However, other nurses found second-wave feminism as antithetical toward their profession of service. Early years of the feminist movement resulted in further divisions within the nursing profession (Malka, 2007). Nurses began to assert themselves with physicians, administrators, and each other.

During the 1970s, many military-trained paramedics (predominately male) entered the nursing profession. Some nursing programs offered for previous military training in order to meet admission criteria.

The 1980s

Health care costs continued to skyrocket during the 1980s, despite a weak economy. More expensive and sophisticated diagnostic equipment and treatments became common as new advances in health care were discovered and consumers demanded them. In 1983, Medicare introduced a prospective payment system known as "diagnosis-related groups." The goal of the program was to reduce cost rate increases for hospital care by reducing the length of hospitalization. Employers selected health insurance programs offering preferred provider organizations that negotiated discounted services from participating health care organizations. By the end of the decade, hospitals experienced decreased profits as beds remained empty. Hospitals consolidated, resulting in a decreased demand for hospital nurses.

In attempts to alleviate the high cost of health care, the nursing profession embarked on expanding the roles of professional nursing. Collegiate nursing programs offered education for nurse practitioners, clinical nurse specialists, and certified nurse midwives along with established advanced education to prepare nursing faculty.

As the number of hospital beds decreased, inpatient acuity increased substantially, thereby requiring that highly skilled nurses care for patients. Primary nursing became the dominant nursing care delivery system and brought the professional nurse back to the bedside. In primary nursing, the RN planned individualized care, implemented the plan, and also provided health education for hospitalized patients and families. Clients were sent home to recover from surgery and illnesses once their condition stabilized. In response, the demand for nurses working in home health care and ambulatory health care increased.

Feminism flourished in the 1980s. Carol Gilligan (1982) published *In a Different Voice*, which highlighted key differences between the communication styles of men and women and in the socialization of boys and girls. Gilligan emphasized that women preferred to be connected to each other. Various approaches to feminism arose. Although devised in the 19th century, the liberal feminist view promoted by Gilligan grew in popularity because of its continued commitment toward achieving equality between men and women. Nursing education embraced feminist traditions. Educators and students alike strove to become their authentic selves, use intuition as one means of clinical decision making, and embark on teaching–learning partnerships (Chinn, 2013; Chinn & Wheeler, 1985; McPherson, 1983; Speedy, 1987).

However, some professional nurses could not accept the feminist movement. Because of the movement's derogatory comments about the nature of the work of nursing, many nursing contributions to client care remained invisible (Malka, 2007). People cannot see nursing assessments and surveillance activities that save lives, but they can see omissions and adverse effects, such as the failure to reposition bedridden patients leading to pressure ulcer development. The feminist movement also devalued nursing as a profession because of nursing's subservient status to the medical profession (Malka, 2007).

The 1990s

The 1990s heralded the movement toward cost containment in health care. By 1990, "95% of insured employees were enrolled in some form of managed care, including fee-for-service plans with utilization management, preferred provider organizations or HMOs" (Bodenheimer & Grumbach, 1995, p. 87). Hospitals, physicians, and insurance companies joined forces and created integrated health care networks. Large surpluses of specialist physicians and a shortage of generalists occurred. Physicians increasingly formed large practices, while large commercial companies dominated the insurance market. For-profit companies took control of many nursing homes, home health care companies, and multihospital system networks. Physicians lost control of their medical practices. Third-party payers dictated reimbursement rates to hospitals. Eighty-five million Americans remained uninsured, underinsured, or enrolled in Medicaid (Ginzberg, 1995). Insurance providers employed tactics to avoid enrolling potentially high users of health care services, expanded managed care, and emphasized case management.

As hospital and home health care agencies' profits declined, efforts to control costs of services led to reductions in professional nursing staff even as the acuity level of inpatients continued to rise. Use of unlicensed assistive personnel (UAP) became popular despite the evidence that RNs improved patient care quality (Brooten & Naylor, 1995). The change in skill mix reduced professional nurse positions, added more delegation responsibilities, and further devalued the contributions of RNs to client care (Buerhaus, 1995).

Patient-focused care and work redesign efforts were developed to increase patient and staff satisfaction. Key elements of patient-focused care included the formation of specialty care units for patients with similar diagnoses, unit-based support services, and cross-training patient care teams (Greenberg, 1994). Critical and acute care staff who were cross-trained would develop an appreciation for all things that occurred across the continuum of care within the hospital.

Work redesign efforts expanded the responsibility and job scope for nonprofessional staff. UAP replaced RNs and licensed vocational (practical) nurses. With minimal on-the-job training, UAP perform the basic tasks of patient hygiene, ambulation, vital signs, and intake–output determination while assuming phlebotomy, electrocardiography, bladder catheterization, and simple dressing changes in some institutions. In addition, some institutions assigned social workers, housekeeping personnel, dietary workers, respiratory therapists, and clinical laboratory staff to a nursing department under the supervision of a nurse manager.

To improve quality of care by minimizing variance in care-providing procedures, hospitals instituted clinical pathways. Clinical pathways outlined standardized plans of care (nursing diagnoses, outcomes, interventions, and projected length of hospital stay) for clients with specific health conditions that required hospitalization. With clinical path implementation, individualization of nursing care declined. However, standardized work processes resulted in superior patient outcomes. Work redesign resulted in a change of the RN role from direct care provider to one that required more delegation and supervision. Nurses focused work efforts at verifying that patient care processes were followed, evaluating patient outcomes, and looking for ways to improve care.

▮ QUESTIONS FOR REFLECTION

1. How do you think the expanded use of unlicensed personnel in health care settings has affected professional nursing practice?
2. What are the consequences for the nursing profession of increased use of unlicensed care providers?
3. What are the consequences for clients of increased use of unlicensed care providers?

To ensure efficient and effective use of health care resources without sacrificing client satisfaction and care quality, health care providers and insurers developed **case management** systems, in order to streamline health care delivery and to assure continuity of care across care settings. Case management systems varied in setting and implementation. Table 2.2 outlines seven components common to all case management models.

Although social workers served as the first case managers, when it became evident that they were unable to see the entire patient situation, health care institutional administration and social workers turned to nurses for assistance. Case management required thought processes frequently used by nurses in clinical practice. Early efforts using nurses as case managers improved patient

TABLE 2.2 Common Components of Case Management Systems

Component	Case Manager Duties
Client identification and outreach	Receive clients through referrals, interviews, and networking
Client assessment and diagnosis	Perform comprehensive holistic client assessments to identify physical, psychological, sociocultural, and spiritual problems
Planning of services and resource identification	Determine what services will be used in collaboration with the client, then assume the responsibility for planning and coordinating the services
Linking clients to required services	Serve as brokers to expedite and follow through with the coordination and planning of services for clients
Coordination and implementation of services	Verify that the identified needs are met and abide by formal agreements made with the service-providing agencies by keeping extensive documentation and records focused on the efficiency, effectiveness, and quality of case-managed care services
Service delivery monitoring	Collaborate with interdisciplinary team members who are providing client services and verify that clients are receiving appropriate, quality services from the agencies
Client advocacy	Work on behalf of clients to ensure clients are receiving services contracted for, making progress in the delineated program, and receiving satisfactory services
Evaluation of services and outcomes	Bear responsibility for specific and general client outcomes; continually monitor and reassess services in order to promptly identify the need for change or problems to ensure timely intervention and replanning

outcomes, increased consumer satisfaction with care, and decreased health care costs (Cohen & Cesta, 2001).

Research in nursing continued to be hampered by inadequate financial support. In 1993, the National Institute for Nursing Research (NINR) was established within the NIH by an act of Congress with the purpose of identifying nursing research priorities, distributing grants to nurse researchers, and disseminating findings of nursing research to the public and other health professions. In 2000, NINR received $90 billion in federal support to achieve its mission.

By the 1990s, the nursing profession continued to have difficulty in attracting the best and brightest women because other professions were now welcoming them. Ironically, successful and highly educated nurses moved away from bedside care. Advanced practice nurses worked in collaborative partnerships with physicians, although some physicians began to see nurse practitioners and certified nurse midwives as competitors rather than partners (Malka, 2007). Nurses attended to all ranges of human responses to health and illness while providing a caring relationship to facilitate health and healing, according to the 1995 ANA *Social Policy Statement* (ANA, 1995).

MEDIA PORTRAYALS OF PROFESSIONAL NURSES

The media plays a key role in public perception of nursing. Some young men and women decide to enter a nursing career based upon what they have read about nurses or have seen in the movies or on television. In general, media portrayals of nurses have been positive and negative. As the profession and the women's movement have gained strength, the media has improved how it portrays nurses in recent years.

During the Great Depression, cinematographers portrayed nurses as attractive young women who placed professional duties over personal desires (Kalisch & Kalisch, 2004). Since the 1960s, television and movies have provided the society with positive and negative images of nurses. In the early 1960s, two fictional medical programs, *Ben Casey* and *Dr. Kildare*, characterized nurses primarily as physicians' handmaidens.

In the 1960s and 1970s, some positive images of nurses surfaced on television shows such as *Julia, Nurse, Emergency,* and *M*A*S*H*. In *Emergency,* Nurse Dixie, a fictional emergency department nurse, had collegial relationships with paramedics, physicians, and fellow nurses; performed telephone triage and complex nursing procedures; and even disagreed with physicians.

However, television and movies also portrayed nurses negatively. Margaret Houlihan of *M*A*S*H* was portrayed as a competent, caring professional who had many personal problems. In the 1975 movie *One Flew Over the Cuckoo's Nest,* nurses were depicted as being rigid and cold.

Media portrayals of nurses in the 1980s were less than flattering. Soap operas and the prime-time television show *Nightingales* depicted nurses and nursing students as sex objects. In a coordinated effort with the

ANA, professional nurses instituted a boycott of sponsors of *Nightingales*, which resulted in its cancellation.

In contrast, the British Broadcasting Corporation's series *Call the Midwife* that first aired in 2012 and ended in 2016, tells the story of a group of competent and caring nurse midwives who safely deliver babies in less than optimal conditions. In one episode, the midwife named Jenny Lee, a highly competent and compassionate nurse midwife, identifies a neurologic condition in a surgeon and reports his substandard skills in order to protect patients. In 2015, Jenny changed positions and moved to hospice nursing. A new main character, Patsy Mount, a competent and dedicated nurse midwife along with other midwife colleagues addressed critical holistic family issues. Although in the series, the other nurse characters tend to defer to physicians for clinical decision-making and orders, this depicts an accurate historical portrayal of nursing practice in the 1950s.

Nurses united in an effort to educate the hosts of the talk show *The View* after Joy Behar and Michelle Collins mocked Kelley Johnson, Miss Colorado, for showcasing her knowledge, skills, and compassion as her talent during the 2015 Miss America Pageant. Her unconventional talent earned her the honor of finishing second. Both hosts wondered what she was doing with a "Doctor's stethoscope." Many furious nurses wrote the show's sponsors who ceased advertisements. As an apology for the ignorant comments of the two hosts, the show hosted a group of nurses from New York University College of Nursing who provided detailed education about what professional nurses do in clinical practice.

An unassuming nurse from Missouri, Janie Harvey Garner started the "Show Me Your Stethoscope" Facebook site. Nurses, physicians, respiratory therapists, and UAP flooded Facebook with photos of themselves and with other nurses to educate the public that nurses routinely use stethoscopes in clinical practice (Spitrey, 2015). For several weeks, the site ranked number one, captured media attention, and has 800,000 united healthcare worker members.

NURSING IN THE EARLY POSTMODERN ERA (2000–2010)

Scholars debate when the postmodern era actually began. Some feel it began in the 1960s; others claim it started with the introduction of the computer and the internet. Another group of scholars heralds the beginning of the postmodern age with questioning of scientific method as the best approach for discoveries

to answer the questions surrounding humanity, the environment, and health-related issues (Watson, 1999). Wilson (1998) introduced the term **consilience** to describe the unity of knowledge. Consilience represents the point where scientific, artistic, ethical, spiritual, social, environmental, and personal knowledge intersect. Some research has discovered that spirituality plays a key role in health and healing, and qualitative research methods hold the same promise as quantitative research in generating health care knowledge.

During the first decade of the 21st century, professional nurses continued to adapt to the changes in practice and the society. Scientific advances increased the complexity and cost of health care. Mandatory use of electronic health records for all health care providers occurred. According to the Centers for Medicare & Medicaid Services (CMS, 2010), health care accounted for 17.6% of the gross domestic product (GDP) at this time. The population of persons over age 65 increased 15.1% from 2000 to 2010 (U.S. Census Bureau, 2011). The CMS estimated that close to 80% of health care resources are used by the persons over age 65. Efforts to contain health care costs resulted in further reduction in inpatient stays, leading to the transfer of health care services from acute care to either the home or rehabilitation setting.

The gap between the rich and the poor continued to widen, resulting in an increase in governmental funding for health care services. Sources of health care insurance include employers, private purchase, or the government. Nearly 50 million Americans joined the ranks of the uninsured and 39 million persons participated in Medicaid programs (Holahan & Chen, 2011).

By virtue of education and practice, nurses demonstrated that they had the best knowledge and skill base to assume the gatekeeper and advocacy roles required of case managers. Nurse practitioners also demonstrated the ability to deliver high-quality health care economically without compromising care quality. Hospitals employed 62.2% of working RNs; many other RNs work in extended-care facilities, homes, clinics, and community health settings (U.S. Department of Health and Human Services, Health Resources and Services Administration, & Bureau of Health Professions, 2010).

The Great Recession that began in 2007 resulted in rises in unemployment (with resultant loss of employer-sponsored health insurance coverage), reduced income for the average American, home foreclosures, and less money to spend on health care (The Kaiser Family Foundation, 2012). Many RNs (especially those over 50 years of age) returned to the active workforce because spouses had lost their jobs (Buerhaus & Auerbach, 2011).

The confluence of economic factors and reduced access to health care for increased numbers of Americans resulted in enactment by Congress in 2010 of the Patient Protection and Affordable Care Act (ACA). This law mandates incremental reforms in the way health care is delivered and financed, and required all individuals to have health insurance by 2014. The law was upheld by the US Supreme Court in 2012.

According to the ACA, employers with more than 50 workers must offer health care insurance. The ACA specifies the following services must be covered by the policy: hospitalization, prescription medications, emergency care, comprehensive pediatric health services (including dental and vision coverage), ambulatory (or outpatient) services; pregnancy, maternity and newborn care, laboratory tests, mental health and substance disorder services, rehabilitative and habilitative (assist the disabled or injured to regain skills for independent living) services and devices, and services for disease prevention, wellness promotion, and chronic disease management (Healthcare.gov, n.d.). Heath insurance exchanges became available to consumers to compare and purchase the best care based on health needs and affordability; and government-financed public health insurance programs were expanded. Programs emphasizing wellness, early detection of illnesses, and disease prevention were established. In addition, programs offering strategies to keep elders at home and out of long-term care institutions were implemented. Health care providers were (and continue to be) held accountable for outcomes based on comparative effectiveness research. Health care providers, including nurses, were (and are) expected to follow evidence-based or best practice guidelines for disease management and prevention.

Reform initiatives, the ever-increasing use by consumers of the internet for health information, and increased use of alternative health care practices created new demands on professional nurses. In some cases, health care consumers (especially those with rare medical conditions) sometimes knew more about their disorders than nurses. Nurses acknowledged that sometimes consumers used sources of unreliable health information and found themselves coaching consumers in strategies to find scientific-based health information.

Because of the ever-increased use of alternative and complementary health care practices, the NIH received funding in 1999 to form the National Center for Complementary and Alternative Medicine (NCCAM) and published its first strategic plan in 2000 (NIH, 2016). In 2008, the NCCAM reported that 38% of Americans used some form of complementary or alternative practices to manage their health (U.S. Department of Health & Human Services, NIH, NCCAM, 2008). The use of natural products was the most often employed by consumers to treat conditions or maintain health (e.g., glucosamine for arthritis, ginseng for mental health and memory). Because of widespread use, many health care organizations added use of complementary and alternative approaches used by consumers to health history forms as some of these practices could result in serious adverse effects when combined with scientific-based Western medicines and surgeries. Nurses also became responsible to know more about alternative and complementary health care practices.

Even though consumers were (and still are) using alternative and complementary practices, the federal government published best-practice protocols for various disease processes. Watson (2012) warned of the possibility of depersonalization of care when nurses may be pressured to abide strictly by rigid policies and protocols required for institutional reimbursement. Nurses had to spend increasingly amounts of time documenting patient care to comply with government-approved protocols (e.g., standardized documentation for influenza vaccines for the Medicare recipients). Electronic health records began to trigger messages to health care providers to alert them to guidelines that needed to be followed to comply with government recommendations in order to maximize reimbursement for rendered services.

NURSING IN THE SECOND DECADE OF THE POSTMODERN ERA AND BEYOND (2010–20 ...)

Along with different settings for professional nurse employment, many nurses have found that the complexity of information in any given practice area required ongoing education. Continuing education and nurse specialty certification persists today. More than 130 professional nursing organizations provide opportunities for further education in such specialized practice fields as critical care, oncology, neuroscience, parish, maternal-child, psychiatric, public health, and administration. Nurse specialty organizations provide certification programs that attest to knowledge and skill in the specialized area of practice. Some professional nursing positions require certification, yet many organizations fail to provide financial rewards for professional certification. Many individuals consider certification prestigious, yet in a 2011 study Kendall-Gallagher and colleagues found that nursing specialty certification had no effect on patient outcome unless the nurse also held a BSN (Kendall-Gallagher, Aiken, Sloane, & Cimiotti, 2011).

Along with specialty certification, nurses in a variety of practice settings participate in health care quality improvement programs. The use of evidence-based standards for client nursing care assessments and interventions reduces client injuries and complications. Regulatory and accrediting agencies such as The Joint Commission (formerly Joint Commission on Accreditation of Healthcare Organizations [JCAHO]) require that certain national and international standards for client care be met before being designating as accredited centers. All Joint Commission–accredited organizations must have quality improvement programs in place (see Chapter 19, "Quality Improvement: Enhancing Patient Safety and Health Care Quality") and meet all requirements to receive reimbursement for rendered services. If an organization fails to meet accreditation criteria, it loses the ability to receive federal monies for delivered health care services. In addition, the CMS has identified hospital-associated conditions for which Medicare and Medicaid may deny reimbursement (see Box 2.1, Professional Building Blocks, "Hospital-Associated Conditions Resulting in Denial of Reimbursement"). The CMS plans to add more conditions to the list in the future.

Since the enactment of the Patient Protection and ACA, more Americans have secured health insurance. The U.S. Census Bureau reported that 89.6% of Americans had healthcare insurance. The sources of health care insurance policies are private 66%, employer-based 55.4%, and government sponsored 36.5%. Many persons, especially those over age 65 have a private Medicare tie-in plan. Only 80.7% of persons living below the poverty level had secured health insurance coverage (Smith & Medalia, 2015). The percentage of GDP consumed by health care was 17.4% in 2013 and is expected to rise to 19.6% in 2024 (Centers for Medicare & Medicaid Services, 2014). The increased reflected increased use of prescription medications and hospitalizations directly linked to the increased numbers of Americans carrying health insurance coverage.

Besides being knowledgeable in a specific practice area, informatics, and quality improvement, today's nurses realize the importance of being well versed in current consumer health care practices. Some complementary therapies, such as aromatherapy, guided imagery, therapeutic touch, and massage may ease some adverse effects of conventional medical and surgical therapies. The NIH has added research on alternative and complementary health care practices to its list of research priorities. In 2015, the NIH renamed the National Center for Complementary and Alternative Medicine to the National Center for Complementary and Integrative Health. The name change more accurately explains how persons use complementary interventions to promote health, prevent illness, and treat mental and physical afflictions (Briggs, 2015). Thus, the knowledge required for effective nursing practice continues to expand and increase in complexity.

Additional projections such as the increasing numbers of the elderly, ever-expanding reliance on technology for health care delivery and general living, political instability, the widening gap between the affluent and poor, natural and manmade ecologic disasters, climate change, emergence of new and once eliminated contagious diseases (some may not have cures) will affect professional nursing practice. Nurses will be there to help persons adapt and adjust to whatever the future may bring. In order to accomplish the task, professional nurses will need to be able to work within complex systems with confidence, competence, and compassion.

The image of nurses in a postmodern society has yet to be elucidated. Current mainstream media tend to ignore the role of nurses in health care delivery, thus continuing the invisibility of the contributions that professional nurses make in health care.

2.1 Professional Building Blocks

Hospital-Associated Conditions Resulting in Denial of Reimbursement

- Foreign object remaining in a patient following surgery
- Infection at surgical site
- Air embolism
- Stages III and IV pressure ulcers
- Transfusion of incompatible blood or blood products
- Falls and trauma that occur as an inpatient
- Manifestations of poor blood sugar control
- Urinary catheter–associated infections
- Intravascular catheter–associated infections
- Deep venous thrombosis or pulmonary embolism

Summary and Significance to Practice

Recognition of nursing as a respected profession continues in the ever-changing, complex, and chaotic world. The existence of three entry levels of education remains a key barrier to nursing attainment of full professional status. Scientific advances are providing an opportunity for the profession to establish its own body of knowledge as well as increasing the need for highly educated nurses. Hard science continues to be intertwined with ethics, spirituality, and philosophy, and points to the validity of individualized holistic nursing care. Professional nurses must focus efforts toward looking at all aspects that affect human health and healing. For many generations, nurses have made remarkable, but invisible, contributions to the delivery of health care. Hopefully, as a result of nurses exhibiting compassion, confidence, and competence, current and future societies will value the contributions of nurses in health care. By showcasing their clinical, cognitive, and communication skills with confidence, today's nurses can shape the image of the nursing profession.

REAL-LIFE REFLECTIONS

Remember Marita, Carol, and Joe from the beginning of the chapter? What topic area should they use for their class presentation? Why do you think this might be a useful topic to be presented? Why is it important for them to have knowledge about nursing history? How might they use history to guide their current and future nursing practice?

From Theory to Practice

1. What are some current issues in health care that might be solved by looking at nursing history?
2. What are the similarities among current and ancient nursing practices?
3. How does current professional practice compare with nursing in various stages of human history?
4. How did the feminist movement affect the nursing profession?

Nurse as Author

This chapter has provided a broad overview of the history of nursing. Visit **www.internurse.com** to view pictures and read more about the nurses who have shaped our profession. Listen to the voice of Florence Nightingale at the following website: **http://publicdomainreview.org/collections/the-voice-of-florence-nightingale/**. Take time to reflect on what you just heard. Then write a paragraph or two describing your thoughts, feelings, and perceptions about nursing history.

Your Digital Classroom

Online Exploration

The American Association for the History of Nursing: **www.aahn.org**
The Center for the Study of the History of Nursing: **www.nursing.upenn.edu/history**
The American Association of Men in Nursing presentation on Men in American Nursing History: **http://www.aamn.org/presentations/Men%20in%20Nursing.pdf**
Women's History: **www.womenshistory.about.com/homework/womenshistory/cs/nurses**
American Nurses Association (ANA): **www.nursingworld.org**
Sigma Theta Tau International: **www.nursingsociety.org**
National League for Nursing (NLN): **www.nln.org**
American Association of Colleges of Nursing (AACN): **www.aacn.nche.edu**
The Truth about Nursing: **www.truthaboutnursing.org**

Expanding Your Understanding

Select a historical era that interests you. Explore nursing and health-related issues encountered during this time in history. Identify at least one issue confronted during this historical time and relate it to current professional nursing practice. What did nurses do during this time to address the identified issue? Is it possible that the same issue might appear again in the future? Do you think that a similar solution that was used during the historical area might be useful? Why or why not?

Beyond the Book

Visit thePoint® **www.thePoint.lww.com** for activities and information to reinforce the concepts and content covered in this chapter.

REFERENCES

African American Registry. (2013). *National Association of Colored Graduate Nurses Founded*. Retrieved from http://www.

aaregistry.org/historic_events/view/national-association-colored-graduate-nurses-founded. Accessed August 30, 2016.

American Nurses Association. (1965). *ANA position paper on education for nursing.* Kansas City, MO: Author.

American Nurses Association. (1995). *Social policy statement.* Kansas City, MO: Author.

Bodenheimer, T., & Grumbach, K. (1995). The reconfiguration of U.S. medicine. *Journal of the American Medical Association, 274,* 85–90.

Bradshaw, A. (2010). An historical perspective on the treatment of vocation in the Briggs Report (1972). *Journal of Clinical Nursing, 19,* 3459–3467. doi:10.1111/j.1365–2702.2010.03359.x

Briggs, J. (2015). *NCAAM has a new name!* Retrieved from https://nccih.nih.gov/about/offices/od/nccam-new-name. Accessed March 14, 2016.

Brooten, D., & Naylor, M. D. (1995). Nurses' effect on changing patient outcomes. *Image, 27,* 95–99.

Brown, E. L. (1948). *Nursing for the future (Brown Report).* New York: Russell Sage Foundation.

Buerhaus, P. I. (1995). Economic pressures building in the hospital employed RN labor market. *Nursing Economic$, 13,* 137–141.

Buerhaus, P., & Auerbach, D. (2011). The recession's effect on hospital registered nurse employment growth. *Nursing Economic$, 29*(4), 163–167.

Burgess, M. A. (1928). *Committee on the grading of nursing schools: Nurses, patients and pocketbooks.* New York: Commonwealth Fund.

Centers for Medicare & Medicaid Services. (2010). *National health expenditure projections 2010–2020.* Retrieved from https://www.cms.gov/Research-Statistics-Data-and-Systems/Statistics-Trends-and-Reports/NationalHealthExpendData/downloads/proj2010.pdf. Accessed May 21, 2013.

Centers for Medicare & Medicaid Services. (2014). *National Health Expenditure Projections 2014–2024 Forecast Summary.* Retrieved from https://www.cms.gov/Research-Statistics-Data-and-Systems/Statistics-Trends-and-Reports/National-HealthExpendData/downloads/proj2014.pdf. Accessed March 14, 2016.

Chinn, P. L. (2013). *Peace and power, new directions for building community* (8th ed.) Burlington, MA: Jones & Bartlett Learning.

Chinn, P. L., & Wheeler, C. E. (1985). Feminism and nursing. *Nursing Outlook, 33*(2), 74–77.

Cohen, E. L., & Cesta, T. G. (2001). *Nursing case management from essentials to advanced practice applications* (3rd ed.). St. Louis, MO: Mosby.

Dock, L. L. (1912). *A history of nursing (Vol. 3).* New York: Putnam.

Flanagan, L. (1976). *One strong voice: The story of the American Nurses Association.* Kansas City, MO: American Nurses Association.

Flexner, A. (1910). *Medical education in the United States and Canada. A report to the Carnegie Foundation for the Advancement of Teaching.* Boston, MD: Merrymount Press.

Gilligan, C. (1982). *In a different voice.* Cambridge, MA: Harvard University Press.

Ginzberg, E. (1949). *A pattern for hospital care.* New York: Columbia University Press.

Ginzberg, E. (1995). A cautionary note on market reforms in health care. *Journal of the American Medical Association, 274,* 1633–1634.

Goldmark, J. (1923). *Nursing and nursing education in the United States.* New York: Macmillan.

Greenberg, L. (1994). Work redesign: An overview. *Journal of Emergency Nursing, 20,* 28A–32A.

Healthcare.gov. (n.d.) *What Marketplace health insurance plans cover.* Retrieved from https://www.healthcare.gov/coverage/what-marketplace-plans-cover/. Accessed August 30, 2016.

Holahan, J., & Chen, V. (2011). *Changes in health insurance coverage in the great recession, 2007–2010.* Retrieved from http://kaiserfamilyfoundation.files.wordpress.com/2013/01/8264.pdf. Accessed May 21, 2013.

Jamieson, E. M., & Sewall, M. F. (1954). *Trends in nursing history* (4th ed.). Philadelphia, PA: WB Saunders.

Kaiser Family Foundation. (2012). *Making sense of the census uninsured numbers.* Retrieved from http://kff.org/health-reform/event/making-sense-of-the-census-uninsured-numbers/. Accessed May 21, 2013.

Kalisch, P. A., & Kalisch, B. J. (2004). *The advance of American nursing* (4th ed.). Philadelphia, PA: Lippincott Williams & Wilkins.

Kendall-Gallagher, D., Aiken, L., Sloane, D., & Cimiotti, J. (2011). Nurse specialty certification, inpatient mortality and failure to rescue. *Journal of Nursing Scholarship, 43*(2), 188–194.

Kjervik, D. K., & Martinson, I. J. M. (1979). *Women in stress: A nursing perspective.* New York: Appleton-Century-Crofts.

Madsen, W. (2005). Early 20th century untrained nursing staff in the Rockhampton district: A necessary evil? *Journal of Advanced Nursing, 51*(3), 307–313.

Malka, S. G. (2007). *Daring to care.* Urbana, IL: University of Illinois Press.

McPherson, K. I. (1983). Feminist methods: A new paradigm for nursing research. *Advances in Nursing Science, 5*(2), 17–25.

Meehan, T. C. (2003). Careful nursing: A model for contemporary nursing practice. *Journal of Advanced Nursing, 44,* 99–107.

Montag, M. (1951). *The education of nursing technicians.* New York: Putman.

National League for Nursing. (1939). More graduate duty nurses. *American Journal of Nursing, 39,* 898.

National Institutes of Health. (2016). *The NIH Almanac: National Center for Complementary & Integrative Health.* Retrieved from http://www.nih.gov/about-nih/what-we-do/nih-almanac/national-center-complementary-integrative-health-nccih. Accessed March 14, 2016.

Nutting, M. A., & Dock, L. L. (1935a). *A history of nursing: The evolution of nursing systems from the earliest times to the foundation of the first English and American training schools (Vol. 2).* New York: Putman.

Nutting, M. A., & Dock, L. L. (1935b). *A history of nursing: The evolution of nursing systems from the earliest times to the foundation of the first English and American training schools (Vol. 3).* New York: Putman.

Roberts, M. M. (1954). *American nursing: History and interpretation.* New York: Macmillan.

Smith, J., & Medalia, C. (2015). *Current population reports. Health insurance coverage in the United States, 2014 (pp. 60–253).* Retrieved from http://www.census.gov/content/dam/Census/library/publications/2015/demo/p60–253.pdf. Accessed March 14, 2016.

Speedy, S. (1987). Feminism and the professionalisation of nursing. *Australian Journal of Advanced Nursing, 4*(2), 20–28.

Spitrey, J. (2015). *Meet the passionate founder of Show Me Your Stethoscope.* Retrieved from http://exclusive.multibriefs.com/content/meet-the-founder-of-show-me-your-stethoscope/healthcare-administration. Accessed March 14, 2016.

Spradley, B. W. (1990). *Community health nursing: Concepts and practice.* Glenview, IL: Scott Foresman/Little Brown.

U.S. Census Bureau. (2011). *Age and sex composition: 2010 Census briefs.* Retrieved from http://www.census.gov/prod/cen2010/briefs/c2010br-03.pdf. Accessed October 22, 2012.

U.S. Department of Health and Human Services, Health Resources and Services Administration, & Bureau of Health Professions. (2010). *The registered nurse population: Findings from the 2008 National Sample Survey of Registered Nurses.* Retrieved from http://bhpr.hrsa.gov/healthworkforce/rnsurveys/rnsurveyfinal.pdf. Accessed October 22, 2012.

U.S. Department of Health & Human Services, National Institutes of Health, & National Center for Complementary and Alternative Medicine. (2008). *The use of complementary and alternative medicine in the United States.* Retrieved from https://nccih.nih.gov/sites/nccam.nih.gov/files/camuse.pdf. Accessed March 13, 2016.

U.S. Public Health Service. (1963). *Toward quality in nursing: Needs and goals. A report of the surgeon general's consultant group in nursing.* Washington, DC: Author.

Watson, J. (1999). *Postmodern nursing and beyond.* Edinburgh, UK: Churchill Livingstone.

Watson, J. (2012). *Human caring science a theory of nursing* (2nd ed.). Sudbury, MA: Jones & Bartlett Learning.

Wheeler, W. (1999). Florence: Death of an icon? *Nursing Times, 95,* 24–26.

Wilson, E. O. (1998). *Consilience: The unity of knowledge.* New York: Alfred A. Knopf.

3

Contextual, Philosophical, and Ethical Elements of Professional Nursing

KEY TERMS AND CONCEPTS

Values

Beliefs

Context

Philosophy

Contextual elements of
  nursing practice

Mission

Morality

Ethics

Principalism

Four phases of caring

Contextualism

Ethical decision-making
  process

Ethical competence

LEARNING OUTCOMES

By the end of this chapter, the learner will be able to:

1. Identify environmental factors that constitute the context for nursing practice.
2. Outline the essential elements of a nursing philosophy.
3. Develop a personal nursing philosophy.
4. Outline key steps for effective analysis of ethical dilemmas.
5. Use a structured method for making ethical decisions.
6. Specify fallacies that might occur when making ethical decisions.
7. Explain how demographic, cultural, economic, environmental, and ethical factors influence professional practice.
8. Incorporate knowledge, freedom, and choice while using nursing process.

REAL-LIFE REFLECTIONS

Jane has been in nursing for 15 years. At times, Jane wonders if she should share her concerns with her unit manager or a trusted nursing colleague. She yearns for the "good old days" when client care was focused on people rather than on business. Jane often feels detached from her clients and perceives herself as a "client care machine." However, she knows in her heart that she does make a difference in her clients' lives, and she derives profound satisfaction from helping others. Jane is considering a career change, but she feels passionate about helping other people.

- *In what ways do you think nursing has become less focused on client care?*
- *What advice would you give to Jane?*

As a science, nursing focuses on humanity in a highly objective manner, using interventions based on scientific evidence. As technologic advances create a more complex world, making sense of the world becomes more important. A well-defined set of **values**

(principles, or what things are important) and **beliefs** (ideas regarded as truths) provides a firm foundation for nursing practice. If nurses relied exclusively on thinking and approached nursing using only hard science, they would appear cold and distant to their clients. However, professional nurses connect emotionally and spiritually with clients, thereby allowing genuine warmth and authentic compassion to guide clinical practice. Values and beliefs influence perceptions, thoughts, and feelings.

Take Note!

Because values and beliefs strongly influence our perceptions, thoughts, and feelings, a well-defined set of values and beliefs provides the best foundation for nursing practice.

Context has been defined as "the whole situation, background, or environmental relationships to a particular event, personality, creation, etc." (Agnes, 2005, p. 315). Environmental and situational conditions create the context of nursing practice. Each nurse brings to the context his or her personal set of beliefs about people, the world, health, and nursing. This set of beliefs constitutes a **philosophy** of nursing. When providing care, nurses interact with the environment, which is composed of contextual factors in which the nurse's philosophy plays a key role.

- The pragmatic professional self seeks cause-and-effect relationships and looks for the practical nature of nursing and how it can be used to solve issues that arise in daily clinical practice.
- The idealistic professional self pays serious attention to the ideal conceptualizations of nursing practice and views nursing as a means for forming authentic and caring relationships with others to help them achieve their maximum health potential.
- The realistic professional self emphasizes facts and scientific principles during nursing practice.
- The existentialist professional self displays great regard for individuals and respects their choices with an acceptance of responsibility for those choices made as nursing care is delivered.

Some degree of congruence with the vastly different worldviews is desirable for authentic, humane, scientific-based, nonpaternalistic nursing practice.

Development of an individual nursing philosophy helps nurses come to terms with diverse worldviews. However, to begin developing a personal nursing philosophy, nurses need to be cognizant of the **contextual elements of nursing practice**. These elements comprise the demographic, economic, environmental, and ethical factors that surround a client care situation. Contextual elements surrounding a clinical situation affect the professional roles assumed by nurses and the clinical decisions they make. Along with a personal nursing philosophy, contextual elements help nurses develop a meaningful and thoughtful practice.

CONTEXTUAL BASIS OF NURSING PRACTICE

What is the world of nursing like today? Before that question can be answered, we must look at the world environment—the place where nursing occurs. Professional nursing practice does not occur in isolation; rather, nursing is embedded in and integral to the complex health care delivery system. When one area of health care experiences a change, all areas of health care delivery undergo change. Dramatic changes in health care over the past two decades have profoundly affected professional nursing practice. Future changes may occur so quickly that nurses (and other health care workers) may have difficulty fully comprehending the effects of change and coping with its implications (Porter-O'Grady & Malloch, 2015).

Professional nursing practice is a complex phenomenon affected by many contextual elements; it is impossible to present all of these elements in a single chapter. To capture an accurate picture of current professional practice, the following discussion focuses on quantum science, which requires relational and whole-systems thinking, technology and consumerism, the global community, communication, and the desire for equality while maintaining personal identity.

Quantum Science: Relational and Whole-Systems Thinking in Health Care

Change is constant; no one can avoid it (Hawking, 2002). To survive change, humans must learn new ways of thinking. The world is a complex place full of chaos, where everything is interconnected. Structure becomes defined by wholes rather than individual parts (Hawking, 2002; Porter-O'Grady & Malloch, 2015). When looking into a hologram, the entire large picture can be seen on any size fraction of the image. Such is the nature of overall structure.

The smallest structural unit of a system mirrors its entire system in terms of organization pattern and behavior. Systems work continuously to renew and reinvent themselves while maintaining their basic integrity. Systems are composed of multiple interacting feedback loops. Structure has disorder, and disorder has structure. Quantum science eliminates dualistic or "either-or" thinking and envisions new possibilities of combining ideas through the use of synthesis.

Synthesis involves putting ideas or things together in a new way. For example, the human body synthesizes food eaten into muscle, fat, energy, and waste products. It takes chemicals from consumed food and transforms them into a new state. In Hegelian philosophy, it means to reconcile two opposites and make a new whole which is a form of dialectical thinking. For the author of this book, work and play are two opposing concepts. Therefore all work and all play would be polar opposites. However, a synthesis of work and play within one's personal life would result in a balance between them. However, if a person immensely enjoys an activity (such as writing) and has a contract to produce a book (work), a synthesis of the two concepts could result in playing while working. The coined terms playwork or workplay could be used to describe this new phenomenon.

Relational thinking involves recognition of the interconnectedness of all things. All things become interdependent. A complex algorithm (series of steps or events) is required for things to occur or exist (Porter-O'Grady & Malloch, 2015). For example, human health is a complex process that involves a safe environment, intact physical and mental capabilities, meaningful interpersonal relationships, and spiritual dimensions. The link between psyche and health has been studied extensively in the field of psychoneuroimmunology. Studies have established relationships among health status, mental outlook, and finding meaning in life (Antonovsky, 1987; Ferreira & Sherman, 2007; Hatala, 2008; Iwarrsson, Horstmann, & Slaug, 2007; Lewis, 2008a, 2008b). As client advocates, caregivers, coordinators, teachers, and counselors, nurses look at the client holistically to determine what resources are required to promote health.

The holistic approach also requires whole-systems thinking, in which many smaller interacting systems that aggregate to create the larger (or whole) system (Porter-O'Grady & Malloch, 2015). For example, a hospital consists of many departments (e.g., surgery, radiology, laboratory, pharmacy, nursing, dietary), each of which assumes responsibility for an integral part of client care. In the case of nursing departments, client care is delivered 24 hours a day, 7 days a week. Thus, different nursing care teams staff the hospital during the different shifts. Each nursing unit represents an additional system. The nursing team on a unit may be broken down even further to represent the professional nurse, a vocational (or practical) nurse, and unlicensed care providers. Each individual providing client care is also a complex system with many personal needs.

When engaging in whole-systems thinking, one must look at the complex nature of all the interacting systems. Consider the hospital as being only one system in the larger health care delivery system. Waste by-products of health care therapies must be either discarded or recycled. The impact of waste affects the global environment.

When nurses use whole-systems thinking in daily clinical practice, they assume the role of care coordinator. They look for ways to use human and material resources optimally to meet client care needs (e.g., staffing nursing units and judicious use of medical supplies). When assuming the role of client advocate, nurses frequently refer clients to community agencies for assistance if needs remain unmet and resources are unavailable in the practice setting.

Take Note!

Whole-systems thinking requires an awareness of the numerous smaller systems that comprise the larger system and note the interrelationships among them.

Because of the complex nature of clinical practice and health care delivery, nurses consider many factors when providing client care. Quantum science and relational and systems thinking provide nurses with the ability to consider the impact of clinical decisions not only on clients but also on the institutional, national, and global communities. Because change remains constant, nurses must stay abreast of factors that influence professional practice. The ability to use relational and systems thinking enables the nurse to appraise the entire client care situation before making decisions focused on the client's best interest. The following discussion provides a broad overview of factors that affect professional nursing practice.

Technology, Communications, Safety, and Consumerism in Health Care

Technology has transformed human lives. Increased use of technology in health care has resulted in people surviving illnesses once thought to be untreatable, enabled instant access to information, increased the cost of health care, and created increasingly savvy health care consumers. In the United States, consumers drive the delivery of health care and frequently rely on information obtained from the internet. Pharmaceutical companies post new information about medications on the internet and target consumers with advertising. When assessing client knowledge of health-related information, nurses must find out what clients know and the sources of their information. As educators, nurses should assist clients in determining the quality of information accessed from the internet (see Chapter 14, "Informatics and Technology in Nursing Practice"). Clients sometimes demand the newest (not always the best) health care treatments from providers (Herzlinger, 2004).

Take Note!
Because of the array of health information found online, nurses must stay abreast of developments in health promotion and disease management to remain effective caregivers and educators.

In some cases, clients may know more about their health problems than health care providers (Herzlinger, 2004). For example, a young woman, newly diagnosed with myasthenia gravis, finds detailed information about her disease from visiting the National Myasthenia Gravis Foundation website. She learns what medications may result in increased muscle weakness. When she needs surgery that requires hospitalization, she brings the long list of medications known to increase muscle weakness in persons with myasthenia gravis to the hospital so that she will not receive them. Although her actions may have been unnecessary because nurses and physicians providing her care have access to the same information, they can save health care providers' time.

Some health care organizations provide nurses with pagers (or cell phones) so they can receive instant messages in case of client emergency or other client needs. These devices can prevent nurses from developing and maintaining therapeutic client relationships (an integral element of professional practice) because of the distraction and interruption they cause. Clients expect nurses to care for them by ensuring their safety, being competent in nursing, taking action that is in their best interests, and listening to them. In addition, some clients become distracted by their cell phones while receiving health care and may miss critical information on how to best manage their health (Herzlinger, 2004). Box 3.1, Professional Building Blocks, "Technologic Devices: Patient Care Enhancement or Distraction?," highlights how technologic devices have the potential of enhancing or distracting nurses and patients in the delivery of care.

Along with the latest developments in traditional medical care, many clients have knowledge of alternative and complementary health care therapies. Some consumers expect health care professionals, including nurses, to have knowledge of, and provide them with, these therapies or to offer advice about them (Dossey & Keegan, 2013; Herzlinger, 2004; Ross, Wenzel, & Mitlyng, 2002). Nurses must inquire as to all health

3.1 Professional Building Blocks

Technologic Devices: Patient Care Enhancement or Distraction?

Device	Enhancement	Distraction
Pager	▪ Increased and immediate awareness of a significant patient care need or another staff member's need for help	▪ Interruption while working with a patient or significant others
Cell phone	▪ Quicker notification of nurse of a significant patient care need, another staff member's need for help or to speak directly to another health care provider or patient's significant others ▪ Access to a variety of clinical resources ▪ Increased availability of health education applications that could be shared with patients and families	▪ Patient distraction while receiving health care services ▪ Nurse interruption during care delivery ▪ Potential for photographing or videotaping care delivery
Personal digital device	▪ Access to a variety of clinical resources	▪ Perceptions of being used for personal rather than professional reasons
Bedside computers	▪ Immediate access to key patient information ▪ Elimination of the need for multiple care providers to ask patients the same questions ▪ Increased safety of care delivery ▪ Instantaneous documentation of nursing assessments, interventions, and evaluations	▪ Focus of getting documentation completed with the potential of ignoring concerns of patient and significant others

care practices used by clients to ensure the safety of prescribed, traditional medical therapies and to determine if any complementary or alternative therapies may pose potential health hazards.

Today, clients and health care providers work as partners toward common goals. Looking out for one's own safety or the safety of a loved one has become a factor in care delivery. Accrediting agencies, health care facilities, and health care professionals provide clients and families with information about how to remain safe while hospitalized by providing them with educational materials about fall prevention and the importance of hand hygiene. The media also share information with consumers about unsafe health care practices. Professional nurses and all health team members strive to keep clients safe. Technologic devices such as bar-coding machines reduce the incidence of errors in medication dosing, and bedside acquisition of blood and body fluid specimens for laboratory testing make the delivery of care quicker, more convenient, and more accurate.

Because of the complex nature of health care delivery, various members of the health care team assume different aspects of care. Breakdowns in communication frequently result in client care errors, and when errors occur, the system involving the entire team bears the blame rather than a single person (Institute of Medicine [IOM], 2000, 2010; Porter-O'Grady & Malloch, 2015).

Take Note!

Effective communication is crucial in ensuring that all health team members involved in the client's care are aware of specific needs and anything that might adversely affect the client.

The Global Community and Health Care

The emergence of a single world economy and the acknowledgment of finite Earth resources have resulted in a changed context for professional practice. Today, the nations of the world are connected as a global economic community (Fig. 3.1). Political and social unrest and economic instability in one nation have the potential to disrupt the economies of many nations.

Various nations have different forms of health care delivery systems. How health care is delivered has an impact on whether people use organized health systems or rely on alternative modes. Developed nations have well-refined health care delivery systems along with access to sophisticated treatments, while undeveloped nations (especially those in political turmoil) may have no organized systems to meet the health care needs of

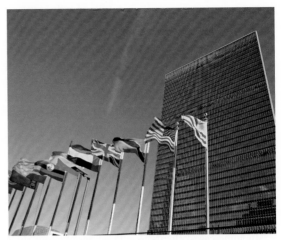

FIGURE 3.1 United Nations Headquarters, New York City, NY.

their residents (Fried & Gaydos, 2002; United Nations Development Programme [UNDP], 2015a; World Health Organization [WHO], 2016a). Other disparities in quality of life and health care are becoming more evident than ever before. Whereas undeveloped and overpopulated nations are looking for ways to combat malnutrition and infectious diseases, citizens of highly developed nations suffer from health problems related to a life of excess, such as obesity, diabetes mellitus, and cardiovascular disease (WHO, 2012).

The United Nations (2015) identified 17 "sustainable development goals" (SDGS) that all 191 United Nations member states have agreed to attain by 2020. The World Health Organization efforts focus on the goals that are related to human health and well-being.

1. No poverty (eliminate all forms of poverty everywhere) (UNDP, 2015b)
2. Zero hunger (eliminate hunger, attain food security and improve nutrition while promoting sustainable agriculture) (UNDP, 2015c)
3. Good health and well-being (ensure healthy lives and promote well-being in all persons) (UNDP, 2015d)
4. Quality education (provide equitable, high-quality education and provide lifelong learning opportunities for all) (UNDP, 2015e)
5. Gender equality (attain gender equality and empowerment for women and girls) (UNDP, 2015f)
6. Clean water and sanitation (ensure access to clean water and effective sanitation for all) (UNDP, 2015g)
7. Affordable and clean energy (ensure access for all to affordable, reliable, and sustainable modern energy) (UNDP, 2015h)

8. Decent work and economic growth (provide inclusive economic growth, employment, and decent work for everyone) (UNDP, 2015i)
9. Industry, innovation, and infrastructure (construct resilient infrastructure, assure sustainable industrialization, and promote innovation) (UNDP, 2015j)
10. Reduced inequalities (reduce economic and power inequalities within and among all nations) (UNDP, 2015k)
11. Sustainable cities and communities (transform and create cities and communities that are resilient, safe, and sustainable) (UNDP, 2015l)
12. Responsible consumption and production (promote sustainable patterns of production and consumption) (UNDP, 2015m)
13. Climate actions (take urgent steps to combat climate change and its impact on the planet and people) (UNDP, 2015n)
14. Life below water (conserve and wisely use the oceans, seas, and marine resources) (UNDP, 2015o)
15. Life on land (manage forests sustainably, reduce desertification, stop and reverse land degradation, and stop loss of biodiverse plants, animals, and organisms) (UNDP, 2015p)
16. Peace, justice, strong institutions (facilitate the development and maintenance of inclusive, just and peaceful societies) (UNDP, 2015q)
17. Partnerships for the goals (develop and renew global partnerships for the achievement of the SDGS) (UNDP, 2015r)

All of the SDGS influence health, and health in turn influences the goals. Other factors that threaten health around the world include war, accidents, community and domestic violence, natural and manmade disasters, human trafficking, health care provider errors, the emergence of drug-resistant infections, obesity, and chemical abuse (see Concepts in Practice, "The Need for Global Cooperation").

Concepts in Practice IDEA → PLAN → ACTION

The Need for Global Cooperation

One of the worst potential threats to global health would be the emergence of a new, highly contagious and highly lethal flu virus. Because of worldwide air travel, such a virus could spread throughout the world in as few as 100 days. Clusters of cases would pop up simultaneously around the world, and hundreds would die as their lungs fill with fluid. Global cooperation among public health officials has been instrumental in preventing such a disaster, including a pandemic of severe acute respiratory syndrome in 2003 (Enserink, 2004), a potential tuberculosis epidemic in 2007, a polio epidemic in the Middle East in 2014, Ebola in 2015, and the Zika virus in 2016. When the World Health Organization (WHO) declares a health emergency, member nations are expected to share data on the incidence of the disease, its health risks and complications; control the vector (if insect-borne or animal-borne illness), issue health-risk warnings, issue travel recommendations and safety measures, and share research findings about the disease and any new products developed to contain, control, or treat the disease (WHO, 2016b).

Desire for Equality While Maintaining a Personal Cultural Identity

Despite globalization and access to information from around the world, people strive to maintain ties to their own culture. Many people immigrate to developed nations to escape political persecution or less-than-ideal economic situations. Others may come to developed nations to secure treatment for health problems. Although they have left their nation of birth, many of these individuals maintain cultural ties and traditions to their homelands. In addition, many of those born in developed nations whose parents or other ancestors came from other countries value their cultural heritage.

Culturally sensitive care enables the health care system to accommodate client needs to abide by specific cultural practices. Some health care facilities use computers that permit printing of discharge instructions in more than one language and have interpreters for staff to use when working with clients from diverse cultures. In some cases, folk healers are permitted to practice in inpatient settings (Dossey & Keegan, 2013). As client advocates, nurses sometimes have to question specific cultural practices that might be detrimental to client health. (More detailed information on multicultural issues in professional practice is presented in Chapter 11, "Multicultural Issues in Professional Practice.")

The ability to determine if and when a client's health practices are questionable depends in part on the individual nurse's knowledge, values, and beliefs. Part of the education involves discovery of things unknown about oneself. The section that follows offers a discussion about philosophy and its significance for professional nursing practice.

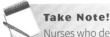

Take Note!
Nurses who deliver culturally sensitive nursing care acknowledge the cultural needs of clients.

NURSING PHILOSOPHY

Philosophy is a conceptual discipline involving things that cannot be directly touched or observed. The word "philosophy" is derived from the Greek *philia* (love or friendship) and *sophia* (wisdom). Philosophers strive for wisdom, not necessarily to possess it. "Wisdom is used inclusively to cover the sustained intellectual inquiry in any area, the understanding and practice of morality, and the cultivation of such enlightened opinions and attitudes as lead to a life of happiness and contentment" (Earle, 1992, p. 2).

People have been searching for meaning and happiness in their lives for centuries (Fig. 3.2). Development of a personal philosophy requires examination of beliefs and values about life and requires a little time. However, development of a collective (group) philosophy requires much time and consolidation of individual beliefs and values. Philosophies may change as people gain new knowledge and skills through life journeys.

Anyone can be a philosopher. Tools used by philosophers include analyzing concepts, doubting everything and determining what it truly means to be human (Earle, 1992). A process known as concept analysis is used to arrive at a clear, concise definition of a concept. During concept analysis, philosophers identify the antecedents (things that must occur prior to something existing or occurring) and consequences (what happens as the result of something existing or occurring). The process then involves the development of a model case of the concept to provide a crystal clear example of the concept.

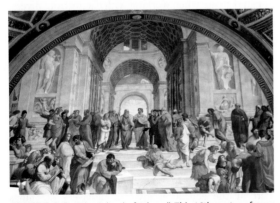

FIGURE 3.2 "The School of Athens". This 16th century fresco by Raphael symbolizes the spirit of philosophical inquiry. "Philosophy" derives from Ancient Greece and means "love of wisdom".

To further clarify the concept, the person conducting the concept analysis designs related and contrary cases (Fitzpatrick & McCarthy, 2016; Walker & Avant, 2011). When philosophers engage in the process of doubting everything, the mere existence of all ideas, events, and tangible objects is questioned (Earle, 1992; Law, 2007). The process of doubting everything enables persons to generate personal or scientific evidence for the existence of things and events. What is deemed to be true for one person, may not be true for another (e.g., religious beliefs, historical events, and even personal strategies that promote health). The variance in beliefs about what is true can be considered a key way of how individuals are unique. People possess common functional and structural elements. However, each person also possesses differences in genetic composition, cultural background, and belief systems. A person's belief system provides a perceptual foundation of what it means to be human. Earle and Law articulate that learning about what it means to be human requires detailed descriptions of human lived experiences and making meaning of one's existence. Finding meaning in one's life enables people to survive harsh conditions (Frankl, 1963) and promotes health (Antonovsky, 1987; Church, 2007; Lewis, 2008b).

Building the Foundation

The Box 3.2, Professional Building Blocks, "Major Disciplines of Philosophy," provides the nine major disciplines of philosophy and the questions each seeks to answer, and can serve as a guide to understanding and developing a philosophy.

Philosophy focuses on conceptual clarity and requires an individual journey while providing a foundation for human action (Earle, 1992; Law, 2007; Reed, 2011). For clarity, nursing philosophy is defined as the intellectual and affective outcomes of the professional nurses' efforts to

1. understand the ultimate relationships between humans, environment, and health.
2. approach nursing as a scientific discipline.
3. integrate a sense of value into practice.
4. appreciate aesthetic elements that contribute to health and well-being.
5. define the mission of nursing.
6. articulate a personal belief system about human beings, environment, health, and nursing.

Significance of Philosophy for Nursing

Over time, the study of philosophy has accrued great benefits for individuals, societies, and, particularly,

3.2 Professional Building Blocks

Major Disciplines of Philosophy

1. **Logic:** Systematic study of arguments for logical or illogical reasoning
   - Does this make sense?
2. **Epistemology:** Study of knowledge
   - What is knowledge? How do people acquire it?
3. **Philosophy of science:** Explanation of the successes of science
   - How is science used? What are the benefits of hard sciences to humans?
4. **Metaphysics (ontology):** Analysis of issues surrounding the ultimate nature of existence, reality, and experience; also addresses the reality of abstractions (from mathematical constructs such as numbers to religious concepts such as God, angels, and the human soul) and the existence of abstractions in the absence of human thought
   - What is there?
5. **Philosophy of mind:** Study of the nature of the mental dimension of people
   - What is the mind? How should we understand intentions, desires, beliefs, emotions, pleasure, and pain? How do mental processes explain human behavior?

6. **Ethics (moral philosophy):** Study of the appropriateness of possible courses of action based on a system of moral principles and values
   - What is morality? What actions are obligatory, morally permissible, or impermissible?
7. **Sociopolitical philosophy:** Study of the control and regulation of persons living in a society, and the means to improve their lives
   - Where do states come from? What does it mean to be a citizen of a state? Must we obey laws, and why? When should laws be changed?
8. **Philosophy of religion:** Study of the meaning of human life
   - Is religious language meaningful? Does God exist? Is there good and evil? What other basis can give meaning to life if the religious assumptions were to be proven false?
9. **Aesthetics:** Study of what constitutes beauty
   - What is beauty? What makes something a work of art? Why are art and other forms of artistic expression important?

specific sciences. Essentially, science benefits from philosophy because philosophy governs scientific methods through logic and ethics.

Pursuing the objectives of philosophy provides individuals with opportunities to develop an understanding of the world around them and to exercise value judgments. Development of a personal system of values requires making ethical and aesthetic decisions. The quest for reason develops understanding. Achievement of intellectual enlightenment is considered better protection against calamitous mistakes than ignorance.

The nursing profession needs philosophers who articulate visions for nursing as a scientific discipline, emphasize concern for the ultimate good of humankind, develop belief systems reflecting sound ethics, reflect on the meaning of nursing, and conduct periodic review of nursing philosophies.

Nurses need personal philosophies that reflect a belief in recasting the health system to benefit all humankind rather than ensuring institutional survival. Nursing philosophers analyze current health care systems and conceptualize the bases for nursing practice, research, and education. These nursing philosophers also concern themselves with moral issues surrounding

nursing and health care while promoting behavior based on a professional code of ethics.

Rafael (1996) coined the term "empowered caring" to denote leadership as a unity of power and caring that values the characteristics and experiences of women, and a system of ethics that "stems from a heightened awareness of interrelatedness and emerges as a sense of responsibility toward others" (p. 15). Rafael's writing demonstrates the work of a nursing philosopher who provides novel thinking and uses this to shift from a hierarchical approach to nursing to one in which nurses and nurse leaders share knowledge and expertise with clients (and each other).

Nurse leaders have identified a system of values to guide the nursing profession. According to the American Association of Colleges of Nursing (AACN) (2008), "professional values and their associated behaviors are foundational to the practice of nursing" (p. 26). AACN (2008) identified "the inherent values of altruism, autonomy, human dignity, integrity, and social justice" (p. 4) as values that underpin the practice of professional nursing. Ethical and honest behavior by professional nurses promote social respect for nurses and enhance patient safety. A strong professional value set facilitates decision making in ethically charged clinical situations.

Developing a Personal Nursing Philosophy

A personal nursing philosophy provides an individualized perspective for nursing practice, research, and scholarship (Salsberry, 1994). Articulation of a personal nursing philosophy enables nurses to make and find meaning about being a professional nurse. Rew (1994) explains that a well-articulated philosophy combines ways of doing with ways of being. Determining ways of being involves an examination of one's personal beliefs and values. For example, how nurses view their professional activities such as doing a job, engaging in a professional career and/or living out one's calling to help other affects how they practice nursing and what it means to be a professional nurse. Marchuk (2014) suggests that a personal nursing philosophy promotes the integration of nursing knowledge into compassionate clinical care. In contrast, Hountras (2015) espouses that having a personal nursing philosophy facilitates personal motivation and provides reasons behind the work of professional nursing for each nurse. A personal nursing philosophy is never complete; rather, it evolves as knowledge and experience expand. Because the nursing profession concerns itself with people, health, nursing, and the environment, most personal nursing philosophies address these key concepts.

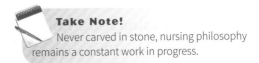

Take Note!
Never carved in stone, nursing philosophy remains a constant work in progress.

Carper (1978) identified four patterns of knowing in nursing: personal knowledge, empirics, aesthetics, and ethics (presented in more detail in Chapter 5, "Patterns of Knowing and Nursing Science"). A well-developed nursing philosophy represents personal knowledge related to professional nursing.

To construct a personal philosophy of nursing, one must engage in reflective thinking about one's relationship to the universe. Discovery of a personal **mission** or goal within the realm of nursing solidifies the decision to practice professional nursing. Because nursing focuses on individuals and the environment, a beginning nursing philosophy should minimally address these concepts (see Box 3.3, Learning, Knowing, and Growing, "Developing a Nursing Philosophy").

The greatest opportunity to begin developing answers to the questions asked in the "Developing a Nursing Philosophy" begins with the first nursing course. Likewise, as nurses attain higher levels of education, beginning a new course becomes an opportune time to evaluate and modify one's professional nursing philosophy. A nurse's professional self-concept is built on the foundation of his

---

3.3 Learning, Knowing, and Growing

Developing a Nursing Philosophy

To develop a nursing philosophy, nurses must examine and answer questions that address the key concepts of professional nursing, elements of nursing as a scientific discipline, and the valuation elements of nursing.

Key Concepts of Professional Nursing

- What is the environment, and what is the nature of the relationship between humans and the environment?
- What is your central belief about the individual person and that person's potential?
- What is your central belief about the family and its potential?
- What is your central belief about the community and its potential?
- What are your central beliefs about the relationship between society and health?
- What is your view on health? Is it a continuum? A state? A process?
- How do illness and wellness relate to health?
- What is the central reason for the existence of nursing?
- Who is the recipient of nursing care?

Nursing as a Scientific Discipline

- Is nursing a science or an art? Or both?
- From what cognitive base does the professional nurse operate?
- What is nursing process? How is it implemented?
- What is necessary to apply nursing knowledge?
- How is the theory base for nursing derived?
- What is the theoretical framework for the profession? Or is there more than one theoretical framework?
- What are the purposes and processes of nursing research?

Valuation Elements of Nursing

- What are the essential rights and responsibilities of the professional nurse?
- What are the essential rights and responsibilities of recipients of nursing care?
- What are the governing ethical principles in the delivery of nursing care and the conduct of nursing research?
- What are your beliefs about the educational requirements for the practice of the profession?
- What are your beliefs about the teaching–learning process?
- What is the ultimate goal of professional nursing care?

or her personal life and educational and clinical practice experiences. As a nurse progresses on his or her life journey, finding meaning in one's personal and professional existence remains a constant challenge.

 Take Note!
Articulation of a personal nursing philosophy helps the nurse find purpose, create meaning, and increase commitment to the profession of nursing.

The Box 3.4, Professional Prototypes, "Sample Professional Nursing Philosophy," presents a brief sample nursing philosophy that employs analogy to present philosophical views about nursing. Analogies can be useful when presenting deeply held beliefs. However, a nursing philosophy does not require using an analogy; statements about personal beliefs serve just as well. As you develop your philosophy, realize that there is no "right" nursing philosophy. You may also find over time that your nursing philosophy may change.

Once you have an established nursing philosophy, you can use it in many ways. When seeking employment, ask to see the potential employer's organizational philosophy and see how closely it matches your own. A recent trend in health care is the development of a unit-based philosophy. To engage in the process, all unit staff meet and draft a philosophy. This process is time consuming and creates some interesting debates among

staff members. When organizational and personal philosophies match, people have a stronger commitment to work processes and increased job satisfaction.

MORALITY AND ETHICS IN NURSING PRACTICE

Within any practice context, nurses feel compelled to do what is "right" for their clients. **Morality**, as defined by O'Neill (1995, p. 224), encompasses "the oughts of a given society." **Ethics** is "the philosophical study of morality" (Noddings, 1984, p. 1). Nurses confront many situations in which they rely on their conscience for decision making. When working with coherent clients, nurses provide information and share decision making with them.

Many nurses acknowledge that a desire to care for others was the impetus for them to enter the nursing profession (Boughn, 1994, 2001; Okrainec, 1994; Streubert, 1994). The science and art of nursing center around the concept of caring. Experts in caring theory emphasize that before one can effectively care for others over a lifetime, one must be able to care for one's self (Benner, 1984, 2000; Benner & Wrubel, 1989; Watson, 1988, 1999, 2005, 2012). Watson (1988, 2005, 2012) called caring a moral imperative. Nurses enter the profession with the intent to care, and society expects them to care.

Changes in health care delivery often prevent nurses from having the time to express caring in practice. Some institutions treat nurses as replaceable technicians who have sophisticated skills. Clients have become consumers. Instead of individualized care, health care consumers receive treatment from standardized plans. Nurses feel pressure to streamline care to maximize the use of health care resources.

The shift of nursing care to a "trade service" is most apparent with the advent of managed care. Managed care looks for cost-cutting measures such as increased use of unlicensed care providers. Health insurers limit covered health care services and an individual's right to choose health care providers. Access to and justification for care supersede the more important, close interpersonal relationships that nurses build with clients. Therefore, the main stimulus for entering nursing—caring—becomes less valued by health care providers, especially administrators whose main concern is financial viability.

3.4 Professional Prototypes

Sample Professional Nursing Philosophy

Nursing is like a diamond. Special conditions must exist for a diamond to be created, and special care must be taken to maximize its luster.

Nurses hold a sacred trust with their clients when clients put their lives in the nurse's hands. The nurse's mission is to focus on what is best for the client when making decisions concerning care. When possible, the nurse and clients work as partners to promote health. Together they carve out a multifaceted plan of care that integrates the needs of body, mind, and spirit. The nurse always considers client choices for care. However, when the client is no longer able to choose, the nurse abides by the information left previously by the client or by the family's wishes. Along with caring for individuals, the nurse cares for families and communities.

A diamond never shows its luster if left in a box. Likewise, a nurse fails to shine when he or she is unable to care for others.

Moral Development

Gilligan (1982, p. 19) identified two ways of thinking about moral development. She associated these concepts of morality with male and female modes of describing relationships between others and self.

1. Fairness: Connecting moral development to the understanding of rights and rules (male mode).
2. Concern with the activity of care: Connecting moral development to the understanding of responsibilities and relationships (female mode).

Traditional views of moral development emphasize "rights" over relationships and responsibilities. In the traditional view of moral development, a person progresses through a series of stages. The first is a preconventional level which encompasses the first two stages with obedience to avoid punishment (stage 1) followed by a self-interest orientation (stage 2). The next level is conventional when people are concerned with interpersonal accord and conforming to expectations (stage 3) and following authority and social orders such as obeying the law (stage 4). The third and final level is the postconventional level in which persons assume a social contract orientation by displaying mutual respect and acknowledging pluralism (stage 5) and then applying universal ethical principles based on conscience and reasoning (stage 6) (Kohlberg, 1981).

Noddings (1984) proposed that morality and ethics should be "rooted in receptivity, relatedness, and responsiveness" (p. 2). Haegert (2004) adapted Noddings' work on the ethics of caring to professional nursing practice. For Noddings, caring involves two aspects of human nature in the embodied self and ethical self. The embodied self describes an idealized self that is "synonymous with caring" and the "vision that implied a picture of goodness toward the one caring (the nurse) and the one cared for (the patient)" (Haegert, 2004, p. 434). Nurses devote energy to the development of authentic, therapeutic, and caring relationships with clients. The ethical self involves nurses considering the legal and institutional standards of care, along with client rights for self-determination and equal access to care. Therefore, nursing presents a unique opportunity for blending different approaches to morality and ethics. However, as long as society values fairness and responsibility over receptivity, relatedness, and responsiveness, contributions made by professional nurses may not be as valued as those made by members of other health professions.

Morality supersedes status when persons entrust their lives to others. Therefore, moral principles guide health care providers in practice. Some of the moral principles central to nursing include beneficence, fidelity, and veracity. According to Flynn (1987), the principle of beneficence is to do only good. This principle also requires that persons act to prevent harm. Aroskar (1987) viewed fidelity as undisputed and primary loyalty and faithfulness to the client. Finally, veracity requires absolute truth telling.

In 1948, the *United Nations Declaration of Human Rights* mentioned human dignity, but failed to define its meaning. Dictionary definitions of dignity mean to be worthy of esteem and honor (Agnes, 2005). Depending upon one's secular or religious views human dignity may mean different things. The Judeo-Christian perspective espouses that humans are made in the image of God. Sulmasy (2008) identified three different ways to conceptualize dignity from a moralistic perspective: attributed (worthiness based on social status, reputation, or merit based upon societal contributions), intrinsic (people have value and worth just because they are human), and inflorescent (the flourishing of the human as he or she acts in manners expressing the intrinsic value of the human).

Fowler (2015) specifies that it is inflorescent dignity that is observed in nurses as they deliver skilled nursing care to others with genuine caring, compassion while displaying the utmost regard for the care recipient's humanness. In the nursing ethical literature, human dignity is inherent (permanently fixed), intrinsic (within and part of the natural innerness and belonging), and inviolable (it must not be violated, broken, or disturbed). By embracing the concept of human dignity as a moral concept, human dignity becomes the foundation for respect, protection, caring, and preservation of human rights of patients.

However, because nurses are also humans, attention needs to be made to the human dignity of the nurse (Fowler, 2015). The recognition of the dignity of the nursing profession is an emerging concept for the profession and is being recognized by society especially with legal efforts to protect nurses from physical and verbal assaults from health care consumers, exploitation from employers, sexual harassment, and lateral violence. A description and model of nursing professional dignity (NPD) has been developed (see the following research box by Sabatino et al., 2014.

Take Note!
Professional nurses use the principles of beneficence, fidelity, and veracity daily when providing care to clients.

FOCUS ON RESEARCH

Nursing Professional Dignity

Nursing professional dignity (NPD) is a concept that has been analyzed only within the last decade. The investigators conducted a meta-synthesis of 12 qualitative and 3 theoretical articles to arrive at a model of this multi-faceted concept. The participants in the article analysis included 322 nurses and 31 physicians. The investigators then carefully read the articles to identify key concepts, themes, and relationships independently then they met as a group and engaged in mutual dialogues to identify them in order to develop a model of NPD.

The derived model (p. 663) posited that nurses as human being possess intrinsic human dignity, possess a subjective perception of their own dignity that consists of a personal identity (self-awareness, self-worth, self-esteem, and self-respect), capable of personal reflection (determine own safety, identify a level of self-control, and possess self-determination) and a professional identity with professional ethical values (possess competencies and capabilities, have autonomy, make decisions, engage in continuous professional development, work-based on professional values, and have professional integrity). Workplace factors that support NPD include intraprofessional relationships (to be respected, mutual communication, shared knowledge, and support of nurse managers); interprofessional relationships (being seen, acknowledged, appreciated, and respected as a person and professional and for competence and personal space by other professional health team members, engaging in reciprocal communication, and being trusted by other professionals); communications with patients and their significant others (mutual effective communication and being appreciated); and organizational characteristics (employed by equal and fair organizations, and adequate financial resources, salary, and workloads).

The investigators outlined strengths of and threats to NPD. The strengths of having NPD included an ability to support patient dignity, improved safety, and quality of care, increased nurse motivation, and effective, ethical interprofessional teamwork. Threats to NPD included denial of the value of professional nursing, change in ethical climate, nurse absenteeism, job abandonment, frustration, depression, loss of self and professional confidence, reduced self-esteem, feelings of solitude, anxiety and helplessness, and dominance of the medical model in practice settings.

The investigators acknowledged several weaknesses in the study including relying on published articles from 11 different countries and working with poorly defined concepts in regards to human characteristics and workplace elements. They proposed needing to analyze more articles addressing NPD from a broader geographical base as the current study may be culturally biased. They also noted that there were no quantitative studies included in the analysis. They suggested that perhaps conducting a longitudinal study on the development of NPD starting at the time a person entered a nursing program through the first few years of professional practice might be useful for model refinement.

The PND model has great significance to the nursing profession. First, it allows nurses to be cognizant of their own worth as persons and professionals. The model also emphasizes the importance of nurses being valued and respected by society, their patients, patient significant others, and other members of the health care team. When professional nurses recognize their own PND, they may be more apt to stand up for themselves and their patients when encountering situations that compromise the nurse's personal and professional values, thereby improving the quality of patient care. There is also the potential for increased nurse retention in the workforce when nurses possess PND. Nurses who are highly motivated, have autonomous decision-making capabilities, know that they have unique skills and capabilities to help others, and can live out their professional and personal values on a daily basis may remain in the workforce for many years because of the financial and personal rewards they experience by being a professional nurse.

Sabatino, L., Stievano, A., Rocco, G., Kallio, H., Pietaila, A.-M., & Kangasniemi, M. (2014). The dignity of the nursing profession: A meta-synthesis of qualitative research. *Nursing Ethics, 21*(6), 659–672. doi: 10.1177/0969733013513215.

Moral and Ethical Dilemmas

Moral and ethical principles create dilemmas for nurses. Disagreements surface regarding what is good for a client, depending on the situation (Flynn, 1987). Individual health care team members may disagree on what is best for a terminally ill person. Fidelity specifies that nurses should always remain loyal and faithful to the client and abide by the client's wishes. Sometimes, nurses encounter situations that require them to deceive clients or withhold information from them to protect the institutions for which the nurses work or the physicians whom they serve. Although most institutions require nurses to report errors using some form of incident reporting, many institutional policies specify that the nurse should not document completion of an incident report.

When nurses encounter situations in which there is no good outcome, the principle of double effect (known as choosing the "lesser evil") guides practice. Burkhardt and Keegan (2013, p. 131) outlined the following four conditions that should be met to justify double-effect actions.

1. The act itself must be morally good or at least indifferent.
2. The good effect must not be achieved by means of the bad effect.
3. Only the good effect must be intended, although the bad effect is foreseen and known.
4. The good effect intended must be equal to or greater than the bad effect.

As client advocates, nurses must act on behalf of clients. To assess a particular clinical situation, nurses use critical thinking skills to collect and analyze information and to formulate possible courses of action. As critical thinkers, nurses also anticipate consequences of actions before choosing the best course to take. Professional nurses use values and philosophical beliefs to set priorities and establish action plans in ethically and morally charged situations (see Concepts in Practice, "An Ethical Dilemma: The Case of Mrs. G").

▌ QUESTIONS FOR REFLECTION

1. How should the nurse respond in this situation?
2. What ethical principles should be applied in this case?
3. What roadblocks might the nurse encounter in providing the best care for Mrs. G?

Concepts in Practice ⸢IDEA⸣→⸢PLAN⸣→⸢ACTION⸣

An Ethical Dilemma: The Case of Mrs. G

Mrs. G, a 96-year-old woman, is comatose due to a head injury from an automobile accident in which she was the driver. Before the accident, she lived independently and volunteered at the library teaching adults to read. Mrs. G has been unresponsive and ventilator dependent for 3 days. She has shown no improvement, but her son is insisting on a tracheotomy so that his mother can be maintained on the ventilator until she regains consciousness.

ETHICAL DECISION MAKING

According to Bandman and Bandman (1995), nursing ethics focus on doing good and avoiding harm. The nurse bears responsibility for valuing choices that clients make. For example, choices may be clearly articulated when people complete living wills before becoming incapacitated. However, when people fail to make their desires known before they are unable to do so, health care professionals rely on families for treatment-related decisions. In the absence of family, moral and ethical tenets guide actions.

Nurses, like scientists and philosophers, base their decisions on outcomes of inquiry. Munhall linked nursing inquiry to ethical reflection, with the ultimate ethical question being "Toward what goal and what end?" (Munhall, 1988, p. 151). Munhall added that "many of our research endeavors focus on facilitating health. The search for a means to produce a desired health outcome requires critical ethical reflection" (p. 152).

Principalism, Care, and Contextualism

Traditionally, three perspectives provide a foundation for and influence ethical thinking: principalism, care, and contextualism.

- Of the three, the most prevalent framework is **principalism**, which can be defined as using a set of principles or general guidelines for analyzing a situation considering general norms that have been derived from common morality. It involves incorporating professional duties rights and principles (Beauchamp & Childress, 2013; Fowler, 2015). Beauchamp and Childress (2013) identify four key ethical principles to guide ethical decision making. Respect for autonomy (an individual's right to self-determination and making his or her own decisions), nonmaleficence (to do no harm), beneficence (to do good), and justice (fairness, impartiality, get what is deserved, and what is right). This perspective values rationalism. However, a health care professional must analyze individual situations, sensitivity to the needs of others, and relationship dynamics when using principalism to guide ethical decision making.

- The care perspective can be used only when the care giver and care receiver have a reciprocal relationship. Fowler (2015) identifies **four phases of caring**: caring about, taking care of, care giving, and care receiving. The four moral elements of an ethic of care are attentiveness, responsibility, competence, and responsiveness. When using the ethic of care, the nurse dialogs with all persons involved in the decision-making process to identify and consider individual needs and preferences. Nursing based on the care perspective recognizes that time must be spent to discover what is meaningful to patients.
- Finally, in **contextualism**, individual situations become the paradigm cases that provide "rules of thumb" to follow. In the contextualist perspective, practical experience in patient care is highly valued (O'Neill, 1995). Nursing based on contextualism supports detailed analysis of individual nursing situations and determines the best approaches to fit each situation.

In a postmodern world, people tend to discount the simpler, monolithic approach to life and prefer pluralism. McCarthy (2006) proposed a pluralistic view of nursing ethics that blends the traditional and theory views of nursing ethics.

The traditional view espouses that nursing ethics is indeed a subcategory of health care ethics. Nurses engage in identifying, analyzing, and making decisions using the concepts of deontology (acting on the basis of moral duty and obligations), utilitarianism (acting to bring about the greatest good), or principalism (using duties, rights, and rules based on truth, laws, or doctrine) to navigate ethical challenges encountered in daily practice.

In contrast, the pluralistic theory view of ethics espouses a nursing-focused, ethical approach based on philosophical approaches derived from "virtue ethics, care ethics, or feminist ethics" (McCarthy, 2006, p. 160). This approach also uses ethical standards developed by international, national, and specialty nursing organizations. The theory view of ethics is contextual and emphasizes the power relationships among persons, societies, and organizations.

In a pluralistic view of nursing ethics, nurses use a combination of approaches to reflect on and make decisions about ethical dilemmas.

In practice, nurses (and other health care professionals) must make decisions with which they can live and, perhaps, make a better decision in the future. However, some people may experience confusion in how to figure out life and find meaning in it when rules are abandoned. They may desire to find the "right" way to approach a given situation and develop radical, steadfast approaches that fuel political debates and conflict.

Consider the debate whether nursing is an art or a science. Emphasis on technology, scientific evidence, and quality improvement suggests that nursing is a science. However, considering the beauty of the deep, meaningful, interpersonal relationship among nurses and clients and capturing how it unfolds suggest that nursing may really be an art. Conventional thinking would require the person to decide whether nursing is an art OR science. A pluralistic view would suggest that, perhaps, nursing could simultaneously be both an art AND a science.

Take Note!

Ethical dilemmas are messy, heart-wrenching situations with no clear-cut answers.

QUESTIONS FOR REFLECTION

1. What are your beliefs and values about human life?
2. How strong are these beliefs and values?
3. What would you do if you encountered a client care situation in which decisions were made that were against your values and beliefs? Why would you act this way?

REAL-LIFE REFLECTIONS

Jane is the charge nurse and Shelia and Ben are working with her today. A 50-year-old patient just received the diagnosis of advanced cancer and the physician told him that he has less than 6 months to live. The patient has three children: 17-year-old John, 15-year-old Ruth, and 12-year-old Daniel. The patient and the family have opted for hospice care and all cancer treatments are being stopped. While the family is at lunch, Ben spends time talking with the patient and learns about his concerns. Because his wife never understood the

(continued on page 76)

financial side of running a household, the patient decided that John should assume this responsibility for the family in anticipation of his death. The patient asks Ben for ideas of how to tell his son about this idea. What would you do if you were in Ben's situation? Why do you think that you would act this way? Is there a correct decision to be made in this situation? Why or why not?

An Ethical Decision-Making Process

Nurses frequently encounter moral and ethical problems in practice, thereby creating a need for a workable method with which to analyze and resolve ethical dilemmas (see Concepts in Practice, "Ethical Decision Making in Action"). Fowler and Levine-Ariff (1987) proposed a systematic **ethical decision-making process** that incorporates principalism, care, and contextualism to help nurses thoughtfully address moral problems in practice (Table 3.1). Consistent use of a sequential process for ethical decision making enables nurses to consider all aspects surrounding a situation before taking action. Once the situation has resolved, engagement in evaluation allows the nurse to reflect on actions taken and to generate ideas for managing a similar situation in the future.

Concepts in Practice [IDEA] → [PLAN] → [ACTION]

Ethical Decision Making in Action

Mary is a nurse who works in night shift on an acute general surgical unit. Because of budget cuts, the hospital has eliminated two night shift professional nursing positions, resulting in a consistent staffing pattern of 1 nurse for 15 patients. Mary has always valued her ability to provide individualized nursing care to postoperative patients. However, under the new staffing pattern, Mary knows that patients are receiving substandard care. She realizes that the hospital has been losing revenue, but she also feels that the staffing pattern is unsafe. Her recent complaints to her nurse manager have been futile. Because of unsafe care situations, Mary knows that she will have to inform her nurse manager's supervisor and possibly the director of nursing and hospital administration to analyze the entire situation. Mary reads current literature, identifies serious gaps in the accepted standards of practice, and examines the effects of the new staffing practice on each ethical principle. After sharing her concerns with her coworkers and manager, Mary and her colleagues work as a team to develop three action plans. They discuss the pros and cons of each plan, and then meet with the director of nursing to share their concerns. The director of nursing thanks the nurses for informing her of the situation and promises action to increase the number of professional nurses for the night shift on the unit. Two months pass with no change in staffing. The nurses decide to meet with hospital administration to voice their concerns.

■ QUESTIONS FOR REFLECTION

1. Can you identify the steps Mary and her colleagues took in their ethical decision-making process?

2. What else could Mary and her colleagues have done to remedy this situation?

Bandman and Bandman (1995, p. 110) discussed the pitfalls—or "fallacies"—that nurses may encounter when using an ethical decision-making process. These errors in reasoning include the following.

1. Arguing that because something (X) is the case, therefore, something else (Y) ought to be the case.
2. Making someone accept the conclusion of another based on force alone (appealing to force).
3. Abusing the person rather than addressing the person's reasons for making a particular decision.
4. Arguing that because everybody does something, that something must be good.
5. Appealing to inappropriate authority to justify a decision.
6. Assuming that if one exception is made to a rule, then uncontrolled events with unwanted circumstances will occur (called the "slippery slope fallacy").
7. Refusing to allow evidence to be shared if it contradicts one's personal position.

Bandman and Bandman (1995) suggested ways to avoid these fallacies by using the following principles for ethical decision making:

1. Valuing and respecting the client's self-determination.
2. Serving the client's well-being in practice in a manner that prevents harm and does good.
3. Treating clients fairly and equally by respecting their rights and treatment options and by making them equal partners in shared health care decisions.

TABLE 3.1 Process for Ethical Decision Making

Steps	Thoughts and Actions
Identify the problem	▪ Analyze the situation to clearly identify the problem ▪ Determine the presence of more than one ethical concern ▪ Look for any conflict of duties with personal or professional values ▪ Determine whether the ethical conflict rightly belongs to you
Identify the morally relevant facts	▪ Examine the complete context of the dilemma (how it occurred, likelihood of arising again) ▪ Identify the key players and their views and vested interest(s) ▪ Identify administrative, political, economic, legal, medical, and aesthetic concerns
Evaluate the ethical problem	▪ Examine the ethical norms by reviewing the literature, code of ethics for nursing, and moral traditions in the profession ▪ Based on this information, identify guides for moral actions that are appropriate for the situation ▪ Consider broader ethical principles, such as justice and autonomy, to provide directions for action ▪ Consider aspects that are unique to the dilemma ▪ Examine the dilemma using each ethical principle ▪ Assign priorities to each of the ethical principles (see Chapter 1) according to professional and personal values
Identify and analyze action alternatives	▪ Determine all possible options for action ▪ Create new options not found elsewhere ▪ Analyze each alternative action for potential harms and benefits ▪ Speculate on the possible outcomes of each action for the key players ▪ Identify which actions will produce subsequent dilemmas ▪ Analyze each alternative according to institutional procedures
Choose and act	▪ Choose a course of action (preferably in consultation with others) ▪ Modify the plan in accordance with legal, institutional, or other values while remaining true to your moral values and norms ▪ Implement the action selected
Evaluate and modify the plan	▪ Identify the result of action taken ▪ Clarify your moral feelings about your actions ▪ Generate modifications to the plan used if you encounter similar situations in the future ▪ Modify the current plan if the ethical dilemma persists

Adapted from Fowler, M. D. M., & Levine-Ariff, J. (Eds.). (1987). *Ethics at the bedside: A source-book for the critical care nurse.* Philadelphia, PA: Lippincott Williams & Wilkins.

Nursing practice, education, and research provide many opportunities for the professional nurse to make ethical decisions and to experience the satisfaction of resolving ethical dilemmas. Situations that generate ethical dilemmas arise from the nurse's efforts to determine what is right. In dealing with each of these ethical issues, the primary responsibility of the nurse in caring for the client is always to respect the person as a unified being. Despite variations in the definition of responsibility in nursing, most nurses would probably agree that the goal for resolving ethical issues is to achieve what is best for clients while attending to the responsibility to self, colleagues, and the profession.

Examples of ethical concerns of nurses include the quality of client care, unfair organizational practices, poor quality work environments, disagreements about end-of-life issues, and conflicts with physicians. When ethical issues arise, nurses may act with power or be powerless. Displays of passivity include silence, "submission, obedience, and powerlessness" (Peter,

Lunardi, & McFarlane, 2004, p. 403). Empowered nurses confront ethical issues directly through the exercise of resistance (e.g., whistle-blowing, refusal to follow physician orders, acts of disobedience, direct confrontation). Failure to abide by one's moral principles has been identified as a reason why nurses leave a job and, in some cases, the profession. Nurses who use resistance to solve ethical dilemmas display great courage because of possible retaliation against them from persons (or the organization) with whom they disagree (Peter et al., 2004).

Achieving Ethical Competence

Achieving ethical competence takes time and practice. **Ethical competence** means that nurses have the knowledge, confidence, and courage to take action to do what is right in an ethically charged situation. In nursing education programs, time is allotted for presentation and discussion of ethical concepts and dilemmas. Consider the situation encountered commonly in practice in emergency departments and how the nurse in the situation possesses a strong knowledge base about escalation of spousal abuse, uses this and a definite value system of keeping patients safe to provide ethically competent care (see Concepts in Practice, "When an Endangered Adult Patient Refuses Help").

Concepts in Practice [IDEA]→[PLAN]→[ACTION]

When an Endangered Adult Patient Refuses Help

A young married woman with injuries consistent with spousal abuse is seen in the emergency department. When the nurse informs the patient that by law the nurses need to contact the local law enforcement agency, the patient pleads with the nurse to keep the suspicious nature of the injuries secret. However, the nurse reports the injuries to the legal authorities who confirm that the injuries are the result of being abused. The woman refuses to file charges, speaks with a social worker who arranges legal aid for divorce assistance, and insists upon returning home with her husband. Knowing that the incidence of spousal homicides greatly increases when a spouse plans to dissolve a marriage, the nurse provides the woman with this information and urges her to go to a shelter for battered women instead of home. What factors should be considered prior to letting this woman return home?

Key concepts related to nursing ethics include understanding basic theoretical approaches to ethics such as principalism, utilitarianism, and deontology. In addition, nurses need to understand the key ethical principles outlined in Table 3.2. Without basic knowledge of ethical principles, nurses may be unaware of ethical dilemmas and how to handle them when they occur.

Before nurses can address ethical dilemmas, they need to have confidence in their nursing knowledge and clinical decision-making skills. They also need to have refined communication skills to collect information about the events and to share professional nursing ideas to manage the ethically charged situation. As nurses gain experience in handling ethical issues, their confidence in their ability to manage them increases. Confident nurses have the courage to tackle ethical issues as they arise in clinical practice.

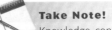

Take Note!
Knowledge, confidence, and courage are the foundations of ethical competence.

MAJOR CONTEXTUAL ELEMENTS AFFECTING NURSING PRACTICE

To understand the moral or ethical dimension of nursing more fully, the nurse needs to understand the contextual elements of nursing practice that either reinforce or challenge belief and value systems. As noted at the outset of this chapter, contextualism refers to the constellation of all factors that impact the current situation. In contextualism, the nurse analyzes a whole situation, including background, environmental and personality factors, and relationships. Box 3.5, Professional Building Blocks, "Five Major Contextual Elements Affecting Professional Nursing Practice," presents selected demographic, economic, cultural, environmental, and ethical factors that characterize the contexts of nursing practice. Public policy, another significant contextual element, is discussed in Chapter 19, "The Professional Nurse's Role in Public Policy."

The following discussion offers a general overview of the factors most influential to professional nursing practice.

Demographics

Americans are growing older and living longer. By 2030, approximately 87.3 million Americans will be 65 years of age or older (Ortman, Velkoff, & Hogan, 2014); the life expectancy for American men and women will be 79.9 and 81.9 years, respectively (Robert Wood Johnson Foundation, 2011). By 2030, the percentage of elderly will also increase in Europe, Asia, and Latin America. The elderly use more health care resources and have different care needs than younger people. Nurses need to consider the specific needs of the elderly when providing care to this population.

The increased elderly population may strain current health care resources because this age group is at increased risk for chronic illness. Persons older than 65 have higher rates of hospital admittance and may have greater need for assistance with activities of daily living. Many people over age 65 have a chronic illness, more than half of which involve some mobility limitations, and 32% with problems performing complex activities. (National Center Health Statistics, 2014). Harrington (2012) notes that over 13 million Americans need

TABLE 3.2 Key Ethical Principles

Principle	Definition	Examples
Nonmaleficence	To do no harm to others	*Due diligence:* Exercise care in a situation so that one does not harm another *Example:* Carefully checking medications before administering them *Double effect:* The outcomes outweigh the potential harm *Example:* Administration of chemotherapy (adverse effects) to kill cancer cells
Beneficence	To do only good for others	*Compassion:* Caring with a desire to help others *Example:* Attending to the psychological needs of a person who has a new colostomy *Veracity:* Being honest and telling the truth *Example:* Informing clients about all options for the treatment of a health condition *Fidelity:* Being faithful in relationships and in matters of trust *Example:* Maintaining the confidentiality of personal health information and disclosing information when obtaining informed consent *Proportionality:* Choosing the option that produces more good than harm *Example:* Determining the best treatment options for clients
Autonomy	The right of people to make free and informed choices	*Privacy:* Respecting another's personal space and business *Example:* Asking for permission prior to touching a client *Confidentiality:* Keeping personal information about clients secret *Example:* Not holding an end-of-shift report within earshot of visitors and other clients *Advocacy:* Hearing and respecting client wishes, needs, and values *Example:* Abiding by a terminally ill client's desires not to be connected to life support *Informed consent:* Ensuring that clients receive all pertinent information surrounding a prescribed treatment so they can make the best possible decision *Example:* Explaining all potential hazards of a surgical procedure
Justice	Fairness and impartiality to provide equality of service according to individual needs and contributions	*Respect:* Preserving or maintaining personal dignity and rights *Example:* Providing equal services for all clients despite their ethnicity or culture *Allocation of resources:* Fairly distributing limited services based on need rather than ability to pay *Example:* Using complex life-saving technology on persons with the potential for survival

Agnes, M. (Ed.). (2005). *Webster's new world college dictionary* (4th ed.). Cleveland, OH: Wiley; Bosek, M., & Savage, T. (2007). *The ethical component of nursing education, integrating ethics into clinical experience.* Philadelphia, PA: Lippincott Williams & Wilkins; Beauchamp, T., & Childress, J. (2013). *Principles of biomedical ethics* (7th ed.). New York: Oxford University Press; and Fowler, M. D. M. (2015). *Guide to the code of ethics for nurses with interpretive statements* (2nd ed.). Silver Springs, MD: American Nurses Association.

3.5 Professional Building Blocks

Five Major Contextual Elements Affecting Professional Nursing Practice

- **Demographic elements** reflect social and economic conditions. The demographics of a population influence the opportunities an individual has to form or maintain cooperative and interdependent relationships with fellow humans.
- **Economic elements** focus primarily on the considerations of costs and return for provided services. In cultures in which health services are viewed as commodities, providers must be reimbursed for their services. However, when societies view health care as a basic right, governments usually provide a national health insurance plan for all citizens.
- **Cultural elements** provide organization and structure for groups of people. Within a culture, people share common values, beliefs, norms, and practices (Giger & Davidhizar, 1999). Culture plays a key role in the development of human behavior patterns. Sometimes cultural beliefs clash with science-based health care practices.
- **Environmental elements** consist of global health influences. Along with safe food sources, humans require clean air and water for survival. Kleffel (1996) presents an ecocentric view of the world by describing that "the environment is considered to be whole, living, and interconnected" (p. 1).
- **Ethical elements** encompass the moral obligations and duties that emerge from an individual's struggle with good and bad, and right and wrong. Ethical nurses act in accordance with approved standards or codes for professional behavior. Nurses confront ethical issues in daily practice. Ethical dilemmas occur when nurses confront situations in which alternatives for action produce unsatisfactory results. Sometimes, what is ethically right can be legally or morally wrong.

assistance with activities of daily living and 92% of these disabled persons rely on family or friends.

The nursing shortage in the United States is a reflection of the worldwide professional nursing shortage. In a February 2016 interview, Pam Cipriano, the president of the American Nurses Association reported that between 2014 and 2016, there will be 1.2 million vacancies for registered nurses that need to be filled. She also specified that an estimated 700,000 registered nurses are expected to retire because many currently working nurses entered the profession in the 1970s. The increased number of the elderly and prevalence of chronic diseases means that there will be an increased demand for registered nurses. The recession that started in 2007 kept many nurses who were expected to retire in the workforce (Grant, 2016).

Perhaps the most important health care need for the American population is for health promotion and disease prevention services. *Healthy People* 2020 is the second decade-long health initiative released by the U.S. Department of Health and Human Services (USDHHS) (2010). *Healthy People* programs measure progress toward strategic health care goals. In addition, the program also sets wellness objectives and targets and examines health progress made in specific populations. *Healthy People* 2020 identified 12 global topic areas to address: "access to health care services; clinical preventive services; environmental quality; injury and violence; maternal, infant, and child health; mental health; nutrition; physical activity and obesity; oral health; reproductive and sexual health; social determinants; and substance abuse and tobacco use" (Office of Disease Prevention and Health Promotion, 2016).

Keeping people healthy reduces long-term health expenditures and increases the quality of life for persons of all ages. Nurses play a key role in imparting health information to clients when they assume client education responsibilities. As the population ages, many middle-aged adults find themselves torn between meeting career obligations, raising teenagers, and caring for aging parents. In the role of counselor, professional nurses can support clients (and their children or spouses) by inquiring about the stresses associated with fulfilling multiple role responsibilities, thus strengthening client mental health.

Culture

The US population is diverse and will continue to become more so (Fig. 3.3). The 2010 census revealed 57 possible multiple racial combinations of American citizens and that 97% of Americans reported that they were of one race. Persons completing census forms sometimes responded positively to more than one category, making data analysis difficult. According to Ortman et al. (2014), the aggregate of all persons identifying themselves as minorities will become the majority of the population in 2043.

The Hispanic population experienced the largest growth among all reported minority groups within the past decade. Texas, California, Hawaii, New Mexico, and the District of Columbia reported minority populations over 50%, with Hawaii having a 77% minority population (Humes, Jones, & Ramirez, 2011). The increasing diversity in the population increases the complexity of providing effective nursing care. Although the heritage profile among nurses is also diverse, it does not mirror the overall population (see Fig. 3.2).

Many immigrant groups tend to settle in a specific community. In such locations, nurses may need to communicate with clients who are not fluent in English. Nurses need to be aware of culturally diverse population clusters and the usual health practices of these groups to provide effective nursing care. Meeting the health care demands of a culturally diverse population means that nurses need to understand the biophysiologic variations related to the risk for specific health problems, development, and medication metabolism, along with specific cultural values, beliefs, and health practices (see Chapter 11, "Multicultural Issues in Professional Practice").

Economics

The economic gap between the wealthy and the poor in the United States continues to expand. Factors associated with increased poverty levels include age, ethnicity, and education. In 2014, the USDHHS reported that 46.7 million Americans, or 14.8% of the population, lived in poverty (26.2% Blacks/African Americans, 23.6% Hispanics, 12.0% Asian Americans, and 10.1% Whites/Caucasians; no data were reported for Hawaiian/Pacific Islanders or Native Americans/Eskimos) (DeNavas-Walt & Proctor, 2015). In 2016, the Assistant Secretary for Planning and Evaluation (ASPE) for the USDHHS set the following poverty guidelines: annual income of $40,890 for a family of eight (an additional $4,160 for each person over 8), $24,300 for a family of four, $20,160 for a family of three, $160200 for two, and $11,880 for one person (ASPE, USDHHS, 2016). Persons living in poverty had a 19.3% rate of not carrying health insurance. In 2014, the uninsured rate for Americans was 10.4% a 1.9% reduction from 2013 (Smith & Medalia, 2015).

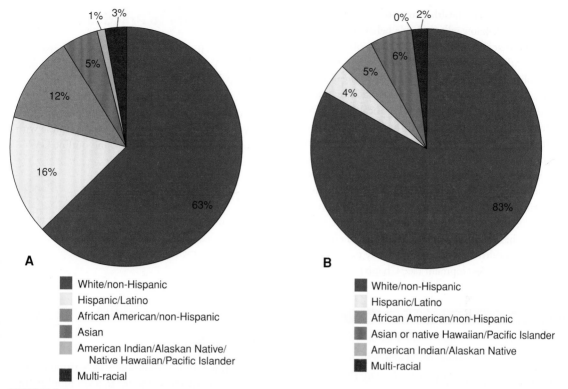

FIGURE 3.3 **A.** Heritage profile of the US population in 2011. (From Humes, K. R., Jones, N. A., & Ramirez, R R. (2011). *Overview of race and hispanic origin: 2010, 2010 census briefs.* Retrieved from www.census.gov/prod/cen2010/briefs/c2010br-2.pdf. Accessed November 9, 2012.) **B.** Heritage profile of US nurses. (From U.S. Department of Health and Human Services, Health Resources and Services Administration. (2010). *The registered nurse population: Findings from the 2008 national sample survey of registered nurses.* Retrieved from http://bhpr.hrsa.gov/healthworkforce/rnsurveys/rnsurveyfinal.pdf. Accessed November 9, 2012.)

Unfortunately, projections for access to health care will be three tiered, with 38% being empowered, 43% being worried, and 28% being excluded (Holahan & Chen, 2011).

- Empowered health care consumers have discretionary income that can be used to cover health care costs. They also tend to be well educated and frequently use technology (especially the internet) as a source for health care information. Empowered consumers often participate in making health-related decisions with physicians and other health care professionals.
- Worried consumers include early retirees and people who are dependent on employer-provided health insurance. As health care expenditures continue to escalate, employers may have to reduce health care benefits or pass on increased costs to employees to afford any form of health insurance coverage.
- Consumers excluded from accessing health care will be the poor, uninsured, unemployed, and uneducated, with the poor and uneducated having the least access.

Health care spending is expected to increase. In 2010, health care expenditures accounted for 7.64% of the gross domestic product (Howden & Meyer, 2011). In 2014, the percent rose to 17.5% (Centers for Medicare and Medicaid Services, 2015), companies providing health care insurance to employees have seen 27% increases in premiums over the past 5 years. Whereas, worker wages have only grown 10% and the inflation rate increased 9% within the same time frame (Kaiser Family Foundation, 2015). Employers have in turn passed the increases on to the employees. When health care insurance premiums become too expensive, employees may opt out of employer-provided insurance plans and instead choose high deductible, less expensive plans. This results in a state of being under-insured, placing these individuals at risk for bankruptcy because of debt incurred for health-related reasons.

The Institute for the Future (2003) identified the following factors that determine personal health status: access to health care (10%), genetics (20%), personal health behaviors (50%), and uncontrollable factors (30%). Uninsured Americans have limited access to health care. Personal health–promoting habits require that individuals know what lifestyle behaviors promote health and that they have the resources to obtain them. Persons without health insurance may use free clinics and public health departments for primary health care services. In these settings, advanced practice nurses frequently assume the role of primary health caregiver. Other clients may prefer a more holistic approach to health care, seeking out nurses rather than physicians for primary care services. As educators, professional nurses can teach clients health-promotion strategies. For clients who do not have the ability to practice these strategies, nurses can refer them to social or governmental agencies that can help (nurse as client advocate). As change agents, nurses can engage in efforts to change the health care system by actively participating in public policy development (see Chapter 19).

REAL-LIFE REFLECTIONS

After reading this chapter, you find yourself talking with Jane. How would you help Jane with her decision making about leaving the profession as a result of shifts in the focus of nursing care? Outline a plan to help Jane make a decision about her future. If she was to decide to leave the profession, how might she best present this to Ben and Sheila, the nursing students getting ready to enter the profession?

Summary and Significance to Practice

Professional nursing centers on caring for others. When delivering care to individuals, groups, and communities, nurses use individual value systems as a basis for some clinical decisions. Many contextual elements affect health care delivery and clinical practice. Sometimes the contextual elements create ethical dilemmas that need to be resolved. Nurses who have examined their beliefs and have developed a personal nursing philosophy have a basis for finding meaning in professional practice. By becoming cognizant of ethical principles and the multiple factors contributing to ethical dilemmas in clinical practice, nurses can readily identify them as they arise. Nurses who have a strong value system and philosophical stance are armed with effective tools to confront ethically charged situations with confidence.

From Theory to Practice

1. What does it mean to be a professional nurse?
2. How do nurses make a difference in the lives of others?
3. Look at your nursing program's philosophy and/or the developmental and organizational philosophies at your place of employment. Compare these with your own personal philosophy, and outline key similarities and differences.

Nurse as Author

Write your own professional nursing philosophy by answering the questions found in Box 3.3 Learning, Knowing, and Growing: Developing a Nursing Philosophy.

Your Digital Classroom

Online Exploration

Visit the International Philosophy of Nursing Society at **http://www.ipons.co.uk/** to learn more about nursing philosophy and philosophical inquiry.

For a sample nursing department vision, mission, and philosophy, visit the University of Mexico hospital website at **http://hospitals.unm.edu/nursing/philosophy.shtml**

For a sample nursing program vision, mission and philosophy, visit the School of Nursing at Ball State University at **http://cms.bsu.edu/academics/collegesanddepartments/nursing/aboutus/missionphilosophy**

For a sample professional nursing organization vision, mission, and philosophy, visit the Philippine Nurses Association of San Diego County, California, at **www.pnasd.org/Philosophy.html**

For another sample professional nursing organization philosophy and mission, visit the Colorado Nurses Association at **http://www.coloradonurses.org/philosophy-and-mission/**

Expanding Your Understanding

1. Search the internet for any college- or university-based nursing program and see if it has the philosophy of its school of nursing posted on the home page.
2. Select a nursing organization that interests you, and visit its website to see whether you can find the organization's values, mission, and philosophy.

Based on a review of available information, outline reasons why you might or might not join the organization.

Beyond the Book

Visit thePoint® **www.thePoint.lww.com** for activities and information to reinforce the concepts and content covered in this chapter.

REFERENCES

Agnes, M. (Ed.). (2005). *Webster's new world college dictionary* (4th ed.). Cleveland, OH: Wiley.

American Association of Colleges of Nursing (AACN). (2008). The essentials of baccalaureate education for professional nursing practice. Retrieved from www.aacn.nche.edu/education-resources/baccessentials08.pdf. Accessed December 29, 2012.

Antonovsky, A. (1987). *Unraveling the mystery of health.* San Francisco, CA: Jossey-Bass.

Aroskar, M. A. (1987). Fidelity and veracity: Questions of promise keeping, truth telling, and loyalty. In M. D. M. Fowler, & J. Levine-Ariff (Eds.), *Ethics at the bedside: A source-book for the critical care nurse.* Philadelphia, PA: Lippincott Williams & Wilkins.

Assistant Secretary for Planning & Evaluation, US Department of Health and Human Services. (2016). *Poverty Guidelines 2016.* Retrieved from https://aspe.hhs.gov/poverty-guidelines. Accessed March 17, 2016.

Bandman, E. L., & Bandman, B. (1995). *Nursing ethics through the lifespan* (3rd ed.). Stamford, CT: Appleton & Lange.

Beauchamp, T., & Childress, J. (2013). *Principles of biomedical ethics* (7th ed.). New York: Oxford University Press.

Benner, P. (1984). *From novice to expert: Excellence and power in clinical nursing practice.* Menlo Park, CA: Addison-Wesley.

Benner, P. (2000). *From novice to expert: Excellence and power in clinical nursing practice* (Commemorative ed.). Menlo Park, CA: Addison-Wesley.

Benner, P., & Wrubel, J. (1989). *The primacy of caring: Stress and coping in health and illness.* Menlo Park, CA: Addison-Wesley.

Boughn, S. (1994). Why do men choose nursing? *Nursing and Health Care, 15,* 406–411.

Boughn, S. (2001). Why women and men choose nursing. *Nursing and Health Perspectives, 22,* 14–19.

Burkhardt, M., & Keegan, L. (2013). Holistic ethics. In B. M. Dossey, & L. Keegan (Eds.), *Holistic nursing: A handbook for practice* (6th ed.). Burlington, MA: Jones & Bartlett Learning.

Carper, B. A. (1978). Fundamental patterns of knowing in nursing. *Advances in Nursing Science, 1,* 13–23.

Centers for Medicare and Medicaid Services. (2015). *National health expenditures highlights: 2014.* Retrieved from https://www.cms.gov/Research-Statistics-Data-and-Systems/Statistics-Trends-and-Reports/NationalHealthExpendData/Downloads/highlights.pdf. Accessed March 17, 2016.

Church, D. (2007). *A vision of the future of medicine, the genie in your genes: Epigenetic medicine and the new biology of intention.* Santa Rosa, CA: Elite Books, Energy Psychology Press.

DeNavas-Walt, C., & Proctor, B. (2015). *Income and Poverty in the United States: 2014,* (2015). U.S. Census Bureau, Current Population Reports, P60–252, U.S. Government Printing Office, Washington, DC. Retrieved from https://www.census.gov/content/dam/Census/library/publications/2015/demo/p60–252.pdf. Accessed March 16, 2016.

Dossey, B., & Keegan, L. (2013). *Holistic nursing: A handbook for practice* (6th ed.). Burlington, MA: Jones & Bartlett Learning.

Earle, W. J. (1992). *Introduction to philosophy.* New York: McGraw-Hill.

Enserink, P. M. (2004). Influenza: Girding for disaster. Looking the pandemic in the eye. *Science, 306,* 392–394.

Ferreira, V., & Sherman, A. (2007). The relationship of optimism, pain and social support to well-being in older adults with osteoarthritis. *Aging and Mental Health, 11*(1), 89–98.

Fitzpatrick, J., & McCarthy, G. (2016). *Nursing concept analysis: Application to research and practice.* New York: Springer Publishing Co. LLC.

Flynn, P. A. R. (1987). Questions of risk, duty, and paternalism: Problems in beneficence. In M. D. M. Fowler, & J. Levine-Ariff (Eds.), *Ethics at the bedside: A source-book for the critical care nurse.* Philadelphia, PA: Lippincott Williams & Wilkins.

Fowler, M. D. M., & Levine-Ariff, J. (Eds.). (1987). *Ethics at the bedside: A source-book for the critical care nurse.* Philadelphia, PA: Lippincott Williams & Wilkins.

Fowler, M. D. M. (2015). *Guide to the Code of Ethics for Nurses with interpretive statements* (2nd ed.). Silver Springs, MD: American Nurses Association.

Frankl, V. (1963). *Man's search for meaning.* New York: Washington Square Press.

Fried, B. J., & Gaydos, L. M. (Eds.). (2002). *World health systems, challenges and perspectives.* Chicago: Health Administration Press.

Giger, J. N., & Davidhizar, R. E. (1999). *Transcultural nursing assessment and intervention* (3rd ed.). St. Louis, MO: Mosby.

Gilligan, C. (1982). *In a different voice: Psychological theory and women's development.* Cambridge, MA: Harvard University Press.

Grant, R. (2016). The U.S. is running out of nurses. The Atlantic Monthly(online). Retrieved from http://www.theatlantic.com/health/archive/2016/02/nursing-shortage/459741/. Accessed March 17, 2016.

Haegert, S. (2004). The ethics of self. *Nursing Ethics, 11,* 434–443.

Harrington, C. (2012). Long-term care policy issues. In S. Mason, J. Leavitt, & M. Chaffee (Eds.), *Policy and politics in nursing and health care* (6th ed.). St. Louis, MO: Elsevier Saunders.

Hatala, A. R. (2008). Spirituality and aboriginal mental health: An examination of the relationship between aboriginal spirituality and mental health. *Advances in Mind-Body Medicine, 23*(1), 6–12 [electronic version].

Hawking, S. (2002). *The theory of everything.* Beverly Hills, CA: New Millennium Press.

Herzlinger, R. (2004). *Consumer-driven health care.* San Francisco, CA: Jossey-Bass.

Holahan, J., & Chen, V. (2011). Changes in health insurance coverage in the great recession, 2007–2010. Retrieved from www.kff.org/uninsured/8264.cfm. Accessed November 9, 2012.

Hountras, S. (2015). What guides your nursing practice? *Journal of Christian Nursing, 32*(3), 179–181. doi: 1:10.1097/CNJ00000000000181.

Howden, L. M., & Meyer, J. A. (2011). Age and sex composition: 2010, 2010 census briefs. Retrieved from www.census.gov/prod/cen2010/briefs/c2010br-03.pdf. Accessed March 14, 2017.

Humes, K. R., Jones, N. A., & Ramirez, R. R. (2011). Overview of race and hispanic origin: 2010, 2010 census briefs. Retrieved from www.census.gov/prod/cen2010/briefs/c2010br-02.pdf. Accessed May 28, 2013.

Institute for the Future. (2003). *Health and health care 2010* (2nd ed.). San Francisco, CA: Jossey-Bass.

Institute of Medicine. (2000). *To err is human: Building a safer health care system.* Washington, DC: National Academies Press.

Institute of Medicine. (2010). *The future of nursing: Leading change, advancing health.* Washington, DC: National Academies Press.

Iwarrsson, S., Horstmann, V., & Slaug, B. (2007). Housing matters in very old age—yet differently due to ADL dependence level differences. *Scandinavian Journal of Occupational Therapy, 14,* 3–15.

Kaiser Family Foundation. (2015). *2015 Employer health benefits survey, summary of findings.* Retrieved from http://kff.org/report-section/ehbs-2015-summary-of-findings/ Accessed March 17, 2016.

Kleffel, D. (1996). Environmental paradigms: Moving toward an ecocentric approach. *Advances in Nursing Science, 18,* 1–10.

Kohlberg, L. (1981). *The philosophy of moral development: Moral stages and the idea of justice.* New York: Harper & Row.

Law, S. (2007). *Eyewitness companions: Philosophy.* New York: DK Publishing.

Lewis, S. (2008a). Helping people live between office visits: An interview with Bernie Siegel, MD. *Advances in Mind-Body Medicine, 23,* 24–27 [electronic version].

Lewis, S. (2008b). The emerging field of spiritual neuroscience: An interview with Mario Beauregard, PhD. *Advances in Mind-Body Medicine, 23,* 20–23 [electronic version].

Marchuk, A. (2014). A personal nursing philosophy in practice. *Journal of Neonatal Nursing, 20,* 266–273. doi: 10.1061/jnn.2014.06.004.

McCarthy, J. (2006). A pluralist view of nursing ethics. *Nursing Philosophy, 7,* 157–164.

Munhall, P. (1988). Ethical considerations in qualitative research. *Western Journal of Nursing Research, 10,* 150–162.

National Center for Health Statistics. (2014). *Health, United States, 2014: With Special Feature on Adults Aged 55–64.* Hyattsville, MD. 2015. Library of Congress Catalog Number 76–641496. Retrieved from http://www.cdc.gov/nchs/data/hus/hus14.pdf#047. Accessed March 16, 2016.

Noddings, N. (1984). *Caring: A feminine approach to ethics and moral education.* Berkeley, CA: University of California Press.

Office of Disease Prevention and Health Promotion. (2016). 2020 LHI topics. Retrieved from https://www.healthypeople.gov/2020/leading-health-indicators/2020-LHI-Topics. Accessed March 17, 2016.

Okrainec, G. D. (1994). Perception of nursing education held by male nursing students. *Western Journal of Nursing Research, 16,* 94–107.

O'Neill, J. (1995). Ethical decision making and the role of nursing. In G. L. Deloughery (Ed.), *Issues and trends in nursing* (2nd ed.). St. Louis, MO: Mosby-Year Book.

Ortman, J., Velkoff, V., & Hogan, H. (2014). *An Aging Nation: The Older Population in the United States, Current Population Reports, P25–1140.* Washington, DC: U.S. Census Bureau 2014.

Retrieved from https://www.census.gov/prod/2014pubs/p25–1140.pdf. Accessed March 15, 2016.

Peter, E., Lunardi, V., & McFarlane, A. (2004). Nursing resistance as ethical action: Literature review. *Journal of Advanced Nursing, 46,* 403–416.

Porter-O'Grady, T., & Malloch, K. (2015). *Quantum leadership: Building better partnerships for sustainable health* (2nd ed.). Burlington, MA: Jones & Bartlett Learning.

Rafael, A. R. (1996). Power and caring: A dialectic in nursing. *Advances in Nursing Science, 19,* 3–17.

Reed, P. (2011). The spiral path to nursing knowledge. In P. Reed, & N. Schearer (Eds.), *Nursing knowledge and theory innovation advancing the science of practice.* New York: Springer Publishing.

Rew, L. (1994). Commentary. In J. F. Kikuchi, & H. Simmons (Eds.), *Developing a philosophy of nursing.* Thousand Oaks, CA: Sage.

Robert Wood Johnson Foundation. (2011). Americans' Life Expectancy Longer Than Government Projections, RWJF Health & Society Scholar Finds. Retrieved from http://www.rwjf.org/en/library/research/2011/09/americans-life-expectancy-longer-than-government-projections-rwj.html. Accessed March 15, 2016.

Ross, A., Wenzel, F., & Mitlyng, J. (2002). *Leadership for the future: Core competencies in healthcare.* Chicago: Health Administration Press.

Sabatino, L., Stievano, A., Rocco, G., Kallio, H., Pietaila, A.-M., & Kangasniemi, M. (2014). The dignity of the nursing profession: a meta-synthesis of qualitative research. *Nursing Ethics, 21*(6), 659–672.

Salsberry, P. J. (1994). A philosophy of nursing: What is it? What is it not? In J. F. Kikuchi, & H. Simmons (Eds.), *Developing a philosophy of nursing.* Thousand Oaks, CA: Sage.

Smith, J., & Medalia, C. (2015). *Health Insurance Coverage in the United States: 2014,* U.S. Census Bureau, Current Population Reports, P60–253. Washington, DC: U.S. Government Printing Office 2015. Retrieved from http://www.census.gov/content/dam/Census/library/publications/2015/demo/p60–253.pdf. Accessed March 17, 2016.

Streubert, H. (1994). Male nursing students' perceptions of clinical experience. *Nurse Educator, 19,* 28–32.

Sulmasy, D. (2008). Dignity and bioethics: History, theory and selected applications. In *Human dignity and bioethics, essays commissioned by the President's Council on Bioethics* (pp. 469–504). Washington, DC: US Government Printing Office. Retrieved from https://repository.library.georgetown.edu/bitstream/handle/10822/559351/human_dignity_and_bioethics.pdf?sequence=1&isAllowed=y. Accessed March 16, 2016.

United Nations Development Programme (UNDP). (2015a). *UN Sustainable Development Goals.* Retrieved from http://www.undp.org/content/undp/en/home/sdgoverview/post-2015-development-agenda.html. Accessed March 15, 2016.

UNDP. (2015b). *Goal 1: No poverty.* Retrieved from http://www.undp.org/content/undp/en/home/sdgoverview/post-2015-development-agenda/goal-1/. Accessed March 15, 2016.

UNDP. (2015c). *Goal 2: Zero hunger.* Retrieved from http://www.undp.org/content/undp/en/home/sdgoverview/post-2015-development-agenda/goal-2.html. Accessed March 15, 2016.

UNDP. (2015d). Retrieved from http://www.undp.org/content/undp/en/home/sdgoverview/post-2015-development-agenda/goal-3.html. Accessed March 15, 2016.

UNDP. (2015e). *Goal 4: Quality education.* Retrieved from http://www.undp.org/content/undp/en/home/sdgoverview/post-2015-development-agenda/goal-4.html. Accessed March 15, 2016.

UNDP. (2015f). *Goal 5: Gender equality.* Retrieved from http://www.undp.org/content/undp/en/home/sdgoverview/post-2015-development-agenda/goal-5.html. Accessed March 15, 2016.

UNDP. (2015g). *Goal 6: Clean water and sanitation.* Retrieved from http://www.undp.org/content/undp/en/home/sdgoverview/post-2015-development-agenda/goal-6.html. Accessed March 15, 2016.

UNDP. (2015h). *Goal 7: Affordable and clean energy.* Retrieved from http://www.undp.org/content/undp/en/home/sdgoverview/post-2015-development-agenda/goal-7.html. Accessed March 15, 2016.

UNDP. (2015i). *Goal 8: Decent work and economic growth.* Retrieved from http://www.undp.org/content/undp/en/home/sdgoverview/post-2015-development-agenda/goal-8.html. Accessed March 15, 2016.

UNDP. (2015j). *Goal 9: Industry, innovation and infrastructure.* Retrieved from http://www.undp.org/content/undp/en/home/sdgoverview/post-2015-development-agenda/goal-9.html. Accessed March 15, 2016.

UNDP. (2015k). *Goal 10: Reduced inequalities.* Retrieved from http://www.undp.org/content/undp/en/home/sdgoverview/post-2015-development-agenda/goal-10.html. Accessed March 15, 2016.

UNDP. (2015l). *Goal 11: Sustainable cities and communities.* Retrieved from http://www.undp.org/content/undp/en/home/sdgoverview/post-2015-development-agenda/goal-11.html. Accessed March 15, 2016.

UNDP. (2015m). *Goal 12: Responsible consumption and production.* Retrieved from http://www.undp.org/content/undp/en/home/sdgoverview/post-2015-development-agenda/goal-12.html. Accessed March 15, 2016.

UNDP. (2015n). *Goal 13: Climate action.* Retrieved from http://www.undp.org/content/undp/en/home/sdgoverview/post-2015-development-agenda/goal-13.html. Accessed March 15, 2016.

UNDP. (2015o). *Goal 14: Life below water.* Retrieved from http://www.undp.org/content/undp/en/home/sdgoverview/post-2015-development-agenda/goal-14.html. Accessed March 15, 2016.

UNDP. (2015p). *Goal 15: Life on land.* Retrieved from http://www.undp.org/content/undp/en/home/sdgoverview/post-2015-development-agenda/goal-15.html. Accessed March 15, 2016.

UNDP. (2015q). *Goal 16: Peace and justice, strong institutions.* Retrieved from http://www.undp.org/content/undp/en/home/sdgoverview/post-2015-development-agenda/goal-16.html. Accessed March 15, 2016.

UNDP. (2015r). *Goal 17: Partnerships for the goals.* Retrieved from http://www.undp.org/content/undp/en/home/sdgoverview/post-2015-development-agenda/goal-17.html. Accessed March 15, 2016.

U.S. Department of Health and Human Services. (2010). Healthy people 2020 [brochure]. Retrieved from www.healthypeople.gov/2020/topicsobjectives2020/pdfs/hp2020_brochure.pdf. Accessed November 9, 2012.

Walker, L. O., & Avant, K. C. (2011). *Strategies for theory construction in nursing* (5th ed.). Upper Saddle River, NJ: Prentice-Hall.

Watson, J. (1988). A case study: Curriculum in transition. In *National League for Nursing. Curriculum revolution: Mandate for change.* New York: Author.

Watson, J. (1999). *Postmodern nursing and beyond.* London: Harcourt Brace.

Watson, J. (2005). *Caring science as sacred science.* Philadelphia, PA: FA Davis.

Watson, J. (2012). *Human caring science, a theory of nursing* (2nd ed.). Sudbury, MA: Jones & Bartlett.

WHO. (2012). Millennium development goals fact sheet. Retrieved from http://www.who.int/mediacentre/factsheets/fs290/en/. Accessed May 24, 2013.

WHO (2016a). *World Health Statistics 2016, Monitoring health for the SDGs.* Retrieved from http://www.who.int/gho/publications/world_health_statistics/2016/en/ Accessed March 14, 2017.

WHO. (2016b). WHO statement on the 2nd meeting of IHR Emergency Committee on Zika virus and observed increase in neurological disorders and neonatal malformations. Retrieved from http://www.who.int/mediacentre/news/statements/2016/2nd-emergency-committee-zika/en/. Accessed March 15, 2016.

4

Establishing Helping and Healing Relationships

KEY TERMS AND CONCEPTS

Helping relationships
Professional boundaries
Communication
Metacommunication
Verbal communication
Nonverbal communication
Interpretation
Perception
Collaborative
  relationships
Principles of
  communication
Presence
Empathy
Respect

Genuineness
Stages of the nurse–
  client relationship
Mutuality
Anxiety
Caring interaction
Therapeutic
  communication
Noncaring
  communication
Healing relationship
Professional
  partnership
Crucial conversation
TeamSTEPPS

LEARNING OUTCOMES

By the end of this chapter, the learner will be able to:

1. Compare and contrast helping and healing relationships.
2. Specify the importance of communication in professional nursing.
3. Outline the major purposes of communication.
4. Discuss principles to establish helpfulness in nurse–client communication.
5. Outline the stages of nurse–client relationship development.
6. Identify the mutuality in helping relationships.
7. Differentiate therapeutic from nontherapeutic communication strategies and relationships.
8. Discuss how nurses use relationships to promote client healing.
9. Explain how health care team members can develop meaningful professional partnerships.
10. Describe strategies that health care team members can use to enhance quality and safety when delivering health care.

REAL-LIFE REFLECTIONS

Marcia, an emergency department nurse, has just arrived at work and is assigned to be the triage nurse. A Latino middle-aged man with severe chest pain and dyspnea arrives with his family. Marcia gets immediate help for the man, who is rushed to the cardiac catheterization lab. Marcia notices that the family members seem very anxious and distressed. When she asks them if they would like anything, they reply, "No," but the wife tries to hold back tears as she wrings her hands, the daughter's hands shake, and the son paces. Marcia notes that the nonverbal behavior of the family seems to be incongruent with their verbal messages. As she interacts with the family, Marcia wonders what would be the best course of action to help this distressed family.

Most nurses enter the profession with a desire to help others, and they do so in many ways.

- Assisting clients in meeting basic physical, psychological, and spiritual needs
- Alleviating pain and suffering
- Imparting health care information
- Doing things for clients that they are incapable of doing for themselves
- Guiding clients and families through the complex health care delivery system
- Advocating for clients
- Helping clients achieve maximal health potentials
- Keeping clients safe
- Using clinical, cognitive, and communication skills to deliver high-quality health care services

Along with helping clients, families, and communities, professional nurses also help each other and other team members. **Communication**—the sharing of information, thoughts, and feelings—is an essential element of helping others. The verbal and nonverbal messages exchanged during human relationships determine the structure and function of interpersonal relationships. This chapter focuses on communication as a key factor for effective nursing practice and an essential element of helping relationships.

COMMUNICATION AS INTERACTION

Nurses establish relationships with clients, each other, and members of the health care team. To participate effectively in all these relationships, nurses must understand the structure and the functions of communication.

The Interpersonal Component of Professional Nursing

In striving to maximize the client's potential for optimal health, nurses must clearly understand the power of communication in shaping professional relationships. Without well-refined communication skills, nurses cannot establish therapeutic relationships with clients. **Helping relationships** are those in which nurses communicate with clients to assist them in attaining optimal health or to support them through difficult situations. The quality of communication between the nurse and the client is an essential determinant of the success of the helping relationship (Fig. 4.1).

Take Note!

Communication is an essential element of helping others. Mutual goals cannot be defined or achieved without effective communication.

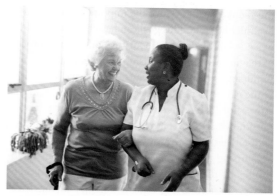

FIGURE 4.1 Careful use of humor enhances the nurse–client relationship.

People are influenced by and in turn influence those whom they encounter. This reciprocal process suggests that the most important human attributes are not only openness to interpersonal experiences but also power to influence self and others. Nurses may be perceived as having power over the persons whom they serve because of their specialized knowledge of and skills in health care. In order to maintain a therapeutic relationship, there needs to be professional boundaries. **Professional boundaries** are imaginary lines that separate the nurse from the patient that occur to maintain the integrity of the therapeutic relationship. Patients possess vulnerability when receiving professional nursing services. Boundary crossings are brief incursions across the invisible barriers. They occur when the nurses use patients for personal gain or when there is confusion about the nature of the special therapeutic relationship either on the nurse's or patient's part. Some examples of boundary crossing are overinvolvement, excessive personal disclosure on the nurse's part, secretive behavior, providing "special treatment" to a single patient, flirtatious actions, and even sexual misconduct. Nurses must be alert to warning signs of potential and actual boundary violations. Careless use of social media increases the likelihood of boundary encroachment. When nurses engage in self-reflection to evaluate patient interactions, they might become more self-aware of the effectiveness of their communication to optimize the nurse–patient relationship (National Council of State Boards of Nursing, 2014).

Humans influence one another primarily through communication, which is defined as the "exchange of meanings between and among individuals through a shared system of symbols that have the same meaning for both the sender and the receiver of the message" (Vestal, 1995, p. 51). Through communication during nurse–client interactions, the nurse hopes to enable the client to acknowledge the importance of and live a healthier lifestyle. This goal can be achieved only if the nurse is knowledgeable about the content and process of the nurse–client relationship. To understand content in nursing situations, the nurse must have knowledge of the person as a complex adaptive human system that strives for "a higher degree of harmony that fosters self-knowledge, self-reverence, self-caring, self-control, and self-healing processes" (Watson, 2012, p. 61).

Nursing has not always been successful in establishing its desired image of autonomy, cohesiveness, and profession. Disagreement among nursing theorists, practitioners, and educators about the purpose and meaning of nursing and key concepts such as nursing diagnosis has led to multiple, and sometimes conflicting, images of nursing. Nurses today generally agree that contemporary nursing practice addresses the client holistically to address the full range of human responses and illness. Nurses also agree that assessment of objective and subjective factors related to client health is essential. They concur that scientific, intuitive, experiential, or mystical evidence may be used to guide practice. However, most nurses in practice acknowledge that establishing authentic, caring relationships with clients is essential to promote health and healing.

Nursing's unique service to society consists of dealing with human responses in health and illness. These responses are the substance of communication. Thus, purposeful communication is an essential dimension in the establishment of effective nurse–client relationships, which should be "characterized by compassion, continuity, and respect for the client's choice. The focus is on the process: the process of the client–environment interaction and the process of the nurse–client relationship" (Newman, Lamb, & Michaels, 1991, p. 406).

The Structure of Communication

Not only does human communication convey information and influence others, but "communication is the relationship" (Sundeen, Stuart, Rankin, & Cohen, 1998, p. 94). It is the dynamic interaction between two or more persons in which ideas, goals, beliefs and values, feelings, and feelings about feelings are exchanged. Even very brief communication exchanges may change all involved parties.

Communication is defined only in the context of process. Holistic communication is "a free flow of verbal and nonverbal interchange between and among people and significant beings such as pets, nature, and God/Life Force/Absolute/Transcendent, that explores

meaning and ideas leading to mutual understanding and growth" (Mariano, 2016, p. 54). Each person is always affected by others and is always affecting others. As one constantly communicates, changes occur in the self, others, and perhaps, the environment.

Although communication is a dynamic process, it is possible to identify components and to analyze the interrelationships among the components. Berlo (1960) traced the various models of communication from the time of Aristotle (circa 350 BCE) to the 1960s. Aristotle identified the related components as the speaker, the speech, and the audience. After analyzing behavioral science research and several points of view, Berlo (1960, pp. 30–32) postulated a communication model that is generally accepted today.

1. **A (interpersonal) source:** Some person(s) with ideas, needs, intentions, information, and a reason for communicating.
2. **A message:** A coded, systematic set of symbols representing ideas, purposes intentions, and feelings.
3. **An encoder:** The mechanism for expressing or translating the purpose of the communication into the message (in people, these are the motor mechanisms—the vocal mechanism for oral messages, the muscles of the hands for written messages, and the muscle systems elsewhere in the body for gestures).
4. **A channel:** The medium for carrying the message.
5. **A decoder:** The mechanism for translating the message into a form that the recipient can use (in people, the sensory receptor mechanisms).
6. **A receiver:** The target or recipient of the message.

In this model, the transmission of meaning occurs via a dynamic transactional process in which:

1. A person has an intention or purpose (the communication source).
2. The purpose is translated into a communicable form by the person's set of motor mechanisms and skills (encoder).
3. The message is transmitted through a channel.
4. The message is translated into receivable form by the recipient's sensory mechanisms and skills (decoder).
5. The recipient receives the message (the communication receiver).

Since Berlo's model was postulated, systems theorists have further explained the reciprocal relationship between participants in the communication process. At any time, the individual person is both an active initiator and a recipient of meanings in an interpersonal situation. Thus, it is important for nurses to understand that they are simultaneously acting and reacting when working with clients and that clients' meanings have an equal effect on the outcome of purposeful relationships.

The dynamic nature of the communication process requires nurses to evaluate their actions and reactions when working with clients. Without such awareness and evaluation, the professional will be less likely to experience the feeling of satisfaction associated with transmitting clear meanings and the validation that the message intended was the message received.

Take Note!
Validation of meanings is essential to achieving any therapeutic goals in helping relationships.

Functions and Types of Communication

Synthesizing from several communication models, Ceccio and Ceccio (1982) proposed four major purposes of communication: to inquire, to inform, to persuade, and to entertain. The nurse may attempt to achieve any of these purposes with clients, the health care delivery system, peers, other health care team members, and even him- or herself. In attempts to achieve one or more of these purposes, the nurse transmits messages.

Messages may be transmitted verbally and nonverbally. Implicit in all models of communication is the concept that communication has two interacting components: the content value of the message and the interactional or perceptual value of the message and its participants. The content value of the message, or its informational aspect, is expressed in verbal or nonverbal forms. The interactional or perceptual value of the message (referred to as **metacommunication**) identifies how participants interpret content and how they perceive the interpersonal relationship. Metacommunication may be expressed in verbal and nonverbal forms.

Verbal Communication

Verbal communication consists of the spoken word and requires functional, physiologic, and cognitive mechanisms that produce, recognize, and receive speech. Although a major influence, specific words are not the *greatest* influences on communication. Language comprises an elaborate system of symbols. Words symbolize actual objects or concepts. Lack of congruence in language between the nurse and the client usually interferes with initiating relationships and creates obstacles to validation of meanings—the essential characteristic of an effective message.

4.1 Professional Building Blocks

Potential Problems in Communication

Nurses need to be aware of three possible types of problems associated with words being symbols of communication (Ceccio & Ceccio, 1982).

1. **The technical problem:** How accurately can one transmit the symbols of communication?
2. **The semantic problem:** How precise are the symbols in transmitting the intended message?
3. **The influential problem:** How effectively does the received meaning affect conduct?

Two primary influences on verbal communications are developmental age and cultural heritage. Developmental age affects verbal ability (the person's physiologic ability to change sounds into words) and cognitive ability (to symbolize through language) (see Box 4.1, Professional Building Blocks, "Potential Problems in Communication"). Through the process of acculturation, an individual develops culture-based variations from others in defining meanings for words. Although denotative (i.e., explicit) definitions of words are the same among different persons, connotative (i.e., associated) meanings often vary because of cultural difference, acculturation, and past experiences.

The verbal content of communication generates the content theme during the communication process. If one evaluates the seemingly varied topics of discussion, the words that underlie or link together several ideas will reflect the "what" (or content) of the communication.

Nonverbal Communication

Nonverbal communication usually exerts more influence on communication than verbal communication. Hunsaker and Alessandra (1980) suggested that 90% of meaning comes from nonverbal communication. **Nonverbal communication** consists of all forms of communication that do not involve the spoken or written word. Perception of nonverbal communication involves all the senses, including hearing, that are used for the perception of verbal communication. Kinesics (facial expressions, gaze, gestures, and all body movements that are not specific signs), objects (all intentional and unintentional display of material things), and proxemics (the use of space) are powerful nonverbal messages perceived by the senses (Hosley & Molle, 2006; Northouse & Northouse, 1998).

Take Note!
Nonverbal communication usually exerts more influence on communication than verbal communication.

Sundeen, Stuart, Rankin, and Cohen (1994, p. 99) identified several purposes of nonverbal communication: expressing emotion and interpersonal attitudes; establishing, developing, and maintaining social relationships; presenting the self; engaging in rituals; and supporting verbal communication.

The tactile senses represent the most primitive sensory process developed by humans. Bonding between the infant and the parent figure (important to infant development) occurs largely through nonverbal tactile communication. As a child develops into an adult, touch as nonverbal communication takes on specific cultural and personal meanings, and remains a powerful communication tool throughout life.

Nurses must understand taboos concerning touch and distance to engage in purposeful communication. For example, a touch on the knee might mean concern to one person but seduction to another. Touch can be a powerful nonverbal tool for the nurse but only when it is used at the proper time and within the context of the client's culture (see Box 4.2, Professional Building Blocks, "Culture and Nonverbal Communication").

All the sensory processes become powerful components of communication throughout life. For example, the olfactory (smell) and gustatory (taste) senses make it possible for people to distinguish pleasant from unpleasant odors and tastes, respectively. Therefore, nurses need to control odors in health care environments.

The sense of hearing the spoken word also has a nonverbal component: interpreting the qualities of the voice. Hunsaker and Alessandra (1980) identified the following voice qualities as strong determinants of effective communication: resonance (the intensity with which the voice fills the environmental space), rhythm (the flow, pace, and movement of the voice), speed (how fast the voice is used), pitch (the highness or lowness of the voice that relates to the tightening of the vocal cords), volume (or loudness), inflection (the change in pitch or volume of voice), and clarity (the articulation and enunciation capacity of the voice).

During communication, people perform various movements of which they may be unaware or have little awareness. Body movements are largely determined through socialization. Developed in a particular psychosocial and cultural setting, motor actions vary according to gender, socioeconomic status, age, and ethnic background. Misinterpretations of culturally

4.2 Professional Building Blocks

Culture and Nonverbal Communication

Culture affects all aspects of nonverbal communication (Hosley & Molle, 2006; Leininger & McFarland, 2006). For example,

- **Proximity/spacing:** People from various cultures define appropriate personal space differently. For example, Americans prefer more personal space (6 in to 4 ft) than Latin Americans. Nurses must acknowledge and respect client preferences for personal space to facilitate effective communication.
- **Touching:** Any physical contact or touching that is part of an individual's communication style can create problems or discomfort for people from many cultures. Nurses need not abandon hands on a shoulder or arm to show support and caring. Rather, clients should feel empowered to tell the nurse if such touching makes them feel uncomfortable.
- **Gestures:** People from some cultures may be more animated than others, using gestures and body language to communicate. Gestures that have a positive meaning in one culture may be considered insulting and rude in another.
- **Eye contact:** Traditionally, Americans have valued direct eye contact as a sign of confidence and respect, whereas not making eye contact has negative connotations. However, in many cultures, making eye contact with an authority Figure is considered an insult.
- **Silence:** People from some cultures prefer active verbal interaction and are uncomfortable with silence. Other cultures may value periods of contemplative silence. Cultural characterizations of the meaning of silence may lead to potential misunderstandings of communication style and motivation.
- **Body language:** The body is one of the more subtle ways people communicate meaning and sincerity. For example, a nurse may say all the right things but communicate tension through his or her body language.

variable kinesthetic behaviors produce barriers to effective communication. For example, eye motions involved with eye contact communicate culturally specific messages. If the nurse and the client assign different meanings to this nonverbal communication, the effectiveness of the nurse–client relationship may be hampered.

Kinesics, the meaning of motor actions, and proxemics, the function of space in nonverbal communication, also play important roles in all aspects of life.

Space is a constant that may be perceived either as surrounding people or existing between them. The nurse can use his or her awareness of what a client perceives as acceptable use of space and how body position and direction affect the meaning of the relationship to create optimal personal and environmental space to enhance nurse–client relationships.

Metacommunication

Occurring on both verbal and nonverbal levels, metacommunication defines the "what," the "who," and the relationship between the "what" and the "who" in the communication process. Because metacommunication is influential in determining the effectiveness of relationships, the nurse must evaluate communication in terms of its context and the relationships among its parts. Understanding themes of the relationship helps the nurse evaluate the metacommunication occurring in the nurse–client interaction.

Three interacting themes occur during metacommunication. The content encompasses the central idea or multiple ideas linked together, that is, the main message being conveyed (the what). The mood theme includes the emotions being communicated during the interaction (the who and how). Finally, the interaction theme involves the dynamics between the participants who are communicating with each other. Metacommunication occurs at all levels of the human experience.

Knowing that change occurs more readily and more effectively if congruence exists between the verbal and nonverbal components of communication, the nurse must be alert to indicators of the degree of agreement on the meaning of the content and on the process of the relationship. When a discrepancy arises between the verbal and nonverbal components, the nonverbal component usually is the more accurate indicator. However, nonverbal behavior is more open to subjective meaning and variations; thus, it must be verbally validated. This validation process plays an important part in effectively using metacommunication in nursing practice.

Take Note!
Communication has both verbal and nonverbal components. When these are not in congruence, the nonverbal components typically dominate the communication.

Interpretation and Perception

The capacity for interpretation makes communication between people possible. When engaged in interpretation, people assign meaning to the interpersonal interaction. Interpretation involves perception, symbolization, memory, and thinking. Perhaps, the most important of these is perception, the basic component from which the others follow. Taylor (1977) described **perception** as the selection and organization of sensations so that they are meaningful. Taylor proposed that humans learn perceptions and that what they learn depends on their socialization experiences. Perceptual expectations are influenced by emotions, language, and attitude and vary widely from one individual to another. Thus, a person's interpretation ability highly depends on his or her individual perceptual ability.

Several factors affect perception in the nurse–client relationship: the capacity for attention (reception of sensations) by the nurse and the client, the perspective each brings to the relationship, and the physical condition of the receptors. Anxiety (the tension state resulting from the actual or anticipated negative appraisal of the significant other in the communication process) in the nurse or the client limits the ability to be attentive in the communication process, interferes with the validation of individual perspectives, and decreases physical capacities. Therefore, anxiety must be controlled in the nurse–client relationship. Validated perceptions between the nurse and the client are essential to goal setting and achievement. The nurse must constantly be aware of the power and influence of perception on the outcomes of a communication, regardless of its form.

Self-Concept and Interpersonal Relationships

The relationships among participants greatly affect communication. The self-concept of each participant largely determines the nurse–client relationship. When nurses and clients have healthy self-concepts, both parties respect each other. Nurses and clients recognize and value the contributions made by each person, thereby setting the stage for true collaboration, mutual goal setting, individualization of nursing interventions, and recognition of the effectiveness of the interpersonal relationship. Clients receiving care from a nurse who has low self-esteem will question the nurse's competence and actions more frequently, whereas clients receiving care from a confident, self-assured nurse will feel more comfortable.

According to Brill (1990, p. 7), "In dealing with people it is essential that workers possess awareness of themselves, their own needs, the ways in which they satisfy these needs, (and) the ways in which they use themselves in relationship with others." In addition to self-awareness, other factors involved in the self-concept are essential to effective communication, including the ability to:

- Share ideas, thoughts, and feelings with individuals (a function of achievement of interpersonal developmental tasks).
- Establish, maintain, and terminate the kind of relationship in which one is comfortable (a function of the human need to perpetuate a personal self-concept).
- Share power (a reflection of the person's view of self and others).

If the major reason for nurses' communication with clients is to influence clients toward better health, nurses must develop concepts of self that are most effective in facilitating the client's growth potential. These concepts include an awareness of one's perceptions of and feelings about the self, the ability to derive satisfaction by sharing with the client the responsibility for the nurse–client relationship, the ability to view the self as a therapeutic tool, and an appreciation for shared power in activities directed toward change.

■ QUESTIONS FOR REFLECTION

1. How do you come across as a professional nurse? (You may have to ask a colleague for the answer to this one; it may surprise you.)
2. Why is it important to know how others perceive you as a professional nurse?
3. What happens to informal communication when the nonverbal behavior is incongruent with what is being said?
4. What occurs when nonverbal behavior contradicts what is being said?
5. Think of the last time that you got angry with or lost patience with a significant other. What happened during the interaction? What verbal and nonverbal behavior cues resulted in anger or lack of patience?

REAL-LIFE REFLECTIONS

Remember Marcia, from the beginning of the chapter? What should she do when the non-verbal behavior of her client's family does not match their verbal message? Why is it important for her to act when she sees this incongruence? How does culture play a role in communication? What aspects of the client's culture might affect the family's reaction to her outreach?

Principles of Communication in Collaborative Relationships

When engaged in communication with clients, nurses empathize with, demonstrate respect for, and respond genuinely to them. When nurses and clients equally share the responsibility and authority for care, they enter into collaborative relationships. During nursing assessments, **collaborative relationships** promote client sharing of all key information and involve nurse verification of interpretations and conclusions based on assessment data. The nurse and the client work together to identify and prioritize nursing diagnoses and determine a plan of care for implementation. They also decide collaboratively how to execute the plan of care. Finally, the client and the nurse evaluate the effectiveness of the care plan and, if it is deemed unsuccessful, explore and propose alternative courses of action. If the plan is successful, the nurse and the client work together to develop another care plan to address a different health concern. Presence, empathy, respect, and genuineness are the **principles of communication** that facilitate successful collaboration.

Presence

Presence is an important part of several nursing conceptual models, including those of Parse (1996), Paterson and Zderad (1988), and Watson (1996, 2012). "The core element in **presence** is 'being there….' It is described as a gift of self and is equated with a use of self that is conveyed through open and giving behaviors of the nurse" (Osterman & Schwartz-Barcott, 1996, p. 24). Table 4.1 describes the characteristics of four ways of "being there." These "reflect degrees of intensity in the context of another" (Osterman & Schwartz-Barcott, 1996, p. 29).

By synthesizing these theoretical conceptions of presence, the nurse focuses all of his or her energy on the client during interactions. The nurse can be present without speaking. Clients and nurses engaged in true presence during an encounter describe an experience that cannot be captured with words and results in a deep, personal connection for both participants with possible resultant personal transformations.

 Take Note!
Presence is integrally related to genuineness and a necessary antecedent to empathy.

■ QUESTIONS FOR REFLECTION

1. Why is it important to be truly present with clients?

TABLE 4.1 Presence: Characteristics of Four Ways of "Being There"

Characteristics of Presence	Presence	Partial Presence	Full Presence	Transcendent Presence
Being there	Physically present in context of another	Physically present in context of another	Physically present (there) (physical attending behavior—eye contact, leaning toward) Psychologically present (with) (attentive listening behavior)	Physically present Psychologically present (metaphysical beliefs) Holistic
Focus of energy	Self-absorbed	Objects or tasks in environment, relevant to the other individual but none of the energy is directed at the other	Self/other (focusing on another influences response)—reciprocal	Centered (drawing from universal energy) Subject/subject—leads to oneness
	Personal, subjective reality	Mechanical/ technical reality	Present oriented (here and now)—anchoring in present reality	Transcending and oriented beyond here and now—sustaining while transforming reality
Nature of interaction	No interaction; self-absorbed, intrapersonal encounter	Interaction with part of other encounter	Interactive; essential communication; boundaries—role constraints; professional relationship; dyad caring	Relationship; high degree of skilled communication; role-free; human intimacy/ love; humanistic caring, no boundaries, monad relationship
Positive outcomes	Reduces stress; reassurance that someone is there; may be quieting and restorative; facilitates creative thinking	Reduces stress; solving a mechanical problem; reduces amount of stimuli in an encounter	Solving of a human problem; relief of a here-and-now distress	Transformations decreased loneliness expansion of consciousness; spiritual peace, hope, and meaning in one's existence (love/ connectedness); nice feeling generated in the environment; transpersonal (oneness)
Negative outcomes	No interpersonal engagement— missed communication; isolation, withdrawn, increased anxiety	No interpersonal connectedness	May be too much energy for recipient or feel negative to a recipient; energy not always available for full presence; increased anxiety	Fusion and possible loss of objective reality; danger of taking on recipient's problems

Osterman, P., & Schwartz-Barcott, D. (1996). Presence: Four ways of being there. *Nursing Forum*, 31, 23–30. Used with permission of the publisher.

2. What factors in your clinical practice setting prevent you from being truly present with clients?

3. How could you proceed with changing the clinical practice setting?

Empathy

Empathy, the ability to understand, sense, share, and accept the feelings of another (Keegan, 1994), enables the nurse to develop helping relationships with clients. Therapeutic, helping relationships focus on change. Understanding the potential impact of change on clients enables the nurse to identify obstacles for clients to change behaviors and attitudes. When using an empathetic approach, the nurse becomes more tolerant of behaviors, attitudes, and values that differ and could impede progress toward goal attainment. Wiseman (1996, p. 1165) identified four defining attributes of empathy: seeing the world as others see it, being nonjudgmental, understanding another's feelings, and communicating the understanding.

Nurses who possess empathy show awareness of the uniqueness and individuality of clients. They listen and respond as clients share feelings and concerns. They care about clients as sentient beings like themselves. If clients perceive that nurses care about them and how they feel, both nurses and clients benefit from (Keegan, 1994):

- More trusting relationships with open communication.
- Increased feelings of being connected to another.
- Enhanced client and nurse self-esteem.
- Genuine acceptance of others just as they are.
- Increased self-awareness for both the nurse and the client.
- Increased self-caring and less self-criticism on the part of the client.

To be truly empathic, nurses as helpers must listen carefully so they can act as intended, perceive and accept the inner feelings and experiences of clients as the clients experience them, and paraphrase feelings, ideas, and intentions accurately. Two essential actions are necessary for a nurse to develop empathy.

1. Awareness and acceptance of self as a feeling person open to one's experiences.
2. Ability to listen to each message of the client, to identify the client's feelings associated with it, and to respond to those feelings.

Thus, empathy involves far more than the cognitive or thinking part of the self. It involves the acceptance that we are *feeling* beings, commonly experiencing multiple emotions simultaneously. In effective communication, the nurse and the client know that the nurse perceives and accepts the client's feelings.

Respect

Respect is "feeling or showing deferential regard or esteem for another" (Agnes, 2005, p. 1221). It is the nonpossessive caring for and affirmation of another's personhood as a separate individual. Respect builds self-esteem and positive self-image. In the nurse–client relationship, respect is demonstrated by equality, mutuality, and shared thinking.

Certain behaviors convey respect toward others. Nurses act respectfully toward clients when they look directly at them when providing care; give them full, undivided attention; maintain eye contact, if culturally appropriate; smile appropriately; determine how each client wants to be addressed and call clients by their preferred means of address; introduce themselves to clients; and make physical contact such as a handshake or gentle touch. Clients who are members of a cultural group unlike that of the nurse may have special needs for respect, and sometimes the aforementioned

actions should be avoided because they conflict with cultural norms and values (Leininger & McFarland, 2006).

According to Bradley and Edinberg (1990, p. 226), clients may view nurses "as being powerful, one-up, and, if from a different racial group, nonempathic. In addition, nurses might view the clients as powerless, one-down, and different." Respecting the client's dignity is critical to therapeutic communication, "even when the client is in dire social, economic, or health circumstances" (Bradley & Edinberg, 1990, p. 226). Respect toward the client facilitates the development of effective helping relationships.

Genuineness

Genuineness is the state of being real, honest, and sincere. Clients readily detect dishonesty and insincerity when interacting with health care providers. Frequently, genuineness is used synonymously with authenticity.

When defining authenticity, phrases such as "being actually and precisely what is claimed," "genuine," "good faith," and "sincere" are used. Nurses who are genuine display their real selves to clients and do not let themselves become distorted or different because of thoughts or emotions. They act from their hearts and do not need to rehearse or contrive actions. In previous times, nurses were expected to be neutral to attain and maintain a helping relationship (Rogers, 1951). However, neutral behavior often seems depersonalized and sends messages of ambiguity. Ambiguous messages may cause client anxiety because clients may not understand their roles or positions in a relationship.

Nurses take risks to be genuine because such behavior frequently involves expressing negative thoughts and confronting others. However, there may be even more risk when incongruence surfaces between nurse intentions and behaviors. When clients detect incongruence in the nurse–client relationship, feelings of distrust, confusion, and suspicion may arise. Clients may begin to question the credibility of the nurse and the value of the health information being shared. They may only believe the nonverbal messages sent and discount the verbal ones. Finally, therapeutic rapport erodes if clients believe that the nurse is attempting to impress them rather than connect with them (Dinc & Gastmans, 2013).

When a nurse is genuine, action occurs spontaneously. "Being real does not mean being overly familiar"; what the client wants "is an emotionally available, calm, caring proficient resource that can protect, care about, and above all, listen to him or her" (Arnold & Boggs, 1989, p. 439).

Internalizing the principles of empathy, respect, and genuineness makes it possible for the nurse to demonstrate these behaviors and experience satisfaction in professional nursing practice. These principles also help nurses to establish healthy, helping relationships with clients and their significant others.

HELPING RELATIONSHIPS: THE NURSE AS HELPER

The nurse–client relationship is a special helping relationship that has the power to transform the lives of both the client and the nurse. Nurses tailor this private, platonic relationship to fit the needs of the individual client. Because the nurse has specialized knowledge and expertise to serve humanity, the nurse assumes the role of helper.

Rogers (1958) set the following essential conditions of a helping relationship, which are applicable to professional nursing.

1. The individual is capable of and expected to be responsible for him- or herself.
2. Each individual (the nurse and the client) has a strong drive to become mature and to be socially responsible.
3. The climate of the helping relationship is warm and permits the expression of both positive and negative feelings.
4. Limits, mutually agreed on, are set on behavior only, not on attitudes.
5. The helper communicates understanding and acceptance.

These characteristics of helping have positively influenced many health care professionals and serve as criteria for nurses as they develop effective helping relationships.

Nurses bear the responsibility to fulfill a helper role, regardless of the specific parameters and purposes of each relationship. The nurse must validate that the client knows why help was sought. The nurse also assumes that both the client and the nurse will share the responsibility for the outcomes of the nursing encounter. The nurse's helping role is viewed as a facilitative one in which the nurse uses self and expertise as therapeutic tools to assist the client to overcome threats to health and well-being or to obtain optimal health.

The nurse and the client bring unique talents, skills, and characteristics that affect the development of a helping relationship (Table 4.2) (Benner, 1984, 2001; Northouse & Northouse, 1998; Riley, 2017). The nurse uses client strengths to facilitate the helping relationship. When the client is confused or unresponsive, his or her significant others (e.g., family members, close friends, those having medical power of attorney) bring these attributes into the therapeutic relationship. At times, as the nurse delivers physical care to the client, efforts are made to fulfill the psychosocial and spiritual needs of the client's significant others.

Theories on Therapeutic Relationship Development

Although the nurse always assumes the roles of facilitator, advocate, and coordinator, his or her specific functions and purposes evolve as the relationship proceeds through predictable sequential stages. **Stages of the nurse–client relationship** vary according to the relationship's helping purpose. For example,

- The facilitator helps the client move toward improved health.
- The advocate protects the client from stress inherent in the petitioner role and acts on behalf of the client in promoting access to and use of health care services.
- The coordinator attempts to organize and articulate all the services related to meeting the client's health care needs.

The knowledge base needed to act as a helper in professional nursing was largely developed by Dr. Hildegard Peplau more than 50 years ago. Her book, *Interpersonal relations in nursing* (Peplau, 1952), presented a thorough analysis of Sullivan's (1953) interpersonal theory in psychiatry and gave nursing a sound conceptual model for practice. Although other nurse scholars have developed models and changed forms of the interpersonal model, Peplau's phases of the nurse–client relationship remain applicable today. Box 4.3, Professional Building Blocks, "Peplau's Phases of the Nurse–Client Relationship," provides associated functions of the nurse in each phase.

Travelbee (1964, 1966, 1971) designated five phases of the nurse-client relationship, starting with the phase of original encounter.

1. During the original encounter, the client and the nurse work to view each other as individual human beings rather than as "nurse" and "client."
2. Once the nurse and the client transcend their respective roles, they enter the phase of emerging identities, in which each perceives the other's uniqueness, values the other, and decides to make an emotional investment to begin the therapeutic relationship.
3. Once the client and the nurse have established their identities in the relationship, they enter the

TABLE 4.2 Interchange of Knowledge, Attitudes, and Skills Between the Client and the Nurse in the Helping Relationship

What the Client Brings to the Relationship	What the Nurse Brings to the Relationship
Cognitive	**Cognitive**
■ Individual ways of perceiving the world	■ Individual ways of perceiving the world
■ Preferred ways of making judgments	■ Preferred ways of making judgments
■ Knowledge and beliefs about health and illness in general	■ Knowledge and beliefs about health and illness in general
■ Specific knowledge related to current personal health status, usual general health status, and meaning of the current particular illness or altered health status	■ Knowledge about his or her clinical specialty
	■ Knowledge about what should help this particular client
■ Knowledge and beliefs about health promotion and maintenance in general and information about own health care routines and activities	■ Knowledge and beliefs about health behaviors that prevent illness and promote, regain, and maintain health
■ Ability to solve problems and knowledge of preferred methods of doing so	■ Ability to solve problems and knowledge of preferred methods of doing so while using nursing cognitive and clinical skills
■ Ability to learn	■ Knowledge about factors that increase client compliance with treatment regimens
■ Preferred ways to learn based on individualized learning style	■ Expectations of client based on previous encounters with other clients
■ Preferred communication patterns	■ Knowledge of available resources to assist client with this particular health problem
■ Knowledge of how current health affects role responsibilities	■ Ability to perceive if help is needed for effective nursing management of client health problem
■ Expectations of encounter with this nurse based on previous encounters with nurses	
Affective	**Affective**
■ Cultural and spiritual values	■ Cultural and spiritual values
■ Self-perceptions	■ Professional nursing values
■ Feelings about seeking help from a nurse	■ Self-perceptions
■ Attitudes toward nurses in general	■ Feelings about being a nurse helper
■ Attitudes related to previous encounters with nurses	■ Attitudes toward clients in general
■ Attitudes toward previous and currently prescribed treatment regimens	■ Attitudes toward this particular client system
■ Values regarding illness prevention	■ Intuitive feelings about the client system
■ Attitude of either being willing to or fighting actions to take the required measures to improve the health status at this time with this particular nurse	■ Biases about nursing treatment regimens
	■ Values placed on being healthy
	■ Values placed on people actively preventing illness or enhancing well-being
■ Personal meaning of current health status and encounter with this nurse	■ Willingness to help client take positive action to improve his or her well-being
	■ Personal meaning of current client encounter
Psychomotor[a]	**Psychomotor**
■ Ability to relate to and communicate with others	■ Ability to relate to and communicate with others using therapeutic communication techniques
■ Ability to carry out own health care management	■ Proficiency in administering general and specialized nursing interventions (in some cases the nurse has developed expertise)
■ Ability to learn new methods of self-care	■ Ability to teach nursing interventions to client

[a]Clients may not always be capable of these if health problem has impaired cognitive or motor abilities.

Adapted from Riley, J. B. (2000). *Communications in nursing* (4th ed.) (p. 28). St. Louis, MO: Mosby. Used with permission of the publisher. Additional information gathered from Benner, P. (1984). *From novice to expert: Excellence and power in clinical nursing practice*. Menlo Park, CA: Addison-Wesley; and Northouse, L. L., & Northouse, P. G. (1998). *Health communication: Strategies for health professionals* (3rd ed.). Stamford, CT: Appleton & Lange.

phase of empathy, during which they predict each other's behavior but fail to genuinely share feelings.

4. After the empathy phase, the nurse and the client enter the phase of sympathy, when the nurse translates sympathy into helpful nursing actions.

5. Following the sympathy phase is the phase of rapport, in which the nurse and the client enter into a personal, meaningful relationship where they genuinely communicate deeply with each other.

Unlike Peplau, Travelbee never addressed the need to end a helping relationship with the client.

Hames and Joseph (1980) outlined the following four stages in the development of a professional helping relationship that is not specific to nursing.

■ **Stage 1: Trust formation.** The client trusts the nurse because the nurse consistently displays honesty, respect, positive regard, and empathy.

4.3 Professional Building Blocks

Peplau's Phases of the Nurse–Client Relationship

Orientation Phase
- Introduction of nurse and client.
- Elaboration of the client's need to recognize and understand his or her difficulty and the extent of help needed.
- Acceptance of the client's need for assistance in recognizing and planning to use services that professional nurses can offer.
- Agreement that the client will direct energies toward the mutual responsibility for defining, understanding, and meeting productively the problem at hand.
- Clarification of limitations and responsibilities in the delivery system environment.

Identification Phase
- Provision of the opportunity for the client to respond to the helper's offer to assist.
- Encouragement for the client to express feelings, reorients those feelings, and strengthens positive forces.
- Provision of the opportunity for the nurse and the client to clearly understand each other's preconceptions and expectations.

Exploitation Phase
- Full utilization of the nurse–client relationship to mutually work on the solution to problems and the changes needed to improve health.
- Provision of opportunities for the client to explore earlier experiences and behaviors and to have emerging needs met.

Resolution Phase
- Provision of opportunity to formulate new goals.
- Encouragement of gradual freeing of the client from identifying with the nurse.
- Promotion of the client's ability to act more independently.

slightly from those of Peplau (1952) and Hames and Joseph (1980). They also proposed that each phase may overlap, depending on various contextual factors.

- **Phase 1: Preparation.** For the nurse, this involves preparing the setting and oneself for client interactions. The client prepares by making plans to actively seek assistance from a health care provider, such as making an appointment or arranging for a hospital stay.
- **Phase 2: Initiation.** The nurse uses a variety of therapeutic communication techniques and demonstrates genuine concern, compassion, and respect for the client. The nurse and the client also clarify client needs and establish mutual agreement on expected outcomes for the professional encounter.
- **Phase 3: Exploration.** The client and the nurse examine and work on client needs and concerns. The nurse creates an environment to foster client sharing of needs and concerns. The nurse also helps the client manage anxiety resulting from discussion of sometimes potentially embarrassing personal issues. The nurse and the client work together to outline a plan to help the client. Finally, the nurse helps the client develop new skills to learn how to live with or resolve the concern (or need) for which the client sought assistance.
- **Phase 4: Termination.** The nurse assesses the client's ability to independently manage and cope with the health-related issues. During this phase, the nurse summarizes client issues and accomplishments. The client and the nurse mutually agree to end the relationship.

> **Take Note!**
> Most of the approaches for developing a helping relationship address the need for the nurse to establish trust with clients by demonstrating the utmost respect for them.

- **Stage 2: Resistance.** The client pulls away from the relationship but the nurse continues to show concern.
- **Stage 3: Working.** The client and the nurse become actively involved in working together to help the client achieve health-related goals.
- **Stage 4: Termination.** The client and the nurse end the relationship by engaging in closure activities, such as saying goodbye, shaking hands, and extending good wishes for the future.

Northouse and Northouse (1998) designated four phases of the nurse–client relationship that differ

Sometimes, the therapeutic relationship has permanent life-changing effects on clients. Occasionally, the nurse may encounter a former client in a social setting or the client may return to the health care setting for a brief visit. When this happens, memories of previous encounters may surface, resulting in an affirmation of the benefits of the helping relationship.

Roles of the Nurse in Therapeutic Relationships

The nurse assumes various roles, depending on the stage or phase of therapeutic relationship development

TABLE 4.3 Roles Assumed by the Nurse During the Therapeutic Relationship

Therapeutic Stage or Phase	Professional Nursing Role
Peplau (1952)	
1. Orientation	Stranger (someone who may or may not be trusted)
2. Identification	Unconditional mother surrogate, resource person, teacher, counselor
3. Exploitation	The above roles plus that of support person or coach
4. Resolution	Primarily a support person as client has attained independence in managing own health
Travelbee (1971)	
1. Original encounter	Stranger
2. Emerging identities	Listener, information giver
3. Empathy	Physical caregiver, but client remains uncomfortable sharing deep personal concerns, early counselor
4. Sympathy	Caregiver, counselor, facilitator, coach, support person, client advocate
5. Rapport	Caregiver, counselor, teacher, facilitator, coach, supporter, client advocate, change agent
Hames and Joseph (1980)	
1. Trust formation	Stranger
2. Resistance	Counselor (especially in offering self-continuously despite rejection)
3. Working	Caregiver, counselor, facilitator, leader, resource person, coach, support person, client advocate, change agent
4. Termination	Counselor, support person
Northouse and Northouse (1998)	
1. Preparation	Critical thinker in deciding how to prepare self and setting for client
2. Initiation	Stranger, counselor
3. Exploration	Caregiver, counselor, resource person, coach, client advocate, change agent, support person, teacher
4. Termination	Counselor and support person

(Table 4.3). Success of the therapeutic relationships relies on nurse consistency in demonstrating deep respect, listening intently, and affirming client thoughts, concerns, and needs throughout all phases. As the relationship unfolds, the client dependence on the nurse decreases, and the nurse's role changes primarily to one of offering supports. The relationship ends when the client assumes independence, responsibility, and accountability for meeting his or her own health care needs.

During the various therapeutic relationship phases, the nurse moves back and forth in some of these roles, depending on the client's needs. The nurse uses client responses as a guide to determine which role to assume at a particular time. Role selection requires that the nurse analyze the client response, weigh the pros and cons of the best role to assume, and anticipate consequences of nursing actions. Thus, the nurse constantly assumes the role of a critical thinker. However, as the client's needs are met, the nurse essentially assumes the roles that promote client independence. The helping roles can be characterized as follows:

- **Stranger:** In the role of stranger, the client perceives the nurse as an unknown individual who may or may not be trustworthy and competent. Peplau

(1952) pointed out that it is essential for the nurse in this role to accord the client respect and convey genuine interest to promote open communication.

- **Surrogate:** A surrogate is a substitute figure who, in the client's mind, reactivates the feeling generated in the earlier relationships. The nurse's responsibility in this role is to help the client to become aware of likenesses and differences and to differentiate the nurse as a person. By permitting clients to reexperience old feelings, the nurse who is acting as surrogate sets up the opportunity for growth experiences.

- **Resource person:** The resource person role involves the nurse providing specific information that has been formulated to address the client's holistic needs. When clients cannot perform activities of daily living or complex care procedures independently, the nurse assumes the role of caregiver.

- **Teacher:** The teacher role involves the nurse sharing information and promoting the client's learning through experience, and requires the development of novel alternatives with open-ended outcomes in the nurse–client relationship.

- **Leader:** The leader role involves the nurse facilitating the client's work in solving problems and coaching the client to continue when obstacles are encountered. (The nurse also assumes the leader role when working with other members of the nursing and interdisciplinary health care teams.) For clients to become independent in meeting their health care needs, they experience change in knowledge, behavior, or attitude.

- **Change agent:** When the nurse facilitates change, the professional role of change agent emerges.
- **Counselor:** The counselor role incorporates all of the activities associated with promoting experiences leading to health. The counselor helps the client to become aware of health behaviors, to evaluate them, and to plan how to improve them. Counseling focuses primarily on how clients feel about themselves and what is happening to them (Peplau, 1952).
- **Critical thinker:** The critical thinker determines what nursing assessment data to collect based upon information shared by the client. The critical thinker also generates multiple approaches to develop and maintain a therapeutic relationship with patients. By using knowledge of and rationale for nursing interventions, the critical thinker anticipates potential complications and then makes clinical decisions based upon consequences of possible actions aimed at achieving optimal care outcomes.

Throughout the entire relationship, nurses frequently assume the counselor and critical thinker roles.

Mutuality in Responsibility and Decision Making

Every person involved in a communication process affects and is affected by every other person involved. Rogers (1970, p. 97) called this phenomenon "reciprocity." Reciprocal relationships are the basis of nursing practice. Having the potential to affect and be affected by the client offers the nurse the potential to assist the client to change behaviors in the direction of improved health. Reciprocity can be a powerful tool in problem-solving and decision-making situations that determine the nature and direction of change.

The concept of reciprocity is similar to that of mutuality. Reciprocity "is characterized as an interpersonal exchange, customarily expected to be symmetrical or equivalent" (Mendias, 1997, p. 435). By contrast, **mutuality** is characterized by having the same relationship toward another person and sharing things in common (Agnes, 2005). Mutuality appears as a concept in Peplau's (1952), Watson's (1996, 2012), and Leddy's (2004) conceptual models in terms of mutual gain in a nurse-client relationship.

Leddy expanded the use of the term "mutual" in terms of shared and connected processes humans have with environments.

Developing these ideas of mutual exchange and gain, Marck (1990, pp. 49, 57) discussed the concept of therapeutic reciprocity as follows:

> "one phenomenon of caring, (which) allows both the nurse and the client to benefit from their relationship in a mutually empowering manner.… Therapeutic reciprocity is a mutual, collaborative, probabilistic, instructive, and empowering exchange of feelings, thoughts, and behaviors between the nurse and client for the purpose of enhancing the human outcomes of the relationship for all parties concerned."

All of the previously specified roles represent elements of presence, empathy, respect, and genuineness. Communication in these role relationships evolves from diagnostic interactions to therapeutic interactions, including education and support, as the client moves toward achievement of optimal health. The absolute element of all these roles is mutuality in responsibility and decision making, if both the nurse and the client are expected to grow and experience satisfaction from the caring experience.

Communication and Anxiety

Nurses facilitate client change. The nature of change includes alternatives of cognitive repatterning (using new information to increase understanding), affective adjustment (using the relationship to become aware of, accept, and express feelings), and synthesis of cognitions and feelings in interpersonal repatterning (using the relationship to learn to interact with others in the social system). The direction of change can be toward health enhancement or deterioration. Obviously, the nurse and the client want to direct change toward enhanced health or a peaceful death.

Every social system has role behaviors for constituents to follow. The way a person communicates is greatly affected by his or her perceived role in the system. Roles "are structures that are imposed on behavior" (Berlo, 1960, p. 153). Three aspects of roles must be understood in trying to positively affect the other person in a relationship.

1. **Role prescription:** The formal, explicit statement of what behaviors should be performed by persons in a given role.
2. **Role description:** A report of the behaviors that are performed by persons in a given role.

3. **Role expectations:** The images that persons have about the behaviors that are performed by persons in a given role ((Berlo, 1960), p. 153; enumeration added).

In the ideal nurse–client relationship, congruence exists among these three aspects. Together, the nurse and the client agree on the structure and dynamics of their purposeful communication. However, when differences arise regarding the prescriptions, descriptions, and expectations of role behavior between the nurse and the client, communication breakdowns can occur, leading to uncertainty. Uncertainty and ambiguity, in turn, create increased tension and discomfort in the interpersonal system. Such tension in the human interpersonal system leads to dissipation of energy and decreased ability to use the energy for healing and growth. In interpersonal systems, this tension is often called "anxiety."

Anxiety (Fig. 4.2) is the tension state resulting from the actual or anticipated negative appraisal regarding uncertainty in any given situation. Prolonged or intense anxiety consumes available energy that could be better used for decision making or problem solving aimed at changing behavior and attitudes toward enhanced health.

Anxiety in one person is readily communicated to others. Sullivan (1953) attributed great power to anxiety and its effect on a person's interpersonal growth, development, and ability in all stages of life. The actual or anticipated negative appraisals by others that lead to anxiety are perceived as threats to one's self-image. If the anxiety is limited in amount and duration, it simply leads to an increased state of alertness, mediated through physiologic reactions and behavior to reduce the tension. However, if the state of anxiety is prolonged or intense, the individual may experience a state of high alert and be unable to engage in successful tension-reducing behaviors.

Sullivan (1953) postulated that learning occurs through an anxiety gradient extending from mild to severe. A client with mild anxiety can focus energy on most of what is really occurring. A client with moderate anxiety has limited ability to focus on what is really occurring and tends to distort reality. A client with severe anxiety cannot focus energy on what is really happening and thus cannot participate effectively in problem solving or decision making. Sometimes nurses encounter anxiety when they feel overwhelmed from heavy workloads, encounter new clinical situations, become uncertain of actions to take in ambiguous situations, or experience communication problems with clients, families, and other health team members. Nurse anxiety hampers effective clinical decision making. Effective health care demands that both the health care provider and the client control anxiety and focus energies upon what is really happening in a particular situation so that optimal decisions can be made.

Nurses have two primary responsibilities in controlling anxiety: (1) to be aware of their own feelings of anxiety and structure interactions in such a way that limited anxiety is transferred to the client; and (2) to use effective strategies for intervening in the client's anxiety. Therapeutic intervention for anxiety relies on the ability of nurses to recognize client anxiety as well as monitor and relieve their own.

Clinical practice settings are often stressful. Clients find themselves on unfamiliar turf when they enter the health care system. Nurses realize the importance of learning stress reduction strategies for themselves that they can share with clients. Techniques to help clients (and nurses) recognize, gain insight into, and cope with threats of anxiety are discussed in the following section.

> **Take Note!**
> Nurses and clients need to control their anxiety so that optimal care decisions can be made.

Caring and Noncaring Nursing Practices: Therapeutic and Nontherapeutic Communication Techniques

Florence Nightingale espoused the importance of caring relationships between nurses and patients, a concept that holds true for today's practice as well (see Focus on Research, "Then and Now: The Critical Nature of Caring").

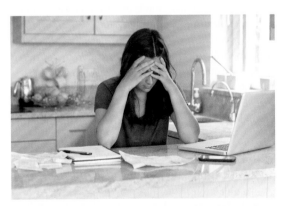

FIGURE 4.2 Anxiety frequently manifests itself in a person's nonverbal behavior.

FOCUS ON RESEARCH

Then and Now: The Critical Nature of Caring

The investigators performed a qualitative historical research study that examined the writings of Florence Nightingale in Victorian times. They read and analyzed Nightingale's work using latent concept analysis (a technique to reflect different traits of an abstract idea) to discover key themes that were indicative of nurses establishing and maintaining caring relationships with patients.

The authors identified the following key themes in Nightingale's writings that represented the nurse's caring relationship.

- "Attend to" referred to the behaviors and actions needed to respond effectively to meet patient and environmental needs.
- "Attention to" defined the nurse's ability to maintain focus and identify the needs of patients using thinking and observation skills.
- "Nurture" meant that the nurse conducted herself in a manner that "cherishes, strengthens, encourages, supports and promotes growth, and protects her patients" (p. 230).
- "Competent" referred to the nurse's ability to provide effective, safe, and excellent care using science and art.
- "Genuine" meant that the nurse had a truthful, honest, and sincere character and was able to display real concern for patients.

Nightingale wrote about the importance of caring in nursing in the same way that many contemporary nursing theorists espouse the critical nature of caring in the development of helping and healing relationships to clients. Today's health care clients expect that nurses genuinely care for them as people and rely on the nurse's ability to remain cognitively focused while engaging in nursing assessments, perform complex nursing skills safely, meet their holistic needs, help them in times or distress, create a safe and therapeutic milieu, and provide education about health issues. Nightingale's caring themes address many key elements of the knowledge, skills, and attitudes presented in the Quality and Safety Education for Nurses (QSEN) competencies.

Wagner, D., & Whaite, B. (2010). An exploration of caring relationships in the writings of Florence Nightingale. *Journal of Holistic Nursing, 28*(4), 225–234.

Because of its abstract nature, the concept of caring is difficult to define. Many nurses identify caring as the essence of nursing. The following actions are frequently used by nurses to show that they care: presence (being physically, emotionally, and spiritually with another to enter the world of the other), sharing (giving of one's skills, thoughts, and knowledge to help another), supporting (providing fortifying help, displaying concern, trusting others, and affirming persons in their actions), and competence (education and clinical skill). A **caring interaction** creates the uplifting effects for persons involved: feelings of being respected, feelings of belonging, personal growth, personal transformation, wanting to learn to care, and desire to care (Beck, 2001). In daily client interactions, nurses primarily use communication to demonstrate caring or noncaring. Caring communication strategies empower clients while being therapeutic. In contrast, **noncaring communication** typically creates a nontherapeutic "power-over" relationship, with the nurse dominating the client. Noncaring communication creates feelings of ill will among clients, nurses, and other members of the health care team. Table 4.4 presents selected differences between therapeutic and nontherapeutic communication strategies.

Sundeen, Stuart, Rankin, & Cohen (1998) stated that it is devastating to the formation of a helpful relationship if the nurse fails to listen. Listening transmits the message "I value and am interested in you." Effective listening requires the use of various techniques (Hosley & Molle, 2006; Schiavo, 2013; Sundeen et al., 1998; Videbeck, 2014), many of which include ignoring internal and external environmental distractions (see Box 4.4, Learning, Knowing, and Growing, "Guidelines for Engaging in Effective Listening").

QUESTIONS FOR REFLECTION

1. As a health care consumer, what caring behaviors have you experienced?
2. What caring behaviors have you experienced as a nursing student from your student colleagues or faculty?
3. What caring behaviors have you seen in a clinical practice setting?
4. What caring behaviors do you display as a nurse?

To listen effectively and to get clients to share thoughts and feelings, the nurse must use verbal communication techniques that facilitate the client's verbal and nonverbal expressiveness. Such techniques, generally referred to as **"therapeutic communication,"**

TABLE 4.4 Therapeutic Versus Nontherapeutic Communication Techniques

Therapeutic Communication Techniques	Description and Outcome(s)	Nontherapeutic Communication Techniques	Description and Outcome(s)
Focused listening	Focusing intently on what the client is saying results in reception of the client's message, equal power, and genuine interest in the client	Inattentive listening	Failure to receive the client's intended message gives the perception of the nurse's disinterest in and power over the client
Silence	Periods of nonverbal communication signify client acceptance	Uncomfortable silence (a prolonged period of silence signifying nothing)	Silence becomes awkward resulting in client feeling very ill at ease
Guideline establishment	Establishing guidelines clarifies roles, responsibilities, purposes, and limitations so the client understands his or her expectations	Nurse constantly talking	When the nurse does not let the client speak, the nurse is perceived as being superior or perhaps even uninterested in what the client has to say
Open-ended questions or broad opening	Comments or questions that require more than one- or two-word responses let client determine what should be shared	Closed-ended questions or comments	One- or two-word responses facilitate data collection but fail to get at the entire story, resulting in the client's impression that the nurse may be rushed
Distance reduction	Decreasing the amount of physical space between the provider and the client conveys desire to become involved	Inappropriate use of space	Being too close invades a client's personal space; being too far away conveys unwillingness to touch or be involved with the client
Acknowledgment or acceptance	Recognition of the client demonstrates the importance of the client in the interaction, thereby equalizing the power balance	False reassurance	Attempting to solve or soothe the client with words or platitudes negates the client's feelings or fears
Restating	Repeating one's perception of the client's main point enhances the validity of the nurse's interpretation of what was said	Parroting	Restating word for word what the client says conveys that the nurse is not listening or may be incompetent with verbal communication skills
Reflection	Stating back client ideas, thoughts, questions, and perceptions shows clients their ideas are important	Rejection	Refusal to discuss topics with clients conveys potential client rejection or that the nurse is disinterested or uncomfortable with the topic of concern, thereby enhancing the nurse's power
Clarification	Requesting more information helps the nurse fully understand the client's views	Giving advice	Telling the client what should be done negates partnership in decision making and emphasizes the nurse's power over the client
Consensual validation	Attempting to attain a mutual direct and underlying meaning of what was said shows the nurse's desire to understand the client more fully	Judging	Approval or disapproval of what is said promotes a client's dependent relationship on the nurse and results in the nurse having power over the client
Focusing	A question or statement that invites client to expand ideas in more detail conveys true interest	Failure to probe	Inadequate data collection results in lack of individualization of client care and increases chance for errors.

Therapeutic Communication Techniques	Description and Outcome(s)	Nontherapeutic Communication Techniques	Description and Outcome(s)
Summarizing	Stating the key points raised in an encounter helps to distinguish relevant from irrelevant information, provides a review, validates the accuracy of interpretation, and closes the interaction	Defensiveness	Protecting someone or something against negative feedback negates the client's right to question, thereby giving the perception that the nurse has power over the client
Collaboration	Mutual decision making about future actions fosters equality	Giving advice	Telling the client what should be done negates client participation in decision making, resulting in shifting power balance to the nurse
Stating direct and implied observations	Stating direct observations or verbalizing what the client says may indirectly remove communication barriers for the client when he or she may be avoiding or may feel fearful of expressing thoughts	Introduction of an unrelated subject or changing topics	When the nurse directs the nature of the interaction, thereby determining what useful information is, and negates the concerns of the client, the nurse is perceived as having power over the client
Offering self	By making oneself available, the nurse presents an unconditional offer to be with, understand, and meet the client's perceived needs and lets the client know that the nurse is available	Patronization Stereotypical comments	Condescending comments by the nurse place the nurse in a superior position Use of trite, meaningless, perhaps fashionable verbal expression negates the importance of what the client has said
General leads	Statements or phrases that invite clients to express ideas or feelings facilitate client sharing of information and ideas	Relentless probing	Insisting that the client talk about a particular issue or concern sets a tone of nurse power over the client and negates the client's right to privacy
Concentrating on a single point	Honing in on a single point focuses the interaction to refine information while preventing the overwhelming nature of the multiple factors contributing to a client care situation	Interpreting	By telling the client the hidden meaning behind the client's thoughts and feelings, the nurse blocks the client's understanding because only the client can identify or confirm his or her thoughts and feelings

Hosley, J., & Molle, E. (2006). *A practical guide to therapeutic communication for health professionals*. Philadelphia, PA: Saunders Elsevier; Schiavo, R. (2013). *Health communication: From theory to practice*. (2nd ed.). San Francisco, CA: Jossey-Bass; Sundeen, S. J., Stuart, G. W., Rankin, E. A. D., & Cohen, S. A. (1998). *Nurse–client interaction: Implementing the nursing process* (6th ed.). St. Louis, MO: Mosby; and Videbeck, S. L. (2014). *Psychiatric-mental health nursing* (6th ed.). Philadelphia: Wolters Kluwer Health/Lippincott Williams & Wilkins.

4.4 Learning, Knowing, and Growing

Guidelines for Effective Listening

- Give the other person your full attention by facing him or her directly.
- Focus solely on the current interaction by resisting all external distractions that cause your mind to stray.
- Listen for central ideas and validate them with the client.
- Ignore gut-feeling traps that confirm prejudices and/or produce biases.
- Do not become defensive.
- Watch for nonverbal and verbal messages.
- Do not prejudge worth based on appearance or delivery of the speaker.
- Listen for ideas and underlying feelings.
- Do not interrupt the person as he or she speaks or when brief pauses in the conversation occur.
- Try to see the situation from the other person's point of view.
- Do not try to have the last word.

facilitate the client's efforts at problem solving, self-expression, and health improvement. Nurses spend time very early in their nursing careers learning caring communication techniques. At first, some nursing students will find the techniques artificial and phony because of current culture values on speed and multitasking. However, nurses must take the time to refine the use of each technique so that it becomes natural and genuine.

To be helpful, the caring nurse must show empathy, attempt to understand the meaning of health and illness for clients, and respond with respect and authenticity.

- *The empathetic nurse* attends carefully and intensely, responds reciprocally to verbal and nonverbal messages, uses appropriate language, time responses appropriately, clarifies and confirms ideas, explores the world from the client's viewpoint, and paces verbal and nonverbal behavior to the client's abilities.
- *The caring nurse* spends time with clients, identifies relationships, makes connections based on knowledge, conceptualizes trends and patterns, summarizes appropriately, explains purposes of activities, and identifies nonverbal meanings while engaging in clinical practice activities. Some nurses, especially in inpatient or residential settings, make unexpected visits to client rooms to offer professional nursing services. Caring nurses make clients feel as though they are the most important people in the world.
- *The respectful nurse* verbalizes a clear commitment to understand, conveys acceptance, and clearly affirms the client's worth as a unique person while affirming the client's strengths and ability to assume self-responsibility. By offering oneself unconditionally and allowing clients when feasible (in situations in which the client is not at risk for harming self or others) to direct the nurse–client interactions, the nurse shares power with the client and enhances client self-worth and personal identity. The nurse who displays the utmost respect toward clients works actively to maintain client dignity at all times.
- *The authentic nurse* consistently responds with genuine thoughts and feelings, resists all urges to playact, assumes ownership of ideas and feelings, and freely shares emotions with clients. Other expressions of authenticity include extending a hand for the client to grasp in times of loneliness or distress, being present with the client in times of need, and connecting with the client on a spiritual level. Authentic nurses do not assume the role of imposter and acknowledge their limitations.

Noncaring or nontherapeutic communication strategies typically make clients feel inferior to the nurse. At times, nurses may demonstrate noncaring behaviors, which communicate the following attitudes: "You have no value," "I am not interested," "I'm bored," or "I have more important things to do than to spend time listening to you." Other nonhelpful nurse behaviors include being judgmental (e.g., putting personal values, beliefs, or expectations above the client's), making stereotypical responses (e.g., negating the uniqueness of the client by using platitudes or clichés as responses), and changing the subject (e.g., verbally directing the interaction to a new topic of importance to the nurse or by nonverbally signaling that the topic being discussed is not important). When nurses distinguish the main differences between caring and noncaring communication strategies, they can determine how to avoid the strategies that disvalue clients (see Table 4.4).

Take Note!
Failing to listen to clients is perhaps the most noncaring behavior a nurse can exhibit.

Nurses display noncaring behaviors for several reasons. In today's health care system, which values cost over care, some nurses find themselves overwhelmed by professional care tasks and have little time to spend engaging in caring interactions with clients. In addition, some nurses may enter the profession with a high need for control. This need, accompanied by increasing anxiety, sometimes leads nurses to adopt an attitude of superiority that is expressed in negative actions, such as moralizing, rejecting, or reacting with hostility.

Defensive behavior commonly occurs in regressive states. For example, a person might demonstrate denial, unconsciously evading or negating the real factors in a situation. Regressive states also may be marked by distortions, rote habitual actions, dogmatic responses, loss of control, invalidated assumptions (jumping to conclusions), parroting, inappropriate timing, and poor judgment. These behaviors represent important components of noncaring and nontherapeutic nursing strategies.

Because therapeutic communication is essential for effective professional nursing practice, nurses should periodically evaluate their communication techniques. This includes reflecting on how and what is said during nurse–client interactions or keeping a written journal. If a pattern of nontherapeutic behaviors is identified, the nurse should seek help from a colleague or counselor, or attend classes or workshops to improve communication techniques. Nurses should let their own feelings be a guide to evaluate the effectiveness of communication during nurse–client interactions. A persistent feeling of anxiety or tension is perhaps the best cue that the nurse may be unwittingly communicating in a noncaring, nontherapeutic, and unhelpful way.

Take Note!

Nurses should periodically evaluate the therapeutic communication techniques that they use in practice to verify how well they work with various clients and their significant others.

Although views vary on the advantages and disadvantages of nurses being characterized as caring persons, the fact is that nurses do care about their fellow humans. One dilemma for nurses is that they are not always permitted to care for clients to the best of their knowledge or ability. Many factors in clinical environments (e.g., short staffing, increased focus on cost reduction, increased turnover, frustration with new technology, and ineffective working relationships with other health care team members) impede the ability of nurses to care for clients as desired and result in feelings of frustration. However, when nurses have the opportunity to share their specialized knowledge and compassion, all involved in health care delivery become enriched as desired outcomes are attained.

■ QUESTIONS FOR REFLECTION

1. As a health care consumer, what noncaring behaviors have you experienced?
2. What noncaring behaviors have you seen in the clinical practice setting?
3. What noncaring behaviors have you displayed as a nurse? What factors contributed to this behavior?
4. How might you change the characteristics of your clinical or practice setting to keep you from displaying noncaring behaviors to clients and families?

Outcomes of Helping Relationships

The nurse–client relationship has three major desired outcomes.

1. Increased client self-awareness and understanding of how to better use personal responsibility to assume accountability for his or her own health (learning).
2. Attainment of optimal health.
3. Perceived satisfaction in the relationships.

Knowing that clients have adequate knowledge and skills to solve problems or take steps to adopt a healthy lifestyle is the goal. Clients who are adequately prepared can make educated choices, expend the required energy, and assume greater responsibility for their own health.

In the nurse–client relationship, change occurs as an outcome of learning in terms of either information gained and understood, or finding meaning in the personal experiences with nurses. The quality of communication plays the paramount role in change. When change and its effects are not communicated clearly, the change cannot be understood. Lack of understanding leads to resistance.

Nurses should continually evaluate their own communication behaviors (see Box 4.5, Learning, Knowing, and Growing, "Self-Evaluation of Communication Patterns"). In addition, feedback should be sought from the client about what has been said and about how the client feels the relationship is going. The value of nurse–client interactions should be explored at intervals to promote mutual benefits to the nurse and the client. A focus on asking the client, "How are we doing in terms of meeting your needs and expectations?" tells the client that the nurse values him or her and cares how the communication affects him or her. In addition, effective therapeutic communication enables clients to feel free to speak out when they have questions or concerns about their care and may result in error reduction (Finkelman & Kenner, 2007).

Along with individual evaluations of nurse–patient relationships, much work needs to be done to validate the benefits of helping relationships built by nurses. Therapeutic communication is an independent nursing intervention. However, nurses frequently fail to make entries in client records such as "therapeutic listening" or "explored feelings about the meaning of (client health concern)" when documenting delivered care. Most nursing research studies addressing caring are qualitative or descriptive in nature. Client satisfaction data offer the potential to identify the benefits of caring communications and helping relationships only from recipients of nursing care. Nursing job satisfaction studies have potential to explore provider benefits of being a helper. Perhaps, a nursing research program exploring the positive outcomes of helping relationships needs to be established.

HEALING RELATIONSHIPS: THE NURSE'S ROLE IN HEALING

A **healing relationship** might be considered a special type of helping relationship. Because "to heal is the activity of becoming whole" (Kritek, 1997, p. 11),

4.5 Learning, Knowing, and Growing

Self-Evaluation of Communication Patterns

Hunsaker and Alessandra (1980) proposed a schema for self-evaluation of communication patterns of persons in management positions that apply equally well to nurses when working with clients. The questions below can be used as a starting point for reflection and journaling.

- Did I comprehend each point made?
- Did I make judgments of the words before the speaker was through speaking?
- Did I make decisions in my own mind while he or she was still speaking?
- Did I hunt for evidence that would prove the speaker right? Wrong?
- Did I hunt for evidence that would prove myself right? Wrong?

- Did I become upset while listening?
- Did I generally jump to conclusions while listening?
- Did I let the client speak at least 50% of the time?
- Did I understand the words in terms of their intended meanings?
- Did I restate ideas and feelings accurately?
- Did I study voice, posture, actions, and facial expressions as the client talked?
- Did I listen between the lines for unspoken meanings behind the words?
- Did I really try to listen to the client?
- Did I really want to listen to the client?
- Did I really show the client I was, in fact, motivated and interested in listening to him?

Adapted from Hunsaker, P. L., & Alessandra, A. J. (1980). *Art of managing people.* Englewood Cliffs, NJ: Prentice-Hall.

healing has been defined as "a lifelong journey into wholeness, seeking harmony and balance in one's own life and in family, community, and global relations…" Healing occurs both within the person and by external interventions that mobilize the client's inner healing resources (Micozzi, 1996). Healing encompasses the improvement of the whole person (body, mind, and spirit). Healing is not synonymous with curing—persons with terminal illness can become whole in the process of dying (Dossey & Keegan, 2016).

Dossey and Keegan (2016) identified many healing modalities used by nurses in practice, including the following.

- Body–mind healing (cognitive therapy, self-reflection, and relaxation techniques).
- Nutritional healing (healthy diets, dietary restrictions, herbs, and vitamin and mineral supplements).
- Exercise and movement therapy (tai chi, walking, dance, and yoga).
- Spiritual healing (faith healing, miracles, play, humor, and use of fine arts).
- Energetic healing (meridians, chakras, aura, smells, sounds, colors, magnets, therapeutic touch, and healing touch).
- Environmental healing (reducing toxins, recycling, and feng shui).

Along with these integrative healing modalities, nurses engage in healing activities based on traditional scientific medicine when administering medications to clients and following pre- and postprocedure protocols.

Lerner (1994) differentiated among universal, common, and unique conditions of healing. Examples of universal conditions are inner peace and a deep experience of love. Attention and care from friends and family, deeply enjoying work, laughter, moving music, and great art are examples of common conditions. However, Lerner indicated that the unique conditions of healing are some of the most important. Unique conditions are those that apply only to a single individual as a result of life experiences or personal relationships. As a healer, the nurse must assess clients as individuals to identify the particular needs that are most meaningful for each client.

Given that healing occurs within the client, the nurse's role as healer is to facilitate another person's growth and life processes toward wholeness or to assist with illness recovery, with a healthier lifestyle, or with transition to a peaceful death (Dossey & Keegan, 2016). The nurse assists and responds to the client, who is the central force in the healing process. "Nurses assume that their actions, as professionals, aim to facilitate wholeness in others through an interaction based on a mutuality of purpose" (Kritek, 1997, p. 14). Kritek (p. 21) stated that four fundamental elements are always present in the healing encounter.

1. Nurse and client interact within a given context.
2. The encounter is in response to a health experience.
3. The nurse works in a pattern of mutuality with the client.
4. Healing is facilitated in response to a client's elicitation of nursing involvement and expertise.

Healing is facilitated within a helping relationship, which is characterized by principles such as presence (being rather than doing), intention and purpose, empathy, guiding, creativity, imagery, and spirituality (Dossey & Keegan, 2016; Keegan, 1994; Lerner, 1994).

As a healer, the nurse must assess all life dimensions for potential positive and negative forces that might influence the energy available to use when healing another. Effective healers have heightened sensitivity and awareness as they act with conscious intent. Nurses must recognize that not only is healing a unique life gift, but it also must be nurtured. Before healing another, some nurse healers practice preparation rituals. Healing fosters personal growth and the ability to live life to its fullest for both the client and the nurse (Conti-O'Hare, 2002; McKivergin, 2005).

Healing relationships produce interpersonal connections. Nurses often display intensity and unconditional love when acting as instruments of healing. Nurse healers usually perceive "that healing does not come from them, but through them" (McKivergin, 2005, p. 243). The potential healing does not come from the healer, but rather it is a mysterious phenomenon involving a higher power and energy within the environment. McKivergin suggested that the following factors may increase the nurse's capacity as "an instrument of healing" (p. 245):

- Self-care in all of life's dimensions to ensure a personal flow of energy and healing
- Personal interpretations of life's lessons and meanings
- Rootedness and expansiveness: balancing grounded approaches with intuitive inspirations
- Understanding the complex dynamics of holographic nature, the systems metaphor, and the essential nature of life, health, and healing
- Expansion of consciousness: broaden one's thinking, shift perspectives, and embrace new approaches to life
- Growth in love
- Courage
- Alignment with the divine
- Openness to being an instrument of the creator's healing grace
- Ability to detach self from the outcomes
- Groundedness and reliability
- Patience
- Authenticity
- Mindfulness
- Integrity

The healing process requires exchange of energy and truth during authentic communication to create an environment of support while helping others become attuned to their own healing capabilities. Outcomes of healing include deep relaxation and the profound change of becoming more whole.

▌ QUESTIONS FOR REFLECTION

1. What types of Keegan's types of healing have you experienced personally?

2. Which of Keegan's factors that may increase your capacity as "an instrument of healing" do you currently use in your life and which might you want to adopt as a professional nurse?

3. Which of Dossey and Keegan's (2016) types of healing, if any, have you used in clinical practice?

4. What would be the potential consequences if you used one of these nontraditional healing techniques with clients?

HELPING AND HEALING RELATIONSHIPS WITH COLLEAGUES AND OTHER HEALTH CARE TEAM MEMBERS

Nurses and other health care team members must work together to achieve the common goal of providing the best possible care for clients. Each member of the interdisciplinary team brings a unique perspective to and skill set for providing health care to clients.

Conflict among the health care team has been present since the beginning of health care delivery. As health care professionals find fewer resources for client care, they sometimes turn against each other instead of working effectively together. Historically and today, physicians have exerted power over nurses. Nurses must compete with other health care team members, such as pharmacists, laboratory technologists, radiology technicians, and dietitians, for scarce resources. Unlicensed assistive personnel may experience lack of respect from professional nurses.

To meet the increasingly complex needs of today's clients, patterns of conflict and competition must end and members of the health care team must establish effective professional partnerships. Currently, many health care organizations do not have healthy working environments. Health care team members tend to blame each other for shortcomings in client care. The needs of the clients, physicians, and organizational administrators frequently supersede the needs of the nursing staff. In today's fast-paced environment, people communicate with each other just to get jobs done.

Civility and politeness have gone by the wayside in an age of instant gratification and ever-present electronic devices as the mainstay for communication.

Professional partnerships help to dispel competition, exploitation, and frustration in the delivery of health care. Early work in the establishment of professional partnerships that are now critical to patient safety occurred in the 1990s. A **professional partnership** is a relationship based on mutual respect to achieve a common mission while each participant lives out his or her life's purpose. "Partnerships join hearts and minds around a common purpose" (Wesorick, Shiparski, Troseth, & Wyngarden, 1997, p. 3). Among health care team members, the common mission is client care and each member plays a key role. For a physician, a life purpose may be curing illness in the sick. For a professional nurse, a life purpose may be to care for and help persons as they respond to health alterations. For an unlicensed nursing staff member, a life purpose may be helping persons incapable of caring for themselves.

The theoretical foundations and concepts related to the development of healthy helping relationships with clients also apply to all health care team members. Healthy working relationships among health care providers require meaningful conversations, which result when people use the following communication principles.

- **Intention:** Creation of a safe place to foster collaborative learning and to share and listen to the thinking of others to connect at a deeply human level (body–mind–spirit).
- **Listening:** Truly hearing oneself and others, using physical, mental, and spiritual connections to learn.
- **Advocacy:** Willingness to share spontaneous personal thinking along with reasons behind the thinking, with the intention only to disclose thoughts, not to defend them.
- **Inquiry:** Willingness to ask others questions to discover new insights and learn by connecting diverse ideas and feelings.
- **Silence:** Time of quiet reflection to learn lessons from unspoken words; personal awareness of "the quiet of the Soul" (Wesorick & Shiparski, 1997, p. 40).

Taking time to abide by these principles could foster the development of more respectful and healthy working relationships among health care team members. Development of professional partnerships might facilitate team members to help each other, bolster team member esteem, and heal wounds. Then, all team members can appreciate each person's contribution to the common mission: excellent client care.

Take Note!
Applying the communication components used for clients to the members of the health care team can lead to respectful, healthy workplace relationships.

■ QUESTIONS FOR REFLECTION

1. How could you develop professional partnerships with your student colleagues and faculty in your nursing program?
2. How can you develop professional partnerships with health care team members in your clinical practice setting?
3. What personal behaviors/attitudes would you have to change to develop these professional partnerships?

In 2002, Patterson, Grenny, McMillan, and Switzler developed a framework for communication when addressing high-stakes issues. They describe this concept as a **crucial conversation**. Characteristics that distinguish a crucial conversation from other forms of discussion are that the participants perceive that they are addressing a high-stakes situation, there is divergence of opinion on how best to handle the situation/problem, and emotions of those involved are highly charged.

Health care team members participate in crucial conversations on a daily basis. Crucial conversations can be used in highly, emotionally charged situations and when disagreements occur related to client care, work processes, and team relationships (Patterson et al., 2002). Figure 4.3 outlines the steps and goals of a crucial conversation using a flow chart format.

Take Note!
Using the crucial conversations framework, health team members can build more effective helping and healing relationships with each other.

Quality and safety for patients rely on effective communication among all health team members. In all health care settings, an ideal situation would place patients first, team members would have equal contribution to care delivery, and the goal of care would be to provide the highest-quality care possible. In 2006, the Agency for Healthcare Research and Quality (AHRQ), a part of the U.S. Department of Health and Human

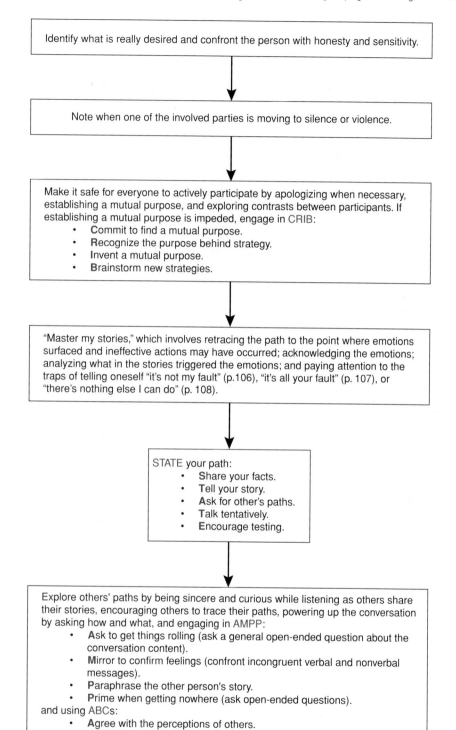

FIGURE 4.3 Flow chart for a crucial conversation. (Adapted with permission from Patterson, K., Grenny, J., McMillan, R., & Switzler, A. (2002). *Crucial conversations: Tools for talking when stakes are high*. New York: McGraw-Hill.)

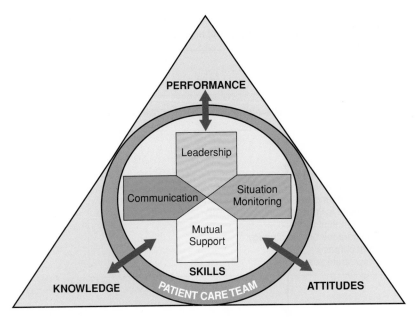

FIGURE 4.4 Improving patient safety and care quality: principles and steps from TeamSTEPPS. (Adapted from Agency for Healthcare Research and Quality. (2008). *Pocket guide: TeamSTEPPS— strategies & tools to enhance performance and patient safety.* AHRQ Publication No. 06–020–2. Retrieved from www.ahrq.gov/instructor/essentials/pocketguide. htm. Accessed November 2, 2012. Used with permission.)

Services, and the U.S. Department of Defense Patient Safety Program released a research-based, team-building, and communication program called **TeamSTEPPS** (Strategies and Tools to Enhance Performance and Patient Safety) in response to dangerous conditions outlined in various reports on patient safety in health care settings. The program offers strategies and tools to enhance health care team performance and meet team competency outcomes of knowledge (a shared mental model), attitudes (mutual trust and team orientation),

and performance (adaptability, accuracy, productivity, efficiency, and safety). Figure 4.3 highlights how knowledge, attitudes, and performance are used by the patient care team to provide safe, effective, high-quality health care services through leadership, situation monitoring, mutual support, and communication. Some of the key principles and strategies from TeamSTEPPS 2.0 are outlined in Table 4.5 and shown in Figure 4.4. A complete description and educational materials can be found at the TeamSTEPPS website (AHRQ, 2015).

TABLE 4.5 Key Principles and Strategies From TeamSTEPPS 2.0

Key Principles	Strategies
Team structure: Determining the fundamentals of team size, membership, leadership, composition, identification, and distribution	■ Identify the core team—the patient, coordinating team, ancillary and support services, and administration—that collaborates with contingency teams when situation arises ■ Clearly delineate all roles and responsibilities of team members
Leadership: Coordinating team member activities by ensuring that team actions are understood, changes in information are shared, and team members have necessary resources	■ Effective team leaders organize the team, articulate clear goals, make decisions using the collective input of members, empower members to speak up and challenge (when appropriate), actively promote and facilitate good teamwork, and are skillful in conflict resolution ■ Team events include planning (short briefing sessions), problem solving (huddling), and process improvement (debriefing to improve performance and effectiveness after the event and during action review)
Situation monitoring: Actively scanning and assessing situational elements to gain information or understanding or to maintain awareness to support team functioning	■ Continuous environmental scanning develops situational awareness (knowing what is going on around you). Along with a shared mental model, all team members are "on the same page" ■ Cross-monitoring is an error-reduction strategy that involves monitoring actions of other team members, providing a safety net within the team, ensuring mistakes or oversights are quickly and easily caught, and "watching each other's back" ■ STEP (**S**tatus of the patient, **T**eam members, **E**nvironment, **P**rogress toward goals) ■ I'M SAFE checklist (check **I**llness, **M**edication, **S**tress, **A**lcohol and drugs, **F**atigue, and **E**ating and elimination)

Key Principles	Strategies
Mutual support: Anticipating and supporting other team members' needs through accurate knowledge about their responsibilities and workload	▪ Task assistance: Team members protect each other from work overload situations, place all offers and requests for assistance in the context of patient safety, and foster a climate in which it is expected that assistance will be actively sought and offered. ▪ Feedback: Information provided for the purpose of improving team performance. Feedback should be timely, respectful (focused on behavior, not personal attributes), specific (outline desired behavior changes), directed toward improvement (specific expectations and direction to meet them), and considerate (consider team member's feeling and deliver negative information with fairness and respect). ▪ Advocacy and assertion: Advocate for the patient whenever a team member's viewpoint is inconsistent with those of the decision maker, and assert corrective action in a firm and respectful manner (make an opening, state the concern, offer a solution, and obtain an agreement). If an initial assertion is ignored, the person with the concern must invoke the two-challenge rule and present the opposing view a second time, while the challenged team member must acknowledge the concern. If the outcome remains unacceptable, the team member who is advocating for the patient should take a stronger action or engage a supervisor and follow up the chain of command. ▪ CUS (I am **C**oncerned, I am **U**ncomfortable, This is a **S**afety issue!) ▪ DESC script for conflict resolution (**D**escribe the situation or behavior using concrete data, **E**xpress how the situation makes you feel/what your concerns are, **S**uggest other alternatives and seek agreement, state **C**onsequences in terms of impact on established team goals); strive for consensus ▪ Collaboration: Achieve a mutually satisfying solution resulting in the best outcome by winning for the patient care team (including patient, team member, and entire team).
Communication: Process by which information is clearly and accurately exchanged among team members	▪ Report critical information that requires immediate attention and action regarding a patient's condition. ▪ SBAR (**S**ituation, **B**ackground, **A**ssessment, **R**ecommendation, and request) ▪ Call-out: Communicates critical information to all team members during emergent situation; helps team members anticipate next steps with a designated person holding the direct responsibility for carrying out this important task (e.g., leader of a Code Blue Team). ▪ Check-back: Closed-loop communication involving the sender initiating the message, the receiver accepting the message and providing feedback, and the sender verifying the accuracy of the message delivered (e.g., read back verification of verbal or telephone orders). ▪ Hand-off: Transfer of information via the I PASS THE BATON strategy (**I**ntroduction [introduce self, including role/job and patient by name]; **P**atient [age, gender, and location]; **A**ssessment [summary of chief complaint, vital signs, symptoms, diagnoses, and concerns]; **S**ituation [current status/circumstances, including code status, level of uncertainty, recent changes, and response to treatment]; **S**afety [critical laboratory values/test reports, socioeconomic factors, allergies, and alerts, such as fall risk, isolation procedures, risk for violence, etc.]; **B**ackground [comorbidities, previous episodes, current medication, and family history]; **A**ctions [what actions were taken or are required along with a brief rationale for each]; **T**iming [level of urgency, explicit timing needed, and prioritization of actions]; **O**wnership [who is the responsible team member/team, including patient/family]; **N**ext [what is scheduled to happen next, including anticipated changes, sharing of plan of care and contingency plans]).

Adapted from Agency for Healthcare Research and Quality. (2015). *Pocket guide: TeamSTEPPS—Strategies & tools to enhance performance and patient safety*. AHRQ Publication No. 14-000-2. Retrieved from http://www.ahrq.gov/sites/default/files/wysiwyg/professionals/education/curriculum-tools/teamstepps/instructor/essentials/pocketguide.pdf. Accessed March 18, 2016. Used with permission.

Standardization of interprofessional health care team communication eliminates oversights related to effective sharing of patient information and conflicts that may arise in the course of providing patient care. When team members follow specific communication guidelines, they verify what is to be done in a given situation as well as being able to anticipate the next steps required for optimal patient outcomes. Any team member is expected to share concerns about a given patient care situation especially if the safety of a patient is questioned (AHRQ, 2008, 2015). Clinical simulations incorporating TeamSTEPPS principles and strategies provide opportunities for health care professionals and students to master essential communication and teamwork skills for optimal patient care (Sweigert et al., 2016).

Summary and Significance to Practice

Professional nurses develop helping and healing relationships with clients. All people have visions of what they would like to accomplish and noble intentions about acting on their dreams. Mastery of communication skills is necessary for carrying out the mission of safe, effective, high-quality health and nursing care to clients, families, and communities.

REAL-LIFE REFLECTIONS

Think about Marcia and the situation encountered at the beginning of the chapter. Which of the communication models you have learned might help her as she works with the patient and family? What would you do if you were the nurse? What would be the consequences of your proposed actions? Are there other actions that you could take?

From Theory to Practice

1. Think about encounters you have had with health care providers as a consumer. Make a list of positive and negative encounters, and compare the lists. What are the characteristics of caring encounters? What are the characteristics of noncaring encounters?
2. Has this exercise changed you as a professional nurse? Why or why not?

Nurse as Author

1. Access the National Council of State Boards of Nursing (2014) Brochure *A nurse's guide to professional boundaries.* **https://www.ncsbn.org/ProfessionalBoundaries_Complete.pdf**. Identity one of the red flags and one example where a nurse might violate a professional boundary. For each identified professional boundary, design a strategy to use for yourself or to help a nursing colleague if it is encountered in your future professional practice.
2. Think about the last time that you encountered a patient care situation that required urgent action. Write about the situation and how it was managed. Compare and contrast the communication that was used with the strategies outlined by

TeamSTEPPS. Write examples of effective and ineffective communication and how a strategy from TeamSTEPPS would have enhanced patient safety and teamwork for the identified patient care situation.

Your Digital Classroom

Online Exploration

American Holistic Nurses Association: **www.ahna.org**
American Psychiatric Association Help Center: **www.apa.org/helpcenter/index.aspx**
American Psychiatric Nurses Association: **www.apna.org**
TeamSTEPPS Pocket Guide: **http://www.ahrq.gov/sites/default/files/wysiwyg/professionals/education/curriculum-tools/teamstepps/instructor/essentials/pocketguide.pdf**
National Council of State Boards of Nursing Resources on professional nurse–patient relationships: Professional Boundaries in Nursing (video): **https://www.ncsbn.org/464.htm**
Social Media Guidelines for Nurses (video): **https://www.ncsbn.org/347.htm**

Expanding Your Understanding

Access the Nurses Association of New Brunswick's (2015) *Standard for the therapeutic nurse–client relationship* at **http://www.nanb.nb.ca/media/resource/NANB-StandardsNurseClientRelation-E-2015–10.pdf**

Outline those that you perceive are unacceptable and list reasons to justify your position. What would you do if you witnessed a nursing colleague engaging in behaviors identified in the document as unacceptable and those that you have identified as unacceptable with a client?

Beyond the Book

Visit thePoint® **www.thePoint.lww.com** for activities and information to reinforce the concepts and content covered in this chapter.

REFERENCES

Agency for Healthcare Research and Quality (AHRQ). (2008). *Pocket guide: TeamSTEPPS—strategies & tools to enhance performance and patient safety.* AHRQ Publication No. 06–020–2. Retrieved from www.ahrq.gov/instructor/essentials/pocketguide.htm. Accessed November 2, 2012.

Agnes, M. (Ed.). (2005). *Webster's new world college dictionary* (4th ed.). Cleveland, OH: Wiley.

Arnold, E., & Boggs, K. (1989). *Interpersonal relationships: Professional communication skills for nurses.* Philadelphia, PA: W. B. Saunders.

Beck, C. T. (2001). Caring within nursing education: A metasynthesis. *Journal of Nursing Education, 40*, 101–109.

Benner, P. (1984). *From novice to expert: Excellence and power in clinical nursing practice.* Menlo Park, CA: Addison-Wesley.

Benner, P. (2001). *From novice to expert: Excellence for clinical nursing practice, commemorative edition.* Upper Saddle River, NJ: Prentice-Hall Inc.

Berlo, D. K. (1960). *The process of communication.* New York: Holt, Rinehart & Winston.

Bradley, J. C., & Edinberg, M. A. (1990). *Communication in the nursing context* (3rd ed.). East Norwalk, CT: Appleton & Lange.

Brill, N. I. (1990). *Working with people: The helping process* (4th ed.). New York: Longman.

Ceccio, J. F., & Ceccio, C. M. (1982). *Effective communication in nursing theory and practice.* New York: Wiley.

Conti-O'Hare, M. (2002). *The nurse as wounded healer: From trauma to transcendence.* Sudbury, MA: Jones & Bartlett.

Dinc, J., & Gastmans, C. (2013). Trust in nurse-patient relationships: A literature review. *Nursing Ethics, 205*(5), 501–516. doi: 10.1177/0969733012468463

Dossey, B., & Keegan, L. (2016). *Holistic nursing: A handbook for practice* (7th ed.). Sudbury, MA: Jones & Bartlett.

Finkelman, A., & Kenner, C. (2007). *Teaching IOM: Implications of the Institute of Medicine reports for nursing education.* Silver Spring, MD: American Nurses Association.

Hames, C. C., & Joseph, D. H. (1980). *Basic concepts of helping: A holistic approach.* New York: Appleton-Century-Crofts.

Healthcare Research and Quality. (2015). *Pocket guide: Team-STEPPS—Strategies & tools to enhance performance and patient safety.* AHRQ Publication No. 14–000–2. Retrieved from http://www.ahrq.gov/sites/default/files/wysiwyg/professionals/education/curriculum-tools/teamstepps/instructor/essentials/pocketguide.pdf. Accessed March 18, 2016.

Hosley, J., & Molle, E. (2006). *A practical guide to therapeutic communication for health professionals.* Philadelphia, PA: Saunders Elsevier.

Hunsaker, P. L., & Alessandra, A. J. (1980). *Art of managing people.* Englewood Cliffs, NJ: Prentice-Hall.

Keegan, L. (1994). *The nurse as healer.* Albany, NY: Delmar.

Kritek, P. B. (1997). Healing: A central nursing construct—Reflections on meaning. In P. B. Kritek (Ed.), *Reflections on healing: A central nursing construct* (pp. 11–27). New York: National League for Nursing.

Leddy, S. K. (2004). Human energy: A conceptual model of unitary nursing science. *Visions: The Journal of Rogerian Scholarship, 12*, 14–27.

Leininger, M., & McFarland, M. (2006). *Cultural care diversity and universality: A worldwide theory for nursing* (2nd ed.). Sudbury, MA: Jones & Bartlett.

Lerner, M. (1994). *Choices in healing: Integrating the best of conventional and complementary approaches to cancer.* Cambridge, MA: MIT Press.

Marck, P. (1990). Therapeutic reciprocity: A caring phenomenon. *Advances in Nursing Science, 13*, 49–59.

Mariano, C. (2016). Holistic nursing: Scope and standards of practice. In B. M. Dossey & L. Keegan (Eds.), *Holistic nursing: A handbook for practice* (7th ed.) (pp. 53–76). Burlington, MA: Jones & Bartlett.

McKivergin, M. (2005). The nurse as an instrument of healing. In B. Dossey, L. Keegan, & C. Guzzetta (Eds.), *Holistic nursing: A handbook for practice* (pp. 233–254). Sudbury, MA: Jones & Bartlett.

Mendias, E. P. (1997). Reciprocity in the healing relationship between nurse and patient. In P. B. Kritek (Ed.), *Reflections on healing: A central nursing construct* (pp. 435–451). New York: National League for Nursing.

Micozzi, M. S. (Ed.). (1996). *Fundamentals of complementary and alternative medicine.* New York: Churchill Livingstone.

National Council of State Boards of Nursing. (2014). *A nurses' guide to professional boundaries.* Retrieved from https://www.ncsbn.org/ProfessionalBoundaries_Complete.pdf. Accessed March 18, 2016.

Newman, M., Lamb, G. S., & Michaels, C. (1991). Nurse case management: The coming together of theory and practice. *Nursing & Health Care, 12*, 404–408.

Northouse, L. L., & Northouse, P. G. (1998). *Health communication: Strategies for health professionals* (3rd ed.). Stamford, CT: Appleton & Lange.

Osterman, P., & Schwartz-Barcott, D. (1996). Presence: Four ways of being there. *Nursing Forum, 31*, 23–30.

Parse, R. R. (1996). The human becoming theory: Challenges in practice and research. *Nursing Science Quarterly, 9*(2), 55–60.

Paterson, J. G., & Zderad, L. T. (1988). *Humanistic nursing.* New York: National League for Nursing.

Patterson, K., Grenny, J., McMillan, R., & Switzler, A. (2002). *Crucial conversations: Tools for talking when stakes are high.* New York: McGraw-Hill.

Peplau, H. (1952). *Interpersonal relations in nursing.* New York: G. P. Putnam and Sons.

Riley, J. B. (2017). *Communication in nursing* (8th ed.). St. Louis, MO: Elsevier.

Rogers, C. R. (1951). *Client-centered therapy: Its current practice, implications, and theory.* Boston, MD: Houghton Mifflin.

Rogers, C. R. (1958). Characteristics of a helping relationship. *Personnel and Guidance Journal, 37*, 6–16.

Rogers, M. E. (1970). *An introduction to the theoretical basis of nursing.* Philadelphia, PA: F. A. Davis.

Schiavo, R. (2013). *Health communication: From theory to practice* (2nd ed.). San Francisco, CA: Jossy-Bass.

Sullivan, H. S. (1953). *The interpersonal theory of psychiatry.* New York: Norton.

Sundeen, S. J., Stuart, G. W., Rankin, E. A. D., & Cohen, S. A. (1994). *Nurse–client interaction* (5th ed.). St. Louis, MO: Mosby.

Sundeen, S. J., Stuart, G. W., Rankin, E. A. D., & Cohen, S. A. (1998). *Nurse–client interaction: Implementing the nursing process* (6th ed.). St. Louis, MO: Mosby.

Sweigert, L. I., Umoren, R. A., Scott, P. J., Carlton, K. H., Jones, J. A., Turman, B., et al. (2016). Virtual TeamSTEPPS® Simulations produce teamwork attitude changes among health professions students. *Journal of Nursing Education, 55*(1), 31–35. doi: 10.3928/01484843–20151212–08

Taylor, A. (1977). *Communicating.* Englewood Cliffs, NJ: Prentice-Hall.

Travelbee, J. (1964). What's wrong with sympathy? *American Journal of Nursing, 64*, 68–71.

Travelbee, J. (1966). *Interpersonal aspects of nursing.* Philadelphia, PA: F. A. Davis.

Travelbee, J. (1971). *Interpersonal aspects of nursing* (2nd ed.). Philadelphia, PA: F. A. Davis.

Vestal, K. W. (1995). *Nursing management: Concepts and issues* (2nd ed.). Philadelphia, PA: J. B. Lippincott.

Videbeck, S. L. (2014). *Psychiatric-mental health nursing* (6th ed.). Philadelphia, PA: Wolters Kluwer Health/Lippincott Williams & Wilkins.

Watson, J. (1996). Watson's theory of transpersonal caring. In P. H. Walker & B. Neuman (Eds.), *Blueprint for use of nursing models: Education, research, practice and administration* (pp. 141–184). New York: National League for Nursing.

Watson, J. (2012). *Human caring science: A theory of nursing* (2nd ed.). Sudbury, MA: Jones & Bartlett.

Wesorick, B., & Shiparski, L. (1997). *Can the human being thrive in the workplace? Dialogue as a strategy of hope.* Grand Rapids, MI: Practice Field Publishing.

Wesorick, B., Shiparski, L., Troseth, M., & Wyngarden, K. (1997). *Partnership council field book.* Grand Rapids, MI: Practice Field Publishing.

Wiseman, T. A. (1996). A concept analysis of empathy. *Journal of Advanced Nursing, 23,* 1162–1167.

Patterns of Knowing and Nursing Science

LEARNING OUTCOMES

By the end of this chapter, the learner will be able to:

1. Discuss the evolution of three systems of thought about how to organize developing knowledge in science.
2. Describe the differences among logical empiricism, historicism, and postmodernism in their philosophical approaches to the development of knowledge.
3. Explain the differences among the patterns of knowing in professional nursing.
4. Compare and contrast concepts, theories, and conceptual models.
5. Identify the four central concepts of nursing that are the focus of scientific inquiry in nursing.

REAL-LIFE REFLECTIONS

Paul, a registered nurse for 7 years, is taking a nursing research course while working on his bachelor of science in nursing degree. He believes that knowledge from "hard science" is the only way nursing can become as respected as other health care professions. He also believes that research is only useful if it directly improves patient care, and he disregards conceptual or explanatory research. Last week, one of Paul's assigned clients with pancreatitis went into shock and was transferred to the intensive care unit. Surprisingly, his colleague Jill (a nurse with 15 years of clinical experience) happened to enter the client's room just as the client started to hemorrhage. At the end of the shift, Paul thanked Jill and asked her how she was able to detect that the client needed help. Jill replied, "I just knew. I cannot explain it other than nurse's intuition. I just get this little voice that tells me to check on clients and I do." Based on this experience, Paul decides to pursue the topic of nurse intuition for his research class.

- *How do you feel about nurse's intuition?*
- *How do you think Paul's feelings about knowledge might change after he researches intuition?*

Understanding nursing's body of knowledge is essential for competent professional practice. Knowledge can be obtained from a number of sources, including experience, reflection, and values. Science is "a unified body of knowledge about phenomena that is supported by agreed-on evidence" (Meleis, 2007, p. 36). For many years, nursing scholars have debated whether professional nursing practice is a science, an art, or both (Chinn & Kramer, 2015; Meleis, 2007, 2012; Rogers, 2005; Roy, 2007; Watson, 2007). According to Rogers (1992, pp. 28–29), "Since nursing is a learned profession, it is both a science and an art. The practice of nurses, [therefore], is the creative use of [this] knowledge in human service."

The science of nursing incorporates the study of relationships among nurses, clients, and environments within the context of health. It also is the result of interrelationships among theory, practice, research, and education. Theory provides the tools to direct nursing practice. Practice provides the professional individual with the setting to apply nursing knowledge and develop and test nursing theories. Research provides the means to test theories. Education provides the means to shape belief systems and to synthesize and disseminate knowledge.

Nursing is emerging as an autonomous, distinctive professional discipline that is valued by society. As an emerging science, the nursing profession uses and builds on knowledge developed from many disciplines through centuries of evolution.

▌ QUESTIONS FOR REFLECTION

1. What are the benefits of establishing a base of nursing science for the profession of nursing?
2. What consequences arise for the nursing profession if it fails to generate a specialized knowledge base?
3. Do you perceive nursing as an art, a science, or both?

THE EVOLUTION OF SCIENTIFIC THOUGHT

Over the course of thousands of years, human life has progressed greatly, due in large part to advances in science. It is impossible to cover each era of human history and the entire evolution of human knowledge. Therefore, this chapter addresses three systems of thought about organizing and developing human knowledge (Spradlin & Porterfield, 1984).

Ancient people understood the world through magical beliefs—people believed they were controlled by forces beyond human understanding or control. A second way of trying to understand the world began during the scientific revolution (around 1500 CE). Science emphasized observations, measurement, and quantification as the means for understanding the world.

With Einstein's discovery of **relativity** in the early 20th century, people began to accept uncertainty and focused on processes that influenced human thought. The 21st century saw a movement toward using complexity theory, which espoused nonlinear interactions, emergent phenomena, continuous and discontinuous change, and unpredictable outcomes (Hazy, Goldstein, & Lichtenstein, 2007; Nicolas & Philippe, 2015; West, 2006).

Ancient Civilizations

The earliest civilizations differentiated the world into two parts: me (internal) and not me (external). They viewed the external world as being populated by spirits, demons, and gods, who directed good and evil in the world. Humans tried to influence gods because they believed that gods were moved to action by whims and passions.

Through trial and error, people discovered that some patterns of action led to predictable outcomes, which could be reproduced as long as the procedure was followed exactly (as one would with recipes from a cookbook). Thus, in an elementary way, humans observed life phenomena sufficiently to gather many isolated facts, which were then used to make decisions about what to do. The earliest "nurses" functioned primarily from protocols and procedures based on tradition.

Because diseases, aches, and pains were assumed to be caused by gods and evil spirits, early medicine was associated with religion or magical beliefs. However, time and attention to cause and effect led to practical approaches and logical sequencing of steps for treatment. Hippocrates (460–377 BCE) was followed by Aristotle (384–322 BCE), who emphasized classification of signs and symptoms. Increasing attention was paid to exploring the mechanisms of the human body (Spradlin & Porterfield, 1984).

▌ QUESTIONS FOR REFLECTION

1. What superstitions have you encountered in your personal or professional life?
2. How do these superstitions affect your life? How might they affect your professional practice?
3. What would be the consequences if you allowed superstitions to guide you in professional practice?

The Search for Certainty

The evolution of mathematics and the ability to count made relationships appear more logical and the world more predictable. By 1500 CE, interest in the scientific study of humans and nature was increasing, and the philosophy of logical positivism was driving the search for **certainty** (undisputed truth). Logical positivism was based on a belief that the world was like a simple machine, but only God understood the laws by which it operated. Time and space were absolute. Time flowed smoothly and uniformly. A reductionist approach was used to identify causes to predict effects. Scientific scholars

"became engulfed in a spiral of logic and increasing certainty about quantification of relationships among absolute entities that led to concepts of truths that could be validated.... We could, with the use of observation, measurement, and logical reasoning, know the laws of nature.... All the entities that composed the whole of nature could be reduced to their smallest parts, studied and understood, and rebuilt" (Spradlin & Porterfield, 1984, p. 106).

The reduction of humans into separate psyche and soma (Cartesian dualism), both of which could be measured physically, was advanced by Descartes (1596–1650) (Fig. 5.1), who saw humans as machines

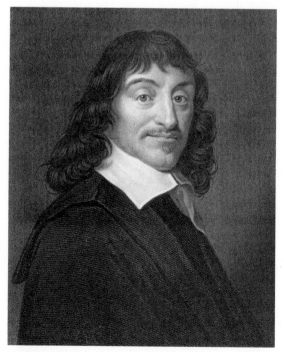

FIGURE 5.1 Engraved Portrait of Rene Descartes (1596–1650) by W. Holl in 1833.

ruled by the same laws as all of nature (Spradlin & Porterfield, 1984, p. 108). The separation of mind from matter (body) and the emphasis on the person as the sum of minute parts dominated medical and nursing science for centuries until the advent (or perhaps re-emergence) of a holistic approach to health in the 20th century.

Four basic assumptions about humans and the universe are inherent in this kind of mechanistic worldview: determinism, quantity, continuity, and impersonality. Leaving no room for uncertainty, the principle of determinism reflects the belief that "nature proceeds by a strict chain of events from cause to effect, the configuration of causes at any instant fully determining the event in the next instant, and so on forever" (Ware, Panikaar, & Romein, 1966, p. 127). The ability to predict comes from this principle, whereas lack of predictability and the presence of uncertainty represent ignorance.

The quantitative principle expresses the exact nature of science. It reflects the belief that science consists of "measuring things and setting up precise relations between the measurements" (Ware et al., 1966, p. 129). In this view, humans and the universe are described by numbers (e.g., spatial coordinates, time, position, amounts, and locations) that quantify physical properties, and by relations among these quantitative characteristics.

Continuity, the third principle, is concerned with the "transitions of nature from one state to another [and] express[es] the sense, deeply engrained in the outlook of the age, that the movements of nature are gradual" (Ware et al., 1966, p. 129). This principle reflects the belief that the processes involving humans and the universe are continuous.

In the fourth principle, impersonality, the scientist is viewed as an instrument, not a person. The scientist uses observation rather than imagination, passively finds order in phenomena rather than creating it, and does not permit personal influence on the phenomena under observation (Ware et al., 1966, p. 129).

Belief in these four principles led Galileo (1564–1642) and Sir Isaac Newton (1642–1727) to develop the scientific method, based on a particular method of reasoning: logic. Logic encompasses principles of reasoning applicable to any branch of knowledge. Because logic is based on reason and sound judgment, it can be convincing.

The scientific method starts with asking questions. Inquiry is a technique of science. It seeks truth, information, or knowledge to solve problems. A problem is any question or matter involving doubt, uncertainty, or difficulty that needs solution. Solution is the act of solving a problem by finding the answer or explanation. The most extensive investigative process of science is the systematic inquiry of research.

◼ Questions for Reflection

1. How do logic, science, and inquiry affect your daily life or professional practice?
2. What are the consequences of using logic, science, and inquiry in the nursing profession?

The Relative World of Process

By the 20th century, scientists realized that the physical world consisted of matter and forces that interact with matter, such as gravity, magnetism, and electricity. By exploring the cell, genetic mechanisms and mechanisms that influenced cellular structure and function were explained. It appeared that "the immutable laws which governed the world" were being discovered.

In the early 20th century, Albert Einstein (Fig. 5.2) demonstrated that the world was composed not of

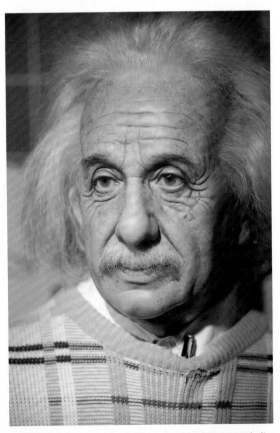

FIGURE 5.2 Waxwork of Albert Einstein (1876–1955) displayed at Madame Tussauds, Bangkok, Thailand, 2005.

events, but of observations, which were relative to the place and velocity of the observer. "Any absolutes or cause and effect sequences [are] illusions . . . testable only in a retrospect organization of events" (Spradlin & Porterfield, 1984, p. vi). Heisenberg's (1971) and Bertalanffy's (1968) work in quantum physics led to the postulation that mass, energy, time, and space coordinates are interchangeable. All systems were considered interrelated and interdependent on a continuum of relativity and probability, and thus uncertainty.

Relativism has varying degrees of forms and degree. Truth may only become apparent when humans have a social structure and accepted methods to allow it to emerge. Thus, what is discovered and known about science relies heavily upon the structure and processes outlined by the scientific process. Moral relativism provides the foundation for tolerance for divergent viewpoints as in the cases of when life begins, when life should end, and all other morally charged issues encountered by persons. New relativism focuses upon the context in which events occur thereby paving the way for different views and actions for doing what is right (Baghramian & Adam, 2016).

The implications of this different conceptual system were enormous. Continuity was replaced by discontinuity, and probability (determined statistically) replaced certainty. Emphasis was placed on patterning rather than on discrete entities, and on interactions rather than on isolated events. The scientist was no longer an isolated objective observer of events. "Man came to be seen not as a detached observer but as an irremovable part of his observations" (Ware et al., 1966, p. 148). In addition, awareness of the limitations and biases of individual perception increased, implying that truth and meaning were not absolute but were relative to history and context. Nonetheless, "while physicists have become increasingly concerned with . . . a relative world of process, biologists have until recently tended to be even more involved in the reductionistic approach to life" (Spradlin & Porterfield, 1984, p. 189).

Complexity Science and Theory

Stephen Hawking (Fig. 5.3) identified the 21st century as the "Century of Complexity." Complexity science values both the quantitative and qualitative approaches to generating knowledge (Linberg, Nash, & Linberg, 2008). As early as the 1980s, multiple disciplines noted that similar observations and discoveries were occurring in their respective fields. There appeared to be some self-organizing framework in nature and human systems; small changes to one thing seemed to

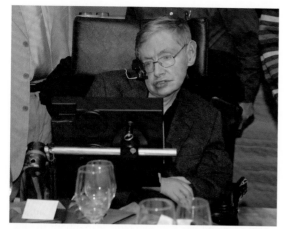

FIGURE 5.3 Physicist, scientist Stephen Hawking (1942–) visiting Tel Aviv University, Israel in December, 2006.

affect the whole; systems engaged in complex adaptation without predictable results; interrelated non-linear dynamics surfaced; and complex response processes resulted in response to changes. Everything in the world apparently appeared to be one. Nicolas and Philippe (2015) provide evidence that there are underlying computations that may indeed mathematically explain the nature of the complexity within the universe. Thus, there is a combination of both relativism and determinism that form the nature of the universe.

▌ QUESTIONS FOR REFLECTION

1. Which theory—relativism or complexity—do you think best applies to the profession of nursing?
2. How do the theories of relativism and complexity apply to your daily life?
3. What future impact do you foresee these theories have on professional nursing practice?
4. How does relativism affect nursing practice? How have you used relativism to justify some of your own personal or professional nursing actions?
5. What are the consequences of the use of relativism for patients, for you as a person and as a nurse, and for the nursing profession?

PHILOSOPHY OF KNOWLEDGE

Because one's belief system is critical to determining sources and methods of discovering knowledge, an understanding of the differing philosophical approaches that currently influence nursing science is critical.

Based on Plato's concepts, knowledge is considered to be the belief that has been justified through reason (Stumpf, 1993). What constitutes adequate justification is the concern of the discipline of philosophy. Philosophy considers questions such as whether there is such a thing as truth and how one can be certain that something is true. It is necessary to accept that some things can be true in order to question the truth or falseness of any particular thing. But must certainty be beyond all possible doubt, or is certainty sufficient if it is beyond logical and reasonable doubt? How does an individual acquire knowledge? What are the roles of intellect, perception, and intuition in the process of knowing?

Processes of Knowing

The three primary processes of knowing are rationalism, empiricism, and intuition. **Rationalism** involves belief in the possibility of knowing truth by thinking and by use of reason that is a priori, or independent of experience. **Empiricism** involves belief that the only source of certainty about knowledge is immediate experience. However, because raw experience is subject to individual perception, the emphasis must be on verification and on confirmation or refutation of observations. **Intuition** is sometimes described as "just knowing." The source of the knowing is internal to the individual and is often perceived as occurring independently of experience or reason. It is subjective and personal in origin, although it can be validated through experience and interaction with others.

Approaches to Knowing

Logical Empiricism

Logical empiricism, a philosophical approach to the development of knowledge accepted since the 16th century, is based on the following assumptions.

1. A body of abstract, general, and universal facts and principles that explain the way the world operates is waiting to be discovered. Theories provide alternative explanations for how the body of facts and principles is ordered and systematically unified.
2. Cause-and-effect (linear) relationships can be established by using deductive processes and experimental methodology. The results are context-free generalizations that can be applied to all individuals. Truth is achieved through sensory data and controlled experiments.
3. It is necessary to control values and biases to achieve "objective" knowledge; therefore, the observer must be separated from the observed world. Science is value free. Social relevance is unimportant.

4. Theoretical reduction is an important scientific goal. It is assumed that the ultimate character of reality is best explained using the logic and simplicity of the fewest possible theoretical concepts and laws.

5. The whole is the sum of its parts. Circumscribing (reducing) observations to small parts of the whole gives better control of the data and stronger explanatory power.

Logical empiricism is synonymous with logical positivism. Logical empiricism provides guidelines for scientific process and criteria for scientific rigor. Under logical empiricism, the goal of science is "to predict, explain, and control" world events, situations, and occurrences. To identify "pure facts," scientists must remain value free while engaging in scientific methods. Nursing knowledge based on the "hard sciences" has its roots in logical empiricism (Rogers, 2005).

REAL-LIFE REFLECTIONS

Think of Paul, from the beginning of the chapter. Explain how Paul's belief in nursing knowledge based on "hard science" relies on the assumptions of logical empiricism. What classes in your nursing program curriculum are based in logical empiricism? How is the content used in these courses applicable to daily life and professional practice?

Historicism

Historicism, advanced since the 1930s under the influence of concepts such as relativity and process, is based on the following assumptions.

1. Because "truth" is dynamic and constantly changing, what is important is the effectiveness of a theory for solving problems.

2. The whole is more than the sum of its parts. Reducing the whole to parts is counterproductive. Interrelationships and interactions are part of what must be studied.

3. An individual or a phenomenon must be studied as a whole in a natural setting. The observer is part of the setting, so interactions between the observer and the setting should be described, rather than controlled. Emphasis is on process rather than fact.

4. Multiple research traditions are desirable (e.g., theories from psychology, physiology, education) to explain different dimensions of the same phenomenon. Synthesis and development of multiple theories are encouraged.

5. Knowledge is related to context. Values, subjectivity, intuition, history, and tradition are useful for discovery.

Unlike logical empiricism, **historicism** emphasizes the "importance of the context and processes in which scientific activity takes place" (Rogers, 2005, p. 99). Truth and knowledge are related to context, and multiple approaches can be used to generate knowledge. Instead of being rigid and stagnant, theories become dynamic (Rogers, 2005; Sitzman & Watson, 2014; Watson, 2007); they are flexible and can be adapted to remain relevant. In professional nursing, historicism specifies that to understand the evolution of nursing knowledge and practice, one must learn about the history of the profession. Interpretation of history relies on the value of the person who reads historical documents and examines artifacts of a specific era. Kuhn's (1970) perspective of science as a way to "solve puzzles" and Laudan's (1981) perspective of science as a means to "solve problems" provide a practical approach to the generation of nursing knowledge. For example, a complete client family history served as the standard for determining client risk for specific diseases prior to the completion of the human genome project. For persons with no access to genetic testing, perhaps a detailed family history may be beneficial in determining future risk of disease.

Postmodernism

Postmodernism is a social movement and a philosophy that originated in Europe in the 1960s (Reed, 1995). Postmodern perspectives on knowledge development are based on the following assumptions.

1. There is a focus on understanding multiple meanings and ways of knowing reality, rather than "a single, transcendent meaning of reality" (Reed, 1995, p. 71). As a result, conceptual models and grand theories are considered irrelevant.

2. Because "multiple truths" are accepted, knowledge is considered to be uncertain and provisional (Holmes & Warelow, 2000). Contradictory positions have value for generating alternative meanings.

3. Statements "reflect a concern for context rather than universality, specificity rather than generalization, uniqueness rather than sameness, and relativism rather than absolutism" (Holmes & Warelow, 2000, p. 90).

4. The emphasis of knowledge development shifts "from concern over the truth of one's findings to concern over the practical significance of the findings" (Reed, 1995, p. 72).

5. Problems are not "solved," but rather are "deconstructed," which means that efforts are made to disentangle or separate concerns from underlying values and beliefs. Language is analyzed for the meanings of words and assumed power structures.

6. With lack of concern about generalization there is a shift toward lived experience and toward "creativity, flexibility, uniqueness, and local value" (Holmes & Warelow, 2000, p. 96). Instead of probable "truth," relevance and usefulness for practice and the potential to generate additional study are the criteria for research.

There is no single definition for postmodernism. Structuralism, a subset of postmodernism, strives to analyze the basic properties of a system. For example, structuralism recognizes the role that language, rituals, social structures (including male and female roles), and traditions play in influencing the discovery of what it means to be fully human. Poststructuralism challenges the dominant thoughts of unity, uniformity, and oneness (Rogers, 2005; Sitzman & Watson, 2014; Watson, 1999). Deconstruction aims to reverse hierarchies and acknowledges the importance of power in relationships. From a poststructuralist view, people have no subjective identity but reveal themselves through various forms of communication along with their actions and behaviors. In postmodernism, "a belief in a single reality that provided a unifying and stable center is discarded" because "it is indefensible" (Rogers, 2005, p. 135). According to a postmodern perspective, everyone has different perspectives and experiences about the world (Rogers, 2005; Watson, 1999).

Until recently, nursing research and theory were dominated by logical empiricism and positivistic philosophy. However, beginning with Rogers (1970) and increasing in the 1980s, nurse scientists incorporated principles of historicism and relativism into theory, research, and practice. In the mid-1990s, principles of postmodernism began to appear in the nursing literature.

Intermodernism

A debate about the appropriate methods for developing nursing knowledge has raged in the nursing literature. Some authors, in support of qualitative methods, maintained that "human behaviors cannot be isolated and quantified and that the attempt to do so results in misleading and dehumanizing outcomes rather than in knowledge that is useful for nursing practice" (Campbell & Bunting, 1991, p. 2). Others suggested that quantitative and qualitative methods can be used at different times to serve different purposes. Meleis

(1997) advocated development of a worldview (Weltanschauung) that includes an integration of norms emanating from all different theories of truth. By combining the rigorous science with personal intuition, information becomes both objective and subjective. Clinical data can be directly observed, but the interpretation of the data relies on the knowledge and values of the health care professional. Thus, the door is opened for nursing to become simultaneously an art and a science.

Such a synthesis of philosophical approaches would encourage various methods for the development of nursing science, thereby capturing the complexity of the discipline of nursing. Beginning in the late 20th century, Reed formulated the concept of **intermodernism**, an unorthodox view of nursing knowledge development that blends nursing science, theory, and practice. In the intermodern approach to knowledge development, all factors entering into the nursing profession (personal values, experiences, worldviews, professional expertise and experiences, and socioeconomic conditions) enrich the knowledge of nursing. Intermodernism differs from postmodernism because it avoids radical extremes and places less emphasis on political philosophy while fostering diversity of ideas. In intermodernism, relativism does not supersede shared values such as "personal autonomy, self-development, agency, humanism, and justice" (Reed, 2011, p. 16).

Reed (2011) uses the acronym INTERMODERN to describe the 11 initial tenets of the intermodern perspective (Table 5.1). From an intermodernist perspective, all things are amenable to change.

PATTERNS OF NURSING KNOWLEDGE

Chinn and Kramer (1999, pp. 1, 7) described knowing as "ways of perceiving and understanding the self and the world.... Nursing's patterns of knowing are interrelated and arise from the whole of experience."

Gender Differences

Gender differences have been identified in the ways in which men and women may develop frameworks for the organization of knowledge. Perry (1970) identified four positions through which men make sense of their educational experiences.

1. **Basic dualism:** Authorities hand down the truth, and subordinates are passive. Choices are perceived as either right or wrong, black or white, good or bad, and we or they.

TABLE 5.1	Tenets of Intermodernism
Tenet	**Brief Description**
In-between-ness	Working outside of traditional methods in between modernism and postmodernism, "between extremes & contradictions" (p. 16)
Nursing	Considers nursing's scientific knowledge and the artistic nature; nursing as a practice discipline and a scientific body of knowledge
Truth	Coordinated, multiple theoretical approaches aimed at addressing similar problems
Empiricism	Nursing evidence that includes subjective and objective data and approaches as well as a network of human, nonhuman, and hybrid elements that constitute the formation of knowledge
Reality	An underlying pattern, diversity, and innovation not totally within or outside the thinker's mind; it emerges through interactions, actions, and knowledge development
Methods	Systematic and chaotic approaches used to discover and generate nursing knowledge (randomized clinical trials, synthesis, and personal professional practice and life experiences)
Openness	The state of being amenable "to critique, self-correction, and change" along with an "ongoing personal reflection on one's theory and practice . . . congruent with the open, self-organizing nature of human systems in process with their environments" (p. 17)
Discovery	Multiple ways of knowing that include the use of dynamic situations and influences that extend empirical knowing; knowledge is constructed out of something such as an experience and combines inductive and deductive logic
Epistemology	The partnership of science and practice for knowledge creation; combines being and doing, thinking and reflecting, technology, and culture, thereby creating a holistic knowledge view
Romanticism	The human quest for goodness, beauty, and meaning; the part of humans that is difficult to explain or study
Nightingale	The symbol of a scholarly practitioner who generated the first nursing-specific knowledge base, proposed the unitary approach of persons and environments, recognized the inner healing capacity, emphasized the importance of caring and vocation, and looked at the entire human life span

Reed, P. G., & Crawford Shearer, N. B. (Eds.). (2011a). *Nursing knowledge and theory innovation: Advancing the science of practice.* New York: Springer Publishing.

2. **Multiplicity:** A personal opinion is acceptable and may be valid. Everyone's opinions may be valid.
3. **Relative subordinate position:** Evidence is sought for opinions. The emphasis is on analysis and evaluation of information.
4. **Full relativism:** Truth is relative. The meaning of knowledge depends on its context.

Perry suggested that the positions occurred in a linear sequence, with each position an advance over the previous one.

In a study of women's perceptions, Belenky, Clinchy, Goldberger, and Tarule (1986) described five major categories used for the organization of knowledge.

1. **Silence:** The individual is subject to the whims of an external authority and perceives herself to be mindless and voiceless.
2. **Received knowledge:** External authority is all-knowing. The individual is capable of receiving and even reproducing knowledge, but not of creating it.
3. **Subjective knowledge:** Truth and knowledge are personal, private, and subjectively known or intuited.
4. **Procedural knowledge:** The individual is invested in learning and in applying objective procedures for obtaining and communicating knowledge.
5. **Constructed knowledge:** The individual experiences herself as a creator of knowledge. She views knowledge as contextual and values both objective and subjective strategies for knowing.

Gender has been linked to the distribution of power and privilege in society (Marecek, 1995). Doering (1992, p. 26) stated that knowledge reinforces and supports existing power relations that "subtly support male dominance and reinforce female submissiveness." "When the male model is assumed to be the human model, women are viewed as the 'other,' deviant from the male norm or prototype" (Doering, 1992, p. 31). However, Doering continued, "since power is always exercised in relation to a resistance" (p. 31), ways of knowing (such as intuitive knowing and contextual, phenomena-centered knowledge) that are not based on a male worldview "may alter the balance of the nursing–medicine power relation" (p. 32).

Think about Paul and Jill from the beginning of the chapter. In what ways do they conform to the male and female frameworks for organizing knowledge? How does Paul's scientific approach to clinical issues affect the balance of power between men and women health care providers? How does Jill's intuition challenge the balance of power between men and women in medicine?

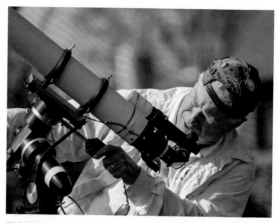

FIGURE 5.4 An amateur astronomer setting up a solar telescope, April 2012. Astronomy, and all other forms of hard science and research findings, constitutes empirical knowing.

In 1978, Carper identified the following four ways of knowing in nursing: Empirical, aesthetic, ethical and personal. Depending upon a nurse's area of clinical practice, different ways of knowing dominate. Even nursing journals prefer publishing articles addressing one pattern of knowing over others (Kearney, 2015). For example, *Nursing Research and Research in Nursing and Health* prefers empirical knowledge; whereas, *Nursing Ethics* tends to publish articles addressing ethical and personal knowing. Nurses have published articles on how they use the patterns of knowing in clinical practice by sharing case studies (Carnago & Mast, 2015).

Empirical Knowledge

The pattern of **empirical knowing** constitutes the science of nursing. It "encompasses publically verifiable, factual descriptions, explanations, and predictions based on subjective or objective group data" (Fawcett, Watson, Neuman, Walker, & Fitzpatrick, 2001, pp. 115–116). "Empirical data, obtained by either direct or indirect observation and measurement … are formulated as scientific principles, generalizations, laws, and theories that provide explanation and prediction" (Carper, 1992, p. 76) or enrich understanding through interpretation or description (White, 1995). **Empirical knowledge** is obtained through the senses, can be verified, is credible, and is used to impart understanding (Fig. 5.4). Processes related to creating empirical knowledge include explaining and structuring (Chinn & Kramer, 1999, 2015).

Aesthetic Knowledge

Aesthetic knowing in nursing "is that aspect of knowing that connects with deep meanings of a situation and calls forth inner creative resources that transform experience" (Chinn & Kramer, 1999, p. 183). This knowledge is not universal but is uniquely experienced and expressed and has subjective meaning (Fig. 5.5). **Aesthetic knowing** involves the creative processes of rehearsing and envisioning (Chinn & Kramer, 1999,

2015). **Aesthetic knowledge** involves the appreciation and understanding the role that creative expression plays in the human experience.

"Art begins with the assumption of a common, generalizable human experience . . . and seeks expression of the infinite creative possibilities for experiencing or responding to the human experience" (Chinn, 1994, p. 30). Intuition, defined as "an immediate apprehension, or the power of gaining knowledge without evidence of rational thought" (Mitchell, 1994, p. 2), can be an important component of aesthetic knowledge in nursing practice.

Benner and Tanner (1987) discussed six aspects of intuitive judgment previously identified by Dreyfus and Dreyfus (1985). These aspects are not sequential but rather are used in combination by the practitioner.

1. **Pattern recognition** is the ability to recognize patterns and relationships without prior consideration of the separate components.

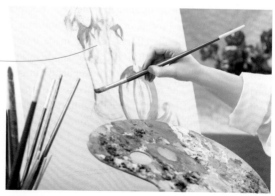

FIGURE 5.5 Painting and all other forms of art are examples of aesthetic knowing.

2. **Similarity recognition** is the ability to see similarities and parallels among patient situations, even when there are marked dissimilarities in objective features.
3. **Commonsense understanding** is "a deep grasp of the culture and language, so that flexible understanding in diverse situations is possible. It is the basis for understanding the illness experience, in contrast to knowing the disease" (Benner & Tanner, 1987, p. 25). It is a way of "tuning in" to the patient and grasping the patient's experience.
4. **Skilled know-how** is based on a combination of knowledge and experience that permits flexibility of actions and judgment.
5. **A sense of salience** makes it possible to differentiate what is particularly significant in a situation.
6. **Deliberative rationality** involves the use of analysis and past experience to consider alternative interpretations of a clinical situation.

Carper (1978) emphasized the importance of integrating aesthetic knowledge into nursing. The experience of helping and caring "must be perceived and designed as an integral component of its desired result rather than conceived separately as an independent action imposed on an independent subject" (Carper, 1978, p. 17). The result is a richness and appreciation of the practice of nursing as an art as well as a science.

Personal Knowledge

Personal knowledge involves a "person's individualized and subjective ways of learning, storing, and retrieving information about the world" (Rew, 1996, p. 96). "The pattern of **personal knowing** refers to the quality and authenticity of the interpersonal process between each nurse and each [client]" (Fawcett et al., 2001, p. 116). Both the nurse and the client are considered to be "integrated, open system(s) incorporating movement toward growth and fulfillment of human potential" (Carper, 1978, p. 19). In the process of mutually establishing a nurse–client relationship, efforts must be made toward "receptive attending" (Moch, 1990, p. 155) and engagement, rather than detachment and a manipulative impersonal orientation. The result is an authentic knowing of an individual apart from the category of nurse or client. The creative processes of personal knowing include opening and centering (Chinn & Kramer, 1999, 2015).

Because personal knowing "concerns the inner experience of becoming a whole, aware, genuine self" (Chinn & Kramer, 1999, p. 5), the individual needs to accept ambiguity, vagueness, and discrepancies in what is essentially a subjective and existential process.

No specific methodology can be used consistently. The individual must be open to experience and intuitive feelings, be honest with self, and make efforts to acknowledge the responses of others. This is an ongoing process because the self is constantly changing.

Belenky et al. (1986) stated that educators can help women develop their own authentic voices if they emphasize connection over separation, understanding and acceptance over assessment, and collaboration over debate; if they accord respect to and allow time for the knowledge that emerges from firsthand experience; if instead of imposing their own expectations and arbitrary requirements, they encourage students to evolve their own patterns of work based on the problems they are pursuing (p. 229).

Moch (1990, pp. 156–159) described three overlapping components of personal knowing.

1. **Experiential knowing** involves becoming aware through participation in which the knower learns through self-observation, by observing others, through feeling, and through sensing.
2. **Interpersonal knowing** is increased awareness through connectedness or interaction, which can involve intense attending, opening oneself to another, and conveying feelings to another.
3. **Intuitive knowing** involves the immediate knowing of something without the use of reason. The knower often describes this as a "hunch" or as a "feeling about something."

Moch (1990, p. 159) believed that personal knowing can be viewed only from within a context of wholeness that "includes a process of encountering, passion, commitment, and integrity; and entails a shift in connectedness at the conscious or unconscious level." Moch saw implications for personal knowing for research and knowledge development, but also recognized key assumptions underlying the capture and transmission of personal knowing. Key assumptions include the following:

1. All perceptions are involved in data gathering.
2. The process of the experience may be more important than the product of knowing.
3. Validation of the product of knowing uses using both internal and external validation criteria.
4. Attempts to reproduce the process or the product are futile because each situation is unique.

"The processing may consist of any combination of human and environmental interaction, rational intuiting, appraisal, active comprehension, and personal judgment" (Sweeney, 1994, p. 917).

Ethical Knowledge

Ethics in nursing focuses on an obligation, or "what ought to be done" (Chinn & Kramer, 1999, 2015, p. 5). Sarvimaki (1995) described four types of **ethical knowledge** that represent different ways of organizing and expressing moral knowledge.

1. Theoretical or ethical knowledge "stands for an intellectual conception of what is good and right. It is organized into concepts and propositions that are formulated into judgments, rules, principles, and theories" (Sarvimaki, 1995, p. 344).
2. Moral action knowledge means "having the skill necessary for performing the act as well as having good judgment. . . . Values and principles are manifested in action" (Sarvimaki, 1995, p. 345).
3. Personal moral knowledge "refers to the way in which morality is organized in the person, that is, in his motives, inclinations, emotions, and commitments" (Sarvimaki, 1995, p. 346).
4. Situational knowledge "means being aware of the moral significance of the situation and being able to identify its morally significant traits" (Sarvimaki, 1995, p. 347).

Biomedical ethics are derived from models of what is good for the patient, rights-based notions of autonomy, or the social contract of medical practice (Fry, 1989). However, it has been argued (Fry, 1989; Sarvimaki, 1995; White, 1995) that nursing ethics should be based on an ethic of caring and must consider the nature of the nurse–client relationship. A caring orientation is based on the moral ideal of doing what is good, rather than that which is just. Mutuality, not autonomy, is foundational (White, 1995). Chinn and Kramer (1999, 2015) specify clarifying and valuing as the creative processes of ethical caring. Thus, **ethical knowing** blends the concepts of biomedical ethics with the ethic of caring enabling nurses to focus on making optimal decisions within the entire context of client care situations.

Other Ways of Knowing

White (1995) proposed that a fifth way of knowing, **sociopolitical knowing**, needs to be added to the original patterns identified by Carper (1978). "The pattern of sociopolitical knowing addresses the 'wherein'" (White, 1995, p. 83), a broader context that includes the context of nurse and client (including cultural identity) as well as the context of nursing as a practice profession. White stated that "a sociopolitical understanding in which to frame all other patterns of knowing is an essential part of nursing's future in an increasingly economically driven world" (p. 85).

Chinn and Kramer (2011, p. 64) suggest a sixth way of knowing, **emancipatory knowing**, which they defined as "the human ability to recognize social and political problems of injustice or inequity, to realize that things could be different, to piece together complete elements of experience and context to change a situation as it is to a situation that improves people's lives." When nurses engage in emancipatory knowing, they become aware of undesirable conditions in practice, analyze who benefits or profits from them, question what is considered knowledge, look for freedom from constraints of current knowledge and conditions, acknowledge that conditions can be improved, demystify the conditions, identify the impediments to freedom, and identify needed changes and what resources would be required to attain and sustain a new desired state. Critical reflection is used to guide action and practice. Formal expressions and creative processes raise critical questions and foster the development of required changes.

In addition, Munhall (1993) proposed "unknowing" as another pattern of knowing in nursing. She argued that the state of mind of **unknowing** is a condition of openness, and "a decentering process from one's own organizing principles of the world" (p. 125). The intent is to "come to know the patient's world" (Munhall, 1993, p. 126), which will "lead to a much deeper knowledge of another being, of different meanings, and interpretations of all our various perceptions of experience" (p. 128).

Garrett and Cutting (2014, pp. 101–102) propose still other ways of knowing. Along with empirical knowing (a posteriori: from science or experience), they suggest nine additional forms of knowing in nursing and in health care. Hallowed knowing described as the knowledge revealed to person via the ancient sacred texts. Esoteric knowing described as knowledge beyond human comprehension that occurs when a person cannot explain it to another. Knowing specified as a coming to know things from a natural curiosity that provides foundation for discovery learning. Visionary knowing explained as the knowledge generated when a person learns something in a dream while sleeping. Luneful knowing identified as knowledge that a person gains from a state of madness. Supernatural knowing stated as knowledge gained from participation in magic or other mystical processes. Lupine knowing attained from an individual from a lycanthrope (werewolf). Satellite knowing discovered when viewing something or a situation from a great height. Other knowing explicated as any other form of knowledge failing to fall in either of the other 10 categories. Although some of these ways of knowing may seem far-fetched, some of the new ways of knowing have application to clinical practice.

▮ Questions for Reflection

1. What ways of knowing have you used in your personal life?
2. How did these ways of knowing guide your personal actions?

3. What ways of knowing have you used in clinical practice?
4. How did these ways of knowing guide your professional nursing actions?

Concepts in Practice, "How Nurses Use the Patterns of Knowing in Clinical Practice," provides examples of how professional nurses use the patterns of knowing in clinical practice. Many years of practice may be needed to develop competence and confidence in using all of the patterns of knowing.

Concepts in Practice

IDEA → PLAN → ACTION

How Nurses Use the Patterns of Knowing in Clinical Practice

Empirical Knowing
- Administering medications and IV therapy safely
- Following isolation procedures for infectious diseases
- Using evidence-based strategies for preventing hospital or treatment complications
- Abiding by principles for hand hygiene
- Adhering to protocols for clinical nursing procedures

Aesthetic Knowing
- Individualizing care for all patients
- Adapting standard procedures to fit a specific clinical situation
- Detecting significant patient pattern changes
- Creating environments to soothe patients and families
- Using art and music as nursing interventions

Personal Knowing
- Using experiential know-how in novel or complex care situations
- Connecting deeply with patients and their significant others
- Opening self to others
- Relying on intuition—a hunch that something is wrong

Ethical Knowing
- Doing what is best for the patient
- Doing what is right and just
- Safeguarding patient rights
- Possessing an altruistic motive when caring for others
- Valuing self and others
- Being aware of moral issues surrounding patient situations

Sociopolitical Knowing
- Understanding legal implications of professional nursing practice
- Using health care resources prudently
- Involving oneself in the political and legislative processes

- Supporting efforts to provide effective health care for all

Emancipatory Knowing
- Raising critical questions
- Noticing undesirable practice situations
- Reporting unsafe and undesirable practice situations
- Working as an equal member of the health care team
- Changing systems for better health care
- Participating in nursing shared governance systems

Unknowing
- Being open to learning
- Quieting oneself to listen
- Learning about the patient's entire story
- Connecting deeply with others to deepen understanding about them
- Acknowledging limitations of one's current knowledge and skills

Hallowed Knowing
- Finding meaning in work from studying a sacred text.
- Using revealed messages from a sacred text to direct work as a nurse

Esoteric Knowing
- Using intuition in practice
- Unexplainably identifying patterns or taking prompt action in a given nursing situation

Visionary Knowing
- Heeding information recovered from a dream when sleeping to guide actions and decisions

Supernatural Knowing
- Permitting or using various religious or cultural healing ceremonies in clinical practice

Satellite Knowing
- Taking a step back to analyze a clinical situation using a global perspective
- Thinking about health care delivery from a macro rather than a micro viewpoint.

Paradigms for Developing Nursing Knowledge

Three different perspectives, each described as reflecting a different point of view (paradigm) of the way to develop nursing knowledge, have been identified (Newman, Sime, & Corcoran-Perry, 1991, p. 4).

1. **Particulate-deterministic perspective:** Phenomena are viewed as "isolatable, reducible entities having definable properties that can be measured." Knowledge includes facts and universal laws that can be used to predict and control change.
2. **Interactive-integrative perspective:** Phenomena are viewed as having multiple, interrelated parts. Reality is assumed to be multidimensional and contextual. Relationships may be reciprocal (rather than linear and causal), and knowledge may be context dependent.
3. **Unitary-transformative perspective:** Each phenomenon is viewed as a unitary self-organizing field embedded in a larger self-organizing field. It is identified by pattern and by interaction with the larger whole. Change is unpredictable. Knowledge is personal and involves pattern recognition. Both the viewer and the phenomenon are involved in a process of "mutuality and creative unfolding."

Patterns as ways of knowing are not mutually exclusive; rather, they "are interrelated and arise from the whole of experience" (Chinn & Kramer, 1999, p. 7). Different ways of knowing are not judged against one another. Each of the ways of knowing and of creating knowledge is useful. Because each pattern adds only one specific component, none alone is a sufficient source of knowledge for **nursing science**. "Nursing depends on the specific knowledge of human behavior in health and in illness, the aesthetic perception of significant human experience, a personal understanding of the unique individuality of the self and the capacity to make choices within concrete situations involving particular judgments" (Carper, 1978, p. 22).

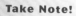

Take Note!

Comprehensive nursing knowledge must be based on an integration of all the ways of knowing.

REAL-LIFE REFLECTIONS

In attending to Paul's patient with pancreatitis, which of the ways of knowing did Jill demonstrate? Which ways of knowing might have aided Paul?

THE DEVELOPMENT OF NURSING SCIENCE

Because of the complexity of the discipline of nursing and competing worldview perspectives (particular-deterministic, interactive-integrative, and unitary-transformative), defining nursing science poses a challenge. However, attaining a clear definition of nursing science would provide a foundation for the profession's unique body of knowledge.

Specialized branches of science develop knowledge and theories. First comes the ideas and theories. Scientists then test and refine the ideas and theories. Nursing contributes uniquely to health care delivery, but failure to articulate exact contributions may place the profession at risk.

Identification of Concepts

For a discipline to have growth of knowledge, the concepts that are important for the discipline must be identified, and there must be a shared acceptance of conceptual definitions. Fawcett (2005) defined the term **"concept"** as "a word or phrase that summarizes ideas, observations, and experiences" (p. 4). She also identified **four central concepts of nursing** that address the key elements of the profession.

1. **Human being:** An individual nurse or client, a family, a group, or a community
2. **Environment:** Alive or inanimate
3. **Health:** Well-being and illness
4. **Nursing:** All the interactions among the nurse, client, and environment in the pursuit of health; as well as what nurses do

These four concepts represent the metaparadigm of nursing that encompasses all phenomena of interest in a value-neutral way to identify a distinctive domain for the nursing profession (Fawcett, 2005; Fawcett & DeSanto-Madeya, 2012).

Since the metaparadigm's creation, various nurse scholars have proposed additional concepts that should be included, such as the concepts of caring. Newman et al. (1991, p. 3) even asserted that "nursing is the study of caring in the human health experience." However, others have expressed concern that "caring is relatively underdeveloped as a concept, has not been clearly explicated, and often lacks relevance for nursing practice" (Morse, Bottorff, Neander, & Solberg, 1991, p. 119). Watson (2011) conceptualized caring as a value and ideal that also encompasses a "philosophy of action" (p. 32).

At least five conceptualizations of caring have been identified: a human trait, a moral imperative, an affect, an interpersonal interaction, and a therapeutic intervention (Morse et al., 1991). Caring seems to be part of content and relationship (Knowlden, 1991) and associated with varying outcomes, such as the client's physical response and the client's or nurse's subjective experience (Morse et al., 1991). When effective, some concepts (including care) can be directly measured using empirical indicators that take the form of clinical practice tools (Fawcett & DeSanto-Madeya, 2012) (such as the McGill pain rating scale) or research instruments.

Meleis (2007, 2012) offered a different approach to the nursing paradigm and proposed the following seven central concepts:

1. **Nursing client:** Recipient of professional nursing services.
2. **Transitions:** Changes in health status, role relationships, expectations, or abilities.
3. **Interaction:** Instrument for assessment and constructing relationships.
4. **Nursing process:** Steps that nurses use to deliver services, including assessment, diagnosis, planning, implementation, and evaluation.
5. **Environment:** Not well defined, but relates to the setting, context, and properties or dimensions of the world that affect human health (see Chapter 6, "Nursing Models and Theories," for various nursing approaches to this concept).
6. **Nursing therapeutics:** Deliberate nursing activities and actions nurses use while caring for clients.
7. **Health:** Goal of nursing services, but not limited to the absence of disease (see Chapter 6, "Nursing Models and Theories," for various nursing approaches to this concept).

Because of their abstract nature, concepts can pose problems within a single discipline or across disciplines. Other issues arise when a particular phenomenon is incompletely understood or lacks procedures to explain or measure it (Fawcett & DeSanto-Madeya, 2012; Meleis, 2007; Rogers, 2005). Because the profession of nursing is highly complex and has various specialty areas of practice, attaining a "single" definition for nursing concepts is extremely difficult. At present, in the absence of a consensus on definitions for the concepts of human beings, environment, health, and nursing, multiple definitions coexist (see Chapter 6, "Nursing Models and Theories").

Theories and Theoretical Frameworks

A theoretical or conceptual framework has been defined as "a logical grouping of related concepts or theories" (Chinn & Kramer, 1999, p. 258). A model is composed of abstract and general concepts and propositions that are linked together in a distinctive way. Fawcett (2000, p. 16) stated that a conceptual model "provides a unique focus that has a profound influence on individuals' perceptions." Theoretical frameworks provide guidance and direction for nursing research endeavors (Meleis, 2007, 2012). Rogers (2005) distinguished theoretical frameworks from theories in that the theoretical framework is broader than a theory and typically has not been validated through scientific testing. Theoretical frameworks tend to address phenomena that are more global in nature. Developing theoretical frameworks for nursing ensures practice that considers the complex nature of profession. Nurses who use theoretical frameworks in professional practice typically have some sort of method to provide holistic care rather than just focusing on client physiologic issues.

Theories communicate links or relationships among concepts in an organized, coherent, and systematic way and vary in levels of abstraction and scope (Fawcett & DeSanto-Madeya, 2012; Meleis, 2012). Theories symbolize reality and can either be discovered or invented (Meleis, 2012). Meleis (2007, p. 37) specified that theories can describe, explain, predict, or prescribe phenomena, including relationships, events, situations, responses, or conditions. Fawcett (2005) explained that propositions are statements that either define or describe a concept (nonrelational) or specify a relationship or linkage between multiple concepts. Grand theories for professional nursing provide a broad characterization of the profession and typically are highly abstract. Thus, they fail to provide specific information to guide research and clinical practice (Fawcett, 2005; Meleis, 2007, 2012; Rogers, 2005; Walker & Avant, 2011). When theories become able to describe, explain, or predict certain relationships between or among concepts, nursing scholars categorize them as middle-range theories, which serve as theoretical frameworks for nursing research and practice (Fawcett & DeSanto-Madeya, 2012; Meleis, 2012; Rogers, 2005; Walker & Avant, 2011). Sometimes, theories can be used for a specific clinical practice situation or to guide a particular research project. Because of the narrow focus in these situations, some nurse scholars refer to these theories as clinical practice theories or microtheories (Peterson & Bredow, 2017). Theories help nurses understand how and why the phenomena of nursing are associated with one another. For example, the gate theory of pain proposes that there is a progression of nerve impulse transmissions from a noxious stimulus outside or within the body that must occur prior to the ability of a person to perceive pain. The impulse transmission may be interrupted if the nerve pathways cannot receive the painful stimulus. A nurse using this theory recognizes that the application of cold or heat to a body part can interrupt the nerve transmission thereby reducing or perhaps even eliminating the patient's perception of pain.

Theories in nursing may be unique to the discipline of nursing, or borrowed from or shared with another discipline that has interest in similar human phenomena (Fawcett, 2000; Meleis, 2007, 2012; Peterson & Bredow, 2017). For example, the concept of self-esteem is borrowed from the field of psychology but plays a key role when nurses establish therapeutic relationships with clients and interprofessional relationships with members of the health care team (see Chapter 4, "Establishing Helping and Healing Relationships"). Before questioning a physician's order, the nurse must have the self-esteem to have confidence in his or her knowledge of pharmacology in order to avoid a serious event for a client. After successfully confronting the situation, the nurse's self-esteem becomes enhanced because he or she did the right thing.

Effectiveness in practice is directly related to the ability to understand, describe, explain, and anticipate human responses concerning health. Theoretically based professional practice enables nurses to anticipate client complications before they occur and determine the best approaches to use in specific client care situations.

Models for Nursing

Several nurse scientists have proposed individual and distinctive models about the interrelationships of concepts that form the nature and processes of nursing. Each nurse scholar who has proposed a conceptual model has based the model on empirical observation, intuitive insights, or deductive reasoning "that creatively combine[s] ideas from several fields of inquiry" (Fawcett, 2000, p. 16). Although they may present diverse views of nursing phenomena, each conceptual model is useful for professional nursing because of the organization it provides for thinking, observing, and interpreting in nursing practice. Some **nursing conceptual models** provide an illustrative diagram to depict relationships among concepts (see, e.g., Fig. 1.1 in Chapter 1, "The Professional Nurse"; Chapter 6, "Nursing Models and Theories" for a discussion of selected conceptual models). Nursing conceptual models identify the interventions that nurses use in practice while explaining the four central concepts of nursing: human beings, environment, health, and nursing (Fawcett, 2005; Fawcett & DeSanto-Madeya, 2012; Meleis, 2007, 2012; Rogers, 2005; Walker & Avant, 2011).

Summary and Significance to Practice

Because of the complexity of client care, nurses use a variety of methods of knowing when they provide professional nursing services. Nursing science encompasses more than the physiologic aspects of client care. Most nurses encounter practice situations in which they rely on personal and ethical knowing to make effective clinical judgments and decisions. Understanding and appreciating the patterns of knowing in nursing sharpen the cognitive skills of professional nurses as they engage in daily practice.

Most nursing scholars have a general agreement on the central concepts of the discipline of nursing. The central concepts help to describe the phenomenon of professional nursing practice and guide nurses in clinical practice, research endeavors, and educational programs. Explication of the central concepts and tenets of professional nursing remain a challenge because of the various approaches to patterns of knowing available to nurses in the postmodern era.

REAL-LIFE REFLECTIONS

Remember Paul, from the beginning of the chapter? What suggestions would you give him as he explores the phenomenon of nursing intuition as the topic of his class research project? How do you think Paul would respond to each of your points? What are the consequences of having a narrowly defined perception of what constitutes nursing knowledge?

From Theory to Practice

1. How do you use the empirical, aesthetic, personal, and ethical ways of knowing in your professional practice? How do your attitudes about the ways of

knowing affect your professional practice? Why are the ways of knowing important for professional nurses?

2. How has reading this chapter affected your views about nursing science and nursing theory?

Nurse as Author

Write an essay about six ways of knowing in your clinical practice. Define each identified way of knowing before you convey information about how you use it in practice. Specify the advantages of using various forms of knowing in your professional or student nursing practice.

Your Digital Classroom

Online Exploration

Nursing Knowledge International: **http://www. nursingknowledge.org/Portal/main.aspx**
Virginia Henderson International Nursing Library: **http://www.nursinglibrary.org/vhl/**

Expanding Your Understanding

Go online and read the article by Angela Hall: Hall, A. (2005). Defining nursing knowledge. NursingTimes. net, 101(48). Available at: **https://www.nursing-times.net/roles/nurse-educators/defining-nurs-ing-knowledge/203491.article**. Answer the following questions and bring the answers to these questions along with your own questions to class.

1. What constitutes nursing knowledge?
2. How is nursing knowledge used in nursing practice and education?
3. How are nurses held accountable for nursing knowl-edge?
4. Provide two examples of how theoretical knowledge differs from practice knowledge.
5. What was done to this article prior to its publication that makes this a reliable, professional reference?

Beyond the Book

Visit **thePoint®** **www.thePoint.lww.com** for activi-ties and information to reinforce the concepts and con-tent covered in this chapter.

REFERENCES

Baghramian, M., & Adam, C. J. (2016). In E. N. Zalta (Ed.), *"Rel-ativism", The Stanford Encyclopedia of Philosophy (Spring 2016* *Edition).* Retrieved from http://plato.stanford.edu/archives/spr2016/entries/relativism/. Accessed on September 25, 2016.

Belenky, M. F., Clinchy, B. M., Goldberger, N. R., & Tarule, J. M. (1986). *Women's ways of knowing: The development of self, voice and mind.* New York: Basic Books.

Benner, P., & Tanner, C. (1987). Clinical judgment: How expert nurses use intuition. *American Journal of Nursing, 87,* 23–31.

Bertalanffy, L. V. (1968). *General system theory.* New York: Braziller.

Campbell, J. C., & Bunting, S. (1991). Voices and paradigms: Perspectives on critical and feminist theory in nursing. *Advances in Nursing Science, 13,* 1–5.

Carnago, L., & Mast, M. (2015). Using ways of knowing to guide emergency nursing practice. *Journal of Emergency Nursing, 41,* 387–390.

Carper, B. A. (1978). Fundamental patterns of knowing in nurs-ing. *Advances in Nursing Science, 1,* 13–23.

Carper, B. A. (1992). Philosophical inquiry in nursing: An appli-cation. In J. F. Kikuchi & H. Simmons (Eds.), *Philosophic inquiry in nursing.* Newbury Park, CA: Sage.

Chinn, P. L. (1994). Developing a method for aesthetic knowing in nursing. In P. L. Chinn & J. Watson (Eds.), *Art and aes-thetics in nursing.* New York: National League for Nursing.

Chinn, P. L., & Kramer, M. K. (1999). *Theory and nursing: Integrated knowledge development* (5th ed.). St. Louis, MO: Mosby-Year Book.

Chinn, P. L., & Kramer, M. (2011). *Integrated theory and knowl-edge development in nursing* (8th ed.). St. Louis, MO: Elsevier Mosby.

Chinn, P. L., & Kramer, M. (2015). *Integrated theory and knowl-edge development in nursing* (9th ed.). St. Louis, MO: Mosby.

Doering, L. (1992). Power and knowledge in nursing: A feminist poststructuralist view. *Advances in Nursing Science, 14,* 24–33.

Dreyfus, H., & Dreyfus, S. (1985). *Mind over machine: The power of human intuition and expertise in the era of the computer.* New York: Macmillan Free Press.

Fawcett, J. (2000). *Analysis and evaluation of contemporary nursing knowledge: Nursing models and theories.* Philadelphia, PA: F.A. Davis.

Fawcett, J. (2005). *Contemporary nursing knowledge: Analy-sis and evaluation of nursing models and theories* (2nd ed.). Philadelphia, PA: F. A. Davis.

Fawcett, J., & DeSanto-Madeya, S. (2012). *Contemporary nursing knowledge: Analysis and evaluation of nursing models and theo-ries* (3rd ed.). Philadelphia, PA: F.A. Davis.

Fawcett, J., Watson, J., Neuman, B., Walker, P. H., & Fitzpat-rick, J. J. (2001). On nursing theories and evidence. *Journal of Nursing Scholarship, 33,* 115–119.

Fry, S. T. (1989). Toward a theory of nursing ethics. *Advances in Nursing Science, 11,* 9–22.

Garrett, B. M., & Cutting, R. (2014). Ways of knowing: Real-ism, non-realism nominalism & a typology revisited with a counter perceptive for nursing science. *Nursing Inquiry, 22*(2), 95–105, doi: 10.1111/nin.12070.

Hazy, J., Goldstein, J., & Lichtenstein, B. (2007). *Complex sys-tems leadership theory: New perspectives from complexity science on social and organizational effectiveness.* Mansfield, CT: ISCE Publishing.

Heisenberg, W. (1971). *Physics and beyond.* New York: Harper & Row.

Holmes, C. A., & Warelow, P. J. (2000). Some implications of postmodernism for nursing theory, research, and practice. *Canadian Journal of Nursing Research, 32,* 89–101.

Kearney, M. (2015). Ways of knowing: A guide to the journal and clinical discipline needs. *Research in Nursing & Health, 38,* 97–99. doi: 10.1002/nur.21649.

Knowlden, V. (1991). Nurse caring as constructed knowledge. In R. M. Neil & R. Watts (Eds.), *Caring and nursing: Explorations in feminist perspectives.* New York: National League for Nursing.

Kuhn, T. (1970). *The structure of scientific revolutions* (2nd ed.). Chicago: University of Chicago Press.

Laudan, L. (1981). A problem solving approach to scientific growth. In I. Hacking (Ed.), *Scientific revolutions.* Oxford: Oxford University Press.

Linberg, C., Nash, S., & Linberg, C. (2008). *On the edge: Nursing in the age of complexity.* Bordentown, NJ: Plexus Press.

Marecek, J. (1995). Gender, politics, and psychology's ways of knowing. *American Psychologist, 50,* 162–163.

Meleis, A. (1997). *Theoretical nursing: Development and progress* (3rd ed.). Philadelphia, PA: Lippincott.

Meleis, A. (2007). *Theoretical nursing: Development & progress* (4th ed.). Philadelphia, PA: Lippincott Williams & Wilkins.

Meleis, A. (2012). *Theoretical nursing: Development & progress* (5th ed.). Philadelphia, PA: Wolters-Kluwer Health/ Lippincott Williams & Wilkins.

Mitchell, G. J. (1994). Intuitive knowing: Exposing a myth in theory development. *Nursing Science Quarterly, 7,* 2–3.

Moch, S. D. (1990). Personal knowing: Evolving research and practice. *Scholarly Inquiry for Nursing Practice, 4,* 155–170.

Morse, J. M., Bottorff, J., Neander, W., & Solberg, S. (1991). Comparative analysis of conceptualizations and theories of caring. *Image, 23,* 119–126.

Munhall, P. L. (1993). "Unknowing": Toward another pattern of knowing in nursing. *Nursing Outlook, 41,* 125–128.

Newman, M. A., Sime, A. M., & Corcoran-Perry, S. A. (1991). The focus of the discipline of nursing. *Advances in Nursing Science, 14,* 1–6.

Nicolas, T., & Philippe, B. (2015). In E. N. Zalta (Ed.), "Propositional Dynamic Logic", *The Stanford Encyclopedia of Philosophy (Spring 2015 Edition).* Retrieved from http://plato.stanford.edu/archives/spr2015/entries/logic-dynamic/. Accessed on September 25, 2016.

Perry, W. G. (1970). *Forms of intellectual and ethical development in the college years.* New York: Holt, Rinehart and Winston.

Peterson, S., & Bredow, T. (2017). *Middle range theories application to nursing research and practice* (4th ed.). Philadelphia, PA: Wolters Kluwer.

Reed, P. G. (1995). A treatise on nursing knowledge development for the 21st century: Beyond postmodernism. *Advances in Nursing Science, 17,* 70–84.

Reed, P. G. (2011). The spiral path to nursing knowledge. In P. G. Reed & N. B. Crawford Shearer (Eds.), *Nursing knowledge and theory innovation: Advancing the science of practice.* New York: Springer Publishing.

Rew, L. (1996). *Awareness in healing.* Albany, NY: Delmar.

Rogers, M. E. (1970). *An Introduction to the theoretical basis of nursing.* Philadelphia, PA: F.A. Davis.

Rogers, M. E. (1992). Nursing science and the space age. *Nursing Science Quarterly, 5,* 27–34.

Rogers, B. L. (2005). *Developing nursing knowledge philosophical traditions and influences.* Philadelphia, PA: Lippincott Williams & Wilkins.

Roy, C. (2007). Advances in nursing knowledge and the challenge for transforming practice. In C. Roy & D. Jones (Eds.), *Nursing Knowledge Development and Clinical Practice.* New York: Springer.

Sarvimaki, A. (1995). Aspects of moral knowledge in nursing. *Scholarly Inquiry for Nursing Practice, 9,* 343–358.

Sitzman, K., & Watson, J. (2014). *Caring science, mindful practice, implementing Watson's human caring theory.* New York: Springer Publishing Company, LLC.

Spradlin, W. W., & Porterfield, P. B. (1984). *The search for certainty.* New York: Springer-Verlag.

Stumpf, S. E. (1993). *Socrates to Sartre: A history of philosophy* (5th ed.). New York: McGraw-Hill.

Sweeney, N. M. (1994). A concept analysis of personal knowledge: Application to nursing education. *Journal of Advanced Nursing, 20,* 917–924.

Walker, L. O., & Avant, K. C. (2011). *Strategies for theory construction in nursing* (5th ed.). Boston, MA: Prentice Hall.

Ware, C. F., Panikaar, K. M., & Romein, J. M. (1966). *History of mankind, cultural and scientific development: Vol. 6.* The twentieth century. New York: Harper & Row.

Watson, J. (1999). *Postmodern nursing and beyond.* Edinburgh: Churchill Livingstone.

Watson, J. (2007). *Nursing human science and human care: A theory of nursing.* Sudbury, MA: Jones & Bartlett.

Watson, J. (2011). *Nursing: Human science and human care.* Sudbury, MA: Jones & Bartlett.

West, B. (2006). *Where medicine went wrong: Rediscovering the path to complexity.* Singapore: World Scientific.

White, J. (1995). Patterns of knowing: Review, critique, and update. *Advances in Nursing Science, 17,* 73–86.

Nursing Models and Theories

LEARNING OUTCOMES

By the end of this chapter, the learner will be able to:

1. Compare and contrast systems, adaptation, caring, and complexity theories.
2. Outline differences in how nursing's metaparadigm concepts are defined in each of the nursing models presented.
3. Explain the key differences among rote, stereotypical, and theoretically based nursing practice.
4. Identify assumptions in the various nursing models presented in the chapter.
5. Determine the strengths and weaknesses of current nursing models and theories.
6. Provide an example of how each presented nursing model and theory might be applied to a clinical practice situation.

REAL-LIFE REFLECTIONS

Nicole and Brianna are two nurses working the night shift. Tonight, Ms. Green uses the call light every 5 minutes because she cannot sleep. Her nurse, Nicole, asks Brianna for help because Brianna always seems to know just what to do. Ms. Green is asleep after Brianna spends 5 minutes with her. Nicole asks, "How do you always know how to help restless patients?" Brianna shares her knowledge about Parse's human becoming theory, emphasizing being truly present with clients. Brianna also summarizes key concepts and approaches presented by other nursing theorists that she learned in her undergraduate nursing program. She mentions that although she prefers to use Parse's model, she finds that other nursing models help in different client care situations.

The discipline of nursing is highly complex. A **metaparadigm** may be defined as a recognizable pattern or model that provides a foundation for a particular discipline used as an overarching framework to describe key organizing concepts related to the field. Over the years, most nursing scholars have adopted the following four key concepts to serve as a metaparadigm: human beings (recipients of nursing care), environment (physical and social), health (a process or state), and nursing (goals, roles, and functions) (Fawcett, 2005). The term metaparadigm comes from the Greek "meta," which means more comprehensive or transcending, and the Greek "paradigm," which means an overall concept accepted by most people in an intellectual community (Agnes, 2005). Hardy (1978) introduced the idea of paradigms to the nursing profession as a means to offer a comprehensive description and possibly a method of unifying the profession (Fawcett, 2005; Meleis, 2007, 2012; Rodgers, 2005; Roy, 2007).

All existing nursing models and theories address these four concepts. In fact, four of the models presented in this chapter contain the word "human" in their titles. Each model also takes a different philosophical view of the world. Although nursing models and theories vary according to philosophical worldviews, all flow from the metaparadigm of professional nursing.

> **Take Note!**
> Most nursing scholars have adopted the following four key concepts to serve as a metaparadigm of professional nursing: human beings (recipients of nursing care), environment (physical and social), health (a process or state), and nursing (goals, roles, and functions).

NURSING MODELS

Prior to 1950, the writings of Florence Nightingale served as the primary source of nursing theory, and nursing science was derived principally from social, biologic, and medical science theories. Nursing science began to emerge as a part of the profession in the 1950s and continues to flourish today. Some nursing theories and models arose when nurses tried to generate a clear, concise definition of nursing; others arose from the need to demonstrate that what nurses do makes a difference in client outcomes.

A model provides a way to visualize reality and simplify thinking. For example, a spaceship model provides a representation of a spaceship. A **conceptual model** gives structure to and shows how various concepts are interrelated. Conceptual models serve as a foundation for theory development; they can also apply theories to predict or evaluate consequences of alternative actions. According to Fawcett (2000), a conceptual model "gives direction to the search for relevant questions about the phenomena of central interest to a discipline and suggests solutions to practical problems" (p. 16). **Nursing models** tend to be more abstract than nursing theory.

Nursing Theory

Chinn and Kramer (2011) defined **theory** as "a creative and rigorous structuring of ideas that project a tentative, purposeful, and systematic view of phenomena" (p. 185). Professional nurses apply concepts, principles, and theories from many disciplines. For example, nurses use physics when placing cardiac electrodes, pharmacology when monitoring results of administered medications, psychology when providing emotional support, microbiology when using aseptic technique, family theory when assessing effective mother–infant bonding, and human development theory when caring for clients of all ages. However, these borrowed theories and principles fail to capture the essence of professional nursing. Theories create a different way of looking at a particular phenomenon by interrelating concepts in a logical manner and provide a framework for describing, explaining, and predicting practice. They also provide a relatively simple yet generalizable view for testable hypothesis development. Once validated through research, theories expand discipline-specific knowledge while identifying other questions for future investigation. Sometimes, research provides evidence for nursing scholars to revise conceptual models and theories. In addition, new advances in clinical management of disease may be the stimulus for refinement of current models and theory or for the development of new ones.

Many nurses base their practice on traditions, experience, or "how I learned it in nursing school." These methods lead to rote and stereotypical practice. Nurses rely on memorization and habit when engaging in rote practice. Rote practice enables nurses to provide care while in an "autopilot" or robotic mode. When nurses use long-standing traditions and incorporate the expectations of others in practice, they engage in stereotypical practice. In the stereotypical practice mode, nurses try to fulfill expectations others may have of them, such as following physician orders without question or willingly assuming the role of the self-sacrificing "angel of mercy."

However, practice based on models or theories allows for hypotheses about practice, which make it possible to derive rationales for nursing actions. When using a specific nursing model or theory, nurses use concepts and relationships to direct client assessments and interventions. Testable theories provide a knowledge base for the science of nursing. As the science of nursing develops, nurses are able to understand and explain events more accurately and provide a basis for predicting and controlling future events. In addition, practice based on science fosters the recognition of nursing as a professional discipline. Looking at the philosophical differences that underlie nursing models and theories helps to explain why they vary in approaches to professional practice.

▇ QUESTIONS FOR REFLECTION

1. How do you rely on family traditions and personal experience when you fall ill or care for a family member?
2. How do you rely on traditions and personal experience when you practice nursing?
3. What consequences have resulted when you used traditions to guide your nursing practice?
4. What is your attitude toward nursing models and theories? Why do you feel this way?

Categories of Nursing Models and Theories

Nursing models and theories categories represent the depth and breadth of how they are used to guide practice, education and research. Theories may either predict or explain phenomena. Nursing theories can also be classified according to their level of abstractness with the most abstract representing the broadest level of theory. When a set of interrelated concepts are linked together and form a visual diagram or picture, a conceptual model has been developed. The Hood Professional Nurse Contributions Model and the Massachusetts Nurse of the Future Nursing Core Competencies serve as examples of conceptual models (see Chapter 1).

Grand theories in nursing articulate attempts to provide a perspective to guide or unite the entire nursing profession. Typically, they address the profession's nature, missions, and goals (Meleis, 2007, 2012). Peterson and Bredow (2017) describe middle-range nursing theories as possessing a narrower scope, addressing fewer, but more specific concepts and propositions; connecting to a particular or limited perspective of nursing; having enough structure to be empirically tested; and being concrete and specific enough for providing explanation to clinical phenomena and for use in clinical practice. Nursing scholars have generated numerous **middle-range theories** through deduction (fusing theoretical concepts and relationships from a grand theory to generate a more specific theory to guide practice), induction (analyzing what occurs in a practice setting and identifying key concepts and their relationships that is frequently done during qualitative research, see Chapter 10), generation by combining ideas, concepts, and relationships from other

disciplines of study (e.g. psychology, medicine, sociology); synthesizing research findings around particular nursing phenomena; and building theory from clinical practice guidelines (Peterson & Bredow, 2017).

Practice theory has been described as micro theory or situation-specific theory in the nursing literature. Practice theory is more concrete than the other forms of theory and frequently provide a theoretical approach to a specific clinical practice situation or a research study. Practice theory provides guidance for nurses encountering culturally diverse situations and specific clinical practice issues (Peterson & Bredow, 2017). Table 6.1 provides examples of some commonly used grand, middle, and practice-specific theories by professional nurses as they engage in clinical practice and nursing research.

This chapter presents the work of nine nursing theorists that provide a foundation for professional practice for individual nurses, nursing research studies, and nursing departments in many health care organizations (Fawcett, 2005; Meleis, 2007, 2012; Watson, 2007). The works selected present a multiplicity of philosophical worldviews to capture reader interest and stimulate dialogue about the essence of professional nursing. To distinguish differences among them, the models and theories have been classified according to the following criteria.

1. The worldview of change reflected by the model (growth or stability)
2. The major theoretical/conceptual classification with which the model seems most consistent (systems, stress/adaptation, caring, or growth/development)

Many nurses fail to appreciate nursing models and theories. Learning the essence of each model or theory, from original sources as much as possible, fosters an appreciation of the similarities and differences among them and identifies points of congruence with the worldviews on which each is based. Some nurse theorists coin words, define familiar words in different ways, and develop new concepts. This chapter clarifies the models, rather than critiquing them or selecting a single best model or theory for use. The selection of a nursing model or theory to guide practice is an individual decision. Interpretations of the professional nursing processes based on these models are presented in Chapter 7, "Professional Nursing Processes."

Take Note!

Nurses make individual decisions when selecting a nursing model or theory to guide their clinical practice.

TABLE 6.1 Examples of Nursing Conceptual Models: Grand, Middle, and Practice Theories Commonly Used by Nurses

Conceptual Models	Grand Theories
Johnson's Behavioral System Model (1959, 1990)	Nightingale's Environmental Model of Nursing (Chapter 2)
King's Systems Interaction Model (1968, 1981) (Chapters 6 and 7)	King's Theory of Goal Attainment (1981, 1996, 1997) (Chapters 6 and 7)
Levine's Conservation Model (1969, 1991)	Leininger's Theory of Culture Care and Universality (1978, 1988, 1995) (Chapter 11)
Neuman's System Model (1982, 1995) (Chapters 6 and 7)	Newman's Theory of Health as Expanding Consciousness (1990, 1994, 1997) (Chapters 6 and 7)
Rogers's Science of Human Beings (1980,1984) (Chapters 6 and 7)	Orem's Self-Care Deficit Theory (1983, 1987, 2000) (Chapters 6 and 7)
Roper-Logan Tierney Model of Nursing (1983, 1996)	Parse's Theory of Human Becoming (1981, 1987, 1992, 1998) (Chapters 6 and 7)
Roy's Adaptation Model (1971, 1999) (Chapters 6 and 7)	Watson's Human Caring Science, a Theory for Nursing (Chapters 6 and 7)
Hood's Professional Nurse Contributions Model (2010, 2014) (Chapter 1)	Peplau's Theory of Interpersonal Relations (Chapter 4)
Leddy's Human Energy Model, (2003, 2004, 2006) (Chapters 6 and 7)	Pender's Health Promotion Model (Chapter 8)

Middle-Range Theories	Practice Theories
Mercer's Maternal Role Attachment-Becoming a Mother Model (1986)	Baird's theory of well-being in refugee women during cultural transitions (2012)
Reed's Self-Transcendence Theory (1989)	Brennan's situation specific theory for crisis emergencies for individuals with severe, persistent mental illness (2012)
Eake, Burke, and Hainsworth Theory of Chronic Sorrow (1998, 2004, 2008)	Broussard's empowerment grounded theory in school nursing practice (2007)
Swanson's Theory of Caring (1991) (Chapter 6)	Bull and McShane's family caregiver perspectives for adults transitioning to adult day care services (2008)
Kolcaba's Theory of Comfort (1994, 2001, 2004)	Clingerman's situation specific theory of migration transitions for migrant farmworker women (2007)
Beck's Postpartum Depression Theory (1993)	Hopia, Paavilainen, and Åstedt-Kurki's practice theory on promoting health for families of children with chronic conditions (2004)
Mishel's Uncertainty in Illness Theory (1988, 1990, 1991, 1999)	Im's situation specific theory of the Caucasian cancer pain experience (2006)
Ray's Theory of Bureaucratic Caring (1989)	Im's situation specific theory of the Asian cancer pain experience (2008)
The American Association of Critical Care Nurses' Synergy Model for Patient Care (1998)	Im, Stuifbergen, and Walker's situation specific theory of midlife women's attitudes toward physical activity (2010)
Tsai's Caregiver Stress Theory (2003)	Lee, Fawcett, Yang, and Hann's practice theory identifying correlates of health promoting behaviors in Korean Americans at risk for or diagnosed with hepatitis b viral infection (2012)
Bergquist and King's Parish Nursing Theory (1994)	Nelson's situation specific theory of the breastfeeding experience for mother and infant (2006)
Weinert and Long's Rural Nursing Model (1991)	Riegel and Dickson's situation specific theory of heart failure self-care (2008)

Masters, K. (2015). *Nursing theories a framework for professional practice* (2nd ed.). Burlington, MA: Jones & Bartlett Learning; McEwen, M., & Wills, E. (2014). *Theoretical basis for nursing* (4th ed.). Philadelphia, PA: Wolters Kluwer Health/Lippincott Williams & Wilkins; Meleis, A. (2012). *Theoretical nursing: Development & progress* (5th ed.). Philadelphia, PA: Wolters-Kluwer Health/Lippincott Williams & Wilkins; and Peterson, S., & Bredow, T. (2017). *Middle range theories application to nursing research and practice* (4th ed.). Philadelphia, PA: Wolters Kluwer.

Growth and Stability Models of Change

Two basic philosophical worldviews exist about the nature of change. Although change remains constant, perceptions of change differ among people. Fawcett (1989) posited two worldviews, each based on its perceptions of change. One worldview recognizes change as continuous, a desired opportunity for growth to attain maximum human potential. The other worldview is persistence, which maintains that humans strive for stability and that endurance results from "a synthesis of growth and stability" (Fawcett, 1989, p. 12). The persistence worldview focuses on continuing and maintaining patterns by emphasizing balance and equilibrium. Although the worldviews differ, they are not mutually exclusive. The selected nursing models in this chapter approach change differently, which provides a means to classify them.

■ QUESTIONS FOR REFLECTION

1. Which worldview seems more compatible with your personal philosophy—change or persistence? Why?
2. Is it possible to embrace both worldviews? Why or why not?

THE STABILITY MODEL OF CHANGE

The **stability model of change** proposes that the natural order of things revolves around consistency.

Although change is inevitable and may be undesirable, it forces adaptation. Once the adaptive adjustment is complete, a state of stability results. Stability means that the organism attains a new and stable equilibrium.

Systems Theory

Systems theory addresses elements and interactions among all the factors (variables) in a situation. Interactions between the person and the environment occur continuously, thereby creating a complex, constantly changing situation. Systems theory provides a way to understand the many influences on the whole person and the possible impact of change on any part of the whole. This theory can help nurses to understand, predict, and control the possible effects of nursing care on the client system and the concurrent effects of the interaction on the nurse system and environment.

Auger (1976) defined a system as "a whole with interrelated parts, in which the parts have a function and the system as a totality has a function" (p. 21). Within the systems framework, single systems (subsystems) form more complex systems (suprasystems) (Fig. 6.1). Subsystems may be smaller than the tiniest cell of an organism. Suprasystems extend beyond what humans know as the universe.

Humans are composed of cells, organs, and physiologic systems. These subsystems are continuously interacting and changing. For example, as a person eats, the blood supply to the gastrointestinal organs increases.

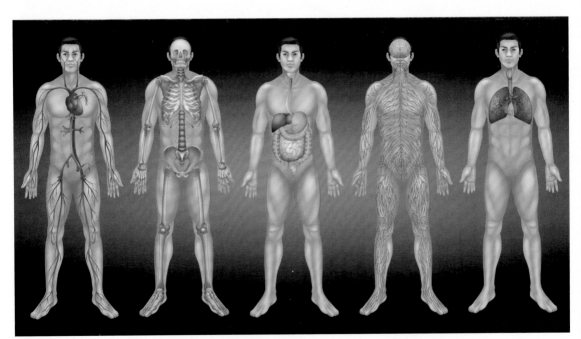

FIGURE 6.1 The human body with its multiple interactive systems provides an example of systems theory.

Absorption of carbohydrates increases the blood glucose level, which results in increased insulin secretion. Simultaneously, changes in the blood circulation and blood glucose level affect the person's attention level and the feeling of hunger. The person may feel satisfied and contented.

The whole person is the suprasystem for multiple interacting subsystems. The person's internal environment consists of interacting subsystems that are contained within bodily boundaries. The person, in turn, will have membership in a subsystem called family (which is a suprasystem of the person, which is a subsystem of the community system, and so on). Subsystems may be isolated for study, but humans are more than and different from the sum of their parts (Rogers, 1970).

A person cannot be characterized by describing physiologic, psychological, and sociocultural subsystems. A person's behavior is holistic, a reflection of the person as a whole. The focus of systems theory is on understanding the interaction among the various parts of the system, rather than on describing the function of the parts themselves (Auger, 1976). Systems analysis assumes that structure and stability can be measured during an arbitrarily frozen period.

Factors from the environment impinge on the system across the system boundary. These factors cause tension, stress, strain, or conflict that may upset system balance. The system seeks equilibrium, or a steady state, in which a balance exists among the various forces operating within and on the system. Change is a process of tension reduction and dynamic equilibrium, which restores a new position of system balance after a disturbance (Chin, 1976).

Because they are open systems, people exchange matter, energy, and information with the environment (Sills & Hall, 1977). A human being's internal environment interacts constantly with an ever-changing external environment. Changes occurring in one affect the other. For example, walking into a cold room (change in the external environment) affects various physiologic and psychological subsystems of the internal environment, which in turn reduces blood flow to the periphery, the ability to concentrate, and the feeling of comfort. Similarly, a person's angry outburst (change in the internal environment) may have a demonstrable effect on the moods of others. It is this openness of human systems that makes nursing intervention possible. Under general systems theory, nurses interact with clients to help them attain homeostasis, defined as the constancy of the internal environment caused by the action of regulatory mechanisms. Constancy

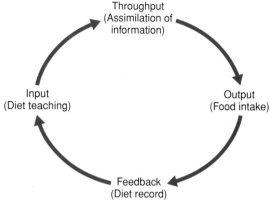

FIGURE 6.2 In this example of systems interaction, information about a therapeutic diet given to a client by the nurse is system input for the client system. What the client eats would be one type of system output, based on the throughput related to assimilation and acceptance of the information originally given. The nurse, using the client's reported food intake as feedback, can help reinforce or modify the client's future behavior.

does not mean that the internal environment is static, but rather that it is constantly changing to maintain its equilibrium. This relative equilibrium is maintained by homeodynamics (Cannon, 1932).

Energy, information, or matter provides system input. The system "transforms, creates, and organizes input in the process known as throughput, which results in a reorganization of the input" (Sills & Hall, 1977, p. 21). Thus, each system modifies its input. Simultaneously, energy, information, or matter is given off into the environment as output. When output is returned to the system as input, the process is known as feedback (Fig. 6.2).

A person can be viewed as "an interrelated, interdependent, interacting, complex organism, constantly influencing and being influenced by (the) environment" (Sills & Hall, 1977, p. 24). Because the person is in constant interaction with the environment, many interrelated factors, including the nurse, affect the person's health status. The person's response, in turn, results in environmental change. Thus, a change in any part affects the entirety of the human–environment system.

Using systems theory to guide nursing process directs assessment of the relationships among all variables that affect the client–environment interaction, including the influence of the nurse. While intervening, the nurse must anticipate the system-wide impact from change in any part of the system and appreciate the simultaneous, rather than cause-and-effect, nature of change in open systems.

Imogene King's Systems Interaction Model (Theory of Goal Attainment)

In her nursing model based on systems theory, King (1981, 1987, 1989) stressed interactions and mutuality. King developed her model when she was trying to outline essential content for a new graduate nursing program (King, 2001). According to **King's systems interaction model (theory of goal attainment)**, the purpose of nursing is to help people attain, maintain, or restore health, primarily by mutual goal setting. King described the nurse–patient interaction as transactional, which involves nurse–patient mutual understanding of events, mutually set goals, and agreement on means to achieve the goal.

King's (1989) model has its roots in sociology and focuses on "individuals whose interactions in groups within social systems influence behavior within the systems" (p. 152). King defined humans as "open systems interacting with environment" (King, 1981, p. 10) and as "rational, sentient, reacting, social, controlling, purposeful, time-oriented, and action-oriented" (King, 1987, p. 107). The human "perceives the world as a total person" (King, 1981, p. 141), resulting in environmental interactions to which he or she must constantly adjust. King (1981) delineated the environment as internal (within the body/person) and external. King proposed that the personal system underlies each person as a whole system who interacts with one or more persons, thereby creating interpersonal systems. When interpersonal systems expand to include large groups of people, social systems are developed. King (1999) emphasized that the three systems (personal, interpersonal, and social) interact with each other and "represent organized wholes in constant interaction in one's environment" (p. 292).

- In personal systems, perception is the comprehensive concept. It is "a characteristic of a human process of interaction and along with communication provides a channel for passage of information from one person to another" (King, 1989, p. 153). Concepts of self, growth and development, learning, body image, time, and space also relate to individuals as personal systems.
- In interpersonal systems, interaction is the comprehensive concept. Related concepts include communication, transactions, roles, stress, and all the concepts identified in personal systems.
- In social systems, organization is the comprehensive concept. Related concepts include power, authority, status, decision making, and control (King, 1989).

As people interact with their environment, their perceptions influence their behavior and health. Nurses interact with clients to facilitate achievement of mutually determined health-related goals.

> **Take Note!**
> According to King's systems interaction model (theory of goal attainment), the purpose of nursing is to help people attain, maintain, or restore health, primarily by mutual goal setting.

Health assumes achievement of maximum potential for daily living and an ability to function in social roles. It is the "dynamic life experiences of a human being, which implies continuous adjustment to stressors in the internal and external environment through optimum use of one's resources to achieve maximum potential for daily living" (King, 1981, p. 5). "Illness is a deviation from normal, that is, an imbalance in a person's biologic structure or in his psychological makeup, or a conflict in a person's social relationships" (King, 1989, p. 5).

"Nursing's domain involves human beings, families, and communities as a framework within which nurses make transactions in multiple environments with health as a goal" (King, 1996, p. 61). Nursing care is accomplished within goal-oriented nurse–client interactions "whereby each perceives the other and the situation, and through communications, . . . set goals, explore the means to achieve them, (and) agree to the means, and their actions indicate movement toward goal achievement" (King, 1987, p. 113).

King (1987, pp. 109–110) identified 10 concepts relevant to understanding the dynamic interacting systems delineated in her model.

1. **Interaction:** A process of perception and communication between person and environment and between person and person, represented by verbal and nonverbal behaviors that are goal directed
2. **Perception:** Each person's representation of reality
3. **Communication:** A process whereby information is given from one person to another
4. **Transaction:** An observable behavior of human beings interacting with their environment … (in which) valuation is a component of human interaction
5. **Role:** A set of behaviors expected of persons occupying a position in a social system
6. **Stress:** A dynamic state whereby a human being interacts with the environment to maintain balance for growth, development, and performance

7. **Growth and development:** Continuous change in individuals at the cellular, molecular, and behavioral levels of activities
8. **Time:** A continuous flow of events in successive order that implies change, a past, and a future
9. **Self:** A personal system defined as a unified, complex whole
10. **Space:** Existing in all directions and the same everywhere

In King's theory (1995), these concepts are interrelated in a number of propositions and hypotheses that indicate "the nature of nurse–client interactions that lead to goal attainment" (p. 27). Decision making (including goal setting) is "a shared collaborative process in which client and nurse give information to each other, identify goals, and explore means to attain goals; each moves forward to attain goals." This is identified in the theory as a critical independent variable called "mutual goal setting" (King, 1989, p. 155). From the theory, a transaction process model has been designed to lead to goal attainment when practiced (King, 1999). Examples of testable hypotheses generated from King's theory include the process of mutual goal setting with clients, the strengths of mutual goal setting, and role conflict between client and nurse in nursing situations (King, 1987).

King's model and the theory of goal attainment provide a "theoretical base for applying the traditional nursing process … aimed at maintaining or restoring health" (Magan, 1987, pp. 129, 132). King's model has provided the theoretical foundation for international nursing practice, nursing departments, nurse empowerment, and client satisfaction (Fawcett, 2005). Studies using King's model have been conducted internationally and include the areas of client decision-making processes, effectiveness of client education, relationships among family coping (including caregiver stress) and health, and effectiveness of nursing and interdisciplinary interventions (Alligood, 2010). King's model also serves as a theoretical foundation for nursing education (undergraduate and programs) and for nursing service departments (Fawcett, 2005). The King International Nursing Group was formed in 1998 and publishes an annual newsletter. Table 6.2 presents the major concepts of this model. Despite being originally conceptualized more than 25 years ago, King's model offers a systems approach that is compatible with the perception of health care delivery as a system with the goal of helping others to attain optimal health status while coping with internal and external stressors by using available resources. When working with persons

TABLE 6.2 Major Concepts as Defined in King's Model

Human being	A personal system that interacts with interpersonal and social systems
Environment	A context "within which human beings grow, develop, and perform daily activities" (King, 1981, p. 18)
Health	"Dynamic life experiences of a human being, which implies continuous adjustment to stressors in the internal and external environment through optimum use of one's resources to achieve maximum potential for daily living" (King, 1981, p. 5)
Nursing	A process of human interaction

recovering from substance abuse or receiving rehabilitation for an injury resulting in permanent disability, King's model provides a theoretical foundation for practice. The following Real-Life Reflection provides an example of how a nurse might use King's model.

REAL-LIFE REFLECTIONS

Ms. Green, the client at the opening of this chapter, has just learned from her physician that she has multiple myeloma (malignant tumor of the bone marrow resulting in abnormal production of plasma cells) and is devastated. She received the news alone and is terrified to break the news to her husband and grown son. Nicole goes to check on Ms. Green to see if she got her lunch and how she is eating. Ms. Green says that anytime she attempts to eat or drink, she chokes because she starts to cry. Nichole offers her an antianxiety pill, but Ms. Green tearfully refuses it and her lunch tray. A few minutes later, Brianna stops by to visit with Ms. Green. Ms. Green shares all of her concerns with Brianna. Brianna expresses concern about Ms. Green's refusal to eat or drink and informs her if she does not at least drink, then she will have to receive intravenous hydration. Brianna asks Ms. Green if she has a favorite food and discovered that she enjoys eating vanilla ice cream. Brianna suggests that Ms. Green should try and eat a small cup of ice cream and promises to get her all

(continued on page 140)

the ice cream that she can eat. Ms. Green laughs and agrees to eat some ice cream, but only if Brianna will stay with her in case she starts to cry. Brianna gets the ice cream and visits with Ms. Green as she eats an entire 4-oz cup.

- *What goals can you identify in these nurse–client interactions?*
- *What goals were attained and why were they attained?*

Betty Neuman's Systems Model

Betty Neuman also used systems theory to provide a foundation for her nursing model, known as Neuman's systems model. Neuman developed her model while attempting to help nursing students organize their thinking and look at clients holistically when teaching mental health nursing (Neuman, 2002). **Neuman's systems model** specifies that the purpose of nursing is to facilitate optimal client system stability by reducing the impact of environmental stimuli or stressors.

Neuman described human beings as having a core that is protected by buffering systems. The following four key concepts describe the interaction of human beings with environmental stressors that determine health status.

1. **Central core:** The basic structure and energy reserves of the human that make life possible
2. **Flexible lines of defense:** Adaptive responses that fluctuate and protect the core from stressor penetration
3. **Normal line of defense:** A conscious adaptation response usually used by an individual to protect the core from stressor penetration
4. **Lines of resistance:** Protection factors, usually unconscious in nature, activated when stressors have penetrated the normal line of defense

Neuman's model focuses on stress reduction, the impact of stress, and how stress and the individual's response to stress affect the development, maintenance, and restoration of health. People are composites of physiologic, psychological, sociocultural, developmental, and spiritual variables that act harmoniously and simultaneously when encountering stressors from either the internal or external environment. Neuman defined clients as individuals, families, groups, or communities who interact constantly with the environment.

Take Note!
Neuman's systems model specifies that the purpose of nursing is to facilitate optimal client system stability by reducing the impact of environmental stimuli or stressors.

The environment includes "all internal and external factors or influences surrounding the identified client or client system" (Neuman, 2002, p. 18).

- The internal environment is composed of interacting elements within the human body.
- The external environment consists of anything outside the human body.
- The created environment encompasses individual perceptions of the internal and external environments.

People constantly encounter stressors from the internal, external, or created environment. Stressors are tension-producing stimuli that have the potential to disturb a person's equilibrium or normal line of defense. This normal line of defense is the person's "usual steady state." It is the way in which an individual typically deals with stressors. Stressors may be positive (eustress) or negative (distress). Stressors may be of three types: intrapersonal (arising from within the person), interpersonal (arising between two or more people), or extrapersonal (arising from the external environment rather than other people).

According to Neuman (1982, 2002), a person's basic structure and energy resources need protection from encountered stressors. Reactions and resistance to stressors are provided by lines of defense. Neuman (1982, 2002) called the outermost line of defense the flexible line of defense. This dynamic protective buffer consists of physiologic, psychological, sociocultural, developmental, and spiritual variables affecting a person at any given moment. These variables may include a person's current physiologic state, mood, beliefs, cognitive state, nutritional status, spiritual beliefs, developmental state, and cognitive ability. If the flexible line of defense is no longer able to protect the person against a stressor, the normal lines of defense work to buffer the effects produced. The normal lines of defense encompass the usual response used by the person, such as exercise, health habits (e.g., basic hygiene), relaxation strategies, and conscious coping methods.

The final protections for the core are the lines of resistance. Examples of lines of resistance include immunologic responses and unconscious emotional defense mechanisms. Obvious reactions to stress become visible when lines of resistance are penetrated.

The reaction to stressors may lead to restoration of balance or to death. Three factors influence a person's reaction to and recovery from encountered stressors: the number and strength of the stressor(s) affecting the person, the length of exposure to the stressor(s), and the meaningfulness of the stressor(s) to the person.

Neuman (1996) intended for the nurse to "assist clients to retain, attain, or maintain optimal system stability" (p. 69). Thus, health (wellness) seems to be related to dynamic equilibrium of the normal line of defense, where stressors are successfully overcome or avoided by the flexible line of defense. Neuman (2002) defined illness as "a state of insufficiency with disrupting needs unsatisfied" (p. 25). Illness appears to be a separate state when a stressor breaks through the normal line of defense and causes a reaction with the person's lines of resistance.

Nurses use primary, secondary, or tertiary prevention to help clients attain optimal wellness. Primary prevention covers interventions to promote health. Secondary prevention occurs once a stressor has penetrated the normal lines of defense or lines of resistance (e.g., pain medication). Tertiary prevention focuses on restoration of balance (e.g., rehabilitation). When restoration is complete, nursing interventions return to primary prevention.

Neuman's systems model is compatible with the traditional medical model. It has been widely used internationally, especially by nurses in the Americas, Pacific Rim, and Europe. The model serves as the framework for the World Health Organization project "Nest of Love" and for delivery of mental health services in Holland (Lowry, 2004). The Neuman Systems Model Organization and Neuman Trustee Group promote utilization of the Neuman's systems model. Table 6.3 summarizes major concepts as defined in Neuman's model. By offering a systems approach, looking for ways to reduce the impact of stressors, and using prevention as intervention, the Neuman health care systems model remains a relevant approach to professional nursing practice. For example, stress has been identified as a major factor contributing to illness and inhibiting healing. Even some nursing students identify high levels of stress as a factor affecting academic performance. The Neuman's systems model provides ways for nurses to examine the level of stress in the lives of care recipients (and even themselves) and look for ways to reduce it as well as develop interventions to promote effective habits to strengthen the normal lines of defense. The following Real-Life Reflection provides an example of how a nurse might use the Neuman's systems model in clinical practice.

TABLE 6.3 Major Concepts as Defined in Neuman's Model

Human beings (client system)	A composite of physiologic, psychological, sociocultural, developmental, and spiritual variables in interaction with the internal and external environment
Environment	All internal and external factors of influences surrounding the client system
Health	A continuum of wellness to illness
Nursing	Prevention as intervention

REAL-LIFE REFLECTIONS

After seeing Brianna's success in using nursing theories as a foundation for her clinical practice, Nicole remembers learning about the Neuman's Systems Model of Nursing. The next day, Brianna is off and Nicole is assigned as Ms. Green's nurse. Upon entering Ms. Green's room, Nicole notices that Ms. Green has been crying again and her hands tremble as she takes her scheduled medications. As she reviews the medical and nursing care plans for the day, Nicole asks Ms. Green if she has any concerns. Ms. Green specifies that she continues to sleep poorly at night and states that she just wants to get a couple of hours of uninterrupted sleep. Nicole thinks of ways to create a quiet physical environment to help Ms. Green nap. Nicole's plan involves keeping the door closed, placing a note on the door for anyone who wants to enter the room to speak first with Nurse Nicole, telling persons wanting to enter the room to return in 3 hours after Ms. Green's nap, providing soft music in the room and informing staff to be quiet when they are close to Ms. Green's room. Nicole remembers how lack of sleep weakens the flexible and normal lines of defense and believes this is affecting Ms. Green's ability to cope with her cancer diagnosis. Ms. Green takes an uninterrupted 3-hour nap and then orders a large lunch that she completely consumes. She also confides in Nicole about how she might lose her

(continued on page 142)

job because of her illness and that she is afraid of dying because her mother died at the same age that she is now.

- *In this situation, how did Nicole use the Neuman's systems model to plan and implement nursing care for Ms. Green?*
- *Were there any unintended benefits that occurred in this nursing situation?*
- *What additional nursing interventions might Nicole consider for Ms. Green?*

Stress/Adaptation Theory as a Framework

In contrast to systems theory, stress and adaptation theories view change in terms of accommodation. People adjust to environmental changes to avoid disturbing a balanced existence. Adaptation theory provides a way to understand both how equilibrium is maintained and the possible effects of disturbed equilibrium. This theory has been widely applied to explain, predict, and control biologic (physiologic and psychological) responses of individuals and serves as traditional medical therapy.

Under stress/adaptation theory, a person's regulatory systems operate by way of compensation. Any change in the internal environment automatically initiates a response to minimize or counteract the change. For example, when the blood glucose level drops, the endocrine system responds with increased cortisol secretion, which decreases the rate at which cells use glucose and stimulates the conversion of amino acids into glucose. These compensatory actions cause the blood glucose level to increase. If it should increase above acceptable limits, insulin secretion would increase the rate of glucose uptake by cells, thus reducing the blood glucose level.

Compensation occurs continuously as the body adjusts to stimuli that tend to disturb equilibrium. Stimuli may be anything that creates change in the internal environment and thus places demands on the body to compensate. Examples of stimuli include changes in environmental temperature or sleep pattern, hunger, joy, and infection. Whether stimuli are beneficial or harmful, all require the body to adapt.

A person's ability to adapt to changes in life events may determine his or her potential for health or disease. One way people adapt is through coping mechanisms that aim "to master conditions of harm, threat, or challenge when a routine or automatic response is not readily available" (Monat & Lazarus, 1977, p. 8). Some regard coping methods primarily as psychological barriers when stimuli are perceived as threats. Thus, a person's reaction to stimuli involves cognitive appraisal and psychological coping methods, in addition to physiologic reactions. One of the best-known nursing models that uses adaptation theory is the model developed by Sister Callista Roy.

Callista Roy's Adaptation Model

Sister Callista Roy developed the **Roy's adaptation model** as a graduate nursing student when confronted with the challenge of defining nursing (Roy, 2002; Meleis, 2007, 2012). Although initially concerned with the focus and target of and indications for nursing care, the model has evolved to incorporate Roy's religious views (Meleis, 2007, 2012). In 2008, Roy (2008, 2011) specified that the philosophical view underlying her model is cosmic unity, which proposes that humans and the earth have three common patterns—"unity, diversity, and self-identity" (2011, p. 346)—and "integral relationships" (p. 139). She also incorporated the concept of veritivity, defined as "a common purposefulness of human existence," which translates into persons finding meaning in life (Meleis, 2007, 2012). Roy viewed purposefulness as meaning that "all persons and the earth have both unity and diversity; all are united in a common destiny; people find meaning in mutual relations with each other and the created world, and most often in acknowledging a creator or God-figure that is the common destiny or final union of all" (Roy, 2011, p. 346). Roy's adaptation model outlines the purpose of nursing as promoting a human being's adaptation in the four adaptive modes (listed below).

Roy used the following five key terms in her model.

1. **Stimulus:** Point of interaction of the human system and environment; stimulus produces a response
2. **Adaptive modes:** Ways in which people adapt (i.e., through physiologic needs, self-concept, role function, or interdependent relations)
3. **Classes of stimuli:** Focal (immediately confronting the person), contextual (all other stimuli present), and residual (nonspecific stimuli, such as beliefs or attitudes)
4. **Adaptation level:** Range of a person's ability to adapt and create changes in the integrated, compensatory, and compromised environments
5. **Coping:** Ways of responding to the changing environment

Roy organized her model around adaptive behaviors that encompass the set of processes by which humans adapt to environmental stimuli. The human being as a unified system is viewed as a "set of parts connected to function as a whole" (Roy & Andrews, 1999, p. 36) through homeostatic and homodynamic systems. Humans constantly interact with an ever-changing environment, and their ability to respond positively reflects their level of adaptation.

Environmental stimuli affect the human being. A focal stimulus is an environmental change that requires an immediate adaptive response from the person. Accompanying the focal stimulus are contextual stimuli (all other stimuli present) and residual stimuli (other relevant factors such as nonspecific stimuli), which mediate and contribute to the effect of the focal stimulus.

The pooled effect of the three classes of stimuli establishes a person's adaptation level. In turn, each individual's adaptation level determines a zone that indicates the range of additional stimulation that will have a positive or adaptive response. If additional stimuli fall outside the zone, the person cannot respond effectively and compromised adaptation ensues. Effective adaptation results in free energy available for use in subsequent adaptation to stimuli.

According to Roy and Roberts (1981, p. 56), "Coping refers to routine, accustomed patterns of behaviors to deal with daily situations as well as to the production of new ways of behaving when drastic changes defy the familiar responses." The two major coping mechanisms for individuals are the regulator subsystem, composed mainly of automatic neural, endocrine, and chemical activity, and the cognator subsystem, which includes cognitive–emotive channels and provides for perceptual and information processing, learning, judgment, and emotion (Andrews & Roy, 1986, p. 7).

In 2008, Roy redefined adaptation as the "process and outcome whereby thinking and feeling persons, as individuals or in groups, use conscious awareness and choice to create human and environmental integration" (p. 138). Roy (1987, 2011) identified the following dimensions of human adaptive modes: physiologic–physical, self-concept–group identity, role function, and interdependence. The desired result is a state in which conditions promote the person's goals, including survival, growth, reproduction, mastery, and personal and environmental transformations.

Health "is viewed in light of human goals and the purposefulness of human existence. The fulfillment of this purpose in life is reflected in becoming integrated and whole" (Roy & Andrews, 1999, p. 54). Thus, health is viewed as both "a state and a process of being and becoming an integrated and whole human being" (Roy & Andrews, 1999, p. 54).

The goal of nursing is "to promote adaptation in the four adaptation modes contributing to health, quality of life, and dying with dignity" (Roy, 2011, p. 346). Nursing assessment and intervention foster the goal of adaptation with the client's active participation. The criteria for goal attainment encompass generally any positive response by the individual that creates free energy that can be used for responding to other stimuli (Riehl & Roy, 1980).

Take Note!
The Roy's adaptation model outlines the purpose of nursing as promoting a person's adaptation in the four adaptive modes: physiologic needs, self-concept, role function, and interdependent relations.

Roy's model provides a classification system for stimuli that may affect adaptation, as well as a system for classifying nursing assessment. The model "has been useful in supporting the traditional concept of nursing practice within the medical model perspective" (Huch, 1987, p. 63). Roy's model has been widely used internationally, revealing its transcultural appeal. The Roy Adaptation Association has chapters in Japan, Columbia, and Mexico. Nurses use Roy's model as a framework for nursing education in baccalaureate and higher-degree programs, as a foundation for health assessment in clinical practice, and as guidance for application in nursing service departments. Roy also advocated the use of the model by other health care professionals (Roy, 2002; Fawcett, 2003). It has been used as a theoretical framework for the development of tools for research and clinical practice, including a foundation for electronic health documentation, development of nursing interventions to promote empowerment, enhanced spirituality, reduced child pain, and factors that influence adaptation and coping; determination of effective coping strategies with impaired activities of daily living; and quality of life in the elderly (Roy, Whetsell, & Frederickson, 2009). Table 6.4 summarizes the major concepts defined in Roy's model. Because of its global nature, the Roy's adaptation model applies across nearly all nursing practice areas, especially when the nurse wants to address recipient needs from a holistic perspective. One example of how a nurse might use the model in practice would be considering the hospitalization of a single-parent with small children. Because of Roy's emphasis on role function, the nurse would analyze the impact of the hospitalization

TABLE 6.4 Major Concepts as Defined in Roy's Model	
Human beings (human system)	"A whole with parts that function as a unity for some purpose" (Roy & Andrews, 1999, p. 31) that shares the patterns of "unity, diversity, and self-identity" (Roy, 2011, p. 346) with the earth. "Each individual contributes to the universe" (p. 346). Human systems include the family, organizations, communities, and global society (Roy, 2011)
Environment	"The world within and around humans as adaptive systems" (Roy & Andrews, 1999, p. 51) and any condition, situation, and influence that affects human behavior and development as an adaptive system
Health	"A state and process of being and becoming an integrated and whole human being" (Roy & Andrews, 1999, p. 54)
Nursing	Manipulation of stimuli to foster successful adaptation in physiologic needs, self-concept, role function, or interdependent relations

TABLE 6.5 A Comparison of Components of Caring	
Swanson's Caring Processes (1991)	**Koldjeski's (1990) Five "Essences" of Caring**
1. Knowing: Striving to understand an event as it has meaning in the life of another	1. Interpersonal valuing and involvement
2. Being with: Being emotionally present for another	2. Being there for and experiencing with another
3. Doing for: Doing for others as they would do for themselves if it were possible	3. Instilling faith
4. Enabling: Facilitating another's passage through life transitions and unfamiliar events	4. Concern and love for another
5. Maintaining belief: Sustaining faith in another's capacity to get through an event or transition and face a future with meaning	5. Actualization

on the parenting role and offer special support (assessing child-care needs, initiating social service consultation early, and making special arrangements so that the children might be able to visit the parent).

THE GROWTH MODEL OF CHANGE

Unlike the models discussed so far, which focus on achievement or restoration of stability, nursing models based on the **growth model of change** tend to focus on helping people grow to realize and attain their full potential. The models of nursing that espouse the growth model of change tend to use caring theory or complexity theory as an underlying framework.

Caring Theory as a Framework

Nursing practice focuses on **caring** for and about others. No single, universally accepted definition exists for caring in the nursing context, as it can be used as a verb or noun (e.g., "The nurse cared for the client," and "Nursing care was given"). Morse, Solberg, Neander, Bottorff, and Johnson (1990, p. 2) found that the literature includes references to care or caring as actions performed (as in to "take care of") as well as concern demonstrated (as in "caring about"). A literature analysis reveals at least five perspectives or categories of caring, including caring as a human trait (Benner & Wrubel, 1989; Gaut & Leininger, 1991), caring as a

moral imperative (Watson, 2007), caring as an interpersonal relationship (Parse, 1987), caring as a therapeutic intervention (Orem, 1980), and caring as an affect (Morse et al., 1990).

Clients perceive as caring "those nursing ministrations that are person-centered, protective, anticipatory, physically comforting, and that go beyond routine care" (Swanson, 1991, p. 161). Kyle (1995, p. 509) concluded that there is a "marked difference between the patients' and nurses' perceptions of caring, with the nurses focusing on the psychosocial skills and the patient on skills that demonstrate professional competency." Caring outcomes may be demonstrated in terms of either subjective experiences or objective client outcomes.

The concept of caring permeates the nursing literature and appears in many nursing models. Table 6.5 compares Swanson's and Koldjeski's theoretical components of caring. Orem's self-care deficit theory uses the term "care" primarily as action, whereas Watson used the term to describe an attitude or display of compassion that is a moral imperative for nurses.

QUESTIONS FOR REFLECTION

1. What characteristics do you identify when you have been the recipient of a caring interaction?
2. What results from a caring interaction between two people?
3. Why is caring an important aspect of professional nursing?

Dorothea Orem's Self-care Deficit Theory

According to **Orem's self-care deficit theory** (1980, 1985, 1990, 1995, 2001), the purpose of nursing is to help people meet their self-care needs. The theory focuses on persons "in society affected by human or environmental conditions associated with their states of health or their requirements for health care that result in inability to provide continuously for themselves the amount and quality of self-care they require" (Orem, 2001, p. 20). When the situation involves children, the nurse provides education and support to parents or guardians. Basically, Orem proposes that nurses do for others what they cannot do for themselves. She observed nurses as they engaged in clinical practice to develop the theory. Orem's theory uses the following five key concepts.

1. **Self-care:** Learned behaviors that a person performs for him- or herself (when able) that contribute to health
2. **Self-care deficit:** A relationship between actions that a person should take for healthy functioning and the capability for action
3. **Self-care requisites:** Needs that are universal or associated with development of or deviation from health
4. **Self-care demand:** Therapeutic actions to meet needs
5. **Agency:** Capability to engage in self-care

The essence of Orem's three-part nursing theory "focuses on a human being in relations. The theory of self-care focuses on the self, the I; the theory of self-care deficit focuses on you and me; and the theory of nursing systems focuses on we, human beings in community" (Orem, 1990, p. 49). Orem's theory integrates each of these theories (Orem, 1995, 2001).

Orem (1995) defined self-care as the "voluntary regulation of one's own human functioning and development that is necessary for individuals to maintain life, health, and well-being" (p. 95). People learn self-care activities as they mature. Culture, society, and family customs play key roles in determining individual self-care activities. Age, developmental state, or health status can affect the ability to perform self-care activities (e.g., parents or guardians must provide continuous care for infants and toddlers).

Orem (1980) specified that nursing is concerned with the individual's need for self-care action to "sustain life and health, recover from disease or injury, and cope with their effects" (p. 6). In Orem's view, nursing

care may be offered to individuals and groups. However, Orem emphasized that only people have self-care requisites. The nurse cares for, assists, or does something for the client to achieve client-desired health outcomes or to meet basic human needs (Orem, 1980, 1985, 1990, 1995, 2001).

> **Take Note!**
> According to Orem's self-care deficit theory, the purpose of nursing is to help people meet their self-care needs.

Orem (1985) implied that health is "a state of a human being that is characterized by soundness or wholeness of developed human structures and of bodily and mental functioning" (p. 179). Orem proposed that individual perception (well-being) affects health. In the self-care deficit theory, human health is a holistic concept.

Orem addressed the physical, psychological, interpersonal, and social aspects of health but indicated that they are inseparable in the human being: "Health describes the state of wholeness or integrity of human beings" (Orem, 1995, p. 96). "If there is acceptance of the real unity of individual human beings, there should be no difficulty in recognizing structural and functional differentiation within the unity" (Orem, 1980, p. 180). Orem viewed individuals as moving "toward maturation and achievement of the individual's human potential" (Orem, 1985, p. 180) rather than as organisms seeking a steady state.

Orem suggested that some people may have self-care requisites (needs) associated with development or health deviations. Self-care requisites are essential enduring needs, whereas other needs may surface because of internal or external conditions that alter the ability to care for oneself. Orem (1980) identified the following universal self-care requisites (p. 42).

1. Maintenance of sufficient air, water, and food intake
2. Provision of care associated with elimination processes and excrements
3. Maintenance of a balance between activity and rest and between solitude and social interaction
4. Prevention of hazards to life, functioning, and well-being
5. Promotion of human functioning and development within social groups in accord with potential, known limitations, and the desire to be normal

Identified self-care requisites require actions known as "therapeutic self-care demands." Therapeutic self-care demands can be determined by the following.

1. Identifying existing or potential self-care requisites.
2. Developing methods for meeting self-care requisites by considering basic factors (e.g., developmental state, general health status, living patterns) that "condition the values of patients' self-care agency and therapeutic self-care demands as well as the means that are valid for meeting self-care requisites and in regulating self-care agency at particular times" (Orem, 1985, p. 78).
3. Designing, implementing, and evaluating a plan of action. Orem tended to use nursing process as a way to develop a system of nursing.

The theory of nursing systems involves "an interpersonal unity at a particular time–space localization. This unity is formed by nurses, persons who have entered into an agreement to accept and participate in nursing, and the relatives or persons who are responsible for the individuals who require nursing" (Orem, 1990, p. 54). Thus, candidates for nursing care are clients who have insufficient current or projected capability for providing self-care. "It is the need for compensatory action (to overcome an inability or limited ability to engage in care) or action to help in the development or regulation of self-care abilities that is the basis for a nursing relationship" (Orem, 1980, p. 58). Other concepts and theories that have been derived from the self-care deficit theory include self-care agency, dependent care, and dependent care agency (Taylor, Geden, Isaramalai, & Wongvatunyu, 2000).

Orem's theory, which is compatible with the traditional medical model, has been widely used in international nursing practice, education, and research (Orem & Taylor, 2011). The International Orem Society publishes the *Self-Care and Dependent Care* nursing journal to promote and validate the use of the model. Table 6.6 summarizes the major concepts defined

TABLE 6.6 Major Concepts as Defined in Orem's Theory

Human being (patient)	A person under the care of a nurse
Environment	Physical, chemical, biologic, and social contexts (including the family) within which human beings exist
Health	"A state characterized by being structurally or functionally sound" (Orem, 2001, p. 96)
Nursing	An art by which practitioners provide specialized assistance to persons with disabilities who require special needs for self-care while participating in the medical plan of care outlined by physicians

in Orem's model. Unlike many of the nursing models and theories, Orem incorporates traditional medical approaches while carving out a unique place for nursing in health care delivery. In practice, Orem's nursing theory has been used as a framework for guiding nursing departments in acute and chronic care settings and health care utilization review programs (Meleis, 2007, 2012). Because Orem emphasizes that the nurse does for the person what he or she cannot do for him- or herself and teaches the patient and/or significant other how to care for the person, Orem's model fits nicely in practice settings in which nurses care for comatose patients, rehabilitation settings, and following any hospital or outpatient visit during which a procedure was performed (educating patients and significant others about how to monitor for complications and when to consult health care providers following the visit). The following Real-Life Reflection provides an example of how a nurse might use Orem's Self-Care Deficit Theory.

REAL-LIFE REFLECTIONS

Ms. Green has finished receiving her first round of chemotherapy and is going to be dismissed from the hospital. She and her husband need to learn about the potential complications of chemotherapy so that they can contact the oncologist if complications arise. Ms. Green's current occupation is manager of a retail clothing store. Using knowledge of basic management skills, Nicole offers suggestions for Ms. Green to chart her daily weight, temperature measurements, food and fluid intake, skin checks for bruising, and scales for rating pain, nausea, sore mouth, mood, and anxiety. Because Ms. Green has a computer at home, Nicole proposes that she develop a flow sheet to record these key assessments for chemotherapy-induced complications. Nicole also proposes that Ms. Green could record results of outpatient lab test results on the flow sheet. She also provides the Greens with medication cards about each of the chemotherapy agents administered, a list of currently ordered medications outlining actions, reasons, and potential side effects, and a dismissal information form specifying activity level, dietary restrictions, and the date for her outpatient follow-up with the oncologist. After reviewing all the information with Ms. Green, Nicole validates Ms. Green's understanding by having her answer a series of questions about medications, activity level, dietary restrictions, and when to contact the oncologist. Ms. Green gives Nicole a hug as she leaves and thanks her for giving her everything that she needed as an inpatient and as a person returning home.

- *Do you think that Nicole was aware that she could be practicing nursing using Orem's Self-Care Deficit Theory? Why or why not?*
- *Outline the factors for self-care covered in this nursing situation. Can you think of other things that Ms. Green might need for safe, effective self-care?*

Jean Watson's Human Caring Science, Theory of Nursing

Jean Watson developed Watson's human science and human care theory while writing a book about a bachelor of science (BSN)–integrated nursing curriculum (Fawcett, 2005; Watson, 2002b). Her work blends Eastern philosophy while representing phenomenologic, existential, and spiritual orientations. Watson proposed that the purpose of nursing is "to help persons gain a higher degree of harmony that fosters self-knowledge, self-reverence, self-caring, self-control, and self-healing processes while allowing increasing diversity" (Watson, 2012, p. 61). In 2012, Watson recognized that her human care theory seemed to be more of a science rather than a nursing theory. Key concepts of **Watson's Human Caring Science, Theory of Nursing** are the phenomenal field (the totality of past, present, and future influences on each human being), "carative" factors (what to do), "carative" processes (how to do), and transpersonal caring (a moral ideal and art). Transpersonal caring occurs when the caregiver and care receiver engage in "a human-spirit-to-spirit connection" (Watson, 2012, p. 85), during which occurs "a special kind of human care relationship—a connection/union with another person, a high regard for the whole person, and their being-in-the-world" forms (Watson, 2012, p. 75). Outcomes of the transpersonal caring interaction include "movement toward greater harmony, spiritual evolution, and omega point/perfection" (Watson, 2012, p. 83).

Watson (2007) stated, "Human life… is defined as (spiritual–mental–physical) being-in-the-world which is continuous in time and space" (p. 47). Although the soul, mind, and body are explicitly identified as spheres of the human being, they are viewed as integrated and inseparable until the time of death, when the soul transcends and continues to exist (Watson, 2012).

> **Take Note!**
> Watson's human science and human care theory proposed that the purpose of nursing is "to help persons gain a higher degree of harmony that fosters self-knowledge, self-reverence, self-caring, self-control, and self-healing processes while allowing increasing diversity."

Watson (2012) described health as "a subjective experience; it can refer to unity of body-mind-spirit" (p. 60). She expanded health to include congruency between the perceived self and the experienced self, and summarized health as "I = Me—Health (harmony, 'in right relation,' with self-world and open to increased diversity)" (Watson, 2012, p. 61). Illness is not always a disease, but rather a "subjective turmoil or disharmony within a person's inner self or soul at some level or disharmony with the person" (Watson, 2012, p. 62). Illness may cause disease. Diseases can be cured, but illness requires healing.

Watson viewed each human being as having a unique phenomenal field that encompasses "the totality of human experience as one's being-in-the-world" (Watson, 2007, p. 55). Although not equivalent to human consciousness, the phenomenal field is the entire constellation of internal and external factors that shape all human experiences (past, present, and future). She described human behavior as being goal directed with the aim of seeking harmony within body, mind, and soul, resulting in self-integration, enhancement, and actualization. When two or more persons come together, they share a phenomenal field and experience a transpersonal event. For a caring event to occur, the nurse and patient must each make a choice to enter the relationship. The nurse enters the experience of the patient and the patient enters into the experiences of the nurse.

Watson (2007) used the word "nurse" as a noun (a person caring for another) and a verb (actions related to caring for another). She described caring as "the moral ideal of nursing" (p. 54) consisting of "transpersonal human-to-human attempts to protect, enhance, and preserve humanity by helping a person find meaning in illness, suffering, pain, and existence; to help another gain self-knowledge, control, and self-healing wherein a sense of inner harmony is restored regardless of the external circumstance" (Watson, 2012, p. 72).

Caring is "a moral ideal, rather than an interpersonal technique" (Watson, 2007, p. 58), which can be demonstrated through the carative factors (nursing interventions) that "allow for contact between the subjective world of the experiencing persons" (Watson, 1989, p. 227). The following carative factors are all presupposed by a knowledge base and clinical competence (Watson, 2012, p. 47).

1. Humanistic-altruistic system of values
2. Faith–hope
3. Sensitivity to self and others
4. Helping–trusting, human care relationship
5. Expressing positive and negative feelings
6. Creative problem-solving caring processes
7. Transpersonal teaching–learning
8. Supportive, protective, and/or corrective mental, physical, sociocultural, and spiritual environment
9. Human needs assistance
10. Existential–phenomenologic–spiritual forces

During the human care process (nursing), the nurse and person engage in a mutual endeavor, a specific level of space and time. The nurse and client together embark on a journey to discover new meanings and understanding that require "serious study, reflection, and action" (Watson, 2007, p. 29). The nurse uses the carative factors to facilitate the human care process.

Watson's theory provides one framework for the study of caring that has served as the foundation for many nursing research studies across the world. Watson (2012) proposed that descriptive phenomenology along with transcendental or depth phenomenology and poetic results may be the most effective ways to generate evidence and knowledge about specific caring processes for professional nursing practice. Despite the abstract nature of caring, 18 instruments have been designed using the human science and human care theory as a theoretical approach to measure caring in studies related to patient satisfaction, nursing student perceptions of caring, intercollegial relationships among professional nurses, and caring behaviors of nursing faculty (Watson, 2002a). Smith (2004) outlined four categories addressed by nurse researchers using Watson's theory: the nature of nurse caring, client and nurse perceptions of the nurse caring experience, human experiences, and human caring needs. Nurses use Watson's theory to measure caring behaviors, attitudes, and efficacy; in practice across various specialty areas; and in nursing education research

TABLE 6.7   Major Concepts as Defined in Watson's Theory

Human beings	Unities of mind, body, soul, and environment with souls that are not confined to the physical world but exist following physical death
Environment	Referred to as the world, described as all universal forces that affect a person, including the person's immediate environment and situation, "be they internal, external, human, human-made, artificial, natural, cosmic, psychic, past, present, or future" (Watson, 2007, p. 56)
Health (healing)	"Unity and harmony with in the mind, body, and soul" that is congruent with the person's perceived and experienced self; "health is I = me" (Watson, 2007, p. 48, 2012, p. 61)
Nursing	A transpersonal process of "human-to-human attempts to protect, enhance, and preserve humanity by helping a person find meaning in illness, suffering, pain, and existence; to help another gain self-knowledge, control, and self-healing within; a sense of inner harmony is restored regardless of the external circumstances" (Watson, 2007, pp. 53–54, 2012, p. 72)

(Smith, 2004). The University of Colorado hosts the Center for Human Caring, where nurses study and practice the human science and human care theory. Table 6.7 summarizes the key concepts defined in Watson's theory. The Watson Human Caring Science Institute serves as the source of an international consortium for her human science and human care theory. The consortium provides consultations to health care organizations for the implementation of her model and theory in practice settings. Human science and human care theory provides a theoretical foundation for nursing service departments, nursing research studies, and nursing educational programs worldwide (Fawcett, 2005). Watson's theory might be used by nurses in any nursing care situation during which a nurse desires to establish a deep, meaningful personal relationship with the persons to whom they provide care.

COMPLEXITY THEORY AS A FRAMEWORK

Like stability theory, complexity theory assumes that reality changes continually. However, change occurs with irregularity and cannot be predicted. **Complexity** theory "emphasizes change over time, long-term unpredictability, and openness to the environment with mutual simultaneous interactions … The complexity perspective seeks to understand patterns of phenomena as wholes within their contexts" (Maliski & Holditch-Davis, 1995, p. 25). In complexity theory, change occurs spontaneously when many individual factors interact interconnectedly and interdependently. Change becomes dynamic and unpredictable and coevolves with the environment (Leddy, 2006). Unlike systems theory, interacting systems cannot be separated because they are one.

Complexity theory replaces the metaphors of separation and interaction (reductionistic) with the metaphor of participation (holistic) (Porter, 1995). The whole cannot be known from the sum of the parts, nor can the sum of the parts be more than the whole because everything is unitary.

Assumptions of complexity theory include the following.

1. Nonlinear change over time
2. Long-term unpredictability
3. Openness to the environment
4. Mutual, simultaneous interactions
5. Continual fluctuations that reveal patterns
6. Variable patterns that appear at critical points

Because the theory assumes mutual change in people and environment, which provides potential for restructuring in new patterns, linear cause and effect is difficult to infer. The theory suggests that multiple, dynamic, mutual relationships, rather than enduring "causes," influence change. Thus, change of an individual, because it is related to initial conditions, is not generalizable.

Nursing models and theories with complexity theory as their foundation emphasize how persons become more fully human (human becoming) in terms of potential for change. Some nurses find models based on complexity theories difficult to understand because complexity theory challenges them to think in multiple dimensions.

Martha Rogers's Science of Unitary Human Beings

Martha Rogers developed **Rogers's science of unitary human beings** while searching for a specific and unique body of knowledge for nursing during the late 1970s (Barrett, Malinski, Ann, & Phillips, 2003). In Rogers's theory, the purpose of nursing is to foster health potential. Rogers incorporates the following three key concepts in her model.

1. **Unitary human being:** An irreducible, indivisible, pandimensional energy field identified by pattern
2. **Unified energy field:** A pandimensional nonlinear domain without spatial or temporal attributes
3. **Mutual process:** Changes within the human and environmental fields that occur simultaneously

Rogers's model builds on an assumption of the human being as a unified energy field that continuously exchanges energy with an environmental energy field. Rogers proposed that "man is a unified whole possessing his own integrity and manifesting characteristics that are more than and different from the sum of his parts" (Rogers, 1970, p. 47). Physical, biologic, psychological, social, cultural, and spiritual attributes are merged into behavior that reflects the total human being as an indivisible whole. Rogers believed that it is impossible to describe humans by combining attributes of each of the parts. Only as the parts lose their particular identity is it possible to describe the human being.

> **Take Note!**
> In Rogers's science of unitary human beings theory, the purpose of nursing is to foster health potential.

The human being is an organized energy field that has a unique pattern. The continuous mutual process of energy field with environmental energy field results in continuous pattern manifestation changes in both the person and the environment (Rogers, 1970). This results in increasing complexity and innovativeness of the human being. Rogers believed that this life process "evolves irreversibly and unidirectionally along the space–time continuum" (Rogers, 1970, p. 59). She conceptualized this unidirectionality as a spiral, with self-regulation "directed toward achieving increasing complexity of organization—not toward achieving equilibrium and stability" (Rogers, 1970, p. 64). The human being is also characterized by "the capacity for abstraction and imagery, language and thought, and sensation and emotion" (Rogers, 1970, p. 73).

Rogers believed that health serves as an "index of field patterning" (Maliski & Holditch-Davis, 1995, p. 27). Health and illness are not separate states, good or bad, or in a linear relationship. "Ease and disease are dichotomous notions that cannot be used to account for the dynamic complexity and uncertain fulfillment of man's unfolding" (Rogers, 1970, p. 42). Thus, observable manifestations are all "manifestations of patterning (that) emerge out of the human/environmental field mutual process and are continuously innovative" (Rogers, 1990, p. 8).

Rogers conceptualized nursing as both an art and a science. Nursing science includes knowledge specific to the domain of nursing that has an abstract nature and has been generated by scientific research and logical analysis. The art of nursing encompasses how nurses creatively use knowledge in professional practice (Rogers, 1992), cited in Fawcett (2005). Nursing intervention is aimed toward promoting the betterment of humans wherever they may be (Rogers, 1992). Rogers also specified that nurses must address health promotion with consumers because disease and pathology may always be a potential manifestation of human patterns. Rogers (1992) viewed caring in nursing as "simply a way of using knowledge" (p. 46).

Rogers (1990, p. 333) described three principles that explain change: integrality, helicy, and resonancy.

1. The principle of integrality emphasizes that the human energy field and the environmental energy field are continuous and must be perceived simultaneously. The relationship is one of constant interaction and mutual simultaneous change. In other words, "they are reciprocal systems in which molding and being molded are taking place at the same time" (Rogers, 1970, p. 97).
2. The principle of helicy predicts that change occurs as a "continuous, innovative, unpredictable, increasing diversity of human and environmental field patterns" (Rogers, 1990, p. 8). The human field becomes increasingly diverse with time. As the person ages, behavior may not be repeated but may recur at evermore complex levels.
3. The principle of resonancy indicates that change in pattern and organization toward increased complexity of the field occurs by way of waves, "manifesting continuous change from lower-frequency, longer wave patterns to higher-frequency, shorter wave patterns" (Rogers, 1980, p. 333).

Rogers believed that an understanding of the mechanisms that affect the life process in humans makes it possible for the nurse to purposefully intervene to affect client pattern manifestations in a desired direction. In the process, the nurse is also changed. Rogers saw the future as "one of growing diversity, of accelerating evolution, and of nonrepeating rhythmicities" (Rogers, 1992, p. 33). Her emphases on holism and on the simultaneity and mutuality of humans and the environment are concepts that have been widely accepted in nursing. Rogers proposed that the science of unitary human beings would serve as a foundation for future theory development to make this abstract science applicable to practice (Fawcett, 2003, 2005). Parse (1987), Newman (1986), and Leddy (2004, 2006) have used the science of unitary human beings as the foundation for practice. Barrett developed a theory of power using the science that nurses use to guide nursing service departments (Barrett et al., 2003).

Nurses use Rogers's theory as a foundation for using complementary and alternative health practices (e.g., therapeutic touch, guided imagery, and other energy therapies). The science of unitary human beings has also been used by nursing scholars to generate practice theories. The following Focus on Research, "Moving Beyond Dwelling in Suffering: A Situation-Specific Theory on Men's Healing from Childhood Maltreatment," provides an example of how the science of unitary human beings has been used to generate a new develop practice (situation specific or micro) theory.

Table 6.8 presents major concepts as defined in Rogers's model. Despite its complexity, the science of unitary human beings provides a theoretical foundation for undergraduate and graduate nursing education programs, guidelines for administration of nursing services in health care organizations, knowledge for the development of clinical practice guidelines, and a foundation for research instrument development. Instruments have been developed for nursing research and clinical practice using the science of unitary human beings (Fawcett, 2005). The Society of Rogerian Scholars offers nursing symposia, networking, and support for nurses who base their scholarly activities on Rogerian science.

TABLE 6.8 Major Concepts as Defined in Rogers's Theory

Human being	A unitary energy field with a unique pattern
Environment	An energy field in mutual process with the human being
Health	An expression of the complexity and innovativeness of patterning of the energy field that is the person
Nursing	Compassionate concern for human beings by using independent science and practice art in which nurses intervene to improve pattern manifestations and the environment to achieve maximum health potentials

FOCUS ON RESEARCH

Moving Beyond Dwelling in Suffering: A Situation-Specific Theory on Men's Healing from Childhood Maltreatment

The investigators used hermeneutical–phenomenologic techniques to uncover the deep personal meaning of the lived experiences of men who survived childhood maltreatment. Following Institutional Review Board approval, 52 men with a history of childhood maltreatment (neglect or physical, emotional, or sexual) and perceived that they had experienced healing were interviewed by a psychiatric mental health nurse. The first interview question asked about the lived experience of healing from their past experiences and they inquired about how each of them moved from living in suffering to a state of well-being. The interviews yielded rich data.

Using an iterative process, the investigative team listened to audiotaped interviews and read interview transcripts. Each member reflected on and then coded the data. The team then engaged in discussion and revised the codes and initial findings. They identified key themes related to healing and then verified their findings with eight of the study participants.

Key themes that were identified were linked to major concepts of science of unitary human beings theory and a specific practice theory was generated for nurses to use to facilitate healing for male childhood maltreatment survivors. They described the findings in terms of pattern manifestations. The first pattern manifestation is the situation which reflected societal view of male childhood maltreatment and how little is known about the phenomenon compared to female childhood maltreatment. The second pattern manifestation was the specific maltreatment event experienced by each participant. Common pattern manifestations occurred for all the participants who had experienced healing.

The first pattern represented helicy and was identified as "moving beyond suffering" (p. 59). The investigators identified the following five dimensions of this pattern: "breaking through the masculine veneer, finding meaning, choosing to live well, caring for self by using diverse healing methods, and engaging in a mutual process perceived as humanizing" (p. 59). The second pattern manifestation desiring release from suffering reflects resonancy and was described as "openness to change, mindfulness, intentions, perseverance, and optimism" (p. 60). The participants' reports of experiences in healing were equated with the principle of integrality. For this aspect of healing, the participants reported experiencing compassion, peace, a mutual process of being one with the universe, and finding a meaning and purpose in their lives.

The situation-specific model generated for the process of male survivor movement from beyond suffering to experiencing well-being proposed that dwelling in suffering has either a negative or no effect on the movement and that desiring release from suffering has a positive effect on the movement toward experiencing well-being. Nurses can use a variety of health patterning modalities such as guided imagery, meditation, rhythmic movement (dance therapy), energy methods (chakra therapy, therapeutic touch), artistic methods for expression (art or music therapy), and creation of a calm, therapeutic environment to facilitate healing in male victims of childhood maltreatment. The researchers recognize that the theory may not apply to other groups of male victims of childhood maltreatment because purposive sampling was used and each participant acknowledged that he had been healed and moved from dwelling in suffering to experiencing well-being.

Willis, D., DeSanto-Madeya, S., & Fawcett, J. (2015). Moving beyond swelling in suffering: A situation-specific theory of men's healing from childhood maltreatment. *Nursing Science Quarterly*, 28(1) 57–63. doi: 10.1177/0894318414558606.

Rosemarie Parse's Human Becoming Theory

Like Rogers, Parse suggested that the purpose of nursing is to improve quality of life for both the client and the nurse. In **Parse's human becoming theory**, she coined three words to describe the essence of nursing.

1. **Coconstitution:** Development of patterning through human–environment interaction
2. **Coexistence:** Dynamic mutual processes between the human and the environment
3. **Situated freedom:** Freedom of choice in a situation

Parse's model incorporates a combination of Rogers's principles and building blocks "with the tenets of human subjectivity and intentionality and the concepts of coconstitution, coexistence, and situated freedom from existential–phenomenologic thought" (Parse, 1987, p. 161). The emphasis is on the meaning and values that influence a person's active choices of behavior. "The human being constructs his or her own meaning" (Parse, 1996, p. 57). The model honors human dignity and freedom (Parse, 2010).

Parse defined the human being as "an open being, more than and different from the sum of parts in mutual simultaneous interchange with the environment who chooses from options and bears responsibility for choices" (Parse, 1987, p. 160). As a person interacts with the environment, patterns of relating are established that provide insight into his or her patterning and values at that moment. Health is viewed as a "nonlinear entity," a constantly changing process of becoming that incorporates values. Because it is not a state, health cannot be contrasted with disease. "The human becoming nurse's goal is to be truly present with people as they enhance their quality of life" (Parse, 1998, p. 69).

Take Note!

Parse's human becoming theory suggests that the purpose of nursing is to improve quality of life for both the client and the nurse.

Parse described her key concepts in a highly paradoxical manner (Parse, 1998, pp. 29–51).

1. **Human becoming:** Human participation with the environment to create health and quality of life
2. **Meaning:** Human interpreted, linguistic, and imaged content of something
3. **Rhythmicity:** The paradoxical patterning of the human–universe mutual process
4. **Transcendence:** "Reaching beyond with possibility—the hopes and dreams envisioned in multidimensional experiences and powering the originating of transforming" (p. 30)
5. **Imaging:** Reflective—prereflective coming to know that explicit-tacit all-at-once
6. **Valuing:** Confirming—not confirming cherished beliefs in light of a personal worldview
7. **Languaging:** Signifying valued images through speaking—being silent and moving—being still
8. **Revealing–Concealing:** Disclosing—not disclosing all-at-once
9. **Establishing–Limiting:** Living the opportunities—restrictions present in all choosings all-at-once
10. **Connecting–Separating:** Being with and apart from others, ideas, objects, and situations all-at-once

11. **Powering:** The pushing–resisting process of affirming—not affirming being in light of nonbeing
12. **Originating:** Inventing new ways of conforming—nonconforming in the certainty—uncertainty of living
13. **Transforming:** Shifting the view of the familiar-unfamiliar, the changing of change in constituting anew in a deliberate way

Parse (1998) combined these 13 concepts into the following 3 principles.

1. **Structuring** meaning multidimensionally is cocreating reality through the languaging of valuing and imaging (p. 35).
2. **Cocreating** rhythmical patterns of relating is living the paradoxical unity of revealing–concealing and enabling–limiting while connecting–separating (p. 42).
3. **Contrascending** (being one) with the possibilities is powering unique ways of originating in the process of transforming (p. 46).

Parse (1996) stated that "the way of living the belief system is through true presence" (p. 57), "which is a nonroutinized, unconditional loving way of being, within which the nurse witnesses the blossoming of others" (p. 57). Practicing within this model, the nurse would provide an empathic sounding board for clients and families to express and therefore uncover the meaning of thoughts and feelings, values, and changing views. In the process of expression through language and movement, and in "dwelling with" the rhythm of the client and family, new possibilities for change in quality of life would become apparent. "The new insights shift the rhythm and all participants move beyond the moment toward what is not-yet. This is mobilizing transcendence" (Parse, 1989, p. 257). In this model, the nurse connects with clients through focused interactions rather than doing things for them (Phillips, 1987). Therefore, Parse blended caring with Rogers's science of unitary human beings.

Parse (1998) also developed a phenomenologic–hermeneutic research methodology to test relationships suggested by the model. The methodology uses "dialogical engagement," a researcher–participant encounter, to uncover the meaning of the live experience being studied (Parse, 1989, p. 256) and serves as the research methodology for many qualitative nursing studies. Parse (2003) expanded her model by introducing the following community change concepts (again using paradoxes): (1) moving–initiating,

TABLE 6.9 Major Concepts as Defined in Parse's Theory

Human being	An open being, more than and different from the sum of parts
Environment	In mutual process with the person
Health	Continuously changing the process of becoming
Nursing	Use of true presence to facilitate the becoming of the participant

(2) anchoring–shifting, and (3) pondering–shaping. She perceived that human becoming could be done at a community level in addition to the individual level.

Parse's theory emphasizes the importance of the meaning that underlies behavior and provides a structure for the identification and clarification of "manifestations of whole people as they interrelate with the environment" (Phillips, 1987, p. 188). Hansen-Ketchum (2004) specified that outcomes for nursing practice using Parse's theory include opportunities for multidimensional client healing, enhanced personal growth (for the client and the nurse), and continued professional growth (for the nurse). Table 6.9 summarizes the major concepts defined in Parse's theory.

Parse's human becoming theory enables nurses to practice differently because it brings a multidimensional approach, incorporates the use of paradoxes, and fosters deep connections among nurses and nursing care recipients. Parse's theory provides a theoretical framework for undergraduate and graduate nursing programs, for individual nurses, and in descriptive applied research projects (Fawcett, 2005). The International Consortium of Parse Scholars offers networking opportunities and support services for nurses interested in Parse's human becoming theory. Parse also is the founder and editor of *Nursing Science Quarterly*, a nursing journal devoted to the advancement of nursing science. When using Parse's human becoming theory, nurses practicing in all areas of practice would aim for achieving deep, personal relationships to persons receiving care with the aim of helping them attain their maximal human potential.

REAL-LIFE REFLECTIONS

Remember Nicole and Brianna, from the beginning of the chapter? In what ways might Brianna have applied Parse's human becoming theory in helping Ms. Green to sleep?

Margaret Newman's Theory of Health as Expanding Consciousness

Like Parse, Newman uses principles from Rogers's science of unitary beings in **Newman's theory of health as expanding consciousness**. The theory states that the purpose of nursing is to promote a higher level of consciousness in both the client and the nurse. Newman used the concept of consciousness as the capacity of the system (human beings) to interact with its environment, the informational capacity of the system in her nursing model.

Newman's theory incorporates Rogers's concept of a unitary human being as a center of energy in constant interaction with the environment. Human beings are characterized by patterning that is constantly changing. According to Newman (1994), "[T]he focus of nursing is the pattern of the whole, health as pattern of the evolving whole, with caring as a moral imperative" (p. 19).

"The total pattern of the human being–environment can be viewed as a network of consciousness" (Newman, 1986, p. 33) that is "expanding toward higher levels: the patterns of interaction of human being–environment constitute health…Health is the expansion of consciousness" (Newman, 1986, pp. 3, 18), and "health and the evolving pattern of consciousness are the same" (Newman, 1990, p. 38). "Consciousness is defined as the information of the system: the capacity of the system to interact with the environment" (Newman, 1994, p. 38).

Health is viewed as a process that encompasses both disease and "nondisease." Instead of the familiar linear relationship between health as good and disease (or illness) as bad, Newman conceptualized disease as a meaningful component of the whole and a possible facilitator of health. "Sickness can provide a kind of shock that reorganizes the relationships of the human being's pattern in a more harmonious way" (Newman, 1994, p. 11). As the person interacts with the environment, "the fluctuating patterns of harmony–disharmony can be regarded as peaks and troughs of the rhythmic life process" (Newman, 1986, p. 21).

Newman posited four major ways in which human being–environment patterning is manifest: movement, time, space, and consciousness. Consciousness is expressed in patterns of rhythmic movement toward higher levels that can be described in time and space. Manifestations of these patterns include exchanging, communicating, relating, valuing, choosing, moving, perceiving, feeling, and knowing

(Newman, 1986, p. 74). The task for nursing intervention is to recognize patterning and relate to it in an "authentic" (genuine, sincere) way.

> **Take Note!**
> Newman's theory of health as expanding consciousness states that the purpose of nursing is to promote a higher level of consciousness in both the client and the nurse.

The new paradigm is relational. The professional enters into a partnership with the client with the mutual goal of participating in an authentic relationship, trusting that in the process of its evolving, both will grow and become healthier in the sense of higher levels of consciousness (Newman, 1986, p. 68).

Nursing facilitates the process of evolving to higher levels of consciousness by "rhythmic connecting of the nurse with the client in an authentic way for the purpose of illuminating the pattern and discovering the new rules of a higher level of organization" (Newman, 1990, p. 40).

Newman's theory contributes to the development of a body of knowledge about manifestations of healthy patterning of unitary human beings. Newman has described a methodology for using practice as the basis for research within the model. Nurses have used this theory in research studies addressing nurses as cancer survivors, effectiveness of nursing spiritual interventions, empowerment of cancer patients, nurse–family relationships with medically fragile children, family caring, and perceived health of men with human immunodeficiency virus.

Table 6.10 lists the major concepts defined in Newman's theory. Along with providing a theoretical framework for graduate and undergraduate nursing programs, Newman's theory guides professional nursing practice in substance abuse settings, pattern recognition for members of a faith congregation, and pattern assessment in a woman with hyperthyroidism. Nurses using Newman's theory strive to help others to understand the holistic impact of a health-related situation. Application of the theory has been useful in the following clinical situations: school-aged children with insulin-dependent diabetes mellitus, the elderly living alone, family caregivers, and persons with cancer (Fawcett, 2005). Nurses who use the model in nursing practice, education, and research can find resources from the Health as Expanding Consciousness Organization.

Susan Leddy's Human Energy Model

Leddy's human energy model was influenced by Rogers's science of unitary human beings, Eastern philosophy, and quantum physics and complexity theories. This model identifies three aspects of universal essence—matter, information, and energy—that constitute an undivided whole. In the human energy model, Leddy (2004) proposed that the purpose of nursing is to facilitate the harmonious pattern of the essence fields of both the client and the nurse. Leddy (2004) used five key concepts in her model.

1. **Self-organization:** The structure of the human being demonstrated by pattern and its manifestations
2. **Energy field:** A dynamic web of energy interactions
3. **Awareness:** An energy that links humans with the environment
4. **Energy:** Manifested by movement and change
5. **Pattern:** A web of relationships

Leddy (1998, p. 192) viewed the human being as "a unitary energy field that is open to and continuously interacting with an environmental universal essence field" that can only be understood as a whole. "Sensitivity to complementary facets and vantage points for observation provides a view of the whole from different perspectives" (Leddy, 1998, p. 192, 2003, p. 68). "Self-organization distinguishes the human energy field from the environmental field with which it is inseparable and intermingled" (Leddy, 2003, p. 68). "Self-organization is a synthesis of continuity and change that provides identity while the human evolves toward a sense of integrity, meaning, and purpose in living" (Leddy, 1998, p. 192). Humans also have awareness that enables the development of self-identity, the construction of meaning, and the capability to influence change by making choices (Leddy, 2004).

TABLE 6.10 Major Concepts as Defined in Newman's Theory

Human beings	"Unitary and continuous with the undivided wholeness of the universe" (Newman, 1994, p. 83)
Environment	"Undivided wholeness of the universe" (Newman, 1994, p. 83)
Health	Expansion of consciousness
Nursing	Facilitating repatterning of the client to higher levels of consciousness

Leddy (2004) viewed the environment as the context in which the human is embedded. People are one with the environment. Change can be partially predicted and is partially unpredictable. She explained that the universal essence environment is ordered and has a rhythmic pattern while constantly changing "through continuous transformation of matter and information" (Leddy, 2004, p. 14). However, change "is also influenced by the inherent order of the universe" (Leddy, 2003, p. 68). History, pattern, and choice also shape change.

Leddy (2003) defined health as being "the pattern of the whole" (p. 68). This pattern is rhythmic, varying in quality and intensity over time. Health is characterized by a changing pattern of harmony and dissonance.

Under Leddy's theory, knowledge-based consciousness in a goal-directed relationship with the client is the basis for nursing. "A nurse–client relationship is a commitment characterized by intentionality, authenticity, trust, respect, and genuine sense of connection. The nurse is a knowledgeable, concerned facilitator. The client is responsible for choices that influence health and healing" (Leddy, 1998, pp. 192–193).

Leddy (2004) derived three theories from her human energy model: the theory of healthiness, the theory of participation, and the theory of energetic patterning.

In the theory of healthiness, healthiness is defined as a manifestation of a health pattern. It is a process characterized by purpose, connections, and power to attain goals. The theory proposes that healthiness acts as a resource that influences the ongoing patterning that is reflected in health (Leddy & Fawcett, 1997). Leddy derived her theory empirically. The pattern of healthiness consists of a constellation of connection, purpose (challenge viewed as change, goals, meaningfulness, choice–possibilities, confidence–competence, and control), and power (choice–creativity, capability, capacity, change–curiosity, and confidence–assurance). The theory emphasizes the importance of goals and meaningfulness in life (Leddy, 2006).

The Leddy Healthiness Scale (LHS) (Leddy, 1997) includes items that measure meaningfulness, connections, ends, capability, control, choice, challenge, capacity, and confidence. In studies using the LHS (Leddy, 1997, 2006; Leddy & Fawcett, 1997), healthiness has been found to be moderately and negatively related to fatigue and symptom experience in women with breast cancer, and moderately and positively related to mental health, health status, and satisfaction with life in a sample of healthy people.

In the theory of participation, participation is defined as the experience of continuous human–environment mutual processes. Leddy (2004) defined participation as the experience of expansiveness (fullness and activity) and ease (smoothness and calmness of the mutual process of the human and environmental fields). The Person–Environment Participation Scale (PEPS) (Leddy, 1995) measures expansiveness and the ease of participation. In studies with PEPS to date, participation has been found to be moderately and positively correlated with healthiness, a sense of coherence (Antonovsky, 1987), and power (Barrett, 1990), and moderately and negatively correlated with fatigue and symptom experience in healthy people.

The theory of energetic patterning proposes that nursing interventions to facilitate the harmonious pattern of both the client and the nurse are accomplished through health pattern appraisal, recognition of patterns, and energy-based nursing interventions (Leddy, 2004, 2006). Nursing healing interventions promote healing by surrounding, supporting, or penetrating the human body. The six domains of energetic patterning are the following.

1. **Coursing:** Reestablishing free flow of energy
2. **Conveying:** Fostering redirection of energy away from areas of excess to depleted areas
3. **Converting:** Augmenting energy resources
4. **Collecting:** Reducing energy depletion
5. **Clearing:** Facilitating the release of energy tied to old patterns
6. **Connecting:** Promoting harmony within the human field and with the environmental field

A number of interventions are consistent with this theory, including nutrition, exercise, touch modalities, bodywork, light therapy, music, imagery, relaxation, and stress reduction (Leddy, 2003, 2004).

Leddy's conceptual model offers a unique and modern perspective for nursing; however, because it is a newer model, its usefulness for practice and research remains to be demonstrated. Table 6.11 presents major concepts defined in Leddy's model. Leddy's model and theories have yet to be empirically tested;

TABLE 6.11   Major Concepts as Defined in Leddy's Theory

Human being	A unitary, self-organized field of matter, energy, and information that constantly interacts with an environmental universal essence field
Environment	A dynamic, ordered, connected web in continuous transformation of energy, matter, and information with the human being (environmental universal essence)
Health	The rhythmic pattern of harmony/dissonance of the whole
Nursing	Knowledge-based consciousness involved in a mutual, connected, and goal-directed relationship with clients

however, they show great promise for providing a framework to guide future research on healthiness and energetic patterning. Professional nurses might use Leddy's model when engaging with persons as individuals or as communities for promoting health and well-being.

NURSING MODELS IN RESEARCH AND PRACTICE

Use of Nursing Models in Nursing Research

Most published nursing research studies fail to use conceptual nursing models as their foundation. Currently, three kinds of research related to nursing models are being conducted: testing the relationships predicted by a model, using a model as a framework for descriptive analysis, and attempting to modify nursing care through use of a model.

For example, Leddy and Fawcett (1997) interpreted the results of a study to explain relationships among theoretical variables (participation, change, energy, and healthiness) derived from the human energy model as being supportive of the model. In another example, Hart (1995), in a study of pregnant women, derived research variables from Orem's general theory and tested the relationships between the variables. The results were interpreted as supporting Orem's model.

Models also have been used as a framework for descriptive analysis. For example, concepts from Watson's science of human caring and Newman's health

as expanding consciousness were used to describe the personal (DeMarco, Picard, & Agretelis, 2004) and professional (Picard, Agretelis, & DeMarco, 2004) experiences of nurses who survived cancer. Picard et al. (2004) demonstrated how nursing models might be used to guide clinical research. Scura, Budin, and Garfing (2004) used the Roy's adaptation model to organize and categorize data in a pilot study using telephone social support and education to promote adaptation in men with prostate cancer. Roy's adaptation model was also used to organize study variables in a study looking at change in exercise tolerance, activity and sleep patterns, and quality of life in cancer patients who participated in a structured exercise program (Young-McCaughan et al., 2003). Brauer (2001) demonstrated how Newman's theory may be helpful in establishing patterns common to human beings with similar health problems.

A few studies have attempted to modify nursing care through use of a model. For example, Kelly, Sullivan, Fawcett, and Samarel (2004) tested the effects of therapeutic touch, quiet time, and dialogue on women's perceptions of breast cancer using Rogerian science. They found that only women receiving therapeutic touch experienced bodily sensations of tingling, magnetic pull, or being touched. Experimental and control groups both found quiet time and dialogue with the nurse to be calming and relaxing, demonstrating that nurses should not overlook the therapeutic results of just spending time with clients.

Use of Nursing Models in Nursing Practice

As more nurses receive BSN degrees and undertake graduate nursing education, the use of models in practice may become more prevalent. Nursing models and theories provide guidance to nurses engaged in practice for holistic assessments, rationales for various nursing interventions, and delineation of professional nursing roles in health care delivery. Some hospitals identify a particular theory as a basis for use of nursing process. For example, nurses at St. Luke's Hospital in Kansas City, Missouri, use Orem's self-care deficit theory as a foundation and guide for nursing practice. The American Nurses Association requests that nursing departments specify the nursing model and theory used by the organization as part of the Magnet hospital application process.

Nevertheless, nursing model (or theory) use in professional practice seems irrelevant to some nurses. Do models make real differences in nursing care delivered to clients? Does it matter if the client need is called a "noxious influence" affecting a behavioral subsystem, a "self-care deficit" leading to a "self-care demand," or a "focal stimulus" that is a stressor? How is the care given any different if its purpose is labeled to "limit self-care deficits," "reduce stressors," or "foster coping"? Why does the profession need specific nursing models and theories?

Although nursing science remains in an early stage of development, nursing scholars agree on categories of concepts (human beings, environment, health, and nursing) that are central to nursing knowledge. Nursing science must attain distinction from medical science. Much discussion about whether there should be one model for nursing has occurred, but the popularity of a growing number of models within different paradigms and frameworks indicates that disagreement still exists about how professional nursing should be described and how its goals can best be achieved.

Professional nursing continues to progress in defining nursing, identifying the unique nursing contributions to health care, developing nursing theory, and using nursing models and theories in practice. As health care evolves, nursing must demonstrate an ability to articulate its important and unique contribution to client care, and perhaps new models and theories may be needed.

■ QUESTIONS FOR REFLECTION

1. What is your attitude toward nursing models and theories? Why do you feel this way?
2. Has your attitude changed since reading this chapter?

3. Do you think that multiple approaches and definitions are advantageous or disadvantageous to the profession of nursing? Provide examples to support your response.
4. What might be the consequences of your attitudes toward nursing models and theories?

Summary and Significance to Practice

The nursing models discussed in this chapter use the metaparadigm concepts of human beings, environment, health, and nursing. Philosophical differences between the change as stability paradigm and the change as growth paradigm are pronounced. Professional nurses have the freedom to select which models to use in clinical practice based on personal philosophy and worldviews. Sometimes, one particular nursing model may fit a clinical situation better than others. Nursing models do not compete with each other but provide a variety of approaches and explanations for the phenomena associated with professional nursing practice.

Table 6.12 compares concepts in selected theories. The major differences and similarities among the models can be seen by comparing Tables 6.13 and 6.14. More research is needed to see if the models provide an effective description of nursing and make differences in client-care outcomes.

REAL-LIFE REFLECTIONS

Consider Brianna and Nicole. Do you believe that Brianna is a better nurse than Nicole because Brianna uses theory to guide her nursing practice? Why or why not?

▌TABLE 6.12 Comparison of Concepts in Selected Theories

Theory	Human	Human–Environment Interaction	Health	Examples of Nursing Implication
Systems	Multiple interacting subsystems that form the human system	Simultaneous change in both systems	Tendency toward increased complexity	Nurse system and client system are mutually affected
Stress and adaptation	Multiple subsystems that share an internal environment	Humans cope and compensate for environmental change	Constancy of the internal environment within normal parameters	Support coping mechanisms of client
Complexity	Unitary whole	Mutual simultaneous interaction; nonlinear	Pattern of the whole	Stimulate repatterning

TABLE 6.13 Similarities and Differences of Conceptualization in Nursing Models within the Change as Stability Paradigm

Model	Person		Health	Environment	Nursing	
	Goal	Composition			Nature	Purpose
King	Functioning in social roles	Open system	Dynamic state of well-being	Internal and external stressors	Goal-oriented interaction	Attainment, maintenance, or restoration of health
Orem	Constancy	Whole with physical, psychological, interpersonal, social aspects	Meeting self-care needs	External forces	An art with systems that address self-care requisites	Help people to meet self-care needs
Roy	Become integrated and whole	System with biopsychosocial components	Adaptation	External and internal conditions	Manipulation of stimuli to foster coping	Promotion of adaptation
Neuman	Balance	Composite of physiologic, psychological, sociocultural, developmental, and spiritual variables	Equilibrium	Internal and external stressors	Stress-reducing activities	Promotion of equilibrium

TABLE 6.14 Similarities and Differences of Conceptualization in Nursing Models within the Change as Growth Paradigm

Model	Person		Health	Environment	Nursing	
	Goal	Composition			Nature	Purpose
Peplau	Equilibrium	System with physiologic, psychological, and social components	Forward movement of the personality	Significant others	Therapeutic interpersonal process	Helping people to meet needs and to develop
Watson	Sense of inner harmony	Integrated and inseparable spiritual, mental, and physical spheres	Unity and harmony	Energy field external to the person	Transpersonal caring	Promoting harmony
Rogers	Increased complexity of pattern	Indivisible energy field	Increasing innovativeness of patterning	Contiguous, continuously interacting energy field	Promotion of repatterning	Facilitating health potential
Newman	Expansion of consciousness	Center of energy	Patterns of person–environment interaction expanding toward higher levels	Energy field in continuous interaction with the person	Repatterning partnership	Promoting higher level of consciousness
Parse	Process of becoming	Open being	Process of becoming	Energy field in continuous interaction with the person	Interpersonal processes	Improving quality of life
Leddy	Harmony, integrity, meaning, and purpose	Unitary energy field	Pattern of the whole	Energy field and person are one	Goal-directed relationship	Facilitation of harmonious health patterning

From Theory to Practice

1. Which of the nursing models or theories presented in this chapter appeals to you the most? How would you incorporate this model or theory into your professional practice?
2. What are the challenges to using a nursing model or theory to guide professional practice?
3. How important is it for all nurses working together in a practice setting to understand and use the same theories when providing care?
4. What strategies would you use to get a group of nurses to select and use the same nursing model or theory in a practice setting?

Nurse as Author

Select one of the nursing models or theories presented in the chapter. Outline the key concepts and propositions of the selected nursing model or theory. Apply the selected model and theory to a clinical nursing situation.

Your Digital Classroom

Online Exploration

Clayton State University School of Nursing's Nursing Theory: **http://www.clayton.edu/health/nursing/nursingtheory**

Health as Expanding Consciousness Organization: **http://currentnursing.com/nursing_theory/Newman_Health_As_Expanding_Consciousness.html**

International Orem Society: **http://oreminternationalsociety.org**

King International Nursing Group: **http://king.clubexpress.com/**

Neuman System Model: **http://www.neumansystemsmodel.org/**

International Consortium of Parse Scholars: **www.humanbecoming.org**

Roy Adaptation Association: **www.bc.edu/schools/son/faculty/featured/theorist/Roy_Adaptation_Association.html**

Society of Rogerian Scholars: **www.societyofrogerianscholars.org**

Watson Caring Science Institute and International Caring Consortium: **www.watsoncaringscience.org**

Expanding Your Understanding

Visit one of the nursing theory websites listed above or found on the Clayton State University Nursing Theory website, and answer the following questions.

1. Which nursing theory are you investigating?
2. Can you contact the nursing theorist?
3. Who maintains the nursing theory website?
4. What materials are available on the website to explain the nursing theory?
5. Where can you go to find additional information about the nursing theory?
6. Would you recommend the website to a colleague interested in the selected nursing theory? Why or why not?

Beyond the Book

Visit **thePoint® www.thePoint.lww.com** for activities and information to reinforce the concepts and content covered in this chapter.

REFERENCES

Agnes, M. (Ed.). (2005). *Webster's new world college dictionary* (4th ed.). Cleveland, OH: Wiley.

Alligood, M. (2010). Family healthcare with King's theory of goal attainment. *Nursing Science Quarterly, 23*(2), 99–104. doi: 10.1177/089431841032553

Andrews, H. A., & Roy, C. (1986). *Essentials of the Roy adaptation model.* Norwalk, CT: Appleton-Century-Crofts.

Antonovsky, A. (1987). *Unraveling the mystery of health: How people manage stress and stay well.* San Francisco, CA: Jossey-Bass.

Auger, J. R. (1976). *Behavioral systems and nursing.* Englewood Cliffs, NJ: Prentice-Hall.

Barrett, E. A. M. (1990). A measure of power as knowing participation in change. In O. L. Strickland & C. F. Waltz (Eds.), *Measurement of nursing outcomes.* New York: Springer.

Barrett, E. A., Malinski, V. M., Ann, M., & Phillips, J. R. (2003). The nurse theorists: 21st-century updates–Martha E. Rogers. Interview by Jacqueline Fawcett. *Nursing Science Quarterly, 16,* 44–51.

Benner, P., & Wrubel, J. (1989). *The primacy of caring: Stress and coping in health and illness.* Menlo Park, CA: Addison-Wesley.

Brauer, D. J. (2001). Common patterns of person-environment interaction in persons with rheumatoid arthritis. *Western Journal of Nursing Research, 23*(4), 414–430.

Cannon, W. B. (1932). *The wisdom of the body* (Rev. ed.). New York: Norton.

Chin, R. (1976). The utility of systems models and developmental models for practitioners. In W. G. Bennis, K. D. Benne, K. E. Corey, & R. Chin (Eds.), *The planning of change* (3rd ed.). New York: Holt, Rinehart & Winston.

Chinn, P. L., & Kramer, M. K. (2011). *Integrated theory and knowledge development in nursing* (8th ed.). St. Louis, MO: Elsevier Mosby.

DeMarco, R. F., Picard, C., & Agretelis, J. (2004). Nurse experiences as cancer survivors: Part 1-personal. *Oncology Nursing Forum, 31*, 523–530.

Fawcett, J. (1989). *Analysis and evaluation of conceptual models of nursing* (2nd ed.). Philadelphia, PA: F. A. Davis.

Fawcett, J. (2000). *Analysis and evaluation of contemporary nursing knowledge: nursing models and theories.* Philadelphia, PA: F. A. Davis.

Fawcett, J. (2003). Conceptual models of nursing: International in scope and substance? The case of the Roy adaptation model. *Nursing Science Quarterly, 16*, 315–318.

Fawcett, J. (2005). *Contemporary nursing knowledge: Analysis and evaluation of nursing models and theories* (2nd ed.). Philadelphia, PA: F. A. Davis.

Gaut, D., & Leininger, M. (1991). *Caring: The compassionate healer.* New York: NLN Press.

Hansen-Ketchum, P. (2004). Parse's theory in practice. *Journal of Holistic Nursing, 22*, 57–72.

Hardy, M. E. (1978). Perspectives on nursing theory. *Advances in Nursing Science, 1*, 37–48.

Hart, M. A. (1995). Orem's self-care deficit theory: Research with pregnant women. *Nursing Science Quarterly, 8*, 120–126.

Huch, M. H. (1987). A critique of the Roy adaptation model. In R. R. Parse (Ed.), *Nursing science: Major paradigms, theories, and critiques* (pp. 47–66). Philadelphia, PA: W.B. Saunders.

Kelly, A. E., Sullivan, P., Fawcett, J., & Samarel, N. (2004). Therapeutic touch, quiet time, and dialogue: Perceptions of women with breast cancer. *Oncology Nursing Forum, 31*, 625–631.

King, I. M. (1981). *A theory for nursing: Systems, concepts, process.* New York: Wiley.

King, I. M. (1987). King's theory of goal attainment. In R. R. Parse (Ed.), *Nursing science: Major paradigms, theories, and critiques.* Philadelphia, PA: W. B. Saunders.

King, I. M. (1989). King's general systems framework and theory. In J. P. Riehl-Sisca (Ed.), *Conceptual models for nursing practice.* Norwalk, CT: Appleton & Lange.

King, I. M. (1995). The theory of goal attainment. In M. A. Frey & C. L. Sieloff (Eds.), *Advancing King's systems framework and theory of nursing.* Thousand Oaks, CA: Sage.

King, I. M. (1996). The theory of goal attainment in research and practice. *Nursing Science Quarterly, 9*, 61–66.

King, I. M. (1999). A theory of goal attainment: Philosophical and ethical implications. *Nursing Science Quarterly, 12*, 292–296.

King, I. M. (2001). The nurse theorists: 21st-century updates–Imogene M. King. Interview by Jacqueline Fawcett. *Nursing Science Quarterly, 14*, 311–315.

Koldjeski, D. (1990). Toward a theory of professional nursing caring: A unifying perspective. In M. Leininger & J. Watson (Eds.), *The caring imperative in education.* New York: National League for Nursing.

Kyle, T. V. (1995). The concept of caring: A review of the literature. *Journal of Advanced Nursing, 21*, 506–514.

Leddy, S. K. (1995). Measuring mutual process: Development and psychometric testing of the person-environment participation scale. *Visions: The Journal of Rogerian Nursing Science, 3*, 20–31.

Leddy, S. K. (1997). Incentives and barriers to exercise in women with a history of breast cancer. *Oncology Nursing Forum, 24*, 885–890.

Leddy, S. K. (1998). *Leddy & Pepper's conceptual bases for professional nursing* (4th ed.). Philadelphia, PA: Lippincott.

Leddy, S. K. (2003). *Integrative health promotion.* Thorofare, NJ: Slack.

Leddy, S. K. (2004). Human energy: A conceptual model of unitary nursing science. *Visions: The Journal of Rogerian Scholarship, 12*, 14–27.

Leddy, S. K. (2006). *Health promotion: Mobilizing strengths to enhance health, wellness and well-being.* Philadelphia, PA: F. A. Davis.

Leddy, S. K., & Fawcett, J. (1997). Testing the theory of healthiness: Conceptual and methodological issues. In M. Madrid (Ed.), *Patterns of Rogerian knowing.* New York: National League for Nursing.

Lowry, L. W. (2004). Conceptual models of nursing: International in scope and substance? The case of the Neuman systems model. *Nursing Science Quarterly, 17*, 50–54.

Magan, S. J. (1987). A critique of King's theory. In R. R. Parse (Ed.), *Nursing science: Major paradigms, theories and critiques.* Philadelphia, PA: W. B. Saunders.

Maliski, S. L., & Holditch-Davis, D. (1995). Linking biology and biography: Complex nonlinear dynamical systems as a framework for nursing inquiry. *Complexity and Chaos in Nursing, 2*, 25–35.

Meleis, A. (2007). *Theoretical nursing development and progress* (4th ed.). Philadelphia, PA: Lippincott Williams & Wilkins.

Meleis, A. (2012). *Theoretical nursing: Development & progress* (5h ed.). Philadelphia, PA: Wolters-Kluwer Health/Lippincott Williams & Wilkins.

Monat, A., & Lazarus, R. (Eds.). (1977). *Stress and coping: An anthology.* New York: Columbia University Press.

Morse, J. M., Solberg, S. M., Neander, W. L., Bottorff, J. L., & Johnson, J. L. (1990). Concepts of caring and caring as a concept. *Advances in Nursing Science, 13*, 1–14.

Neuman, B. (1982). *The Neuman systems model: Application to nursing education and practice.* Norwalk, CT: Appleton-Century-Crofts.

Neuman, B. (1996). The Neuman systems model in research and practice. *Nursing Science Quarterly, 9*, 67–70.

Neuman, B. (2002). The Neuman systems model. In B. Neuman & J. Fawcett (Eds.), *The Neuman systems model* (4th ed.). Upper Saddle River, NJ: Prentice Hall.

Newman, M. A. (1986). *Health as expanding consciousness.* St. Louis, MO: Mosby.

Newman, M. A. (1990). Toward an integrative model of professional practice. *Journal of Professional Nursing, 6*, 167–173.

Newman, M. A. (1994). *Health as expanding consciousness* (2nd ed.). New York: National League for Nursing.

Orem, D. E. (1980). *Nursing: Concepts of practice* (2nd ed.). New York: McGraw-Hill.

Orem, D. E. (1985). *Nursing: Concepts of practice* (3rd ed.). New York: McGraw-Hill.

Orem, D. E. (1990). A nursing practice theory in three parts, 1956–1989. In M. E. Parker (Ed.), *Nursing theories in practice.* New York: National League for Nursing.

Orem, D. E. (1995). *Nursing: Concepts of practice* (5th ed.). St. Louis, MO: Mosby.

Orem, D. E. (2001). *Nursing: Concepts of practice* (6th ed.). St. Louis, MO: Mosby.

Orem, D. E., & Taylor, S. G. (2011). Reflections on nursing practice science: The nature, the structure and the foundation of nursing sciences. *Nursing Science Quarterly, 24*(1), 35–41. doi: 10.1177/0894318410389061

Parse, R. R. (1987). *Nursing science: Major paradigms, theories, and critiques.* Philadelphia, PA: W. B. Saunders.

Parse, R. R. (1989). Man-living-health: A theory of nursing. In J. P. Riehl-Sisca (Ed.), *Conceptual models for nursing practice.* Norwalk, CT: Appleton & Lange.

Parse, R. R. (1996). The human becoming theory: Challenges in practice and research. *Nursing Science Quarterly, 9,* 55–60.

Parse, R. R. (1998). *The human becoming school of thought.* Thousand Oaks, CA: Sage.

Parse, R. R. (2003). *Community: A human becoming perspective.* Sudbury, MA: Jones & Bartlett.

Parse, R. R. (2010). Human dignity: A human becoming ethical phenomenon. *Nursing Science Quarterly, 23*(3), 257–262.

Peterson, S., & Bredow, T. (2017). *Middle range theories application to nursing research and practice* (4th ed.). Philadelphia, PA: Wolters Kluwer.

Phillips, J. R. (1987). A critique of Parse's man-living-health theory. In R. R. Parse (Ed.), *Nursing science: Major paradigms, theories, and critiques.* Philadelphia, PA: W. B. Saunders.

Picard, C., Agretelis, J., & DeMarco, R. F. (2004). Nurse experiences as cancer survivors: Part II—professional. *Oncology Nursing Forum, 31,* 537–542.

Porter, E. J. (1995). Non-equilibrium systems theory: Some applications for gerontological nursing practice. *Journal of Gerontological Nursing, 21,* 24–31.

Riehl, J. P., & Roy, C. (1980). *Conceptual models for nursing practice.* New York: Appleton-Century-Crofts.

Rodgers, B. L. (2005). *Developing nursing knowledge: Philosophical traditions and influences.* Philadelphia, PA: Lippincott Williams & Wilkins.

Rogers, M. E. (1970). *An introduction to the theoretical basis of nursing.* Philadelphia, PA: F. A. Davis.

Rogers, M. E. (1980). Nursing: A science of unitary man. In J. P. Riehl & C. Roy (Eds.), *Conceptual models for nursing practice.* New York: Appleton-Century-Crofts.

Rogers, M. E. (1990). Nursing: Science of unitary, irreducible human beings: Update 1990. In E. A. M. Barrett (Ed.), *Visions of Rogers' science-based nursing.* New York: National League for Nursing.

Rogers, M. E. (1992). Nursing science and the space age. *Nursing Science Quarterly, 5,* 27–34.

Roy, C. (1987). Roy's adaptation model. In R. R. Parse (Ed.), *Nursing science: Major paradigms, theories, and critiques.* Philadelphia, PA: W. B. Saunders.

Roy, C. (2002). The nurse theorists: 21st-century updates—Callista Roy. Interview by Jacqueline Fawcett. *Nursing Science Quarterly, 15,* 308–310.

Roy, C. (2007). Advances in nursing knowledge and the challenge for transforming practice. In C. Roy & D. Jones (Eds.), *Nursing knowledge development and clinical practice.* New York: Springer.

Roy, C. (2008). Adversity and theory: The broad picture. *Nursing Science Quarterly, 21,* 138–139.

Roy, C. (2011). Research based on the Roy adaptation model: Last 25 years. *Nursing Science Quarterly, 24*(4), 312–320. doi: 10.1177/0894318411419218

Roy, C., & Andrews, H. A. (1999). *The Roy adaptation model* (2nd ed.). Stamford, CT: Appleton & Lange.

Roy, C., & Roberts, S. L. (1981). *Theory construction in nursing: An adaptation model.* Englewood Cliffs, NJ: Prentice-Hall.

Roy, C., Whetsell, M., & Frederickson, K. (2009). The Roy adaptation model and research. *Nursing Science Quarterly, 22*(3), 209–211.

Scura, K. W., Budin, W., & Garfing, E. (2004). Telephone social support and education for adaptation to prostate cancer: A pilot study. *Oncology Nursing Forum, 32,* 335–338.

Sills, G. M., & Hall, J. E. (1977). A general systems perspective for nursing. In J. E. Hall & B. R. Weaver (Eds.), *Distributive nursing practice: A systems approach to community health.* Philadelphia, PA: Lippincott.

Smith, M. (2004). Review of research related to Watson's theory of caring. *Nursing Science Quarterly, 17*(1), 13–25.

Swanson, K. M. (1991). Empirical development of a middle range theory of caring. *Nursing Research, 40,* 161–166.

Taylor, S. G., Geden, E., Isaramalai, S., & Wongvatunyu, S. (2000). Orem's self-care deficit nursing theory: Its philosophic foundation and the state of the science. *Nursing Science Quarterly, 13,* 104–110.

Watson, J. (1989). Watson's philosophy and theory of human caring in nursing. In J. P. Riehl-Sisca (Ed.), *Conceptual models for nursing practice.* Norwalk, CT: Appleton & Lange.

Watson, J. (2002a). *Assessing and measuring caring in nursing and health science.* New York: Springer.

Watson, J. (2002b). The nurse theorists: 21st-century updates—Jean Watson. Interview by Jacqueline Fawcett. *Nursing Science Quarterly, 15,* 214–219.

Watson, J. (2007). *Nursing human science and human care: A theory for nursing.* Sudbury, MA: Jones & Bartlett.

Watson, J. (2012). *Human caring science, a theory of nursing* (2nd ed.). Sudbury, MA: Jones & Bartlett.

Young-McCaughan, S., Mays, M. Z., Arzola, S. M., Yoder, L. H., Dramiga, S. A., Leclerc, K. M., et al. (2003). Research and commentary: Change in exercise tolerance, activity and sleep patterns, and quality of life in patients with cancer participating in a structured exercise program. *Oncology Nursing Forum, 30,* 441–454.

Professional Nursing Processes

LEARNING OUTCOMES

By the end of this chapter, the learner will be able to:

1. Outline the cognitive processes that nurses use in clinical practice.
2. Specify the steps of nursing processes.
3. Appraise the strengths and weaknesses of using nursing process in practice.
4. Discuss variances in the use of nursing process when practice is based on a selected nursing model.
5. Compare and contrast critical thinking, reflection, and intuition.
6. Differentiate among the stages of the novice-to-expert model of clinical practice.
7. Distinguish between linear and integrated cognitive nursing processes.
8. Discuss interpersonal nursing processes consistent with selected nursing conceptual models.
9. Outline psychomotor processes for patterning of health.

REAL-LIFE REFLECTIONS

Carol, a nurse employed in a university-based health clinic, serves as a preceptor for community-health nursing students from a local baccalaureate nursing program. Today is her first day working with Jane, a senior nursing student. Carol receives a telephone call from the university campus police informing her that they are bringing in an obese student who fell and has a very swollen ankle. Before the student arrives, Carol asks Jane, "What is the first thing we should do when the injured student arrives?" Jane replies, "We should find out her name and how the accident happened." Carol responds, "OK. What other information do we need?" Jane becomes nervous and answers, "I never had a client with an orthopedic problem, so I really don't know where to begin. I always get confused in the clinical setting about what I should do first. Maybe I shouldn't be a nurse."

Knowing the frustration she experienced as a nursing student, Carol replies, "Once I understood nursing process, it seemed as though what to do in the clinical setting fell into place for me when I was a nursing student. Can you tell me the steps of nursing process and what nursing theory you use?"

"I get the steps of nursing process confused all the time, and the program has us use Rogers' nursing theory," replies Jane.

Carol sighs and thinks to herself, "How can a nursing student get this far in her education without understanding how to use nursing process? What can I do to help Jane master nursing process quickly?" Carol instructs Jane just to observe while she handles the injured student and tells Jane that the two of them will talk about nursing process and Rogers' nursing theory later.

- *How should Carol explain the nursing process to Jane?*
- *Why is nursing process important to practice?*

Beliefs about nursing shape the way nurses practice. When nurses engage in practice using the medical model, they pay more attention to disease processes, pharmacology, and surgical and other invasive procedures. A medically oriented approach to nursing is common in acute care settings. The physician does the assessment, determines the diagnosis, and issues orders. To provide safe, effective client care, nurses use knowledge from other disciplines (e.g., pharmacology, medicine, social work, rehabilitation) while also considering the physical, mental, social, and spiritual aspects of the client's response to illness.

Nursing practice focuses on human responses to health status and the medical plan of care. Nurses practice autonomously by diagnosing and treating human responses to protect, promote, and optimize a client's well-being, health, and abilities. Nurses focus on injury and illness prevention, alleviating suffering, assessing for adverse effects of prescribed therapies, and advocating for persons, families, communities, and populations (American Nurses Association, 2015). Nursing knowledge includes detailed understanding of the client as a whole person, health and the factors that promote it, the environment and its impact on health, the mutual and ongoing interaction between humans and the environment, and the purpose and functions of nursing. Nurses perform their own client assessments, gathering information about each client's well-being, including the following.

1. Strengths and weaknesses
2. Whole responses to health concerns
3. Analysis of circumstances associated with well-being status
4. Knowledge related to health and well-being
5. Beliefs and values about health
6. Lifestyle
7. Health-related goals
8. Support systems

Because nurses view clients as whole persons and consider themselves key partners in an interdisciplinary health care team, they also have knowledge about the care regimens of other providers, such as physicians, pharmacists, and physical therapists. Understanding care regimens outlined by other health team members helps nurses to appreciate the global health care plan and acknowledge its impact on the whole client. By sharing knowledge about the plan, nurses help clients assume mutual and equal responsibility for setting health-related goals and participating as equal members of the health care team.

The knowledge projected by the model of nursing, accepted by the nurse, provides the basis for all nursing processes. Skill in the integrated use of cognitive, interpersonal, and psychomotor processes in client care is basic to the practice of professional nursing. This chapter emphasizes the relationship between nursing processes and the practice of professional nursing according to the nursing models discussed in Chapter 6, "Nursing Models and Theories."

CRITICAL THINKING

Many definitions of critical thinking appear in the nursing and higher education literature (Table 7.1). Although they vary somewhat, some elements are common to most definitions of **critical thinking**.

- Critical thinking is a highly complex thinking pattern that requires higher-order thinking.
- Persons who think critically take time to examine situations in terms of content and context, instead of jumping into action to make personal judgments and clinical decisions or to solve problems.
- Critical thinkers take time to examine the consequences of anticipated actions.
- Critical thinking demands that persons have solid, logical reasons for judgments and actions.

Scholars debate whether critical thinking is a general life skill. If viewed as a general life skill, critical thinking must be learned by everyone to survive in a rapidly changing world (Paul, 1993). Fortunately,

TABLE 7.1 Commonly Used Definitions of Critical Thinking

Author(s)	Definitions
Bandman and Bandman (1995)	"The rational examination of ideas, inferences, assumptions, principles, arguments, conclusions, ideas, statement, beliefs, and action" (p. 7)
Brookfield (1987)	"Reflecting on the assumptions underlying our and others' ideas and action and contemplative alternative ways of thinking and living" (p. 18); reflective skepticism
Turner (2005)	"A purposeful self-regulatory judgment associated with clinical decision making, a diagnostic reasoning, the nursing process, clinical judgment and problem solving, characterized by reasoning, inference, interpretation, knowledge, and open-mindedness" (p. 276)
Kennedy, Fisher, and Ennis (1991)	"Reasonable and reflective thinking that is focused upon deciding what to believe or do" (p. 46)
Facione (2006)	"The process of purposeful self-regulatory judgment . . . gives reasoned consideration to evidence, context, conceptualization, methods, and criteria" (p. 21)
Kurfiss (1988)	"An investigation whose purpose is to explore a situation, phenomenon, question, or problem to arrive at a hypothesis or conclusion about it that integrates all available information and that, therefore, can be convincingly justified" (p. 37)
McPeck (1981)	"The propensity and skill to engage in an activity with reflective skepticism" (p. 8)
National League for Nursing Accrediting Commission (2000)	"The deliberative nonlinear process of collecting, interpreting, analyzing, drawing conclusions about, presenting and evaluating information that is both factual and belief based" (p. 8)
Paul (1993)	"A unique kind of purposeful thinking in which the thinker systematically and habitually imposes criteria and intellectual standards upon the thinking, taking charge of the construction of thinking, guiding the construction of the thinking according to the standards, and assessing the effectiveness of the thinking according to the purpose, the criteria, and the standards" (p. 21)
Scheffer and Rubenfeld (2000), Rubenfeld and Scheffer (2015)	"In nursing . . . an essential component of professional accountability and quality nursing care" that displays "confidence, contextual perspective, creativity, flexibility, inquisitiveness, intellectual integrity, intuition, open-mindedness, perseverance, and reflection." Critical thinkers use "the cognitive skills of analyzing, applying standards, discriminating, information-seeking, logical reasoning, predicting, and transforming knowledge." (pp. 357, 7)
Watson and Glaser (1990)	Problem definition; decision making about pertinent information for problem solving; identifying and recognizing overt and covert assumptions; hypothesis formation and selection; drawing valid conclusions and judging validity of inferences (p. 1)

skills can be taught. However, basic elements of critical thinking may have to be altered to "fit" the context of the situation (Paul, 1993). When a nurse encounters a person without a pulse or respirations, spending time critically thinking about the situation would cause great harm; instead, immediate action is warranted. After the emergency has been handled, the nurse could spend some time engaged in critical reflection about why the arrest occurred, how it could have been avoided, and the effectiveness of professional actions.

In contrast to Paul (1993), Facione (2006) and Facione, Facione, and Sanchez (1994) proposed that critical thinking may be a personal quality that relies on attitude in addition to cognitive skills. Before persons can engage in regular critical thinking, they must value truth-seeking, open-mindedness, analyticity (recognizing potential problems, anticipating results, and prizing the use of reason), systematicity (the orderly, focused approach to inquiry), and inquisitiveness (natural curiosity) while having the maturity to make honest, reflective judgments and self-confidence in reasoning processes (Facione, Facione, & Giancarlo, 1996). This view of critical thinking fits well with Benner's novice-to-expert model (Benner, 1984, 2000), which illustrates the idea that experts develop certain characteristics related to practice (confidence, competence, and maturity) that enable them to quickly make correct clinical judgments that seem to simultaneously spring into action. Critical thinking is integrated throughout the cognitive nursing processes.

COGNITIVE NURSING PROCESSES

Clinical Decision-Making

Nurses make numerous clinical decisions when engaging in professional practice. Whenever nurses encounter situations that require them to select from several

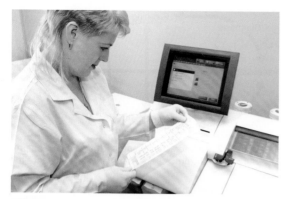

FIGURE 7.1 A nurse reviewing blood test results in order to have solid evidence to back a clinical decision.

7.1 Professional Building Blocks

Steps of Nursing Process

Step 1. Assessment: Collect comprehensive data regarding the factors related to client health status.

Step 2. Diagnosis: Identify actual or potential client health strengths and weaknesses.

Step 3. Planning:

a. Determine health-related goals (or outcomes).

b. Specify a series of actions to be taken to attain the identified goals.

Step 4. Implementation: Execute the action plan outlined in Step 3.

Step 5. Evaluation: Determine the effectiveness of the implemented action plan to either make needed revisions or restart the process with Step 1.

courses of action to manage a clinical situation, they engage in clinical decision making (Fig. 7.1). Before settling on a final course of action, nurses consider the personal, environmental, and contextual elements of a specific clinical situation. Clinical decision making contains the following key attributes: "intuition, analysis, heuristics, experience, knowledge, clinical reasoning, and critical thinking" (Johansen & O'Brien, 2015, p. 43). After making clinical decisions, nurses have to accept decisions that were made, the consequences that resulted and reflect on the processes used and the outcomes. Reflection-on-action enables nurses to determine if they made optimal decisions. Reflection also provides nurses the opportunity to improve their knowledge and skills in the clinical decision-making process.

Nursing Process

Clients rely on nurses to make effective clinical decisions. Kataoka-Yahiro and Saylor (1994), Banning (2006), Huckabay (2009), Shoulders, Follett, and Eason (2014), and Turkel (2016) suggest that the **nursing process**, as a method for problem solving and decision making in nursing practice, represents a discipline-specific version of critical thinking. Huckabay (2009) proposed that the critical thinking elements embedded within nursing process and clinical judgments are (1) identifying purposes, goals, and objectives for care, (2) identifying a problem to solve or question to answer, (3) sorting and distinguishing relevant from irrelevant information, (4) considering conceptual dimensions underlying a nursing situation (concepts, principles and theories), (5) examining different points of view, (6) identifying assumptions, (7) making interpretations and inferences, and (8) considering implications and consequences of various action options (see Box 7.1, Professional Building Blocks, "Steps of Nursing Process").

Nursing process began in the late 1950s and basically mirrors the scientific method. In its early stage it was a four-step process (assessment, planning, implementation, and evaluation) for nurses to use to identify and solve patient problems. Using a standardized process for nursing gained momentum in the 1960s. By the 1970s, nursing process became a pivotal part in the scope and standards of professional nursing and the professional nursing licensure exam contained test items to verify that program graduates could use it effectively.

Effective problem solving relies on extensive data collection for proper problem identification. Nurses assess clients holistically to determine actual and potential health-related problems or strengths (nursing diagnoses). Problem solving, the scientific method, and nursing process incorporate planning as a key step. When determining ways to solve a problem, test hypotheses, or deliver individualized nursing care, people generate action plans consisting of a desired goal and steps for attaining that goal. After executing action plans, nurses use problem solving, scientific method, and nursing process to evaluate the effectiveness of the action plans in meeting the desired outcome (or goal).

The nursing process provides a logical and rational way for the nurse to identify actual and potential problems and make decisions to resolve them. Nurses use critical thinking skills in all steps of the nursing process to

- collect relevant data from a variety of sources, sift out irrelevant data and determine which data are important, and validate the meaning of data with others if uncertain.
- organize data into meaningful patterns, determine if more data are required, compare data patterns with norms and known theories, examine assumptions about the client situation, and identify the major client health concerns to arrive at a nursing diagnosis.
- set safe care priorities and realistic care outcomes, determine appropriate nursing interventions, and generate a rationale for interventions while considering client needs and concerns.
- apply knowledge for intervention performance, test the efficacy of interventions, update and revise care plans as needed, noting changes in client status, and determine when to consult other health team members.
- evaluate the effectiveness of the care plan, determine alternative approaches and interventions, monitor the quality of care delivered, track client progress toward desired outcomes, and revise the plan as needed.

Although nursing process has its roots in the scientific process, nurses execute it in a sensitive and caring manner when working with people. Nurses consider individual client needs and preferences when providing care. Nurses use creativity to individualize nursing care for clients. Thus, the nursing process is both an artistic and scientific process.

> ### Take Note!
> Nursing process steps come from the steps of the scientific process, but when nurses individualize client care, nursing process becomes artistic in nature.

Invariably, the nursing process is presented as a series of four or five phases, with a number of steps within each phase. The net effect is a procedure that appears linear (or, at best, overlapping or circular) and cumbersome. However, all parts of the process are interrelated and influence the whole. The steps or phases of the nursing process occur sequentially, but they are not linear. Planning may lead to interventions for implementation or outcomes for evaluation. However, nurses continually assess clients when using all steps of the nursing process and make needed changes based on assessment findings. Figure 7.2 depicts the nursing process viewed from an interactional perspective. The following discussion presents an overview of each step of the nursing process.

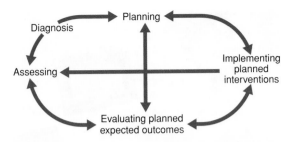

FIGURE 7.2 An interactional approach to the nursing process. All parts of the process are interrelated and influence the whole.

Step 1: Assessment

During **assessment,** nurses collect subjective and objective data about the client's health status (Fig. 7.3). Subjective data (e.g., the presence of pain, its location, its intensity, and aggravating and alleviating factors) are provided by the client or significant other. Objective data can be directly measured or observed (e.g., test results, increased blood pressure, pulse, and respiratory rates). Nurses collect data systematically and verify the accuracy with clients. If unable to collect the desired data, nurses use critical thinking to determine the reasons for obstacles and devise alternative approaches to collect it. When working with clients, nurses continuously collect and analyze data to make nursing decisions. Nurses document the data collected to provide a legal record of their surveillance activities and so that members of the interprofessional health care team have access to it.

Before nurses can begin collecting data, clients must trust them. Usually nurses initiate client relationships. When possible, nurses and clients work together as partners to outline specific care goals and specify responsibilities and ways to tailor nursing care to meet individual client needs. Nurses use critical thinking to

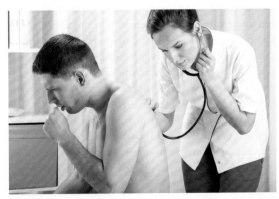

FIGURE 7.3 A nurse using a stethoscope to auscultate breath sounds is one example of how nurses collect patient data for the assessment step of the nursing process.

evaluate client responses and determine ways to facilitate communication.

Most nurses use an organized process for data collection. They decide which data are desirable and significant to collect in a particular situation and determine what sources and methods would be best to obtain these data. First, the nurse must know who the client is, why the client needs nursing care, and what factors currently influence the client's health status. Therefore, the nurse must collect key data such as the client's name, age, gender, marital status, occupation, education, economic status, existing knowledge about health–illness status, and family (and significant other) attitudes toward health care. Second, to individualize care, the nurse collects data regarding the client's personal habits, communication styles, cultural influences, growth and development status, learning capacity, supports and resources, previous experience with the health care system, medical diagnosis and regimen, coping patterns, personal values, and desired changes. Finally, the nurse uses a preferred conceptual nursing model to guide and organize data collection using the suggestions outlined in Table 7.2.

As data are collected, the nurse validates the findings with the client and other sources and clarifies any discrepancies. Nurse evaluation of the data should consider accuracy and whether all relevant factors have been included. As data collection continues, the organization and analysis of patterns within the data proceed concurrently, which may identify additional data collection needs. Nurse-collected data should supplement, rather than duplicate, data collected by other health care professionals (e.g., history) and should focus on information needed for nursing care. During data collection, nurses review all data to determine if more information is needed. If more information is needed, data collection is continued until the nurse decides that all relevant information has been collected. After deciding that the assessment is completed, the nurse moves to the second step of the nursing process.

Step 2: Diagnosis

Nurses derive nursing **diagnoses** from client data. Nurses organize collected data during assessment into clusters and interpret what the data reveal about the client. Effective data analysis and synthesis require that nurses remain objective, engage in thoughtful deliberation, make sound judgments, and discriminate relevant from irrelevant information. Nursing diagnoses represent the professional nurse's judgment about human responses within a contextual situation that may either threaten or strengthen health and well-being. Nursing diagnoses exclusively address care situations for which the professional nurse has responsibility. Although

TABLE 7.2 Implications for Data Collection in Selected Nursing Models Organized by Theoretical Frameworks

Nursing Model	Implications for Data Collection
Systems Theory	
King	Perceptions of self, level of growth and development, stress level, abilities to function in usual role, make decisions, and communicate
Neuman	Stressors, indications of disruption of the lines of defense, resistance factors
Stress/Adaptation	
Roy	Adaptation level (related to three classes of stimuli), coping in relation to modes of adaptation, position on the health–illness continuum
Caring	
Orem	Therapeutic self-care demand, presence of self-care deficits, ability of clients to meet self-care requisites
Watson	Phenomenal field (self within life space and motivational factors for health), values, needs for information, problem-solving abilities, developmental conflicts, losses, feelings about the human predicament
Complexity	
Peplau	Physiologic and personality needs, illness symptoms, relationships with significant others, influences on establishment, and maintenance of the nurse–client relationship
Rogers	Characteristics of patterning, health potential, rhythms of life, simultaneous states of the individual and environment
Parse	Thoughts and feelings about the situation, the synchronizing rhythms in human relationships, personal meanings, ways of being alike and different, and values
Newman	Person–environment interactions, patterns of energy exchange, client's responses to symptoms, transforming potential, client's feelings and what he or she does because of those feelings, patterns of life
Leddy	Characteristics of human universal essence field and environmental essence field

nursing practice may vary across state and national boundaries, nurses make independent judgments when clustering data to formulate nursing diagnoses. Professional nursing responsibility means that the nurse has the legal qualifications and accountability to take action. Nursing diagnoses may apply to individuals, families, or communities (Carpenito-Moyet, 2010; Hardman & Kamitsuru, 2014).

The concept of **nursing diagnosis** started in professional nursing practice in the early 1970s (Webber, 2008) in North America and has now expanded to all continents. The North American Nursing Diagnosis Association International (NANDA-I) (Hardman & Kamitsuru, 2014) identified five types of nursing diagnoses: actual, wellness, risk, for, syndrome, and possible.

1. When defining characteristics of a nursing diagnosis are present, nurses work with an actual nursing diagnosis. Actual nursing diagnoses are written using a three-phrase clause: the client problem, followed by the words "related to," then the etiology. Proper formatting of actual nursing diagnoses forbids the use of disease names or surgical procedures as the related-to clause.
2. Wellness diagnoses occur when a person, family, or community experiences a transition to a higher level of wellness.
3. At-risk nursing diagnoses are used when a particular person or group have characteristics that increase the likelihood that a specific human response is apt to occur, but the signs and symptoms (diagnostic cues) are absent.
4. Nurses use a syndrome diagnosis when a particular clinical situation results in a predictable cluster of commonly encountered actual or at-risk nursing diagnoses.
5. A possible nursing diagnosis is identified when nurses encounter a clinical situation in which insufficient data are present to designate an actual, risk for, wellness, or syndrome diagnosis. The possible nursing diagnosis provides a nurse with an option to address a human response despite insufficient client data.

When nurses monitor for possible complications from medications or an invasive procedure, they use collaborative problem statements (Hardman & Kamitsuru, 2014; Carpenito-Moyet, 2010). The number of clauses in a nursing diagnosis varies according to its classification. Table 7.3 offers definitions, specific formats, and examples of the various classifications of nursing diagnoses.

Ideally, nurses develop nursing diagnoses in collaboration with clients. When nurses involve clients in generating nursing diagnoses, clients validate that the nurse has the complete story, become more aware of the goals, and have the opportunity to determine the desired outcomes of nursing care. Human response patterns, functional health patterns, and health perceptions provide different ways for nurses to collect and organize data to compile a nursing diagnosis. Gordon's (1995) 11 functional health patterns provide an internationally coherent method to identify nursing diagnoses.

1. Health perception—health management
2. Nutritional—metabolic
3. Elimination
4. Activity—exercise
5. Sleep—rest
6. Cognitive—perceptual
7. Self-perception—self-concept
8. Role—relationship
9. Sexuality—reproduction
10. Coping—stress tolerance
11. Value—belief (Hardman & Kamitsuru, 2014)

Although the more commonly used nursing diagnoses tend to be problem oriented only, nurses also identify nursing diagnoses for enhancing client wellness and to prevent potential health complications. For example, a hospitalized person with a new diagnosis of insulin-dependent diabetes has many problems to confront in order to manage and cope with the change in health. Immediate concerns include learning how to administer insulin injections and to comply with recommended dietary changes. The client also needs to know the long-term complications associated with the disease.

Because nurses may also work with well persons in the community, NANDA-I identifies nursing diagnoses that focus on enhancing wellness. These wellness nursing diagnoses enable nurses to identify ways to enhance wellness and prevent potential health problems in risk clients (e.g., persons with an inherited risk to develop diseases such as cardiovascular disease or cancer). Most wellness diagnoses enable nurses to focus on client strengths and use them to improve client health.

Nursing diagnoses have created a unique language for professional nurses. However, recent patient safety and interprofessional team collaboration initiatives emphasize the importance of all health team members speaking a common language when discussing patient care issues. Box 7.2, Professional Building Blocks, "Strengths and Limitations of Using NANDA-I Nursing Diagnoses in Clinical Practices," outlines reasons for and against using NANDA-I nursing diagnoses in clinical practice. To date, there is no research-based evidence that demonstrates that the use of nursing diagnoses improves client outcomes.

TABLE 7.3 Definition, Format, and Examples of Nursing and Collaborative Diagnoses

Nursing Diagnosis Classification	Definition	Format	Examples
Actual	A clinical judgment identifying a problem with major defining characteristics being present with identified contributing factors influencing the health status change	Three clauses: 1. The human response 2. Etiology (or contributing factors) 3. Clinical signs and symptoms	Altered nutrition less than body requires (1) related to persistent nausea and vomiting (2) as evidenced by no food intake for 1 wk, refusal to eat, weight loss of 4.53 kg (10 lb) within 2 wks, (3) prealbumin of 14.8 mg/dL and complaints of "I feel tired all the time" and statement "I am afraid to eat because I will throw up"
Risk	A clinical judgment identifying a potential problem because of increased vulnerability to developing it	Two-clause statement designating the potential human response and the etiology	Risk for infection related to compromised host defenses from the potentially immunosuppressive effects of chemotherapy and the presence of a central venous catheter
Syndrome	A clinical judgment identifying a health-altering situation resulting in the likely presence of multiple nursing diagnoses	One-clause statement designating the type of altered health	Battered child syndrome
Wellness	A clinical judgment identifying a transition from a current wellness level to a higher one	One-clause statement designating a human response with the possibility of moving toward greater wellness	Potential for enhanced spiritual well-being
Possible	A clinical judgment describing a suspected problem not validated by the available data	Two-clause statement designating the human response and possible etiology	Possible death anxiety related to recent cancer diagnosis
Collaborative problems and diagnostic statements	Potential complications arising from a disease process or medical interventions	Two-part phrase including the words "potential complication"	Potential complication: hemorrhage secondary to cardiac catheterization

Adapted from Carpenito-Moyet, L. J. (2010). *Nursing diagnosis application to clinical practice* (13th ed.). Philadelphia, PA: Wolters Kluwer Health/Lippincott Williams & Wilkins; and North American Nursing Diagnosis Association International. (2012). *Nursing diagnoses: Definitions and classification, 2012–2013.* Philadelphia, PA: Author.

Take Note!
Safe effective health care requires clear, concise communication among all health team members so that everyone understands the client situation.

QUESTIONS FOR REFLECTION

1. How do you think that nurses might best communicate the patient's actual and potential problems with each other?
2. Why do you think this method would be best?
3. What has been your nursing education or professional experiences with nursing diagnoses?

Step 3: Planning

Once a comprehensive list of nursing diagnoses has been generated, nurses develop a plan of care to communicate specific client care needs to other nursing personnel so that desired outcomes are attained. Care plans guide and direct client care efforts to ensure continuity of care when different nurses assume care responsibilities. In addition, care plans designate specific interventions to meet client care goals. Finally, nursing care plans outline contributions that nurses make to client health care delivery.

Nurses follow certain guidelines to generate effective nursing care plans. When **planning** client care, nurses establish a set of nursing diagnoses in priority

7.2 Professional Building Blocks

Strengths and Limitations of Using NANDA-I Nursing Diagnoses in Clinical Practices

Strengths

- Provides a common language for nurses to communicate to the client the actual and potential problems
- Improved client–nursing assessments (Müller-Staub, Lavin, Needham, & von Achterberg, 2006)
- Increased continuity of nursing care among members of the nursing care team during client handoffs when shifts change
- Increased client satisfaction
- Improved documentation of assessments
- Provides a possible organizational system for nursing documentation on electronic health records

Limitations

- Rigid formatting of diagnostic statements increase the time to write them
- Other health professionals, especially physicians, find nursing diagnostic terminology confusing and impede effective interprofessional communication in and across health care settings (Gordon, 2005; Finkelman & Kenner, 2007; Webber, 2008)
- Failure of interprofessional health team members to understand each other may delay emergent medical intervention (Finkelman & Kenner, 2007)
- Increased risk for errors (sometimes fatal ones) (Finkelman & Kenner, 2007)
- Exclusive use of NANDA-I approved nursing diagnoses may limit nurse's individual thinking when a client situation falls outside of a typical clinical situation
- NANDA-I terminology is difficult to understand across cultures (Gordon, 1995)
- A diagnosis should be a true problem and cannot be a potential one (Zanotti & Chiffi, 2015)
- Nursing diagnoses are based exclusively on clusters of data and are not confirmed or justified by actual diagnostic testing (Zanotti & Chiffi, 2015)

order, designate desired nursing goals and client outcomes, and prescribe specific nursing interventions. Nurses set priorities based on preserving client functional status (except in the terminally ill), promoting client comfort, and meeting mutually agreed-on client goals.

Because of the need to streamline care and improve client outcomes, some nurses rely on standardized care plans. Standardized nursing care plans provide less variance in care delivered to clients with similar health problems and theoretically improve quality. They address all critical assessments and customary interventions for medical therapies, invasive procedures, and diagnostic tests. When nurses follow standardized care plans, they may forget to include clients in care decisions or neglect client preferences.

The nursing care plan includes the priorities and the prescribed nursing interventions to achieve the desired **goals** (the global desired state) derived from the nursing diagnoses. Ideally, nurses and clients work together to develop the desired goals and outcomes of nursing care. Once the goals are defined, specific outcomes can be generated. **Outcomes** are end results that, when measured, determine client progress toward resolution of the nursing diagnosis. These expected outcomes must be realistic and stated clearly and concisely as they provide the basis for evaluating nursing care plan effectiveness. Table 7.4 presents broad guidelines for goal setting in selected nursing models. Because nursing models vary, the foci of nursing goals differ.

Nursing Outcomes Classification

Nurses must demonstrate that what they do makes a difference in client outcomes and find ways to determine the effectiveness of nursing care. The **Nursing Outcomes Classification (NOC)**, developed by nurse researchers at the University of Iowa in 1988, offers an approach for developing measurable client outcomes. Currently, the NOC provides nurses with more than 300 scales to measure outcome. Each outcome is defined and has a list of key indicators for use in evaluation, a target outcome rating, a place to identify each data source, a scale to measure patient status, and a list of references that provides evidence substantiating the validity and reliability for each identified outcome (Center for Nursing Classification and Clinical Effectiveness, n.d.). For example, the NOC has a scale to measure personal safety behaviors. A nurse can use this scale to identify client risk for injury. After educating the client about, for example, personal safety or correction of metabolic disorders, the nurse can reassess the client using the scale to determine if improvement in behavior has occurred.

NOC facilitates the development of computerized information systems for tracking nursing care outcomes across health care settings. NOC also facilitates comparable data collection, substantiates nursing care contributions, creates uniform nursing data sets, provides nurses with outcome measurement tools, facilitates electronic documentation of client care, improves reimbursement for nursing services, and standardizes

TABLE 7.4 Broad Guidelines for Goal Setting in Selected Nursing Models Organized by Theoretical Frameworks

Nursing Model	Broad Guidelines for Goal Setting
Systems Theory	
King	Achieve goals and solve problems related to personal, interpersonal, and social systems
Newman	Maintain or restore dynamic equilibrium by reducing stressor penetration or strengthening the normal line of defense
Stress/Adaptation	
Roy	Promote adaptation from successful coping
Caring	
Orem	Restore external and internal constancy
Watson	Meet human needs and solve problems in a caring interpersonal relationship
Complexity	
Rogers	Help people design ways to attain optimal rhythmic patterns
Parse	Illuminate meaning, synchronize rhythms, and mobilize transcendence
Newman	Transform patterns of life and facilitate evolving consciousness
Leddy	Mutual process to define meaningful goals to attain an optimal pattern of the whole

the ways nurses can evaluate nursing care innovations. Through the process of determining measurable, standardized outcomes, nurses clearly articulate the contributions they make to client care while developing a unique body of nursing knowledge (Johnson, Maas, & Moorhead, 2000).

Not all nurses use the NOC in clinical practice. However, the planning phase requires that long-term goals and desired outcomes (short-term or immediate goals) are determined within the client plan of care. After goals and outcomes have been established, priorities must be set. When survival is threatened, physical needs must take precedence. Cost, available personnel, and resources (including time) may influence priorities. The theory or model being used to organize care can also influence the determination of priorities. For example, the use of Maslow's (1962) theory would assign higher priority to physiologic, safety, and security needs, and lower priority to love, self-esteem, and self-actualization needs. In addition, as always, the client must be closely involved in priority setting.

Once the priorities among goals and outcomes have been determined, alternative options for care can be generated and their probability for success predicted. The possible solutions or approaches are heavily influenced by availability of resources and by factors in the client's lifestyle and cultural background. The NOC provides a standardized method to track client progress toward care objectives across inpatient, community, and home settings (Johnson et al., 2000) (see Concepts in Practice, "Nursing Outcomes Classification in Action").

Concepts in Practice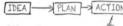

Nursing Outcomes Classification in Action

NOC aids nurses with the challenge of delineating client goals and outcomes, including setting priorities, identifying potential barriers, and choosing interventions that have the best likelihood of success. Consider, for example, the client whose story opened this chapter: an overweight teen who has a broken leg. Although weight loss may be considered an important goal for this teen, the more important goal is immediate mobility. Therefore, teaching the teen how to use crutches safely is a higher priority. Once that is accomplished, the goal of weight loss can be addressed. This goal could be achieved by 2 weeks of residence at a health spa or a self-monitored weight reduction program consisting of weighing portions of food, keeping a diary of food intake, and following a prescribed exercise program. However, financial constraints may make the spa trip unfeasible, and time and lifestyle constraints may influence the desirability of the exercise or food-weighing approach. With NOC, nurses working with the client would look at adherence to the outlined dietary regimen, compliance, knowledge and use of health-promoting behaviors, knowledge about the prescribed diet, and specific weight control behaviors, along with weight reduction measurements, to help this client meet her weight loss goal once her leg has healed.

Today's nurses care for clients with increasingly higher levels of acuity, spend much of their time documenting care rendered, and pay close attention to safety considerations. Time pressures prevent nurses from developing multiple approaches to address client situations (Finkelman & Kenner, 2007; Gordon, 2005). As a result, nurses may quickly generate a plan of care without taking the time to analyze interventions for appropriateness and likelihood of success in a particular clinical situation.

Nurses must make a conscious effort to avoid choosing a prescribed "cookbook" approach to delineating care outcomes. To preserve nursing as a collaborative partnership with clients, the nurse and the client together must determine goals and select interventions that have the best likelihood of success. The individualized and collaborative approach can then be translated into specific actions, the desired frequency of the actions, who will be assigned to carry out those actions (e.g., the nurse, the client, or other health team members), and the timetable for expected achievements.

Along with establishing goals and outcomes (or objectives) for nursing care, the nursing care plan outlines specific nursing interventions. Nursing interventions are the actions nurses take to attain care goals and outcomes. Frequently, nursing students find written nursing care plans challenging and complex. Unlike the care plans written by practicing nurses, student care plans usually require written rationales for proposed nursing interventions. However, even experienced nurses must conscientiously take time to reflect and recall the rationales behind clinical interventions. Nurses determine priority lists for each identified nursing diagnosis, determine expected outcomes and goals, and prescribe specific interventions (with established frequencies and time for each action). Computerized software for care plan generation offers nurses a series of checklists to complete individualized care plans.

As part of the care plan, the nurse can prescribe independent interventions (those not requiring a physician's order, such as using a pillow under a client's foot to keep the heels off the mattress), designate collaborative interventions (those requiring a physician's order, such as the administration of prescription medications), and outline specific interventions to screen for potential complications associated with medical or surgical treatments. Ideally, other nurses should be able to follow the care plan exactly as written by the nurse who developed it. Nurses can find published care plans in books and journal articles, in computer programs, and on the internet.

> **Take Note!**
> Nursing interventions are actions nurses take to attain care goals and outcomes.

Nursing Interventions Classification

In 1987, the University of Iowa developed the **Nursing Interventions Classification (NIC)** system as a means to standardize all possible nursing interventions. The NIC contains over 540 standard nursing interventions and outlines more than 12,000 nursing activities. Most interventions contain 10 to 30 specific activities that include information related to client assessment, safe care environment maintenance, health education strategies, psychological and spiritual support techniques, interprofessional consultations, and client and family referrals. The NIC facilitates nursing professionalism by standardizing nursing treatment nomenclature; strengthening links between nursing knowledge, diagnoses, interventions, and outcomes; facilitating electronic documentation of nursing care; assisting in determining costs and resources needed for nursing interventions; providing a theoretical foundation to help beginning nurses learn clinical decision making; and increasing nursing-specific knowledge (Dochterman & Bulechek, 2004).

Concepts in Practice, "Nursing Interventions Classification in Action," applies the use of the NIC as it pertains to the overweight client with the broken leg presented at the outset of this chapter.

Concepts in Practice IDEA → PLAN → ACTION

Nursing Interventions Classification in Action

The NIC contains two interventions related to weight reduction and management. The NIC uses the label "weight reduction assistance" for the nursing intervention for the following nursing diagnosis—alteration in nutrition: more than body requires, related to reduced activity secondary to nonbearing weight status for fractured leg.

Nursing Activities for the Intervention
- Assessment of eating patterns
- Reasons for overconsumption
- Weekly weight determinations
- Development of weight loss goals, an exercise program, and a daily eating plan with the client

Teaching Activities for the Intervention

- Appropriate energy-expending activities
- Nutritional needs to promote fracture healing without increasing caloric intake
- Calculation of fat content in food

Desired Client Outcomes

- Food selections staying within predetermined daily caloric limit when eating out or participating in social gatherings.

The NIC suggests other tips, such as posting weekly weight loss goals in a strategic location (such as the refrigerator), referring to community weight reduction support groups, and rewarding the client for meeting goals. Because the NIC designates a framework for nursing interventions that can be computer coded (and clients can be charged for them), NIC use in clinical practice has become standard in some health care organizations. Evaluation of the care plan occurs by using NOC (Dochterman & Bulechek, 2004).

Concept Mapping

Some nurse educators have replaced traditional nursing process papers (including written care plans) with **concept mapping**, which enables students to draw connections among assessment data, multiple nursing diagnoses, pathophysiology, nursing interventions, and desired client outcomes (Carpenito-Moyet, 2010; Fonteyn, 2007; Rubenfeld & Scheffer, 2015; Schuster, 2016; Shelton, 2008; Taylor & Wros, 2007). Concept mapping was started in the 1960s by Dr. Joseph Novak at Cornell University as a way to promote meaningful learning, which requires well-organized, relevant knowledge structures, and a personal commitment to integrate new with existing knowledge (Novak & Cañas, 2008). A concept map is a diagram resulting from analytical thought that depicts relationships among important pertinent concepts related to a clinical situation. Creating a concept map incorporates multiple areas of the brain, including areas for affect, motor function, and memory (short term, long term, and working) (Novak & Cañas, 2008). Concept maps may be generated by using a prescriptive template or developed freely with few guidelines. The center of the map typically specifies the major concept of interest (central concept). The nurse (or student) then identifies supporting data and the relationships between that data and the central concept. Many concepts in professional nursing can serve as a central concept (e.g., client strengths or weaknesses, a medical or nursing diagnosis, a desired

outcome). Figure 7.4 provides a sample concept map. Computer software programs and online resources are available for generating concept maps. Nurses rarely use concept mapping in clinical settings unless they are explaining complex processes to nursing students. Nevertheless, concept mapping may have value in facilitating client understanding of diseases and health management regimens.

> **Take Note!**
> Concept mapping enables students to make connections among assessment data, multiple nursing diagnoses, pathophysiology, nursing interventions, and desired client outcomes.

Client Care Paths

Since the 1990s, client care paths have outlined standardized care plans for commonly encountered illnesses, surgeries, and procedures in outpatient and inpatient health care settings. Client care plans address nursing diagnoses, outline evidence-based interventions, and specify observations for and prophylactic treatment of potential complications. Standardized client care paths reduce variation in nursing care received by clients with the same clinical problem, streamline care to reduce costs, reduce care errors and oversights, and decrease care documentation (paths frequently contain checklists, instead of requiring nurses to write detailed narrative notes). Clients receive a copy of the care path so they know what to expect, learn about how they can facilitate care, have written instructions for self-care, and can track their own progress toward health restoration. Most care paths accommodate instances when care delivery fails to follow the path exactly because of an unexpected client response. Criticisms of care paths include reduced individualization of client care plans and decreased critical thinking by nurses because of the perceived pressure to follow the path exactly as outlined.

Step 4: Implementation

During **implementation**, nurses execute proposed nursing care plans (Fig. 7.5). Nursing actions support and complement the medical plan of care. Ideally, professional nurses use interventions based on scientific evidence. Nurses use the following skills for successful care plan implementation: teaching clients (and significant others), managing others, facilitating group process, resolving conflicts, performing technical skills, and, above all, communicating effectively.

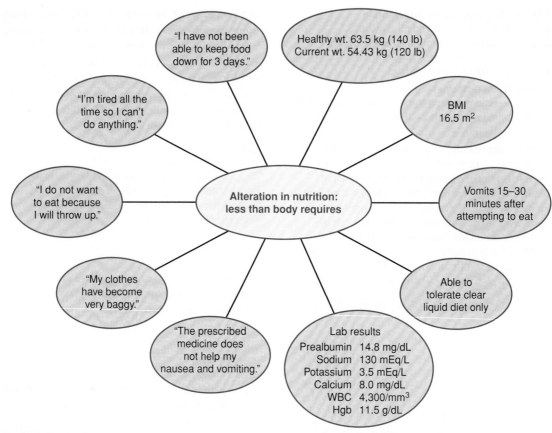

FIGURE 7.4 Sample concept map showing the relationship between assessment data and nursing diagnosis.

All client–nurse interactions should be goal directed and purposeful. As nursing actions are performed, nurses collaborate with the clients and their significant others to involve them appropriately in the care. Nurses perform interventions with sensitivity to the client's feelings and individual preferences. Conceptual models play a role in the organization of nursing care. Table 7.5 outlines how conceptual models may be used to organize care along with possible implications for nursing interventions.

An important part of implementation is the documentation of nursing interventions and their results. Documentation provides a means to track client progress toward desired outcomes as well as a legal record of rendered health care services. More importantly, documentation serves as a key method for communication among interprofessional health team members. Nurses continually assess clients to determine responses to nursing and medical interventions. When interventions are determined to be ineffective, the nurse revises the nursing care plan. Changes in a client's condition may mean an alteration in the frequency of prescribed interventions, modification of the current interventions, prescription of new interventions, or consultation with other health care professionals. The process of intervention is integrally involved with the final phase of the nursing process—evaluation.

FIGURE 7.5 Preparing to administer an intravenous infusion while wearing a mask and gloves for a patient in isolation is an example of the implementation step of the nursing process.

TABLE 7.5 Implications for Nursing Interventions in Selected Nursing Models Organized by Theoretical Frameworks

Nursing Model	Implications for Nursing Interventions
Systems Theory	
King	Emphasis is on exploration of the situation, shared information, mutually set goals, and explored means to resolve problems, achieve goals, and move forward
Neuman	Emphasis is on primary, secondary, or tertiary prevention to reduce stressors or strengthen the lines of defense
Stress/Adaptation	
Roy	Emphasis is on increasing, decreasing, or maintaining focal, contextual, or residual stimuli
Caring	
Orem	Emphasis is on self-care actions for or with the client if the client is unable to perform them for him- or herself
Watson	Emphasis is on caring that reflects interpersonal teaching–learning, mutual formulation of the problem, joint appraisals, shared need for problem solving, joint planning, provision of cognitive information, and evaluation of helpfulness for learning and coping
Complexity	
Rogers	Emphasis is on mobilization of the client's resources and repatterning of the human–environment interaction
Parse	Emphasis is on guidance to relate the meaning of the client's situation, to share thoughts and feelings with one another, and to change the meaning of the situation by making it more explicit
Newman	Emphasis is on the process of growth in which the nurse focuses on the client's evolving capacities, diversity, and complexity in the process of expanding consciousness
Leddy	Emphasis is on the mutual process of transforming energy to create change

Step 5: Evaluation

During evaluation, nurses and clients collaborate to determine whether progress is being made toward the attainment of desired health-related goals. Processes in the evaluation of care include reassessing, reviewing, and reordering (if necessary) care priorities; establishing new goals; and revising the care plan. Evaluation occurs continuously throughout each phase of the nursing process. However, the main purpose of evaluation is to compare changes in client behavior or health status with the determined goals or expected outcomes specified in the nursing care plan. Results of evaluation may reveal one or a combination of the following.

- **Goals and outcomes were fully met** and the determination of future client contacts are needed to reaffirm that the health status change remains permanent.
- **Goals and outcomes were partially met,** revealing that the health problem or the desired health status change has not been resolved. However, progress continues. Continued monitoring is warranted; more time may be needed with the current plan before considering modification.
- **Goals and outcomes were not met.** The client has little or no evidence of change in health status or health problem since the initial assessment. The care plan needs revision.

- **New problems have emerged** and the entire care plan needs to be revised to address them.

Not all client-related health goals are amenable to quantification, so nurses sometimes have difficulty finding valid and reliable tools to objectively measure progress. It may be helpful to consider what appropriate tools are available to measure progress toward goals when the goals are established. For example, weight loss and blood pressure reduction are easily validated. However, it is difficult to assess improved self-concept or attitudes toward a more healthful lifestyle. Sources for instruments to measure progress may be found in the NOC, journal articles, websites, and instrument handbooks.

Because the nursing process is systematic, logical, and goal directed, nurses assume that adherence to the process should result in desired goal attainment. When evaluation indicates that the problem is not resolved, other possible reasons must be considered through collaborating with clients, their significant others, nursing colleagues, and other interprofessional health care team members.

If the goals have been met and no new ones have emerged, the nurse and the client may terminate the relationship, which may be difficult for both parties. Clients may be unsure of their ability to maintain the changes in health behavior or well-being status independently. The nurse may have ambivalence about not being needed any longer. Being aware of and openly sharing these feelings can lead to satisfaction in having accomplished the desired goals and acceptance of the need to end the relationship.

> **Take Note!**
> Nursing process provides a logical, sequenced, and rational way for nurses to identify potential and actual patient problems, develop a plan to address them, and then evaluate the effectiveness of nursing actions on achieving desirable patient outcomes.

Despite the extensive attention given to nursing process, many experienced nurses continue to intervene using standardized procedures based on medical diagnoses. Efforts to standardize client care have resulted in the development of client care paths. In many institutions, professional nurses helped develop client care paths that incorporate nursing assessments and interventions to address commonly encountered nursing diagnoses for specific health problems.

The use of client care paths can lead nurses to engage in rote practice. However, when nurses use nursing models to guide care, they engage in critical thinking because models provide solid reasoning behind clinical practice. In the following section, two brief examples illustrate that nurses can approach the nursing process differently when they use conceptual nursing models to guide practice.

> **Take Note!**
> Nursing process provides an organized way of thinking about client care and fosters deliberate nursing actions.

▉ QUESTIONS FOR REFLECTION

1. Based on the information you have read related to nursing process, list and define each step. How do you think nursing process will help you as you engage in clinical practice as a nursing novice?
2. How does your clinical practice setting promote or discourage the use of nursing process?
3. What are the barriers to developing individualized nursing care plans for clients in your current practice setting?
4. Why do you perceive these as barriers?
5. How can you change your practice setting to facilitate individualization of client care?
6. What are the consequences of not individualizing client care in practice?

Conceptual Models Emphasizing the Nursing Process

Roy and Neuman addressed nursing process specifically in their nursing models. Instead of keeping with the five-step process, however, they refined it. Roy and Andrews (1999) kept nursing process focused on nursing practice, whereas Neuman and Fawcett (2002) proposed the use of nursing process for all health care professionals because it is based on the scientific method.

The Roy Adaptation Model

In the Roy adaptation model, the goal of the nurse is to manipulate stimuli to move the client in the desired direction of change toward adaptation. The process of nursing is described as a six-step problem-solving method (Roy & Andrews, 1999).

1. First-level assessment: Examine client behaviors in the four adaptation modes and make a judgment about whether the behaviors are adaptive or ineffective.
2. Second-level assessment: Analyze stimuli that influence ineffective behaviors and determine nursing care priorities.
3. State problem areas as nursing diagnoses.
4. Determine specific goals.
5. Determine interventions.
6. Evaluate as behavior changes, and modify as needed.

The Neuman Systems Model

In the Neuman systems model, the purpose of nursing action is "to best retain, attain, and maintain optimal client health or wellness using the three preventions as intervention to keep the system stable" (Neuman & Fawcett, 2002, p. 25). Client stability depends on the depth of stressor penetration. Nurses assess for actual and potential effects of environmental stressors before making judgments or taking action. Neuman proposed a modification of the nursing process to incorporate the following three steps.

1. Determine a nursing diagnosis.
2. Establish nursing goals.
3. Determine nursing outcomes with interventions classified as primary (wellness retention), secondary (attainment of health), or tertiary (maintenance of health) prevention.

Benefits and Criticisms of Nursing Process

The American Nurses Association, the National Council of State Boards of Nursing, and other nurse specialty organizations incorporate the five phases of nursing process in professional nursing practice standards. Many professional nurses use nursing process daily in clinical practice, and many organizations have documentation forms based on the steps of nursing process. Nursing process provides an organized way of thinking about client care and fosters deliberate nursing actions.

Nevertheless, some nurses report that they do not use nursing process in daily practice (Webber, 2008). Benner (1984, 2000) suggested that many nursing experts do not follow the steps of nursing process as they engage in professional nursing practice. Henderson (1987), Lindsey and Hartrick (1996), Rew (1996), Varcoe (1996), and Webber (2008) offered the following concerns that the nursing process

- is inconsistent with real-world practice because it is a linear, rational problem-solving process.
- is focused on problems rather than client strengths and potential.
- is time-consuming and requires elaborate nursing jargon.
- prefers rules over interaction.
- is antithetical to a holistic approach to client care.
- labels clients by nursing diagnoses.
- minimizes disallowance of nursing intuition.
- is a questionable approach for expert nursing practice.

The formulaic structure of nursing process has been useful to teach rules to novice learners, and the National Council of State Boards of Nursing Licensing Exam uses it as a means for demonstrating minimal competence to begin a professional nursing career. However, many nurses treat the nursing process as if it were the only process in nursing practice. Research has demonstrated that the nursing process is inadequate "when sensory data are changing rapidly or are ambiguous, uncertain, or conflicting" (Rew, 1996). Benner, Tanner, and Chesla (1996) found that clinically proficient and expert nurses use intuitive cognitive processes, rather than rule-based thinking, to make clinical judgments. Turkel, Ray, and Kornblatt (2012) stated that the current labels for the steps of nursing process fail to embrace the unitary-transformative approach to nursing practice. They propose renaming the steps as follows.

- **Recognizing:** Incorporating deeper assessment that involves intentional listening to recognize the health issue being encountered by the client.
- **Connecting:** Expanding planning to integrate the client, client patterns, and client meaning into the

plan and involve the client's significant others in determining what could be done.
- **Partnering:** Including a process where the nurse and the client work collaboratively while they connect to live out a mutual process in which both parties constantly recognize issues and address new ones as they arise.
- **Reflecting:** Where evaluation becomes a collaborative process between the nurse and the client to verify that the implemented interventions were successful.

Integrated Models for Clinical Judgment

Along with nursing process, nurses use other models to make clinical judgments. Benner et al. (1996, p. 1) suggested that "the clinical judgment of experienced nurses resembles much more [the] engaged, practical reasoning . . . than the disengaged, scientific, or theoretical reasoning . . . represented in the nursing process." Experienced nurses tend to bypass some steps of nursing process, whereas novice nurses comply with each of the five steps.

Intuition

Studies of expert clinical practice have identified intuition, knowing the patient, and reflection as important characteristics. **Intuition** has been described as "another way of knowing wherein facts or truths are known or felt directly rather than arrived at through a linear process of rational analysis" (Rew, 1996, p. 149) (see Chapter 5, "Patterns of Knowing and Nursing Science"). In a study that supported the novice-to-expert model, Polge (1995, p. 8) found that "as the level of nursing proficiency increases from advanced beginner to expert, there is a significant increase in the use of intuitive critical thinking to make clinical nursing judgments." Young (1987) proposed that intuition is multidimensional. The functional dimension of intuition is composed of cues and judgment, in which actions do not have a logical link with data. Intuition as a personal way of knowing relies on direct patient contact, self-receptivity, experience, energy, and self-confidence. Many nurses have saved lives by acting on intuitive feelings. In some cases, physicians have been known to come and see hospitalized clients because the nurse identified intuition as the reason for contacting the physician.

▮ Questions for Reflection

1. How have you used intuition to guide personal or professional actions? What were the consequences?

2. What advice would you give to someone about using intuition to guide action?

3. Would the advice you give be different for a professional colleague than for a friend? Why or why not?

Reflection

Reflection is a process of thinking about the concerns associated with an experience. Reflection develops the affective domain of learning and allows nurses to relate to the aspects of their experience that are the most profound at the time. Consequently, reflection has the potential to provide for personal growth. Reflective learning is multidimensional and may be triggered by a sense of inner discomfort. When things do not go according to plan, nurses engage in reflection to identify and clarify concerns surrounding a clinical situation. Effective reflection requires that the nurse be open to new information that may arise from nonempirical sources. Sometimes reflection results in the resolution (or "aha moment") of confounding situations or with the feeling that one has learned something that is personally significant. Reflection may result in profound changes in attitudes or behaviors.

The Pew Health Professions Commission (1998) identified reflection as one essential skill that health professionals must be able to perform along with critical thinking and rational problem solving. Health care professionals need to develop skills in reflective and critical thinking to identify and respond to new situations and practice dilemmas. Professionals also use reflection during practice and afterward to evaluate professional performance.

Schon (1987) identified two ways in which professionals use reflection: reflection-in-action and reflection-on-action. During **reflection-in-action**, health care practitioners think about the purposes and reasons behind the actions being performed. **Reflection-on-action** is a self-evaluative process in which practitioners analyze personal performance in a given clinical situation, think of what could have been done better, and determine plans to improve performance the next time a similar clinical situation is encountered.

Take Note!
Health care professionals need to develop skills in reflective and critical thinking to identify and respond to new situations and practice dilemmas.

7.3 Learning, Knowing, and Growing

Developing Skills in Reflection

A variety of tools can help you to develop your skills in reflection:

- Write your autobiography.
- Keep professional logs.
- Self-audit your performance.
- Construct criteria for role model profiles.
- Develop survival advice memos.
- Videotape yourself in professional action.
- Undergo peer evaluations.
- Identify critical incidents.
- Engage in meaningful dialog with others.

Brookfield, S. D. (1995). *Becoming a critically reflective teacher.* San Francisco, CA: Jossey-Bass.

Brookfield (1995, p. 8) proposed that reflection becomes critical reflection when it questions "assumptions and practices" as well as seeks to understand the power forces behind current practice. Reflection also provides opportunities for professionals to find meaning in practice (Brookfield, 1995; Schon, 1987). Reflection takes time to master, especially in today's fast-paced society (see Box 7.3, Learning, Knowing, and Growing, "Developing Skills in Reflection," for actions you can take to improve your skills).

Clinical Judgment

Tanner (2006) reviewed over 200 studies that addressed clinical judgments made by nurses in practice that substantiate the use of intuition and reflection by professional nurses. According to Tanner, what nurses bring to practice situations may be more important than the objective data available to the nurse when clinical judgments are made. Tanner developed a **research-based model of clinical judgment** which is described in the following paragraphs.

Professional nurses bring knowledge and experience to clinical practice situations. As nurses gain more experience, they learn to identify the patterns that indicate impending deterioration in client status requiring rapid action. Quick pattern identification occurs rapidly and sometimes intuitively. Most nurses who work in clinical settings typically reflect on what they are currently doing and the outcomes of interventions. When a situation fails to unfold as planned, many nurses review their actions (or lack of action) to see what went wrong. Thus, reflection-on-action becomes a mechanism for nurses to refine clinical practice strategies.

Within the practice context, experienced nurses notice (i.e., perceptually grasp) the global situation. Nurses interpret the situation by using reasoning, pattern identification, analysis, intuition, and personal narratives. They then respond by taking action to help clients. Immediately following action, they assess the client outcomes. The process of interpreting and responding requires reflection-in-action. The final step in the clinical judgment model is reflecting, in which the nurse reflects-on-action and solidifies the knowledge learned from the clinical experience.

INTERPERSONAL PROCESSES

As noted above, intuition and reflection are professional nursing processes that integrate experience with cognition. Cognitive processes receive more attention during discussions related to nursing process, intuition, and reflection.

Professional nursing practice, particularly the nurse–client relationship, requires the use of interpersonal processes. **Interpersonal processes** can be defined as interactions between two or more persons. Without attention to interpersonal processes, nursing practice may become impersonal, dominated by technology, and self-serving. The following section provides brief examples of different approaches used by selected nursing conceptual models and theories in the use of interpersonal processes.

King's Theory of Goal Attainment

In King's (1995) theory (discussed in Chapter 6, "Nursing Models and Theories"), the goal of nursing is to help individuals maintain their health so they can function in their roles. Nursing is a process of action, reaction, and interaction that results in goal attainment. Although the process proposed by King's theory is classified according to the steps in the nursing process, the emphasis is on interpersonal processes within the steps. Assessment incorporates perception, communication, and interaction of the nurse and the client. Planning includes mutual determination of goals and agreement on the means to attain them. Implementation is the process in which transactions are made. Finally, evaluation is the process in which nurses ask, "Was the goal attained?"

Peplau's Interpersonal Relations Model

In Peplau's model (Reed, 1996) (discussed in Chapter 4, "Establishing Helping and Healing Relationships"), nursing is a therapeutic, interpersonal process. Nurses use the interpersonal process as an educative instrument, a maturing force that aims to promote forward movement of the personality. The interpersonal process is the method by which nurses facilitate useful transformation of the client's energy or anxiety. The interpersonal process is based on a participatory relationship between the nurse and the client, in which the nurse governs the purpose for and the process in the relationship and the client controls the content. The process consists of the following four phases:

1. **Orientation:** Clients become aware of the availability of and trust in the nurse's abilities.
2. **Identification:** The nurse facilitates expression of feelings without rejection.
3. **Exploitation:** The client derives the full value from the relationship.
4. **Resolution:** The client no longer needs the professional nurse and is independently capable of meeting his or her needs.

Paterson and Zderad's Humanistic Theory

In humanistic nursing practice theory, nursing is perceived as a lived experience between human beings. "Nursing is a response to the human situation. One human being needs a kind of help and another gives it" (Paterson & Zderad, 1988, p. 11). The humanistic nursing effort is directed toward increasing the possibilities of making responsible choices. The process, which is labeled the "phenomenologic method of nursology" (science of nursing), consists of five phases:

- **Phase I:** The nurse knower prepares for coming to know
- **Phase II:** The nurse intuitively knows the "other"
- **Phase III:** The nurse scientifically knows the other by:
  - Analyzing the situation
  - Considering the relationships between components
  - Synthesizing themes or patterns
  - Conceptualizing or symbolically interpreting a sequential view of this postlived reality
- **Phase IV:** The nurse complementarily synthesizes known others by:
  - Comparing similarities and differences
  - Synthesizing the similarities and differences to create an increased knowing
- **Phase V:** Succession occurs within the nurse from the many to the paradoxical one—"a conception or

abstraction that is inclusive of and beyond the multiplicities and contradictions" (Paterson & Zderad, 1988, p. 74)

Parse's Human Becoming Theory

In Parse's (1996) theory (discussed in Chapter 6, "Nursing Models and Theories"), the goal of practice is quality of life from the client's perspective, with the focus on the meaning constructed by the client. The nurse is present in a nonroutine, unconditional, loving way of being with the client. The full attention of the nurse is with his or her clients "as they move beyond the moment." The methodology in this theory consists of three processes.

1. **Explicating (illuminating meaning):** Making clear what is appearing now through languaging.
2. **Dwelling with (synchronizing rhythms):** Giving of self over to the flow of the struggle in connecting–separating.
3. **Moving beyond (mobilizing transcendence):** Propelling with envisioned possibles in transforming.

Newman's Theory of Health as Expanding Consciousness

In the Theory of Health as Expanding Consciousness (discussed in Chapter 6, "Nursing Models and Theories"), Newman described nursing as "caring in the human health experience" (Newman, 1994, p. 139). "The responsibility of the nurse is not to make people well, or to prevent their getting sick, but to assist people to recognize the power that is within them to move to higher levels of consciousness" (Newman, 1994, p. 15). The focus of nursing in this theory is the pattern of the whole that is clarified through a praxis (practice) method. The method starts with the establishment of a partnership with the client with a mutual goal of participating in an authentic relationship that requires meeting and forming connections. The nurse and the client then form a shared consciousness that serves as the basis for increasing awareness. When client and nurse goals are met, the client and the nurse move apart. Each participant in the nursing encounter tells his or her story in his or her own way.

The nurse is free to be authentic and fully present. "Awareness of being, rather than doing, is the primary mechanism of helping" (Newman, 1994, p. 104). To develop a sequential pattern over time, the nurse organizes data in chronologic order as a narrative.

Focus on Research, "Cognitive, Interactive, and Intuitive Elements of 'Making Sure'," outlines how the cognitive and interactive processes used by nurses help keep clients safe in inpatient settings. Hospital nurses engage in surveillance, a nursing intervention that requires systematic data collection (assessment) and analysis to detect changes in client condition; and in vigilance, the mental work of nursing that results in attention to and identification of significant observations, cure, or signals that need decisive action. Surveillance and vigilance represent key elements of clinical decision making that result in nurses taking action (Schmidt, 2010).

FOCUS ON RESEARCH

Cognitive, Interactive, and Intuitive Elements of "Making Sure"

Using a grounded theory (collecting data using multiple methods to identify key concepts and relationships of a situation) methodology, the investigator identified and outlined a basic social process called "making sure," a key element of professional nursing practice that hospital nurses use to verify that they are making accurate assessments, interpreting assessment data correctly, and taking appropriate professional action. Fifteen registered nurses employed in the intensive care unit of a university medical center or community hospital participated in the study. Participants were interviewed in person or via telephone using a semi-structured interview format. Interview data were transcribed verbatim. Follow-up interviews were conducted based on coding results from the first interviews.

Results of the interview transcripts revealed that the core concept and basic social process was "making sure," which involved assuming responsibility that encompassed being in control of the clinical situations of all assigned patients for a given shift. To meet their assigned patients' needs, the nurses needed to have confidence and comfort in their clinical abilities Making sure started with "knowing what's going on" (p. 403), which involved having a global picture of the client and his or her assigned care needs as well as an awareness of all the other care dimensions from all the specialty interprofessional team members. The next major category of "making sure" involved "being close" (p. 403) to assigned patients, which meant being in close physical proximity and being intellectually connected to them. The third element involved "watching," or close, direct, frequent patient observations, including physiologic monitoring, but more importantly watching the entire person with frequent checking to "see how they were doing" (p. 404). The fourth phase was "not taking anything for granted" (p. 404), which involved nurse alertness and attentiveness in order to sense when things were not right and therefore be able to catch things prior to patient deterioration. These four concepts were fundamental to the nurse in "taking action" (p. 405) in order to protect patients.

This study is clinically significant because it outlines the cognitive, interactive, and intuitive processes that professional nurses use on a daily basis in the acute care setting to keep patients safe. Some of the concepts identified have been addressed by nursing theorists. Further research is needed to see if the process of "making sure" would apply to other settings besides acute care and to identify ways to measure the four elements of "making sure" in order to provide quantitative evidence to substantiate the theory outlined in the study.

Schmidt, L. A. (2010). Making sure: Registered nurses watching over their patients. *Nursing Research*, *59*(6), 400–406.

TABLE 7.6 Noninvasive Nursing Interventions that Promote Self-Patterning	
Intervention	**Example(s)**
Imagery	Guided imagery in which client visualizes healing occurring
Relaxation	Progressive relaxation exercises or warm bath
Affirmations	Positive self-talk
Sound	Listening to music at 60 beats/min
Exercise	Yoga or tai chi
Wave modulation	Color or light therapy
Nutrition	Special diet or herbal, vitamin, or mineral supplements
Meaningful presence	Being with another
Humor	Clowning, sharing appropriate jokes
Authentic dialog	Guided reminiscence
Wellness counseling	Health education
Therapeutic touch	Centering and altering energy fields
Movement therapy	Dance or imposed motions
Journaling	Diary writing or critical incident written records
Balancing	Finding balances between activity, rest, work, and fun
Bibliotherapy	Reading self-help or inspirational literature
Body therapy	Acupressure, massage, or healing touch

PSYCHOMOTOR PROCESSES

In addition to cognitive and interpersonal processes, nursing care includes psychomotor processes. **Psychomotor processes** are defined as manual dexterity, coordination, and the ability to use equipment effectively while performing nursing procedures. Skill in the performance of physician-ordered, often invasive, disease- or problem-related interventions is a key part of nursing clinical practice. Associate degree programs emphasize these technical aspects of nursing, whereas baccalaureate and higher-degree programs focus on cognitive and interpersonal processes. Health care consumers and organizations expect nurses to be able to carry out complex procedures smoothly and efficiently.

PATTERNING NURSING PROCESSES

Patterning nursing processes use energy to enhance health and well-being. Patterning processes have compatibility with a unitary approach to nursing. Some complementary and alternative health care interventions incorporate manipulation of human–environment energy fields. Table 7.6 presents some noninvasive nursing interventions that promote self-patterning.

Rogers's Science of Unitary Human Beings

Nursing from an interaction perspective delineates structure in qualities and persons in the environments. Rogers' science of unitary human beings proposes that separations do not exist, but rather all things form a single constellation. Rogers (1988, 1992) specified that the purpose of nursing is to create optimal health and well-being for all persons. The science of unitary human beings defines health not as a separate state or as the result of lifestyle choices or an encounter with illness, but rather as "an index of field patterning" (Malinski, 1986, p. 27). "Pattern is concerned with qualities and is expressed by the map of the configuration of relationships" (Bartol, 2016, p. 225). Only manifestations of patterns can be accessed by humans (Leddy, 2004, 2006).

In Rogerian science, behavior patterns are viewed as manifestations of the human–environment field. Field manifestations may include lifestyle parameters such as nutrition, work, and play; exercise; sleep–wake cycles; safety; interpersonal networks; and decelerated–accelerated field rhythms.

Examples of field rhythm manifestations might include diversity (from greater to lesser), motion (from slower to seemingly continuous), time (from slower to timelessness), and creativity (from pragmatic to visionary). The client is a knowing participant in change in this model. Through being aware, having choices and the freedom to act intentionally, and being involved in creating changes, the client is a mutual participant with the nurse in the patterning process. A healing relationship is characterized by certain principles:

- The focus is on strengths and skills.
- The nurse and the client are involved in creating changes and influencing outcomes.
- The nurse and the client are equal partners, but the client has the major responsibility for changing decisions.
- A balance of exchange or reciprocity occurs.
- Presence and involvement or connectedness emerge.
- Flow and harmony exist.

The patterning process has two phases, appraisal and deliberative. The elements of appraisal in Phase I include the following:

- Using multiple modes of awareness, including recognizing, being aware, and being sensitive.
- Tuning into a person's unique patterns.
- Appreciating manifestations of the human field in the form of experience, perception, and expressions.
- Constructing pattern knowing through synthesis.
- Verifying with the client.

Phase II involves the mutual deliberative patterning of behavior, which is possible because of the integral connectedness of the person–environment. Although diversity is considered a norm, patterning of each individual is unique. Each person has an intrinsic potential for growth, which can be identified by exploring the meaning of experiences for the individual. The client and the nurse are viewed as connected, and the healing milieu is as important as the treatment modality. Because change is viewed as inevitable, the challenge is to reframe problems into opportunities for positive becoming. By tuning in to the client's rhythms, the nurse can help the client to free energy for self-patterning through a number of possible noninvasive interventions:

- Imagery
- Relaxation
- Affirmation
- Sound (music)
- Exercise
- Color/light (wave modalities)
- Nutrition (diet, vitamins, minerals, and herbs)
- Meaningful presence
- Humor
- Authentic dialog (guided reminiscence)
- Wellness counseling (health education)
- Therapeutic touch (centering)
- Movement (dance, imposed motion)
- Journal keeping
- Balance between activity and rest
- Bibliotherapy
- Acupressure
- Bodywork (massage, touch for health)

The science of the unitary human being seems highly compatible with traditional and integrative approaches to health care. As clients become more aware of complementary and alternative health care treatments, professional nurses need the knowledge to help them make wise choices for health enhancement.

QUESTIONS FOR REFLECTION

1. How do you feel about using energy to promote healing and health?
2. Which of the patterning processes would you like to try to enhance your health? Why would you like to try that one?

REAL-LIFE REFLECTIONS

Remember Carol and Jane from the beginning of the chapter? If you were Carol, how would you respond to Jane's difficulty using nursing process? Why is it so important that beginning nurses understand nursing process?

Summary and Significance to Practice

Cognitive, interpersonal, and patterning nursing processes provide methods by which the nurse sensitively and systematically approaches practice to achieve mutually determined health goals with the client. Nurses use a variety of cognitive skills (knowledge, nursing process, intuition, and reflection) when delivering client care. Critical thinking enables nurses to effectively use nursing cognitive processes in clinical practice. Although nursing process arises out of scientific foundations, nurses can be artistic when developing individualized client care plans.

In addition to nurse cognitive processes, the nurse–client relationship facilitates data collection (assessment) and collaborative goal setting. Recent efforts to standardize nursing diagnoses, outcomes, and interventions may interfere with the ability to provide individualized client care developed in partnership with clients.

The use of interactive processes may provide enriching relationships for the client and the nurse because authenticity provides the basis for therapeutic partnerships. Patterning processes provide a complex holographic approach to nursing care, in which nurses focus on maximizing client–human potential. The various nursing models and theories presented in this chapter guide nursing practice. However, the individual nurse decides the approaches and processes used to implement nursing care effectively and in collaboration with clients and interprofessional health team members.

From Theory to Practice

1. Why is it important for professional nurses to use cognitive, interactive, and patterning processes when engaging in clinical practice?
2. Which nursing process do you use most frequently in clinical practice? Why? What assumptions underlie your most frequently used professional nursing process?

Nurse as Author

1. Obtain a clinical path (or standardized care plan) from a clinical setting. Make a list of all the steps contained within it. Analyze it for the presence of all steps of the nursing process. Outline the rationale behind all the nursing interventions. Write a brief summary of how the path or standardized care plan facilitates and hinders the delivery of patient-centered nursing care. Specify how you would revise the path (or care plan) to individualize the plan for a person with special needs not included in the plan.

2. Take a moment to reflect about how you use nursing diagnoses in clinical practice. Write a brief essay about the strengths and weaknesses of using nursing diagnoses using in-text citations and your personal clinical experiences. Based upon your analysis about the strengths and weaknesses of nursing diagnoses in practice, make a recommendation for its continued use or elimination as a step of nursing process.

Your Digital Classroom

Online Exploration

Foundation for Critical Thinking: **www.criticalthinking.org**
How to Construct a Concept Map (University of Delaware): **http://www.udel.edu/chem/white/teaching/ConceptMap.html**
Insight Assessment: **www.insightassessment.com**
North American Nursing Diagnosis Association-International (NANDA-I): **www.nanda.org**
The Concept Mapping Homepage: **http://users.edte.utwente.nl/lanzing/cm_home.htm**
University of Iowa College of Nursing Center for Nursing Classification and Clinical Effectiveness: **http://www.nursing.uiowa.edu/center-for-nursing-classification-and-clinical-effectiveness**

Expanding Your Understanding

1. Visit the North American Nursing Diagnosis Association International website and answer the following questions.
   a. Browse the site to determine the cost of being a full member of the organization and what benefits the membership offers. Would you consider becoming a member? Why or why not?
   b. Find the newly approved nursing diagnoses. Identify the ones that you would use in clinical practice to generate nursing care plans for your clients. Would the current care planning program in your practice support using one of these new diagnoses? If not, how would you proceed to make a clinical practice change so that you could use one of these new diagnoses?
   c. Access the process for submitting a new nursing diagnosis. What do you think would be the barriers for proposing and submitting a new nursing diagnosis? Why do you think that the process is so detailed and prescriptive?

Beyond the Book

Visit thePoint® **www.thepoint.lww.com** for activities and information to reinforce the concepts and content covered in this chapter.

REFERENCES

American Nurses Association. (2015). *Nursing: Scope and standard of practice* (3rd ed.). Silver Spring, MD: Nursebooks.

Bandman, E. L., & Bandman, B. (1995). *Critical thinking in nursing* (2nd ed.). East Norwalk, CT: Appleton & Lange.

Banning, M. (2006). Nursing research perspectives on critical thinking. *British Journal of Nursing, 15*(2), 458–461.

Bartol, G. M. (2016). The psychophysiology of body mind healing. In B. Dossey, L. Keegan, (authors). C. C. Barrere, M. A. Blasko-Helming, D. A. Shields, K. Avino, & C. Guzzetta (Eds.), *Holistic nursing: A handbook for practice* (7th ed., pp. 221–238.). Burlington, MA: Jones & Bartlett Learning.

Benner, P. (1984). *From novice to expert*. Menlo Park, CA: Addison-Wesley.

Benner, P. (2000). *From novice to expert: Excellence and power in clinical nursing practice* (commemorative ed.). Menlo Park, CA: Addison-Wesley.

Benner, P., Tanner, C. A., & Chesla, C. A. (Eds.). (1996). *Expertise in nursing practice: Caring, clinical judgment, and ethics*. New York: Springer.

Brookfield, S. D. (1987). *Developing critical thinkers: Challenging adults to explore alternative ways of thinking and writing*. San Francisco, CA: Jossey-Bass.

Brookfield, S. D. (1995). *Becoming a critically reflective teacher*. San Francisco, CA: Jossey-Bass.

Carpenito-Moyet, L. J. (2010). *Nursing diagnosis application to clinical practice* (13th ed.). Philadelphia, PA: Wolters Kluwer Health/Lippincott Williams & Wilkins.

Center for Nursing Classification and Clinical Effectiveness. (n.d.). Overview: Nursing outcomes classification. Retrieved from http://www.nursing.uiowa.edu/cncce/nursing-outcomes-classification-overview. Accessed November 29, 2012.

Dochterman, J., & Bulechek, G. (Eds.). (2004). *Nursing Interventions Classification (NIC)* (4th ed.). St. Louis, MO: Mosby.

Facione, P. A. (2006). *Critical thinking: What it is and why it counts*. Millbrae, CA: California Academic Press.

Facione, P. A., Facione, N. C., & Giancarlo, C. A. (1996). *The California Critical Thinking Disposition Inventory Test Manual*. Millbrae, CA: California Academic Press.

Facione, N. C., Facione, P. A., & Sanchez, C. A. (1994). Critical thinking disposition as a measure of competent clinical judgment: The development of the California Critical Thinking Disposition Inventory. *Journal of Nursing Education, 33,* 345–350.

Finkelman, A., & Kenner, C. (2007). *Teaching IOM: Implications of the Institute of Medicine Reports for Nursing Education*. Silver Spring, MD: American Nurses Association.

Fonteyn, M. (2007). Concept mapping: An easy teaching strategy that contributes to understanding and may improve critical thinking. *Journal of Nursing Education, 46*(5), 199–200.

Gordon, M. (1995). *Manual of nursing diagnosis, 1995–1996*. St. Louis, MO: Mosby-Year Book.

Gordon, S. (2005). *Nursing against the odds*. Ithaca, NY: Cornell University Press.

Hardman, T. H., & Kamitsuru, S. (Eds.). (2014). *NANDA-International Nursing Diagnoses Definitions & Classification 2015–2017*. Oxford: Wiley Blackwell.

Henderson, V. (1987). Nursing process: A critique. *Holistic Nursing Practice, 1,* 7–18.

Huckabay, L. M. (2009). Clinical reasoned judgment and the nursing process. *Nursing Forum, 44*(2), 458–461.

Johansen, M. L., & O'Brien, J. L. (2015). Decision making in nursing practice: A concept analysis. *Nursing Forum, 5*(11), 40–48.

Johnson, M., Maas, M., & Moorhead, S. (2000). *Nursing Outcomes Classification (NOC)*. (2nd ed.). St. Louis, MO: Mosby.

Kataoka-Yahiro, M., & Saylor, C. (1994). A critical thinking model for nursing judgment. *Journal of Nursing Education, 33,* 351–356.

Kennedy, M., Fisher, M. B., & Ennis, R. H. (1991). Critical thinking: Literature review and needed research. In L. Idol & B. F. Jones (Eds.), *Educational values and cognitive instruction: Implications for reform* (pp. 11–40). Hillsdale, NJ: Lawrence Erlbaum.

King, I. M. (1995). The theory of goal attainment. In M. A. Frey & C. L. Sieloff (Eds.), *Advancing King's systems framework and theory of nursing*. Thousand Oaks, CA: Sage.

Kurfiss, J. (1988). *Critical thinking, theory, research and possibilities*. Washington, DC: Association for the Study of Higher Education.

Leddy, S. (2004). Human energy: A conceptual model of unitary nursing science. *Visions: The Journal of Rogerian Scholarship, 12,* 14–28.

Leddy, S. K. (2006). *Health promotion mobilizing strengths to enhance health, wellness, and well-being*. Philadelphia, PA: F. A. Davis.

Lindsey, E., & Hartrick, G. (1996). Health-promoting nursing practice: The demise of the nursing process? *Journal of Advanced Nursing, 23,* 106–112.

Malinski, V. M. (1986). *Explorations on Martha Rogers' science of unitary human beings*. Norwalk, CT: Appleton-Century-Crofts.

Maslow, A. H. (1962). *Toward a psychology of being*. Princeton, NJ: Van Nostrand.

McPeck, J. E. (1981). *Critical thinking and education*. New York: St. Martin's Press.

Müller-Staub, M., Lavin, M. A., Needham, I., & von Achterberg, T. (2006). Nursing diagnoses, interventions and outcomes—application and impact on nursing practice: Systematic review. *Journal of Advanced Nursing, 56*(5), 514–531.

National League for Nursing Accrediting Commission. (2000). *Guidelines for nursing program accreditation*. New York: Author.

Neuman, B., & Fawcett, J. (2002). *The Neuman systems model* (4th ed.). Upper Saddle River, NJ: Prentice Hall.

Newman, M. A. (1994). *Health as expanding consciousness* (2nd ed.). St. Louis, MO: Mosby.

Novak, J., & Cañas, A. (2008). The Theory Underlying Concept Maps and how to Construct and use Them [Technical Report IHMC Cmap Tools 2006–01 Rev 2008–01]. Retrieved from http://cmap.ihmc.us/publications/researchpapers/theorycmaps/theoryunderlyingconceptmaps.htm. Accessed November 29, 2012.

Parse, R. R. (1996). The human becoming theory: Challenges in practice and research. *Nursing Science Quarterly, 9,* 55–60.

Paterson, J. G., & Zderad, L. T. (1988). *Humanistic nursing.* New York: National League for Nursing.

Paul, R. (1993). *Critical thinking: What every person needs to survive in a rapidly changing world* (3rd ed.). Santa Rosa, CA: Foundation for Critical Thinking.

Pew Health Professions Commission. (1998). *Recreating health professional practice for a new century.* San Francisco, CA: University of California, San Francisco Center for the Health Professions.

Polge, J. (1995). Critical thinking: The use of intuition in making clinical nursing judgments. *Journal of the New York State Nurses Association, 26,* 4–9.

Reed, P. G. (1996). Peplau's interpersonal relations model. In J. J. Fitzpatrick & A. L. Whall (Eds.), *Conceptual models of nursing: Analysis and application* (3rd ed.). Stamford, CT: Appleton & Lange.

Rew, L. (1996). *Awareness in healing.* Albany, NY: Delmar.

Rogers, M. E. (1988). Nursing science and art: A prospective. *Nursing Science Quarterly, 1,* 99–102.

Rogers, M. E. (1992). Nursing science and the space age. *Nursing Science Quarterly, 5,* 27–34.

Roy, C., & Andrews, H. A. (1999). *The Roy adaptation model* (2nd ed.). Stamford, CT: Appleton & Lange.

Rubenfeld, M., & Scheffer, B. (2015). *Critical thinking TACTICS for nurses.* (3rd ed.). Burlington, MA: Jones & Bartlett Learning.

Scheffer, B. K., & Rubenfeld, M. (2000). A consensus statement on critical thinking in nursing. *Journal of Nursing Education, 39,* 352–359.

Schmidt, L. A. (2010). Making sure: Registered nurses watching over their patients. *Nursing Research, 59*(6), 400–406.

Schon, D. A. (1987). *Educating the reflective practitioner: Toward a new design for teaching and learning in the professions.* San Francisco, CA: Jossey-Bass.

Schuster, P. (2016). *Concept mapping: A critical-thinking approach to care planning* (4th ed.). Philadelphia, PA: F. A. Davis.

Shoulders, B., Follett, C., & Easonk, J. (2014). Enhancing critical thinking in clinical practice: Implications for critical and acute care nurses. *Dimensions of Critical Car Nursing, 33*(4), 207–214. doi:10.1097/dcc.0000000000000053

Shelton, D. (2008). Beyond tests: Other ways to evaluate learning. In B. Penn (Ed.), *Mastering the teaching role: A guide for nurse educators.* Philadelphia, PA: F. A. Davis.

Tanner, C. (2006). Thinking like a nurse: A research-based model of clinical judgment in nursing. *Journal of Nursing Education, 45*(6), 204–211.

Taylor, J., & Wros, P. (2007). Concept mapping: A nursing model for care planning. *Journal of Nursing Education, 46*(5), 211–216.

Turkel, M., Ray, M., & Kornblatt, L. (2012). Instead of reconceptualizing the nursing process let's re-name it. *Nursing Science Quarterly, 25*(2), 194–198.

Turkel, M. C. (2016). Describing self-reported assessments of critical thinking among practicing medical-surgical registered nurses. *MEDSURG Nursing, 51*(4), 244–250.

Turner, P. (2005). Critical thinking in nursing education and practice as defined in the literature. *Nursing Education Perspectives, 26*(5), 272–277.

Varcoe, C. (1996). Disparagement of the nursing process: The new dogma? *Journal of Advanced Nursing, 23,* 120–125.

Watson, J. M., & Glaser, E. M. (1990). *The Watson-Glaser critical thinking appraisal manual.* San Antonio, TX: The Psychological Corp., Harcourt, Brace, Jovanovich, Inc.

Webber, P. (2008). Facilitating critical thinking and effective reasoning. In B. Penn (Ed.), *Mastering the teaching role: A guide for nurse educators.* Philadelphia, PA: F. A. Davis.

Young, C. E. (1987). Intuition and nursing process. *Holistic Nursing Practice, 1,* 52–62.

Zanotti, R., & Chiffi, D. (2015). Diagnostic frameworks and nursing diagnoses: a normative stance. *Nursing Philosophy, 16,* 64–73. doi: 10.1111/nup.12074.

The Health Process and Self-Care of the Nurse

LEARNING OUTCOMES

By the end of this chapter, the learner will be able to:

1. Differentiate wellness from health.
2. Distinguish illness from disease.
3. Compare and contrast the interaction and integration worldviews of health.
4. Identify factors that contribute to individual variability in wellness.
5. Describe how health/illness can be explained as a unitary concept.
6. Differentiate health protection from health promotion.
7. Outline strategies for changing lifestyle behaviors and health patterning in clients and nurses.
8. Identify signs and symptoms of work-related stress, role underload, role overload, and burnout.
9. Describe strategies for managing work-related stress and enhancing personal wellness.

REAL-LIFE REFLECTIONS

After an exhausting shift, two nurses, Michael and Nadine, discuss how ironic it seems that they have worked all day to help others get better at the expense of their own health. Michael states, "The hospital doesn't seem to care about the health and well-being of the staff. We never have time to eat or even take bathroom breaks. Within a few months we'll all be ready to occupy one of the beds." Nadine continues the discussion, "You know, I never thought about the toll this job is taking on my health. I wonder what we could do to make this a more healthful place in which to work?"

Most nurses enter the nursing profession "to help people." One key way that nurses do this is by supporting and educating clients as they embark on their journeys to enhanced health and well-being. Unfortunately, nurses sometimes neglect their own health because of the perception that professional obligations supersede their personal needs.

Curing disease remains the major focus of medicine despite high costs and sometimes futile efforts. Americans are inundated with public service announcements regarding the importance of good nutrition, regular exercise, and routine disease screenings. Reports on the role of nutrition and exercise in preventing debilitating and fatal illness permeate the airways, internet, and print media. The Patient Protection and Affordable Care Act (ACA) of 2010 endorses health promotion and primary care services as a way to reduce health care expenditures while improving quality of life. Professional nurses have the opportunity to expand their scope of influence on society by (1) reinforcing the importance of health promotion, (2) promoting health and well-being, and (3) reinforcing client strengths by sharing nursing knowledge and expertise. Health promotion is an essential nursing activity in all nursing care settings, including acute care.

This chapter presents the interaction and the integration worldviews of health, organizing frameworks for alternate views of the concepts of health, well-being, wellness, disease, illness, and sickness. Models and nursing interventions for the protection, promotion, and patterning of health are outlined, and strategies for nurses to attain optimal health are presented.

WORLDVIEWS OF HEALTH

Basic philosophical assumptions about the nature of reality, including humans and the human–environment relationship, are referred to as worldviews. Nursing scholars have described several approaches to worldviews of health, including change/persistence (Hall, 1981), totality/simultaneity (Parse, 1987), particulate-deterministic/interactive-integrative/unitary-transformative (Newman, 1992), and reaction/reciprocal interaction/simultaneous action (Fawcett, 1993). The interaction and integration worldviews of health presented here synthesize elements of these approaches.

The Interaction Worldview of Health

In the **interaction worldview**, as in the totality worldview (Parse, 1987), the individual is conceptualized as a whole, comprised of parts, who interacts with a physically separate environment. The environment exerts stressors on people to which they must react. The interaction worldview supports a belief in linear, predictable, and quantifiable cause-and-effect relationships.

In the interaction worldview, people strive to maintain a balance or state of stability. When the environment changes, people must change. Effective reactions to environmental changes result in personal changes without negative effects on well-being, wellness, or

health. However, ineffective reactions may negatively affect personal well-being, resulting in disease, illness, or sickness.

Disease

Disease is a medical term consistent with the interaction worldview of health. Benner, Tanner, and Chesla (1996, p. 45) defined **disease** as a "dysfunction of the body." Medical interventions seek to cure diseases. Many nursing interventions support the medical regimen as nurses administer medications, perform treatments, encourage rest, and evaluate the effects of the interventions.

A variety of factors related to the person (host), agent, and environment are considered interrelated in the cause and effective treatment of disease. These interactions must be considered in determining a plan of care.

Illness

Illness is a subjective feeling of being unhealthy that may or may not be related to disease. A person may have a disease without feeling ill and may feel ill in the absence of disease. For example, a person may have hypertension (a disease), controlled with medication, diet, and exercise, and be symptom-free (no illness). Another person may have pain and feel ill but may not have an identifiable disease. What is important is how people feel and what they do as a result of those feelings.

Nursing interventions address the human response to illness, the identification of reasons for symptoms, and efforts to decrease symptoms, if possible. In contrast, medical interventions focus on efforts to label and treat symptoms and cure disease. When a person's illness is accepted by society and thus given legitimacy, it is considered a "sickness."

Sickness

According to Twaddle and Hessler (1977, p. 97), **sickness** is "a status, a social entity usually associated with disease or illness, although it may occur independently of them." Once a person fulfills criteria for being sick, others condone various dependent behaviors that otherwise might be considered unacceptable. Nurses assist people who are sick until they can reassume responsibility for independent decision making or functioning.

Well-Being

Well-being is a subjective perception of vitality and feeling that is a component of health within the interaction worldview. Although well-being is a variable subjective trait, it can be described objectively, experienced, and measured. Experienced at the lowest degrees, people might feel ill. Experienced at the highest levels, people perceive maximal life satisfaction, feel in perfect harmony with the universe, and believe they have made a significant contribution to humanity.

Health as Wellness

Health is difficult to define. Various nurse scholars describe it as a value judgment, a subjective state, a relative concept, a spectrum, a cycle, a process, and an abstraction that cannot be measured objectively (Dossey & Luck, 2016; Leddy, 2006; Mariano, 2013; McElligott, 2013). In many definitions, physiologic and psychological components of health are dichotomized. Other subconcepts that might be included in definitions of health include environmental and social influences, freedom from pain or disease, optimum capability, ability to adapt, purposeful direction and meaning in life, and a sense of well-being.

In the interaction worldview of health, **health** indicates the absence of disease and the ability to function independently and perform one's life roles. In this book, health is defined as a state or condition of integrity of functioning (functional capacity and ability) and perceived well-being (feeling well). As a result, a person is able to

- function adequately (can be observed objectively).
- adapt adequately to the environment.
- feel well (as assessed subjectively).

Wellness, as defined in the literature, is similar to the open-ended and eudemonistic models of health described in this chapter, and in this book it is considered synonymous with health. Dunn (1977, p. 9), in his classic work on high-level wellness, described wellness as "an integrated method of functioning which is oriented toward maximizing the potential of which the individual is capable, within the environment where he is functioning." Others characterize wellness–illness as "the human experience of actual or perceived function–dysfunction" (Jensen & Allen, 1994, p. 349). Indications of wellness (health) might include the following.

- A person's capacity to perform to the best of his or her ability.
- The ability to adjust and adapt to varying situations.
- A reported feeling of well-being.
- A feeling that "everything is together."

Smith (1981, p. 47) presented four models of health consistent with the interaction worldview that "can be viewed as forming a scale—a progressive expansion of the idea of health": The clinical model, the role performance model, the adaptive model, and the eudemonistic model.

The clinical model is the narrowest view. People are seen as physiologic systems with interrelated functions. Health is identified as the absence of signs and symptoms of disease or disability. Thus, health might be defined as a "state of not being sick" (Ardell, 1979, p. 18) or as a "relatively passive state of freedom from illness . . . a condition of relative homeostasis" (Dunn, 1977, p. 9). The current health care delivery system, which is based on this model of health, is designed to deal with disease and illness after they occur. In the clinical model of health, the opposite end of the continuum from health is disease.

Next on the scale is the idea of health as role performance. This model adds social and psychological dimensions to the concept of health. The critical criterion for health is that the person has the ability to fulfill societal roles effectively. If a person becomes unable to perform expected roles, this inability can mean illness, even if the individual appears clinically healthy. For example, "Somatic health is . . . the state of optimum capacity for the elective performance of valued tasks" (Parsons, 1958, p. 168). In the role performance model of health, the opposite end of the continuum from health is sickness.

In the adaptive model, which combines the clinical and role performance models, health is perceived as a condition in which the person can engage in effective interaction with the physical and social environment. This model addresses continuous and simultaneous growth and change in people and the environment. For example, McWilliam, Stewart, Brown, and Coderre (1996, p. 1) defined health as "the individual's ability to realize aspirations, satisfy needs, and respond positively to the challenges of the environment." The adaptive model suggests that health may be a process rather than a state of being. In the adaptive model of health, the opposite end of the continuum from health is illness.

The eudemonistic model provides an even more comprehensive conception of health. In this model, health is "the actualization of inherent and acquired human potential" (Pender, Murdaugh, & Parsons, 2002, p. 22). Health "transcends biologic fitness. It is primarily a measure of each person's ability to do what he wants to do and become what he wants to become" (Dubos, 1978, p. 74). In the eudemonistic model, health is consistent with high-level wellness and at the opposite end of the continuum from disabling illness.

Examples of nursing conceptual models that are consistent with the interaction worldview are King's systems interaction model, Neuman's health care systems model, Roy's adaptation model, and Orem's self-care deficit model (see Chapter 6, "Nursing Models and Theories").

> **Take Note!**
> In the interactive worldview of health, effective reactions to change promote a state of well-being; ineffective reactions lead to a state of disease, illness, and sickness.

The Integration Worldview of Health

In the **integration worldview**, as in the simultaneity worldview (Parse, 1987), individuals are considered to be unitary, indivisible wholes, embedded in and inseparable from their environments. Because the person is in mutual process with the environment, multiple "causes" and "effects" and nonlinear changes make prediction probabilistic and sometimes imprecise.

In the integration worldview, the goal is for people to develop their potential toward increased diversity (becoming the fully unique person that they are meant to be). Change is inevitable and provides an opportunity for growth. Health is viewed as a unitary pattern. A pattern can be described as a "configuration of relationships" (Crawford, 1982, p. 3) or a consistency in all the interconnections among all energy processes that are not detectable through human perception processes (Leddy, 2006). Thus, a person's health (critically ill to optimally well) is a manifestation of the energy patterns that reflect the whole of the person.

Disease and Illness as Manifestations of Health

In the integration worldview, health is viewed as encompassing both disease and "nondisease" (Newman, 1994). Disease can be considered "a manifestation of health . . . a meaningful aspect of health" (Newman, 1994, p. 5) and "a meaningful aspect of the whole" (p. 7). Illness and health are viewed as a single process of ups and downs that are manifestations of varying degrees of organization and disorganization. Disputing that death is the antithesis of health, Newman (1994, p. 11) proposed that disease and nondisease are not opposites, but rather are complementary, to determine health, a unitary process. Illness, like health, simply represents a pattern of life at a particular moment. The tension characteristic of disease throws one off balance, which promotes growth toward a new level of evolving

capacities, personal uniqueness, and complexity. The person may transform into a new pattern of being.

Therefore, health can be conceptualized as an actively continuing process that involves initiative, ability to assume responsibility for health, value judgments, and integration of the total person. It is a goal, a fluid process, rather than an actual state. Thus, health is difficult to quantify for objective evaluation. In clinical practice, nurses collaborate with clients while trying to help them attain optimal health. Nurses help clients by focusing on client strengths while getting them to acknowledge the factors impeding growth toward maximal health potential. Client goals and feelings direct nursing interventions.

Nursing models and theories that are consistent with the integration worldview include Rogers' science of unitary human beings, Parse's theory of human becoming, Neuman's theory of health as expanding consciousness, and Leddy's human energy model (see Chapter 6, "Nursing Models and Theories"). These models and theories describe health as an evolving or emerging process, a forward movement with mutual person–environment patterns.

> **Take Note!**
> In the integration worldview of health, health can be conceptualized as an actively continuing process that involves initiative, ability to assume responsibility for health, value judgments, and integration of the total person.

QUESTIONS FOR REFLECTION

1. Which of the worldviews on health appeals to you the most? Why?
2. Do you view health as a state or a process?
3. How do your views about health affect your professional practice or your life? Can you provide an example from your professional or personal experiences?

HEALTH PROTECTION AND PROMOTION

Health promotion has been defined as "activities directed toward increasing the level of well-being and actualizing the health potential of people, families, community, and society" (Hravnak, 1998, p. 284). Pender et al. (2002) and Pender, Murdaugh, and Parsons (2006) distinguished health promotion from disease prevention, stating that health promotion is the process of increasing well-being and actualizing an individual's maximal health potential. Individual motivation plays an important role in health promotion. Whereas **health protection** focuses on active avoidance of disease or injury and early detection or optimal functioning within the confines of an illness, health promotion expands the potential for health.

Goals for Health Promotion and Protection

The U.S. health care system remains disease oriented, despite increased efforts toward health promotion and fitness. With its goal of curing and controlling illness, the United States spends more on health care than all other nations. Health promotion, disease prevention, and health education receive less funding, and health education efforts mainly address illness prevention. For example, children are taught to brush their teeth to avoid cavities (not because the mouth will feel, look, taste, and smell better) and to eat properly and exercise to prevent diabetes (rather than because they will feel better).

In the 1990s, recognizing the need to promote the health of Americans, the federal government initiated Healthy People 2000. In 2000, the U.S. Department of Health and Human Services (USDHHS, 2000) issued its *Healthy People 2010 report*, which described national objectives for health promotion and disease prevention, including "increase quality and years of healthy life" (p. 8) and "eliminate health disparities" (p. 11). The outcomes of *Healthy People 2010* were mixed. Between 2000 and 2010, the incidence of Americans dying from heart disease and stroke declined, overall life expectancy rose, and access to and acceptance of mental health services increased, but health disparities for socially, economically, or environmentally disadvantaged persons rose 13%, millions of Americans lost health insurance coverage, and obesity rates increased dramatically (the percentage of obese individuals increased by 54.5% for children ages 6 to 11 years, 63.6% for adolescents ages 12 to 19 years, and 48% for adults) (USDHHS, 2011).

In 2011, the federal government completed work on Healthy People 2020, a collaborative process among the USDHHS, other federal agencies, members of the public, and an advisory committee. No nurse was part of the development of the program. Healthy People 2020 envisions a society in which all citizens can "live long, healthy live" (USDHHS, 2017, para 3). Features in Healthy People 2020 include increased emphasis on health equity that considers the social determinants of health, increased attention to health promotion across the lifespan, and an interactive website that permits users to tailor information based on their health individual needs so that they can explore evidence-based health resources to improve their health.

The mission of Healthy People 2020 is fivefold:

1. Identify priorities for American health improvement.
2. Increase awareness and understanding of health, disease, and disability determinants and inform person of the opportunities for improvement.
3. Identify and provide measurable and applicable goals and objectives for all levels of government.
4. Engage multiple sectors of society to improve policies and practices to use the best available knowledge and evidence for health promotion.
5. Identify the critical areas for data collection, research, and evaluation.

Box 8.1, Professional Building Blocks, "Goals, Measurement Categories, and Progress Measures for Healthy People 2020 and Professional Nurse Roles" summarizes the program's highlights and the professional nurse's role in relation to them. Some of these areas are embedded in the 2010 ACA. The program identifies 42 topics, including such areas as health services access, growth and development across the lifespan, genomics, health care–associated infections, injury and violence prevention, food and medical product safety, optimal nutrition and weight, sleep health, and use of tobacco and substance abuse. In the future, the federal government may require health care providers to address these determinants of health with each health care consumer.

The next section discusses various models and strategies for use in clinical practice to guide nurses in interventions targeted for health promotion and protection.

Take Note!

Concepts of health protection and promotion are consistent with the interaction worldview.

▌ QUESTIONS FOR REFLECTION

1. Think about the last time you engaged in clinical practice as a student or registered nurse. Write down examples of when your practice focused on health protection and health promotion. Why is it important for nurses to engage in client health protection and promotion?

2. Do you have any of the unhealthy conditions or habits outlined in the Healthy People 2020

8.1 Professional Building Blocks

Goals, Measurement Categories, and Progress Measures for Healthy People 2020 and Professional Nurse Roles

Overarching Goal	Measurement Category	Progress Measures	Professional Nurse Roles
Attain high-quality, longer lives free of preventable disease, disability, injury, and premature death	General health status	■ Life and healthy life expectancy ■ Number of physical and mental unhealthy days ■ Self-reported health status ■ Activity limitations ■ Prevalence of chronic diseases ■ International comparisons if available	■ Inquire about client perception of health status ■ Assess all clients for mobility limitations ■ Provide education and support on how to enhance health through optimal nutrition, exercise, and ways to avoid chronic illness
Achieve health equity, eliminate disparities, and improve the health of all groups	Disparities and inequality	■ Assessment of disparities using the following criteria: race/ethnicity, gender, socioeconomic status, disability statistics, gender preference and transgender status, and geographical location	■ Assess clients' socioeconomic status, disabilities, gender preference, and location of primary residence ■ Advocate for clients when disparities are identified ■ Create a health delivery environment that provides equal care to all persons ■ Use community activism to remove social and economic disparities
Create social and physical environments that promote good health for all	Social determinants of health	■ Social and economic factors ■ Natural and manmade environments ■ Educational status ■ Current policies and programs	■ Develop and implement healthy environmental policies in health care organizations and educational facilities ■ Perform detailed environmental assessments in homes, workplaces, schools, neighborhoods, and in public and private facilities
Promote quality of life, healthy development, and healthy behaviors across all life stages	Health-related quality of life and well-being	■ Self-reports of well-being and life satisfaction ■ Physical, mental, and social health-related quality of life ■ Participation in common activities	■ Assess client growth and development levels ■ Educate clients on developmentally appropriate health promotion, disease prevention, and early detection of illness based on age ■ Perform detailed sociocultural assessments that include participation in some form of community involvement

Adapted from *Healthy People 2020*. Retrieved from http://www.healthypeople.gov.

initiatives? How can you work to become a role model of health for your clients?

3. How do you and your family focus on health protection currently? Where did you get these ideas for health protection?

Models for Changing Lifestyle Behavior

Health Belief Model

Why do people behave in certain ways in certain situations? What kinds of nursing intervention would

be most effective in modifying a person's behavior to reduce the risk for disease? Rosenstock's (1966) "health belief" model still has relevance for today's health care situations. The model includes the following factors.

1. Perceived susceptibility: The client's perception of the likelihood of experiencing a particular illness.
2. Perceived severity: The client's perception of the seriousness of the illness and its potential impact on his or her life.

3. Benefits of action: The client's assessment of the potential of the health action to reduce susceptibility or severity.
4. The client's perception of the threat of disease.
5. Costs of action: The client's estimate of financial costs, time and effort, inconvenience, and possible side effects, such as pain or discomfort.
6. Cues that trigger health-seeking behaviors, such as information in newspapers or on television; internal signals, such as symptoms; and interpersonal relationships with the health care provider and significant others.

The health belief model, called a "rational model," explains how people work toward improving their general well-being and health. The model assumes that all people value well-being and that different actions taken to promote health and well-being vary according to individual perceptions, beliefs, interactions, and motivations. Kasl and Cobb (1966) extended the basic model by specifying a relatively positive variable, the "perceived importance of health matters," in addition to perceived value and perceived threat. Becker and Maiman (1975) expanded the model further by including positive health motivation. In 1988, Rosenstock, Strecher, and Becker (1988) urged incorporation of self-efficacy into the model. In a review of 10 years of studies related to the model, Janz and Becker (1984) concluded that only two of the model components, perceived barriers and perceived susceptibility, explained or predicted preventive behaviors. Perceived susceptibility has been found to be strongly related to compliance with medical advice (Vincent & Furnham, 1997).

Revised Pender Health Promotion Model

The health promotion model (HPM) (Pender et al., 2002, 2006; Pender, Murdaugh, & Parsons, 2011), developed in the early 1980s, has undergone several revisions based on research. The HPM provides a framework for combining professional nursing and behavioral science outlooks on various determinants of health behaviors. Pender categorized the determinants of health-promoting behavior into cognitive-perceptual factors (individual perceptions), modifying factors, and variables affecting the likelihood of action. Pender distinguished the HPM from other models explaining health action because it eliminates the "fear" and "threat" perceptions for health action.

Based on extensive research, the HPM was revised in 1996 (Fig. 8.1) (Pender, 1996; Pender et al., 2002, 2006, 2011). The revised model proposes that health-promoting behavior is related to direct and indirect influences among the 10 determinants of individual characteristics and experiences (e.g., previous related behavior and personal factors), behavior-specific cognitions and affect (e.g., perceived benefits of action, perceived barriers to action, perceived self-efficacy, activity-related affect, interpersonal influences, and situational influences), commitment to a plan of action, and immediate competing demands. Pender (1996) considered the behavior-specific cognitions and affect category of variables "to be of major motivational significance . . . [and to] constitute a critical 'core' for intervention, because they are subject to modification through nursing actions" (p. 68).

A review of studies testing the revised HPM by Pender et al. (2002, 2006, 2011) reveals that the following factors contribute to health-promoting behaviors.

1. Perceived benefits of action
2. Perceived barriers to action
3. Perceived self-efficacy
4. Interpersonal influences
5. Situational influences

Additional research is needed to validate Pender's HPM. Identified areas for future research include how mood and attitude affect success of health-promoting activities, the effects of commitment level to successful health promotion, and the relationship between competing demands and personal preferences when determining specific health promotion actions to take (Pender et al., 2011).

The Transtheoretical Model

The transtheoretical model assumes that change requires movement through discrete motivational stages over time, with the active use of different processes of change at different stages. The model has been supported in the studies of a number of lifestyle behaviors, including smoking cessation, weight control, sunscreen use, exercise acquisition, mammography screening, and condom use (Prochaska et al., 1994b).

According to Prochaska, Redding, Harlow, Rossi, and Velicer (1994a), the stages of change in this model represent a continuum of motivational readiness for behavior change. The stages include the following.

1. **Precontemplation:** Not intending to change
2. **Contemplation:** Intending to change within 6 months
3. **Preparation:** Actively planning change
4. **Action:** Overtly making changes
5. **Maintenance:** Taking steps to sustain change and resist temptation to relapse

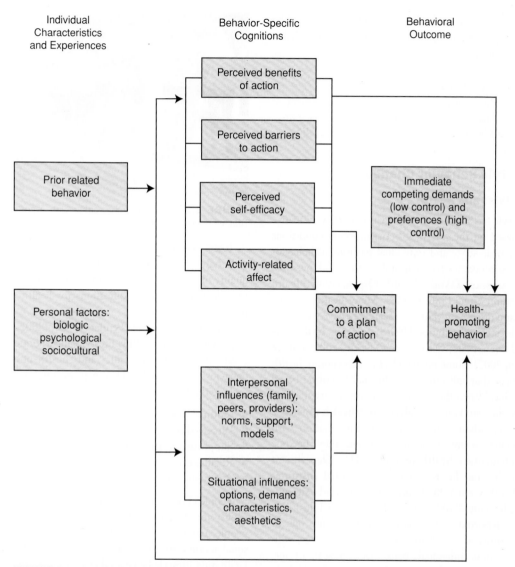

Individual Characteristics and Experiences	Behavior-Specific Cognitions	Behavioral Outcome

FIGURE 8.1 The health promotion model. (From Pender, N. J., Murdaugh, C. L., & Parsons, M. A. (2011). *Health promotion in nursing practice* (6th ed.). Upper Saddle River, NJ: Prentice Hall. © Reprinted with permission from Pearson Education, Inc., Upper Saddle River, NJ.)

Westberg and Jason (1996, p. 147) described the steps of successful change that are consistent with the stages of the transtheoretical model. These steps are as follows:

1. Acknowledging that something is not right in one's life
2. Deciding that a change is wanted
3. Setting one or more goals
4. Exploring options for the achievement of goals
5. Deciding on and trying to implement a plan
6. Assessing progress
7. Guarding against backsliding

Also included in the transtheoretical model is the concept of decisional balance. The model proposes that part of the decision to move toward the action stage of change is based on the relative weight given to the pros and cons of changing behavior to reduce risk. "The pros represent the advantages or positive aspects of changing behavior, and may be thought of as facilitators of change. The cons represent the disadvantages or negative aspects of changing behavior, and may be thought of as barriers to change" (Prochaska et al., 1994a, pp. 478–479).

This model provides a rationale for individualizing interventions based on a client's readiness for change. It remains to be demonstrated whether stage-appropriate interventions are effective not only in encouraging behavior change progress but also in promoting maintenance of the desired change.

Take Note!
The effectiveness of interventions to modify an individual's lifestyle behavior will depend on the individual's perceptions, values, beliefs, and motivations.

Lifestyle Behavior Change

Lifestyles and Health

Lifestyle has been described as a "general way of living based on the interplay between living conditions in the wide sense and individual patterns of behavior as determined by sociocultural factors and personal characteristics" (World Health Organization Health Education Unit, 1986, p. 118). Many health promotion and disease prevention researchers have suggested that lifestyle contributes 33% to a person's health status (Logan, 2007; O'Keefe & O'Keefe, 2006; Rau & Wyler, 2007). Some people elect to incorporate health practices that fall outside traditional scientific-based medicine. When these health practices are used exclusively, they are known as **alternative health practices**. However, when they are used in combination with traditional scientific-based medicine, they become **complementary health practices** (U.S. Department of Health and Human Services, National Institutes of Health Center for Complementary and Alternative Medicine 2008). Cuellar, Rogers, and Higshman (2007) reported that 2.1% of Americans use one or more forms of complementary health practices, with 88% of these individuals being over 65 years of age. Examples of complementary health practice include the following (Rau & Wyler, 2007).

- Isopathic remedies (disarming viruses and bacteria by pairing them up with a neutralizing agent).
- Chelation therapy (giving intravenous medication that binds body toxins to the blood for renal excretion).
- Ozone therapy (exposing the client's own blood to ozone and reinfusing it).
- Chiropractics (spinal manipulation).
- Myoreflex therapy (acupressure points and meridian theory).
- Homeopathy (usually diluted organic substances to stimulate the immune system).
- Cleanses (detoxifying programs with specific diets, juices, and colonic irrigations).
- Hyperthermia or sauna treatment.

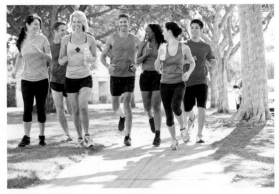

FIGURE 8.2 Regular exercise, either with a group or by yourself is a key component of a healthy lifestyle.

Recent evidence reports that modifying simple lifestyle habits can increase the length and improve the quality of life. Table 8.1 presents attainment strategies for selected lifestyle modifications for health protection and promotion.

Pender (1996) and Pender et al. (2002, 2006) suggested that a healthy lifestyle incorporates both health-protecting behaviors and health-promoting behaviors (Fig. 8.2). Health-protecting behaviors include the following.

- Optimal nutrition
- Perceived self-efficacy
- Supportive relationships
- Regular exercise
- Adequate sleep

People choose their lifestyles. Many assume responsibility for their own lifestyle choices; however, some people may refuse to accept the consequences of personal actions resulting in an unhealthy lifestyle. Before facilitating lifestyle behavioral changes, the nurse must assess the client's perceived interpretation of what it means to live a healthy lifestyle, perception of health promotion, current health promotion behaviors, level of motivation to change, and expected outcomes of lifestyle changes. The client and the nurse collaborate to determine what changes need to be made and how the nurse can facilitate and support identified changes, thereby shifting thinking from using professional expertise to overcome client weaknesses to empowering clients to help themselves by building on their strengths.

Health Strengths

A large body of literature associates stress with illness. Stress is assumed to arise when a situation is appraised as threatening or otherwise demanding and an appropriate coping response is not immediately available (Lazarus & Folkman, 1984). When an event

TABLE 8.1   Lifestyle Modifications and Attainment Strategies

Lifestyle Modification	Attainment Strategies
Get adequate sleep (7–8 h nightly)	■ Establish a sleep routine ■ Use the bed and bedroom exclusively for sleeping
Maintain a body mass index between 19 and 25 m²	■ Weigh at least on a weekly basis ■ Monitor food intake and exercise patterns on a daily basis ■ Chew each bite of food 20–30 times before swallowing it ■ Use any opportunity available to engage in physical activity ■ Avoid eating before retiring for sleep
Consume a healthful diet containing at least nine servings of fruits and vegetables daily that includes breakfast	■ Strive to eat mainly fresh produce ■ Bake or poach foods rather than frying them ■ Avoid fast food or eating on the run ■ Avoid bringing calorie-dense foods into the house—consider going out for sweet treats rather than storing them at home ■ Schedule meal times and eat with another person
Exercise on a regular schedule	■ Determine what form of exercise gives you pleasure ■ Schedule exercise time daily ■ Seek out companionship during exercise ■ Engage in aerobic exercise (e.g., walk 10,000 steps per day, run, or dance) for at least 5 days a week ■ Lift weights every other day ■ Perform flexibility (stretching) exercises after each exercise routine
Participate in recreational activities	■ Discover what you like to do ■ Make time to play each day ■ Try something new and different
Drink 64 or more ounces of water daily	■ Drink water instead of soda, fruit juice, dairy drinks, or caffeinated beverages ■ Get a water bottle or commuter cup, and wash it daily ■ Consume a glass of water between other beverages
Schedule quiet time for reflection, prayer, or relaxation techniques	■ Schedule quiet time by learning to say "no" ■ Turn off cell phones and other paging devices ■ Inform other household members of the need for quiet time alone
Brush teeth twice and floss them once daily	■ Establish the routine of brushing your teeth each morning on arising and each evening before bed ■ Keep toothbrush, toothpaste, and dental floss in a visible location ■ Floss either in the morning or in the evening
Maintain an optimistic attitude	■ Try to always look at the bright side of life ■ Take time to inventory life's pleasures
Secure an integrated approach between allopathic and complementary health practices	■ Follow governmental guidelines for health screenings ■ Communicate all health-promoting and health-protecting practices to health care providers ■ Practice skepticism of any health care device or preparation that makes unsubstantiated claims to improve health and well-being
Keep in touch with social support network	■ Schedule time to meet with persons who uplift you ■ Establish meaningful relationships with family and friends

Leddy, S. K. (2006). *Health promotion: Mobilizing strengths to enhance health, wellness, and well-being*. Philadelphia, PA: F.A. Davis; Logan, A. C. (2007). *The brain diet, revised and expanded*. Nashville, TN: Cumberland House; O'Keefe, J., & O'Keefe, J. (2006). *The forever young diet & lifestyle*. Kansas City, MO: Andrews McMeel; Pender, N. J., Murdaugh, C. L., & Parsons, M. A. (2011). *Health promotion in nursing practice* (6th ed.). Upper Saddle River, NJ: Prentice Hall; and Rau, T., & Wyler, S. (2007). *The Swiss secret to optimal health*. New York: Berkeley.

is appraised as stressful, emotionally linked responses occur that result in vulnerability to illness.

Certain characteristics, including social support, self-efficacy, and internal locus of control, seem to decrease the relationship between stress and illness. Two models explain the process by which these characteristics might influence well-being. One model

suggests that the person is protected, or buffered, from the potentially pathogenic influence of stressful events. In this case, these characteristics would be related to well-being only (or primarily) for persons under stress (Cohen & Wills, 1985, p. 310). The alternative model suggests that health strengths have a beneficial effect, regardless of whether the person is under stress.

Some research suggests that certain personality characteristics reduce the perception of stress or increase resistance to stress and thus may be considered health strengths. In her theory of hardiness, Kobasa (1979) assumed that life is always changing and thus is inevitably stressful. However, people who have a sense of commitment (an overall sense of purpose), control (a belief that one can influence the course of events), and challenge (a view of change as opportunity and incentive for personal growth) are thought to be more resistant to stress. In the sense of coherence theory, Antonovsky (1987) proposed that confidence in comprehensibility (a cognitive sense that information is consistent, clear, and ordered), manageability (a belief that resources are adequate to meet demands), and meaningfulness (a motivational commitment and engagement) provides generalized resistance resources and promotes health.

Strategies for Lifestyle Behavior Change

A **lifestyle behavior change** means that people assume different activities in multiple aspects of their lives. The idea of changing health behavior is uncomfortable for many people. Deeply ingrained habits, even harmful ones, can be difficult to change, and most people have difficulty making even minor changes. According to Westberg and Jason (1996, pp. 147–148), people tend to resist change because change of behavior may

- require giving up pleasure (e.g., eating high-fat ice cream).
- create an unpleasant feeling (e.g., doing certain exercises).
- cause overt pain (e.g., discontinuing addictive substances).
- produce stress (e.g., facing social situations without alcohol).
- jeopardize social relationships (e.g., engaging in unprotected adolescent sex).
- seem unimportant anymore (e.g., in the case of older individuals).
- require alteration in self-image (e.g., in the case of a hard-working executive learning how to play).

As a result, giving up long-standing habits and attitudes is not easy for most people.

Given that health behavior change is difficult for most people, Westberg and Jason (1996, pp. 148–150) suggested that to promote "what it takes" to make meaningful, lasting changes in lifestyle, the individual should

- endorse the need for change.
- have "ownership" of the need for change.

- feel that there is more to gain than to lose.
- develop an enhanced sense of self-worth.
- identify realistic goals and workable plans.
- seek gradual change, rather than a "quick fix."
- have patience.
- address starting new behaviors, instead of just focusing on what behaviors should be stopped.
- practice new behaviors.
- seek the support of family, friends, colleagues, and/or health professionals.
- gain positive reinforcement for the desired behavior.
- have a strategy for monitoring progress and making needed changes.
- seek constructive feedback.
- have a mechanism for follow-up to reduce backsliding.

Learning how to help people adopt and sustain healthy attitudes and habits is a challenge for health professionals. "There are no miracle drugs available for helping people change long-standing patterns of living. Simply telling people to stop smoking, eat less fat, have safe sex, exercise more, discontinue their abusive practices, or reduce their life stresses seldom works" (Westberg & Jason, 1996, p. 146). Clients often do not follow the advice of nurses or physicians, particularly when authoritarian "orders" are given. Clients must be actively involved as collaborative partners who assess their current health, develop a health promotion plan, and monitor plan effectiveness. Rewards facilitate adherence to health promotion plans. The nurse can best assist in promoting and changing health behaviors by providing education (see Box 8.2, Professional Prototypes, "Teaching the Benefits of Exercise"), facilitating changes (e.g., positive reinforcement for adhering to a plan), and sustaining positive health behaviors (e.g., reminding clients of how they were before they started the health promotion plan).

According to Prochaska et al. (1994a), some of the most frequently replicated strategies and techniques to help clients modify their behavior include the following.

- Consciousness raising
- Self-reevaluation
- Environmental reevaluation
- Self-liberation
- Social liberation
- Helping relationships
- Stimulus control
- Counterconditioning
- Reinforcement management

8.2 Professional Prototypes

Teaching the Benefits of Exercise

Disease Prevention/Treatment

Exercise ...

- Reduces the lipids and lipoproteins that are associated with atherosclerosis development, helping prevent cardiovascular disease and stroke.
- Has anti-inflammatory effects by reducing C-reactive protein and white blood cells associated with cardiovascular disease.
- Reduces fibrinogen levels, thereby reducing thrombus formation.
- Is associated with a reduced incidence of some types of cancer (colon, breast, endometrial, lung) and cancer recurrence (breast).
- Stabilizes the release of insulin and reduces the risk for type 2 diabetes mellitus and metabolic syndrome.
- Increases bone density.
- Slows the loss of bone density.
- Reduces pain associated with arthritis.

Health Promotion

Exercise ...

- Improves muscle strength and flexibility.
- Helps maintain physical functioning status.
- Improves cognitive function.
- Releases endorphins, resulting in increased feeling good (could become addictive if exercise is extreme).
- Reduces body mass index and core body fat, enhancing appearance.
- Increases endurance, leading to improved sustainability of independent execution of activities of daily living.
- Improves strength and balance, reducing the risk for fall and injury.
- Increases longevity (persons who are physically active for 7 h a week have a 40% lower risk for dying early).

Centers for Disease Control and Prevention. (2011). Physical activity and health. Retrieved from http://www.cdc.gov/physicalactivity/everyone/health/index.html. Accessed December 5, 2012; and Lewis, H. H. (2012). Physical activity is the key to cardiac health. *Primary Health Care*, 22(1), 16–21.

During the contemplation stage of behavior change, consciousness raising occurs as the individual seeks information. Nurses can help this process by providing informational resources so that the individual can make informed decisions and consider incentives for and barriers to change. In addition, nurses can help assess the knowledge and interest of family members (significant others) to ensure support for the client about to make a lifestyle change. It may also be helpful for the individual to talk with others who have successfully made the contemplated changes.

As movement occurs toward the preparation and action stages of change, individuals assess and evaluate themselves and their environments. They consider how the current behavior (negative or problem) affects their physical well-being, interpersonal relationships, and personal values and aspirations. Questions that might arise include "Will I like myself better as a (thinner, nonsmoking, less stressed) person?" "Is my environment supportive of the proposed changes?" and "Do I believe that I am able to make and continue the changes needed?" The assumption is that changes will not occur unless they are congruent with a person's self-concept. For some people, introduction of a new lifestyle change produces anxiety and they may turn to nurses for guidance and support.

A strategy that can assist with self- and social liberation is cognitive restructuring. "Cognitive restructuring focuses on client's thinking, imagery, and attitudes toward the self and self-competencies as they affect the change process" (Pender, 1996, p. 171). The nurse's role is to help clients clarify the messages clients give themselves about their health and health-related behaviors. Certain beliefs can be irrational. Positive affirmations and imagery, repeated several times daily, can assist clients in believing and thinking positively that they have the power to make desired lifestyle changes.

Helping relationships with family members, friends, colleagues, or health care professionals can be critical in helping to move the individual through the preparation, action, and maintenance stages of change. For some people, self-help groups have been instrumental in modeling, supporting, and reinforcing desired behavior.

Controlling stimuli that precede previous behavior and newly acquired desired behavior helps the action and maintenance stages of change. These activities must be personally relevant for the individual client, such as a postcard reminder for a mammography screening, a personal call from the nurse to encourage continued exercise, or a scheduled group meeting to practice relaxation. Consistency of setting, context, and time facilitates the development of a new habit. For example, the client can be encouraged to exercise in a consistent place, early each morning before starting other daily activities.

Counterconditioning to break an undesirable association between a stimulus and a response can be desirable during the latter part of the action stage and during the maintenance stage. Undesirable associations can occur that create a negative emotional response to the new behavior. For example, many people indicate that exercising can become boring. The nurse can encourage a varied routine, walking outside when the weather permits, and at least occasional exercise with a partner to counteract boredom.

Reinforcement management is an effective strategy, especially during the preparation and action stages of change. "It is based on the premise that all behaviors are determined by their consequences. If positive consequences occur, the probability is high that the behavior will occur again. If negative consequences occur, the probability is low for the behavior's being repeated" (Pender, 1996, p. 172). Immediate reinforcement of the desired behavior is important, especially in the early phases of change. Personalized attention and positive verbal feedback are helpful. Eventually, a desirable consequence of the behavior can become an intrinsic reward. For example, a weekly scale reading indicating decreasing weight can be a reward in itself for continuing a weight reduction diet.

The objective of these strategies is to decrease barriers and increase incentives to change behavior. Table 8.2 summarizes barriers and incentives to change.

The nurse and the client should base the choice of appropriate strategies on fostering incentives and reducing barriers, thereby promote behavior change. Concepts in Practice, "Weight Management Success for Night Shift Nurses," demonstrates how one group of nurses applied these strategies to their own behaviors.

Concepts in Practice [IDEA]──▶[PLAN]─▶[ACTION]

Weight Management Success for Night Shift Nurses

Four nurses, Maria, James, Carol, and Rachel, have worked the night shift for 2 years together with nursing assistants Derek and Chris. They established a monthly potluck to celebrate holidays and birthdays. The monthly festivity involves everyone bringing his/her favorite foods. On other days, one of them makes a trip to the hospital cafeteria at 5:30 AM to get everyone breakfast. Since working together, all of them have gained at least 9.07 kg (20 lb) each.

Maria and James, who have gained the most weight, report that they are having difficulty sleeping during the daytime. Derek and Carol have two young children at home resulting in frequent sleep interruptions. One night, Rachel complained that she was going to have to purchase another even larger set of work clothes. The others also mentioned that they were going to have to do this too.

After analyzing what they had been doing, the six of them decided to stop the monthly potluck and take turns bringing in one dessert rather than everyone bringing something. They also agreed that on days off each of them would start some type of exercise program. Rachel created a spreadsheet for weekly weigh-ins and compliance to exercise. By the end of 6 months, each of them lost at least 2.27 kg (5 lb).

TABLE 8.2 Changing Behavior

Barriers	Incentives
Inaccurate knowledge	Expectation of benefit
Perceived lack of skills or abilities	Sense of personal responsibility
Perception of control	Enjoyment of the activity
Lack of access to facilities	Previous experience
Failure to acquire needed materials	Guilt
Inability to set clear goals	Support from family, peers, and/ or professionals
Lack of social support	Willingness to and capability of acquiring new attitudes and required resources to change
Lack of time	Carving out time for change
Lack of motivation	Being motivated

Leddy, S. K. (2006). *Health promotion: Mobilizing strengths to enhance health, wellness, and well-being*. Philadelphia, PA: F.A. Davis; Leddy, S. K., & Fawcett, J. (1997). Testing the theory of healthiness: Conceptual and methodological issues. In M. Madrid (Ed.), *Patterns of Rogerian knowing*. New York: National League for Nursing; Pender, N. J., Murdaugh, C. L., & Parsons, M. A. (2011). *Health promotion in nursing practice* (6th ed.). Upper Saddle River, NJ: Prentice Hall; Clark, C. C., & Paraska, K. K. (2014). *Health promotion for nurses, a practical guide*. Burlington, MA: Jones & Bartlett Learning.

This section has addressed models and strategies for health promotion consistent with the interaction worldview of health. In the next section, models and strategies for health patterning consistent with the integration worldview for health are discussed.

Take Note!

Modifying simple lifestyle habits, incorporating health-protecting and health-promoting behaviors, and an individual's "health strengths" can increase the length and improve the quality of life. Family members, friends, colleagues, or health care professionals can provide critical support in this process.

▋ QUESTIONS FOR REFLECTION

1. Take a moment to think about your lifestyle habits during the past month. What are your current health promotion strategies? What are some of your not-so-healthy habits?
2. Outline a plan to improve one of your identified unhealthy habits.

HEALTH PATTERNING

Models for Health Patterning

For centuries, the concept of vital life energy, or chi, has been a part of Eastern religion and culture. For example, the ancient Chinese originated the belief that chi circulates through invisible channels called meridians that can be blocked by stressors or by living excesses. A blockage in energy flow results in energy imbalances and areas of the body with energy deficits, producing symptoms or disease. **Health patterning** involves interventions aimed at targeting any or multiple energy sources within the body, mind or spirit to promote optimal health and healing (Leddy, 2004, 2006).

Leddy's (2004, 2006) practice theory of energy (see Chapter 6, "Nursing Models and Theories") proposed that consciousness or focused attention by the nurse can pattern client–nurse energy by clearing (transforming), conveying (carrying), coursing (reestablishing free flow), conserving (decreasing disorder), converting (amplifying resonance), or connecting (promoting synchronization to promote harmony) energy.

Rogers introduced the concept of the person as an energy field interacting with an environmental energy field (see Chapter 6, "Nursing Models and Theories"). She theorized that health patterning of the human energy field occurs simultaneously and mutually with changes in the environmental energy field. The nurse (part of the environmental energy field) can influence the client's health by redistributing energy and thus repatterning the client's energy field. Nurses work with manifestations of health patterns (Leddy, 2003). Viewing persons as energy fields provides a rationale for nontraditional healing modalities that enhance health patterns.

Health-Patterning Modalities

Leddy (2003, 2006) identified integrative nursing interventions to promote health and healing. The following interventions act on the human energy field and can be used by nurses in clinical practice.

- **To release bound energy:** Herbal preparations and aromatherapy.

- **To reestablish energy flow:** Physical activity, tai chi, qigong (chi gung), and aerobic and strengthening exercises.
- **To release blocked energy:** Touch, massage, acupressure, reflexology, applied kinesiology (touch for health), jin shin do, self-massage, the Alexander technique, the Feldenkrais method, the Trager psychophysical integration, and structural integration (Rolfing).
- **To reduce energy depletion:** Meditation, autogenic training to elicit the relaxation response, progressive muscle relaxation, deep-breathing exercises, yoga, biofeedback, and guided imagery.
- **To regenerate agent's optimal nutrition:** Vitamin and mineral supplements, a high-fiber diet, ingestion of phytonutrients (soy, garlic, onions, and deep-colored fruits and vegetables), and antioxidants (vitamins A, C, and E; selenium; coenzyme Q 10; and beta-carotene).
- **To restore energy field harmony:** Centering, chromotherapy (color therapy), music therapy, polarity therapy, prayer, Reiki, and therapeutic touch.

Other complementary interventions aimed at strengthening or restoring energy harmony include feng shui and life energy therapies such as yoga and chakra cleansing, strengthening, and healing. Healing modalities using interventions to balance, release, or restore energy have been used for centuries in Eastern cultures (Fig. 8.3). Feng shui works on the assumption that

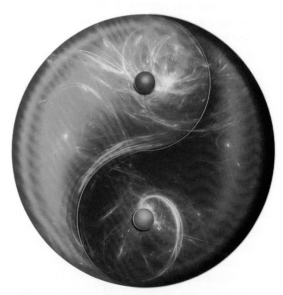

FIGURE 8.3 The balance of hot and cold energy fields represented by the yin-yang symbol is an example of viewing health from an energy field perspective and provides the basis for many complementary health-promoting and curing practices.

TABLE 8.3	The Seven Chakras		
Name	**Location**	**Color**	**Influences**
Crown	Top of head	Pale violet	Spirituality, peace, bliss, and enlightenment
Brow or midbrain	Between the eyebrows	Indigo	Intelligence, inspiration, intuition, insight, and wisdom
Throat	Throat	Blue	Expression in all forms, integrity, creativity, and listening
Heart	Center chest	Green	Emotional feelings, giving and receiving love, empathy, compassion, acceptance, and forgiveness
Solar plexus or stomach	Midway between the chest and navel	Yellow	Responsibility, motivation, power, prosperity, and gut feelings
Sacral or abdomen	8 cm (3 in) below the navel	Orange	Vitality, sexual pleasure, generation of new ideas, flexibility, and ability to give and receive nurturance
Root or reproductive organs	Spinal base near genitals	Red	Survival, stability, assertiveness, self-worth, good judgment, desire, and grounding

Gerber, R. (1988). *Vibrational medicine: New choices for healing ourselves*. Rochester, VT: Bear & Co; Brown, S. (2005). *The feng shui bible: The definitive guide to improving your life, home, health & finances*. New York: Sterling Publishing; and Rosen, B. (2007). *A Gaia busy person's guide: Chakras: Finding balance and serenity in everyday life*. London: Gaia.

persons have an emotional energy field running through and around their bodies, thereby creating an external aura and concentrated internal energy centers called chakras. Chakras within the human body flow with energy outside the human body. Personal ideas, thoughts, and feelings mix with the world, and the energy fields interact and become one. Feng shui incorporates chi ("the subtle change in electromagnetic energy that runs through everything, carrying information from one thing to another"; (Brown, 2005, p. 25)). Brown (2005) and Rosen (2007) explained that the chi in the seven chakras relates to the aspects of a person's character. The locations of the chakras are presented in Table 8.3 along with a color that may be used for the strengthening or healing of each chakra (Brown, 2005; Rosen, 2007). People also have an aura or outer energy field that projects the energy within the inner body, thereby enabling the life energy within to connect with the world and "tap into the vast array of cosmic information" (Brown, 2005, p. 26).

Chi has two opposing but complementary forms: yin and yang. Yin is slower, cooler, and more dispersed, whereas yang is hotter, faster, and more compressed. Most of the time, it is healthy to be more of one form than the other. However, if one form becomes too dominant, an imbalance occurs that results in health problems. Chi energies interact with each other in a positive or negative manner. In feng shui, complex interactions (e.g., a person's position, the location of objects within the environment [such as a room or even a building], and the magic nine patterns of chi [the magic square determines the flow of chi]) serve as the basis for timing events, arranging a home or work space, decorating, and remediating personal problems (Brown, 2005).

Concepts in Practice, "Using the Human Energy Field," demonstrates how awareness of your energy field can affect your daily life and may even help accomplish goals.

Concepts in Practice [IDEA]→[PLAN]→[ACTION]

Using the Human Energy Field

Geena, a nursing student, is trying to start a written assignment for a class, but is suffering from writer's block. Using information about the chakras, she pushes her chair back from her computer, closes her eyes, and visualizes her throat chakra. During the visualization, Geena sees the chakra turn from a pale to a vivid, iridescent peacock blue. She speaks aloud the idea generated immediately after the chakra changed colors, then types what she said into the computer. After reviewing what has been entered, Geena is pleased with the results and continues working on the assignment until it is completed.

Geena's fellow nursing student, Minh, uses a different technique when she has a difficult writing assignment. Minh always makes certain that she is facing north as she writes. According to feng shui, facing north is a good position to access deep creativity and to produce individualistic, original work.

Many of the interventions that act on the human energy field have yet to be scrutinized through double-blind controlled scientific studies. In 2007, the National Institutes of Health's Center for Complementary and Alternative Medicine reported that

38% of American adults and 12% of American children used some form of complementary or alternative medical therapy. Because of the prevalence of use, the National Institute of Health Center for Complementary and Integrative Health provides research grants for basic and applied research to substantiate the use of complementary healing modalities. One grant-funded study found that mindfulness mediation reduces pain levels while bypassing human opioid receptors (Chen, 2016). In 2012, only 33.2% of American adults and 11.6% of American children reported using some form of complementary or alternative medical therapy (Clarke, Black, Stussman, & Nahin, 2015; Black, Clarke, Barnes, Stussman, & Nahin, 2015).

Additional published studies contain contains increasing evidence that noninvasive complementary therapies, especially those that require the client's active participation, have tangible and highly desirable outcomes for health and healing. In fact, nursing licensing examinations in Europe contain information about the safe use of herbs and essential oils. Before using complementary interventions with clients, however, the nurse must be educated about how each may affect physiology and potential adverse effects (Dossey & Keegan, 2016). In the future, nurses will be increasingly expected to incorporate patterning methods as an integral part of clinical practice.

Take Note!

A focus on client energy fields provides a rationale for nontraditional healing modalities that enhance health patterns.

IMPLICATIONS OF THE NURSE'S VIEW OF HEALTH FOR ROLE PERFORMANCE

A positive model of health emphasizes personal strengths and power that are resources for health, wellness, and well-being. Personal strengths include having meaning, goals, and connections (with other persons or a higher being) in life. Personal power includes self-perceptions of capability, control, choice, and the capacity to cope with life challenges with confidence (Leddy, 2006). The integrative worldview supports the belief that nurses work with persons who display areas of strength and weakness in health pattern manifestations at a specific time. The effects of the nurse on client manifestations of patterns are complex and nonlinear. Persons entrenched in reductionism or who espouse an interaction worldview may find this approach confusing, and perhaps even nonscientific.

In trying to improve the quality of health of clients and self, the nurse is obligated to fulfill roles that incorporate promoting health, systematically and strategically planning changes, and using the strengths displayed by the client. Note that the term "promotion and maintenance of health" was missing. "Maintenance" is an obsolete concept because wellness (health) is an active process in which life moves forward, and the client is always evolving. The nurse may promote well-being and may restore perceptions of well-being, but the process of health does not permit the status quo that maintenance implies.

If health is a process, and if nurses believe that nursing focuses on the person's responses, as a whole, to the environment and to a perception of well-being, then nurses have a basis for a variety of professional roles when clients perceive a sense of harmony, vitality, and ability; when they can learn most effectively how to enhance their personal strength and gain greater control of their lives; and when they perceive a lack of harmony, feel consumed by weakness, and feel vulnerable (the illness state).

SELF-CARE OF THE NURSE

This chapter has described strategies the nurse can use to help promote or protect the health of the client. In the next section, the emphasis is on self-care strategies nurses can use to promote their own health.

The Stressful Work Environment

A stressful work environment refers to the pressure that is put on nurses by the external organizational forces that determine work conditions. The health care system contributes to nurse burnout through multiple regulations, inadequate staffing, heavy workloads, mandatory overtime, reimbursement issues, inadequate professional input into work processes, and lack of perceived administrative and interprofessional team support. Sometimes, a nurse may feel as though patient care is occurring similar to assembly line work, with the goal of moving clients in and out of the system as quickly as possible to reduce costs. Client care protocols that streamline care and reduce chances for error leave little room for individualization of nursing care. Little time is available to develop therapeutic client relationships and do the small things for clients that make big differences. With reduced client contact, nurses frequently cannot see the outcomes of nursing interventions. Nurses sometimes compromise values and beliefs about what constitutes safe, high-quality, effective care by being pressured to focus on employer financial agendas (especially in for-profit organizations). Nurses become distressed when they cannot deliver the type of care they want to provide. If left alone, the distress becomes the state of emotional and physical apathy and exhaustion known as **burnout**.

The more conscientious nurses, who have a need to give their very best, are most vulnerable to burnout. Cullen (1995) suggested that one of the two things happens when nurses work in a system in which they are never able to give their best. Either the nurses lower their standards and work apathetically, or they continue trying to give their best while constantly bucking a system that fails to have excellence in nursing as a top priority, until they finally experience burnout.

Stress and Burnout

A person becomes overstressed when demands exceed perceived resources. Some stress is inevitable and even positive in energizing the person. However, more stress than can be managed may be associated with physical, mental, emotional, and behavioral symptoms in health care providers. Some of the more common symptoms of stress in nurses and other practitioners include the following.

- Sleep disturbance and fatigue
- Appetite changes: increases or loss
- Reduced abilities to think and concentrate
- Frequent tardiness or absences from work
- Overeating or increased smoking
- Sudden mood swings
- Deep resentment of clients (Bartholomew, 2006; Gordon, 2005; Mitchell & Cormack, 1998)

If a nurse is constantly exposed to a situation in which demands exceed resources, the nurse's energies gradually becomes depleted, culminating in burnout. Stressful events may be perceived as either challenges that lead to positive growth or threats that can lead to negative consequences (Wells-Federman, 1996). Escalating and continual emotional overload is a common factor in burnout (Bartholomew, 2006; Gordon, 2005; Kahn & Saulo, 1994; Sutton, 2006). When nurses experience constant exposure to clinical practice situations that demand that they continually work in overloaded and stressful conditions, they experience reduced efficiency, irritability, a sense of constant pressure against time, diminished motivation, poor judgment, accidents, and care errors. In professional nursing practice, care errors may sometimes be fatal. The threat of potentially making a fatal error exacerbates stress levels in clinical practice.

The best time to think about burnout is before it happens. Answers to questions such as "Do I feel little enthusiasm for doing my job?" "Do I feel tired even with adequate sleep?" and "Do I have too much to do and too little time in which to do it?" can help the nurse identify symptoms and sources of job stress and signs of impending burnout (Davis, Eshelman, & McKay, 2000). Box 8.3, Learning, Knowing, and Growing, "Managing Job Stress," provides suggestions for the ways to manage nursing job stress. Many of the strategies require that the nurse take time to assess current working conditions, determine possible action, and make attitudinal and/or behavioral changes.

Techniques to Enhance Well-Being

Some nurses have innate or learned resilience. **Resilience** is another personality characteristics that help nurses adapt to change and bounce back repeatedly after exposure to multiple, stressful situations. Characteristics of resilient nurses include an internal locus of control, highly social behavior, very empathetic, positive self-image, and an optimistic approach to life (Turner & Kaylor, 2015). Methods to develop resilience are also health-enhancing techniques can be used to avoid burnout, promote health and well-being, and reframe stressors into challenges. These techniques include stress management, affirmations, refuting irrational ideas, social support, values clarification, and taking care of oneself.

Stress Management

In life (and nursing practice), perfection is impossible. However, given that stressors are an inevitable part of personal and professional interactions, a number of techniques have been proposed in the literature as positive ways to build strengths, avoid burnout, and promote well-being. First, it is necessary to identify sources of stress and be aware of tension buildup and situations that are likely to prove stressful. Nurses should try to get in touch with their bodies and learn their bodily reactions to and manifestations of stress (e.g., sweaty palms, tightening of back and neck muscles, dry mouth). If signs of stress are recognized early, it is possible to start stress-relieving exercises that can keep the effects of stress from increasing (Eliopoulos, 1999) (see Box 8.4, Learning, Knowing, and Growing, "Stress Reduction and Supportive Noninvasive Modalities").

8.3 Learning, Knowing, and Growing

Managing Job Stress

- Identify sources of job stress.
- Set realistic goals and priorities.
- Avoid procrastination.
- Say "no" when offered special projects or opportunities.
- Remove workplace clutter.
- Develop and maintain trusting, mutual, and meaningful collegial relationships with coworkers (and persons outside the work setting).
- Adopt an attitude that change is a challenge rather than an inconvenience.
- Cast off the perception that nurses are victims.
- Inject fun and humor in the work setting.
- Create a positive environment by looking at the bright side of adversity.
- Take control over nursing work processes.
- Participate in decision making.

- Schedule time to eat a healthy meal or snacks each day while at work.
- Consume a healthy diet (a balanced diet with moderation in refined sugars).
- Take responsibility for successes and failures.
- Take a 15- to 20-minute mini-vacation daily while on the job by going to a quiet place to relax (progressive relaxation, deep breathing exercises, meditation, or prayer with your beeper and/or cell phone turned off).
- Confront work issues directly with persons involved.
- Engage in a daily regimen of enjoyable physical exercise.
- Take vacations and personal days when needed.
- Get adequate sleep (7 to 8 hours per night for most people).
- Balance your work and personal life.

Sources: Clark, C. C., & Paraska, K. K. (2014). *Health promotion for nurses, a practical guide.* Burlington, MA: Jones & Bartlett Learning; Davis, M., Eshelman, E. R., & McKay, M. (2000). *The relaxation and stress reduction workbook* (5th ed.). Oakland, CA: New Harbinger; Dossey, B. M., & Keegan, L. (2016). In C. C. Barrere, M. A. Blasko-Helming, D. A. Shields, & K. Avino (Eds.), *Holistic nursing, a handbook for practice* (7th ed.). Burlington, MA: Jones & Bartlett Learning; Ellis, A., & Harper, R. (1961). *A guide to rational living.* North Hollywood, CA: Wilshire Books.

It is important for nurses to take care of themselves first before attempting to meet someone else's needs (Elder, 1999; Turner & Kaylor, 2015). Optimal time management allows people to focus on the most important goals (see Box 8.5, Learning, Knowing, and Growing, "Time Management Strategies to Achieve Goals"). Goal achievement requires setting time aside to set realistic goals, determining an action plan, using personal values to determine priority goals, and delegating tasks to others.

Affirmations

Use of **affirmations**—positive declarations that facilitate identification of personal value and enhancement

8.4 Learning, Knowing, and Growing

Stress Reduction and Supportive Noninvasive Modalities

- Make the environment conducive to relaxation, rather than overstimulation, by adjusting the noise, room temperature, and lighting.
- Follow good health practices by eating nutritious foods; avoiding excessive caffeine, simple carbohydrates ("junk food"), and food additives; and taking supplemental vitamins (A, C, E, and the B-complex group).
- Engage in regular physical activity (exercise).
- Get ample and regular rest and sleep.
- Instead of coffee and cigarette breaks, enjoy short relaxation exercises, recline in a quiet area, or listen to relaxing music.
- Have a pet.
- Practice mindfulness and relaxation.
- Get in touch with nature.

- Build leisure activities into the day, such as engaging in a hobby.
- Take vacations and breaks from routine work.
- Use alternative therapies, such as therapeutic massage, guided imagery, progressive relaxation, meditation, yoga, herbs, or aromatherapy.
- Use herbs (e.g., echinacea, ginseng) to protect the immune system.
- Learn how to center. "The skill of relaxing in the face of stress, taking a deep breath, loosening some of the tension in your neck and shoulders, and quieting your mind for a few moments is called centering. Centering is simply regaining your physical, mental, and emotional balance in order to proceed with the task at hand" (Achterberg, Dossey, & Kolkmeier, 1994, p. 62).

8.5 Learning, Knowing, and Growing

Time Management Strategies to Achieve Goals

- Control situations as much as possible; plan your schedule to avoid too many changes or events happening at the same time.
- Organize your time to accomplish the most important goals; identify values and goals and set daily priorities.
- Set limits; be assertive.
- Say "no" to unrealistic and low-priority demands; imagine yourself protected inside a bubble.
- Reduce tasks into smaller parts to allow mastery and feelings of competence.
- Delegate responsibilities and enlist the assistance of others; never try to be "all things to all people"; differentiate between time urgencies that are valid and others that are needlessly created; overinvolvement leaves little time for fulfillment of personal needs and often leads to resentment and blame (Wells-Federman, 1996).

Enhancing self-esteem is another way to avoid burnout and promote well-being. Increasing self-awareness of one's positive characteristics can enhance self-esteem. Additional strategies for preventing burnout include assertive expression of thoughts and feelings, sharing with others, accepting personal shortcomings and imperfections, and maintaining a positive and tolerant attitude toward others and the world at large. One way to do this is to change the way a stressor is viewed by putting it in proper perspective to help make the stressor manageable.

To help avoid worrying, it may be helpful to practice the serenity prayer, authored by a medieval monk, St. Francis of Assisi: "God grant me the serenity to accept the things I cannot change, the courage to change the things I can, and the wisdom to know the difference" (quoted in Mauk and Schmidt (2004, p. 98)). In addition,

it is helpful for the nurse to try to reduce the "shoulds" and "should nots." It is reasonable, legitimate, and healthy for clients to express their needs and do what is best for themselves; why do nurses perceive themselves as being different (Eliopoulos, 1999, p. 311)?

Box 8.4, Learning, Knowing, and Growing, "Stress Reduction and Supportive Noninvasive Modalities," presents stress reduction strategies that can be helpful in achieving balance and relieving stress. Many of these modalities fall within the realm of health-promoting behaviors and require that the nurse ask for help from others.

Strategies to Balance Threatening and Challenging Stress

- Develop a sense of balance among physical, mental, and spiritual dimensions.
- Get personal and social support during times of stress and distress; develop personal support systems at work.
- Find ways to maintain interest, enthusiasm, and knowledge at work by remaining alert to new ideas, learning new things, attending conferences and discussing your practice with others, giving honest positive feedback to colleagues, hearing and accepting praise from clients and colleagues.
- Leave work behind when you go home.
- Set limits and have priorities other than work.
- Be interested. "Everyone wants to be interesting, but the vitalizing thing is to be interested. . . . Keep a sense of curiosity. . . . Discover new things" (Gardner, 1996, p. 11).
- Avoid unfulfilling or burdensome relationships; minimize contact with the people who add more stress, rather than joy, to your life.
- Risk failure.

of self-esteem (Carter, 2006; Dossey & Keegan, 2016)—can serve as healthy alternatives to negative self-talk. An affirmation is simply a positive thought, a short phrase, or a saying that has meaning for the person. It can help change assumptions and beliefs that have negative consequences. Affirmations are important in reinforcing new ways of thinking and behaving from moment to moment. They are statements that can be selected to reaffirm new intentions, increase the clarity of goals, and help the nurse assume responsibility for actions. When starting to feel upset, anxious, frustrated, sad, or overwhelmed, the nurse can stop and examine his or her internal monolog and simply challenge that monolog with

language that is more affirming, such as the following.

- I can ask for what I need.
- I can take care of myself.
- I'm doing the best I can.
- I can find alternatives to problems.
- I can meet my needs.
- I care for myself, and I care for others.

Initially, using affirmations may seem superficial and uncomfortable, but as the internal monolog is changed, you will begin to notice changes in behavior and in the environment (Carter, 2006; Wells-Federman, 1996). Negative thought patterns of others may derail efforts

8.6 Learning, Knowing, and Growing

Guidelines for the Use of Affirmations

1. Find a calm, quiet location away from the hectic environment. Turn off all portable electronic devices. Take three to five deep breaths, breathing slowly with maximal inspirations and blowing out through pursed lips. Use the statements to name, claim, frame, and aim one's roles/concerns/issues. It is critical to use the first person singular pronoun "I" in all generated statements.
   - Naming (identifying roles/concerns/issues)
     - What occurred that triggered the negative reaction of stressful situation?
     - What is the issue precisely?
     - "I am a good, kind, compassionate nurse with special knowledge and skills to share with others."
     - "I can remain calm and in control when I disagree with others."
   - Claiming (clarifying role/concerns/issues)
     - "By taking care of myself, I can provide better care to the persons whom I serve."
     - "By confronting issues that impact the quality of nursing care, I am a better nurse."
     - "My loving kindness to others is a sign of personal and professional strength."
   - Framing (specifying the importance of what you do)
     - "I provide essential services to clients, colleagues, and other health team members."
     - "My contributions are as important as everyone else's."

   - "I provide great value to all care situations."
   - "I am a valued member of the health care team."
   - Aiming (positive action to attain the desired target outcome)
     - "I am becoming more comfortable in acknowledging the strengths I bring to the table as a team member."
     - "It is easier for me to see the differences that I make in the lives of others."
     - "I am able to do my job/fulfill my role at a very high level with ease."

2. Select one of the affirmations, and say it to yourself or write it 10 to 20 times daily while listening to your internal gut response to it.

3. Carry your chosen affirmation with you (e.g., on video, in your smart phone, on an index card, posted on your car dashboard, formatted into your computer screensaver) so that you can read it throughout the day.

4. Build in a healthy, personal reward for using the affirmations on a daily basis.

5. Do not become frustrated by unrealistic expectations for positive results because effective use of affirmations takes much time and practice.

6. You can substitute any personal role for your role as a professional nurse.

Clark, C. (1996). *Wellness practitioner: Concepts, research and strategies* (2nd ed.). New York: Springer; Clark, C. C., & Paraska, K. K. (2014). *Health promotion for nurses, a practical guide*. Burlington, MA: Jones & Bartlett Learning; Dossey, B. M., & Keegan, L. (2016). In C. C. Barrere, M. A. Blasko-Helming, D. A. Shields, & K. Avino (Eds.), *Holistic nursing, a handbook for practice* (7th ed.). Burlington, MA: Jones & Bartlett Learning; Jackson, C. (2012). Ballistic holistic nurses: Developing ourselves as healers. *Holistic Nursing Practice, 26*, 117–119. doi:10.1097/HNP.0b013e318252e6e0

of effective affirmation use. Box 8.6, Learning, Knowing, and Growing, "Guidelines for the Use of Affirmations," provides guidelines for the use of affirmations for personal and professional growth.

> **Take Note!**
> Constant exposure to situations in which demands exceed resources will culminate in burnout. Practicing self-care through stress reduction, life balance, affirmations, and other modalities can mitigate the risk of burnout.

Refuting Irrational Ideas

In a system called rational emotive therapy, Ellis and Harper (1961) proposed that emotions are not caused

by actual events. In between the event and the emotion, they identified realistic or unrealistic self-talk that produces negative or irrational emotions. Accordingly, the person's own thoughts, directed and controlled by the individual, are what create anxiety, anger, and depression. However, irrational self-talk can be changed, and the stressful emotions change with it (Davis et al., 2000).

At the root of all irrational thinking is the assumption that things are done to someone. Statements that interpret experience as catastrophic (e.g., a momentary chest pain is a heart attack) or absolute (e.g., I should, must, ought, always, or never) are examples of irrational thinking. Other examples are presented in Box 8.7, Learning, Knowing, and Growing, "Examples of Irrational Ideas."

8.7 Learning, Knowing, and Growing

Examples of Irrational Ideas

- It is possible to please all persons all of the time.
- Complete competence and perfection are possible in everything.
- Things can always be as I want them to be.
- Misery is created from external factors.
- The unknown, uncertain, and potential dangers instill great fear in me.
- I need to rely on others at all times.
- Avoiding life's difficulties and responsibilities is easier than facing them.
- The past directs the present and the future.
- Constant relaxation and leisure lead to happiness.

- I am the only one capable of doing the job properly.
- Life situations and other persons are the source of pressure.
- It is possible to have it all, all the time.
- I am responsible for everything that happens.
- Genetics dictate my reactions and life outcomes.
- It is impossible to control my emotions.
- Just getting over things is easy.
- Contributions I make to the world are unimportant.
- All my problems are my fault.
- There is one single best approach to life.

Davis, M., Eshelman, E. R., & McKay, M. (2000). *The relaxation and stress reduction workbook* (5th ed.). Oakland, CA: New Harbinger; Dossey, B. M., & Keegan, L. (2016). In C. C. Barrere, M. A. Blasko-Helming, D. A. Shields, & K. Avino (Eds.), *Holistic nursing, a handbook for practice* (7th ed.). Burlington, MA: Jones & Bartlett Learning; Ellis, A., & Harper, R. (1961). *A guide to rational living.* North Hollywood, CA: Wilshire Books; McGraw, 2004.

Irrational ideas can be disputed and eliminated through a process of rational thinking that includes the following (Davis et al., 2000; Ellis & Harper, 1961).

- Writing down the objective facts of the event.
- Writing down your self-talk, rational and irrational.
- Focusing on your emotional response.
- Questioning the rational support (e.g., evidence) for and against an irrational idea.
- Identifying the worst and best things that could happen.
- Substituting alternative self-talk.

Social Support

Colleagues can provide the insights and perspectives necessary to cope with commonly shared experiences. "Acknowledging the pain and seeking support from others are the most enduring long-term coping strategies. Practicing collegiality is a way of fostering this social support network. It is a way of building an atmosphere at work where you can support your colleagues and they you" (Wells-Federman, 1996, p. 15).

Building a supportive work environment requires conscious awareness of and action toward valuing yourself and your colleagues. Following are some suggestions (Turner & Kaylor, 2015; Wells-Federman, 1996) for shaping the quality of the atmosphere in which you work and developing a stronger support network.

- Find someone doing something right, and acknowledge him or her.

- Expect the best from yourself and those with whom you work.
- Model the values you believe. Take responsibility for your health and well-being, and encourage others to do the same.
- Establish a mentoring or buddy system.
- Make decisions based on nursing's ethical values.
- Establish a support group to help deal with the feelings that can arise from professional practice.
- Be supportive, but refer colleagues to professional support when needed.

Values Clarification

It may be helpful to consider why, despite the drawbacks, nursing can be so rewarding. Editors at *Nursing 2000* magazine (Nursing Top Ten Rewards, 2000) compiled the following list of 10 values, or "qualities that make nursing great," based on the interviews with 20 seasoned nurses. Some of these values may be helpful in considering personal strengths of practicing nursing.

- A way to make a difference
- The human connection
- Flexibility
- The chance to use all of yourself
- Long-term security
- The chance to mentor
- A connection between technology and humanity
- Respect
- Personal growth
- Personal rewards

A procedure known as **values clarification** can be used to try to identify the values that are most significant for an individual (Clark, 1996, p. 19). Being able to practice nursing without compromising personal values fosters satisfaction for many nurses (Turner & Kaylor, 2015). Spending time clarifying personal and professional values enables nurses to identify self-care priorities.

1. Prizing and cherishing
   - Learn to set priorities, become aware of what you are for or against, begin to trust your inner experiences and feelings, and examine why you feel as you do.
   - Clearly communicate personal values and actively listen to others as they share theirs.
2. Choosing
   - Choose freely by examining values that others have imposed on you.
   - Choose thoughtfully between alternatives by examining the process by which you choose and by considering the possible consequences of each choice.
3. Acting
   - Try out the value choice by developing a plan of action and implementing it.
   - Evaluate what happened when you took action, and make plans to reinforce actions that support your values.

Taking Care of Oneself

Nurses have a responsibility to take care of themselves because they can be in a position to give only when their own needs have, at least to some extent, been acknowledged and satisfied. The American Nurses Association recognized the importance of nurses taking care of themselves and declared 2017 as the Year of the Healthy Nurse (ANA, 2017). Mitchell and Cormack (1998, p. 142) have suggested ways for nurses to protect themselves from burnout, including the following.

- Do some honest soul searching to determine whether you're the kind of nurse who needs to express creativity and excellence, and who values and displays originality and enthusiasm in the work.
- Objectively evaluate your workplace and respond proactively to achieve a more positive outcome for yourself.
- Don't assume responsibility where you have none.
- Be honest about what you can and can't do in your role, given the constraints on your time and resources.
- Remember that you're not on duty 24 hours a day and that nursing is one part of your life.
- Remember that a good job doesn't love you back, and get your priorities straight.

- Find your own outlets for creativity.
- Don't stay in a situation that consistently fails to meet your needs; give yourself permission to leave.
- Give yourself a break.
- Create support for yourself.
- Love yourself; heal your wounds.
- Use food for physical nourishment, not as a stress reliever. Although carbohydrate-rich, protein-poor foods stimulate serotonin production, a poor diet is associated with oxidative stress and inflammation, which contribute to numerous disorders.
- Get enough sleep. Chronic stress interferes with sleep, and sleep deprivation alters a person's moods and cognitive processes (Logan, 2007; O'Keefe & O'Keefe, 2006).
- If the problem is a feeling of helplessness, the solution is to develop personal power.
- Try approaching each task as a challenge.
- Remember that you are here to serve, not to rescue.

Focusing on the positive sides of giving care to others can be helpful. Helping others as professional nurses provides great rewards. The work is challenging and fulfilling, especially when nurses can see the effects of interventions. Some nurses find problem solving thrilling, especially when they have success with creative methods never used. Some nurses derive a deep intrinsic pleasure just by knowing that they helped another person. The personal pleasure becomes enhanced when clients express gratitude, and nurses see the results of efforts to reduce human suffering (Mitchell & Cormack, 1998; Sacco, Ciurzynski, Harvey, & Ingersoll, 2015; Turner & Kaylor, 2015).

Barriers to Self-Care

One example of a barrier to self-care is the belief that "it can't happen to me," in which nurses may feel that they will not be in danger of burnout because they are too smart or too aware to let negative feelings progress to burnout. Another issue may be rooted in the altruistic nature of many nurses, in which the client or the job may take precedence over the nurse's own health.

In recent years, nurse scholars have identified and studied the concept of compassion fatigue that happens when nurses become tired of caring for others. **Compassion fatigue** has been described to be a state of emotional, physical, social, and spiritual exhaustion that consumes a person resulting in a pervasive decline in the desire, ability, and energy to care for others. Compassion fatigue occurs when health care professionals consistently care for traumatized persons and arises as a vicarious trauma in which the care provider shares in the psychological and spiritual distress of the persons for whom they provide services. When compassion fatigue arises, nurses lose their ability to feel and display genuine concern for others (Clifford, 2014). A tool measuring compassion fatigue contains items related to burnout and secondary traumatic stress (Sacco et al., 2015).

In contrast, a concept of compassion satisfaction has emerged recently. **Compassion satisfaction** is a sense of fulfillment that health care professional experience after helping persons through traumatic events (Sacco et al., 2015). To understand the magnitude of compassion satisfaction and compassion fatigue in professional nursing Sacco et al. (2015) conducted a study on the incidence of compassion satisfaction and compassion fatigue in intensive care nurses (see the following research box).

FOCUS ON RESEARCH

Compassion Fatigue and Compassion Satisfaction in Critical Care Nurses

The investigators were curious as to the incidence of compassion fatigue and compassion satisfaction among practicing critical care nurses in a large tertiary medical center. Two hundred twenty-one intensive care unit (ICU) nurses responded to a survey that consisted of items inquiring about nurse demographic and organizational characteristics, and the Professional Quality of Life (ProQOL), an instrument that measures compassion satisfaction and compassion fatigue.

The investigator compared mean scores on the ProQOL with nurse age, gender, educational level, type of critical care unit, and organizational characteristics. They found statistically significant differences in compassion satisfaction scores in several areas. Female nurses had higher compassion satisfaction scores than male nurses. Nurses between the ages of 40–50 years of age had lower compassion satisfaction scores than nurse of other ages. Nurses working in ICUs devoted to a single specialty had higher compassion satisfaction scores compared to nurses employed in multi-specialty ICUs. Lower compassion satisfaction scores were found in nurses who had experienced a recent managerial change. Nurses with associate's or master's degree in nursing had higher compassion satisfaction scores compared to nurses with baccalaureate degrees, Nurses aged 40 to 49 years working on mixed-acuity units had higher burnout and higher secondary traumatic stress scores than other nurses in the study. Finally, nurses aged 50 years or older had the highest compassion satisfaction scores and lower scores on burnout and secondary traumatic stress scales than nurses in other age groups.

The investigator's suggested that the older nurses' higher compassion satisfaction and lower compassion fatigue scores could be the result of them being better equipped to cope with the challenges of critical care nursing because they have more life and professional nursing experience. They also proposed that managerial change is a key factory to the development of burnout of staff within a unit and may be a contributing factor to compassion fatigue and that a major systems or practice change may be a contributing factor to compassion fatigue.

The investigators outlined the following study limitations: (1) the cross-sectional nature of the study and perhaps nurses completed surveys when they were having a bad day, (2) low survey response rate (38%), and low reliability of the secondary trauma subscale of the ProQOL for this sample.

The investigators outline the several clinical implications for the study. Personal nurse circumstances and the populations for which they provide care directly affect professional nurse burnout, compassion satisfaction and compassion fatigue. Therefore, nursing administration should examine workplace environments to see what can be changed to facilitate the work of nurses as well as to recognize nurses for the work that they perform. Nurses should be given a voice in professional practice issues in which they are directly involved. Efforts should be made to create a healthy work environment in which there is effective communication among all interprofessional health team members, increased authentic collaboration, no tolerance of intimidation, provision of safe staffing patterns, meaningful recognition of nurses, and leaders who promote a caring culture, professional development, individual nurse recognition, and debriefing.

Sacco, T. L., Ciurzynski, S. M., Harvey, M. E., & Ingersoll, G. L. (2015). Compassion satisfaction and compassion fatigue among critical care nurses. *Critical Care Nurse, 35*(4), 32–44. doi: http://dx.doi.org/10.4037/ccn2015392

Take Note!
Nurses must take care of themselves first. By doing so, they will be better able to continue to deal with the stresses of the work environment, and advocate for the needs of their clients.

Summary and Significance to Practice

In American society, responsibility for illness has been delegated to health care professionals who have been prepared and are rewarded for delivering care to the sick. Short-term incentives and rewards to maintain health do not exist for the recipient of such care; in addition, the health care system is not organized to reward health care providers for keeping clients well.

Clients must be encouraged to assume an increased concern and responsibility for their health potential. Nurses can support, facilitate, and encourage those positive skills, qualities, and plans that will promote health. The client and the nurse, based on goals and a timetable determined by the client, can then devise interventions collaboratively.

In addition, nurses need to take responsibility for self-care. Approaches to managing job stress and techniques such as stress management, affirmations, refuting irrational ideas, social support, values clarification, and taking care of oneself are positive techniques that can be used to avoid burnout, reframe stressors into challenges, and enhance well-being.

REAL-LIFE REFLECTIONS

Think about Nadine and Michael from the beginning of the chapter and identify the factors in their work environment that are not health promoting. What are the stressors in your school or work environment? Why is having a colleague to share common experiences important for promoting health? What steps can you take in the short term to alleviate stress in your life? What long-term strategies can you employ to ensure you don't experience burnout in your career?

From Theory to Practice

1. Identify the factors within your lifestyle that fall into the categories of health promotion and health protection. What are the consequences of a lifestyle focused on health protection rather than health promotion?
2. Did you find some of the tips for caring for yourself helpful? If so, which ones do you plan to use? If not, why not?

Nurse as Author

Use a mobile app or **https://www.supertracker. usda.gov/** to track your food and activity level for a week. Also, make a record of your social and religious activities for the same week. Take time and reflect on your psychological behavior for the same week paying close attention to when you may have felt bad about yourself, gotten angry at others, experienced stress (at work and at home), felt excited or happy, and experienced a sense of calmness and tranquility. Based on your personal assessment, create a holistic plan to improve your health and well-being (using the Neuman System Model dimensions of health: physiologic, psychological, sociocultural, developmental and spiritual or another nursing theorist who addresses health from a holistic perspective).

Your Digital Classroom

Online Exploration

American Association of Retired Persons: **www.aarp.org**. Access information related to healthy living and aging and a wide array of information addressing the special sociocultural concerns of the elderly.

American Heart Association: **www.heart.org**. Visit this site to learn the latest on cardiovascular disease, and refer clients and their families to this client-oriented site.

The American Holistic Nurses Association: **www.ahna.org**.

American Institute for Cancer Research: **www.aicr.org**. Consult this site for research-based information for the prevention of cancer and healthy lifestyle information.

Association for Applied and Therapeutic Humor: **http://www.aath.org**. Tickle your funny bone by visiting this website, and link to other health care humor sites to lift your spirits.

Healthy People 2020: **www.healthypeople.gov/ 2020**.

National Center for Chronic Disease Prevention and Health Promotion: **www.cdc.gov/nccdphp**. Learn the latest about the prevention of communicable diseases along with health promotion information to reduce the incidence of chronic diseases.

National Institute of Health Center for Complementary and Integrative Health **https://nccih.nih.gov/**

National Institutes of Health: **www.nih.gov**. Read about the latest government-sponsored health research along with opportunities for funding health promotion research.

National Health Information Center: **http://health. gov/nhic/** Learn about special days to increase awareness about important health topics

Federal Health Information Centers and Clearinghouses at **http://health.gov/nhic/pubs/clearing houses/** Here you can obtain educational materials for your clients and yourself. Health topics are listed in alphabetical order so click on the first letter of what you want to find.

Wellness, Self-care, and Relationship Resources: **www.carolynchambersclark.com**. This site offers books, ebooks, and articles related to wellness. Get a free subscription to *The Wellness Newsletter*, a research-based e-newsletter.

Expanding Your Understanding

1. Visit the American Holistic Nurses Association (AHNA) website, and read the "About AHNA" section. Would you be interested in joining the AHNA? Why or why not?

2. Search online for one of the nursing interventions for the human energy field identified by Leddy (2003, 2006). Prepare for a class discussion about the information you find. Do you think other health team members would agree that the identified intervention would be beneficial to clients? Why or why not?

Beyond the Book

Visit thePoint® **www.thePoint.lww.com** for the activities and information to reinforce the concepts and content covered in this chapter.

REFERENCES

Achterberg, J., Dossey, B., & Kolkmeier, L. (1994). *Rituals for healing: Using imagery for health and wellness*. New York: Bantam.

American Nurses Association (2017). 2017—The Year of the Healthy Nurses. Retrieved from http://www.nursingworld.org/MainMenuCategories/ThePracticeofProfessionalNursing/2017-Year-of-Healthy-Nurse. Accessed March 26, 2017.

Antonovsky, A. (1987). *Unraveling the mystery of health*. San Francisco, CA: Jossey-Bass.

Ardell, D. B. (1979). The nature and implications of high level wellness or why "normal health" is in a rather sorry state of existence. *Health Values, 3*, 17–24.

Bartholomew, K. (2006). *Ending nurse-to-nurse hostility: Why nurses eat their young and each other*. Marblehead, MA: HCPro.

Becker, M. H., & Maiman, L. A. (1975). Sociobehavioral determinants of compliance with health and medical care recommendations. *Medical Care, 13*, 10–24.

Benner, P., Tanner, C. A., & Chesla, C. A. (Eds.). (1996). *Expertise in nursing practice: Caring, clinical judgment, and ethics*. New York: Springer.

Black, L. I., Clarke, T. C., Barnes, P. M, Stussman, B. J., & Nahin, R. L. (2015). Use of Complementary Health Approaches Among Children Aged 4–17 Years in the United States: National Health Interview Survey, 2007–2012. *National Institutes of Health National Health Statistics Report, 78* (February 10, 2015). Retrieved from http://www.cdc.gov/nchs/data/nhsr/nhsr078.pdf. Accessed April 2, 2016.

Brown, S. (2005). *The feng shui bible: The definitive guide to improving your life, home, health & finances*. New York: Sterling Publishing.

Carter, D. (2006). *10 Smart things women can do to build a better life*. Eugene, OR: Harvest House.

Chen, W. (2016). Mindfulness meditation reduces pain, bypasses opioid receptors. *NIH Research Blog*. Retrieved from https://nccih.nih.gov/research/blog/mindfulness-meditation-pain. Accessed April 2, 2016.

Clark, C. (1996). *Wellness practitioner: Concepts, research and strategies* (2nd ed.). New York: Springer.

Clarke, T. C., Black, L. I., Stussman, B. J., & Nahin, R. L. (2015). Trends in the Use of Complementary Health Approaches Among Adults: United States, 2002–2012, *National Health Statistics Report 79* (February 10, 2015). Retrieved from http://www.cdc.gov/nchs/data/nhsr/nhsr079.pdf. Accessed April 2, 2016.

Clifford, K. (2014). Who cares for the carers? Literature review of compassion fatigue and burnout in military health professionals? *Journal of Military and Veteran's Health, 22*(3), 53–63.

Cohen, S., & Wills, T. A. (1985). Stress, social support and the buffering hypothesis. *Psychological Bulletin, 98*, 310–357.

Crawford, G. (1982). The concept of pattern in nursing: Conceptual development and measurement. *Advances in Nursing Science, 5*, 1–6.

Cullen, A. (1995). Burnout: Why do we blame the nurse? *American Journal of Nursing, 95*, 22–28.

Cuellar, N., Rogers, A., & Higshman, V. (2007). Evidence-based research of complementary and alternative medicine (CAM) for sleep in the community-dwelling older adult. *Geriatric Nursing, 28*(1), 46–51.

Davis, M., Eshelman, E. R., & McKay, M. (2000). *The relaxation and stress reduction workbook* (5th ed.). Oakland, CA: New Harbinger.

Dossey, B. M., & Keegan, L. (2016). In C. C. Barrere, M. A. Blasko-Helming, D. A. Shields, & K. Avino (Eds.), *Holistic nursing, a handbook for practice* (7th ed.). Burlington, MA: Jones & Bartlett Learning.

Dossey, B. M., & Luck, S. (2016). Chapter 30: Self assessments. In B. M. Dossey, & L. Keegan (authors); C. C. Barrere, M. A.

Blasko-Helming; D. A. Shields, & K. Avino (Eds.), *Holistic nursing, a handbook for practice*. (7th ed.). Burlington, MA: Jones & Bartlett Learning.

Dubos, R. (1978). Health and creative adaptation. *Human Nature, 1*, 74–82.

Dunn, H. H. (1977). What high-level wellness means. *Health Values, 1*, 9–16.

Elder, A. (1999). Nurturing the caregiver in today's health care arena. *Advance for Nurses, 7*.

Eliopoulos, C. (1999). *Integrating conventional and alternative therapies: Holistic care for chronic conditions*. St. Louis, MO: Mosby.

Ellis, A., & Harper, R. (1961). *A guide to rational living*. North Hollywood, CA: Wilshire Books.

Fawcett, J. (1993). *Conceptual models of nursing* (3rd ed.). Philadelphia, PA: F.A. Davis.

Gardner, J. W. (1996). Self-renewal. *The Futurist, 30*, 9–12.

Gordon, S. (2005). *Nursing against the odds*. New York: Cornell University Press.

Hall, B. A. (1981). The change paradigm in nursing: Growth versus persistence. *Advances in Nursing Science, 3*, 1–6.

Hravnak, M. (1998). Is there a health promotion and protection foundation to the practice of acute care nurse practitioners? *AACN Clinical Issues, 9*, 283–289.

Janz, N. K., & Becker, M. H. (1984). The health belief model: A decade later. *Health Education Quarterly, 11*, 1–47.

Jensen, L. A., & Allen, M. N. (1994). A synthesis of qualitative research on wellness-illness. *Qualitative Health Research, 4*, 349–369.

Kahn, S., & Saulo, M. (1994). *Healing yourself: A nurse's guide to self-care and renewal*. Albany: Delmar.

Kasl, S., & Cobb, S. (1966). Health behavior, illness behavior and sick role behavior. *Archives of Environmental Health, 12*, 246–266.

Kobasa, S. C. (1979). Stressful life events, personality and health: An inquiry into hardiness. *Journal of Personality and Social Psychology, 37*, 1–11.

Lazarus, R. S., & Folkman, J. (1984). *Stress appraisal and coping*. New York: Springer.

Leddy, S. K. (2003). *Integrative health promotion: Conceptual bases for nursing practice*. Thorofare, NJ: Slack.

Leddy, S. K. (2004). Human energy: A conceptual model of unitary nursing science. *Visions: The Journal of Rogerian Nursing Science, 12*, 14–27.

Leddy, S. K. (2006). *Health promotion: Mobilizing strengths to enhance health, wellness, and well-being*. Philadelphia, PA: F.A. Davis.

Logan, A. C. (2007). *The brain diet, revised and expanded*. Nashville, TN: Cumberland House.

Mariano, C. (2013). Chapter 2: Holistic nursing: Scope & standards of practice. In B. M. Dosesy & L. Keegan (Eds.), *Holistic nursing, a handbook for practice* (6th ed.). Burlington, MA: Jones & Bartlett Learning.

Mauk, K., & Schmidt, N. (2004). *Spiritual care in nursing practice*. Philadelphia, PA: Lippincott Williams & Wilkins.

McElligott, D. (2013). The nurse as an instrument of healing. In B. M. Dosesy & L. Keegan (Eds.), *Holistic nursing, a handbook for practice* (6th ed.). Burlington, MA: Jones & Bartlett Learning.

McWilliam, C. L., Stewart, M., Brown, J. B., Desai, K., & Coderre, P. (1996). Creating health with chronic illness. *Advances in Nursing Science, 18*, 1–15.

Mitchell, A., & Cormack, M. (1998). *The therapeutic relationship in complementary health care*. Edinburgh: Churchill Livingstone.

Newman, M. A. (1992). Prevailing paradigms in nursing. *Nursing Outlook, 40*, 10–13, 32.

Newman, M. A. (1994). *Health as expanding consciousness* (2nd ed.). St. Louis, MO: Mosby.

Nursing Top Ten Rewards. (2000). *Nursing 2000, 30*(5), 42–43.

O'Keefe, J., & O'Keefe, J. (2006). *The forever young diet & lifestyle*. Kansas City, MO: Andrews McMeel.

Parse, R. R. (1987). *Nursing science: Major paradigms, theories, and critiques*. Philadelphia, PA: W.B. Saunders.

Parsons, T. (1958). Definitions of health and illness in the light of American values and social structure. In E. G. Jaco (Ed.), *Patients, physicians, and illness*. Glencoe, IL: Free Press.

Pender, N. J. (1996). *Health promotion in nursing practice* (3rd ed.). Stamford, CT: Appleton & Lange.

Pender, N. J., Murdaugh, C. L., & Parsons, M. A. (2002). *Health promotion in nursing practice* (4th ed.). Upper Saddle River, NJ: Prentice Hall.

Pender, N. J., Murdaugh, C. L., & Parsons, M. A. (2006). *Health promotion in nursing practice* (5th ed.). Upper Saddle River, NJ: Prentice Hall.

Pender, N., Murdaugh, C., & Parsons, M. A. (2011). *Health promotion in nursing practice* (6th ed.). Upper Saddle River, NJ: Pearson Education.

Prochaska, J. O., Redding, C. A., Harlow, L. L., Rossi, J. S., & Velicer, W. F. (1994a). The transtheoretical model of change and HIV prevention: A review. *Health Education Quarterly, 21*, 471–486.

Prochaska, J. O., Velicer, W. F., Rossi, J. S., Goldstein, M. G., Marcus, B. H., Rakowski, W., et al. (1994b). Stages of change and decisional balance for 12 problem behaviors. *Health Psychology, 13*, 39–46.

Rau, T., & Wyler, S. (2007). *The Swiss secret to optimal health*. New York: Berkeley.

Rosen, B. (2007). *A Gaia busy person's guide: Chakras: Finding balance and serenity in everyday life*. London: Gaia.

Rosenstock, I. M. (1966). Why people use health services. *Milbank Memorial Fund Quarterly, 44*, 94–127.

Rosenstock, I. M., Strecher, V. J., & Becker, N. H. (1988). Societal learning theory and the health belief model. *Health Education Quarterly, 25*, 175–183.

Sacco, T. L., Ciurzynski, S. M., Harvey, M. E., & Ingersoll, G. L. (2015). Compassion satisfaction and compassion fatigue among critical care nurses. *Critical Care Nurse, 35*(4), 32–44. doi: http://dx.doi.org/10.4037/ccn2015392

Smith, J. A. (1981). The idea of health: A philosophical inquiry. *Advances in Nursing Science, 3*, 43–50.

Sutton, R. (2006). *The no asshole rule*. New York: Warner Business Books.

Turner, S. B., & Kaylor, S. D. (2015). Neuman Systems Model as a conceptual framework for nurse resilience. *Nursing Science Quarterly, 28*(3), 213–217. doi: 10.1177/0894318415585620

Twaddle, A. C., & Hessler, R. M. (1977). *A sociology of health*. St. Louis, MO: Mosby.

U.S. Department of Health and Human Services. (2000). *Healthy People 2010*. Boston, MD: Jones & Bartlett U.S. Department of Health and Human Services.

U.S. Department of Health and Human Services, National Institutes of Health Center for Complementary and Alternative Medicine (2008). *The use of complementary and alternative medicine in the United States.* Retrieved from https://nccih.nih. gov/sites/nccam.nih.gov/files/camuse.pdf. Accessed April 2, 2016.

U.S. Department of Health and Human Services. (2017). About Healthy People 2020. Retrieved from https://www.healthy-people.gov/2020/About-Healthy-People. Accessed March 26, 2017.

U.S. Department of Health and Human Services. (2011). HHS Releases Assessment of Healthy People 2010 Objectives. Retrieved from http://www.healthypeople.gov/2020/about/ HP2010PressReleaseOct5.doc. Accessed January 15, 2016.

Vincent, C., & Furnham, A. (1997). *Complementary medicine: A research perspective.* Chichester, UK: John Wiley & Sons.

Wells-Federman, C. L. (1996). Awakening the nurse healer within. *Holistic Nursing Practice, 10,* 13–29.

Westberg, J., & Jason, H. (1996). Fostering healthy behavior: The process. In S. H. Woolf, S. Jonas, & R. S. Lawrence (Eds.), *Health promotion and disease prevention in clinical practice.* Baltimore, MD: Williams & Wilkins.

World Health Organization Health Education Unit. (1986). Lifestyles and health. *Social Science and Medicine, 22,* 117–124.

THE CHANGING HEALTH CARE CONTEXT

Providing access to health care for all people, delivering nursing care based on strong science and evidence, addressing specific cultural preferences when providing care, balancing accountability and quality of care in the era of cost containment, creating healthy environments, and using technology effectively are challenges for today's professional nurses. In addition, spiraling health care costs have led to increased consumer discontent with the health care system, thus placing health care providers at risk for litigation. Current laws to improve health care access for Americans have created improved health care delivery for some while creating discontent in others. This section provides an overview of these challenges while reinforcing professional nursing's goal of doing what is best for clients.

Health Care Delivery Systems

KEY TERMS AND CONCEPTS

Primary care

Secondary care

Tertiary care

National health service
  insurance model

Medicare

Medicaid

Children's Health
  Insurance Program
  (CHIP)

Mandated insurance
  model

Entrepreneurial
  insurance model

Prospective payment

Patient Protection and
  Affordable Care Act of
  2010

American Health Care
  Act (ACHC)

Interdisciplinary/
  Interprofessional
  health care team

Nursing care delivery
  model

LEARNING OUTCOMES

By the end of this chapter, the learner will be able to:

1. Explain the differences among primary, secondary, and tertiary care.
2. Identify key concerns and pressures for all health care delivery systems.
3. Specify the three major ways in which health care is financed.
4. Compare and contrast the American, Canadian, and Mexican health care systems.
5. Explain the major forces that influence change in the health care system.
6. Identify the impact of changes in health systems on nurses.
7. Explore practical and ethical issues associated with health care delivery systems on professional nurses.

REAL-LIFE REFLECTIONS

Maria is a registered nurse employed by a hospital owned by a for-profit company. When Maria's father had hip replacement surgery, he received generic medication instead of his regular medicines during his hospital stay. He got quite upset because he was convinced that he was receiving the wrong medication. Two days after surgery, the case manager informed Maria's parents that her father would be transferred the next day to an extended-care facility for rehabilitation. Maria's parents became distraught because they had promised each other they would never put each other in a nursing home. Maria's parents bombarded her with questions about why her father did not receive the same medications that he took at home and why he had to leave the hospital before he was well enough to care for himself.

In recent years, health care delivery has undergone radical transformation as a result of the explosion of scientific knowledge, technologic advances, emphasis on health promotion, resource limitations, and shortages of health care professionals (especially professional nurses, primary care physicians, and pharmacists) (United States Bureau of Labor Statistics [USBLS], 2012). Health care delivery systems provide **primary care** for health promotion and illness prevention, **secondary care** for early detection and cure of illness, and **tertiary care** for chronic disease management, rehabilitative, and end-of-life services. These changes impact the availability of and access to health care for many people. This chapter explores current challenges for health care delivery, highlights selected countries that use different strategies to provide health care services, and outlines specific challenges for professional nurses in today's health care arena.

CHALLENGES OF HEALTH CARE DELIVERY IN THE 21ST CENTURY

All health care delivery systems in the world struggle to provide optimal services for the people they serve (see Box 9.1, Professional Building Blocks, "Challenges for Today's Health Care Delivery Systems"). Access, cost, quality, and safety seem to be the most prevalent issues today. Approaches to health care delivery vary across the globe because of differing values, beliefs, economic resources, history, and politics.

9.1 Professional Building Blocks

Challenges for Today's Health Care Delivery Systems

- Ensuring access to care for all
- Operating within the confines of available health care resources
- Providing both preventive and curative services
- Determining the optimal balance among health promotion, disease prevention, illness treatment, and quality of life
- Attaining an effective system using governmental support and private resources
- Providing and maintaining a qualified, competent health care workforce
- Achieving a balance between health care needs and all other human needs
- Optimizing the use of technology for efficient care delivery while maintaining consumer privacy
- Providing coordinated health care delivery across inpatient, outpatient, home, and rehabilitation settings
- Coordinating public and private resources for optimal care delivery
- Responding to actual and future epidemics and other potential health threats
- Allowing consumer participation in the provision of health care services
- Enabling optimal health essential for a high quality of life

Andersen, R., Rice, T., & Kominski, G (2007). *Changing the U.S. health care system* (3rd ed.). San Francisco, CA: Wiley; Yarbrough, A. Y. & Erwin, C. O. (2015). Organization of medical care. In J. R. Knickman & A. R. Kovner (Eds.), *Jonas & Kovner's health care delivery in the United States* (11th ed.). New York: Springer; Fried, B. J., & Gaydos, L. M. (2002). *World health systems: Challenges and perspectives*. Chicago: Health Administration Press.

Health Care Access

When the United Nations (UN) was chartered in 1945, its aim was to provide a global agency for international cooperation and collaboration. World health and the provision of health care services quickly emerged as key issues. The World Health Organization (WHO) was established as a UN unit whose early efforts included the eradication of infectious diseases and provision of health services for mothers and children (Jamieson & Sewall, 1954). By the middle of the 20th century, WHO's focus broadened to include the provision of essential health services to all.

By the late 1970s, the need to change global health care delivery became apparent (Zakus & Cortinois, 2002). In 1978, WHO and the United Nations Children's Fund (UNICEF) issued a joint declaration that affirmed that health and health care were fundamental human rights, and that social and economic development were keys to supporting health care initiatives. In 1981, the World Health Assembly expanded the initiatives to foster and coordinate social and economic efforts to promote the general health and welfare of all people (Zakus & Cortinois, 2002). WHO continues to monitor the progress of nations around the world with regard to the status of health care delivery and outcomes of health care services.

The 2010 *World Health Report* identified several leading sources of inefficiency in health care, including issues with medications (underuse of generics, use of substandard or counterfeit medications, inappropriate and ineffective use of medicines); overuse of health products, investigations, and procedures; inappropriate mix and unmotivated health care workers; inappropriate use of health care services (such as overuse of emergency rooms and underutilization of primary care providers); and inefficiencies or inappropriate levels of health interventions (WHO, 2010).

Despite international efforts to secure health care services for all, serious gaps persist. Wealthier nations tend to have fully developed health care systems, while many poorer countries lack basic infrastructures for health care delivery. The affluent can always access and receive health services because of their ability to purchase such services as needed. Typically, people living in rural areas in both developed and undeveloped nations have less access to health care services.

Countries differ in their approach to health care access. Some nations aspire to a free enterprise or business/market approach that relies on an individual's ability to pay for health care services rendered. Other nations use government-sponsored programs, viewing health care as a basic human right that the government has the obligation to provide. Although access is guaranteed under this approach, health care may be delayed because of government funding shortfalls; this may occur in cases of high unemployment (decline in income tax revenue), reduced sales (or value-added) taxes, or reduced price of a government-controlled commodity (such as oil revenues in Nigeria (Lacey, 2002)). Whichever approach is used, funding is needed to provide the basic infrastructure and qualified health care professionals.

Health Care Funding

The American culture values individualism, independence, innovation, and capitalism. In the United States, health care is a big business. Pharmaceutical and health care equipment vendors bombard the public with advertisements for the newest medications and therapies. Because American health care delivery has been based on a free enterprise system, some Americans believe that if the government were to control the system, the quality of and access to health care services might be compromised (Fifer, 2007; Sanders, 2002). In contrast, Canada and many European countries hold the belief that health care is the right of all citizens and fair access should be provided to all (Andersen, Rice, & Kominski, 2007; Fried & Gaydos, 2002; McIntyre & Thomlinson, 2003; Storch, 2005).

How to fund health care delivery is a challenge for many nations (Andersen et al., 2007; Gantz et al., 2012; Knickman, 2015; O'Donnell, Smyth, & Frampton, 2005; Rosen & Haglund, 2005). Three different models of funding health care expenditures dominate.

The National Health Service Insurance Model

The **national health service insurance model** guarantees access to health care services through a national health insurance plan, usually funded by general tax revenues. The citizens or government either own or control the factors for health care delivery and/or production of health care goods (Andersen et al., 2007; Sanders, 2002). The United Kingdom, Australia, Canada, and Japan are among the nations that have adopted this model (Fried & Gaydos, 2002). Canadians value equal access to care, and in some cases Canadians may be prohibited from purchasing private health insurance (McIntyre & Thomlinson, 2003; Sanders, 2002; Storch, 2005). Other countries, such as Australia, enable citizens to purchase private insurance in addition or as an alternative to the national plan.

A citizen's right to choose drives the justification for permitting private insurance purchase even though disparities in services may result (Fifer, 2007).

The United States has partially adopted the national health service model by offering tax-funded health insurance plans funded to the elderly, the disabled, and to people who meet strict income and asset guidelines.

- **Medicare** is a federal program funded by income taxes that provides health care insurance for elderly and disabled Americans. Many elderly also purchase private insurance known as "tie-in" plans to eliminate the gaps in Medicare coverage.
- **Medicaid** offers health care insurance coverage to people who qualify for federally supported, but state-managed, welfare programs. Individual states determine Medicaid eligibility requirements, but all states must provide coverage for families and children who receive federal aid.
- The **Children's Health Insurance Program (CHIP)** covers health care costs for children from low-income families who do not meet individual state guidelines to receive Medicaid.

Other tax-supported health care insurance programs cover public employees, military personnel and families, veterans, Native Americans, and Alaskan Natives (Knickman, 2015).

The Mandated Insurance Model

The **mandated insurance model** requires compulsory universal health care insurance. Nonprofit insurance funds provide resources for individuals and employers to purchase health insurance (Andersen et al., 2007; Knickman, 2015). Nations that have adopted this model include Germany, Brazil, Italy, Jamaica, and South Africa (Fried & Gaydos, 2002). In the United States, the mandated health insurance model is part of the Patient Protection and Affordable Care Act (ACA) (Billings, Cantor, & Clinton, 2011; Knickman, 2015; U.S. Supreme Court, 2012).

The Entrepreneurial Insurance Model

The **entrepreneurial insurance model** consists of voluntary health insurance coverage that relies on purchase of health insurance by individuals. In this model, employment-based insurance is common. Employers provide group coverage and employees pay part of the insurance premium (Andersen et al., 2007; Feldstein, 2016 & Longest, 2016). The United States, China, South Korea, Mexico, Nigeria, and India espouse this model (Fried & Gaydos, 2002).

QUESTIONS FOR REFLECTION

1. What experiences have you had with the different insurance models?
2. If you were designing an insurance model, what components would you incorporate and why? Would your model be feasible to implement? Why or why not?

Health Care Workforce

The *World Health Statistics 2015 report* documented an estimated global shortage of health care professionals (WHO, 2015), including estimated critical shortages of physicians (defined as less than one physician per 1,000 citizens) in 66 of 195 reporting countries, and 41 nations reporting less than one nurse/midwife per 1,000 citizens (WHO, 2015).

There is a shortage of registered nurses (RNs) in the United States. In 2014, there were slightly more than 2.75 positions for RNs (excluding advanced practice nurses). By 2014, there will be slightly more than 3.29 RN positions (USBLS, 2015a). American hospitals employ close to 61% of all working RNs. Seven percent of nurses work in outpatient settings such as physician offices and another 7% work in the long-term care facilities. Six percent of nurses have jobs in home health care or serve in the government positions (USBLS, 2015b). Of working RNs, 58.4% work full time (with 12% of these having more than one job) and 74.2% work more than 32 hours per week. Because of the projected growth in the elderly population, a shift to health promotion and disease prevention and increased number of persons with chronic conditions within the next decade, 16% additional professional nurses will be needed by 2024 (USBLS, 2015a). Even more may be needed because in 2015, 50% of nurses are currently over the age of 50 years and some of these nurses may need to cut the number of their working hours or might opt for early retirement (National Council of State Boards of Nursing, 2016).

As a global phenomenon, the current nursing shortage differs from cyclical shortages of the past. Nursing traditionally has been considered women's work. Since the women's movement, however, more career opportunities have become open to women, resulting in younger women pursuing more lucrative and respected careers. Today's worldwide nursing workforce, comprising 13 million nurses (International Council of Nurses [ICN], 2012), is also aging. As these RNs retire, there are not enough entering the profession to replace them. Along with the nursing shortage, the need for American physicians is expected to grow: about 14% more physicians will be needed by 2024 (USBLS, 2015c). There are currently 708,300 practicing physicians in the United States; of these, 40.7% practice primary care, with 12.8% engaged in general/family practice. Median salaries for American physicians range from $241,273 (primary care) and $411,852 (specialists) (USBLS, 2015d). High physician salaries increase health delivery costs and open the door for increased use of nurse practitioners (NPs) for primary and specialty care services.

In most nations, well-equipped and well-staffed hospitals, when available, are located in larger urban areas. Rural areas have special challenges to overcome to attract qualified health care personnel. Some countries (and states) pay for the education of health care professionals and expect a tour of service in an underserved area for a designated time frame. Despite such incentive programs, health care professionals (including nurses) prefer to work in environments that offer them a voice in decision-making processes, provide support for continued professional development, and pay a life-sustainable wage (ICN, 2012).

Take Note!
The shortage of nursing professionals is a global phenomenon that is expected to worsen in the coming decades.

QUESTIONS FOR REFLECTION

1. Why do you think that there is a shortage of professional nurses and physicians?
2. What would you do to combat the national and global professional nurse shortage?
3. Do you think your plan would be feasible? Why or why not?

SELECTED CURRENT HEALTH CARE DELIVERY SYSTEMS

Health care delivery systems arose as people identified a need to care for the infirmed and injured. Societal beliefs about the nature of the world provided for early health delivery systems and guided their evolution. Because it is not feasible to cover all systems within a single chapter, selected nations representing various geographical locations with different approaches to health care delivery are covered here.

The U.S. Health Care Delivery System

The health care delivery system in the United States was largely influenced by Europe because European immigrants quickly became the dominant cultural group in the United States. The evolution of the U.S. health care delivery system explains its emphasis on market competition and individualism.

The Roots of the U.S. Health Care Delivery System

In the United States in the late 18th and early 19th centuries, philanthropy and the government were the leading sources for health care funding. No organized health care programs existed because the predominant ethic of the time was that of self-sufficiency, and accepting charity was seen as a sign of grave weakness (Torrens, 1978). Thus, the seeds for the American value of independence were sown into its health care delivery system.

Most early hospitals in the United States were actually almshouses or pesthouses where the socially marginal fragments of society resided (Vogel, 1979). Because hospitals were supported by the philanthropy of the wealthy, class distinctions were considered to be justified. Hospital patients were stigmatized as dependent and somehow unworthy of society membership.

By 1873, the United States had 178 established hospitals (Jonas, 1998) and formal education in nursing began (Torrens, 1978). In the mid-to-late 1800s, scientific discoveries also began to revolutionize health care. Anesthesia was introduced in 1847 and antisepsis became prevalent by 1865, leading to the need for centralized facilities to support expensive equipment for surgery. Germ theory became accepted for the transmission of infectious diseases, and the typhus vaccine became available in 1896. By 1860, the thermometer, ophthalmoscope, and laryngoscope were in use, joined by the gastroscope, cystoscope, hypodermic needle, and sphygmomanometer by 1883. X-rays were discovered in 1895. Hospitals improved hygiene measures. People went to hospitals for advanced diagnostic tests and treatment and hospitals became places of healing rather than death (Jamieson & Sewall, 1954).

The Growth of the Health Care Industry and Insurance Systems

As urbanization increased, hospitals flourished. Hospital-owned schools of nursing provided an inexpensive source of nursing care. Hospitalized patients provided rich learning experiences for nursing and medical students. An apprenticeship approach dominated nursing and medical education. Medical education moved to university settings and developed independent prestige based on increased scientific knowledge, whereas nursing became associated with a medically dependent scope of practice, with an apprenticeship-type of education completely dominated by hospitals.

By the early 20th century, hospitals and physicians enjoyed high profits by providing services to wealthy patients who could afford them. However, "the poor and penniless, whom the institution had originally been meant to serve, became a liability" (Vogel, 1979, p. 115). A two-tier system of private and public institutions arose. Public institutions met the health care needs of the poor, while physician-dominated private hospitals met the needs of the affluent. As the nuclear family replaced the extended family, health care moved from being home-oriented and family-centered to institutionally centered. Health care became a stratified and localized system administered by municipalities (as in the British and French traditions).

In 1901, the American Medical Association (AMA) was restructured, and "doctors sought to assure their financial security and power through their own organization and reform of medical education" (Markowitz & Rosner, 1979, p. 186), thereby eliminating competition from other persons as health care providers. Private foundations supplied additional resources to the AMA, creating a central power source for medical practice and education. Efforts focused on replacing the haphazard art of medical practice with new scientific-based knowledge. As new treatments and technology developed, more hospitals were needed. By 1910, the number of hospitals in the United States had expanded to 4,400 (Jonas, 1998).

In 1910, concerned with the impact of illness on worker productivity, Montgomery Ward and Company provided group insurance to its employees for illness and injury. This plan frequently is regarded as the first group health insurance coverage in the United States. The Ladies' Garment Workers' Union provided the first union medical care services after a fatal fire that killed 146 women (Public Broadcasting Service [PBS], 2007). Between 1915 and 1920, 16 states introduced, debated, and rejected legislation mandating health insurance coverage for all (PBS, 2007).

The global influenza epidemic of 1918 and pneumonia killed more soldiers than combat did. Because of contagious disease fatalities, public health efforts focused efforts on containing and preventing infectious diseases. Hospital overcrowding forced families to assume responsibility for nursing care at home and physicians made home visits (Jamieson & Sewall, 1954).

The Great Depression of the 1930s devastated the developing American health care system. Without employment, many could not feed or clothe their families, much less even think about paying for health care services if needed. Increasingly, the government assumed responsibility for providing and funding health care services, and illness prevention and health promotion became top priorities for government-sponsored health programs (Jonas, 1998). In 1935, the Social Security Act included provisions for financially supporting the indigent and the infirmed elderly, carving out for the first time a role for the federal government in providing health care services (PBS, 2007).

Accident and life insurance companies started offering insurance covering hospital services. In 1929, the first hospitalization insurance plan, Blue Cross, provided coverage for a group of teachers from Dallas, Texas (Scofera, 1994). In 1939, a Blue Shield plan for medical and surgical expenses was sponsored by the California Medical Society.

Prior to World War II (WWII), less than 20% of Americans had any form of health care insurance (Scofera, 1994). During WWII, the War Labor Board froze wages to divert resources to the war effort. To appease unions and workers, employers added health insurance to fringe benefit packages (PBS, 2007). To assume responsibility for war-related injuries (physical or psychological), the federal government established the Veterans Administration (VA) program (Jamieson & Sewall, 1954). The VA health care system still offers extensive rehabilitation programs and health care services to all veterans.

Following WWII, workers came to expect reasonable wages and hospitalization insurance. In response to problems arising in the growing health insurance industry, the McCarran–Ferguson Act was enacted to provide state regulation of all forms of insurance (PBS, 2007). By 1951, 100 million Americans had some form of health care insurance coverage (Scofera, 1994), enabling many people to reap the benefits of newly developed medications and surgical interventions. Because of the technical skills required to administer new therapies, hospitals expanded and became places where people got well.

Health Care in the Mid- to Late 20th Century

Health care changed dramatically in the mid- to late 20th century. Increased scientific knowledge resulted in an information explosion that led to the era of specialization for health care delivery, which resulted in fragmentation and increased cost (Jonas, 1998; Knickman & Kovner, 2015). Deaths from infectious diseases lessened and the need for treatment for chronic diseases became more prevalent, along with complex regimens to control chronic illness.

"The percentage of Americans covered by some form of health insurance rose from less than 20% prior to WWII to more than 70% by the early 1960s" (Torrens, 1978, p. 13). The increased demand for health care resulted in the passage of the Hill–Burton Act (1946), which stimulated hospital construction. The U.S. Department of Health, Education, and Welfare (now the U.S. Department of Health and Human Services) was formed in 1953 to provide a mechanism to coordinate health research and service programs. The Civil Rights Movement espoused the belief that equal health care is a basic right and encouraged the government to became more involved in health care. In 1965, Congress amended the Social Security Act to create the Medicare and Medicaid programs, thereby creating a role for the federal government in health care delivery for the elderly and poor.

By 1960, 120 million Americans were covered by some form of health insurance (Scofera, 1994). Whereas the 1960s had emphasized equity and cohesion of services, the 1970s concentrated on access, with tremendous growth in the number of hospitals, ancillary services, and sophisticated technology available. The emphasis on research and technology led to specialization and depersonalization, as well as rapidly escalating expenses (Jonas, 1998; Knickman & Kovner, 2015). Health care expenditures were essentially unmonitored. Increased demand for services led to more hospitals, extended-care facilities, and health-related research facilities.

By the late 1970s, spiraling health care costs became impossible to ignore. The federal government established new regulations to monitor delivered services along with reductions in federal funding. The changes rewarded efficiency over equity, quality, and access. Prospective payment reimbursement of hospital expenses for Medicare patients was introduced in 1981 in an effort to reduce hospital costs. **Prospective payment** established prearranged reimbursement amounts (by diagnostic category known as diagnosis-related groups [DRGs]) that the federal government paid hospitals for care given to Medicare recipients. The hospital received a prearranged amount, regardless of accrued costs.

Under the prospective payment system, big profits could be made, resulting in a business approach to health care. Detailed documentation of medical services provided and supplies used became crucial as insurance providers looked for reasons to deny reimbursement. For-profit insurance companies and hospital chains grew. Not-for-profit hospitals invested increased profits back into expanding and improving hospital services for the community, thereby increasing consumer access to sophisticated health care. However, by the late 1980s, the federal government progressively reduced the amount of reimbursement for specific DRGs, adding financial pressure to struggling smaller (and usually rural) hospitals.

Managed care plans started in the 1970s and flourished as health care costs continued to rise. Enrollment in managed care plans rose from 2 million people in 1970 to more than 39 million people in 1992. Managed care proponents believed these plans could reduce health care costs by promoting health (Andersen et al., 2007; Scofera, 1994). Three models of managed care emerged: health maintenance organizations (HMOs), preferred provider organizations (PPOs), and point-of-service (POS). Table 9.1 highlights the differences among the plans.

In the economic downslide of the 1980s, many people lost their jobs and consequently their health care coverage. In 1985, the Consolidated Omnibus Budget Reconciliation Act (COBRA) was enacted. It requires that employers with more than 20 workers partially subsidize the health insurance coverage offered to former employees (and their dependents) for 18 months after termination of employment. Because of the high costs associated with COBRA, however, many of those unemployed could not afford to continue health care coverage (Andersen et al., 2007; Knickman, 2015).

Health care expenditures rose at close to twice the rate of inflation between 1990 and 1995. Between 1995 and 2000, health care costs rose, on average, 3.4%. At the same time, inflation rose 2.5%. In response to spiraling health care costs, the Clinton administration, in the early 1990s, tried unsuccessfully to enact health care reform legislation. Since 2003, expenditures for health care in the United States continue to outpace the rate of inflation and consumed $2.5 trillion (combined public and private funds) in 2009 (Center for Medicare & Medicaid Services, 2011). The Center for Medicare & Medicaid Services (2014) predicts that by 2024, health care expenditures will account for 19.6% of the gross national product.

TABLE 9.1 Differences in Managed Care Models

Health Maintenance Organization	Preferred Provider Organization	Point-of-Service Plan
Group-model HMOs contract directly with a single medical group to care for members. Staff-model HMOs contract with individual physicians to serve members. Network HMOs contract with a network of physicians to provide services for members.	Network of preferred health care providers contained within an insurance plan who agree to follow the insurance company's utilization guidelines and accept deeply discounted fees for provided services.	Network of preferred providers who contract to provide services for a managed care company and follow guidelines set by the insurance carrier while accepting discounted fees for rendered services.
Open-panel HMOs permit physicians to treat non-HMO members. Closed-panel HMOs require physicians under contract to see members only.	Members can access physicians not on the list of preferred providers, but they have substantially higher co-payments for services.	Members select their level of managed care services: 1. Use of a primary care provider gatekeeper for specialist referrals 2. Self-referral to specialists within the provider network 3. Self-referral to specialist of choice
Cheapest of all forms for consumer because of limitations in covered services.	Costs for co-payments higher than those for HMOs.	Graduated co-payments, with members using a gatekeeper having the lowest out-of-pocket expenses and members with the ability to self-refer to their specialist of choice having the highest co-payment.
Members must receive authorization for care from a specialist, usually a primary care physician.	Members can self-refer for specialist services.	
In the 1990s, some HMOs offered self-referral to specialists, but members had higher co-pays.	Higher co-pays for members seeing specialists if they see a specialist within the preferred providers list and if a specialist not listed as a preferred provider, even higher co-payments.	

Adapted from Andersen, R., Rice, T., & Kominski, G. (2007). *Changing the U.S. health care system* (3rd ed.). San Francisco, CA: Wiley.

Multiple efforts in hopes to contain health care costs in the late 20th century included reductions in prospective payments, consolidation of health care services, and hospital closures. Hospital costs fell because of reduced lengths of inpatient stays. Only the medically unstable were hospitalized. Once stabilized, people were expected to leave the hospital. Medicare and insurance companies provided coverage for rehabilitation in extended-care facilities (if patients were too weak to return home safely). When possible, family members would provide care to relatives at home. Insurance companies also shifted the burden of rising health care costs to consumers by increasing premiums, co-payments, and deductibles (Andersen et al., 2007).

Increased competition as a cost-containment mechanism provided an opportunity for NPs to expand their provision of primary and secondary health care services despite opposition by many physicians.

Health Care Costs in the United States Today

The free market approach dominated the health care industry in the 20th century and continues to do so today (Jonas, 1998; Knickman, 2015). Many health care leaders debate the benefits of a market-driven health care system that is based on the premise that competition controls the costs of health care delivery. These changes have resulted in a highly complex, multifaceted health care delivery system in the 21st century, which has led to the United States spending over 17% of its gross domestic product for health care (Centers for Medicare & Medicaid Services, 2014).

According to the Centers of Medicare and Medicaid Services, health care expenditures fall into the following categories: health-related research, facility construction, and payment for personal health care services and supplies. Costs for individual health care services and supplies supersede those of new construction or research, with hospital costs comprising the greatest single health care expense (Slavitt & Burwell, 2016).

Provider Costs

The late 20th century saw an explosion of technology and scientific advances. Today, American hospital costs surpass those of all developed nations. The amount of money charged for an acute-care hospital patient day in the United States is more than twice that of Canada and three times higher than that of most other developed countries. Hospitalized Americans undergo more sophisticated diagnostic procedures and intensive medical regimens. The increased use of highly technical equipment and expensive medications fuels these rising costs. Because of the litigious nature of

the American culture, the ever-present threat of malpractice suits adds to the costs (Bodenheimer, 2005; Knickman, 2015).

Physician income in the United States is (on average) 1.5 to 3 times higher than that of physicians in other developed countries. The United States tends to have a surplus of specialist physicians because they earn substantially more than general practice physicians (Bodenheimer, 2005; Knickman, 2015).

Advanced practice RNs offer an alternative to the high costs of physician services. Despite resistance by organized medicine, in 1996 all states allowed third-party reimbursement to advanced practice RNs (Sultz & Young, 2004). Services rendered by advanced practice RNs cost substantially less, and consumers report high satisfaction.

Insurance

In 2011, 49.9 million Americans did not have health insurance in 2010 and 31% of Americans relied on some form of government health insurance program. In 2011, the number of uninsured Americans fell to 48.6 million largely due to changes in coverage of younger Americans on parent insurance policies (DeNavas-Walt, Proctor, & Smith, 2012). The rate of uninsured Americans tends to fluctuate with the unemployment rate.

In 2010, employer-based health insurance coverage fell to 55.3% of the population from a high of 69.2% in 2000. That same year, the average cost of an employer-sponsored family health insurance plan rose to $13,770 annually (Gould, 2012). One in four workers could not afford to purchase health insurance (De-Navas-Walt et al., 2012).

Corporations represent the largest purchasers of private health insurance. To contain costs, companies have

- limited consumer choice of providers through HMOs or PPOs
- increased premiums, deductibles, and out-of-pocket charges
- required authorization for hospitalizations and second opinions
- substituted ambulatory and home care to reduce hospital stays
- encouraged reduced use of services

Patient Protection and Affordable Care Act of 2010

Because of escalating health care costs, increased numbers of uninsured Americans (as a result of increased unemployment), and the inability of many American workers to purchase expensive private and employer-based health insurance plans. President Obama signed the **Patient Protection and Affordable Care Act (ACA) of 2010** into law in 2010. Under the ACA, federal and state governments assume a larger role in providing health insurance to all Americans. Table 9.2 highlights some of the key provisions of the ACA. The ACA sets new requirements on individuals and employers; requires insurance plans to include coverage for periodic screenings for diseases; eliminates the barrier of no coverage for pre-existing conditions; removes lifetime coverage limits; and offers health-promotion strategies. Provisions of the law are being implemented over time, and the entire law should be enacted by January 2018 (Kaiser Family Foundation, 2012). With final rules and regulations in place, the essential health services covered by the ACA are ambulatory, emergency, maternity and newborn care, mental health services including substance use and behavioral disorder care (including treatment of behavioral health issues), devices and services for rehabilitation and activities of daily living, lab tests, prevention and wellness care (with no costs to patients), and pediatric care (medical, dental, and visual services) (Stapleton & Skinner, 2015).

The ACA develops some new programs and renames others. Changes include the following.

- **Bundled payment:** A new approach to reimbursement for treatment received from a hospital or physician for a fixed amount for episodic care received over time if a person has a chronic condition (Knickman, 2015).
- **Medical home:** A medical practice directed by a physician that consists of a provider team in which a patient has an ongoing relationship with a personal physician who coordinates care (Knickman, 2015).
- **Accountable Health Care Organization (ACHCO):** A group of health care providers (nonprofit or for profit) across the continuum of care that have legal agreements with each other and have aligned their incentives to provide and promote quality care while containing costs. An ACHCO may be an HMO, a PPO, or an integrated health care system (IHCS) that contracts with external insurance providers or self-insures (Knickman, 2015).
- **Insurance exchange:** A marketplace administered through a government agency or nonprofit organization that consumers can use to compare health insurance plans, choose a desired plan, and purchase health insurance (Kaiser Family Foundation, 2011).
- **Comparative effectiveness research:** Studies comparing the outcomes of two or more health care technologies, services, or products (including medications) either against each other or with conventional treatment to compare their costs relative to benefits (Knickman, 2015).

The Congressional Budget Office projects that the ACA will provide an additional 32 million Americans with health insurance coverage. Projected costs of the new law are estimated to be $938 million and will reduce the budget deficit by $124 billion. Costs are to be funded by reductions in Medicare and Medicaid expenditures, new taxes (excise taxes on high-cost insurance and medical devices), and fees for noncompliance by health care organizations and individuals (Knickman, 2015).

Implementation of the ACA has resulted in some positive and negative outcomes for Americans. Benefits from ACA implementation for individuals and families vary according to state of residency, type of community (urban versus rural), and annual income. Some health care organizations have reaped benefits, but others have experienced financial difficulty because of increased complexities associated with administrative costs (Geyman, 2015; Haeder & Weimer, 2015; Maizel, Bernadino, Caine, & Garfinkle, 2015). In addition, some small businesses have had to close because of requirements to provide health insurance coverage for employees. Within the first 5 years, there have been substantial increased costs for prescription medication use, administrative costs for organizations providing health care, and federal administration of required programs for law implementation (Geyman, 2015). Table 9.3 presents some of the positive and negative outcomes that have been identified in the literature during the first 5 years of ACA implementation.

Because of some mandates contained within the ACA and other shifts in American viewpoints, Americans elected Donald Trump as President of the United State as well as more Republicans to the legislative governmental branches. In early 2017, legislation known as the **American Health Care Act (ACHC)** was introduced early into the Trump administration. Initial efforts to pass this legislation failed. Some legislators could not support it because provisions would eliminate insurance coverage for some citizens as well as cutting services for health promotion and access to care. Other legislators failed to support the bill because provisions contained in the bill failed to eliminate aspects of the ACA that reduced state rights to designate health care benefits at the state level including covered services that are financed at the state level of government. Because of the complexity of the American

TABLE 9.2 Key Provisions and Processes of the 2010 Patient Protection and Affordable Care Act

Provision	Process
Expanded access to health care insurance coverage	■ Set up state-based health insurance exchanges with cost-sharing credits for purchase of insurance based on family income.
Individual mandate that all Americans have health insurance coverage	■ Individuals without coverage will pay a fine. ■ Provisions provided for hardship and other exemptions such as religious beliefs.
Employers required to offer health insurance coverage	■ Employers with more than 50 employees will be required to offer health insurance to employees or face a fine. ■ Tax credits will be offered to employers providing coverage. ■ Employers can provide free choice vouchers. ■ Employees who work for a company with more than 200 employees may opt out of coverage.
Medicaid expanded	■ Federal tax subsidies to states as they enroll more people into Medicaid programs. ■ The percentage of subsidy decreases over time. ■ Increased payment to primary care service providers. ■ No penalties to the states if they do not expand Medicare.
Children's Health Insurance Plan (CHIP) expanded	■ Increases state reimbursement for CHIP and sets enrollment caps on CHIP. ■ Eligibility for tax credits through the state insurance exchanges for children unable to enroll in CHIP.
Premium and cost-sharing subsidies to individuals	■ Eligibility rules for immigrants and employees with access to employer-based insurance. ■ Income sliding-scale cost-sharing subsidies and premium credits. ■ Proof of legal citizenship or immigrant status. ■ Verification of income. ■ No subsidies can be used for abortions except in cases of mother's life being threatened, or incidences of rape or incest.
Small business tax credits	■ Two phases and tax credits reimburse 35–100% of the employer's contribution to employee health insurance premiums. ■ Amounts vary based on number of employees and the average employee wage.
Reinsurance program for employers providing health insurance to retirees over 55 yrs of age and ineligible for Medicare	■ Reimbursement to these employers of 80% of retiree claims for costs incurred ranging from $15,000 to $90,000 to reduce the costs for employees enrolled in the provided employer plan.
Tax changes related to health insurance	■ Tax persons without coverage $695 up to, three times that amount ($2,085) or 2.3% of household income for annual incomes less than $90,652. Once annual income exceeds $90,652 then the person will be fined 2.3% of annual income. ■ Allow purchase of over-the-counter medications using tax-free health spending accounts. ■ Increase taxes on unused funds from tax-fee health spending accounts. ■ Limit contributions to tax-free health spending accounts to $2,500. ■ Increase the allowable deduction to 10% of health care expenses for persons who itemize deductions on income tax forms. ■ Increase taxes on Medicare Part A rate on wages. ■ Impose an excise tax on employer health plans, with aggregate values of $10,200 for individuals and $27,500 for families. ■ Eliminate tax deductions for employees receiving Medicare Part D.
Tax changes to finance health care reform	■ Impose new annual fees on pharmaceutical manufacturing and health insurance sectors. ■ Impose a 2.3% excise tax on the sale of taxable medical devices. ■ Limit compensation deductibles to $5,00,000 for health insurance sector executives and employees. ■ Charge a 10% tax on indoor tanning fees.

Provision	Process
Health insurance exchanges	■ Health insurance exchanges may be developed regionally and cross state lines. ■ Only legal citizens and residents can be covered by exchanges. ■ Incarcerated people cannot be covered by an exchange. ■ One plan must be nonprofit. ■ One plan must not cover abortions beyond federal guidelines. ■ Create a consumer-operated and consumer-oriented plan to stimulate development of nonprofit member-run health insurance companies. ■ Catastrophic coverage for persons under 30 yrs of age and those who are exempt from the mandate. ■ Create four plans: bronze, silver, gold, and platinum (percentage of coverage increases with each level, with bronze covering 60% and platinum covering 90% of costs for covered health care services). ■ New limits on out-of-pocket expenditures.
Private insurance changes	■ Establish a national medical high-risk pool and limit the amount that can be charged to cover these individuals. ■ Require health plans to report the amount spent in proportion to premium dollars received. ■ Establish a process for approving rate increases. ■ Simplify the administration process especially those for claims. ■ No lifetime limits for coverage. ■ Extend coverage to adult children to age 26 yrs. ■ Impose the same insurance marketing regulations regarding guarantee issue, premium rating, and prohibitions on pre-existing conditions. ■ Provide bronze, silver, gold, and platinum plans. ■ Limitations of deductibles. ■ Finance the reinsurance program. ■ Allow states to merge small markets. ■ Establish a website so consumers can compare plans. ■ Develop standards to provide information on benefits and coverage. ■ Allow states to participate in state insurance compacts. ■ Establish the Health Insurance Reform Implementation Fund within the U.S. Department of Health and Human Services and allocate $1 billion to implement health care reform policies.
Changes for the states	■ Create American Health Benefit Exchange and a Small Business Health Options Program Exchange for small businesses and individuals to purchase health insurance. ■ Enroll newly eligible Medicaid enrollees by January 2014. ■ Establish an office of health insurance consumer assistance or an ombudsman program to advocate for persons with private coverage in the individual and small business markets. ■ Create a basic health plan for all uninsured people with incomes between 133% and 200% of the federal poverty limit.
Cost-containment strategies	■ Administration simplification by developing a single set of rules for eligibility and status of claims. ■ Medicare and Medicaid reforms to reduce costs to include primary care delivery in "medical homes" and expand use of bundled payment strategies for health care provider reimbursement. ■ Reduce the time for FDA approval of generic medications to 12 yrs. ■ Implement plans to reduce waste, fraud, and abuse.
Improvement in health care quality and outcomes	■ Establish a nonprofit "Patient-centered Outcomes Research Institute" that would establish research priorities and determine the effectiveness of available medical and surgical treatments. ■ Results of comparative studies would not become mandates for care delivery. ■ Abolish the Federal Council for Comparative Effectiveness Research.
Reduce costs of medical malpractice	■ Provide grants for demonstration projects to design and implement alternatives to medical malpractice litigation. ■ Preferential grant awards to projects that include methods to improve patient safety such as reducing medical errors and adverse events.

(continued on page 226)

TABLE 9.2 Key Provisions and Processes of the 2010 Patient Protection and Affordable Care Act *(continued)*

Provision	Process
Medicare	■ Institute a pilot program to develop and evaluate a bundled payment program for the following services: acute, inpatient hospital care; physician care; outpatient services; and postacute care 3 days after an acute-care event. ■ Develop Independence at Home program for primary care in the home. ■ Establish a value-based purchasing program based on performance measures for hospital reimbursement.
Dual Medicare and Medicaid beneficiaries	■ Create the Federal Coordinated Health Care Office to integrate Medicare and Medicaid benefits more effectively. ■ Improve coordination between the federal government and states to facilitate access to and improve the quality of care.
Medicaid	■ Medical health homes for recipients with two or more chronic conditions or one condition and a high risk for developing another, or a persistent chronic mental disorder. ■ Funding for the development of demonstration projects to develop and establish and determine efficacy of new bundled payment programs for care received across the health care continuum in Accountable Care Organizations. ■ Expand the Medicaid and CHIP Payment Access Commission to include assessment of services provided to adult recipients.
Primary care	■ Provide 100% reimbursement for care received from primary care providers. ■ Award primary care doctors a 10% bonus in Medicare payments from 2011 to 2015.
National quality strategy	■ Develop and establish a national quality improvement strategy that sets priorities for health care improvement, health care delivery, health outcomes, and population health.
Financial disclosure	■ Reports indicating financial relationships between health entities (e.g., physicians, hospitals, pharmacists, and other providers) and manufacturers and distributors of pharmaceuticals, medical devices, and supplies.
Disparities in health care delivery	■ Required data collection and reporting of demographic data including race, ethnicity, gender, primary language, disability status, and location of primary residence.
Prevention and wellness strategies	■ National strategy to include development of the National Prevention, Health Promotion, and Public Health Council to coordinate efforts of wellness and disease prevention. ■ Establish a Prevention and Public Health fund to pay for wellness and disease prevention programs. ■ Improve coverage of prevention and health-promotion services. ■ Support the use of comprehensive health risk assessment and the development of a personalized health-promotion plan. ■ Require health care plans to cover wellness and disease prevention programs. ■ Permit employers to offer rewards for healthy lifestyle behaviors. ■ Provide technical assistance to small employers to develop health and wellness programs. ■ Require disclosure of nutritional content of foods served in vending machines and at chain and fast food restaurants.
Long-term care strategies	■ Establishment of a voluntary insurance program to purchase community living assistance and supports through voluntary payroll deductions, with vested services after 5 yrs of contributions. ■ Provide states with funding for offering home and community-based services. ■ Establish the Community First Choice Option for Medicaid that would provide support and services to persons with disabilities who require institutional care. ■ Creation of the State Balancing Incentive program to increase federal matching funds to eligible states to increase the number of non-institutionally based long-term care services. ■ Mandatory reporting of ownership, accountability requirements, and expenditures by skilled nursing facilities. The report data would be published on a website so Medicare participants can compare facilities.

Provision	Process
Other investments	■ Improvements to Medicare. ■ Workforce development grants to educate primary care physicians and advanced practice nurses and create career ladders for seamless education for unlicensed nursing personnel to become nurses; professional nurses to become advanced practice nurses; public health, mental health, and oral health workers to become professional and potentially advanced practitioners in these fields of health care. ■ Improve school-based and community health care centers. ■ Establish a new national trauma center program to strengthen emergency departments in handling traumas. ■ Establish a commissioned Regular Corps and Ready Reserve Corps for deployment in times of national disasters. ■ Require nonprofit hospitals to perform community assessments every 3 yrs and then adopt an implementation strategy to meet the identified community needs. They must also widely publicize financial assistant policies (a $50,000 fine will be incurred for noncompliance with these new regulations).

Kaiser Family Foundation. (2011). Focus on health reform: Summary of new health reform law. Retrieved from http://www.kff.org/healthreform/upload/8061.pdf. Accessed December 12, 2012.

health care delivery and the importance of health care access for all, the administration and legislators have opted to take ample time to develop legislation to better meet health care needs for all Americans. Whatever occurs, there will need to be some form of incremental implementation from ACA to its replacement (Kaiser Family Foundation, 2017).

Canada's Health Care Delivery System

Like the United States, Canada enjoys much wealth. The countries share a similar history, but different historical events resulted in Canada adopting a very different form of health care delivery.

Historical Development of Canada's Health Care System

The French established some of the earliest colonies in Canada. In May 1639, Madame de la Peltrie, along with Augustinian and Ursuline sisters, established a trading post infirmary. The Augustinian sisters established the Hôtel-Dieu in Quebec City, Quebec in 1639, where they dispensed medications and offered cheerful encouragement to ill persons who preferred to stay at home. In 1645, Jeanne Mance established the Hôtel Dieu in Montreal as a hospital for wounded French and British soldiers during the Seven Years' War. In 1693, the Jesuits built another hospital in Canada using the support of the wealthy Duchesse d'Aiguillon, who obtained land and permission to establish a hospital (Jamieson & Sewall, 1954).

The Canadian Fathers of Confederation laid out terms of the British North America Act of 1867 that specified responsibilities of the Canadian government, which included taking a census, collecting vital statistics, determining quarantine regulations, providing hospitals for persons in quarantine, and caring for Canadian natives. Along with these basic responsibilities, a section of the act provided for the establishment of provincial hospitals, asylums, and charities (Goldsmith, 2002; McIntyre & Thomlinson, 2003; Storch, 2005).

In the 20th century, as in the United States, rising health care costs became an issue in Canada, resulting in federal efforts to provide coverage for health expenditures for everyone. In 1947, the Province of Saskatchewan enacted the Hospital Insurance Act, which provided hospital insurance for all its residents. At the same time, the Canadian government offered grants to the provinces and public health agencies for hospital construction and provision of health care services. In the 1960s, Saskatchewan expanded insurance coverage to include outpatient health care, and by 1968 the Medical Care Act was enacted, providing national health insurance for all Canadians (Goldsmith, 2002; McIntyre & Thomlinson, 2003; Storch, 2005).

In the 1980s, paralleling the trend in the United States, Canada also experienced problems with skyrocketing health care costs and limited public funding. In response, the Canada Health Care Act of 1984 resulted in provincial administration of health care programs. All Canadians have equal access to a specific list of health care services under provincial policy plans. Additional costs cannot be incurred by citizens for services covered by these plans. Finally, the Canadian plan is portable and covers citizens if they move from province to province or travel abroad. However, nonemergency and out-of-province services require preauthorization (McIntyre & Thomlinson, 2003; Storch, 2005).

TABLE 9.3 Positive and Negative Outcomes of the Affordable Care Act—Five Years into Implementation

Positive:
- 24 of 50 states expanded Medicaid coverage resulting in 7 million persons having Medicaid coverage for health care costs (Geyman, 2015)
- Development of government-sponsored health care exchanges where the all Americans who do not have health insurance can shop and purchase health insurance (Geyman, 2015)
- 8 million Americans have been able to secure health insurance and 57% of new insurance enrollees have obtained insurance for the first time (Geyman, 2015)
- More than 3 million young adults from ages 19 to 26 yrs had insurance by staying insured on the health insurance policy of their parents (Geyman, 2015; Wong, Ford, French, & Rubin, 2015)
- A 6.7% rise in young adults with dental insurance following the implementation of young adult coverage on parent health insurance policies with the sharpest increase in middle income families (Shane & Ayyagari, 2015)
- Temporary increases in reimbursement for primary care physicians (Geyman, 2015)
- Opening of multiple free-standing specialty outpatient surgery centers resulting in decreased health care costs, fewer infections, and improved outcomes (Maizel et al., 2015)
- New federal funding for community health centers (Geyman, 2015; Haeder & Weimer, 2015)
- Increased opportunities for nurse practitioners to meet the primary care needs of the newly insured
- All insurance plans must cover essential health benefits (Stanley, 2015; Stapleton & Skinner, 2015)
- Contraceptive coverage included in all insurance policies offered by federal and state exchanges (Mulligan, 2015)
- Federal government grants available for implementation of the law (Haeder & Weimer, 2015)

Negative:
- 26 of 50 states failed to expand Medicaid coverage for persons with incomes 100–400% of the federal poverty level leaving 4.8 million people without access to health insurance coverage (Geyman, 2015; Haeder & Weimer, 2015)
- Sometimes citizens experienced time during which the government-sponsored exchange websites would not function properly
- Some employees are being shifted to a defined contribution from a defined benefit policy and others are being required to purchase coverage from an exchange either because of increased premium costs or employer dropping health insurance benefits (Geyman, 2015; Lahm, 2015; Maizel et al., 2015)
- Insurance providers increased rates for coverage for policies and/or providing less benefits per policy (Geyman, 2015; Lahm, 2015)
- Expansion of consolidated health care systems to gain market share in a geographical locale (Geyman, 2015; Maizel et al., 2015)
- No substantial evidence that pay for performance improves health care outcomes (Geyman, 2015)
- Exponential increases in administrative bureaucracy and costs especially for private sector health care organizations and business (Geyman, 2015; Lahm, 2015; Maizel et al., 2015)
- Closure of smaller health care providing organizations resulting in some Americans needing to travel longer distances to access emergency and primary care services (Maizel et al., 2015)
- Shortage of primary care physicians to meet the needs of the newly insured (Geyman, 2015)
- Perception of the health care industry of being a new, profitable market and a good investment that has resulted in increased prices and costs in a free-market system (Geyman, 2015)
- Perceptions of or actually being underinsured for a significant illness or injury due to high deductibles ($8,000–10,000) or percentage of coverage for rendered services (60% bronze plan, 70% silver plan) (Geyman, 2015)
- An estimated 36 million of uninsured Americans (5 million in the Medicaid gap) because of the inability to afford health insurance (Geyman, 2015)
- Limited choice of provider in many insurance plans (Geyman, 2015)
- Accountable Care Organization definition changed to require an organization that serves at least 5,000 persons thereby limiting opportunities for smaller organizations to become one (Geyman, 2015)
- The Patient-Centered Outcomes Research Institute has no authority to determine reimbursement policies for evidence-based best practices (Geyman, 2015)
- Reductions in federal reimbursement to states for Medicaid expansion to 90% of incurred costs not enough for some states and facilities where profit-margins for health care services is less than 10% resulting in bankruptcies in state-funded and managed health insurance exchanges (Maizel et al., 2015)
- Investors buying and selling hospitals and health systems to turn a quick profit (Maizel et al., 2015)
- Increased costs of care for the uninsured (Maizel et al., 2015)
- Hospitals being penalized for readmission rates (patient re-admitted 30 days or less from a stay) despite there might issues about the patient that they cannot control (Maizel et al., 2015)
- Reimbursement tied to patient surveys measuring satisfaction with care (Maizel et al., 2015)
- Loss of stand-alone physician practices with many physicians becoming employees of a hospital or health system (Maizel et al., 2015)
- Lack of recognition for the complexity of patients for care is being provided (Maizel et al., 2015)
- Wide variance in coverage for various services such as for complementary and alternative health care strategies with one state covering them and another state denying coverage (Haeder & Weimer, 2015; Stanley, 2015)
- No coverage assistance for non-American citizens if they need health care (Geyman, 2015; Haeder & Weimer, 2015)

Principles of the Canadian Health Care System

Health care in Canada is directed by five key principles.

1. A public, nonprofit authority administers provincial health insurance plans and answers to the provincial government.
2. Each insurance plan covers all eligible residents using uniform terms and conditions.
3. Canadians have health insurance coverage when they travel abroad or across provinces. However, the plans have limited out-of-country coverage and provincial plan approval is required for nonemergency services when receiving care out of the province in which a citizen resides.
4. Each plan covers "all medically necessary services" citizens may need from physicians and hospitals.
5. The plans provide reasonable access to health services without discrimination. Provincial plans may require premiums from citizens, but care cannot be denied based on inability to pay for coverage (Goldsmith, 2002).

Funds for the Canadian health care system come from taxes (primarily payroll), health insurance premiums, and consumer out-of-pocket expenses. Tax credits offer relief for high out-of-pocket health care expenditures. For services not covered by government plans, some Canadians may purchase private health care policies. Approximately 65% of Canadians have private insurance that covers dental, chiropractic, and some complementary health care services (Goldsmith, 2002; Jost, 2005).

Because of citizens' complaints about accessing required health care in a timely fashion, the provincial premiers agreed to the Health Renewal Accord in 2003. Principles outlined by the accord include 24/7 access to a health care provider; timely access to diagnostic and treatment procedures; elimination of the need to repeat health histories or diagnostic tests for each provider seen; and access to home and community health care. Although the Canadian health care system is perceived as being efficient, it responds slowly in addressing needed reforms. Increased collaboration among the federal and provincial governments and the sharing of best practices based on solid evidence has resulted in improvement of Canadian health care outcomes (Storch, 2005).

Mexico's Health Care Delivery System

Mexico has less wealth than Canada or the United States. Rapid industrialization with increasing environmental pollution, along with increasing tobacco and alcohol use, poor diet, sedentary lifestyle, and infectious diseases (in crowded urban areas) pose challenges to the health of Mexicans.

Not all Mexicans have equal access to health care services. The affluent purchase private health insurance plans and have access to the same quality of care and services enjoyed by Canadians and Americans. Workers are covered through a social security system or purchase employment-based health insurance, and the poor rely on a public services system. The Ministry of Health manages health promotion and disease prevention for Mexican citizens. The Ministry of Health also monitors and tests medications made by and sold in Mexico for quality, safety, and efficacy (Johnson, Carillo, & Garcia, 2002).

The Mexican health care system consists of hospitals, outpatient facilities, and long-term care facilities. Modern medical centers are located in urban areas. Health care facilities in rural areas are often understaffed and rely on medical students as providers. In recent years, health care delivery to Mexicans covered by public services has become decentralized, and emphasis has been placed on a healthy municipalities program. Shifting the emphasis to health promotion rather than disease treatment for public health services has increased access to health care services for the poor (Johnson et al., 2002).

Comparing and Contrasting the Selected Health Care Delivery Systems

Access to a clean water source, effective sanitation, and adequate food supply clearly separate health care needs for developed and undeveloped nations. In developing nations, malnutrition, infant and child mortality, and communicable diseases are often the major health concerns. In wealthy, developed nations, diseases of affluence (e.g., obesity, diabetes mellitus, degenerative joint disease) emerge as major health concerns.

National wealth also dictates the funding available to build and maintain health care facilities, along with providing the facilities with adequate human and material resources. Wealthy persons have resources to spend on health care services even if they live in undeveloped countries. Not all citizens of a wealthy nation have resources to access and receive required health care services.

The *World Health Statistics 2012* report revealed that the United States spends 17.9% of its gross domestic product on health care, significantly more than either Canada (9.0%) or Mexico (6.5%) (WHO,

2012). Governmental support comes from local and state taxes. The Canadian government pays the largest share of the health care bill (70.6%), followed by the Mexican government (48.3%). Combined government support for American health care expenditures is 45%. Nations with a history of British or communist influences tend to approach health care delivery as a state, rather than a personal, responsibility.

The number of health care professionals also varies according to the development and financial status of a country. The United States reported the highest concentration of physicians, pharmacists, and managerial and support staff (WHO, 2012). Fifer (2007) and Bodenheimer (2005) proposed that the high level of management and support staff greatly increases the cost of American health care delivery. Canada ranks highest in the concentration of nurses and midwives at 104.3 nurses/midwives per 10,000 people; the United States has 98.2 per 10,000 persons, and Mexico has less than one nurse/midwife per 10,000 people. Although the United States and Canada offer similar health care services, albeit with different sources of funding, citizens of both nations tend to be satisfied with the services that they receive. Focus on Research, "Health Care Quality and Satisfaction in the United States Versus Canada," details a landmark study comparing the health status between these two countries.

FOCUS ON RESEARCH

Health Care Quality and Satisfaction in the United States Versus Canada

Fifteen years ago, a landmark multinational study compared health care quality and satisfaction with health care delivery in the United States and Canada. In 2002 and 2003, a random sample of 5,000 Americans and 3,500 Canadians participated in telephone interviews.

The study revealed that Canadians and Americans have similar access to a variety of health care services. Citizens of both countries rely on insurance for dental care. Eighty-five percent of Americans and 88% of Canadians described their health as being good or excellent. Persons with low incomes in both countries reported poorer health status. Ninety percent of Americans and 87% of Canadians reported being very or somewhat satisfied with their current health care. Similarities in health status were noted in mobility, depressive episodes within the past 12 months, percentage of persons seeing a physician within the previous 12 months, number of dental visits, and dental insurance coverage. Differences occurred in the following areas.

- Canada had a slightly higher percentage of daily smokers.
- More Americans were found to be obese.
- Poor persons in the United States reported more difficulty accessing health care services.
- More Canadians reported having regular medical appointments.

- American women of ages 50 to 69 years were more likely to have had annual mammograms.
- Americans between the ages of 45 and 64 reported using more prescription drugs.

The investigators reported the following study limitations: data collected exclusively at the national level, participants had household telephones, potential inaccuracies from self-reported information, potential misinterpretation of survey questions by respondents, potential sampling error, and no available data on characteristics of nonparticipants.

This study clearly highlights the perceived high levels of satisfaction and health status of Americans and Canadians. However, low-income citizens of both nations had perceived levels of reduced health status. The study findings could be used to improve the health care delivery systems of both nations. Implications for professional nursing practice vary for Canadian and American nurses. American nurses may need to improve efforts aimed at obesity prevention and treatment, the dangers of using multiple prescription medications, and advocating for health care services for Americans with low incomes. Canadian nurses might want to look for ways to plan and execute smoking cessation programs. The study could be repeated to see if any changes in satisfaction or health status have occurred in relation to changes in health care policies.

Sanmartin, C., Ng, E., Blackwell, D., Gentleman, J., Martinez, M., & Simile, C. (2004). *Joint Canada/United States survey of health, 2002–2003*. Washington, DC: Centers for Disease Control and Prevention. Retrieved from http://www.cdc.gov/nchs/data/nhis/jcush_analyticalreport.pdf. Accessed December 12, 2012.

QUESTIONS FOR REFLECTION

1. Think about your current health care insurance plan and coverage. How do you think that coverage may change based on your reading of phased-in changes required by the Affordable Care Act?

2. What current disparities in health care access exist in your community? Outline some suggestions for ways to improve health care access in your community. Analyze each of your suggestions for feasibility. What actions would you need to take to implement one or more of your suggestions?

HEALTH CARE DELIVERY SETTINGS

In the United States, health care services can be obtained in a variety of settings (Table 9.4). Organizations offering health care services differ according

TABLE 9.4 Settings for Health Care Delivery

Setting	Definition
Public hospital 1. Federal hospital 2. Nonfederal hospital	Nonprofit, government-owned institution that provides inpatient care 1. Owned and operated by the US government 2. Owned and operated by a state or local government
Community hospital	Locally owned institution that offers short-term services that are accessible to the public
Specialized hospital	Institution that offers services in one specialty area of health care (e.g., oncology, mental health, orthopedics, maternal–child health, children's services)
General hospital	Institution that offers a full scope of short-term services, including obstetric care
Teaching hospital	Institution that provides medical education to undergraduate or graduate medical students, residents, or postgraduate medical fellows
Extended-care facility	Institution that offers long-term care, also known as nursing home (75% owned by for-profit companies)
Long-term care home	Small group home that provides a homelike setting for persons with chronic mental illness or dementia
Rehabilitation center	Institution that offers services to help disabled persons become independent
Chemical dependence center	Institution that offers detoxification and rehabilitation for persons with drug or alcohol addiction
Neighborhood health center	Outpatient facility offering comprehensive primary care health services
Retail store–based health clinic	Clinic designed for episodic care of frequently occurring illnesses staffed by nurse practitioner; care recipient frequently able to purchase treatment for the illness in the store where the clinic is located
Private physician office	Comprehensive ambulatory patient medical care provided by a single physician
Physician partnership office	Comprehensive ambulatory medical care provided by a pair of physicians
Group physician office practice	Comprehensive ambulatory medical care services provided by a group of three or more physicians
Managed care clinic	Comprehensive ambulatory medical care provided within the confines of an office or clinic operated by a managed care company
Public health clinic	State-, county-, or city-funded health service that focuses primarily on preventing or controlling communicable diseases
Community health center	Neighborhood center that offers integrated primary care, education, and social services using a community-oriented, culturally sensitive approach; receives federal financial support
Ambulatory surgery center	Outpatient center where minor surgical procedures are performed
Specialty care center	Outpatient office or center that offers full scope of ambulatory care services to persons with specific health problems (e.g., renal failure, cancer, diabetes, pain); may have for-profit status
Emergency department	Outpatient facility linked to a hospital where life-threatening health problems can be managed. Some emergency facilities have designated trauma center certification. Frequently used by persons to receive health care after office or clinic hours

(continued on page 232)

TABLE 9.4 Settings for Health Care Delivery *(continued)*

Setting	Definition
Urgent care center	Outpatient facility (may be linked to a hospital) where people receive medical care services for health-related problems when clinics or offices are closed or when the person does not have an established health care provider. Usually have for-profit status. Some emergency rooms may dedicate a specific location to provide urgent care for non–life-threatening health problems
Hospital-based clinic	Outpatient comprehensive medical care service linked with a specific hospital. Many teaching hospitals hold resident clinics to provide health care to the poor
Hospital outpatient department	Ambulatory diagnostic testing or rehabilitation service that has connections to a specific hospital
Diagnostic testing center	Ambulatory diagnostic testing service. Some have connections to nonprofit hospitals; others are run by for-profit companies
Industrial health service unit	Employment-based health service to address job-related illnesses and injuries. Some units provide health-promotion activities and health screenings for employees
School health clinic	Health care service offered to students in academic settings (e.g., health rooms in primary or secondary schools or university health clinics)
Home health care	Medical care and nursing services offered for persons who are homebound
Hospice	Comprehensive service to assist persons in receiving a "good" death. Services may be given in the home or in extended-care or acute-care facilities

Jonas, S. (1998). *An introduction to the U.S. health care system* (4th ed.). New York: Springer Publishing; Knickman, J. R., & Kovner, A. R. (Eds.). (2015). *Jonas & Kovner's health care delivery in the United States* (11th ed.). New York: Springer; McGinn, D., & Springen, K. (2007). Express-lane medicine. *Newsweek*, (4), 44; and Sardell, A. (2012). Community health centers: Successful advocacy for expanding health care access. In D. Mason, J. Leavitt, & M. Chaffee (Eds.), *Policy & politics in nursing and health care* (6th ed.). St. Louis, MO: Elsevier Saunders.

to mission and philosophy. Although they all exist to offer health care services, some organizations may be proprietary (privately funded and for profit) and governmental (publicly funded and not for profit), while others are voluntary (privately funded and not for profit) (Jonas, 1998). For-profit organizations tend to emphasize providing services while achieving a high-profit margin.

To mitigate the high costs associated with hospital-based care, individuals are able to access alternative ambulatory care systems, including diagnostic, urgent care, surgery, birthing, substance abuse, and rehabilitation centers. Health care consumers can also receive health care services in outpatient clinics and urgent care centers located in shopping malls or pharmacies. Some clinics may be affiliated with an integrated health care delivery system or hospital. Annual influenza vaccinations are now routinely made available at retail and grocery stores, pharmacies, and/or places of employment. In addition, home health agencies and hospice services provide in-home nursing care. Recognizing the need to offer more outpatient services, some hospitals have built plush outpatient centers complete with food courts and small shops. To promote health within the community, hospitals hold classes on health-promotion topics, such as smoking cessation, weight reduction, safety, physical exercise, and basic lifestyle changes.

Primary Care Options

Persons seeking allopathic medical care typically consult physicians. Physicians tend to practice in either individual practice associations (IPAs) or PPOs. IPAs consist of a group of physicians who independently negotiate for set fee schedules with hospitals and insurance providers. Physicians employed in an IPA enjoy freedom to practice medicine as they desire; in contrast, physicians working in PPOs who must follow specific fee payment schedules and clinical utilization guidelines determined by the PPO. Integrated health care delivery systems employ physicians and some may even own the group practice.

HMOs were designed to focus efforts and resources on health promotion, preventive care, and consumer education to reduce health care costs. HMOs provide capitated payments (a set amount of money) for each member rather than paying only for rendered services. The traditional group- or staff-model HMO is a vertically integrated organization that operates its own physical facilities in various geographical locations and whose salaried physicians work solely for the HMO. A physician group may also contract services to an HMO. To increase practice revenues, some HMO physicians employ NP and physician assistants (PAs). The practice gets to keep surplus payments when care is delivered below the capitated payment (Gabel, 1997).

Growth in health care clinics in retail establishments continues to expand. NPs provide health care services in clinics located in drug, grocery, and discount chain stores. NPs treat common illnesses that can be diagnosed by simple tests (e.g., strep throat, urinary tract, and ear infections) following standardized care regimens. In 2005, only a handful of convenience clinics existed; by 2007, there were 500; and today they number in the thousands. Consumers appreciate the convenience of securing a diagnosis and treatment in one location (McGinn & Springen, 2007).

Many consumers opt to receive routine vaccinations at public health departments or immunization clinics held in faith-based facilities, retail establishments, or shopping centers. Local public health departments may waive fees for local residents who are unable to pay for services or if local taxes cover immunizations. Sometimes fees may be reduced if the health department has a fee schedule based on resident incomes.

The Hospital Industry

Hospitals provide acute inpatient and outpatient services. Inpatients often undergo expensive (and frequently invasive) procedures for diagnosis and treatment. Highly technical equipment and qualified nurses monitor patients to detect abnormal conditions, progress of ordered treatments, and potential complications associated with diagnostic procedures and therapies. The hospital industry employs more than 50% of RNs. Although hospital occupancy rates have been decreasing, the severity of illness of clients who are admitted to hospitals has been increasing.

Hospitals vary in size and scope of service. Large medical centers may have hundreds (or thousands) of inpatient beds, whereas small community hospitals may have fewer than 50 beds. Hospitals may be owned by for-profit corporations, nonprofit organizations, or the government (state, military, or U.S. Department of Veterans Affairs). Some hospitals are part of a larger integrated health care delivery system. Along with providing inpatient care, hospitals offer emergency services for persons who sustain traumatic injuries or become seriously ill. Sometimes people without health insurance or a primary care provider use emergency rooms for routine health care needs that arise. Inappropriate

use of emergency rooms increases the cost of health care delivery (Andersen et al., 2007).

Some hospitals also offer outpatient services such as surgery and specialized diagnostic testing. Hospitals may specialize in a single service, such as cancer care, orthopedic surgery, burn care, pediatrics, or rehabilitation. Acute-care hospitals provide services to people who have episodic health care needs. Subacute-care hospitals care for patients who no longer need the intensity of care provided by acute-care hospitals but have complex medical needs above the services offered by extended-care or rehabilitation facilities. The intensity of required nursing care is less acute, but professional nursing care services are still needed.

▊ QUESTIONS FOR REFLECTION

1. Do you think that the average person without exposure to delivering health care could navigate through the current system without assistance? Why or why not?
2. What are the benefits and potential conflicts of quick care health clinics based in retail establishments that also sell prescription medications?
3. Have you ever used a retail quick care health clinic? What was your experience? Would you use one again? Why or why not? If you have never received health care from a retail quick care health clinic, why have you not done so?

Integrated Health Care Delivery Systems: A Choice for Today's Consumer

Integrated health care delivery systems provide consumers with high continuity of care by providing primary, secondary, and tertiary health care services within a single health care system. The health care system combines dimensions of consumer preference, expert providers, and economic reimbursement into a single package. The system offers a variety of local health care centers that are typically linked to a large urban health care center that offers comprehensive, sophisticated therapies. Some systems may offer complementary therapies. The system may be part of a national proprietary (for-profit) chain, a national or regional nonprofit organization (frequently faith based), or an arm of the local, state, or federal government.

To provide effective health care today, three factors are key: cost, access, and quality. In the United States, health care costs continue to rise and outpace the rate of inflation. High costs result in consumer inability to access needed health services. Some consumers with low-paying jobs cannot afford the co-payments on health insurance offered by their employers. Some health care organizations charge higher fees for rendered services when consumers do not have health care coverage. When consumers know that they bear the responsibility for full payment of medical services, they frequently hesitate to seek care until a condition becomes life-threatening, impedes the ability to engage independently in activities of daily living, or prevents their ability to work.

Take Note!

Cost, access, and quality are the three key factors in providing effective health care.

THE INTERDISCIPLINARY/ INTERPROFESSIONAL HEALTH CARE TEAM

The science behind health care is highly specialized. To best meet the physical, psychological, social, and spiritual health care needs of persons seeking care, a multidisciplinary approach is commonly used. Table 9.5 specifies the various members of the **interdisciplinary/ Interprofessional health care team** and the contributions of each member. Sometimes, care is coordinated by a case manager (CM), who may be a nurse or social worker. Professional nurses usually coordinate care delivery in inpatient care environments.

As members of the interdisciplinary health care team, nurses provide key information for holistic client

TABLE 9.5 The Interdisciplinary Health Care Team

Member	Role
Client (consumer or patient)	▪ Seeks out various health care services and makes decisions related to plan of care.
Board of directors (or trustees)	▪ Responsible for organizational mission, service quality, strategic planning, medical staff credentialing, evaluation and selection of the chief executive officer, self-evaluation and education, and financial status. ▪ For-profit companies report to stockholders. ▪ Nonprofit organizations usually have a variety of persons from the community with specialized expertise (e.g., lawyers) and philanthropists as board members.
Chief executive officer (or administrator)	▪ Responsible for overall daily operation of the organization, including implementing board policies, addressing health care concerns within the local community, and preparing and delivering board reports.
Administrative staff (managers or directors)	▪ In large organizations, each department usually has someone responsible for its overall daily operations. ▪ In nursing, the head of the nursing department has the title chief nursing executive or director of nursing.
Medical staff	▪ Medical doctor, doctor of osteopathy, dentist, podiatrist, advanced practice nurse (nurse practitioner, certified registered nurse anesthetist, certified nurse midwife, or clinical nurse specialist), physician's assistant, clinical social worker, registered nurse, dietitian or nutritional professional, who may be an independent practitioner or organizational employee, diagnoses and treats clients using medical therapies. ▪ To become a member of the medical staff the health care professional must go through a credentialing and approval process of the health care organization.
Nursing staff (registered nurses, licensed practical/vocational nurses [LPN/LVN], unlicensed assistive personnel [UAP; care assistants], clerical assistants [unit clerk, secretaries])	▪ Responsible for execution of direct and indirect client care services. ▪ RNs assess clients, diagnose human responses to illness, outline a care plan, implement the plan (including the delegation of tasks to others), and evaluate the effectiveness of nursing care. ▪ LPN/LVNs implement the care plan outlined by the RN, administer medications, and perform sterile procedures. ▪ UAPs perform basic care tasks under the supervision of RNs or LPN/LVNs. In long-term care facilities, a UAP with state certification may act as a medication technician and administer routinely ordered medication (excluding most parenteral medications). ▪ Clerical assistants enter orders into computers, order supplies, and compile reports for patient charges.
Case manager (for managed care organizations)	▪ Advanced practice nurse or social worker who follows clients across the spectrum of health care settings. Most start the discharge process as soon as clients are admitted to acute-care facilities.
Dietitians	▪ Baccalaureate-prepared nutritionists who have had internships to learn clinical nutrition. They outline specific client therapeutic diets, verify that client nutritional needs are met, and provide client and family education related to therapeutic diets. ▪ Inpatient facilities have food service departments that prepare client and cafeteria meals.

Member	Role
Pharmacists	■ Prepare and dispense medications, educate other team members about medications, monitor-controlled substance use, monitor client allergies, work to prevent medication errors, and monitor potential drug interactions.
Paramedical personnel or technologists	■ Highly trained professionals with specialized education or training. ■ Examples include medical technologist (lab tests), radiology technologist (e.g., X-ray, CT scan, PET scan), and respiratory therapist (breathing therapies, ventilator management, oxygen therapy)
Social workers	■ Assist clients with social concerns that arise from illness, injury, or surgery. ■ Help clients with financial issues resulting from disruption of work and insurance benefit gaps. ■ Refer clients to community support agencies.
Therapists	■ Physical therapists assess function and provide restorative therapy for body movement, ambulation, and safety. ■ Occupational therapists assess and provide restorative therapy for problems with activities of daily living as well as skills for employment. ■ Speech therapists assess for swallowing difficulties and speech problems, and provide restorative therapy related to these areas.
Medical records or health information services	■ Keep detailed and accurate medical records on clients.
Business manager or office staff	■ Coordinates client appointments (outpatient settings) and keeps financial records for services rendered.
Central supply or central products services	■ Warehouse and distribute client care products (not pharmaceuticals) per ordered request.
Linen services	■ Provide client linen and gowns.
Environmental or housekeeping services	■ Maintain a clean, safe physical environment.
Biomedical engineering services	■ Maintain proper functioning of electronic client care machines (e.g., IV pumps, bedside monitors, thermometers). ■ Verify electrical safety of client care equipment.
Information services	■ Develop integrated computer systems and provide user support services (some may offer computer and software staff education).
Quality management personnel	■ Monitor the quality of rendered services. ■ Outline a plan for continuous quality improvement. ■ Includes the risk management department, which monitors actual and potential client care errors and financial losses.
Third-party payers	■ Pay for all or part of health care services used by the consumer. ■ Various levels of government are third-party payers for tax-supported health insurance plans. ■ Private insurance companies provide funding for plan enrollees. ■ Frequently audit client records to verify rendered services.
Utilization review	■ Set up in the late 1970s by the federal government to verify effective utilization of health care resources and avoid fraud.
Spiritual support services (chaplain)	■ Inpatient settings usually have chaplain support services to provide spiritual and other support to clients and their significant others.
Human resources (personnel department)	■ Hires new employees, tracks employee incidents, and coordinates employee fringe benefits. ■ Payroll departments that issue employee paychecks may fall under this category.
Foundation	■ Nonprofit organizations usually have services to coordinate private donations to the organization.
Alternative care providers	■ Persons who provide alternative or complementary therapy (e.g., chiropractors, herbalists, acupuncturists, massage therapists, reflexologists, folk healers).

Adapted from Center for Medicare & Medicaid Services. (2011). CMS Manual System Pub. 100–07 State operations provider certification, Transmittal 78, Retrieved from http://www.cms.gov/Regulations-and-Guidance/Guidance/Transmittals/downloads/R78SOMA.pdf; Jonas, S. (1998). *An introduction to the U.S. health care system* (4th ed.). New York: Springer Publishing; Knickman, J. R. & Kovner, A. R. (Eds.). (2015). *Jonas & Kovner's health care delivery in the United States* (11th ed.). New York: Springer; and American Hospital Association. (1999). *Welcome to the board: An orientation for the new health care trustee*. Chicago: AHA Press.

care. When clients and families become overwhelmed with the complexity of health care, nurses guide them through the system while offering them emotional support. For example, "nurse navigator" programs have surfaced in the field of oncology nursing. The nurse navigator meets with clients on a regular basis to discuss questions about and barriers to care, provide individualized client education, offer special emotional support, and facilitate referrals to needed community resources and other health care professionals. Identified strengths of nurse navigator programs include facilitation of continuity across the continuum of care, and timely treatment and prevention of complications in today's ever complex delivery of health care (Bruce, 2007).

NURSING CARE DELIVERY MODELS

Management of nursing care for clients has always fallen within the purview of professional nurses. On a daily basis, nurses make decisions about how to organize client care. They consider a variety of factors when choosing the best way to deliver care to a group of clients, including client factors (acuity and specialized needs), staff factors (number of available staff, licensure status, clinical experience, and staff preferences), and organizational factors (the usual nursing care delivery system). A **nursing care delivery model** is a system used by nurses to organize and deliver nursing services to best meet client care needs. Effective nursing care delivery models match client care needs with available human resources to attain the best possible outcome (Porter-O'Grady & Malloch, 2007).

Traditional methods of nursing care delivery models include case method (total patient care), functional nursing, team nursing, district nursing, primary nursing, case management, and client-focused (patient-focused or modular) care. Table 9.6 outlines the origins and rationale of each model, describes clinical decision making, outlines the scope of responsibility and authority, delineates team titles (when appropriate), presents the level of nurse and client satisfaction, and identifies major advantages and disadvantages of each model. Prior to industrialization and employer-based insurance, professional nurses practiced case nursing, during which they performed all intervention, to meet all the client's needs. The case method is still used in home health and private duty nursing as well as in clinical nursing education when faculty assign beginning nursing students to care for a client.

In the functional team and district nursing care models, nursing staff members with different skills and licensure status care for a group of patients. Functional

and team nursing models work well when there is a shortage of nursing staff. When either model is used, however, care may become fragmented, and without effective communication, little attention is paid to client needs for rest and privacy.

During the 1980s, job satisfaction among nurses plummeted and nurse turnover in hospitals was high (McGillis-Hall, Doran, & Petch, 2005). Increased responsibility for supervision of others for direct client care was cited as a major factor. Primary nursing emerged as a way to reconnect professional nurses with direct client care. A primary nurse for each patient develops and revises the nursing care plan. In the event of the primary care nurse's absence, nursing care is delivered by another RN, who is the designated associate nurse. Continuity of client care is also increased because the same nurses provide care services to the client. However, some nurses and hospital administrators frown on using professional nurses to perform tasks that could be done by unlicensed assistive personnel (UAP).

The economic crunch of the early 1990s experienced by acute-care facilities gave rise to redesigned care delivery systems. Quality improvement efforts focused on optimal client outcomes and satisfaction. Work redesign efforts resulted in a model that placed the client (or patient) in the center. The model has been identified as client-focused care, patient-focused care, or modular nursing. Some institutions expanded the roles of UAP and provided them with intensive on-the-job training so that they could perform sterile urinary catheterization, phlebotomy, and electrocardiograms. Professional nurses were then free to engage in holistic assessment, advanced nursing procedures, and client education. However, supervision of UAPs was added to the professional nurse's role.

Modular nursing represents a unique form of client-focused care. In modular nursing, UAPs and professional nurses receive assignments to work continuously as "care partners." Care partners receive cross-training to perform basic respiratory therapy treatments, physical therapy, phlebotomy, and electrocardiography. Under this delivery system, clients receive almost instantaneous therapy as they do not have to wait for ancillary personnel to arrive.

Case management provides a system of patient care delivery that focuses on the achievement of outcomes within effective time frames and with appropriate use of health care resources. Key elements of case management involve a CM (who may be a bachelor's-prepared RN, advanced practice nurse, or social worker) and a standardized method for managing a particular

TABLE 9.6 Comparison of Nursing Care Delivery System Models

Nursing Care Delivery Model	Case Method (Total Patient Care)	Functional Nursing	Team Nursing	District Nursing	Primary Nursing	Case Management	Client-focused Care (Patient-Focused or Modular)
Date of origin and reason designed	1880s; patients were at home	1940s in response to nursing shortage	1950s in response to movement in management away from tasks to human relations	1950s–1960s to decrease the amount of leg work required for team nursing	1960s to facilitate movement of nurses toward independence and autonomous practice	1980s in response to diagnosis-related grouping (prospective payment system), budget awareness, and total quality management philosophy	1990s in response to increased efficiency with escalating costs and as a response to the nursing shortage
Clinical decision making	Done per shift	Done per shift	Shift based	Shift based	24-h accountability of the primary nurse	24-h accountability of the case manager	Shift based
Responsibility and authority	One or a small group of patients	Autonomous to a large group of patients	Large group of patients	Group of patients located in close proximity to each other	Autonomous for a small group of patients as a primary nurse	Coordination of care with members of the interdisciplinary health care team	Coordination with case manager common for plan of care Individual actions are autonomous and shift based for a large group of patients
Work allocation	Total care to all assigned patients	Each member assigned specific tasks for all patients	Tasks for entire team, with some being assigned according to skills or license requirements	Same as in team nursing	Total care of own primary patients along with care of small number of patients with a different primary nurse	May serve as coordinator or actual provider of direct client care May be required to see caseloads of clients with similar health problems at more than one clinical site	Tasks assigned according to on-the-job training and licensure requirements
Nursing team title(s)	Nurse	Charge nurse Medicine nurse Treatment nurse Education nurse Admissions and discharge nurse Nurse's aide Orderly	RN becomes team leader and delegates tasks to team members Team members: licensed practical nurses (LPNs)/ licensed vocational nurses (LVNs), and unlicensed assistive personnel (UAP)	RN becomes the district nurse Team members have the same titles as in team nursing	Primary nurse Associate nurse No LPN or LVN Nursing assistants and orderlies assigned to unit to help RNs	Case managers Care manager RNs and LPNs are nurses UAP titles may be the same as in team nursing or client-focused care	Care pairs or care partners consisting of an RN with a UAP (who is called a patient care technician) or patient service associate

(continued on page 238)

TABLE 9.6 Comparison of Nursing Care Delivery System Models *(continued)*

Nursing Care Delivery Model	Case Method (Total Patient Care)	Functional Nursing	Team Nursing	District Nursing	Primary Nursing	Case Management	Client-focused Care (Patient-Focused or Modular)
Professional nurse satisfaction	Yes	No	Yes	Yes	Yes	High for the case manager and nursing staff	Mixed for nurses; Higher for UAP than for team
Client satisfaction	Yes	No	Yes	Yes	Yes	Mixed	Yes
Major advantages	Care received from one nurse per 8-h shift; Holistic care provided; Clear lines of responsibility; No complex assignment planning required	Highly cost-effective; Clear lines of responsibility; Development of technical experts if assigned the same tasks daily; Useful with severe staffing shortages	Cost-effective and staff satisfaction with working with small patient groups; Comprehensive holistic care possible; Development of better staff relationships	Same as with team nursing, except less exhaustion by nursing staff from reduced walking	Very satisfied nurses and patients; Comprehensive holistic nursing care delivered	Cost-effective care coordinated to achieve client outcomes; Holistic care orientation; Continuity of care across the spectrum of health care settings; Client knows whom to call for assistance	Cost-effective and clients seem to be satisfied; Clients can ask anyone for help; Staff develop technical competence in a variety of skills
Major disadvantages	No continuity of care; Very expensive by today's standards; Potential overloading of ancillary departments with multiple requests for the same supplies in a short time frame	Task-oriented system resulting in fragmentation of care; Staff boredom from repetitive work; Limited communication among staff members	Team leaders may not be available to lead the team; Poor communication may lead to tasks being omitted; Team leader needs time to supervise team members, which decreases time available for clients	No district nurse available to lead team; Same as in team nursing	Not cost-effective to have all-RN staffing; Some primary nurses not available 7 days a week for 24-h-a-day consultation; Not all nurses want to assume primary nursing responsibilities; Requires large numbers of RNs; Sense of loss by ancillary workers	High costs required for successful implementation; Critical pathways reduce individualization of client care; Physician resentment about being called for consultation by a nurse; Chief executive officer complaints of expenditures requested for care by case managers	Expensive to develop and provide technologic support; Blurs the distinctions of nursing roles from those of other interdisciplinary team members; Nurses may lose essential elements of nursing practice
Areas where currently used	Home care; Private duty; Intensive care units; Nursing student assignments	Hospitals; Extended-care facilities; Rehabilitation centers; Operating rooms; Outpatient surgical centers; Physician offices	Hospitals; Extended-care facilities; Rehabilitation centers; Home health agencies	Hospitals; Extended-care facilities; Rehabilitation centers	Hospital intensive care units; Specialty centers such as dialysis, oncology, and diabetes outpatient centers; Hospice; Home care	Hospitals; Home health agencies; Health departments; Anywhere managed care is practiced	Hospitals; Home health agencies; Transport teams

Adapted from Manthey, M. (1991). Delivery systems and practice role models. *Nursing Management, 22*(1), 28–30; Sportsman, S. (2014). Care delivery strategies. In P. S. Yoder-Wise (Ed.), *Leading and managing in nursing* (6th ed.). St. Louis, MO: Elsevier Mosby; and Tappen, R. M. (2001). *Nursing leadership and management: Concepts and practice*. Philadelphia, PA: F. A. Davis.

disease process. The predetermined path for specific care delivery (critical path, clinical path, or care map) is followed for the duration of client care. The path outlines typical interdisciplinary clinical problems with desired outcomes, maps out daily expected interventions, and specifies discharge client instructions and education. Staff nurses and the CM frequently monitor client progress toward desired outcomes. Some paths cross the health care settings, enabling a seamless continuum of care. The CM assumes responsibility for matching client care needs so that appropriate services are rendered. The CM may use standardized clinical protocols, guidelines, and third-party payer criteria to ensure optimal outcomes with the most efficient use of resources.

The CM executes multiple roles that require critical thinking. As a clinician, the CM communicates effectively with the multidisciplinary health care team. The CM also coordinates care among all professionals and consultants. To ensure that economic constraints do not affect quality of client care, the CM justifies expenditures and care variances. The CM sometimes troubleshoots conflicts that might arise between health care providers, third-party payers, and consumers, and acts as a client advocate. Some CMs maintain an ongoing relationship with clients using the telephone or internet (Mahn-Dinicola & Zazworsky, 2005).

Innovative Patient Care Delivery Systems

Porter-O'Grady and Malloch (2007) specified that delivery of patient care encompasses more than nursing care and proposed that the care delivery system models should encompass the entire multidisciplinary patient care team. Such models have the client at the center of the circle and the interdisciplinary care team surrounding the client. The direct client caregivers (the nursing staff) constitute the first tier of service. Surrounding the nursing team and providing direct patient care are nursing support systems, including nursing directors, resource nurses, rapid response teams (to support nurses with patient care crisis situations), phlebotomy services or admissions staff, clinical nurse specialists, and staff development personnel. The outermost circle includes all other members of the interdisciplinary client care team.

Donlevy and Pietruch (1996) developed a model of nursing known as the connection delivery model. The connection delivery model provides an interdisciplinary team approach to chronic disease management. For acute-care nurses, this model provides cross training for them to work effectively in patient homes. This model has been associated with high levels of patient satisfaction because they are followed by nurses who cared for them in the hospital who are familiar with their cases. Nurses also report high level of satisfaction with the model because they follow patients across the continuum of care, establish long-term relationships with patients and engage in independent clinical decision-making outside of the hospital setting.

Nursing care delivery models affect health care delivery in several dimensions including cost, safety, efficiency, patient satisfaction with care and nurse job satisfaction (Allen & Vitale-Nolen, 2005; Donlevy & Pietruch, 1996; Fernandez, Johnson, Tran, & Miranda, 2012; Wells, Manuel, & Cunning, 2011). Nurses become empowered when they have a voice in how they deliver nursing care (see Focus on Research, "Changing the Model of Care Delivery: Nurses' Perceptions of Job Satisfaction and Care Effectiveness").

NURSING CHALLENGES RELATED TO HEALTH CARE DELIVERY SYSTEMS

Each health care delivery system possesses different challenges for professional nursing practice. For example, nurses working in a system based on a free-market, encounter challenges when clients are unable to pay for rendered health care services. Nurses working a government-based universal care system may experience challenges with adequate staffing and supplies to provide high-quality, effective care. Because professional nurses play a key role in health delivery, they encounter practical and ethical challenges on a daily basis.

Practical Challenges

Two key practical challenges encountered by nurses involve the shortage of professional nurses and changes in the structure of the work environment.

The Nursing Shortage

There are currently an insufficient number of nurses to meet the health care needs of clients, and the shortage is expected to worsen. The USBLS (2015a) reported that from 2014 to 2024, the number of professional nurses needed will rise from 2.75 to 3.24 million. Because many nurses over the age of 65 years remain working, it is difficult to project exactly how many nursing positions will need to be filled within the next decade.

FOCUS ON RESEARCH

Changing the Model of Care Delivery: Nurses' Perceptions of Job Satisfaction and Care Effectiveness

The investigators combined qualitative and quantitative research methods to examine the effects of changing from a team nursing care delivery model to a modified total patient care model on nurse perceptions of job satisfaction and the effectiveness of nursing care. They employed a longitudinal descriptive, mixed methods research design. After securing approval from an ethics board, the nurses were informed of the purpose of the study, data collection methods, received education of the new delivery model and then surveys were distributed to the RNs and licensed practical nurses (LPNs) working on an acute-care unit in a Canadian hospital.

Before the nursing care delivery model was changed to a modified total patient care approach (TPC), baseline data were collected using Stamps's 1997 Index of Work Satisfaction (IWS), 2 subscales of Roller's 1999 Perceptions of Empowerment (POE), and Hastings's (1995) Care Delivery Effectiveness Tool (CDET). Thirty-eight (30 RNs and 8 LPNs) completed the baseline surveys (32% response rate). The nurses were then sent the same surveys at 3 months (31% response rate) and then 12 months (27% response rate) after the delivery model had been changed. At the 12-month data collection point, the researchers included a 3-item open-ended question survey inquiring about the positive aspects and challenges that they had encountered with TPC along with an item requesting suggestions to address any identified challenges.

Data were analyzed using percentages, means, standard deviations on the IWS, POE, and CDET scores to describe findings and *independent t-tests* were run to detect differences in scores across the baseline, 3-month, and 12-month time frames. Mean scores on the total IWS remained basically unchanged (3.64 to 3.66) for all three measurements. There were no statistically significant changes in the POE scores (4.61 at baseline, 4.51 at 3 months, and 4.66 at 12 months). Participant mean scores changed at a statistically significant level ($p < 0.05$) on the CDE with the baseline score being 2.62, at 3 months 3.14, and at 12 months 3.40. The

researchers used content analysis thematic analysis for the responses to open-ended questions.

Findings from the analysis revealed that the nurses who responded ($n = 8$) that participants perceived better care coordination, improved professional practice and enhanced nurse–patient relationships, especially having the time to "really know the client". They also perceived less responsibility because the nurse to patient ratio dropped from 1:28 to 1:4–6. Along with more time for care prioritization activities, they also reported improved nurse–physician relationships. Challenges identified were lack of organizational support, some staff support for TPC, updated care plans, and delayed nursing interventions. In addition, some replacement nurses were unfamiliar with TPC and the organization replaced RNs with LPNs. Suggestions to handle these challenges included improving staff orientation to TPC, requiring all nurses to perform chart audits to verify that all interventions had been completed, having the charge nurses complete assignments, employing a ward clerk after 1600, and developing and implementing a career development and maintenance plan for all nurses.

Clinical implications for this study include that TPC may improve the effectiveness of patient care delivery because nurses who work on the front lines perceives that it does. The nurses in this study perceive that TPC enables them to deliver holistic care and that improves care coordination. TPC most likely does not directly improve nurse job satisfaction, but it does give some nurses enhanced professional practice. Results of this study should be interpreted with caution because of the low sample size with substantially more RNs completing surveys than LPNs, and the confounding variables that occurred during the study (use of float nurses on the unit, nurse attrition, hiring new staff without orienting them effectively to TPC, staff shortages, and informing staff that they would have to work more over the Christmas holidays). More research is needed to see what nurse care delivery model enhances patient care outcomes, professional practice environments and nurse job satisfaction.

Wells, J., Manuel, M., & Cunning, G. (2011). Changing the model of care delivery: Nurses' perceptions of job satisfaction and care effectiveness. *Journal of Nursing Management, 19,*777–785. doi: 10.1111/j.1365–2834.2011.01292.x

According to a Robert Woods Johnson Study conducted in 2014, they found that 74% of RNs are working beyond age 62 years and 25% of RNs working are at least 69 years old. Eight percent of RNs and 17% of advanced practice RNs remain working past the age of 65 years. Some of the older nurses transition to part-time employment. There are more nurses working that are over the age of 60 years than nurses who are less than 30 years of age. Of the nurses working in hospitals, 80% are 30 years old or less and 35% are 65 years old or older. Eventually, the older nursing workforce will retire. However, exactly when remain elusive. Earlier predictions assumed that older nurses would retire when they reached 65 years of age. These earlier prediction projected that the United States would need more than 1.2 million more professional nurses to meet the demand for nursing services (712,000 nurses to fill new positions and an additional 495,000 to fill nursing positions vacated by retiring nurses) (USBLS, 2012).

The supply of professional nurses also looks bleak in Canada, where the Canadian Nurses Association (2009) reported an 11,000 full-time equivalent (FTE) professional nursing shortage in 2007. FTE is defined as 2,080 clock hours of employment. The Canadian Federation of Nursing Unions (2014) reported that for each RN under the age of 35 years there are two RNs over age 50. They also reported that the average age of RN retirement in Canada is 56 years. In 2014, Canada needs to replace 12,000 RNs annually to keep up with the demand for and retirement of RNs. However, Canadian nursing programs graduated only 10,074 new nurse resulting in a shortfall of 1,926 new nurses. (Canadian Federation of Nursing Unions, 2014). The Canadian Nurses Association also predicted a shortfall of 60,000 FTEs by 2022. Many factors contribute to the current global nursing shortage, including the following.

- Reduced number of young persons (18 to 24 years) entering the profession
- Decreased interest in a professional nursing career because of other career options for women (91% of the current nursing workforce is female)
- Compressed salary and fewer promotions throughout a nursing career
- Increased labor intensity from increased client acuity and numbers of clients
- Chronic understaffing in acute- and extended-care settings
- Poor collegial relationships with other health team members

- Widespread fear of contracting medication-resistant infectious diseases
- Increased chance of sustaining musculoskeletal injuries because of increased client body mass index (in the United States) and lack of enforceable policies related to lifting limitations for nursing staff
- Reduced job satisfaction
- High turnover
- Unfavorable stories about the profession being shared with potential nursing recruits
- Nursing faculty shortage
- Aging workforce (in 2014, the average age of an RN in the United States was 50 years (American Nurses Association, 2014))

If the RN shortage persists, health care facilities will be forced to explore other staffing mix options, which may mean having RNs assume more supervisory responsibilities (ICN, 2006; Porter-O'Grady & Malloch, 2007; Seago, Spetz, Chapman, & Dyer, 2007). Historically, the nursing shortage has been perpetuated by external factors such as problems with recruitment, retention, negative image, and poor working environments. In addition, internal factors such as job dissatisfaction, role overload, poor collegial relationships, and professional disillusionment exacerbate the shortage (West, Griffith, & Iphofen, 2007). However, the current projected nursing shortage is linked to the aging nursing workforce and a reduced number of persons entering the nursing profession (ICN, 2006).

Alleviating the nursing shortage requires that the nursing profession attack all associated factors. Nurses must believe they have the power to change work environments to promote professional autonomy and safety. Empowering nurses begins with nursing education programs and continues through an entire career. All areas of nursing (practice, administration, and education) must collaborate rather than compete with each other to shape the nursing profession.

Challenges Resulting from Changes in the Structure of the Work Environment

Hospitals have implemented numerous changes over the past decade. In many facilities, when people are admitted to the hospital, a hospitalist rather than their private physician manages their stay. Hospitalists are physicians (some of whom have direct employment status or contracts with the hospital) who manage client care in acute-care settings for primary care physicians (and NPs). After dismissal from the hospital, health care management is resumed by the primary care provider (physician or NP). Some acute-care facilities have reported reduced inpatient length of stay and substantial cost savings since introducing the hospitalist role (McDonald, 2001).

The emergence of hospitalists has created the need for professional nurses in hospitals to educate clients about the advantages of receiving medical care from a physician who specializes in the complex nature of acute care. Sometimes, clients and their significant others inquire if the physician whom they see in the outpatient setting will be seeing them in the hospital. In recent years, very few primary care physicians make hospital visits. Nurses reassure recipients of hospital care that their primary care physician will receive a detailed report about what transpired during the hospitalization.

Some health systems, hospitals and hospitalist physician groups have hired acute-care NPs to follow hospitalized clients. Thus, hospitalized clients may be seen more often by an acute-care NP than a physician. Health care systems, hospitalist physician groups and hospitalist care teams use a developed list of evidence-based protocols that include a list of standardized orders for the management of commonly encountered reasons for and health problems arising from hospitalization (e.g., electrolyte replacement and constipation). Because of the transfer of patient care to hospitalists, who may be unfamiliar with the patient history, nurses have experienced increased workload demands such as medication reconciliation as part of the routine hospital admission process. Medication reconciliation requires that the admission nurse makes certain that the list of medications a patient is taking at home exactly matches or there is a specific reason to add or to discontinue a medication during the hospital stay upon hospital admission. Because hospital nurses, acute-care NPs, and hospitalists work closely with each other on a regular basis, they sometimes develop close, truly collaborative working relationships.

Business managers and facility administrators continue to have powerful voices in health care delivery. Recent reductions in the length of hospitalization mean that nurses care for more acutely ill clients. Nurses must be more vigilant to notice small changes in client status that may foreshadow a catastrophic health event. They also must have detailed knowledge about potential adverse effects of complex interactions among medications. Nurses also must possess the capability to perform sophisticated procedures such as central line management, intravenous medication drips, and complicated dressings. Finally, nurses must document patient care activities using electronic documentation systems; forgetting to document something may result in reduced hospital reimbursement from governmental and private health care insurance plans. New medications and technology demand increased knowledge, skills, and time.

■ QUESTIONS FOR REFLECTION

1. What changes have you seen (if you are a practicing nurse) or have you heard about (if you are a nursing student with no practice experience) in clinical nursing practice within the past 2 years? How do these changes impact your ability to provide safe, effective nursing care to patients and families?

2. What areas of professional nursing practice do you see expanding based on current changes to government funding of health care?

3. What has been your personal experience as a patient or family member of a patient with the current changes in hospital care?

4. What changes in professional practice do you foresee occurring as a result of increased governmental influences in health care delivery?

5. What strategies may be helpful for nurses to cope with current and future changes in health care delivery? Design a plan for helping current and future professional nurses. Determine the feasibility of this plan.

Ethical Challenges

Ethical concerns have been raised by an increasing life span, the development of health care technology, and the increasing cost of health care delivery. For decades, the ability of persons to pay for health care has determined who has access to services and the quality of service that can be received (Andersen et al., 2007; Curtin, 1996; ICN, 2006; WHO, 2012).

Because it is not possible to meet all goals of accessibility, equity, and quality given available resources, difficult choices must be made among competing values and multiple desirable alternatives. One basic issue is the relative valuing of containment of health care costs versus access to health care for all persons.

Ethical questions raised by these choices include the following.

1. What will some people have to do to absorb the costs of health care for those who are unable to pay so that quality health care is available to everyone?

2. Is health care a basic right or a privilege?

3. What is the basic acceptable level of health care?

4. Who has priority for health care services if there are access limitations and finite resources for health care delivery?

5. What governmental and/or social programs should be cut to increase health care resources for better access to health care?

6. How much choice should people have in deciding from whom and where they can receive health care?

7. Should the wealthy be able to purchase private health care services or insurance coverage?

8. How should rationing of health care be determined?

9. Who should determine rationing criteria?

10. What criteria should be used for rationing of health care services?

11. Should expensive technology and advanced life support measures be made available to all persons?

12. What (and when) is death?

13. How much is the prolongation of life worth?

14. What rights do clients have?

15. Is cure of all disease possible and desirable?

16. Who needs professional nursing services?

17. How do we use health care resources and personnel for the best interest of the human race?

"Treating health care primarily as a business and a commodity to be sold like cars is an impoverished notion of health care in relation to the concept of health care as a human service created by society to meet the needs of vulnerable people who are ill or at risk of becoming ill" (Aroskar, 1987, p. 65). It is critical that the voice of the nursing profession be added to that of the public in discussions of the philosophical considerations and values that will shape the decisions concerning the size, shape, and direction of all future health care delivery systems.

Summary and Significance to Practice

As a result of significant demographic, economic, attitudinal, and available manpower forces, health care delivery systems are in the process of massive structural reorganization, raising multiple ethical and practical considerations. Health care delivery systems are shaped primarily by history, cultural values, and resource availability. Nurses should assume leadership in shaping future health care delivery by using their cognitive skills and compassion so that all persons will have access to optimal health care services.

REAL-LIFE REFLECTIONS

Recall Maria and her parent from the beginning of the chapter. How should Maria explain to her father the benefits of receiving generic medication and a temporary stay in an extended-care facility on his recovery? How would you explain the complex web of health care delivery to elderly clients? What type of help do they need to navigate their way through the health care system?

From Theory to Practice

1. Identify the strengths and weaknesses of the American and Canadian health care delivery systems. Explain why you consider the items in your list strengths or weaknesses.

2. How can nurses work to improve health care delivery? What are the consequences if nurses do not get involved with changes in the health care delivery system?

Nurse as Author

Write a 2- to 3-page essay on how you think that the American health care system could be improved. For each of your key ideas, provide a reference citation from a peer-reviewed journal. Include a reference list at the end of your essay.

Your Digital Classroom

Online Exploration

Agency for Healthcare Research and Quality:
www.ahrq.gov
American Association of Retired Persons:
www.aarp.org
American Hospital Association: **www.aha.org**
American Medical Association: **www.ama-assn.org**
American Nurses Association Nursing World:
www.nursingworld.org
America's Health Insurance Plans: **www.ahip.org**
Centers for Medicare & Medicaid Services:
www.cms.hhs.gov
International Council of Nurses: **www.icn.ch**
National Health Information Center:
www.health.gov/nhic

Expanding Your Understanding

1. Visit the America's Health Insurance Plans website to learn about the complexities of the health insurance industry. The website contains the latest updates on legislative efforts to reform health insurance and provides consumers with information about the types of health insurance plans and how to enroll in them.
2. Visit the American Medical Association website to learn about issues confronting physicians in today's health care environment. While there, look for the listing of a physician you know.
3. Visit the American Nurses Association Nursing World website to learn about issues confronting professional nurses in the health care system.
4. Please visit the Kaiser Family Foundation to compare the Affordable Care Act with a proposed replacement in 2017. **http://kff.org/interactive/ proposals-to-replace-the-affordable-care-act/** List how the replacement for the Affordable Care Act will affect you or your family.

Beyond the Book

Visit thePoint® **www.thePoint.lww.com** for activities and information to reinforce the concepts and content covered in this chapter.

REFERENCES

Allen, D., & Vitale-Nolen, R. (2005). Patient care delivery model improves nurse job satisfaction. *Journal of Continuing Education in Nursing, 36*(6), 277–282.

American Nurses Association. (2014). *Fast facts: The nursing workforce 2014, growth, salaries, education, demographics and trends.* Retrieved from http://www.nursingworld.org/MainMenuCategories/ThePracticeofProfessionalNursing/workforce/Fast-Facts-2014-Nursing-Workforce.pdf. Accessed April 16, 2016.

Andersen, R. M., Rice, T. H., & Kominski, G. F. (2007). *Changing the U.S. health care system: Key issues in health services policy and management* (3rd ed.). San Francisco, CA: John Wiley.

Aroskar, M. A. (1987). Fidelity and veracity: Questions of promise keeping, truth telling, and loyalty. In M. D. M. Fowler & J. Levine-Ariff (Eds.), *Ethics at the bedside: A sourcebook for the critical care nurse.* Philadelphia, PA: J.B. Lippincott.

Billings, J., Cantor, J., & Clinton, C. (2011). Access to care. In A. Kovner & J. Knickman (Eds.), *Jonas & Kovner's health care delivery in the United States* (10th ed.). New York: Springer.

Bodenheimer, T. (2005). High and rising health care costs: Part 3: The role of health care providers. *Annals of Internal Medicine, 142,* 996–1002.

Bruce, S. D. (2007). Taking the wheel, oncology nurses help patients navigate the cancer journey. *ONS Connect, 22*(3), 8–11.

Canadian Federation of Nursing Unions. (2014). *The nursing wordforce, Canadian Federation of Nursing Union backgrounder.* Retrieved from https://nursesunions.ca/sites/default/files/2012.backgrounder.nursing_workforce.e_0.pdf. Accessed April 16, 2016.

Canadian Nurses Association. (2009). Tested solutions for eliminating Canada's registered nurse shortage. Retrieved from http://www2.cna-aiic.ca/CNA/documents/pdf/publications/RN_Highlights_e.pdf. Accessed February 17, 2013.

Center for Medicare & Medicaid Services. (2011). CMS Manual System. Pub. 100-07 State Operations Provider Certification, Transmittal 78. Retrieved from http://www.cms.gov/Regulations-and-Guidance/Guidance/Transmittals/downloads/R78SOMA.pdf. Accessed February 17, 2013.

Center for Medicare & Medicaid Services. (2014). National Health Expenditure Projections 2014–2024, Forecast Summary. Retrieved from https://www.cms.gov/Research-Statistics-Data-and-Systems/Statistics-Trends-and-Reports/NationalHealthExpendData/downloads/proj2014.pdf. Accessed April 10, 2016.

Curtin, L. L. (1996). The ethics of managed care—part I: Proposing a new ethos. *Nursing Management, 27,* 18–19.

DeNavas-Walt, C., Proctor, B., & Smith, J. (2012). Income, poverty & health insurance coverage in the United States: 2011. Retrieved from http://www.census.gov/prod/2012pubs/p60–243.pdf. Accessed February 17, 2013.

Donlevy, J. A., & Pietruch, B. L. (1996). The connection delivery model: Care across the continuum. *Nursing Management, 27*(5), 34–36.

Fernandez, R., Johnson, M., Tran, D. T., & Miranda, C. (2012). Models of care in nursing: A systematic review. *International Journal of Evidence-Based Healthcare, 10*(4), 324–337. doi: 10.1111/j.1744–1609.2012.00287.x

Fifer, J. J. (2007). A healthcare mystery. *Healthcare Financial Management, 61*(2), 28.

Fried, B. J., & Gaydos, L.M. (Eds.). (2002). *World health systems: Challenges and perspectives.* Chicago: Health Administration Press.

Gabel, J. (1997). 10 ways HMOs have changed in the 1990s. *Health Affairs, 16,* 134–135.

Gantz, N., Sherman, R., Jasper, M., Choo, C. G., Herrin-Griffith, D., & Harris, K. (2012). Global nurse leader perspectives on health systems and workforce challenges. *Journal of Nursing Management, 20*(4), 433–443.

Geyman, J. P. (2015). A five-year assessment of the Affordable Care Act: Market Forces Still Trump the Common Good in U.S. Health Care. *International Journal of Health Services, 45*(2) 209–225. doi: 10.1177/0020731414568505

Goldsmith, L. (2002). Canada. In B. J. Fried & L. M. Gaydos (Eds.), *World health systems: Challenges and perspectives.* Chicago: Health Administration Press.

Gould, E. (2012). A decade of declines in employer-sponsored health insurance coverage. Retrieved from http://www.epi.org/publication/bp337-employer-sponsored-health-insurance/. Accessed February 10, 2013.

Haeder, S. F., & Weimer, D. L. (2015). A federalism perspective on the affordable care act. *Journal of Health Politics, Policy and Law, 40*(2), 281–323.

International Council of Nurses. (2012). About ICN. Retrieved from http://www.icn.ch/about-icn/about-icn/. Accessed February 10, 2013.

Jamieson, E. M., & Sewall, M. F. (1954). *Trends in nursing history* (4th ed.). Philadelphia, PA: W. B. Saunders.

Johnson, A., Carillo, A., & Garcia, J. (2002). Mexico. In B. J. Fried & L. M. Gaydos (Eds.), *World health systems: Challenges and perspectives*. Chicago: Health Administration Press.

Jonas, S. (1998). *An introduction to the U.S. health care system* (4th ed.). New York: Springer.

Jost, T. (2005). Chaoulli v. Quebeck: Charter rights, private health insurance and the future of Canadian Medicare. *Health Affairs, 25*(3), 878–879.

Kaiser Family Foundation. (2011). Focus on health reform: Summary of new health reform law. Retrieved from http://www.kff.org/healthreform/8061.cfm. Accessed December 7, 2012.

Kaiser Family Foundation. (2012). Implementation timeline for new health reform law. Retrieved from http://www.healthreform.kff.org/timeline.aspx. Accessed December 12, 2012.

Knickman, J. (2015). Chapter 11: Health care financing. In J. Knickman & A. Kovner (Eds.), *Jonas & Kovner's health care delivery in the United States* (11th ed., pp. 231–252). New York: Springer.

Kaiser Family Foundation (2017). Compare proposals to replace the Affordable Care Act. Retrieved from http://kff.org/interactive/proposals-to-replace-the-affordable-care-act/ Accessed April 1, 2017.

Knickman, J. R., & Kovner, A. R. (Eds.). (2015). *Jonas & Kovner's health care delivery in the United States* (11th ed.). New York: Springer.

Lacey, L. (2002). Nigeria. In B. J. Fried & L. M. Gaydos (Eds.), *World health systems: Challenges and perspectives*. Chicago: Health Administration Press.

Lahm, R. J. (2015). Small business and Obamacare: Ripple effects when the cost is "too high". *Academy of Entrepreneurship Journal, 21*(2), 25–40.

Mahn-Dinicola, V., & Zazworsky, D. (2005). The advanced practice nurse case manager. In A. Hamric, J. Spross, & C. M. Hanson (Eds.), *Advanced practice nursing: An integrative approach* (3rd ed.). St. Louis, MO: Elsevier-Saunders.

Maizel, S., Berandino, C., Caine, M., & Garfinkle, J. (2015). Corporate bankruptcy panes the healthcare industry post-Affordable Care Act: A bankruptcy perspective. *Emory Bankruptcy Development Journal, 31*(2), 249–272.

Markowitz, G. E., & Rosner, D. (1979). Doctors in crisis: Medical education and medical reform during the Progressive era, 1895–1915. In S. Reverby & D. Rosner (Eds.), *Health care in America: Essays in social history*. Philadelphia, PA: Temple University Press.

McDonald, M. D. (2001). The hospitalist movement: Wise or wishful thinking? *Nursing Management, 32*(3), 30–31.

McGillis-Hall, L., Doran, D. M., & Petch, T. (2005). Measurement of nurse job satisfaction using the McCloskey/Mueller Satisfaction Scale. *Nursing Research, 55*, 128–136.

McGinn, D., & Springen, K. (2007). Express-lane medicine. *Newsweek, 150* (5), 44.

McIntyre, M., & Thomlinson, E. (2003). *Realities of Canadian nursing: Professional, practice and power issues*. Philadelphia, PA: Lippincott Williams & Wilkins.

Mulligan, K. (2015). Contraception use, abortions, and births: The effect of insurance mandates. *Demography, 52*, 1195–1217. doi: 10.1007/s13524-015-0412-3

National Council of State Boards of Nursing. (2016). *National nursing workforce study*. Retrieved from https://www.ncsbn.org/workforce.htm. Accessed April 16, 2016.

O'Donnell, J., Smyth, D., & Frampton, C. (2005). Prioritizing health care funding. *Internal Medicine Journal, 35*, 409–412.

Porter-O'Grady, T., & Malloch, K. (2007). *Managing for success in health care*. St. Louis, MO: Mosby.

Public Broadcasting Service. (2007). The Online News Hour: The uninsured in America—Timeline: Insurance in the U.S. Retrieved from http://www.pbs.org/newshour/indepth_coverage/health/uninsured/timeline/index.html. Accessed December 12, 2012.

Robert Woods Johnson Foundation. (2014). Older nurses push retirement envelope. Retrieved from http://www.rwjf.org/en/library/articles-and-news/2014/12/older-nurses-push-retirement-envelope.html. Accessed April 16, 2016.

Rosen, M., & Haglund, B. (2005). From healthy survivors to sick survivors—Implications for the 21st century. *Scandinavian Journal of Public Health, 33*, 151–155.

Sanders, J. (2002). Financing and organization of national health systems. In B. J. Fried & L. M. Gaydos (Eds.), *World health systems: Challenges and perspectives*. Chicago: Health Administration Press.

Scofera, L. (1994). The development and growth of employer-provided health insurance. *Monthly Labor Review, 117*(3), 3–10.

Seago, J., Spetz, J., Chapman, S., & Dyer, W. (2007). Can the use of LPNs alleviate the nursing shortage? *American Journal of Nursing, 106*(7), 40–49.

Shane, D. M., & Ayyagari, P. (2015). Spillover effects of the Affordable Care Act? Exploring the impact on young adult dental insurance coverage. *Health Sciences Research, 50*(4), 1109–1124. doi: 10.1111/1475–6773.12266

Slavitt, A. M., & Burwell, S. (2016). Basic health program; federal funding methodology for program years 2017 & 2018. *The Federal Register*. Retrieved from https://www.federalregister.gov/articles/2016/02/29/2016–03902/basic-health-program-federal-funding-methodology-for-program-years-2017-and-2018. Accessed April 10, 2016.

Stanley, C. (2015). The patient protection and affordable care act: The latest obstacle in the path to receiving complementary and alternative health care? *Indiana Law Journal, 90*(2), 879–900.

Stapleton, P., & Skinner, D. (2015). The Affordable Care Act and assisted reproductive technology use. *Politics and the Life Sciences, 34*(2), 71–90. doi: 10.1017/pls.2015.13

Storch, J. L. (2005). Country profile: Canada's health care system. *Nursing Ethics, 12*(4), 413–418.

Sultz, H. A., & Young, K. M. (2004). *Health care USA: Understanding its organization and delivery* (4th ed.). Sudbury, MA: Jones & Bartlett.

Torrens, P. R. (1978). *The American health care system: Issues and problems*. St. Louis, MO: Mosby.

United States Bureau of Labor Statistics (USBLS). (2012). *Employment projections 2010–2020*. Retrieved from http://www.bls./gov/newsrelease/ecopro.t06.htm. Accessed February 17, 2013.

USBLS. (2015a). U.S. Department of Labor, *Occupational Outlook Handbook, 2016–17 Edition*, Registered Nurses, Summary. Retrieved from http://www.bls.gov/ooh/healthcare/registered-nurses.htm. Accessed April 16, 2016.

USBLS. (2015b). U.S. Department of Labor, *Occupational Outlook Handbook, 2016–17 Edition,* Registered Nurses, Work Environment. Retrieved from http://www.bls.gov/ooh/healthcare/registered-nurses.htm#tab-3. Accessed April 16, 2016.

USBLS. (2015c). U.S. Department of Labor, *Occupational Outlook Handbook, 2016–17 Edition,* Physicians and Surgeons, Summary. Retrieved from http://www.bls.gov/ooh/healthcare/physicians-and-surgeons.htm#tab-1. Accessed April 16, 2016.

USBLS. (2015d). U.S. Department of Labor, *Occupational Outlook Handbook, 2016–17 Edition,* Physicians and Surgeons, Pay. Retrieved from http://www.bls.gov/ooh/healthcare/physicians-and-surgeons.htm#tab-5. Accessed April 16, 2016.

U.S. Supreme Court. National Federation of Independent Business et al. v. Sebelius, Secretary of Health and Human Services, et al., 567 U.S. _____ (2012).

Vogel, M. J. (1979). The transformation of the American hospital, 1859–1920. In S. Reverby & D. Rosner (Eds.), *Health care in America: Essays in social history.* Philadelphia, PA: Temple University Press.

Wells, J., Manuel, M, & Cunning, G. (2011). Changing the model of care delivery: Nurses' perceptions of job satisfaction and care effectiveness. *Journal of Nursing Management, 19,* 777–785. doi: 10.1111/j.1365–2834.2011.01292.x

West, E., Griffith, W., & Iphofen, R. (2007). A historical perspective on the nursing shortage. *MEDSURG Nursing, 16,* 124–130.

Wong, C. A., Ford, C. A,, French, B., & Rubin, D. M. (2015). Changes in young adult Primary care under the Affordable Care Act. *American Journal of Public Health, 105,* S680–S685. doi:10.2105/AJPH.2015.302770

World Health Organization (WHO). (2010). The world health report, health systems: Finding the path to universal coverage. Retrieved from http://www.who.int/whr/2010/10_summary_en.pdf. Accessed February 17, 2013.

World Health Organization (WHO). (2015). *World health statistics 2015.* Retrieved from http://apps.who.int/iris/bitstream/10665/170250/1/9789240694439_eng.pdf. Accessed April 10, 2016.

Zakus, D., & Cortinois, A. (2002). Primary healthcare and community participation: Origins, implementation and the future. In B. J. Fried & L. M. Gaydos (Eds.), *World health systems: Challenges and perspectives.* Chicago: Health Administration Press.

Chapter 10

Developing and Using Nursing Knowledge Through Research

KEY TERMS AND CONCEPTS

Research
The research process
Quantitative research
Qualitative research
Research critique
Variable
Independent variable
Dependent variable
Research ethics
Informed consent
Anonymity
Institutional review
  board (IRB)
Research utilization
Evidence-based practice
Diffusion

Innovation
Diffusion of
  innovations
Research utilization
  and evidence-based
  practice facilitators
Research utilization
  and evidence-based
  practice barriers
Stetler model of
  Evidence-Based
  Practice
Scholar
National Institute of
  Nursing Research
  (NINR)

LEARNING OUTCOMES

By the end of this chapter, the learner will be able to:

1. Describe how professional nurses contribute to research in nursing.
2. Outline the sequential steps of the research process.
3. Differentiate qualitative and quantitative research.
4. Debate the ethical considerations of nursing research.
5. Compare and contrast research utilization and evidence-based practice (EBP) models.
6. Discuss the key elements of a research study critique.
7. Identify barriers to research utilization by nurses in the clinical setting.
8. Identify strategies to facilitate clinical research utilization.
9. Differentiate research utilization from EBP.
10. Specify how using nursing research affects the public image of professional nursing.

REAL-LIFE REFLECTIONS

Jessica and Malika work together on a surgical unit. Malika, who has been a nurse for 12 years, takes pride in her expertise and practices nursing "the way that I was taught." Jessica has read several research articles substantiating the effectiveness of noninvasive nursing interventions on reducing client need for narcotics for postoperative pain control. Jessica is unsure about whether she should use these findings in practice and how Malika will react if she suggests implementing these findings on a unit-wide scale. Jessica also knows that current federal guidelines related to postoperative pain control specify that nurses should use other methods besides pain medication. Both nurses wonder what they might need to do to change practice on their unit. What steps should these nurses follow to validate the benefits of various, available nonpharmacologic techniques for postoperative pain control? What barriers might they encounter as they explore this practice change? Why would these be considered barriers? How might they go about attaining support from their manager and peers to change unit practice?

- *Does the idea of conducting research intrigue you or intimidate you?*
- *What research-based interventions have you used in clinical practice?*

Interprofessional health care team members and consumers rely on research-based interventions (including medication) to help them provide safe, high-quality health care. Discipline-specific research enables a profession to develop and validate its unique knowledge base. Research also validates principles and techniques of clinical practice. Because nursing is primarily a practice discipline, nurses must understand basic research principles, critically analyze research study results, and use research findings to guide client care.

Although nursing research has been part of the profession since its inception, serious efforts to conduct research and develop theory to guide practice only began about 50 years ago, when nursing scholars drove the pursuit of establishing theoretical- and factual-based nursing practice instead of perpetuating nursing practice based on personal opinions, long-standing traditions, and prescribed protocols from other disciplines. Even up until the mid-1990s, however, a study of medical-surgical nurses found that many relied on information from individual patients, personal experience, and information gained during nursing school far more than on facts from journal articles (Baessler et al., 1994). Today, nurses must appreciate that incorporating research findings into practice is not an optional activity in which to engage when there is time but rather a critical element of professional practice (Fig. 10.1).

Science seeks the truth, and humans create science through research (Barrett, 2002). Therefore, nursing research should result in the creation of nursing science. **Research** is "a careful, systematic inquiry that uses disciplined methods to answer questions or solve problems. The ultimate goal of research is to develop, refine, and expand knowledge" (Polit & Beck, 2012, p. 3). Nursing research focuses on generating knowledge for and solving encountered problems within the profession and practice of nursing. When research-generated nursing knowledge results in improved client outcomes, enhances the professional practice environment, or contains health care costs, the research has practical applications for client care. When unresolved client care or professional nursing issues arise, nurses can conduct research to solve the problem. Therefore, research guides practice and practice generates new ideas for research.

Take Note!
Incorporating research is not optional; it is a critical part of the profession.

According to the American Nurses Association (2010), nurses integrate research into professional practice by the following.

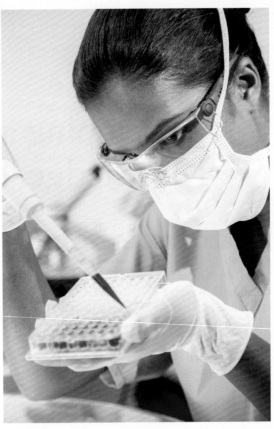

FIGURE 10.1 Nurses interested in expanding knowledge in the hard sciences engage in laboratory experimentation.

1. Utilizing current evidence-based nursing knowledge, including research findings, to guide practice.
2. Incorporating evidence when initiating changes in nursing practice.
3. Participating, as appropriate to education level and position, in the formulation of evidence-based practice (EBP) through research.
4. Sharing personal or third-party research findings with colleagues and peers.

Baccalaureate nursing programs provide a natural forum for the incorporation of research into practice. One of the hallmarks of a Bachelor of Science in Nursing (BSN) degree is a research course that prepares graduates for engagement in scholarly endeavors and for EBP (American Association of Colleges of Nursing, 2008). Typical educational activities include the following.

1. Reading and critiquing nursing research studies effectively.
2. Using nursing research findings to guide practice.
3. Valuing a sense of inquiry about the phenomena of nursing.

4. Participating in research projects when opportunities arise.
5. Distinguishing the quality of evidence.
6. Learning the processes of collecting, organizing, categorizing, and analyzing data.
7. Identifying nursing research and evidence-based questions.
8. Obtaining information and develop an evidence-based or nursing research project.
9. Disseminating information from a research or evidence-based project with others.
10. Initiating evidence-based changes in clinical practice.

To meet the rigor of using research and other forms of evidence effectively in practice, nurses should possess a solid understanding of the research process, a keen ability to critique research studies, comprehensive analysis skills, the creative capability to synthesize evidence from a variety of sources, and effective strategies to overcome obstacles to facilitate using research and other forms of evidence in practice.

THE RESEARCH PROCESS IN NURSING

The research process consists of a series of rigorous, logical steps of inquiry. Nurses must be familiar with the research process to critique nursing research studies effectively. Complete understanding of and comfort with the research process develop with time and practice.

The research process starts with a nurse's query about some aspect of nursing that might arise during clinical practice or that seems interesting (see Box 10.1, Professional Building Blocks, "Raising Questions for Research"). **The research process** structures the systematic investigation of that question, discovers answers, reports findings, and generates future questions on the topic. The process follows scientific methods, so that nursing research

- has an identifiable order.
- includes controls over factors not being investigated.
- includes gathering of evidence about the question.
- is built on a theoretical framework.
- operates for the purpose of applying results to improve nursing practice, generating theory, or expanding nursing science.

Take Note!

The purposes of nursing research are to improve nursing practice, generate new nursing theory, and expand nursing science.

10.1 Professional Building Blocks

Raising Questions for Research

The most significant step in the nursing research process may be the first one—the identification and articulation of a question. When nurses seek to find the best way to practice, they become accountable for asking questions that reflect the sensitivity needed to better understand all that falls within the domain of nursing. Nurses identify potential research questions when they encounter clinical practice problems. Because nursing theory and practice are deeply intertwined, research questions also may arise when nurses identify a gap in theory and practice. Some potential areas for research studies include the following.

- Nursing assessments, interventions, characteristics, and responsibilities.
- Facilitating factors for nurse–client relationships.
- Environmental factors to promote and maintain health and well-being, health and disease trajectories, and client adjustment to illness and other life transitions.

Clearly and concisely stated questions are essential to provide direction for studies. The successful execution of clinically relevant nursing research studies is most likely when clinical nurses and nurse researchers collaborate.

Quantitative and Qualitative Approaches

Two research approaches to developing nursing knowledge have emerged in recent years: the quantitative approach and the qualitative approach. In the earliest years of nursing research, valuing of the scientific method led to the use of quantitative approaches primarily. However, nurse researchers use qualitative approaches to develop subjective information when investigating human emotional, social, and existential responses to factors affecting well-being, such as illness, life transitions, or lifestyle changes.

According to Haase and Myers (1988), quantitative and qualitative research approaches have a common purpose: to gain understanding. The difference between the approaches is one of emphasis. **Quantitative research** focuses on the "confirmation of theory by explaining," demonstrating an empirical analytical emphasis, while **qualitative research** focuses on the "discovery and meaning of theory by describing," demonstrating a human science emphasis (Haase & Myers, 1988, p. 131). Because nursing addresses

TABLE 10.1   Quantitative and Qualitative Assumptions in Nursing Research

	Research Approach	
Assumption	**Qualitative**	**Quantitative**
View of reality	Researcher focuses on subjective realities seen as multiple and related; the process for understanding reality is ecologic, which suggests that "the whole is greater than the sum of its parts" (p. 132).	Researcher focuses on objective reality seen as singular; the process for discovering reality uses reductionism, which proposes that knowledge of the whole can be gained through knowledge of the parts.
View of relationships	Researcher interacts with the subject and believes that a unity exists between them and that both are integral to the research process.	Researcher distances self from subjects and believes that boundaries must exist to ensure objectivity.
View of truth	Researcher sees the world as dynamic and believes that truth is discovered in the changing patterns of the world; the researcher's goals are to discover uniqueness, valuing differences as well as similarities.	Researcher sees the world as stable and predictable and believes that the truth is discovered in common laws, principles, and norms; the researcher's goal is generalization.

Haase, J. E., & Myers, S. T. (1988). Reconciling paradigm assumptions of qualitative and quantitative research. *Western Journal of Nursing Research, 10,* 128–137.

subjective and objective phenomena, both approaches contribute equally to nursing science.

According to Guba and Lincoln (reported by Haase & Myers, 1988), the differences between the two approaches can be categorized in three ways based on the assumptions made by each approach: the nature of reality, the nature of relationships, and the nature of truth (Table 10.1).

Appreciating the complexity of nursing phenomena and valuing subjective experiences as legitimate foci of nursing research, Artinian (1988) noted that nurses use various qualitative approaches, including participant observation and in-depth interviewing. Cohen and Tripp-Reimer (1988, p. 226) supported ethnography as a significant qualitative research approach to help nurses understand cultural differences, stating that "ethnography is a method designed to describe a culture. The ethnographer seeks to understand another way of life from the native's point of view."

Grounded theory methodology, a qualitative approach, seeks to outline a basic social process or generate a new theory based on participant data. Using grounded theory methodology, Artinian (1988) described four modes of inquiry the qualitative researcher can use. These are highlighted in Box 10.2, Professional Prototypes, "Artinian's Four Modes of Qualitative Inquiry."

The researcher decides which of the four modes of inquiry to use only after clarifying the purpose of the research and evaluating available knowledge on the topic.

Qualitative research enables nurses to discover individualized and human phenomena surrounding health

10.2 Professional Prototypes

Artinian's Four Modes of Qualitative Inquiry

1. **Descriptive mode:** "Presents rich detail that allows the reader to understand what it would be like to be in a setting or to be experiencing the life situation of a person or group" (p. 139). For example, What it like to be a professional nurse?

2. **Discovery mode:** "Enables the researcher both to identify patterns in the life experiences of the subjects and to relate the patterns to each other" (p. 141). For example, What are the patterns associated with the development of a meaningful nursing career?

3. **Emergent fit mode:** "Used when a substantive theory has already been developed about the phenomenon under study" from which a research question "is formulated to extend or refine the previously developed theory" (p. 142). For example, How might Benner's Novice to Expert Theory fit with nurses currently undergoing the transition from nursing program graduate to a fully seasoned professional nurse?

4. **Intervention mode:** The researcher tries to answer the fundamental question of how to make something happen after the "phenomenon has been adequately conceptualized so that the conditions under which the basic social process takes place are understood" (p. 139). For example, Nurse residency programs facilitate the ease of transition that a nursing program graduate assumes the roles and responsibilities of independent nursing practice.

and illness. For example, phenomenology looks at the "lived experience" of a particular life transition, a clinical experience, or a specific illness or surgery. Hermeneutic inquiry seeks to find the deep, personal meaning of an experience. Historical studies examine artifacts from a particular era to determine what persons did in the past that may be applicable today.

Steps in the Research Process

Whether the nurse researcher chooses a qualitative or a quantitative approach, the overall steps in the research process are essentially the same. The study question determines which approach would be best.

The process is a sequence of 11 steps during which researchers make decisions to plan and execute a study. While engaged in the research process, the investigator may not necessarily complete a step, but rather may revisit it while planning and executing a study. Knowledge of the research process steps discussed in the subsequent sections will facilitate the nurse's use of findings in practice.

Step 1: Focus on the Clinical Problem Area

All nurses can identify problems in professional practice. Whenever a nurse identifies a gap between what is and what could be in practice, a clinical problem has arisen. Nursing research is one option to resolve such clinical problems.

Once a problem area has been identified, nurses can discover the state of knowledge about the problem by reviewing current practice protocols, research, and other forms of information on the identified topic. They can derive questions from the theories or conceptual models used to guide practice in their clinical setting or educational program, or by seeking out ideas from external sources such as faculty, peers, or the nursing research priorities published by the **National Institute of Nursing Research (NINR)** or professional nursing organizations (see Box 10.3, Learning, Knowing, and Growing, "Identifying Priority Areas for Research").

According to Polit and Beck (2012), the development of the research problem incorporates the following sequence of events.

1. Select a general area of interest about which you have questions.
2. Narrow and evaluate the topic with a mentor or expert.
3. Establish the benefits of the investigation. (Who would benefit? What relevance and/or applications would the study have to the profession? How important would the findings be? In other words, so what?)
4. Ensure that the selected problem is amenable to either quantitative or qualitative methodology (or both).
5. Verify that the problem is not primarily a moral issue.
6. Critique the feasibility of studying the problem in terms of time, subject and resource availability, and costs (actual and potential).

10.3 Learning, Knowing, and Growing

Identifying Priority Areas for Research

Many professional associations and governmental agencies have designated priority areas for research. For example,

- **Oncology Nursing Society:** Ongoing research initiatives on pain control, prevention of nausea, optimal nutrition, and fatigue in persons with cancer (www.ons.org) and has established a research agenda for 2009–2013 (www.ons.org/media/ons/docs/research/2009–2013onsresearchagenda.pdf).
- **American Nurses Association:** Ongoing studies related to workplace hazards for nurses (www.nursingworld.org) and an established research agenda (http://nursingworld.org/MainMenuCategories/ThePracticeofProfessionalNursing/Improving-

Your-Practice/Research-Toolkit/ANA-Research-Agenda/Research-Agenda-.pdf).
- **American Association of Critical Care Nurses:** Clinical research focuses on client pain, nosocomial infections, and ventilator weaning (www.aacn.org) and information about AACN research priorities (http://ajcc.aacnjournals.org/content/21/1/12.full).
- **National Institute of Nursing Research** sets research priorities for American nurses on a variety of topics of interest (www.ninr-nih.gov) and has published research priorities in its 2011 strategic plan (https://www.ninr.nih.gov/sites/www.ninr.nih.gov/files/ninr-strategic-plan-2011.pdf).

Visiting their websites or those of other nursing organizations may help inspire your research efforts.

Step 2: Perform an Initial Literature Review

An initial review of the literature enables nurse researchers to obtain a broad understanding and general background on the problem to be studied. Once the researcher has raised a question, this initial review of the literature is helpful in

- identifying the major variables in the area of interest.
- finding out what is already known.
- gathering feasibility data on the needs for problem investigation.
- sharpening the focus of the problem to be investigated.

A literature review should make the researcher aware of all the possible relevant materials available regarding a problem of interest. Tips for searching for information about the problem include typing in key terms contained within the problem statement using a computerized data base of scientific and research literature. Expanding the search to include literature from other disciplines besides nursing facilitates finding more relevant literature (medicine, psychology, social work, or business depending upon the nature of the problem). Nurse investigators frequently consult research librarians to assist in this step (and step 4) of the research process. Along with reading the existing literature, researchers must appraise each research study by assessing its strengths and weaknesses. A **research critique** points out the strengths and weaknesses of a study and helps researchers discover gaps in the current literature.

Helpful sources for locating resource materials include indexes from nursing, related disciplines, and popular literature; abstracting services from nursing and related disciplines; computer searches of appropriate databases; dictionaries; encyclopedias; guides; and directories. Most reference librarians can provide tremendous help to nurse researchers in locating and using these materials (Fig. 10.2).

Frequently, those conducting qualitative research avoid reviewing the literature before collecting data to avoid developing preconceived ideas about the topic area. In quantitative research, such a knowledge base makes it possible for the researcher to proceed to the next stage of research: specifying the problem and defining the variables.

> **Take Note!**
> The initial literature review should answer some questions about the topic of interest, identify others who are interested in the topic, and help the researcher develop a knowledge base of what is currently known about the topic.

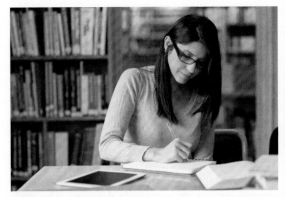

FIGURE 10.2 Sometimes nurses must make a trip to the library to review printed materials in order to conduct a comprehensive literature review.

Step 3: Specify the Problem and the Defining Variables

Researchers must specify a problem and identify key variables or phenomena within the nursing domain to be investigated. The nurse researcher may investigate a client aspect that affects the nurse–client therapeutic relationship, a phenomenon that impacts client health, ways to enhance client care quality and safety, the effectiveness of a specific nursing intervention, any aspect of the delivery of nursing care services, environmental elements influencing health and well-being, professional practice issues, or any combination of these factors.

Clear articulation of the problem incorporates the identification of the phenomenon to be investigated. In quantitative research, a phenomenon of interest generally is called a "variable." A **variable** is a characteristic, trait, property, or condition. If a variable is purposefully manipulated by the researcher to have a direct effect on another variable, it is an **independent variable**. A variable that is observed, measured, and presumed to be influenced by or related in some special way to the independent variable is a **dependent variable**. Quantitative studies may have one or more independent and dependent variables (see Box 10.4, Professional Prototypes, "Variables in Quantitative Research"). Variables do not exist in qualitative research because the purpose may be to identify key phenomena surrounding a client or nurse experience.

Step 4: Establish Tentative Propositions— Hypotheses and Second Literature Review

After the nurse researcher has clarified the problem under investigation, studied the available data, and recalled observations from professional experience, he or she may formulate a hypothesis, a formal statement

10.4 Professional Prototypes

Variables in Quantitative Research

Following is an example of a study with one variable that is manipulated and another that is observed and measured.

What is the relationship between specific parenting guidance by the professional nurse and the development of positive nutritional habits of the toddler? In this investigation, the independent variable is the specific parenting guidance, the dependent variable is the toddler's nutritional habits, and the approach to studying the variables is quantitative.

To make these variables measurable, the researcher must determine exactly what is meant by each variable, that is, what constitutes parenting guidance and what constitutes positive nutritional habits in the toddler. The statement of the problem may be in the form of a question or a declaration. In both the cases, this problem statement must also clearly identify who and what are to be studied.

that predicts or explains the relationships between two or more variables (Polit & Beck, 2012). Not all studies require that the researcher generates a hypothesis; for example, questions of a descriptive, qualitative, and exploratory nature do not need hypotheses, but instead generate questions. However, for studies requiring manipulation of an independent variable with the purpose of influencing a dependent variable, hypotheses must be stated and tested.

Nurses have excellent opportunities to form hunches about the relationships among variables they observe in practice. The hypothesis is like a bridge—it connects theory with those observations and is derived from observations, reasoning, and theoretical bases.

Hypotheses in quantitative studies are tested statistically in relation to the laws of chance. Thus, they are based on statistical probability and incur an element of risk of reaching an incorrect conclusion. How much risk can be afforded is a judgment of the investigator, but when permanent or serious consequences are involved, the investigator cannot afford to take too many risks. Because hypotheses sometimes force the investigator to infer from the sample findings an interpretation about the population, the researcher uses probability statistics (level of significance) to determine the likelihood that the relationship between the variables results from something other than chance.

When the researcher is determining hypotheses, additional review of the literature is used to evaluate testing procedures and to project a research design

appropriate for investigating the variable(s). The literature review can be used to learn what investigative methods have been used, how data have been collected and analyzed, and what has and has not been successful in previous research.

> **Take Note!**
> In quantitative studies, hypotheses declare the researcher's proposition about the relationship between variables and then serve as the means for testing the proposed relationship.

Step 5: Determine a Suitable Research Design

The nurse researcher selects the type of research design suitable for the study based on the research questions or hypotheses.

- A descriptive design answers questions about the nature of presently occurring events.
- An experimental design tests the effects of manipulating one or more specific variables on other variables.
- An historical design is based on the desire to describe or evaluate past events.
- In ethnographic research, the researcher frequently acts as a member of or observes a group. Detailed interviews followed by participant validation of data serve as the means to capture the essence of an experience in phenomenology.

Step 6: Develop a Research Methodology: Data Collection Methods and Instruments

After the approach is selected for a particular study, the nurse researcher decides on the appropriate method for gathering data, and then selects instruments for data collection depending on the purpose of the research. Instruments generally are categorized under three methods: observation, questioning, and measurement.

Examples of data collection instruments include critical incidents, tests, interviews, questionnaires, checklists, records, scales, and physical measurement techniques. The researcher strives to select a measurement tool that is appropriate to answer the research question, is unbiased, and has precision in measuring the variables being studied. For quantitative studies, the researcher carefully analyzes available measurement tools to determine instrument validity (the extent to which the tool actually measures the variable of interest) and reliability (consistency of variable measurement). In qualitative studies, the researcher exercises caution to eliminate any personal biases that could interfere with objective data collection. The quality of data generated for a study relies on careful selection of data collection methods.

Knafl and Webster (1988) pointed out how the researcher's data collection, analysis of those data, and reporting are likely to vary according to the purpose of the study. They described four purposes of qualitative research.

1. **Illustration:** The researcher aims to identify qualitative examples of specific quantitative variables.
2. **Instrumentation:** The researcher aims to collect data that serve as the basis for developing an instrument to describe and measure perceptions of some phenomenon of interest to nursing.
3. **Description:** The researcher aims to "translate the data into a form that would facilitate an accurate, complete description" (p. 200) of a phenomenon of interest to nursing by identifying and delineating the major themes.
4. **Theory building:** The researcher aims to conceptually explain the phenomenon under study.

Mixed methods research studies (also called triangulated, multi-method, or integrated designs) combine quantitative and qualitative research methods within a single study. Blending quantitative and qualitative approaches emerged in the early 21st century in the field of nursing. By integrating the two approaches, researchers can capitalize on the strengths of each approach while minimizing their weaknesses. Typically, one method (qualitative or quantitative) dominates the study when mixed methods are used (Burns, Grove, & Gray, 2013; Polit & Beck, 2012). For example, a nurse studying the effects of nurse job satisfaction on patient care outcomes (quantitative approach), the researcher might want to know about the lived experiences of the nurse working on a specific unit that have enhanced or reduced the nurse's job satisfaction (qualitative approach).

In addition to selecting instruments for data collection during this stage of research, the nurse must determine the composition of the sample (persons who will participate in a study), establish a process for collecting data from the sample, and prepare a format for data collection (which may include designing specific forms), data classification, and data storage for later analysis. The criteria for inclusion in a sample must be clearly described, and the method for selecting subjects must be appropriate. The number of sample subjects must meet statistical requirements for the nurse to draw appropriate conclusions about the findings (for quantitative studies).

Step 7: Ensure an Ethical Process

Research requires honesty and integrity. Research ethics are principles by which researchers abide to ensure truth in scientific studies, protect the human rights of participants, balance risks and benefits of a study, and prevent exploitation of vulnerable persons. The importance of **research ethics** came to the forefront after reports of inhumane and unethical treatment sustained by prisoners during medical experiments in Nazi Germany. In 1949, the Nuremburg Code was established to protect human subjects in biomedical experiments. The researcher bears the responsibility for protecting human rights when persons participate in a research study. This protection process is achieved primarily through **informed consent** and protection from harm.

- **Informed consent** means that the researcher provides subjects with a clear description about the study, how they meet study criteria, requirements for participation, information of study withdrawal, and potential hazards. Subjects must understand study details so that they can freely consent to participate. Even after giving informed consent, a subject can decide to withdraw from a study at any time.
- **Protection from harm** means just that the investigator will not knowingly do anything that will harm or abuse the subjects. Investigators also work to preserve subject **anonymity** (keeping the identification of all subjects confidential).

Most research institutions have a formal process for approving research proposals before implementation. An **institutional review board (IRB)** meets on a regular schedule to review research proposals, verify that investigators have fully considered the ethics involved, and ensure that the study meets scientific standards. In health care settings, nurses sometimes hold IRB membership. Because they are client advocates and have holistic views of health care, nurses sometimes identify potentially harmful research treatments that other IRB members may overlook. A research study must always be subjected to IRB review. Depending on the potential for harm, coercion, and loss of anonymity, some EBP, research utilization, and quality improvement projects may also need IRB scrutiny (Burns et al., 2013; Melnyk & Fineout-Overholt, 2011; Polit & Beck, 2012).

To ensure truth in research, the researcher assumes responsibility for honesty when collecting and analyzing data and when reporting research findings.

For-profit and nonprofit organizations frequently fund research studies. Corporations fill gaps in research funding to bring new health products to the market. The investigator bears the responsibility for using the highest standards of scientific inquiry and reporting findings honestly at all time. When extramural funding (public, nonprofit, or for-profit organizations) has been received for the research study, the investigator has an obligation to report the source of funds within the written report (Blumenstyk, 2001; Burns et al., 2013; Polit & Beck, 2012).

Step 8: Collect Data

After protection of human rights and well-being for all subjects has been ensured, data collection can begin. However, before any subject associated with an institution can be approached, the researcher must have approval from appropriate agency personnel. The subjects of the research must also sign an informed consent form that they have received information about the purpose of the study, their role in study participation, how they can cease participation, and any potential ill effects from participation.

The researcher or a specified data collector orients each subject clearly and concisely to the data collection method, and then administers the data collection instrument to each subject in the same manner. Throughout this implementation stage, the researcher follows the written proposal (in the methodology) as closely as possible. While collecting data, the researcher records the data on the prepared forms. The data are then classified and organized for analysis.

Step 9: Analyze Data and Report Findings

Once data are collected, the researcher organizes them in a manner that makes them amenable to analysis. If the researcher's goal is simply to display the data collected, no analysis other than a narrative description and display tables is needed. However, if the researcher aims to infer some characteristics about a population or to evaluate some relationship among variables, the organized data must be subjected to statistical analysis. Many researchers consult a statistician for help with this step. Computations are done. If hypotheses have been stated, statistical testing, by hand or by computer, of those hypotheses must be done.

Based on accurate data analysis, the researcher reports and summarizes the findings exactly as they occurred. All data collected for purposes of testing the hypotheses must be reported. Tables, charts, and graphs used to present data should be pertinent, clear, and well labeled, and should be discussed in the text of the research report. The reports of the findings are then used to draw conclusions.

Step 10: Make Conclusions and Outline Implications

For quantitative research studies, the researcher must determine the meaning of the findings, articulate their value to nursing, and link them to the theoretical foundation(s) guiding the study. Findings are analyzed first by inspecting the statistical tests performed to test the hypotheses or evaluate the data. The researcher then interprets the numerical analysis. With hypothesis testing, the findings may support the predicted relationship with demonstrated statistical significance (the findings were not attributable to chance alone), may not be in the predicted direction, may be contradictory, or may indicate an unpredicted relationship. Sometimes statistical significance has little practical significance. Practical significance indicates that the results add to the body of nursing knowledge or lead to major changes in clinical outcomes. For example, the tobacco industry has argued in the court system that the link between cigarette smoking and lung cancer is not statistically significant. However, research studies reveal a high degree of correlation (strong relationship) between smoking and the development of lung cancer.

For qualitative studies, the researcher determines the meaning of the study and its value to professional nursing by identifying the impact of the new knowledge generated by the study. The conceptual overview generated by a qualitative study may have profound importance to those working with clients with similar conditions. Qualitative studies frequently provide a foundation for hypothesis generation and research instrument development for future quantitative research studies.

Based on the analysis and interpretation of data, the researcher might make generalizations about what the data mean and whether the data can be applied to groups that differ from the sample. Generalizations should emerge only from the findings, and the researcher should not go beyond the data as a result of the excitement generated by scientific discovery.

Study implications usually relate to one of the four aspects of professional nursing: clinical practice with clients, professional education, clinical practice environments, and ideas for additional nursing research. In a section of the research study called "Recommendations," the implications for practice (i.e., how the findings affect the nursing process with clients) should be discussed. Recommendations for the education of practitioners and for future research are also usually given. If the recommendations are clearly and concisely stated and derived logically, clinical nurses can find the study valuable and incorporate the findings in practice.

Step 11: Disseminate Findings: The Written Report and Professional Presentations

Research completed but not compiled into a report is wasted. Some experts argue that the research process is not complete until it is shared in writing or some other public medium. Characteristics of an effective research report are brevity, clarity, and complete objectivity.

Although faculty or other institutional requirements, or a particular style manual, may influence the form of the report, research reports usually follow the outline of the research process presented in this chapter. Most outlines include the problem statement, review of literature, methods of investigation, presentation of findings, discussion of analyses and conclusions, bibliographic data, and appendices. The reader is directed to a nursing research book or a writing style manual for specific guidance in developing each part of the written research report. Sometimes space limitations in journals prevent authors from including details about studies accepted for publication.

In addition to written reports, nurse researchers present study findings by giving oral presentations and presenting posters. Like the written report, posters and presentations describe the research methodology, present findings, articulate the significance to practice, and generate ideas for future study on the topic.

> **Take Note!**
> An effective research report is one that is brief, clear, and completely objective. Its recommended practice changes must stay within the confines of the data collected. A good research study outlines study limitations and suggests areas for further research on the study topic.

▌ QUESTIONS FOR REFLECTION

1. What questions do you have related to the research process and how to critique nursing research studies?
2. Referring back to the vignette, do you think Jessica would be able to better convince Malika of the value of the studies she had read if they were qualitative or if they were quantitative? Why?
3. Would you be interested in starting or participating in a nursing research journal club? Why or why not? If so, how could you make journal club participation a reality?

NURSING RESEARCH UTILIZATION AND EVIDENCE-BASED PRACTICE

Nurses use many forms of evidence to guide clinical practice, including nursing research. Over the past two decades, nurses have made great progress in increasing the use of scientific evidence in clinical practice. Sherwood and Barnsteiner (2009) define **evidence-based practice** as "practice based on the best available evidence that also incorporates patient values and preferences and clinician judgment and expertise" (p. 134). Polit and Beck (2012, p. 28) identify the following seven levels of evidence ranked from the least to most rigorous.

- **Level 7:** Opinions of authorities or expert committees
- **Level 6:** A single descriptive/qualitative/physiologic study
- **Level 5:** Systematic review of descriptive/qualitative/physiologic studies
- **Level 4:** Single correlational/observational study
- **Level 3:** Systematic review of correlational/observational studies
- **Level 2:** A single randomized or nonrandomized clinical trial
- **Level 1:** Systematic review of randomized or nonrandomized clinical trials

Polit and Beck fail to specify professional nurse and patient opinions as a level of evidence. Nurses sometimes base care strategies on client preference or the successful past use of a nursing assessment or intervention. Table 10.2 compares and contrasts the processes of nursing research utilization and EBP. Nursing research utilization is used by nursing, whereas EBP ideally includes all interprofessional team members.

A clinically relevant question initiates the processes of EBP and research utilization. Melnyk and Fineout-Overholt (2011, 2015) propose a standardized question format that will result in retrieval of the most compatible information when conducting a literature search on a clinical topic. They suggest using the acronym PICOT.

> "**P**atient population
> **I**ntervention or issue of interest
> **C**omparison intervention or status
> **O**utcome
> **T**ime frame for the [I] to achieve the [O]" (p. 579)

In most research utilization and EBP projects, the goal is to improve client outcomes, professional nurse work environments, or cost-effectiveness of care delivery.

TABLE 10.2   Comparison of Nursing Research Utilization and Evidence-Based Practice

	Nursing Research Utilization	Evidence-Based Practice
Purpose	Establish nursing practice based on scientific evidence	Establish best practice guidelines for various clinical problems
Participants	Professional nurses	Interdisciplinary health team
Sources of evidence	Quantitative or qualitative research study findings	Research study findings Quality improvement data Retrospective and concurrent chart audits Risk management data Infection control data Local, national, and international standards Pathophysiology of clinical problem Cost-effectiveness data Benchmarking data Expert opinions Logical reasoning Clinical experience Individual patient situations Client preference data
Processes	Critiques of research reports of topic of interest Integrative review of research reports Innovation subjected to a planned change process Evaluation of results of care innovation	Group meetings of one component of the health care team for issues related to a specific discipline Group meetings of interdisciplinary health team members to develop critical paths or other care pathways Interdisciplinary review of current clinical needs, practices, established guidelines, and care principles Extensive systematic review of published research on issue to be addressed from all health care disciplines if the guideline will be interdisciplinary or from one health care discipline if guideline will be specific to a special group Guideline review by experts, clinicians, and clients Guidelines tested for effective clinical use Guidelines subjected to continuous review
Outcomes	Improved client outcomes Improved professional practice Research-based nursing care and clinical practice protocols	Improved client outcomes Clinical guidelines for client care based on solid evidence that yields the most benefit for the least possible cost
Dissemination of information	Agency newsletter Letters to staff Staff email Electronic or printed agency clinical policy manual Staff in-services Nursing publications Nursing specialty organization websites	Agency newsletter Staff email Electronic or printed agency policy manuals Professional publications Websites of professional organizations, large health care agencies, Agency for Healthcare Research and Quality, the National Guideline Clearinghouse American Medical Association, American Association of Health Care Plans

Burns, N., Grove, S. K., & Gray, J. (2013). *The practice of nursing research: Appraisal, synthesis & generation of evidence* (7th ed.). St. Louis, MO: Elsevier Saunders, Glanville, I., Schirm, V., & Wineman, N. M. (2000). Using evidence-based practice for managing clinical outcomes in advanced practice nursing. *Journal of Nursing Care Quality, 15*(19), 1–11; Goode, C. J., & Piedalue, F. (1999). Evidence-based clinical practice. *Journal of Nursing Administration, 29*, 15–21; and Jennings, B. M., & Loan, L. A. (2001). Misconceptions among nurses about evidence-based practice. *Journal of Nursing Scholarship, 33*, 121–127.

Research Utilization

Research utilization is a systematic process to incorporate research study findings into clinical practice. Polit and Beck (2012) view research utilization as a narrow term and define it as "the use of findings from a study or series of studies in a practical application that is unrelated to the original research" (p. 26). However, nurses have been using research findings in practice for decades (see Box 10.5, Professional Prototypes, "The Origins of Nursing Research Utilization").

Every medication that nurses administer on a daily basis is an example of research utilization. The U.S.

10.5 Professional Prototypes

The Origins of Nursing Research Utilization

Florence Nightingale instituted utilization of nursing research more than a century ago. Using a systematic approach, Nightingale collected data and presented detailed results in bar graphs, pie charts, and color-coded tables to highlight how improving sanitation and using trained nurses reduced mortality of ill and wounded soldiers during the Crimean War. She presented her findings, published in *Notes on Nursing* (Nightingale, 1860), to the British government, which subsequently increased funding for the care of soldiers so that Nightingale's methods could be implemented (McDonald, 2001).

10.6 Professional Building Blocks

Benefits of a Research Bases for Clinical Nursing Practice

- A solid, sound, scientific foundation for practice.
- Enhanced self-confidence, autonomy, critical thinking skills, and professional self-concept.
- Cost-effective patient care.
- Increased patient and job satisfaction and quality of care.
- Improved patient outcomes.
- A stimulus for collaborative practice, retention, and recruitment.
- An improved image of nursing.
- An ever-increasing scientific nursing knowledge base (Goode et al., 1991).

Food and Drug Administration requires that the efficacy of a medication has been substantiated through a series of randomized clinical trials. A randomized clinical trial is a research design in which subjects are randomly assigned to experimental (to receive the investigational drug) and control (to receive a placebo) groups, with stringent control of variables outside the study, to determine whether a medication produces its stated therapeutic effects. Medical devices also undergo a series of scientific tests. Because health care is a scientifically based discipline, all health care team members use research on a daily basis. To stay abreast of practice changes, professional nurses must read the current nursing research literature and apply new findings to their practice as appropriate (see Box 10.6, Professional Building Blocks, "Benefits of a Research Bases for Clinical Nursing Practice").

Research utilization may be as simple as one nurse changing the way in which care is given (Gennaro, 1994) or as complex as changing nursing practice standards. Although many research findings are printed and posted within a given month, there is a delay between study completion and dissemination. In addition, there are barriers for research utilization in practice settings (see Concepts in Practice, "Making a Case for Research Utilization in Practice").

Research findings can be used in many ways in professional practice. An individual nurse could read a qualitative nursing research article exploring fatigue in persons receiving hemodialysis and incorporates the finding by being more attentive and sensitive to increased needs for uninterrupted rest periods when planning and implementing care with these clients. Nurses also perform quality improvement studies

within health care organizations using new research findings (see Chapter 18, "Quality Improvement: Enhancing Patient Safety and Health Care Quality"). Many nurses opt to use published models for research

Concepts in Practice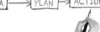

Making a Case for Research Utilization in Practice

Tony works on a rehabilitation unit with many clients who, when first admitted, cannot turn themselves. Over the past year, he and several of his coworkers have experienced increased back pain as a result of lifting and turning immobile patients. Tony decides to conduct a literature review to see if any new equipment might be available to facilitate turning immobile clients in bed. He discovers that new slider sheet systems (sheets made of slick, parachute-like material) have the potential to reduce muscular and perceived nurse effort while turning patients in bed (Theou et al., 2011). When Tony suggests using the slider sheets to see if they reduce back strain on the unit, his colleagues tease him and call him "professor." His work setting does not permit him time to prepare a proposal for using research-based findings on the job.

- What barriers to research utilization does Tony face?
- How might he address the situation to ameliorate the issue of back pain among the health care team?

Later in this chapter, we will revisit Tony and see how implemented research utilization and EBP resolve the issues he faces.

10.7 Professional Building Blocks

Models for Nursing Research Utilization and Evidence-Based Practice

- ACE STAR Model of Knowledge Transformation (Academic Center for Evidence-Based Practice, 2009)
- Advancing Research and Clinical Practice Through Close Collaboration (ARCC) Model (Melnyk & Fineout-Overholt, 2011)
- Diffusion of Innovations (Rogers, 1995)
- Iowa Model of Evidence-Based Practice to Promote Quality Care (Titler et al., 2001)
- Stetler Model of Evidence-Based Practice (Stetler, 2010)
- Disciplined Clinical Inquiry (Malloch & Porter-O'Grady, 2006)

utilization and EBP. A review of the literature for this chapter revealed over 50 models for research utilization and EBP, with some being solely nursing focused and others having an interprofessional approach. Some models can be readily accessed on the internet and others require user registration and fees. Box 10.7, Professional Building Blocks, "Models for Nursing Research Utilization and Evidence-Based Practice," provides a brief list of models for professional consideration. Research utilization, EBP, and quality improvement all begin with the identification of actual or potential clinical problems or issues.

Evidence-Based Practice

EBP has nearly become a standard mode of care delivery. Evidence-based medicine, evidence-based physical therapy, evidence-based nutrition, and evidence-based nursing provide mechanisms for the delivery of best practices for health care. Nursing research provides nurses with the opportunity to supply their own body of evidence for clinical practice guidelines. However, the support for EBP does not rely solely on research findings but includes clinical experience, quality improvement data, logical reasoning, recognized authority, and client satisfaction, situation, experience, and values (Boswell & Cannon, 2007; Burns et al., 2013; DiCenso, Guyatt, & Ciliska, 2005; Glanville, Schirm, & Wineman, 2000; Malloch & Porter-O'Grady, 2006; Melnyk & Fineout-Overholt, 2015; Polit & Beck, 2012).

Some health care organizations encourage and support nurses in implementing evidence-based nursing projects. Malloch and Porter-O'Grady (2006) outlined

a model of disciplined clinical inquiry to guide the process of evidence-based patient care (EBPC). The EBPC model, which is patient centered, resource efficient, knowledge driven, and clinically appropriate, includes the following five phases (Malloch & Porter-O'Grady, 2006, p. 37).

- **Phase 1:** Needs assessment and environmental scan
- **Phase 2:** Learning and knowledge generation
- **Phase 3:** Knowledge assimilation
- **Phase 4:** Knowledge application
- **Phase 5:** Appraisal/evaluation

Melnyk and Fineout-Overholt (2011, p. 10) outlined a different approach to EBP consisting of the following seven critical steps. Melynk and Fine-Overholt's process requires a highly refined question to be answered. The question must contain a population (P), intervention (I), comparison (C), outcome (O), and optional timing (T). Here is an example of a PICOT question: In new graduate nurses (P) what is the effect of nurse residency programs (I) on retention rate (O) compared with no nurse residency program participation (C) for the first 2 years?

- **Step 1:** Cultivate a spirit of inquiry.
- **Step 2:** Ask the burning clinical question in PICOT format.
- **Step 3:** Search for and collect the most relevant, best evidence.
- **Step 4:** Critically appraise the evidence (i.e., rapid critical appraisal, evaluation, and synthesis).
- **Step 5:** Integrate the best evidence with one's clinical expertise and patient preferences and values in making a practice decision or change.
- **Step 6:** Evaluate outcomes of the practice decision or change based on evidence.
- **Step 7:** Disseminate the outcomes of the EBP decision or change.

Ironically, both approaches appear to be congruent with steps of problem-solving strategies. Malloch and Porter-O'Grady (2006) emphasized the importance of creating an organizational culture that supports nurses as they embark on learning how to assess evidence and execute EBP clinical practice changes.

Proponents of EBP view it as a means to solve clinical practice problems by making the best possible decisions related to care based on client reports, clinician observations, and research data. Systematic review of all research literatures on a particular health topic provides the best form of evidence for clinical practice (Boswell & Cannon, 2007; DiCenso et al., 2005; Malloch & Porter-O'Grady, 2006; Melnyk & Fineout-Overholt,

2011, 2015; Polit & Beck, 2012). Clinical practice guidelines fall into this category. In the United States, the Agency for Health Care Research and Quality (AHRQ; formerly the Agency for Health Care Policy and Research) created the National Guideline Clearinghouse (NGC) in 1998 to offer interprofessional health team members a rich source of evidence-based clinical practice guidelines. NGC publishes free guidelines on disease management and prevention that have been generated through synthesis of recent, valid research findings along with expert commentary for each guideline. Some health care insurance companies use NGC as a basis for reimbursement (NGC, 2008).

The Cochrane Collaboration is an international organization that also provides information for health care providers based on systematic integrative reviews of controlled clinical trials. The Cochrane Collaboration charges a fee to access evidence based solely on disease management.

Currently, many health care professionals use EBP guidelines developed by the AHRQ for the treatment of urinary incontinence, low back problems, pain, depression, and prevention and treatment of pressure ulcers (Boswell & Cannon, 2007; DiCenso et al., 2005; Malloch & Porter-O'Grady, 2006). When research data are not available on a specific clinical problem, experts who specialize in a specific area develop practice guidelines by consensus. EBP also enables health care providers to use objective and subjective ways of knowing when making client care decisions and revising clinical procedures.

EBP opponents in medicine and nursing suggest that the development of clinical practice guidelines, critical care pathways, and protocols entices practitioners to adopt a "cookbook recipe" approach to client care. The basic tenet of quality improvement initiatives specifies that elimination of variation in practice decreases the chance for error and improves quality (Glanville et al., 2000). However, quality improvement has its roots in industrial production and such standardization may not be as desirable in the health care setting because clients have unique characteristics and needs that may be overlooked when practitioners adhere strictly to clinical practice guidelines. In addition, consumers and third-party payers may hold health care providers accountable for actions in addition to or for not strictly following established clinical practice guidelines (Glanville et al., 2000; Goode & Piedalue, 1999).

Health care organizations and individual health team members hold the key to the successful implementation of EBP. Organizations must display commitment to developing evidence-based care pathways and provide health care team members with the time and required resources. Up to 6 months may be required for the development of a single evidence-based pathway (Kirrane, 2000; Malloch & Porter-O'Grady, 2006).

▋ QUESTIONS FOR REFLECTION

1. What forms of evidence do you use as a basis for clinical decision making?
2. How are client care policies, protocols, and pathways developed where you engage in clinical practice?

Models to Guide Research Utilization and Evidence-Based Practice

Since the 1970s, professional nurses have used models to guide the movement of research and evidence into practice. Some of the successful models have been borrowed from the corporate world (Rogers's Diffusion of Innovations), developed by nurse researchers (Stetler Model for Evidence-Based Practice and Advancing Research and Clinical Practice Through Close Collaboration), or designed using interprofessional collaboration (Ottawa Model of Research Use). Some nursing research utilization models, such as the Iowa Model, contain paths for nurses to follow when they cannot find adequate research on which to base practice changes (Melnyk & Fineout-Overholt, 2011, 2015; Polit & Beck, 2012; Rycroft-Maline & Bucknall, 2010). Because no single model fits each practice setting and needs, nurses can find a variety of models for use in nursing research textbooks, in professional journals and publications, and in postings on nursing specialty organization, academic health center, hospital, and corporate websites.

The following key elements appear in most of the nursing research utilization models.

1. Identifying a gap in desired outcome.
2. Articulating the clinical problem clearly and concisely.
3. Reviewing research literature.
4. Preparing a comprehensive report outlining key research findings.
5. Selecting from one of the research-based innovations found in the literature review.
6. Developing specific practice outcomes for the proposed innovation.

7. Establishing an implementation plan for the innovation.
8. Creating an evaluation plan development to assess the effects or practice outcomes of the innovation.
9. Implementing the innovation within a practice setting.
10. Evaluating the clinical effects of the innovation.

Concepts in Practice, "Nursing Research Utilization in Action," returns to the example of Tony and his colleagues and shows how these elements may be implemented.

8. Create an evaluation plan to assess the effects or practice outcomes of the innovation (keep daily staff logs documenting incidences of back strain).
9. Implement the innovation within a practice setting (use the slider sheet system to turn patients at all times for 1 month).
10. Evaluate the clinical effects of the innovation (compare incidences of back strain before and after implementation of the slider sheet system).

Concepts in Practice IDEA ⟶ PLAN ⟶ ACTION

Nursing Research Utilization in Action

Recall Tony and his colleagues, who experienced back pain from turning immobile patients in the rehabilitation unit. The following list illustrates the key elements specified by many nursing research utilization models and how Tony might use them to help institute new evidence-based guidelines on the unit.

1. Identify a gap in desired outcome (skin integrity maintenance).
2. Articulate the clinical problem clearly and concisely (increased back strain and perceived nurse effort when turning clients in bed).
3. Review research literature (secure, read, and critique the literature based on nurse and unlicensed assistive personnel risk factors for back strain).
4. Prepare a comprehensive report outlining key research findings (prepare a table outlining the research findings from literature reviewed on risk factors for back strain and available turning devices, along with drawing conclusions and forming clinical implications for the rehabilitation unit).
5. Select from one of the research-based innovations found in the literature review (select the slider sheet system for reduction of back strain and increased perception of effort to turn clients while in bed).
6. Develop specific practice outcomes for the proposed innovation (incidence of back strain will be reduced by 50% within 1 month of using the slider sheet system to turn patients).
7. Establish an implementation plan for the innovation (educate staff on the use of the slider sheet system, and secure staff acceptance of the system).

Once the effectiveness of the innovation has been demonstrated, agency policy and procedures may be revised to make using the innovation standard practice.

Many nurses looking to facilitate change and innovation in practice find theories and models of research utilization helpful.

Rogers' Theory of Diffusion of Innovations

According to Rogers (1983, p. 5), "**diffusion** is the process by which an innovation is communicated through certain channels over time among the members of a social system." Rogers (1983, p. 11) defined **innovation** as "an idea, practice, or object that is perceived as new." In the example of Tony and his colleagues used earlier in this chapter, changing the method that nursing personnel would use to turn clients in bed (the slick sheet system) would be considered an innovation.

Rogers (1983) suggested that diffusion of innovations is useful for deciding whether to adopt an innovation (something perceived as new by those who are considering adoption). **Diffusion of innovations** is a five-stage process.

- **Stage 1—Knowledge:** Becoming aware of the existence of the innovation
- **Stage 2—Persuasion:** Forming an attitude toward the innovation
- **Stage 3—Decision:** Making the choice for adoption or rejection of the innovation
- **Stage 4—Implementation:** Using the innovation
- **Stage 5—Confirmation:** Seeking reinforcement of the decision

Reversal of the decision can occur at any time during the implementation and confirmation stages. Concepts in Practice, "Rogers' Diffusion of Innovations Process in Action," returns to the example of Tony and his colleagues and shows how these elements may be implemented.

Concepts in Practice [IDEA]──→[PLAN]──→[ACTION]

Rogers' Diffusion of Innovations Process in Action

Tony incorporates Roger's diffusion of innovations theory in his quest to determine whether the slick sheet system will help relieve the back pain that results from turning immobile patients.

- **Knowledge:** Tony becomes aware of the slick sheet system, a research-validated method for patient turning.
- **Persuasion:** Tony asks his colleagues what they would think about trying the slick sheet systems for turning for a month.
- **Decision:** Tony's staff decides to give the slick sheet system a try to see if it makes a difference.
- **Implementation:** Staff members use the slick sheet system and keep a log about how their backs feel at the end of each shift.
- **Confirmation:** Staff reports a reduced incidence of back strain.

For an individual to consider adoption of an innovation, he or she must be aware of the innovation. Rogers (1983) used the term "diffusion" to describe the dissemination of an innovation. The theory proposes that diffusion of an innovation is enhanced by face-to-face and mass media communication channels, time, and interaction within the social system. Adoption of an innovation is enhanced by persuasion by a peer colleague or by influence from opinion leaders within the social system. An outside change agent also may facilitate diffusion and adoption of an innovation.

The perceived characteristics of the innovation affect favorable or unfavorable attitudes toward adoption. The probability and speed of adoption are enhanced if the staff perceives the innovation as being superior to current practice; the innovation is consistent with current values, experience, and priorities; the innovation is easy to learn, understand, or use, or can be tried out on a limited basis with the option of returning to previous practices; and the innovation causes visible results.

The Stetler Model of Evidence-Based Practice

Although Rogers' theory addresses the structure of diffusion of any innovation, including research findings, Stetler and Marram were early developers of models for incorporating research into clinical practice, and in 1976 developed the original Stetler/Marram Research Utilization Model. This model provided a decision tree for nursing students and nurses to follow before using research findings in practice (Stetler, 1994, 2001, 2010). The latest version of the model, which has been

renamed the **Stetler Model of Evidence-Based Practice** (Stetler, 2010), refers to a five-phase critical-thinking and decision-making process to assist the individual practitioner in using published research (Fig. 10.3).

Stetler (2010) describes each phase as follows:

- **Phase I—Preparation:** *Purpose, Context and Sources of Evidence*
  - **Potential Issues/Catalysts** = a problem, including unexplained variations; less-than-best practice; routine update of knowledge; validation/routine revision of procedures, etc.; or innovative program goal.
  - **Affirm/clarify perceived problem/s, with internal evidence** re: current practice [baseline]
  - **Consider other influential internal and external factors,** e.g. timelines
  - **Affirm and focus on high priority issues**
  - **Decide if need to form a team, involve formal stakeholders, and/or assign project lead/facilitator**
  - **Define desired, measurable outcome/s**
  - **Seek out systematic reviews/guidelines first**
  - **Determine need for an explicit type of research evidence, if relevant**
  - **Select research with conceptual fit**
- **Phase II—Validation:** *Credibility of Evidence and Potential for/Detailed Qualifiers of Application*
  - ***Critique & synopsize essential components, operational details, and other qualifying factors, per source**
    - *See instructions for use of utilization-focused review tables,* with evaluative criteria, to facilitate this task; fill in the tables for group decision making or potential future synthesis*
  - **Critique *systematic reviews and guidelines**
  - **Re-assess fit of individual sources**
  - ***Rate the level and quality of each individual evidence source per a "table of evidence"**
  - **Differentiate statistical and clinical significance**
  - **Eliminate non-credible sources**
  - **End the process if there is clearly insufficient, credible external evidence that meets your need**
- **Phase III—Comparative Evaluation/Decision Making:** *Synthesis and Decisions/Recommendations per Criteria of Applicability*
  - ***Synthesize the cumulative findings:**
    - *Logically organize display the similarities and differences across multiple findings, per common aspects or sub-elements of the topic under review*

---

*Stetler, Morsi, Rucki, et al. (1998). Utilization-focused integrative reviews in a nursing service. *Applied Nursing Research; 11*(4): 195–206 for noted tables, reviews, & synthesis process.

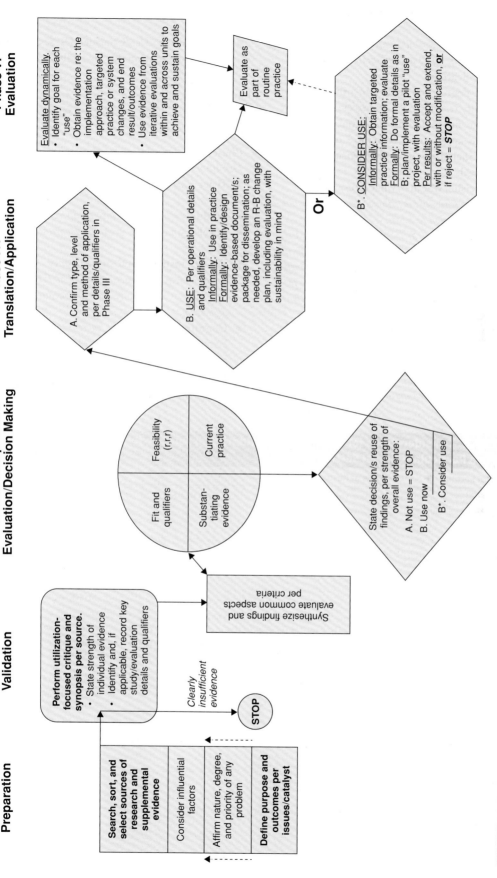

FIGURE 10.3 The Stetler model of evidence-based practice. (From Rycroft-Malone, J., & Bucknall, T. (Eds). (2010). *Models and frameworks for implementing evidence-based practice: Linking evidence to action* (1st ed.). Chichester, West Sussex, UK: Sigma Theta Tau International and Wiley-Blackwell. © Reprinted with permission from Cheryl Stetler.)

- *Evaluate degree of substantiation of each aspect/ sub-element; reference any qualifying conditions* **for application**
- **Evaluate degree and nature of other criteria: **feasibility (r, r, r = risk, resources, readiness); pragmatic fit, including potential qualifying factors to application; & nature of **current practice, including the urgency/risk of current issues/needs**
- **Make decision whether/what to use:**
  - **Can be a personal practitioner-level decision or a recommendation to others.*
  - **Judge strength of decision; indicate if primarily "research-based" (R-B) or, per hi use of supplemental info, "E-B"; note level of strength of recommendation/s per related* table; note any qualifying factors that may influence individualized variations*
- **If decision = "Not use" research findings:**
  - *May conduct own research or delay use till additional research done by others*
  - *If still decide to act now, e.g., on evidence of consensus or another basis for practice, consider need for similar planned change and evaluation*

- **If decision = "Use/Consider Use," can mean a recommendation for or against a specific practice**

(Table 10.3 presents considerations for examining the fit, flow, and feasibility of reported research that fit with phases II and III.)

- **Phase IV—Translation/application:** *Operational Definition of Use/Actions for Change*
  - **Types** = *cognitive/conceptual, symbolic and/or instrumental*
  - **Methods** = *informal or formal; direct or indirect*
  - **Levels** = *individual, group or department/organization*
  - **Direct instrumental use:** *change individual behavior (e.g., via assessment tool or Rx intervention options); or change policy, procedure, protocol, algorithm, program, etc.*
  - **Cognitive use:** *validate current practice; change personal way of thinking; increase awareness; better understand or appreciate condition/s or experience/s*
  - **Symbolic use:** *develop position paper or proposal for change; or persuade others regarding a way of thinking*

TABLE 10.3 Considerations for Preliminary Evaluation of Nursing Research for Use in a Particular Clinical Setting

Fit to Clinical Setting	Flow of Research Study	Feasibility of Adoption
The purpose of study fits the clinical area where findings may be adopted.	Research questions or hypothesis flows from the study's stated purpose.	The proposed innovation is legally permitted by the state nurse practice act.
The study sample represents clientele of the clinical setting.	Researcher follows all steps outlined in the research process.	The innovation is ethical practice.
Sample size is appropriate.	Variables are well defined.	Costs are acceptable to clients, third-party payers, or the institution.
The study enhances the fulfillment of the clinical area's mission.	Measurements for the variables make sense. Validity and reliability of variable measurements are presented. Efforts are made to control factors that might affect the results. Data are presented accurately. The correct statistics are used to answer the research question(s) or test the hypothesis(es): ■ Research purpose ■ Number and type of variables ■ Level of measurement for each variable The sample size is large enough to support the statistical test or researcher reports power level. Weaknesses of the study are reported. The study generates logical and accurate conclusions. Implications for practice logically flow from findings.	There is enough staff and time to fully execute the proposed innovation. The innovation is congruent with the nursing philosophy of the organization or unit. Risks to clients, nurses, and organization are considered. Needed resources are obtained. Staff is ready to adopt the proposed innovation.

Important Note: Do not change practice on the basis of the findings of one study. Similar findings from multiple studies indicate that the findings were more likely not to be the result of chance.

Burns, N., Grove, S. K., & Gray, J. (2013). *The practice of nursing research: Appraisal, synthesis & generation of evidence* (7th ed.). St. Louis, MO: Elsevier Saunders; Liehr, P., & Houston, S. (1993). Critiquing and using nursing research: Guidelines for the critical care nurse. *American Journal of Critical Care, 2,* 407–412.

- **CAUTION: Assess whether translation/product or use goes beyond actual findings/evidence:**
  - *Research evidence may or may not provide various details for a complete policy, procedure, etc.; indicate this fact to users, and note differential levels of evidence therein*
- **Formal dissemination and change strategies should be planned per relevant research and local barriers:**
  - *Passive education is usually not effective as an isolated strategy. Use Dx analysis** and an ***implementation frame work to develop a plan. Consider multiple strategies; e.g., opinion leaders, interactive education, reminders, and audits.*
  - *Focus on context[&] to enhance sustainability of organizational-related change*
- **Consider need for appropriate, reasoned variation**
- **WITH B, where made a decision to use in the setting:**
  - *With formal use, may need a dynamic evaluation to effectively implement and continuously improve/refine use of best available evidence across units and time*
- **WITH B', where made decision to** consider use **and thus obtain additional, pragmatic info before a final decision:**
  - *With formal consideration, do a pilot project*
  - *With a pilot project, must assess if need IRB review, per relevant institutional criteria*
- **Phase V—Evaluation:** Alternative Evaluation
- **Evaluation per type, method, level: e.g., consider conceptual use at individual level****
- **Consider cost-benefit of change + various evaluation efforts**
- **Use RU-as-a-process to enhance credibility of evaluation data**
- **For both dynamic and pilot evaluations, include:**
  - ***formative, regarding actual implementation & goal progress*
  - *Summative, regarding identified end-goal and end-point outcomes*
- **NOTE:** Model applies to all forms of practice, i.e., educational, clinical, managerial, or other; **to use effectively read 2001 & 1994 model papers.**

**Stetler et al. (2006) re: dx analysis

***E.g.: Rogers' re: implications of attributes of a change; Rycroft-Malone et al. & PARIHS (2002) & Green & Krueter's PRECEDE (1992) models re: implementation ^{&&}Stetler, 2003 on context & ^{&&}Stetler & ^{&&}Caramanica (2007) on outcomes.

Concepts in Practice, "Stetler Model of Evidence-Based Practice in Action," returns to the example of Tony and his colleagues and shows how these elements may be implemented.

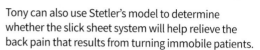

Concepts in Practice

Stetler Model of Evidence-Based Practice in Action

Tony can also use Stetler's model to determine whether the slick sheet system will help relieve the back pain that results from turning immobile patients.

- **Phase I:** Tony identifies the problems of increased back strain, reviews reasons for it within his institution, networks with nurses who work elsewhere, clarifies the problem and surrounding factors, decides that reducing back strain is a very high priority, forms an EBP team that includes coworkers, conducts a literature search, and selects relevant sources to review and critique.
- **Phase II:** Tony's team analyzes acquired resources, critiques the research studies, and based on the findings, identifies the slick sheet system as a feasible way to reduce back strain as staff turns clients in bed.
- **Phase III:** Tony and the team prepare a proposal to administration to support the evidence-based way to move patients differently. The manufacturer of the slick sheet system agrees to provide a unit demonstration and several sheet systems for the staff to use during the evidence-based project.
- **Phase IV:** Tony and his team decide that the slick sheet system should become the policy when turning patients in bed. The manufacturer provides six slick sheet systems for the unit to use in its pilot project and educates the staff on safe, effective use of the product. The team develops a daily log for the staff to complete regarding how frequently they turn patients with and without the slick sheet system and their level of back strain after turning patients. Before implementing the project, they submit a proposal to the IRB, which expedites the process because it identifies no potential harm to patients. The pilot study is implemented.
- **Phase V:** Tony and the team have unit staff use the slick sheet system for 2 months and provide data. They analyze the data and discover that when staff uses the slick sheet system for turning bedridden patients, they report a 50% reduction in back strain. The decision is made by the nurse manager to extend the pilot study to other units of the hospital to see if similar results occur before implementing the process of changing clinical practice policies and procedures through the established shared governance processes.

Facilitators of Research Utilization and Evidence-Based Practice

The process of research utilization is a continual one. Advances in the health science arena mean that nurses must stay abreast of changes in their clinical practice areas. New theoretical developments in nursing result in different approaches to client assessments, nursing interventions, and outcome evaluation. Nursing research utilization success relies on a variety of factors that facilitate use of research findings in practice.

Many factors influence the utilization of nursing research in clinical practice. **Research utilization and EBP facilitators** are any factors that promote the use of research-based knowledge and other forms of evidence in clinical practice. Individual nurse and employing organization factors can facilitate research utilization and EBP in the clinical practice setting. Estabrooks, Floyd, Scott-Findlay, O'Leary, and Gushta (2003)

identified six categories of possible individual nurse factors that promoted research utilization and EBP from a review of 22 studies (Table 10.4).

In 2007, Estabrooks and colleagues developed a three-tier multilevel model to predict research utilization and again noted that individual nurse factors contributed to research utilization. Cultivating these characteristics in all professional nurses remains a challenge for the profession. They also discovered that nurses employed in larger hospitals tended to use research more than nurses employed in other settings (Estabrooks, Midodzi, Cummings, & Wallin, 2007).

Organizational factors also serve as facilitators to research utilization by nurses. Research utilization efforts are time intensive and require use of human and financial resources. Nursing research utilization also requires organizational commitment. The following strategies to facilitate research utilization and EBP in nursing departments have been used with some success.

TABLE 10.4   Individual Nurse Facilitators for Research Utilization and Evidence-Based Practice

Main Category	Facilitator
Beliefs and attitudes toward nursing research	Positive attitude toward nursing research Self-expectation to use nursing research in practice Interest in nursing research Lower levels of emotional exhaustion
Involvement with research activities	Perceived availability of research findings Current collaboration or past participation on a research project Collecting data for other researchers Participation in a research study as a subject or participant Previous use of nursing research Experience with the research process
Information-seeking behaviors	Reading nursing journals as the top information source to stay current in practice Regular reading of professional journals (*Nursing Research, American Journal of Nursing*) Subscribing to professional journals More time spent studying while off duty Use of nursing school as a resource for nursing research materials and information Increased use of the internet
Education level	Education preparation in the research utilization process Attendance at professional nursing conferences Attendance at more staff in-services BSN or higher degree Perception of being well prepared in the education process Completion of a research and/or statistics course
Professional characteristics	Perceived organizational support for research utilization activities Perception of an organizational policy for research use Increased number of years' experience in a nursing specialty area or clinical unit Nursing leadership or advanced practice nursing role Membership in the American Nurses Association Certification from the Oncology Nursing Society
Socioeconomic factors	Younger age

Adapted from Estabrooks, C., Floyd, J., Scott-Findlay, S., O'Leary, K., & Gushta, M. (2003). Individual determinants of research utilization: A systematic review. *Journal of Advanced Nursing, 43,* 506–520; Estabrooks, C., Midodzi, W., Cummings, G., & Wallin, L. (2007). Predicting research use in nursing organizations: A multilevel analysis. *Nursing Research, 56*(4, Suppl. 1), S7–S23.

- Clear expectation of research utilization as part of a job description.
- Staff educational programs on the process of research utilization.
- Incentives, such as promotions or salary increases.
- Formation of nursing research/research utilization committees.
- Provision of time for nurses to read research reports while on duty.
- Clinical career ladders requiring research utilization as criteria for promotion and maintenance of organizational position.
- Organizational support to defray expenses for research utilization projects.
- Formalized collaboration between nursing service and academia.
- Library services for nurses to use to perform computerized literature searches and access needed materials.
- Nursing unit–based libraries and nursing journal subscriptions.
- Sponsorship of nurses to attend professional nursing conferences.

Characteristics of published research studies also serve as facilitators of research utilization and EBP in nursing. Because many nurse researchers may not engage in clinical practice on a regular basis, performing clinically relevant studies may be challenging. However, nothing captures the interest of professional nurses better than a study that demonstrates substantial improvements in client outcomes or working environments. A well-written research study using clear, concise language enhances the ability of all nurses to read and understand published nursing research studies.

Barriers to Research Utilization and Evidence-Based Practice

Research utilization and EBP barriers are any factors that block or impede the use of research findings in clinical practice. Abrahamson, Fox, and Doebbeling

FOCUS ON RESEARCH

Facilitators and Barriers to Research Utilization in Practice

The investigators of this study sought to identify nurse perceptions of the facilitators and barriers to using evidence-based clinical practice guidelines in Veterans Administration Medical Centers. They used free-text responses to two open-ended survey questions asking the nurses about facilitating factors and barriers to using clinical practice guidelines on a daily basis. They received 575 completed surveys from the nurses.

Results of the study included the identification of internal and external factors that either promoted or obstructed the use of clinical practice guidelines. The researchers defined nurse attitude as an individual nurse's perception that guidelines facilitated clinical decision making or that the nurse did not have the willingness or flexibility to change practice habits and only five nurses in the study indicated this a reason for not using clinical practice guidelines. Information overload was identified as an internal barrier to guideline use. External factors that impeded use identified by 15% or more of the nurses included workload and staffing issues, lack of education and training opportunities, inadequate communication, and lack of administrative support. External factors that promoted research utilization identified by 15% of more of the nurses included effective education/training/orientation, good communication, accommodations to workload, time and staffing to implement new guidelines, administrative support, and staff input into the development of clinical practice guidelines. Other supportive factors included the assistance of other health team members, a perception that guidelines were current and accurate, having the required resources for implementation, and ease of access to the practice guidelines.

The facilitators and barriers to clinical practice guideline use in this study closely mirror the results of previous research. The clinical significance of this study reveals that nurses need education, time, resources, and support for implementing evidence-based clinical guidelines in daily practice. If research utilization is to be implemented successfully, communication of changes in clinical practice guidelines and attention to work and information overload issues are essential.

Abrahamson, K., Fox, R., & Doebbeling, B. (2012). Facilitators and barriers to clinical practice guideline use among nurses. *American Journal of Nursing, 112*(7), 26–35.

(2012), Goode et al. (1991), Rutledge, Mooney, Grant, and Easton (2004), and Funk, Champagne, Wiese, and Tornquist (1991) identified a number of barriers to research utilization and EBP, including barriers from researchers, practicing nurses, and the health care agency administration (Focus on Research, "Facilitators and Barriers to Research Utilization in Practice").

Researchers

Barriers to research utilization which result from the nature of disseminated research studies include the following.

- Insufficient current research with solutions to address today's complex clinical problems.
- Failure of replicated research studies.
- Research reports that are difficult to read.
- Many unpublished or nondisseminated research reports (especially studies done to meet graduate and postgraduate program requirements).
- Lack of a central repository for nursing research studies.

Nursing practice should not be changed on the basis of a single study because of potential confounding factors that may have caused the study results. Unfortunately, few replication studies appear in the nursing literature. Either nurses are not performing replication studies or they are not being accepted for publication when they are submitted.

Practicing Nurses

Barriers to research utilization and EBP based on characteristics of practicing nurses include the following.

- Lack of education in how to read, critique, conduct, and use research.
- Negative attitudes among practicing nurses about using research findings in practice.
- Not enough time or commitment to implement research utilization projects.
- Failure of nurses to read nursing research articles or journals.
- Inability of nurses to understand statistical analyses contained within studies.
- Comfort with practice based on tradition, which is difficult to change, even if it is ineffective.
- Difficulty determining whether studies are well designed and scientifically sound.
- Isolation from knowledgeable colleagues who could assist them in understanding research studies.

Nursing research utilization and EBP require much time and deep commitment. In today's society, many nurses assume multiple roles that compete for their attention. Even though practice based on sound science is preferred, changing personal attitudes and the status quo remains difficult.

The Nurse Researcher

Barriers arising from nurse researcher characteristics include the following.

- Submission of studies for publication to journals not read widely by most nurses.
- Use of research jargon in publications which is not understood by practicing nurses.
- Failure to offer realistic implications for clinical practice because of either lack of patient care experience or current clinical experience.
- Presentation of findings in a format not conducive to clinical implementation.

Failure to understand statistics serves as another barrier to research utilization and EBP. Researchers sometimes manipulate statistics to distort the truth (Abrahamson et al., 2012; Best, 2001). Because the average nurse does not comprehend statistical tests presented in a research study, the nurse accepts the studies' reported findings, even though the authors might have made implausible claims. A common misconception related to statistics is that they "prove" something. A critical approach to statistics avoids the extremes of naïve acceptance and cynical rejection. When reading statistics, the research consumer must realize that researchers choose variable definitions, instruments for data collection, and samples for a variety of reasons (Best, 2001). Reported statistics represent a compromise among various choices that researchers make during a study (see Box 10.8, Professional Building Blocks, "Analyzing the Reliability of Research Study Data").

Take Note!
Statistics found in research reports must be analyzed critically before they are accepted as truth.

Health Care Agency Administration

Barriers to research utilization and EBP from the health care agency administration include the following.

- Minimal value placed on research by administrators and managers.
- No provision made for resources such as time, financial support, and education.

10.8 Professional Building Blocks

Analyzing the Reliability of Research Study Data

To determine whether the findings of a research study are reliable, ask yourself the following questions about the statistics used.

- Do they answer the question or issue outlined in the purpose of the study?
- What is the level of measurement of the research variables contained in the study?
- How many independent and dependent variables appear in the study?
- Is the sample size large enough to effectively use the statistical test?
- What instruments were used to collect data, and what is the level of measurement that these instruments generate?
- How might the sampling techniques affect the study results?
- Are comparisons appropriate if comparisons are being made?
- How have the figures been generated, and have any techniques been used to alter the appearance of the data?
- What stakes does the researcher have if the statistical tests used are not significant?

Instead of being awestruck or overwhelmed by complex statistical tests found in research reports, nurses should read for logical, feasible, and appropriate findings. Many advanced practice nurses find great rewards in helping staff nurses understand research reports.

- Lack of nursing autonomy within a bureaucratic structure to implement data-based solutions to problems.
- Lack of incentives for nurses to participate in research utilization activities.
- Reliance on established policy and procedures, rather than openness to change.
- Lack of support for implementation of research findings by physicians and other staff.

Strategies to Facilitate Research Utilization and Evidence-Based Practice

In BSN programs, students are exposed to the basic steps of the research process and how to effectively critique studies for use in clinical practice. Most BSN graduates have a basic understanding of research terminology, and some (though not all) can read and understand published research reports containing basic statistical analysis techniques (Hunt, 2001). Nursing students and professionals gain confidence and expertise in reading and understanding research with continual practice. Graduate nurses focus on acquiring clinical competence and spend little or no time reading nursing research reports. Rutledge et al. (2004) found that when oncology nurses received formal education in research utilization, they could master the process well enough to design and implement nursing research utilization projects in clinical settings.

Researchers should make an effort to write for practicing nurses and to emphasize the meaning of the findings for practice in language that is understandable by most nurses (Hunt, 2001). Consultation with a nurse holding a master's or doctorate degree serves as a useful method for understanding and interpreting complex statistical analyses. Some clinical agencies employ a nursing research facilitator for staff consultation. Nursing faculty and graduate students may also be a source of research consultation services. A team of nurses could work together with a consultant in locating and interpreting relevant literature to address a clinical issue or to answer a PICOT question. Finally, some institutions have implemented a clinical scholar program that pairs staff nurses with research mentors to develop and implement nursing research studies or research utilization and EBP projects.

To use research findings, practicing nurses must read professional journals, including academic research journals (Box 10.9, Professional Building Blocks, "Nursing Journals That Emphasize Research"). Other means of finding research articles pertinent to one's areas of nursing practice is to use electronic databases such as Medline or the Cumulative Index of Nursing and Allied Health Literature (CINAHL). Many hospitals have a basic medical (or health sciences) library that includes a core collection of nursing journals. Nurses also may visit local college, university, or public libraries. To save time, nurses should look for integrative reviews or meta-analyses that review a number of studies and provide information about the quality of the results.

Nurses can also obtain access to research findings through research bulletin boards, newsletters, or research grand rounds, but these strategies need to be organized, maintained, and supported. Many institutions have a research committee that can take responsibility for coordinating the review of literature, exploring ideas, pilot-testing innovations, and developing and disseminating research-based protocols and policies.

10.9 Professional Building Blocks

Nursing Journals that Emphasize Research

The following publications are excellent sources of nursing research and associated content.

Research Findings and Methodologic Issues

- *Nursing Research*
- *Western Journal of Nursing Research*
- *International Journal of Nursing Research*

Publication of Research and Nursing Theory

- *Journal of Nursing Scholarship*
- *Journal of Advanced Nursing*
- *Nursing Science Quarterly*
- *Advances in Nursing Science*

Evidence and Research for Clinical Nursing Practice

- *Nursing in Research and Health*
- *International Journal of Nursing Studies*
- *Clinical Nursing Research*
- *Applied Nursing Research*
- *Evidence-Based Nursing*

General Nursing Journal with Research as a Regular Feature

- *The American Journal of Nursing* (official publication of the American Nurses Association)

Nurses also may find the in-service education or nursing staff development departments useful when seeking to establish nursing practice based on research. Master's-prepared clinical educators could evaluate and synthesize knowledge across studies and provide direction for clinicians. Some agencies offer nurses continuing education on research processes; developing a research, research utilization, or EBP project; performing effective literature searches; evaluating the quality of research; understanding data analysis; and determining the relevance of research findings for EBP nursing policies and procedures.

Even where resources are readily available to nurses, agency managers and administration must create an atmosphere where nurses are encouraged and supported to question and evaluate current practice protocols, to use research study findings as a basis for protocol revisions, and to be valued (and even rewarded) for using research in practice. Without a supportive environment, nurses who use research in practice may become discouraged and rely on agency traditions, or they may leave the work setting for an agency that supports research utilization. Managers and administrators who use research and current literature in their positions serve as role models for research utilization and EBP.

When research utilization and EBP become valued as a way of knowing, positive attitudes and tangible resources for research utilization become standard practice. To show that they value research utilization and EBP, managers and administrators must provide the resources to nurses to develop and conduct studies. Required resources depend upon the type of study to be conducted. Nurses planning and conducting studies need access to computerized databases, financial support for consulting with nurse researchers and statisticians, and release time from patient care duties. Incentives and rewards for risk taking and creativity promote research utilization. Fostering peer collaboration and networking with other colleagues also provide impetus for research use in practice. Most of all, the atmosphere must be one of respect and encouragement for professional practice and delegation of authority so that nurses control nursing practice.

In the final analysis, the clinician has to value the use of research as the basis for practice enough to put forth the time and effort required for research utilization activities. Only when a significant number of nurses value scholarship enough to participate in its creation, dissemination, and utilization will nursing be viewed as a true profession.

CREATING A PUBLIC IMAGE OF THE NURSE AS SCHOLAR

A **scholar** is an intellectual who has undertaken advanced study in a given field. Public perceptions of nurses tend toward the nurse as a person with technical expertise, a subordinate to physicians, and as one who cares for others. However, a visit to a college or university today reveals the strides the nursing profession has made in developing a unique research base and expert researchers.

Advanced technology offers great support for today's nurse researcher. The storage, retrieval, and analysis of data afforded by computer support make conducting research much faster and more achievable by nurses. Many professional nursing journals are published in print and electronic (online) versions. In most educational and practice settings, a researcher should not have to manage data manually. Computer programs can be used to manipulate numbers, facilitating almost unlimited analysis of data and the ability to use research findings to a fuller capacity. Laptops, smart phones, and the internet facilitate the rapid sharing and dissemination of research findings with those in practice.

Traditionally, nurses have not been viewed as scholars. Some nurses fail to acknowledge the advanced education of colleagues. Some health care agencies refuse to place academic credentials on nurses' employment name badges. The public perception of nursing is highly affected by individual experience with nurses. With approximately 60% of nurses having less-than-BSN preparation, nurses remain among the least educated members of the interdisciplinary health care team. Nurses and clients tend to value clinical practice over nursing scholarship. However, when (and if) nurses communicate to others the contributions of nursing research to health outcomes, the nursing profession will attain recognition as a scholarly, rather than an exclusively practice, discipline.

As nursing has developed its own theory base during the past 50 years, nurses have begun to value nursing scholarship. Most nurses today probably would agree that a practice based on research is desirable. Capitalizing on that consensus, the profession can begin to present a different image to the public. To help actualize the motivation to base nursing practice on research, educational programs need to prepare students in scientific inquiry while preparing them to apply theory in professional practice.

In 1993, the NINR was established, replacing the National Center for Nursing Research. Separating the NINR from the National Institutes of Health and making it a free-standing institute acknowledges the unique contribution of nursing science and research to the health of American citizens.

"The mission of the NINR is to promote and improve the health of individuals, families, communities, and populations. The institute supports and conducts clinical and basic research and research training on health and illness across the lifespan to build the scientific foundation for clinical practice, prevent disease and disability, manage and eliminate symptoms caused by illness, and improve palliative and end-of-life care. NINR's goal is to enhance nursing science and health care by integrating the biologic and behavioral sciences, applying new technologies, promoting health equity, and developing scientists of the future." (NINR, 2011a, p. 4)

The NINR identifies nursing research priorities, distributes grants to nurse researchers, and disseminates nursing research findings to health professionals and the public.

Current focus areas for research for the NINR include health promotion, disease prevention, quality-of-life improvement, health disparities elimination, and directions for end-of-life research (NINR, 2011b). Funding for the NINR has risen steadily since its inception. The NINR is funded through Section 301, Title IV of the National Public Service Act. For fiscal year 2016, the NINR received $146.485 million in federal funding (NINR, 2016). Public funding of nursing research acknowledges the valuable contributions it makes to all Americans.

As nurses begin to feel and act like scholars, the public will acknowledge the scholarly side of nursing. If the profession nourishes this scholarship in nurses, it undoubtedly will help change the image of the nurse. Because scholars accept that research is a vital component of nursing, the development of scholars will increase the supply of researchers to better serve the profession and the public.

QUESTIONS FOR REFLECTION

1. How can you promote the image of nurses as scholars?
2. What are the potential consequences of changing the image of the nurse from caregiver to scholar?

Summary and Significance to Practice

From the 1960s to 1990s, many researchers and scholars generated clinically relevant research for use in practice. Nurses gradually saw the benefits of using research findings in practice. By the early 21st century, nurses began to routinely incorporate research findings and other form of evidence to improve client outcomes and contain costs. Nurses use multiple cognitive skills to navigate the vast web of information and decide how to use available research findings and various forms of evidence in clinical practice. With practice, nurses gain confidence in their ability to analyze, critique, and decide how and when to use evidence in clinical practice. Qualitative and quantitative research findings provide evidence that captures the complex, holistic nature of clients, nurses, and health care delivery. Recent public funding of nursing research initiatives shows that the public values nursing research. As nurses assume the roles of researcher and scholar, they make discoveries, generate evidence, and determine how to incorporate the best possible evidence to guide and change clinical practice in today's complex and sometimes chaotic health care delivery systems.

REAL-LIFE REFLECTIONS

Recall Jessica and Malika from the beginning of the chapter. What strategies would you suggest for Jessica to use in her attempts to integrate research-based knowledge about alternative forms of pain control on her unit? Outline a research utilization project for Jessica to follow.

From Theory to Practice

1. What forms of evidence are used as a foundation for current clinical policies and procedures in your area of clinical practice?
2. Has your perception as a nursing student changed about the profession of nursing now that you have read about all the evidence and research behind clinical practice? Why or why not?
3. How would you differentiate research utilization from EBP?
4. In addition to your instructor, who might you turn to for help or what resources might you use if you had difficulty making sense of a published research study?

Nurse as Author

Identify a clinical problem that you have encountered in practice. Using the PICOT format presented in the chapter, generate a question for an EBP project. Perform a literature using a computerized literature database and enter the search terms by combining the terms outlined in your PICOT question. Write a one-page paper describing the literature search terms that you entered, which computerized literature database that you used and how many articles you obtained when you completed the search.

Your Digital Classroom

Online Exploration

Agency for Healthcare Research and Quality: **www.ahrq.gov**
American Nurses Foundation: **www.anfonline.org/**
Canadian Foundation for Healthcare Improvement: **www.cfhi-fcass.ca/Home.aspx**
Centers for Disease Control and Prevention: **www.cdc.gov**
Midwestern Nursing Research Society: **www.mnrs.org**

National Guideline Clearinghouse: **guideline.gov/**
National Institute of Nursing Research: **https:www.ninr.nih.gov**
Nursing Health Services Research Unit: **http://fhs.mcmaster.ca/nru/mission.htm**
Southern Nursing Research Society: **www.snrs.org**
The Cochrane Collaboration: **www.cochrane.org**

Expanding Your Understanding

1. Visit the NINR website, and read about the group's mission and strategic plan. Identify the research priorities of the NINR and bring them to class for discussion.
2. Peruse the online version of the journal Evidence-Based Nursing (**http://ebn.bmj.com/**). Read one or two free selections from the journal, and answer the following questions.
   a. Do you believe the content contained in the summary of each research article and the commentary that follows it?
   b. What are the advantages of reading an entire research report?
   c. What are the disadvantages of reading an entire research report?
   d. Would you use information found in this journal in your clinical practice? Why or why not?
3. Visit the Integrity in Science website at **www.cspinet.org/integrity/**. Find a list of what corporations are currently funding or have funded research in nursing and health care.

Beyond the Book

Visit **thePoint® www.thePoint.lww.com** for activities and information to reinforce the concepts and content covered in this chapter.

REFERENCES

Abrahamson, K., Fox, R., & Doebbeling, B. (2012). Facilitators and barriers to clinical practice guideline use among nurses. *American Journal of Nursing, 112*(7), 26–35.

Academic Center for Evidence-Based Practice. (2009). ACE star model of knowledge transformation. Retrieved from http://www.acestar.uthscsa.edu/acestar-model.asp. Accessed December 15, 2012.

American Association of Colleges of Nursing. (2008). The essentials of baccalaureate education for professional nursing practice. Retrieved from http://www.aacn.nche.edu/education-resources/BaccEssentials08.pdf. Accessed December 15, 2012.

American Nurses Association. (2010). *Nursing scope and standards of practice* (2nd ed.). Silver Spring, MD: Author.

Artinian, B. A. (1988). Qualitative modes of inquiry. *Western Journal of Nursing Research, 10,* 138–149.

Baessler, C. A., Blumberg, M., Cunningham, J. S., Curran, J. A., Fennessey, A. G., Jacobs, J. M., et al. (1994). Medical-surgical nurses' utilization of research methods and products. *Medsurg Nursing, 3,* 113–117, 120–121, 141.

Barrett, E. A. M. (2002). What is nursing science? *Nursing Science Quarterly, 15,* 51–60.

Best, J. (2001). Telling the truth about damned lies and statistics. *The Chronicle of Higher Education, 47,* B7–B9.

Blumenstyk, G. (2001). A new web site details the corporate ties of some researchers. *The Chronicle of Higher Education, 47,* A25.

Boswell, C., & Cannon, S. (2007). *Introduction to nursing research: Incorporating evidence-based practice.* Sudbury, MA: Jones & Bartlett.

Burns, N., Grove, S. K., & Gray, J. (2013). *The practice of nursing research: Appraisal, synthesis & generation of evidence* (7th ed.). St. Louis, MO: Elsevier Saunders.

Cohen, M. Z., & Tripp-Reimer, T. (1988). Research in cultural diversity: Qualitative methods in cultural research. *Western Journal of Nursing Research, 10,* 226–228.

DiCenso, A., Guyatt, G., & Ciliska, D. (2005). *Evidence-based nursing: A guide to clinical practice.* St. Louis, MO: Elsevier/ Mosby.

Estabrooks, C., Floyd, J., Scott-Findlay, S., O'Leary, K., & Gushta, M. (2003). Individual determinants of research utilization: A systematic review. *Journal of Advanced Nursing, 43,* 506–520.

Estabrooks, C., Midodzi, W., Cummings, G., & Wallin, L. (2007). Predicting research use in nursing organizations: A multilevel analysis. *Nursing Research, 56*(4, Suppl 1), S7–S23.

Funk, S. G., Champagne, M. T., Wiese, R. A., & Tornquist, E. M. (1991). Barriers to using research findings in practice: The clinician's perspective. *Applied Nursing Research, 4,* 90–95.

Gennaro, S. (1994). Research utilization: An overview. *Journal of Obstetric, Gynecologic, & Neonatal Nursing, 23,* 313–319.

Glanville, I., Schirm, V., & Wineman, N. M. (2000). Using evidence-based practice for managing clinical outcomes in advanced practice nursing. *Journal of Nursing Care Quality, 15,* 1–11.

Goode, C. J., Butcher, L. A., Cipperley, J. A., Exstrom, J., Gosh, B., Hayes, J., et al. (1991). *Research utilization: A study guide [video recording].* Ida Grove, IA: Horn Video Productions.

Goode, C. J., & Piedalue, F. (1999). Evidence-based clinical practice. *Journal of Nursing Administration, 29,* 15–21.

Haase, J. E., & Myers, S. T. (1988). Reconciling paradigm assumptions of qualitative and quantitative research. *Western Journal of Nursing Research, 10,* 128–137.

Hunt, J. (2001). Research into practice: The foundation for evidence-based care. *Cancer Nursing, 24,* 78–87.

Kirrane, C. (2000). Evidence-based practice in neurology: A team approach to development. *Nursing Standard, 14,* 43–45.

Knafl, K. A., & Webster, D. C. (1988). Managing and analyzing qualitative data: A description of tasks, techniques, and materials. *Western Journal of Nursing Research, 10,* 195–218.

Malloch, K., & Porter-O'Grady, T. (2006). *Introduction to evidence-based practice in nursing and health care.* Sudbury, MA: Jones & Bartlett.

McDonald, L. (2001). Florence Nightingale and the early origins of evidence-based nursing. *Evidence-Based Nursing, 4,* 68–69.

Retrieved from http://ebn.bmjjournals.com/content/vol4/ issue3/. Accessed December 15, 2012.

Melnyk, B., & Fineout-Overholt, E. (2011). *Evidence-based practice in nursing and healthcare: A guide to best practice* (2nd ed.). Philadelphia, PA: Lippincott Williams & Wilkins.

Melnyk, B., & Fineout-Overholt, E. (2015). *Evidence-based practice in nursing and healthcare: A guide to best practice* (3rd ed.). Philadelphia, PA: Wolters-Kluwer.

National Guideline Clearinghouse (NGC). (2008). Help & About. Retrieved from http://guideline.gov/about/index. aspx. Accessed December 15, 2012.

National Institute of Nursing Research. (2011a). Mission and strategic plan. Retrieved from https://www.ninr.nih.gov/ aboutninr/ninr-mission-and-strategic-plan#.VxQYsfkrLrc Accessed April 17, 2016.

National Institute of Nursing Research. (2011b). Bringing science to life, NINR strategic plan. Retrieved from https://www. ninr.nih.gov/sites/www.ninr.nih.gov/files/ninr-strategic-plan-2011.pdf Accessed April 17, 2016.

National Institute of Nursing Research. (2016). FY 2017 Budget. Retrieved from https://www.ninr.nih.gov/sites/default/files/ NINR_CJ_FINAL.pdf. Accessed April 17, 2016.

Nightingale, F. (1860). *Notes on nursing.* New York: Appleton.

Polit, D. F., & Beck, C. (2012). *Nursing research: Generating and assessing evidence for nursing practice* (9th ed.). Philadelphia, PA: Wolters Kluwer Health/Lippincott Williams & Wilkins.

Rogers, E. (1983). *Diffusion of innovations* (3rd ed.). New York: Free Press.

Rogers, E. (1995). *Diffusion of innovations* (4th ed.). New York: Free Press.

Rutledge, D., Mooney, K., Grant, M., & Easton, L. (2004). Implementation and refinement of a research utilization course for oncology nurses. *Oncology Nursing Forum, 31,* 121–126.

Rycroft-Maline, J., & Bucknall, T. (Eds.) (2010). *Models and frameworks for implementing evidence-base practice: Linking evidence to action.* Chichester, West Sussex: Sigma Theta Tau International and Wiley-Blackwell.

Sherwood, G., & Barnsteiner, J. (2009). *Quality and safety in nursing a competency approach to improving outcomes.* West Sussex: Wiley-Blackwell.

Stetler, C. B. (1994). Refinement of the Stetler/Marram model for application of research findings to practice. *Nursing Outlook, 42,* 15–25.

Stetler, C. B. (2001). Updating the Stetler model of research utilization to facilitate evidence-base practice. *Nursing Outlook, 49,* 272–279.

Stetler, C. B. (2010). Stetler model. In J. Rycroft-Maline & T. Bucknall (Eds.), *Models and frameworks for implementing evidence-base practice: Linking evidence to action.* Chichester, West Sussex: Sigma Theta Tau International and Wiley-Blackwell.

Theou, O., Soon, Z., Filek, S., Brims, M., Leach-Macleod, K., Binsted, G., et al. (2011). Changing the sheets: A new system to reduce strain during patient repositioning. *Nursing Research, 60,* 302–308. doi: 10.1097/NNR.0b013e-318225b8aa.

Titler, M., Kleiber, C., Steelman, V., Rakel, B. A., Budreau, G., Everett, L. Q., et al. (2001). The Iowa model of evidence-based practice to promote quality care. *Critical Care Nursing Clinics of North America, 13,* 497–509.

11

Multicultural Issues in Professional Practice

LEARNING OUTCOMES

By the end of this chapter, the learner will be able to:

1. Discuss diversity and assimilation issues for a shrinking world.
2. Compare and contrast theoretical frameworks addressing cultural competence in nursing practice.
3. Differentiate between transculturalism and multiculturalism.
4. Specify strategies to address special cultural needs of nursing care consumers.
5. Outline strategies to foster a multicultural nursing profession.
6. Specify ways to enhance working relationships among multicultural health team members.

REAL-LIFE REFLECTIONS

Judy, a hospital nurse administrator, cannot get US-born nurses to work in the small rural hospital where she's employed. The hospital has decided to send her and a group of nurses to the Philippines to recruit Filipino nurses. Although she has reservations about hiring Filipino nurses and paying them for relocation, education, and licensure expenditures, Judy knows that she needs more registered nurses (RNs) to provide effective client care. Judy wonders how her current RNs will respond to having to work with nurses from another country, especially after they discover that the hospital has spent a lot of money to attract and hire the Filipino nurses. She also worries about the potential language and cultural barriers that might surface.

- *How do you think Judy should address the concerns about her staff working with the Filipino nurses?*
- *What might Judy do to ensure that the Filipino nurses feel welcome in the hospital and in the local community?*

Technology and transportation systems create opportunities for people to experience the world. Technology enables instant communication despite vast differences in locale. Modern transportation systems allow people to travel halfway around the world in a day, allowing individuals from different nations to meet each other easily and for the breakdown of cultural barriers.

Health care in the United States is highly consumer driven. In 2000, the Office of Minority health published the first National Standards for Culturally and Linguistically Appropriate Services for Health Care (the national CLAS standards) in response to the increasingly diversity of the American people. They became part of a requirement for Joint Commission Accreditation of Health Care Organizations standards of accreditation in 2006. In 2010, the standards underwent revisions to enhance cultural sensitive health care delivery with a specific aim to reduce disparities in health and access to services. These standards require health care organizations (HCOs) to provide culturally sensitive health care, including foreign language interpreters for people who do not speak or fully comprehend English. In addition, HCOs must also periodically survey the communities they serve and strive to employ health care providers (HCPs) that mirror the local community demographics. The national CLAS standards also holds HCOs accountable for educating staff about culturally sensitive care, posting signs in the languages of frequently encountered clients, working toward promoting people from diverse backgrounds into leadership positions, and monitoring the effectiveness of culturally sensitive and interpreter services. These standards also set criteria for the involvement of people from local cultural groups to assist in designing and implementing cultural and linguistic services. HCOs are required to inform the culturally diverse consumer about available language interpretation services, including written materials about available services and how to initiate conflict resolution and grievance processes if culturally insensitive care or inappropriate situations should arise (U.S. Department of Health and Human Services, 2010). Effective nursing care includes meeting the special cultural care and language needs of clients.

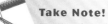

Take Note!
Meeting the cultural care and language needs of clients is essential for effective nursing care.

DIVERSITY AND ASSIMILATION IN A SHRINKING WORLD

American culture values unity and equality. The United States consists of many immigrants who assimilated into one culture. In the United States, people tend to identify themselves in terms of economic status and geographical locale. However, sometimes as people lose their ethnic identity they yearn for it more. Some people from immigrant backgrounds often speak their native language when they are at home, when they are with people from the same cultural background, and when they encounter stressful situations.

Historically, people from all parts of the world have sought refuge or a new home in the United States. In the first half of the 20th century, immigrants fled from religious persecution and economic and political turmoil in Eastern Europe, often hiding their ethnic roots by anglicizing their names. After World War II, many people from Eastern Europe and the Soviet Union came to the United States to escape communism. The American withdrawal from Vietnam resulted in increased immigration from Southeast Asian nations.

In recent years, people from Mexico and South America have sought economic refuge in the United States. Figure 11.1 outlines the cultural diversity in the United States according to the U.S. Census Bureau (2011). From 2000 to 2010, the populations of all ethnic groups grew in the United States, with Asians having the fastest growth rate (43%) and the Caucasian/white group having the slowest growth rate (12%). The exclusively Caucasian group lost 3% in terms of proportion of the total population, and growth in all other groups accounted for this proportional loss. The Black/African American population had the smallest percentage growth (1%), and the Hispanic/Latino group accounted for the second largest percentage increase (4.9%). According to the U.S. Census Bureau (2016), there is one birth every 8 seconds, one death every 12 seconds, and one international migrant entering the nation every 28 seconds.

The cultural background of HCPs does not mirror the demographics of American citizens. In recent years, strides are being made to improve the cultural diversity of health care professionals. The Sullivan Commission (2004) on Diversity in the Healthcare Workforce identified that only 9% of nurses, 6% of physicians, and 5% of dentists came from diverse cultural groups. According to the 2013 *National Workforce Survey of Registered Nurses* conducted by the National Council of State Boards of Nursing and the Forum of State Nursing Workforce Centers, 83% of all American RNs are Caucasian/white; the remainder are from minority groups (1% American Indian/Alaskan Native, 6% Black/African American, 3% Hispanic/Latino, 6% Asian or Native Hawaiian/Pacific Islander and 1% reported other) (National Council of State Boards of Nursing & The Forum of State Nursing Workforce Centers, 2013). Preliminary findings of the 2015 *National Workforce Survey of Registered Nurses* specify that 19.5% of licensed RNs reported themselves as being a member of an ethnic minority group with more newly licensed nurses reporting coming from an ethnic minority background.

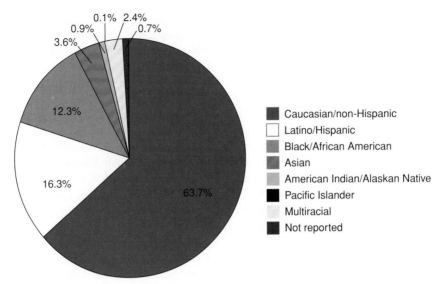

FIGURE 11.1 Cultural diversity in the United States, 2010. (Adapted from U.S. Census Bureau. (2011). Overview of race and Hispanic origin. U.S. Hispanic population surpasses 45 million. Retrieved from http://www.census.gov/prod/cen2010briefs/c2010br-02.pdf. Accessed December 21, 2012.)

The survey also noted that 6.7% of licensed RNs have been educated outside of the United States and that 14.1% of RNs are male (National Council of State Boards of Nursing, 2016). Because many people feel more comfortable with people like themselves (especially when sharing sensitive information), the nursing profession must find ways to recruit and retain people from different cultural backgrounds. The goal is for the profession to attain a cultural profile that mirrors population demographics. Until that happens, nurses must understand cultural and ethnic factors when providing care to clients from many diverse cultures.

Take Note!
Ideally, the cultural profile of the nursing profession should match that of the population being served.

Basic Terminology to Understand Culture

In 1871, British anthropologist Sir Edward Taylor first used the term **culture** to refer to the complex whole, including knowledge, belief, art, morals, law, custom, and any other abilities and habits people acquired as societal members. In 1935, anthropologist Margaret Mead expanded the definition of culture to include technologic systems, political practices, and habits of daily life. Culture serves as a guide for determining the values, beliefs, and practices of individuals or groups of people.

Transcultural nursing uses the Latin prefix "trans," which means *across*, thereby referring to nursing across cultures. **Multicultural nursing** uses the Latin prefix "multi," which means many, denoting nursing of many different cultures. Finally, **intercultural nursing** uses the Latin prefix "inter," which means between, denoting nursing between cultures (Andrews & Boyle, 2016). Box 11.1, Professional Building Blocks, "Understanding the Terminology of Culture," defines additional terms critical to this discussion.

Culture may include large numbers of people, as in the global or national culture, or it may incorporate small numbers of people, such as a single-family unit or gang. Culture also can be differentiated by age (youth culture) or gender preference (gay, lesbian, bisexual, or transgender cultures). Cultural analysis enables HCPs to understand the impact of lifeways (a way of life distinctly different in anthropology from lifestyle), rituals, and taboos when providing care.

Madeline Leininger, a nurse with advanced education in anthropology, started the transcultural nursing movement and founded the Transcultural Nursing Society. Leininger (1995, p. 4) defined **transcultural nursing** as "a formal area of study and practice in nursing focused upon comparative holistic cultural care, health, and illness patterns of individuals and groups with respect to differences and similarities in cultural values, beliefs, and practices." The goal of transcultural nursing is "to provide culturally congruent, sensitive, and competent nursing care to people of diverse

11.1 Professional Building Blocks

Understanding the Terminology of Culture

- **Acculturation:** Blending of two cultures by taking the best of each and combining them into one
- **Cultural accommodation:** Allowing specific cultural practices within another culture
- **Cultural assimilation:** Adoption of group culture by a member or members of a different culture
- **Cultural blindness:** Ignoring cultural differences or acting as though they do not exist
- **Cultural competence:** Integration of knowledge, attitudes, and skills that enable effective and appropriate communications and behaviors when working with people from one or more cultures different from one's own
- **Cultural diffusion:** Spreading out of cultural traits, patterns, and beliefs
- **Cultural diversity:** Differences within groups
- **Cultural empathy:** Expressive concern and the ability to see experiences as the client sees them
- **Cultural group:** Two or more people sharing the same ancestry, nationality, values, beliefs, or behavior
- **Cultural identity:** Professed membership within a group
- **Cultural imposition:** Forcing cultural beliefs, values, and patterns onto someone from a different background
- **Cultural lifeways:** Group beliefs about activities of daily living, inherited traits, and behaviors
- **Cultural maintenance:** Continued practice of a specific culture
- **Cultural negotiation:** Working with a person from another culture to determine what cultural practices can be used without jeopardizing effects
- **Cultural norms:** Acceptable behaviors and practices
- **Cultural pluralism:** Maintaining cultural differences after being assimilated into another culture
- **Cultural preservation:** Continued practice of a specific culture
- **Cultural relativism:** Acknowledging that other ways of doing things are different, but they are valid and may be superior

- **Cultural repatterning (or restructuring):** Changing unhealthy cultural behavior patterns to promote better health
- **Culture shock:** State in which one feels totally disconnected from a group because of extreme differences
- **Cultural values:** Prevalent, powerful forces that provide meaning and direction to group actions, decisions, and lifeways
- **Culture:** An integrated pattern of socially transmitted behaviors, including all products of human work and thoughts specific to a group of persons, that guides formulation of worldviews and decision-making processes
- **Emic perspective:** An insider's view
- **Enculturation:** Attempting to get one group to accept the ways of another group
- **Ethnicity:** Sharing the same ancestral, physical, racial, and national origins along with the same language, lifestyle, religion, or other characteristics
- **Ethnocentrism:** Believing that one's way is best
- **Etic perspective:** An outsider's view
- **Generalization:** Oversimplified assumption about a group of persons
- **International nursing:** Providing nursing care services outside one's country of legal residence
- **Rituals:** Routine practices
- **Stereotype:** Oversimplified idea, opinion, or belief about all members of a particular group
- **Taboo:** A practice that is absolutely forbidden by a group
- **Transcultural nursing:** Providing physical, psychological, and spiritual nursing care to clients from a different cultural background while considering the clients' cultural beliefs and practices
- **Worldview:** Personal perception of the universe that provides a foundation for values and beliefs about the world and life

Adapted from American Association of Colleges of Nursing. (1998). *The essentials of baccalaureate education for professional nursing practice.* Washington, DC: Author; Andrews, M. M., & Boyle, J. S. (Eds.). (2008). *Transcultural concepts in nursing care* (5th ed.). Philadelphia, PA: Lippincott Williams & Wilkins; Giger, J. N., & Davidhizar, R. E. (2008). *Transcultural nursing assessment and intervention* (5th ed.). St. Louis, MO: Mosby; Leininger, M. (1995). *Transcultural nursing* (2nd ed.). New York: McGraw-Hill; Leininger, M., & McFarland, M. (2006). *Cultural care diversity and universality: A worldwide theory for nursing* (2nd ed.). Sudbury, MA: Jones & Bartlett; Pedersen, P. B., Dragunus, J. C., Lenner, W. J., & Trimble, J. E. (Eds.). (1996). *Counseling across cultures* (4th ed.). Thousand Oaks, CA: Sage; Purnell, L. (2014). *Transcultural health care, a culturally competent approach* (3rd ed.) Philadelphia, PA: F. A. Davis; and Purnell, L. D., & Paulanka, B. J. (2008). *Transcultural health care: A culturally competent approach* (3rd ed.). Philadelphia, PA: F. A. Davis.

cultures" (Leininger, 1991, p. 4). Leininger's writing justifies transcultural nursing by saying that people have rights and expectations to have their cultural values and beliefs respected and that nurses are obligated to meet clients' cultural needs. Leininger suggested that being kind, relying on common sense, and ignoring prejudices do not foster culturally relevant care to clients. She proposed that nurses should receive formal education in transcultural nursing that begins with an analysis of one's own cultural values and beliefs.

Transcultural nursing blends nursing and anthropology in theory and practice. A provision of culture-specific care and culture-universal care serves as the aim of transcultural nursing. "Care" refers to providing nursing services with consideration to particular values, beliefs, and behavior patterns unique to a specific group. These tend not to be shared with people from other cultures. **Culture-universal care** denotes the commonly shared values, behaviors, and life patterns that appear among most cultures (Andrews & Boyle, 2016; Leininger & McFarland, 2002, 2006). Examples of culture-universal care include the formation of family, the socialization of children into society, and the basic physical survival needs.

Culture-Specific and Culturally Congruent Care

Most people use a culture-based health practice before entering the formal health care system (Andrews & Boyle, 2016; Giger, 2013; Giger & Davidhizar, 2008; Leininger, 1995; Leininger & McFarland, 2002, 2006). Professional nurses must understand the concept of **cultural relativism**, which encompasses a profound respect for all cultures, an acknowledgment that all cultures are equal, and an understanding that what is ethically and morally correct for each person is determined by his/her culture. **Culture-specific care** includes the specific practices of a particular cultural group. Culture-specific care practices may be similar across groups, but each group has slight differences in either the manner in which practices are implemented or the meaning behind them. **Culturally congruent care** incorporates aspects of a specific cultural group practices while adding other remedies or healers that do not conflict with a culture's morals beliefs and practice.

For example, individuals from many cultural groups use folk (or generic) remedies and healers before or in conjunction with seeking care from the health care system (Fig. 11.2). A culture-specific practice would invite a shaman of a hospitalized Native American client to perform a specific healing ceremony immediately following surgery. An example of culturally congruent care would be the nurse serving "hot" and "cold" foods and beverages to a Chinese woman (cultural health practices) who is hospitalized for a cervical radiation implant (a culturally acceptable medical intervention for cancer). Table 11.1 provides a summary of the culture of the American health care system, then lists traditional culturally based healers and folk remedies for various populations.

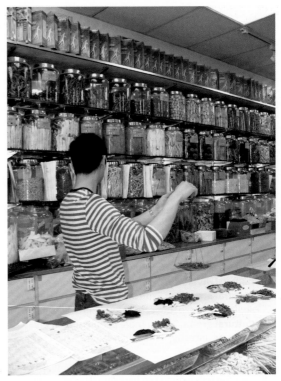

FIGURE 11.2 A herbalist uses plant life to enhance health and healing, which may either be a form of culture-specific or culturally congruent health care.

Great differences may occur across various ethnic groups. Health care practitioners frequently impose their own cultural values, beliefs, and practices on clients receiving care. However, competent transcultural care blends culturally based practices with empirically based medical practices. When these practices conflict with each other, the nurse (or other HCP) works with the client from another culture to accommodate cultural practices with the medical plan of care so that the combination of remedies does not cause harm (Andrews and Boyle, 2016; Giger, 2013; Leininger & McFarland, 2002, 2006).

QUESTIONS FOR REFLECTION

1. Have you used folk healers or healing practices to enhance your health or recover from an illness or injury? How did you learn about these practices?
2. Have you ever encountered a folk healer in your professional practice? How did you react? How would you react if one of your clients (or a client's family member) insisted that a folk healer practice folk medicine as part of his or her treatment?
3. What are the policies related to the use of folk healers in your clinical practice setting?

TABLE 11.1 Examples of Traditional Cultural Healers and Folk Remedies

Cultural Group	Healers	Folk Remedies
American health care system	Physician Nurse practitioner Nurse Physical, occupational, and respiratory therapists Social worker Chaplain	Scientifically validated medication and therapies Complex technologic equipment for diagnosis and treatment Some reliance on intuition Effectiveness based on cost–benefit ratio High degree of concern for timeliness of treatments and appointments Spiritual needs of clients usually referred to chaplain
Amish	Brauch or brauch-doktor Lay midwife	Combination of many modalities, including manipulation of body parts, massage, herbs, herbal teas, reflexology, and other folk healing remedies Midwife provides prenatal, birthing, and postpartum care
Caribbean and African	Extended family members, friends, and neighbors Old Lady (experienced woman who successfully raised a family) Folk practitioners Faith healer (spiritualist) Hougan (Voodoo priestess or priest)	Health clinic and physician visits occur when all folk remedies have been exhausted Herbal remedies, potions, applications of heat and cold, crystals, massage, meditation, oils, powders, tokens, rites, and ceremonies Oils, candles, soaps, and aerosolized sprays are used to repel evil forces
Chinese (traditional)	Physician Acupuncturist Herbalist	Physician diagnoses health problems by listening, questioning, and palpating, including feeling quality of pulse and sensitivity of body parts Acupuncture Herbal preparation (have used 5,767 documented herbs)
Eastern Indian	Ayurvedic healer	Remedies used come from vegetable and mineral raw materials Yoga Meditation Herbal preparations
Filipino	Family traditions Folk healer	Based on hot/cold theory that requires people to consume hot foods for a cold illness and cold foods for a hot illness Widely use herbal remedies Very quiet and passive when seeking health care
Greek	Magissa Bonesetters Greek orthodox priest	Magician, usually a woman, who cures "evil eye" and other disorders caused by spells Bonesetters specialize in setting uncomplicated fractures Ordained priest consulted for advice, direct healing, or exorcism
Japanese	Kampo practitioners Family members	Kampo is a holistic approach to illness and uses acupuncture, herbal medicines, moxibustion, and spiritual exercises For colds, use of ginger, sake, and egg; herbal teas for "cure-all"; headaches are treated by rubbing the head with sesame or ginger oil; finger massage and exercise are used to stay well Hot/cold (yin and yang) theory applies to health-related situations
Mexican	Family member Curandera Sobadora (massage and bone and joint manipulation specialist) Espiritualista (spiritualist) Yebero (herbalist)	Curanderismo is an eclectic, holistic, and syncretic compilation of beliefs from the Mesoamerican Spanish, spiritualistic, homeopathic, and modern medical beliefs System is based on herbal preparations, Spanish prayers, altered states of consciousness, and healing rituals that blend Indian traditions and Catholic rituals Herbal teas, ingestion or application of powdered substances, massage with warm oils, and skin popping on the small of the back

(continued on page 280)

TABLE 11.1 Examples of Traditional Cultural Healers and Folk Remedies *(continued)*

Cultural Group	Healers	Folk Remedies
Native American and Alaskan Native	Shaman Singer or chanter (highest position in the Navajo tribe) Crystal gazer, hand trembler, or diagnostician (one step below singer in the Navajo tribe) Singer for healing ceremonies Medicine man (Hopi tribe) Herbalist Nuclear and extended family (Muckleshoot tribe, some Northwest Native Americans, and Alaskan natives)	Sweating and purging usually done in a lodge Herbal remedies from local environment Healing ceremonies using the medicine wheel, sacred hoop, and singing (Lakota, Dineh, and Navajo tribes) Stargazing and hand trembling for diagnosis (Navajo) Herbalist prescribes herbs for symptomatic relief while members await healing ceremony (Navajo) Mothers, grandmothers, and aunts may be key sources of health information related to pregnancy, birth, and childhood illnesses Health care decisions may be made by familial consensus.
South and Central American	Curanderismo	Foods with qualitative (not literal) properties of "hot" and "cold" Persons with "hot" diseases should receive "cold" foods and vice versa to restore a balance of hot and cold
South African	Medicine man Isangoma (diagnostician) Inyanga (healer) Midwife Herbalist	Ukincinda (licking), ukubhema (inhalation of snuffing substances), ukuhlanza (emetics), ukuchatha (enemas), ukugguma (steaming), and ukugcaba (incisions made and medicine rubbed into them) are forms of traditional healing methods Herbal preparations Spiritual ceremonies and sacrifices to spirits Goal of health is to achieve a balance with nature
Southeast Asians	Shaman	Serves as the mediator between people and the spiritual world to prevent, diagnose, and treat health problems Principles of yin and yang (hot and cold) Infections are hot and should be treated with a cold food such as fruit; cancers are cold and should be treated with hot food such as chicken soup Strong herbal teas that may be dangerous if concurrently used with Western medicine Dermabrasion, massage, acupressure, acupuncture, and moxibustion Spiritual healing rituals (more commonly used by Vietnamese)
Puerto Rican	Santiguadora Spiritual healers	Herbal teas Massage with warm oils Spiritual rituals

Andrews, M. & Boyle, J. (Eds.) (2008). *Transcultural concepts in nursing care* (5th ed.). Philadelphia, PA: Wolters Kluwer Health/ Lippincott Williams & Wilkins; Andrews, M., & Herberg, P. (1999). Transcultural nursing care. (pp. 23–77). In M. M. Andres & J. S. Boyle (Eds.), *Transcultural concepts in nursing care* (3rd ed.). Philadelphia, PA: Lippincott Williams & Wilkins; Dayer-Berenson, L. (2011). *Cultural competencies for nurses, impact on health and illness*. Sudbury, MA: Jones & Bartlett; and Purnell, L., & Paulanka, B. (1998). *Transcultural health care, a culturally competent approach*. Philadelphia, PA: F. A. Davis.

ESTABLISHING CULTURAL COMPETENCE

Attainment of cultural competence is a lifelong journey that requires the elimination of **ethnocentrism** (belief that one's way is best) and an unconditional acceptance of cultural diversity unless the practice places another person in harm's way. Establishment of cultural competence requires contact and interaction with people from other cultures.

Minority Populations

Kavanagh and Kennedy (1992) proposed that minority status be assigned to those who do not have power, status, and wealth within a given society (or situation), rather than being established by sheer numbers. However, some persons who do not have societal power may find the term "minority" offensive because the term might lead to perceptions of diminished status by the majority or dominant group. Perceptions of reduced status (being less than a full person who deserves respect, dignity, and equality) may move the dominant group to exclude others unlike themselves from full participation in society.

Those with power, status, or wealth frequently may be viewed as being worthy of receiving health care services. In American culture, the ability to pay defines who is given access to health care services. Some HCPs may view the working poor as being more worthy of health care than the nonworking poor, because the working poor contribute beneficial services to society and pay taxes.

Health care professionals often expect minorities to adapt to the established norms and policies of the institution, rather than the institution adapting to the needs of minorities. To become minority friendly, health care institutions must have their professionals learn about the social organization and processes of each minority group served (Kavanagh & Kennedy, 1992).

Steps to Acquiring Cultural Competence

Becoming culturally competent does not happen overnight, but rather takes time and commitment. Burchum (2002) defined **cultural competence** as a developmental process that builds continuous increases in knowledge and skill development in the areas of cultural awareness, knowledge, understanding, sensitivity, interaction, and skills. The following six steps outline a process for nurses to follow to acquire cultural competence.

Step 1: Examine Personal Values, Beliefs, Biases, and Prejudices

The journey to cultural competence begins with an examination of attitudes, which reflect personal values, beliefs, biases, and prejudices. Attitudes result from evaluative judgments that may have developed over time, either during childhood or from life experience. A variety of self-report tools can be used to measure cultural sensitivity (the degree to which someone has awareness and demonstrates positive responsiveness to cultural differences); these tools include the Cultural Attitude Scale, developed by Bonaparte in the late 1970s and modified by Rooda in 1991 and 1992 (Giger, 2013; Giger & Davidhizar, 2008), the Cultural Self-Efficacy Scale, developed by Forman in 1987 (Giger, 2013; Giger & Davidhizar, 2008), Randall-Davis's checklist *How Do You Relate to Various Groups of People in the Society?* (Andrews & Boyle, 2016), and Terrence Freeman's 1987 Cross-Cultural Interaction Scale (Hughes & Hood, 2007). People are often unaware of their own values, beliefs, biases, and prejudices, as well as those of the dominant culture. For self-report tools to be effective, the people completing them must be honest in their answers rather than answering the question items in a socially acceptable manner. Once a person identifies areas for attitudinal and/or behavioral change, even longstanding negative attitudes and beliefs may be changed. However, sometimes a personal experience

with one or more people from a cultural group may be required to eliminate individual biases and prejudices (Giger, 2013; Giger & Davidhizar, 2008; Purnell, 2014; Purnell & Paulanka, 2008).

Step 2: Build Cultural Awareness

To several transcultural nursing specialists, cultural awareness serves as an antecedent toward obtaining specific communication strategies and knowledge about other cultures (Andrews & Boyle, 2016; Giger, 2013; Giger & Davidhizar, 2008; Purnell, 2014; Purnell & Paulanka, 2008). Results of the self-report methods presented in Step 1 provide a means for people to become more aware of values, beliefs, biases, and prejudices that may be culturally induced. Nurses who understand how their cultural beliefs affect care delivery can change their behavior and attitudes toward clients from other cultures.

In order to build cultural awareness, nursing students typically provide inpatient client care for persons who are from different cultures in clinical settings. Other opportunities to increase cultural awareness for students include clinical experiences such as providing health screenings and education in a neighborhood community center, administering injections at a health department–sponsored immunization clinic, and participating in national or international mission trips. Nursing students can also interact with classmates, clinical agency staff, and school employees who have a cultural background different from their own.

Step 3: Learn Culturally Specific Communication Strategies

Once health team members are aware of key cultural differences, they can develop specific communication strategies to tear down barriers and provide culturally and linguistically appropriate health care. Learning and implementing culturally specific communication strategies affirm respect for diversity and serve as the third step toward attainment of cultural competence. Verbal and nonverbal communication patterns are a key part of understanding cultural nuances when serving people from different cultural backgrounds (Andrews & Boyle, 2016; Kavanagh & Kennedy, 1992; Leininger, 1995; Leininger & McFarland, 2006). For example, principles of therapeutic communication suggest that making direct eye contact facilitates client assessment, shows genuine compassion, and cues people engaged in a conversation when it is each person's turn to speak (DeVito, 2004). However, some cultures (e.g., Asian, Native American) believe that making direct eye contact is rude and demonstrates a lack of respect.

A key way to foster communication with clients from other cultures is to approach them in a manner that displays authentic empathy and deep respect (Pullen, 2007). Some organizations provide nurses with information about various cultural groups in print (books, pamphlets) or digital (software programs or access to online information) format. The nurse's body language also plays a big role in displaying confidence when working with people from other cultures. A calm, cheerful, unhurried approach displays a sense of concern across most cultures. When nurses hurry while working with clients from another culture, clients may perceive that the nurse is indifferent to or biased against them (Pullen, 2007).

Speaking even a few words in the client's native language conveys awareness and respect for his or her culture. Some nurses find using gestures and pantomimes effective to get key assessments completed and to meet clients' basic needs.

Step 4: Interact with People from Different Cultures

Interacting with people from different cultures is the fourth step in cultural competence. This requires risk taking. People sometimes avoid others who differ from themselves. This practice minimizes or denies differences that exist across various groups, such as race, class, nationality, or gender (to name a few broad differences). Such avoidance enforces the invisibility of sensitive issues (Kavanagh & Kennedy, 1992). Respectful engagement during interactions with members of another culture or group provides an opportunity to develop the personal and professional expertise needed to work effectively with culturally diverse clients and colleagues.

Most people from different cultures send cues to each other during interactions. If heeded, the cues can guide the transcultural interaction, and errors can be avoided (Andrews & Boyle, 2016; DeVito, 2004; Giger, 2013; Giger & Davidhizar, 2008; Grossman, 1996; Yoder, 1996, 1997). Asking questions before acting also serves as a useful tool. For example, personal space needs to be respected when working with all people. The definition of personal space varies across cultures, with people from North American backgrounds requiring the most distance. In contrast, people from Middle Eastern, Latin American, and Japanese cultures feel quite comfortable being close to others, and the closeness indicates interest and concern. Nurses who are uncertain whether a clients' cultural mores permit touching by a person other than a family member should ask the client's permission before touching him or her.

Some nurses and health team members may consider themselves to be bilingual or multilingual.

However, the true extent of the provider's language proficiency may be more appropriate to social conversational use. Some nurses may speak enough of the client's language to perform a physical assessment and meet the client's basic care needs.

Occasionally, professional nurses and other health team members rely on families, friends, or nonprofessional members of the health care team who speak the client's language to explain medical procedures to non–English-speaking clients. However, reliance on people who do not have the educational background to fully comprehend the implications of complex health care tests and interventions limits full disclosure of potential complications and accurate client education. The National Standards for Culturally and Linguistically Appropriate Services in Health Care (NSCLASHC) requires the use of a qualified interpreter, rather than a translator, when clients and HCPs speak different languages (Office of Minority Health, 2007; United States Department of Health and Human Services, Office of Minority Health, 2010). To avoid legal and ethical issues related to protected health information and privacy concerns, family members and friends may be used as interpreters only with client permission.

■ QUESTIONS FOR REFLECTION

1. In either your practice or your daily activities, how much opportunity do you have to interact with those from other cultures? How do you usually handle communicating with those who do not speak English or whose cultural norms differ from yours? Do you think you conduct yourself in a culturally competent manner in such interactions? Why or why not?

2. In interacting with persons from different cultures in clinical or other settings, what resources, policies, and procedures might you draw upon?

Step 5: Identify and Acknowledge Mistakes

Mistake identification and acknowledgment serve as the fifth step toward cultural competence. Because literature on culturally diverse practices places people into various groups, resulting in large clumps of cultural categories, errors of similarities may occur, with devastating effects (Leininger, 1995; Leininger & McFarland, 2002, 2006). For example, demographics related to Pacific Islanders represent 40 different cultural groups who speak 23 languages (Farella, 2001). Within this cultural group, health practices and taboos differ greatly.

Along with errors of similarity, errors of assumption are common. People assume things about others based on outward appearances. Racial profiling results when people assume that people who look alike share specific traits and behaviors. The US population is a melting pot, and citizens often refer to themselves as African American, Japanese American, Italian American, Native American, Mexican American, or some other "American" designation. A person's physical appearance, however, is not an accurate indicator of beliefs or practices. Second- or third-generation immigrants may or may not abide by the cultural practices of their ancestral homelands (Leininger, 1995; Leininger & McFarland, 2006). Likewise, as people learn about health practices from other cultural groups, culturally based folk practice may become intertwined with traditional Western medicine, resulting in an inability to know what individuals do to achieve and maintain health. For example, an American of Latin American or Asian descent may or may not abide by the hot and cold food theory for illness treatment, although this is common practice among these cultural groups. The best way to avoid errors of similarity and assumption is to perform a detailed, individually focused client health assessment.

Most people accept sincerely offered apologies when HCPs inadvertently commit a cultural faux pas. Valuable lessons can be learned from such communication and behavioral mistakes. Concepts in Practice, "The Value of an Apology," provides an example of how effective a professional apology can be when an error occurs.

Concepts in Practice [IDEA] → [PLAN] → [ACTION]

The Value of an Apology

Alice is a professional nurse who works on a cardiac unit. During a busy day, she was assigned to provide care to an elderly Chinese man with a suspected heart attack. Following her usual patient care routine, she entered the room and made complete eye contact as she introduced herself. Alice proceeded to speak English as she shared her intentions to perform a head-to-toe assessment before the client went for an invasive cardiac procedure. As she moved to touch the man, he grabbed her hand and stopped her. Startled, Alice realized that the man did not understand English and that this action was his way of protecting himself. She immediately apologized and then dialed the phone to reach the language interpreting services. Once securing the services of a Chinese interpreter, she explained the situation, requested that the interpreter apologize to him for her and then gave the telephone to the man. After speaking with the interpreter, he smiled and chuckled while baring his chest so that Alice

could listen to his heart. Alice used the interpreter during her nursing assessment. The man went for his cardiac procedure.

Upon return to the unit following his procedure, the man asked for Alice by name. Alice entered the room and the man immediately threw off his blanket, motioned for Alice to come to his side, showed her the pressure dressing on his groin, and pantomimed for Alice to touch the dressing. Alice called the interpreter to translate postprocedure care to the man. The man gave the telephone to Alice so that the interpreter could tell her that the man was very pleased with her nursing care and that he only wanted her to care for him because she displayed great respect toward him. The interpreter also told Alice that, should the man offer her some food, Alice should take it and eat it in front of him because sharing food with another person would be the utmost compliment for his subcultural group.

Along with errors of assumption, nurses and other HCPs must understand that they hold membership in the American (or other national) HCP culture. In the United States, health care delivery organizations value efficiency, quality, and empirical evidence. This culture often expects consumers to hold the same (or similar) values (Andrews & Boyle, 2016; Giger, 2013; Giger & Davidhizar, 2008; Leininger, 1995; Leininger & McFarland, 2002, 2006). Some clinics that serve diverse client populations hold clients to standards determined by the values of HCPs (e.g., a well-baby outpatient clinic has an established policy that specifies that patients must arrive 15 minutes prior to a scheduled appointment to check in and complete paperwork. If a mother and infant fail to arrive early, the appointment is immediately cancelled. If they arrive later than specified appointment guidelines, the mother and infant will be "worked in" to be seen. If a mother is late for appointments more than three times, the clinic reserves the right to refuse to schedule appointments).

▮ QUESTIONS FOR REFLECTION

1. Do the health care settings in which you've worked or received care reflect the cultural values of the populations they serve? Provide examples of how they are or might become culturally sensitive.

2. What policies have you encountered in health care settings that reflect a foundation of the American health care system values? How do such policies obstruct the provision of culturally sensitive care?

Step 6: Remediate Cultural Mistakes

Remediation for cultural mistakes serves as the final step toward cultural competence. Correcting mistakes requires communication between people as well as groups. Genuine dialogues result in the development of ideas for cultural accommodation and preservation. Because nursing focuses on client comfort, culture-specific care nursing interventions enhance client comfort by fostering maintenance of client cultural identity. When members of a cultural group receive culturally sensitive care, they may share this information with other members of their group, resulting in positive advertising for a particular HCO.

Hallmarks of Culturally Congruent Care

Once transcultural communication has been established, nurses and other HCPs can expand their knowledge related to culture-specific care practices. Andrews and Boyle (2008, 2016) identified several areas about which nurses should know to provide transcultural nursing care, including assessment, communication, hygiene, activities of daily living, and religious practices.

- **Assessment:** Nurses must consider biologic variations in signs of illness and health, avoid potential cultural taboos in such routine activities as measuring the heads of infants, modify childhood developmental screening tools, and use appropriate ways to conduct gynecologic examinations of women from various cultures.
- **Communication:** Transcultural communication skills include speaking in the client's native language, providing health care information in the client's native language, and providing a language interpreter for clients.
- **Hygiene:** Nurses must be cognizant of specific hair and skin care needs of clients of various ethnic backgrounds.
- **Activities of daily living:** Nurses must be aware and capable of coaching clients who require special needs for activities of daily living (such as eating with chopsticks or using special assistive devices such as the West African "chewing stick" for oral hygiene). Nutrition also plays a key role in health care. Providing hot and cold foods to clients whose cultures abide by this practice instills trust between nurses and clients.
- **Religious practice:** Permitting clients to engage in their religious practices enhances spiritual well-being. Some religious ceremonies include the anointing of the sick (among Roman Catholics), the reciting of psalms and prayers for healing (among those of the Jewish faith), and cleansing before daily prayer (among practicing Muslims).

Several theories related to transcultural nursing have been published. Cultural phenomena that address the culturally unique individual vary slightly across these theories (Table 11.2). Reference works by the theorists cited in Table 11.2 provide more detailed descriptions of cultural traditions and taboos related to health protection, maintenance, and restoration.

Nurses are members of the culture of HCPs; thus, value conflicts frequently occur between nurses and health care consumers (Giger, 2013; Giger & Davidhizar, 2008; Leininger, 1995; Leininger & McFarland, 2006; Spector, 2012). At times, nurses may be unaware to cultural issues surrounding a client care situation. Failure to acknowledge and incorporate culture into client care increases the likelihood of distrust on the part of the health care consumer and antagonism on the part of the HCP. Conversely, the client's trust and comfort increase when nurses consider cultural preferences during client care. However, transcultural care considerations should not supersede the need for safe, effective client care (Andrews & Boyle, 2016).

Assessment

Identification of cultural nursing considerations begins with the nursing assessment. An individualized cultural assessment prevents the nurse from making cultural errors based on client appearance and provides the nurse with the opportunity to learn about the client's way of life. Elements of the **cultural assessment** include family and kinship systems, social life, political systems, language, traditions, perceptions of the world, values orientation, cultural norms, religious and health beliefs, and health practices. Table 11.3 presents information on each of these elements and suggests ways for nurses to collect data that may be relevant for nursing care. While performing a cultural nursing assessment, nurses must observe clients for cues that indicate misunderstanding or discomfort with any questions asked. Before involving family members in health care communications, the nurse should receive permission from the client to involve family members. Family involvement may be necessary when a particular family member serves as the patriarch or matriarch who makes health care decisions for a family. However, to verify complete understanding of questions, use of a specially educated medical interpreter is the best course of action.

■ TABLE 11.2 Comparison of Transcultural Nursing Theories

Theory	Background and Goals	Key Cultural Elements

Leininger's sunrise model and theory of culture care diversity and universality (Leininger & McFarland, 2006)	Describes, explains, and predicts factors for nurses to address when providing nursing care services to people from different cultures
	Sets the goal of providing culturally congruent care for all clients
	Enables high flexibility for use with individuals, families, groups, communities, and institutions across diverse health care settings
	Examines the culture of individuals, families, groups, institutions, local communities, societies, nations, and all humankind
	Outlines three phases for obtaining and using transcultural nursing knowledge:
	Cultural awareness
	Use of theory to guide cultural research and explain cultural behaviors
	Use of cultural knowledge in nursing practice to provide culturally congruent care
		1. Interacting and influential factors for client holistic well-being: available technology, religion, client personal philosophy, kinship and social relationships, cultural values and lifeways, political and legal factors, educational background, and economic forces
		2. Professional nurse roles to provide culturally relevant care:
		  ▪ Mediator between the Western health care system and the folk health care system used by the client
		  ▪ Advocate for maintenance of the client's culture by accommodating folk practices that do not interfere with Western health care system treatments
		  ▪ Educator who assesses, plans and implements teaching for individual clients (or community) to establish different patterns and structures to enhance health and general well-being

Purnell's model for cultural competence (2008, 2014)	Cultural competence requires that the health care provider master the following tasks: 1. Develop a deep self-awareness of personal existence, feelings, ideas, and emotions and hold these from influencing actions and attitudes when working with persons from a different culture 2. Learn and understand the culture of the health care client 3. Accept and respect cultural differences (2008, p. 2) 4. Adapt usual care practices to become congruent with the culture of the client Cultural competence is seen as a nonlinear conscious process The individual is seen as the core of an ever-expanding network that includes the family, community, and global society Theory acknowledges that health care providers' cultural competence falls into four categories: unconsciously incompetent, consciously incompetent, consciously competent, and unconsciously competent Emphasizes the use of interpreters over translators when clients do not speak the same language as the health care provider The 12 key elements of culture provide a comprehensive assessment of cultural care considerations	1. Cultural overview and heritage includes the country of origin (climate and topography), heritage, residence, reasons for migration, economic factors, educational level, and occupation. 2. Communication encompasses the dominant group language, cultural communication patterns (eye contact, space, touch, facial expressions, separate ways to greet outsiders), temporal relationships (time orientation, social and clock time differences, importance of punctuality), and format for names (formal and informal use, sequencing of family and individual names). 3. Family roles and organization include gender roles, accepted head of household, behaviors that are accepted or restricted, taboos, familial roles, familial priorities, alternative lifestyles, and nontraditional families. 4. Workforce issues includes permanent and temporary immigration, multicultural workplace considerations, acculturation into the work group, native health care practices, issues related to professional autonomy, cultural gender roles, religious issues, perception of authority figures, and language barriers. 5. Biocultural ecology includes skin color, biologic variations, culturally prevalent diseases, ethnic health conditions, and variances in medication metabolism. 6. High-risk behaviors include use of tobacco, alcohol, and illegal drugs; sedentary lifestyle; and failure to use protective devices. 7. Nutrition considers the meaning of food, commonly consumed food, rituals, health-promoting dietary practices, nutritional deficiencies, and alterations in food metabolism. 8. Pregnancy and childbearing practices include cultural views and practices related to fertility control, culturally specified practices, restrictions, or taboos related to pregnancy and childbearing.

(continued on page 286)

TABLE 11.2   Comparison of Transcultural Nursing Theories *(continued)*

Theory	Background and Goals	Key Cultural Elements
	Acknowledges workplace issues and the potential value conflicts between clients and providers and conflicts among health team members	9. Death rituals encompass cultural expectations of death, purposes behind death and mourning rituals, burial practices (including cremation), cultural expectations of grief, and cultural meanings about death and afterlife. 10. Spirituality considers the influence of the dominant religion on persons and families, the meaning of prayer, other religious rites and rituals, faith-based symbols (such as icons, statues, medallions), meaning of life, personal sources of strength, and the linkage of spiritual beliefs with health practices. 11. Health care practices encompass predominant cultural beliefs that influence health promotion, disease prevention, curative practices, payment for services, use of nonmedically prescribed preparations, definition of who is responsible for health care, folk, folk practices, health care barriers, cultural responses to health/illness/and rehabilitation, cultural perceptions of the "sick role," and acceptance of blood transfusion and organ donations. 12. Definition of health care practitioners includes an exploration of the roles of traditional, folk, and religious health care providers, acceptance of Western medicine health care providers, significance of health provider age, perception of various members of the health care team, status of various health team members, and perceptions of health team members of each other.
Spector's model of heritage consistency (2012)	Socialization is the focal point of the model. Heritage consistency refers to the degree that a person's lifestyle reflects his or her traditional culture. Factors indicating heritage consistency: 1. Childhood development within the country of origin or other persons sharing same country of origin 2. Extended family participation in cultural or religious activities 3. Return visits to country or neighborhood of birth 4. Regular contact with extended family 5. Extended family homes within the same community 6. Participation in cultural and religious events 7. Engagement in social activities with others from the same ethnic background 8. Personal knowledge of culture and language of origin 9. Deep personal pride about heritage 10. Surname not Americanized 11. Extended family engaged in childrearing Heritage consistency occurs as a continuum.	1. Culture is a complex phenomenon that includes a connected web of symbols, a means for making and limiting human decisions, an extension of biologic capabilities, a medium for social relationship, and personhood. Only part of culture is conscious and exists in a person's mind as well as in the environment. 2. Ethnicity is the condition of belonging to a particular group that shares common characteristics, such as geographic origin, race, migratory status, religion, kinship, geographic locale, traditions, symbols, institutions, literature and other fine arts, values, food preferences, race, language, and dialect. Ethnicity provides an internal sense of distinctness as well as an external perception of distinctiveness. In the United States, a person may belong to different ethnic groups simultaneously. 3. Religion is the belief in a higher power to be obeyed and to worship that also provides a foundation for beliefs, practices, and ethics. 4. Socialization is the process by which persons are raised within a group and acquire group characteristics. Socialization results from the interactive effects of culture, ethnicity, and religion.

Theory	Background and Goals	Key Cultural Elements
	Uses Giger and Davidhizar's six cultural phenomena that affect health: environmental control, biologic variations, social organization, communication, space perception, and time orientation Views health providers as a special cultural group with values that frequently conflict with those of health care consumers	
Giger and Davidhizar's Transcultural Assessment Model (2008)	Provides a systematic approach for assessing culturally diverse clients	1. Communication is language spoken, voice quality, pronunciation, use of silence, and nonverbal behavior. 2. Space perception involves action with personal space invasion, conversation distance, body movement, role of objects, and perception of space. 3. Social organization is the culture, ethnicity, race, role and function of family, work, leisure, religious practices, and friends. 4. Time includes how time is spent, measurement, definition, social, work, and orientation (future, past, or present). 5. Environmental control is cultural health practices (efficacious, neutral, harmful or uncertain effects), values and cultural definitions of health and illness. 6. Biologic variations include body structure, skin color, hair color, genetic makeup, enzymatic deficiencies, increased susceptibility to disease and chronic illness, nutritional preferences (and if these result in deficiencies) and psychological characteristics, including coping strategies and social support.

Along with verbal communication, the nurse can scan the environment for clues related to culture. In the home and also in inpatient settings, many people display symbolic objects to signify their beliefs. Sometimes, items such as charms or religious medals are worn; such items should not be removed without first asking permission of the client. Displayed objects, such as statues, prayer beads, shrines, or special candles, may provide clues to nurses that special cultural health needs may surface. Polite inquiries related to unfamiliar objects may begin a dialogue about culture (Grossman, 1996).

Sometimes a nurse and client may share the same religious beliefs but come from different cultural groups. For example, an Irish Roman Catholic nurse performing spiritual assessments on clients of Hispanic or African descent might discover that although she and the clients come from different cultural backgrounds, they share common religious beliefs. In this example, clients who know that their beliefs are acknowledged and understood may feel more at ease when receiving care (see Concepts in Practice, "Shared Beliefs"). Institutional chaplains serve as invaluable resources for information regarding religious differences and accessing services for various religious rites and practices.

Concepts in Practice [IDEA]──▶[PLAN]──▶[ACTION]

Shared Beliefs

Juanita is a night nurse who practices Roman Catholicism. Frequently, she notices various religious artifacts that patients bring to the hospital. Juanita received a report about an elderly woman of German descent who has a terminal condition and does not respond to questions. Upon entering the woman's room, Juanita notices that the woman has her eyes closed and is moving her lips while touching beads. Juanita recognizes the beads as a rosary. She decides to join the woman in her prayers. As Juanita speaks the words of one of the prayers, the elderly woman opens her eyes and smiles. Juanita asks the woman if she is having pain. The elderly woman says "No." and reaches out to Juanita. Juanita takes the woman's hand and gently squeezes it. Juanita asks the woman if she needs anything. The woman replies, "I would like to see a priest." Juanita makes a call to the Roman Catholic priest on call. Upon learning this, the elderly woman relaxes and asks Juanita to stay and pray until the priest arrives.

TABLE 11.3   Elements of Cultural Assessment

Cultural Element	Description	Suggestions for Data Collection
Family and kinship system	Family structure, roles, and relationships	Describe your family to me. Who lives in your home? Describe the roles of each family member. Who provides support to you in the home? Observe the client as he or she interacts with family members.
Social life	Daily routine, group memberships, and recreation	Describe your typical day/week for me. To what groups do you belong? How do you spend your free time?
Political systems	Government, organizational, and economic affiliations	What support systems do you use outside the home? Describe your work environment. What are your feelings about the government? Do you have any economic concerns related to this illness/injury or seeking health care? What type of support do you need at home?
Language	Language spoken inside and outside the home	What is your native language? Do you speak more than one language? What language do you speak at home?
Traditions	Nonverbal communications, personal space, and other rituals that may have been passed down from previous generations	Is there anything that I should share with other health team members with regard to your personal space or other aspects of communication? Do you have any rituals or habits that we need to consider in providing health care to you?
Perceptions of the world	Viewpoints on the meaning of existence and how the world operates	How do you view the world and your place in it?
Values orientation	What the person considers the most important things in life	What things in life matter the most to you? How can we see that these things are preserved for you?
Cultural norms	Cultural attitudes about food, time, work, and leisure	What are your attitudes about food, time, work, and leisure? (It may be useful to separate this into four separate questions.)
Religion	Spiritual beliefs, including special beliefs and rituals surrounding life, health or illness, and death	Do you have any special spiritual needs related to your life, health, or illness? If you were to have a terminal illness, do you have a living will or advance directive?
Health beliefs	Group attitudes about health and illness	What are your beliefs about health and illness?
Health practices	Behaviors and rituals surrounding health and illness, including the use of folk healers and remedies	Tell me about the things you do at home to maintain your health. What type of measures did you take to cope with this health problem before you sought health care?

Andrews, M. M., & Boyle, J. S. (Eds.). (2008). *Transcultural concepts in nursing care* (5th ed.). Philadelphia, PA: Lippincott Williams & Wilkins; Dayer-Berenson, L. (2011). *Cultural competencies for nurses, impact on health and illness*. Sudbury, MA: Jones & Bartlett.

Provision of Culturally Congruent Care

Once the assessment is complete, the nurse proceeds with planning culturally congruent care. This may require referring to resources related to specific cultures and detailed information about the medical plan of care. Sometimes, traditional folk remedies may interfere with ordered medications. When this occurs, the nurse must find ways to work with clients so that they understand the hazards of using folk remedies along with prescription medications. Some special rituals, such as providing clients with water for cleansing themselves before daily prayer, present no harm.

However, the use of marijuana tea as a treatment for asthma poses great harm (Pachter, 1994). By engaging in respectful conversations, nurses and clients work together to make decisions related to accommodating lifeway practices with health care treatments.

Linguistically appropriate care serves as the final hallmark of culturally congruent care for clients who do not speak the language of HCPs. When possible, interpreters should be used for health teaching unless the provider is fluent in the client's language. Conversational foreign language provides the nurse with an ability to meet the client's basic needs. Most people who speak English as a second language find comfort with providers who speak to them in their primary language. However, mistakes can be made by the provider, so interpreters are essential when sharing critical information. If an interpreter happens to know the client or is part of a small, local community, preservation of client confidentiality might become an issue.

International Nursing Opportunities

Nurses can enhance their culturally competence by taking advantage of nursing opportunities outside of their home country. Governmental, private, and religious organizations offer opportunities for international nursing practice. The United Nations has nursing opportunities in various areas, including refugee support, immunization programs, AIDS prevention and treatment, and health promotion in developing countries. The Peace Corps offers nurses an opportunity to improve health in developing countries under the sponsorship of the US government. The U.S. Public Health Service offers assignments abroad. Private organizations, such as Doctors Without Borders, CARE, Catholic Relief Services, and Project HOPE (Health Opportunities for People Everywhere), seek the services of professional nurses for long- and short-term programs. The International Red Cross offers worldwide disaster relief, for which nursing services are needed. Various organized religions offer opportunities for missionary nursing.

The nursing shortage in the United States is shared with other countries. Saudi Arabia frequently recruits professional nurses from around the world. Nurses must be aware, however, that when accepting employment for a foreign assignment, they become bound by the host country's laws, cultural values, and norms. Therefore, before embarking on an international nursing experience or career, the professional nurse (or student) should read extensively about the culture, politics and economics, religions, health care system, and laws of the destination country. Scholarly journals and popular media provide sources for this information. If possible, the nurse should meet with host country residents to learn more about the culture. Some nurses find it very useful to develop fluency in the country's language(s) and visit the country as a tourist.

Upon arrival to the host country, the nurse should visit his or her native country's embassy or consulate (Herberg, 2008). Lack of knowledge serves as no excuse for breaking laws, and in some cases nurses have been subjected to corporal punishment for failure to abide by laws related to dress and for being in public without escorts.

STRATEGIES AND CHALLENGES FOR MULTICULTURAL NURSING PRACTICE

Nurses who care for clients from multiple cultural backgrounds must treat each person as an individual with unique personal needs. Some people become assimilated to the culture of the nation in which they reside while others do not. Not only are there international differences, but there also may be geographical differences within a country. Differences also may occur within a state (or province), county, or city. Taking time to listen to clients as care is delivered and having a broad knowledge base of cultural preferences enable the nurse to increase client comfort.

Health Disparities

The governmental publication *Healthy People 2020* (U.S. Department of Health and Human Services, 2010) examines disparities in the quality of health across various cultural groups in the United States, most of which arise from poverty, limited education, and lack of access to health care. *Healthy People 2020* defines a **health disparity** as

> "a particular type of health difference that is closely linked with social, economic, and/or environmental disadvantage. Health disparities adversely affect groups of people who have systematically experienced greater obstacles to health based on their racial or ethnic group; religion; socioeconomic status; gender; age; mental health; cognitive, sensory, or physical disability; sexual orientation or gender identity; geographic location; or other characteristics historically linked to discrimination or exclusion." (U.S. Department of Health and Human Services. The Secretary's Advisory Committee on National Health Promotion and Disease Prevention Objectives for 2020. Phase I report: Recommendations for the framework and format of Healthy People 2020. Section IV. Advisory Committee findings and recommendations. Available at: http://www.healthypeople.gov/hp2020/advisory/PhaseI/sec4.htm#_Toc211942917. Accessed 1/6/10.)

Healthy People 2020 has set target goals for eliminating health disparities (see Chapter 8, The Health Process and Self-Care of the Nurse).

With regard to health promotion among various cultural groups, knowledge of specific disease risks across those groups provides useful information to the professional nurse. Table 11.4 summarizes some health risks and diseases that occur with higher incidence in various cultural groups in the United States.

TABLE 11.4 Common Health Risks and Diseases Encountered by Various Cultural Groups in the United States

Cultural Group	Health Risks	Diseases
African American	Higher incidence of homicide Lower physical activity levels Obesity Cigarette smoking Alcohol abuse Incarceration Unintended pregnancy Untreated dental caries Sexually transmitted infections HIV/AIDS	Heart disease Stroke High blood pressure Chronic renal disease Cancer Premature death associated with breast and prostate cancer Cirrhosis of the liver Arthritis Asthma Blackout[a] Low blood[a] High blood[a] Thin blood[a]
Native American or Alaskan Native	Highest infant death rate among cultural groups in the United States Unintentional injuries Suicide Cigarette smoking Alcohol abuse Lack of health insurance coverage (38%)[c] Home fire deaths Gingivitis	Heart disease Cancer Diabetes Chronic liver disease Cirrhosis of the liver Pneumonia/influenza Chronic renal disease Ghost affliction[a]
Pacific Island/Asian American	Cigarette smoking	Heart disease High blood pressure Diabetes Cancer Cervical cancer (Vietnamese) Hepatitis Arthritis[b] Koro[a] (Southeastern Asian) Wagamama[a] (Japanese) Hwa-byung[a] (Korean)
Hispanic American	Low birth weight Lower physical activity levels Obesity Cigarette smoking Lack of health insurance coverage (33%)[c] Unintended pregnancy Sexually transmitted infection HIV/AIDS Home fire death Untreated dental caries Gingivitis	High blood pressure Diabetes Tuberculosis (20% higher rate than European Americans) Cancer, particularly cervical, esophageal, gall bladder, and stomach Increasing rates of breast and lung cancer Asthma Empacho[a] Fatigue[a] Mal ojo (evil eye)[a] Pasmo[a] Susto[b]
European American	Lower physical activity levels Obesity Alcohol abuse Cigarette smoking Sexually transmitted infections HIV/AIDS	Heart disease Arthritis Osteoporosis[b] Asthma Anorexia nervosa Bulimia[a] Hysteria[a] (Eastern European, Mideast cultures) Evil eye[a] (Eastern European)

[a]Culturally based syndromes.

[b]Health problem identified in elderly women of specified cultural group.

[c]Holahan, J. & Chen, V. (2011). Medicaid and the uninsured. Kaiser Family Publication 8264. Retrieved from www.kff.org/pub8264. Accessed February 25, 2013.

Adapted from Andrews, M. M., & Boyle, J. S. (Eds.). (2008). *Transcultural concepts in nursing care* (5th ed.). Philadelphia, PA: Lippincott Williams & Wilkins; Andrews, M., & Herberg, P. (1999). Transcultural nursing care. In M. M. Andrews & J. S. Boyle (Eds.), *Transcultural concepts in nursing care*. Philadelphia, PA: Lippincott Williams & Wilkins; Burggraf, V. (2000). The older woman: Ethnicity and health. *Geriatric Nursing*, 21,183–187; and U.S. Department of Health and Human Services. (2001). National standards for culturally and linguistically appropriate services in health care. Retrieved from http://www.minorityhealth.hhs.gov/assets/pdf/checked/Executive%20Summary.pdf. Accessed December 21, 2012.

Attitudes and Behaviors Toward Health Care

As noted through this chapter, health beliefs vary across cultures. Burggraf (2000) noted that elderly persons of non-European backgrounds have different attitudes and behaviors about health care. These include the following.

- General distrust of health care systems, societal disadvantages, language problems, reliance on traditional or spiritual healing practices, and discrimination based on race, ethnicity, gender, or age.
- Reduced satisfaction with health care plans and providers.

Burggraf (2000) also noted that language barriers may be a deterrent to seeking health care in populations of older Hispanics and elderly Asian women. These groups of elderly women tend to rely on folk and spiritual healing practices before entering the health care system (Burggraf, 2000). Young immigrant women (IW) receiving obstetrical care services in Canada have experienced issues with maternity care because of language barriers and lack of social support from their extended families who stayed in their homeland. Specific challenges to them are presented in Higginbottom et al.'s (2016) "An ethnographic investigation of the maternity health care experience of immigrants in rural and urban Alberta, Canada": in the Focus on Research Box below. The United States

FOCUS ON RESEARCH

Cultural Care Considerations for Nurses Working with Immigrants

An ethnographic investigation of the maternity health care experience of immigrants in rural and urban Alberta, Canada

Using individual and focus group semi-structured interviews, the investigators wanted to discover what issues were being encountered by immigrants in accessing and receiving health care services. Data were collected over a time frame of 2.5 years from 34 IW who received obstetrical care, 29 HCPs, and 23 social workers (SWs). They used purposive sampling techniques for each group included in the study.

Perceived personal barriers to access to effective maternity services by the IW were communication barriers (not fluent in English or French), lack of social support (extended family not available to help new mother), incongruent cultural beliefs (e.g., childbirth as a natural process not requiring

medical care services), and lack of information about available services. The IW identified the following structural barriers to services: inadequate health care and high cost of prescription medications. Factors identified by the IW as reducing satisfaction with rendered care services included: experiencing culture shock, feeling as being stereotyped, being discriminated against by HCPs, having to be dismissed from the hospital too soon, having too short of visits with HCPs, misunderstanding the process of informed consent and listening to HCPs violate their confidential issues.

Some HCPs expressed concern about the IW not fully understanding patient education and treatment plans. Other HCPs expressed disdain for some IW who expected medical care to be provided like concierge services in a hotel. The cultural dissonance between childbirth as a medical versus a natural event proved to be a source of distress for some HCPs. Cultural clashes also occurred during prenatal care (diet and exercise expectations), postnatal care (early hospital dismissals vs. a 72-hour stay), and newborn care (infant staying in mother's room).

Generalizing the study findings to other situations must be done with caution because it was conducted in one Canadian province, poor language fluency on the part of the IW, varying stages of the immigration process among IW, and some IW participants may have been reluctant to criticize services because of a previous history of civil strife in their homeland.

This study has clinical and health policy implications. In a health care system that strives for equality for all, persons who are different may experience discrimination and receive care based upon stereotypes of a particular ethnic group. Personal attributes of HCPs may reduce the adequacy and acceptability of care. Health information education material must be provided in multiple languages and media based upon the population service by a particular organization. HCPs caring for diverse populations should be educated about cultural competence, monitored for culturally sensitive delivery of care and evaluated for their performance. Programs to ameliorate system and personal discrimination need to be developed and maintained.

Higginbottom, G. M., Safipour, J., Yohani, S., O'Brien, B., Mumtaz, Z., & Paton, P. (2016). An ethnographic investigation of the maternity healthcare experience of immigrants in rural and urban Alberta, Canada. *BioMed Central Pregnancy and Childbirth 16*, 20. doi: 10.1186/s12884-015-0773-z and Canada frequently receive immigrants for politically unstable countries which may result in immigrant recipients of health care services to refuse to criticize health services rendered. Nurses need to tailor client health assessments to collect all culturally relevant data for using when planning, implementing, and evaluating care. Despite cultural differences regarding perceptions and beliefs of body parts and certain types of illness, all humans have similar biologic structure and basic physiology and some aspects of nursing care can be considered culturally neutral care.

Folk Illnesses

In addition to different risks for specific illnesses based on ethnicity, some cultures have **folk illnesses** that may require the use of culturally based healers. For example,

Empacho is a gastrointestinal condition that persons from some Mexican cultures believes occurs in infants. The belief proposes that empacho results in a backup of food and other matter within the walls of the stomach or intestines. Empacho is believed to occur if the child swallows too much saliva during teething or when parents change formulas that do not mix well with each other. Symptoms include abdominal distention, pain, poor appetite, perceived stomach lump, and diarrhea. Infants are placed on a regimen of clear liquids and herbal teas to "refresh the stomach" (Pachter, 1994, p. 692). If the infant loses too much weight, the parents may consult a physician to avoid being perceived by others as being neglectful.

Culturally competent care blends conventional medical therapy with folk remedies. For example, some people with medical illnesses go to physicians but may seek the advice of a folk healer to discover why the illness occurred. Some people view medical illnesses as the result of an evil spell and need to seek treatment from a spiritual healer to be fully well (Andrews & Boyle, 2016; Giger, 2013; Giger & Davidhizar, 2008; Pachter, 1994).

Physical Assessment Challenges

Along with increased specific health risks, people from different ethnic backgrounds have variations in physical appearance (Andrews & Boyle, 2016; Giger, 2013; Giger 2013; Pachter, 1994). The transculturally competent nurse considers **variations in physical appearance** when performing health assessments. A general appearance scan reveals information related to gender, age, skin color, body structure, consciousness level, facial features, clothing, and behavior. Initial interaction

with the client permits the nurse to collect information regarding orientation, speech patterns, facial expression, mood, and cognition. Clothing choice shows the nurse whether the person is able to select appropriate clothing for the weather and social situation. Although grooming is often a matter of personal preference, it can provide the nurse with cues related to the client's culture.

Clothing styles vary widely across cultures. Amish women usually wear solid-color dresses, held together by pins or snaps, and a bonnet. Mennonite women wear similarly styled clothing, but the dresses may be of printed material and have buttons. Islamic women may wear clothing to cover all extremities and cover their hair and sometimes their faces with a veil or scarf. Islamic men sometimes wear a cloth headdress (burka or hijab) and long robe. Depending upon the sect of Islam, clothing may be all black or very high fashion. Some Indian women wear saris. In certain instances, cultural and religious clothing may be concealed, as in the case of special white undergarments known as "temple garments" that are worn by members of the Church of Jesus Christ of Latter Day Saints (Mormons) (Andrews & Boyle, 2016). Roman Catholics often wear religious medals or pictures of Jesus and the Blessed Virgin encased in plastic around their necks (scapulars). When providing physical care to clients, the nurse should ask permission before removing specific items of clothing or jewelry. Attention should be paid to problems with caregiver gender, with alternate staffing arrangements made when feasible.

Skin color varies among all persons and depends on melanin concentrations. Because everyone (other than true albinos) has some level of melanin in the skin, all persons are people of color. When assessing for skin changes, the nurse must determine what the usual healthy shade is for the individual, rather than for the ethnic group. Specific skin variations for various ethnic groups may be found in physical assessment and transcultural nursing textbooks. Table 11.5 provides a brief summary of some key aspects for nursing assessments related to variations in ethnic descent. If the nurse relies on assessment data based on the skin color of those considered as "white," critical errors could occur.

Physiologic Variances

In addition to skin color, genetic traits result in **variations in physiology** across ethnic groups such as the adjustment in "normal" reference laboratory values for blood tests. For example, the hemoglobin levels of African Americans tend to be lower than those of

TABLE 11.5 Nursing Assessment Considerations Based on Ethnicity

Ethnic Group	Assessment Considerations
African	Mongolian spots and vitiligo more common Higher carotene levels in sclerae may give them a yellow appearance Pallor appears as ashen or gray Erythema difficult to see, but inflammation is more detectable by palpation for warmth, edema, and hardness Hard and soft palates may be the best place to see a macular rash Petechiae cannot be seen in some cases and, if seen, can be found on the buccal mucosa, conjunctiva, abdomen, buttocks, and volar forearm surface Tend to have stronger body odor Hair and scalp tend to be dry Copper-colored hair in children is an indication of severe malnutrition Less susceptible to noise-induced hearing loss Increased incidence of oral hyperpigmentation in older age Increased periodontal disease Highest bone density of all groups
Native Americans and Alaskan Natives	Mongolian spots and vitiligo more common Pallor appears yellow-brown Mild or absent body odor 18% have cleft uvula Alaskan Native populations have the largest teeth 30% of Navajo women have longitudinal vascular pattern on chest Alaskan Native populations have lower bone density than do whites
Asian	Mongolian spots and vitiligo more common Areola and genitalia are darker Pallor appears as pasty or nearly white Mild to absent body odor Hair usually silky, black, and straight Delayed hair graying Highest incidence of myopia (Japanese and Chinese) 10% have cleft uvula Lower bone density than whites
European	Persons of Mediterranean descent frequently have bluish lips, thereby negating reliance on circumoral cyanosis as a reliable indicator of poor oxygenation Pallor appears pasty or nearly white Skin wrinkles appear at a younger age Tend to have more moles than other groups Tend to have stronger body odor Hair turns gray at an earlier age Smallest teeth, resulting in more tooth loss
Pacific Island	Higher carotene levels in sclerae may give them a yellow appearance Pallor appears yellow-brown
Middle Eastern	Vitiligo more common Persons of Mediterranean descent frequently have blue lips, thereby negating reliance on circumoral cyanosis as a reliable indicator of poor oxygenation Pallor appears yellow-brown
Hispanic	Pallor appears yellow-brown Hair may have more natural oils

Andrews, M. M., & Boyle, J. S. (Eds.). (2016). *Transcultural concepts in nursing care* (5th ed.). Philadelphia, PA: Lippincott Williams & Wilkins; Andrews, M., & Herberg, P. (1999). Transcultural nursing care. In M. M. Andrews & J. S. Boyle (Eds.), *Transcultural concepts in nursing care*. Philadelphia, PA: Lippincott Williams & Wilkins; Purnell, L. (2014). *Transcultural health care, a culturally competent approach*. (3rd ed.) Philadelphia, PA: F. A. Davis; and Purnell, L., & Paulanka, B. (1998). *Transcultural health care, a culturally competent approach*. Philadelphia, PA: F. A. Davis.

their African counterparts; Native, Japanese, and Hispanic Americans have higher blood glucose levels than do European Americans. African Americans tend to have higher baseline levels of high-density lipoproteins (HDLs) than do persons of European descent, and Hispanic Americans have lower HDL levels. The source of these variations may be genetic or environmental. The federal government has identified medical research across gender and ethnic groups as a research priority (Jarvis, 2016; U.S. Department of Health and Human Services, 2010).

Pharmacogenetics (or pharmacogenics) is the field of study that describes metabolic variations that result in different responses to pharmacologic agents. Some of the known responses are summarized in Table 11.6. Some variations result from an inherited enzyme deficiency, whereas the source of other variations remains unknown. When providing care for a culturally diverse client population, professional nurses should be aware of differing responses to medications to anticipate potential adverse effects and different therapeutic responses that may require dosage alterations (Andrews & Boyle, 2016).

Take Note!

When performing health assessments, culturally competent nurses take into account variations in cultural beliefs, physical appearance, and physiology among specific ethnic groups.

TABLE 11.6 Cultural Variations in Response to Pharmacologic Agents

Cultural Group	Pharmacologic Agent	Variations
African Americans	Analgesics	Reduced sensitivity to therapeutic effects Increased gastrointestinal adverse effects, especially with acetaminophen
	Antihypertensives	Blood pressure responds better to single-agent therapy Less responsive to beta-blockers and angiotensin-converting enzyme inhibitors Increased mood responses to thiazide diuretics
	Mydriatics	Less pupil dilation
	Psychotropics	Increased risk for extrapyramidal side effects
	Steroids	Increased risk for steroid-induced diabetes (especially with methylprednisolone in renal transplantation)
	Tranquilizers	15–20% poorly metabolize diazepam
Arab Americans	Antiarrhythmics	Some dose reduction may be needed
	Antihypertensives	Some dose reduction may be needed
	Neuroleptics	Some dose reduction may be needed
	Opioids	Higher doses may be required because this group may have diminished ability to metabolize codeine to morphine
	Psychotropics	Some dose reduction may be needed
Native Americans	Muscle relaxants	Alaska Natives may have prolonged muscle paralysis with succinylcholine administration during surgery and may need mechanical ventilation for respiratory support
Chinese Americans	Narcotic analgesics	Less sensitive to respiratory depressant and hypotensive effects Have a higher clearance of morphine
Asian Americans	Antihypertensives	Best response with calcium antagonists
	Neuroleptics	May need reduced dosage
	Psychotropics	May need reduced dosage and up to one half the normal dose for tricyclic antidepressants and lithium
	Fat-soluble drugs	Increased dosages of fat-soluble drugs needed because of reduced percentages of body fat (especially vitamin K for warfarin reversal)
Hispanic Americans	Psychotropics	May need to reduce dosage as this group frequently has a higher incidence of adverse effects with tricyclic antidepressants
Americans of Mediterranean descent with glucose-6-phosphate dehydrogenase deficiency	Oxidating medications	Precipitation of a hemolytic crisis with primaquine, quinidine, thiazolsulfone, nitrofurazone, furazolidone, naphthalene, toluidine blue, phenylhydrazine, chloramphenicol, and aspirin
Jewish Americans (Ashkenazi)	Psychotropics	20% experience agranulocytosis with clozapine treatment for schizophrenia

Andrews, M., & Herberg, P. (1999). Transcultural nursing care. In M. M. Andrews & J. S. Boyle (Eds.), *Transcultural concepts in nursing care*. Philadelphia, PA: Lippincott Williams & Wilkins; Munoz, C., & Hilgenberg, C. (2005). Ethnopharmacology: Understanding how ethnicity can affect drug response is essential to providing culturally competent care. *American Journal of Nursing, 105*(8), 40–48.

CREATING A MULTICULTURAL NURSING PROFESSION

To offer health care services to a diverse population, a **multicultural nursing profession** must be created (Fig. 11.3). Attracting persons from different cultural backgrounds to the nursing profession remains a challenge. Nursing competes with other professions for the same students. Unfortunately, the best and the brightest students often prefer to enter other professions because nursing sometimes is perceived by outsiders as an oppressed profession that holds a status subservient to physicians. Adding membership to one more oppressed group may be more than a person can bear.

In addition to the perception of nurses as being less powerful members of the health care team, white women traditionally have dominated nursing. This dominance brings with it values, beliefs, and practices that reflect the socialization of white women. Current efforts to increase cultural diversity in the nursing profession include minority nursing scholarships, grant programs, and targeted recruitment efforts. Gordon and Copes (2010) describe success in the recruitment and retention of minority students by offering a year-round program to 8th to 12th grade minority students that highlights the rigors and benefits of pursuing a professional nursing career. The program includes academic remediation activities, mentoring, tutoring, counseling, and advisement along with learning activities in a nursing program lab and clinical experiences in a hospital with assigned preceptors. The National Coalition of Ethnic Minority Nurses serves as a clearinghouse for information related to nursing education, leadership, practice, research, and health care policy initiatives (Farella, 2001). According to the U.S. Bureau of Health Professions (2010), graduation rates for professional nursing programs 2001 to 2008 reveal that 22% of new graduates were from a minority group (7.3% African American, 6.6% Latino, 5% Asian/Pacific Islander, 3% multiracial, less than 0.1% Native American/Alaskan Native).

Once accepted into a nursing program, some minority nursing students experience **culture shock** (feelings of alienation, difficulty in relationships, loss of excitement, and a general dislike of the nursing program). This is exacerbated when some programs do not have a culturally diverse student body. Some minority students may become isolated because of an inability to interact with others like themselves or feel uneasy when interacting with students who are not like themselves. Most nurse educators come from the dominant group of nurses (Caucasian) and students of color may have difficulty connecting with them and finding professional role models who look like them.

Health care system and professional nursing values align with those of middle class, European-based values such as assuming responsibility for one's actions, being proactive rather than reactive, assuming the Protestant work ethic, meeting deadlines, and arriving on time. Nursing programs expect students to abide by these traditional cultural values of nursing. For example, punctuality is a highly valued work practice in nursing and education. Students sometimes receive a grade penalty for arriving to class late or submitting assignments late, especially when faculty fail to explore reasons for a late assignment or neglect to explain the reasons why punctuality is valued.

Faculty may make errors when working with students from various cultural groups. Nursing students from different cultures may use different nonverbal

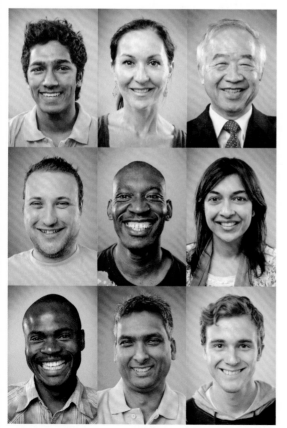

FIGURE 11.3 A team of culturally diverse persons provides varying views of how best to plan culturally specific and congruent health care services.

behaviors than their instructors expect when conversing with persons of authority. For example, students from Asian countries tend to not make eye contact when conversing with teachers, supervising staff nurses, physicians, and older persons. Although for the student this practice is a way of conveying respect, some faculty and staff may label the student as being cold and distant and question the student's ability to practice nursing with genuine compassion.

Upon graduation from a nursing program, nurses from perceived minority or "foreign" cultures may fall victim to racism and stereotyping, especially in stressful working relationships (Farella, 2001). Leininger (1995) and Farella (2001) reported incidents in the 1980s in which Filipino nurses who accepted offers of employment in the United States fell victim to racial slurs and stereotyping. Sometimes, clients and relatives falsely accuse health team members from ethnic backgrounds different than their own of theft of personal belongings. Professional nurses have an obligation to be hospitable to nurses and other health team members who are from different ethnic backgrounds.

Platz and Wales (1999) outlined various methods to make others feel welcome. First, culturally competent nurses make all clients and colleagues feel cared for and appreciated. Second, standards for business etiquette include greeting colleagues and all persons with each encounter; respecting the time of others; being prompt for meetings and appointments; calling to inform others if delayed for more than 5 minutes; sending thank-you notes; listening actively to others; respecting the religion and culture of others; and considering the privacy of others and the right to a neat, clean, and safe working environment.

Strategies for Working in Multicultural Health Care Teams

The influx of persons from other cultures as health care team members is expected to increase with increased

---

11.2 Learning, Knowing, and Growing

Guidelines for Working Successfully with Health Team Members from Other Cultures

Cultural Issue	Suggested Guidelines
English as a Second Language (ESL)	Have direct care givers being supervised repeat instructions back to validate that they understand what needs to be done. Have physicians, APRNs, and other health professionals repeat what was said to validate that they understood what was reported to them. Learn a few phrases to converse with team members in their native language. Inform team members of the importance of speaking English in clinical practice areas unless the patient and family speak the same language as the team member.
Cultural Group Membership that Differs from the Professional Nurse's Cultural Group	Become aware of your own biases and prejudices. Deal with personal biases, prejudices, and stereotypes openly. Get to know team member as an individual rather than a member of a specific cultural group. Learn about cultural group values and practices of all team members. Organize and hold cultural celebrations of all team members. Offer to work for team members when they want to take time for cultural holidays or religious celebrations. Develop deep, meaningful relationships with health team coworkers as client care is executed.
Internationally Educated Nurses	Learn about professional nursing practice in the nurse's country of origin. Orient the nurse to state professional nursing practice laws and institutional practice guidelines. Trust the nurse to provide safe, effective client care. Correct social and nursing care errors with sensitivity. Invite the nurses to attend a local professional nursing organization meeting. Invite the nurses to participate in facility governance meetings when available. Offer to work on days when national holidays are celebrated in the internationally educated nurse's homeland. Inquire about life in the nurse's homeland. Plan and execute social events for the nurses. Provide emotional support during times of homesickness if the nurse is away from family. Develop deep, meaningful working relationships as client care is executed.

cultural diversity in the population. Lack of adequate representation of various cultural groups in health care teams has been linked to disparities in access to care services and health care outcomes. Culturally diverse people have a key role to play in filling the projected vacancies in the health care team of the future. Professional programs, especially nursing programs, need to recruit culturally diverse students, commit to admitting them, and offer services to facilitate program success.

Effective health and nursing care requires a multidisciplinary effort and includes work efforts of licensed professionals and technicians. Unlicensed assistive personnel frequently perform the less mentally challenging and more physically demanding work associated with inpatients in acute or long-term care facilities. Many professional nurses encounter different cultural groups as they work with various members of the health care team. Principles of cultural competency used with clients foster effective teamwork.

As noted earlier in this chapter, the majority (83.2%) of practicing professional nurses in the United States are Caucasian with members of culturally diverse groups being underrepresented in the profession (U.S. Bureau of Health Professions, 2010). Unlicensed care providers (UCPs) and licensed practical/vocational nurses (LPN/ LVNs) frequently hail from more diverse backgrounds. Technical education programs frequently attract people who cannot afford a 4-year college education. Therefore, nurses from a middle class, Caucasian cultural background find themselves supervising nursing care delivered by members of a different cultural group. Box 11.2, Learning, Knowing, and Growing, "Guidelines for Working Successfully with Health Team Members from other Cultures," provides suggestions for easing this process.

▉ QUESTIONS FOR REFLECTION

1. What are the benefits of having people from different cultural backgrounds and identities serving on the health care team?

2. What are the values promoted by the health care system in terms of work habits? Do you see a potential conflict with these values based on your cultural background? Why or why not?

Summary and Significance to Practice

As the US population grows more diverse, professional nurses need knowledge and skills to provide culturally relevant care. Some professional nurses unfortunately cling to personal biases and misconceptions related to cultural differences when providing health care services to culturally diverse populations. The reluctance to abandon negative attitudes towards persons different from the care provider's cultural group creates a climate of distrust and discrimination which increases the likelihood of negative health care outcomes.

Genetic differences and predispositions among various cultures increase the complexity of medical decision making and mandate careful consideration be given to the optimal strategies for health promotion and disease prevention as nurses encounter culturally diverse clients.

In addition to the challenges of working with culturally diverse populations, the nursing profession faces challenges in developing a workforce that mirrors the population demographics of the clients served.

To establish cultural competence in clinical practice, professional nurses must first become cognizant of personal biases; this requires the cognitive skill of honest self-reflection. Establishing cultural competence requires an attitude of genuine caring toward all humankind as well as personal commitment to make the time to learn about client cultural care considerations. Nurses should take the time to ask questions related to cultural preferences, listen to individuals, consider cues given to them by people from a different culture, and analyze the benefits (or hazards) of generic (or folk) health practices before outlining care plan strategies. Interacting with people from cultural backgrounds different from their own sometimes means that nurses must take risks, but nurses can learn from their mistakes. Nurses serve as client advocates when they see that individual client cultural needs are met. Authentic caring and effective communication skills enhance the development of therapeutic relationships with clients and collegial relationships with colleagues from different cultural backgrounds.

REAL-LIFE REFLECTIONS

Recall Judy from the beginning of the chapter. What do you think Judy could do to facilitate the teamwork for a multicultural nursing care team? Why is it important that team members of diverse cultural groups understand each other?

From Theory to Practice

1. Think of a time when you worked with someone who was from a different cultural background than your own. What did you learn from this person? Did your personal encounters with this person result in any changes in your thoughts, values, or beliefs? Why or why not?

2. Outline a plan of how you might resolve a dispute in a clinical situation with either a client or coworker. How would your plan change if the person were from a cultural background different from your own?

Nurse as Author

Think about your own level of cultural competence. Write a short essay about your level of cultural competence. Include information about your strengths and your areas for further growth to become a cultural competent professional nurse.

Your Digital Classroom

Online Exploration

International Council of Nurses: **www.icn.ch**
MinorityNurse.com: **www.MinorityNurse.com**
National Association of Hispanic Nurses:
   http://www.nahnnet.org/
The American Folklife Center: **www.loc.gov/folklife**
The National Black Nurses Association, Inc.:
   www.nbna.org
Transcultural Nursing Society: **www.tcns.org**
United States Department of Health and Human Services, Office of Minority Health:
   https://www.thinkculturalhealth.hhs.gov

Expanding Your Understanding

1. Search online using the terms "Living in (*specify the country or countries of your heritage*)," and read a description of the daily life and any legal or cultural issues that you might encounter if you lived or visited there. Note any specific laws to which you would be accountable for following. Bring these to share with your classmates.

2. Visit the United States Department of Health and Human Services Health Resources and Service Administration's website for Culture, Language, and Health Literacy at https://www.hrsa.gov/cultural competence/index.html. Select two resources that you found interesting and relevant to your future nursing practice. Explain why you think this is important to your future practice and how you might use these resources to guide your future professional practice. Bring these to share with your classmates.

3. Visit the website for the United States Department of Health and Human Services, Office of Minority Health at **http://www.minorityhealth.hhs.gov/,** and find a variety of resources to facilitate culturally sensitive and linguistically appropriate nursing care. Select two resources that you found interesting and relevant to your future nursing practice. Explain why you think this is important to your future practice and how you might use these resources to guide your future professional practice. Bring these to share with your classmates.

Beyond the Book

Visit the**Point®** **www.thePoint.lww.com** for activities and information to reinforce the concepts and content covered in this chapter.

REFERENCES

Andrews, M. M., & Boyle, J. S. (Eds.). (2008). *Transcultural concepts in nursing care* (5th ed.). Philadelphia, PA: Lippincott Williams & Wilkins.

Andrews, M. M., & Boyle, J. S. (Eds.) (2016). *Transcultural concepts in nursing care* (8th ed.). Philadelphia, PA: Wolters Kluwer.

Burchum, J. (2002). Cultural competence: An evolutionary perspective. *Nursing Forum, 37*, 5–15.

Burggraf, V. (2000). The older woman: Ethnicity and health. *Geriatric Nursing, 21*, 183–187.

DeVito, J. (2004). *The interpersonal communication handbook* (10th ed.). Boston, MA: Pearson.

Farella, C. (2001). How we hurt our own. *Nursing Spectrum, 2*(2), 12–13.

Giger, J. N. (2013). *Transcultural nursing assessment and intervention* (6th ed.). St. Louis, MO: Elsevier/Mosby.

Giger, J. N., & Davidhizar, R. E. (2008). *Transcultural nursing assessment and intervention* (5th ed.). St. Louis, MO: Mosby.

Gordon, F. C., & Copes, M. A. (2010). The Coppin Academy for pre-nursing success: A model for the recruitment and retention of minority students. *The ABNF Journal: The Official Journal of the Association of Black Nursing Faculty in Higher Education, 21*(1), 11–13.

Grossman, D. (1996). Cultural dimensions in home health nursing. *American Journal of Nursing, 96*, 33–36.

Herberg, P. (2008). Perspectives on international nursing. In M. M. Andrews, & J. S. Boyle (Eds.), *Transcultural concepts in nursing care* (5th ed.). Philadelphia, PA: Lippincott Williams & Wilkins.

Hughes, K., & Hood, L. (2007). Teaching methods and an outcome tool for measuring cultural sensitivity in undergraduate nursing students. *Journal of Transcultural Nursing, 18*(1), 57–62.

Jarvis, C. (2016). *Physical examination and health assessment* (7th ed.). St. Louis, MO: Elsevier.

Kavanagh, K. H., & Kennedy, P. H. (1992). *Promoting cultural diversity: Strategies for health care professionals.* Newbury Park, CA: Sage.

Leininger, M. (1991). *Transcultural nursing.* New York: McGraw-Hill.

Leininger, M. (1995). *Transcultural nursing* (2nd ed.). New York: McGraw-Hill.

Leininger, M., & McFarland, M. (2002). *Transcultural nursing: Concepts, theories, research and practice* (3rd ed.). New York: McGraw-Hill.

Leininger, M., & McFarland, M. (2006). *Cultural care diversity and universality: A worldwide theory for nursing* (2nd ed.). Sudbury, MA: Jones & Bartlett.

National Council of State Boards of Nursing and the Forum of State Nursing Workforce Centers. (2013). *The NCSBN and the Forum of State Nursing Workforce Centers 2013 National Workforce Survey of Registered Nurses.* Retrieved from https://www.ncsbn.org/2013_Poster_graphics.pdf. Accessed April 24, 2016.

National Council of State Boards of Nursing. (2016). *2015 National Workforce Survey.* Retrieved from https://www.ncsbn.org/workforce.htm. Accessed April 24, 2016.

Office of Minority Health (2007). *National standards on culturally and linguistically appropriate servies (CLAS).* Retrieved from http://minorityhealth.hhs.gov/templates/browse.aspx?lvl=2&lvlID=15, Accessed December 21, 2012.

Pachter, L. M. (1994). Culture and clinical care: Folk illness beliefs and behaviors and their implications for health care delivery. *Journal of the American Medical Association, 271,* 690–694.

Platz, A., & Wales, S. (1999). *Social graces: Manners, conversation and charm for today.* Eugene, OR: Harvest House.

Pullen, R. (2007). Tips for communicating with a patient from another culture. *Nursing, 37*(10), 48–49.

Purnell, L. D., & Paulanka, B. J. *Transcultural health care: A culturally competent approach*, (3rd ed.). Philadelphia: F.A. Davis.

Purnell, L. D. (2014). *Transcultural health care: A culturally competent approach* (4th ed.). Philadelphia, PA: F. A. Davis.

Purnell, L. D., & Paulanka, B. J. (2008). *Transcultural health care: A culturally competent approach* (3rd ed.). Philadelphia, PA: F. A. Davis.

Spector, R. E. (2012). *Cultural diversity in health and illness* (8th ed.). Upper Saddle River, NJ: Pearson Prentice Hall.

Sullivan Commission. (2004). Missing persons: Minorities in the health professions, a report of the Sullivan Commission on diversity in the healthcare workforce. Retrieved from http://health-equity.pitt.edu/40/. Accessed December 21, 2012.

U.S. Bureau of Health Professions. (2010). *The registered nurses population: Finding from the 2008 National Sample Sruvey of Registered Nurses.* Retrieved from http://bhpr.hrsa.gov/workforcestudies/rnsurvey2008.html. Accessed December 21, 2012.

U.S. Census Bureau. (2011). Overview of race and Hispanic origin. US Hispanic population surpasses 45 million. Retrieved from http://www.census.gov/prod/cen2010/briefs/c2010br-02.pdf. Accessed December 21, 2012.

U.S. Census Bureau. (2016). United States Population: Components of population change. Retrieved from https://www.census.gov/data.html. Accessed April 24, 2016.

U.S. Department of Health and Human Services. (2010). Healthy people 2020 [brochure]. Retrieved from http://www.healthypeople.gov/2020/TopicsObjectives2020/pdfs/HP2020_brochure_with_LHI_508.pdf. Accessed December 21, 2012.

United States Department of Health and Human Services, Office of Minority Health. (2010). National standards on culturally and linguistically appropriate services (CLAS) in health and health care. Retrieved from https://www.thinkculturalhealth.hhs.gov/pdfs/enhancednationalclasstandards.pdf Accessed April 24, 2016.

Yoder, M. K. (1996). Instructional responses to ethnically diverse nursing students. *Journal of Nursing Education, 35,* 315–321.

Yoder, M. K. (1997). The consequences of a generic approach to teaching nursing in a multicultural world. *Journal of Cultural Diversity, 4,* 77–82.

Professional Nurse Accountability

LEARNING OUTCOMES

By the end of this chapter, the learner will be able to:

1. Differentiate accountability from autonomy and authority.
2. Identify the essential questions the professional nurse must answer to be accountable to the client and public.
3. Relate current standards of professional nursing practice to accountability.
4. Identify some of the positive outcomes of nurses becoming accountable to clients, profession, self, employing institution, managed care networks, and third-party payers.
5. Evaluate oneself on professional accountability, using the checklist provided.

REAL-LIFE REFLECTIONS

Carol is a charge nurse on a neuroscience unit. Mr. Jones, a frail 90-year-old, has been admitted for altered level of consciousness. Mrs. Jones wants absolutely everything done to make her husband well. She insists that the nursing assistant, Gloria, give him food and fluid to drink. When Gloria refuses, Mrs. Jones insists on seeing the charge nurse. Carol is busy and cannot talk to Mrs. Jones immediately. Mrs. Jones grows impatient and fixes coffee for her husband, then holds the cup to his mouth for him to take sips. Mr. Jones chokes violently. Carol runs into the room and finds that there are no suction catheters for the wall unit suction apparatus. As she delivers the Heimlich maneuver to Mr. Jones, she sends Gloria to the supply cart to get suction catheters; none are found there. Mr. Jones stops breathing, and Carol "calls a code." Unfortunately, Mr. Jones dies.

- *List the mistakes made in this scenario and who made them.*
- *What are the potential consequences of Mr. Jones' death?*
- *How would you feel if a similar situation happened while you practiced nursing?*

In early writings about the nursing profession, the term *responsibility* meant duty. In *Notes on Nursing* (1946/1859), Florence Nightingale frequently outlined the responsibilities of professional nurses, from the state of the sick room to the need for careful observation on the part of the nurse to avoid patient accidents. She also noted, "I have often seen really good nurses distressed, because they could not impress the doctor with the real danger of their patients" (p. 68).

In the early 1900s, private-duty nursing represented the epitome of nursing accountability to clients: a nurse took a "case," lived with the client, and remained until the client no longer needed nursing services. The nurse assumed responsibility and was held accountable for the client's life, space, and nursing care.

After the Great Depression of the 1930s, health care moved from the home to institutions and fewer nurses chose to practice private-duty nursing. They opted instead for employment as staff nurses in hospitals or public health agencies (Dachelet & Sullivan, 1979). Nurses focused on specific care tasks, and duties were assigned according to functions outlined by job descriptions. The professional nurse supervised other staff and assumed accountability for the actions of self and others.

The notion of accountability also began to evolve; it became tied to negative situations and carried a punitive connotation. Although often unaware, nurses were legally liable for their actions or their lack of action. Many nurses believed that the ultimate liability remained with the institution, which would "cover" them in the event of a lawsuit.

Accountability in the professional sense did not exist until the 1970s, when nurses' and society's view of nurses as holding subservient roles and merely following physician orders began to change. True professional accountability in nursing surfaced in the late 1970s (Clifford, 1981). In 1980, accountability first appeared as a free-standing topic heading in the Cumulative Index of Nursing and Allied Health Literature.

DEFINITION OF ACCOUNTABILITY AND RELATED CONCEPTS

To assume accountability, nurses must understand its definition. As an adjective, the word *accountable* means being required to explain actions or decisions to another party or required to be responsible for the outcomes of actions and decisions (Merriam-Webster, 2015a). Therefore **accountability** is the state of being responsible or answerable for one's decisions and actions. In contrast, **responsibility** is defined as the state of being

the person who caused something to happen, a task or duty that someone is expected to accomplish, or a moral, legal, or ethical requirement (Merriam-Webster, 2015b). Accountability and responsibility differ in that responsibility arises within the nurse and accountability comes from others (employers, clients, society). For example, a professional nurse assumes responsibility for providing safe effective, client care and society holds the nurse accountable for actions taken (or not taken) while providing client care.. Although not part of its definition, the term *accountability* carries a negative connotation in today's business environment because the question "Who's accountable or responsible?" tends to surface only when things go wrong (Armstrong, 2011; Dethmer, 2006a; Miller, 2004). Accountability "is increasingly confused with and used in place of autonomy and authority, although it is synonymous with neither, but related to both" (Batey & Lewis, 1982, p. 13).

Accountability

By dividing the term *accountability* in two parts, Dethmer (2006a) simplified its definition. Dethmer's (2006a) first aspect of accountability incorporates the concept of responsibility, which basically means "to account for what has been done" (p. 46). Accountability for an outcome is assessed by the questions "Who did it?" "Who participated in it?" and "Who started it?" In contrast, the term *responsibility* means "to be able to respond" (Dethmer, 2006a, p. 50). Dethmer (2006a) took the concept of accountability one step further and devised the term *radical responsibility*, which is to take full responsibility for whatever happens in one's life rather than blaming others, while being committed to learning from each personal experience. The beauty of this interpretation of accountability is that people must take credit for successes and failures.

The second aspect of Dethmer's (2006b) conceptual approach to accountability includes making and keeping agreements that he calls "impeccable agreements." He defined an agreement as anything people say they will or will not do. An impeccable agreement involves a deep personal commitment to doing what the person wants to do, fully aligned with the person's values, completely connected to something over which the person has control, personal acknowledgment of importance, and detailed record keeping to document completion. Whenever an agreement is made, people are to keep it or renegotiate it should something interfere with its execution because "broken agreements damage trust" (Dethmer, 2006b), p. 80).

Clear agreements involve facts (exactly what the agreement contains), feelings (emotional reactions to agreeing), and reasons (the specific rationale behind the agreement). Renegotiating a deadline involves just giving plain, simple facts and works best if the renegotiation occurs prior to the deadline. When an agreement is broken, all involved parties must acknowledge that the agreement was broken and communicate it to all involved people. The person breaking the agreement needs to take responsibility for the action without providing excuses, justifications, or explanations and also listen to the responses of the affected person(s). The person breaking the agreement should inquire about what can be done to address the consequences of the broken agreement. Finally, when agreements are broken, all involved people should take the time to analyze what happened, learn from it, and not repeat the same mistake (Dethmer, 2006b).

Thus, accountability is the state of being responsible for agreements and answerable for the behaviors and their outcomes that fall into the realm of one's professional role. The American Nurses Association (ANA)'s *Nursing Scope and Standards of Practice* (2015b) and all nurse practice acts (NPAs) consider that a binding agreement has been made when a nurse establishes a relationship with a person to provide professional nursing services. Nurses become accountable for implementing these established agreements with clients. They also become accountable to employers when providing nursing services to clients. When working for an agency, professional nurses agree to abide by the agency's policies and procedures. Nurses are accountable to interprofessional colleagues for reporting changes in the physical and mental conditions of clients that they note when providing nursing care services. They are accountable to each other when working as a team to provide care to client groups. Nurses also are held accountable for their social media posts. In fact, some nurses and nursing students have lost positions for posting client confidential information, photos of themselves with clients, and negative comments about employers. Finally, society holds nurses accountable for harmful acts that occur during clinical practice.

Responsibility and Answerability

Ethical codes for nurses published by national and international nursing organizations contain information related to professional accountability (ANA, 2015a; International Council of Nurses [ICN], 2012). Under these, accountability continues to retain its original meaning of responsibility but has an added dimension—**answerability**—which is the requirement to offer answers, reasons, and explanations to certain others. As the ANA *Code of Ethics for Nurses* defines, accountability as "being answerable, or to give an account or defense to oneself or others for one's own choices, decisions and actions as measured against a standard…" (Fowler, 2015, p. 59). Examples of standards to which nurses are held accountable include the *ANA's Nursing Scope and Standards of Practice,* the ANA and ICN Code of Ethics for Nurses, state NPAs where they practice, and standards determined by specialty professional nursing organizations (e.g., American Association of Critical Care Nurses, Oncology Nursing Society, etc.).

In 2010, the ANA revised its *Nursing's Social Policy Statement,* which specified that a social contract provides the basis for the authority of professional nursing practices (2010). The contract gives the nurse professional rights and responsibilities for all actions taken while engaged in clinical practice, such as following the scope and standards for professional and specialty nursing practice; using the best evidence to provide safe, high-quality care; abiding by legal rules and regulations for practice designated by the state or national professional organizations; following institutional policies and procedures; and making independent decisions for self-determination about practice situations. Protection of the public from unscrupulous and unsafe nurses is afforded by legal mechanisms, including civil and criminal laws and penalties, as well as various laws that govern professional nursing licensure. In the United States, state governments set rules and regulations for professional nursing licensure and practice. When credentialing health care professionals, state governments consider the potential for public harm if the professional fails to follow safe, acceptable practice standards as well as how much autonomy and accountability for decision making are assumed by the professional (Milstead, 2008).

Currently, discussions of accountability for professional nursing revolve around client assessments, interventions (nursing care), outcomes (results), and costs (expenditures). Because of legal, accreditation, third-party payer, and managed care requirements, documentation frequently serves as evidence that nurses either performed or did not perform specific nursing assessments and interventions. The health care delivery industry has higher error rates today than other industries. Estimates suggest that 3% to 4% of all hospital patients experience a medical care error and tens of thousands of persons die annually as a result of care errors (Sherwood, 2012).

In the early 21st century, many efforts to improve the safety and quality of health care emerged. Examples of safety initiatives include those of the U.S. Agency for Healthcare Research and Quality (www.ahrq.gov); the Joint Commission (www.jointcommission.org) revised annual National Patient Safety Goals; the Institute for Healthcare Improvement's (www.ihi.org) "5 Million Lives Campaign" (December 2006 to December 2008) (Berwick, 2010) and "10,000 Lives Campaign" (January 2005 to June 2006) (McCannon, Schall, Calkins, & Nazem, 2006); the Institute of Medicine (IOM)'s Quality Chasm series of reports on improving the safety and quality of health care in America (www.iom.edu); and Quality and Safety Education for Nurses (QSEN) efforts to increase nurse awareness of patient-safety needs (www.qsen.org). QSEN developed competencies, knowledge, skills, and attitudes for undergraduate nursing education initially and later added graduate education competencies. QSEN has evolved and is now known as the QSEN Institute. It is managed by a faculty team at Case Western Reserve University and offers free resources to nurses and nursing faculty that require no user account (The QSEN Institute, 2013). Findings from these initiatives have been incorporated into the Patient Protection and Affordable Care Act of 2010 (see Chapter 9, Health Care Delivery Systems). The expectation of higher-quality and safer health care based on scientific evidence may result in increased areas of professional nurse accountability. Professional nurses display accountability each time they answer questions about the reasons behind actions, document interventions and outcomes of delivered care, and participate in clinical competency programs.

> **Take Note!**
> Accountability is the state of being responsible and answerable for actions and client outcomes that fall under the auspices of one's professional role.

Autonomy and Authority

Although related to the concept of accountability, the concept of autonomy should be seen distinct, as it refers to independence of functioning. **Autonomy** means that one can perform one's total professional function on the basis of one's own knowledge and judgment and that one is recognized by others as having the right to do so. Obviously, autonomy is related to accountability because a person who functions autonomously must be accountable for his or her behavior (Holden, 1991; Hylka & Shugrue, 1991).

Another term closely related to yet distinct from accountability is authority. **Authority** can be defined as being in a position to make decisions and to influence others to act in a manner determined by those decisions. Authority is certainly related to accountability because those who are in authority are accountable for the decisions they make and for both their own actions and those of others who act on the basis of their decisions. Authority also relates closely to autonomy, because those in authority often act autonomously in performing all or part of their respective roles.

Professional autonomy has been incorporated as an essential element of a magnetic work environment for nurses. According to Kramer et al., "Autonomy is the *freedom* to act on *what you know,* to make independent clinical decisions that *exceed standard nursing practice,* in *the best interest of the patient.*" *Freedom* is about trust and organizational sanction for autonomous practice (Kramer, Schmalenberg, & Maguire, 2008, p. 25). Kramer et al. (2008) developed their definition for "clinical autonomy" using transcripts of recorded interviews with 289 nurses employed in Magnet hospitals.[1] In the 2015 version of the *ANA's Nursing Scope and Standards of Practice,* autonomy is defined as "The capacity of a nurse to determine her or his own actions through independent choice, including demonstration of competence, within the full scope of nursing practice" (p. 85).

This definition of autonomy empowers nurses to act on all forms of nursing knowledge to provide optimal client care. Nurses practicing in hospitals with Magnet status are expected to use evidence-based practice as the standard for professional practice. When nurses encounter a situation that is not based on evidence or is counterintuitive, they are expected to take steps to verify that the proposed therapeutic interventions are in the best interest of their clients before proceeding. To question physician orders, nurses must have the cognitive skills to recognize a discrepancy, the solid knowledge (or evidence) to justify questions, and the confidence to know that they must consult with a physician prior to action. When nurses exercise autonomy,

---

[1]Magnet is a special recognition accorded to hospitals by the American Nurses Credentialing Center (a subsidiary of the ANA) and designates a hospital that practices transformational leadership, provides mechanisms for structural empowerment, displays exemplary professional practice, has commitments to discovering new knowledge, practices innovations while continuously improving quality, and possesses a record of high rankings on empirical quality outcomes (ANA, 2008) (see Chapter 13, Environmental and Global Health, for more information about the Magnet recognition program).

they become accountable for the results (either positive or negative).

Delegation

Professional nurses need to understand that being able to provide for every single client care need by themselves is an impossibility. Understanding the division of tasks that can be accomplished by unlicensed assistive personnel (UAP) and licensed/vocational nurses (LPN/LVNs) enable others to assume responsibility for executing some of the most rewarding aspects of professional practice (basic hand-on physical care). Delegating of tasks enables professional nurses to focus on care coordination and education of clients and their significant others (White, Jackson, Bessner, & Norris, 2015). **Delegation** is the act of transferring a task that one would do (if time permitted) to another person who is capable of performing the task.

Because professional nurses frequently delegate nursing responsibilities to UAPs and LPN/LVNs, professional nurses become accountable for the outcomes of the actions of others. Delegation of tasks requires that nurses use professional judgment to decide what tasks can be performed safely by another member of the nursing team. Before delegating any task, the nurse must ascertain that the person has the **competence** (or ability) to perform the task. Most state NPAs address the delegation process. Many of the directives regarding delegation leave room for the professional nurse to decide what tasks can be safely delegated to others (see Box 12.1, Professional Building Blocks, "Considering the Safety of Delegation").

In 2016, the National State Boards of Nursing developed a national set of evidence-based guidelines for effective delegation. The Delegation Guidelines emphasis the importance of effective communication between delegators and delegatees, assessing the competence of the person accepting the delegated tasks, for tasks to be done, availability of the delegator to the delegate, and ongoing education and training. Once a delegated task is accepted, the delegate assumes accountability for the results and the responsibility for completing the task. In addition, the delegator must provide directions and communication about the task to be completed and verify that the task is completed through effective supervision and evaluation. (Right task, right circumstance, right person, right directions and communication, and right supervision and evaluation which are known as the traditional five rights of delegation) (National Council of State Boards of Nursing, 2016).

When UAP or LPN/LVN accepts delegated tasks, they assume responsibility for completing them. In

12.1 Professional Building Blocks

Considering the Safety of Delegation

The questions that follow can help nurses decide what tasks can be safely done by another member of the nursing care team:

1. Are there laws that support delegating the task?
2. Is the task within the scope of the professional nurse's practice?
3. Does the delegating nurse have the knowledge and skill to make competent decisions about delegation (such as determining client risk for each delegated task)?
4. Does the task meet all conditions and criteria for delegation to an unlicensed care provider (i.e., guidelines are within the NPA; task routinely recurs in daily work, needs no modification, has a predictable outcome, and does not require ongoing assessment, interpretation, or independent decision making)?
5. Does the unlicensed care provider have the knowledge, skill, and ability to perform the task effectively?
6. Do the skills of the unlicensed care provider match with client care needs?
7. Does the agency have policies, protocols, and procedures in place for the proposed delegated task?
8. Will appropriate supervision be available during task completion?

American Nurses Association and the National Council of State Boards of Nursing. (2005). Joint statement on delegation. Retrieved from https://www.ncsbn.org/Delegation_joint_statement_NCSBN-ANA.pdf. Accessed March 5, 2013; National Council of State Boards of Nursing (2016). National guidelines for nursing delegation, *Journal of Nursing Regulation, 7*(1), 7–14.

some instances, such as delegation of a bedbath, UAP can make simple decisions about whether to use commercially prepackaged baths or traditional soap, water, and washcloths (unless the agency has set a policy on how to perform bedbaths). When administering medications, an LPN/LVN can make decisions about whether or not to administer unscheduled medications that are ordered as needed (e.g., pain medication) At times, nurses may opt to perform a task usually delegated to an unlicensed care provider or LPN/LVN when client situations reveal a high potential for harm and quick independent decision making is required to avert a serious complication. For example, a registered nurse (RN) may decide to feed a newly admitted client who has difficulty speaking because the nurse can assess for safe swallowing and intervene quickly should the client choke or administer and monitor the effects

FOCUS ON RESEARCH

RNs, UAP, and Pressure Ulcers

In seeking to identify how hospital "RNs perform, document, and reflect on pressure ulcer prevention," the investigators observed RNs as they worked on acute care units for 24 to 25 hours, conducted semi-structured interviews with the RNs, and reviewed patient records over a 4-month period. Nine female nurses from three units (geriatric, orthopedic, and medical) participated in the study. Using the Modified Norton Scale, which has scores ranging from 4 to 28 with persons scoring 20 or less being at increased risk for pressure ulcer formation, the nurses identified a total of 32 patients having an increased risk. Twenty-eight patients had scores between 7 and 11 and four additional patients were considered to be at risk because of immobility issues.

The investigators observed nurses as they provided care. The investigators reported one instance of an RN who failed to perform assessments of one of the patient's heels, pressure ulcers, and Modified Norton Scale during the time of data collection. RNs used air mattresses on 6 patients, relieved heel pressure twice, and changed patient position 16 times. They assessed nutritional and fluid status once and provided nutritional support six times. The RNs communicated patient-reported concerns to UAP about pressure ulcers twice, discussed the issue of pressure ulcer once with another RN, and informed a physician of increased risk for pressure ulcer once. The UAP reported pressure ulcers to RNs three times. The RNs inquired about nutritional intake or nutrition support once. There was one instance of an RN delegating heel pressure relief and reporting concerns about nutrition to UAP.

Interview transcripts revealed that RNs relied on UAP to inform them of skin issues if found when bathing patients and had high trust and confidence in the ability of UAP to position patients, perform basic skin care, and inform the RN of any issues regarding skin integrity, nutrition, and mobility. As leaders of the nursing care team, the RNs also reported that they frequently discussed high-risk patient needs with UAP. RNs on one of the units aimed for consistent use of evidence-based guidelines. Explanations for not using an evidence-based protocol included disorganized work, the belief that experience was a better guide than a standardized tool for identifying patients at risk for pressure ulcer, and interference with turning due to the presence of relatives. Reviews of documentation revealed that risk assessment occurred 13 times, skin inspection happened 17 times, and care plans for patients at high risk for pressure ulcers were created 6 times.

The results of this study are clinically significant because they demonstrate RN reliance on UAP for reporting changes and concerns about patients as well as RN comfort in delegating basic patient care tasks to UAP. However, the investigators did note that RN attention to pressure ulcer prevention on the nursing units was deficient. More research is needed to determine whether evidence-based protocols for pressure ulcer prevention are being used in practice, identify the barriers and facilitators to evidence-based protocol use, and explore the working relationships between RNs and UAP.

Sving, E., Guningberg, L., Hogman, M., & Mamhidir, A. (2012). Registered nurse' attention to and perceptions of pressure ulcer prevention in hospital settings. *Journal of Clinical Nursing, 12,* 1293–1303. doi:10.1111/j.1365–2702.2011.04000.x

of oxygen therapy and bronchodilators for a patient who is experiencing respiratory difficulty. The following Focus on Research, "RNs, UAP, and Pressure Ulcers," demonstrates how heavily professional nurses rely on UAP for basic nursing care.

Agencies that use UAP are responsible for verifying that the UAP received adequate education and training before assuming work duties. Part of this education includes when to report problems to nurses. Nurses who fail to respond to client problems reported by subordinates typically fail to comply with their job descriptions and may be violating their state NPA.

Unit charge nurses have a duty to report any conditions that keep them from effectively performing their designated roles.

The related concepts of accountability, responsibility, and autonomy project an image of responsible, independent individuals, capable of making decisions and influencing others to act on them. They answer for their own behaviors as well as the behaviors of their associates. In the professional nursing context, the nurse becomes an autonomous practitioner who brings a different perspective and fulfills a particular role in the interdisciplinary health team. The nurse assumes responsibility for professional activities (including using research-based nursing actions, maintaining clinical competence, and staying abreast of new developments) and is held accountable for the outcomes of client care. This evolving image of a professional nurse demonstrates how increased accountability for the outcome of actions moves nursing toward the status given to other health care professions.

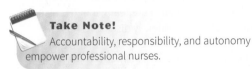

Take Note!
Accountability, responsibility, and autonomy empower professional nurses.

■ QUESTIONS FOR REFLECTION

1. Do you agree with the definitions of responsibility, accountability, autonomy, and authority presented in this chapter. Why or why not?

2. What would you do if you saw another nurse engage in dangerous practice? What is your responsibility to the patients? To your coworkers? To your manager? To your clinical faculty member?

3. Do you feel that nurses possess the authority and autonomy to change practice protocols and policies? Why or why not?

4. As a professional nursing student, what are the things to which you are held accountable? Are they the same in the clinical setting as they are in the classroom? Outline the similarities and differences. Why do you think there are differences?

PROFESSIONAL ACCOUNTABILITY

Porter-O'Grady and Malloch (2015) suggested replacing "responsibility" with "accountability" in professional practice because responsibility historically has been tied to tasks and work processes, rather than outcomes. To be responsible, workers need to arrive for work and fulfill outlined job activities. Responsibility focuses on processes, action, work, task performance, functions, and jobs. Accountability emphasizes products, results outcomes, accomplishments, differences, and roles (Porter-O'Grady & Malloch). Responsibility-based work means having to report to someone else (usually a supervisor), who typically evaluates the worker's performance and determines how well the person met expectations. The supervisor, rather than the worker, determines when exceptional or excellent work occurred. In contrast, accountability facilitates self-assessment of professional role performance. Responsibility is externally generated;

whereas, "Accountability is internally generated" (Porter-O'Grady & Malloch, 2015, p. 472).

Ideally, all people in a living system such as a workplace assume ownership of job roles and responsibilities that contribute to desired outcomes. In health care, all members of the health care team work toward providing the best care possible to attain optimal outcomes for the patients. Each person is designated to fulfill a particular role, and also has the authority to design their work, has clear expectations of their contributions, and strives to do their absolute best. Through increased authority, the worker assumes accountability for outcomes of his or her work. Coworkers develop relationships and create meaningful partnerships with each other to fulfill specified outcomes. Sustainable changes occur when those changes are generated by people engaged in the actual work. With this new approach, workers become empowered, shape the workplace, and experience higher job satisfaction (Porter-O'Grady & Malloch, 2015). Empowered persons experience higher levels of job satisfaction and frequently work to exceed expectations.

Professional Standards of Practice

As nurses assume more leadership and advanced practice, interest in and concern with accountability has surfaced. Flexner (1915) identified accountability as a key characteristic of a profession. He also indicated that professions are likely to be more responsive to public interest than are unorganized and isolated individuals. Therefore, nurses must work together professionally to develop practice standards and policies on which all can agree.

In terms of nursing's involvement with its professionalization in the 1950s and 1960s, Bixler and Bixler (1959) specified that professions function autonomously to carve out a scope of practice, develop professional standards, and institute policies that control professional activity. McGlothlin (1961) explained that a profession undertakes tasks that require the exercising of judgment in applying knowledge to the solutions of problems and accepts responsibility for the results. To be accountable, however, a profession must know that for which it is accountable. To that end, nursing organizations have established and work to enforce professional standards. **Professional standards** outline the guidelines and principles of a specific line of work or career. The ANA, nursing's major professional organization, has done this with its *Scope and Standards of Professional Nursing*, which specifies the professional standards of nursing practice, service, and continuing education. Using the standards of practice (ANA, 2015a) as a guide, nurses can identify the scope and limits of professional nursing practice, and internalize that for which they are accountable. By establishing standards, the ANA has complied with one of the functions of a professional organization—that is, of providing the means by which members of the profession can judge the competence of its members (Merton, 1958).

The National Council of State Boards of Nursing sets standards for "safe nursing practice." Individual state boards of nursing develop standards for professional practice and monitor professional nurse performance. In addition, individual nursing service departments monitor their collective accountability through the process of peer review. For example, Nolan, Burkard, Clark, Davidson, and Agan (2010) reported that initiation of morbidity and mortality peer review conferences improved patient care quality, as evidenced by the following outcomes: (1) nurse compliance with an evidence-based protocol for ventilator patients increased from 90.1% to 95.2%, (2) cases of ventilator-acquired pneumonia decreased from six cases to two cases after 2 months, and (3) nurses reported increased levels of accountability.

Take Note!
Through its standards, the ANA has contributed greatly to the ability of the nursing profession to be accountable.

Nurses monitoring of their own practice for effectiveness has increased dramatically in recent years through the introduction of systematic nursing quality improvement activities with active participation by staff nurses in many institutions and agencies. In 1991, the Joint Commission on Accreditation of Healthcare Organizations (now the Joint Commission) moved from reactive quality assurance programs to proactive quality improvement programs as mandated criteria for health care agency accreditation. This move hastened the process of operationalizing the concept of accountability as quality assurance at the nursing service department level (see Chapter 18, "Quality Improvement: Enhancing Patient Safety and Health Care Quality"). Thus, nurses become accountable for continuously improving the quality of health care for consumers.

Nurses have another document to guide them for practice accountability. The *Code of Ethics for Nurses* (2015a), also developed by the ANA, outlines terms for **ethical accountability** for professional nurses. **Nurses as client advocates** base professional decisions on what is best for clients. The *Code of Ethics for Nurses* provides a clear framework within which nurses can seek to uphold the standards of care and protect the clients they serve. The code lays to rest any doubt about accountability of the nursing profession by directly confronting the issue. As stated in item 4 of the code, "The has authority, accountability, and responsibility for nursing practice; makes decisions and takes action consistent with the obligation to promote health and provide optimal care" (ANA 2015a, p. 15). Other items in the code do not address the area of accountability directly but, by discussing various factors that are necessary underpinnings for accountability, indirectly support the concept. These factors include the presumed competence of the nurse, the use of informed judgment, and the use of nursing research.

Because society holds individual nurses accountable for professional actions, the nursing profession is accountable for establishing and monitoring standards for safe practice. Only nurses can determine the definition of "safe practice" and care standards. In some states, physicians routinely testify in court proceedings that a nurse displayed unsafe practice or deviated from the standard of care. Obviously, nursing is accountable as a profession and its individual practitioners also are accountable. It has been implied throughout this discussion that nurses are accountable to the public and to the profession itself. In addition, with most nurses employed by health care agencies rather than engaging in totally independent practice, nurses are also accountable to their employers (Copp, 1988; Vaughn, 1989). In the current climate of cost control, nurses must understand the delicate balance of being accountable to their employers (cost-containment strategies resulting in rapid patient turnover or abiding by outdated care polices) and being accountable to themselves (delivering patient-focused care based on current, best evidence, and blowing the whistle on substandard care).

Accountability to the Public and Clients

Although it may be personally and intellectually stimulating, gratifying, and exciting to execute professional roles and responsibilities, the ultimate reason for the existence of any profession is to provide service to the public. Thus, almost by definition, a profession must be accountable to the public. Consumers have the right to receive the safest, best possible quality of care from nurses who use a specialized knowledge base while applying sound judgment and utilizing a professional value system to make clinical decisions. To provide the best possible care, nurses must stay abreast of current best practices by remaining employed in the field, attending continuing education seminars, completing required competency tests, and reading professional literature.

As consumers become more knowledgeable about health care through formal education and access to information from many media formats, they sometimes know a great deal about what the profession is supposed to be doing. This increased knowledge empowers consumers to demand more and to make those demands openly. Nurses must be aware of increased consumer knowledge and sophistication and be prepared to respond to it in an equally knowledgeable and sophisticated manner. Instead of assuming positions of authority, nurses work collaboratively with clients to determine and attain health-related goals. Nurses must demonstrate clearly the principles and concepts on which practice is based. They also need to access current information, use problem solving to effectively evaluate outcomes of care, and revise care strategies if desired outcomes are not achieved (see Concepts in Practice, "Working Collaboratively with Empowered Clients").

Concepts in Practice [IDEA] → [PLAN] → [ACTION]

Working Collaboratively with Empowered Clients

Josiah is a nurse who works on a cardiac unit. He cares for persons who frequently receive six or more medications to control their heart disease. When working one day, one of his male patients requests not to take the ordered statin to reduce cholesterol. After inquiring as to the reason why, the man responds "There was a research study finding on the news today that reported that taking statins causes more health problems for persons taking them than they do in the prevention of another heart attack. I am just tired of taking all these prescribed pills, racking up a large monthly pharmacy bill and feel like the medical profession treats all patients like lab rats." Josiah mentions to his patient that he has not heard about the study. He holds the man's medication per request and states that he will return with more information.

Josiah goes online and reads the study. He discovers that the study compared persons receiving statins to persons adhering strictly to a Mediterranean diet. He makes a copy of the research study, which was conducted in Great Britain, Ireland, Scotland, and Wales. Josiah realizes that if his patient refuses to take the ordered statin, he will have to notify the cardiologist.

In addition to the study information, Josiah gathers detailed information about the Mediterranean diet for his patient. After presenting all the information to his patient, the patient turns up his nose when he learns about all of the fruits and vegetables that he would have to eat, and that he would have to limit consumption of red meat, and no longer eat fast foods. He asks Josiah if he still has the statin for him to take.

Society holds nurses legally accountable for professional practice. Every state has a board of nursing that monitors practice according to the state's NPA. A state's NPA defines professional nursing practice, specifies the scope of practice, and distinguishes professional nursing from other health professions. Nurses must practice within their state NPA guidelines.

State NPAs hold professional nurses to a standard of safe and prudent practice, which means that the nurse must exercise reasonable judgment and deliver reasonable care (Kopp, 2001; Milstead, 2008). Reasonable actions and judgments include being competent in the area of current practice, securing help for situations one is unqualified to manage, and fulfilling professional duties as a nurse.

> **Take Note!**
> Securing a copy of the NPA for states in which you practice is essential. You can use the internet, telephone, or postal service to secure a copy of your state NPA.

When nurses hold professional nursing licenses, they have a duty to provide health care services (either as an employee or volunteer). Negligence occurs when a nurse commits a breach of duty; an example of this would be falling short of an acceptable standard of care through an action or omission (Kopp, 2001; Watson, 2014). "**Liability** refers to the responsibility of one person or entity to another person or entity" (Anselmi, 2012, p. 45). Legal nurse scholar Anselmi describes the following two forms of liability.

1. **Strict liability** occurs when a person (or entity) is responsible "for damage or harm without having to prove fault" (p. 45), such as when a hospital uses explosive gases or other dangerous chemical and an accident occurs.
2. **Vicarious liability** occurs when one person assumes accountability for the actions of another (Box 12.2).

12.2 Professional Building Blocks

Forms and Examples of Vicarious Liability

- *Respondeat superior* means "let the superior answer." Thus a hospital can be held accountable for any action performed by staff nurses or UAP. For example, if a staff nurse fails to follow the policies and procedures outlined for a sterile procedure such as changing a central line dressing and the patient contracts a bloodstream infection, the hospital can be held accountable for the nurse's action.
- The *most distant relationship* liability occurs between an employer and an independent contractor in a situation when the independent contractor requires no supervision when performing work duties. For example, a hospital that uses physician or advanced practice nurse contractors could be held vicariously liable because patients perceived that the contractors were part of the hospital staff.
- *Negligent entrustment or supervision* arises when supervising physicians are held liable for the actions of medical students, advanced practice nurses, or residents.
- *Joint enterprise or venture* would apply when two or more individuals "form a limited liability partnership or other protective business structure" (p. 46) for a specific business purpose or a specified time frame. All parties in the joint venture share liability. For example, two nurses set up a home infusion business and hire four nurses. As a health care entity, both nurses would be liable for any errors that cause harm.

Anselmi, K. (2012). Nurses' personal liability vs. employer's vicarious liability. *Medsurg Nursing, 27*(1), 45–48.

Legal actions against nurses must contain the following elements: a breach of duty (may be an omission or incorrect action), foreseeability (a specific result could be predicted from the action or omission), causation (the omission or action directly resulted in injury). Recipients of inappropriate nursing services may suffer physical, emotional, or financial losses and deserve compensation when losses occur (Watson, 2014).

When nurses deviate from approved policies, procedures, or standards, they are at increased risk of being accused of malpractice or negligence. For example, if a nurse fails to perform routine circulation, movement and sensation checks for a client who has returned from orthopedic surgery per standardized postoperative protocols and the person ends up with having a permanent loss of function, the nurse places himself/herself at risk. However, before legal action is taken, the plaintiff (individual or group originating the legal action) must demonstrate that the event caused some form of injury.

Documentation of care delivered serves as legal evidence in the nurse's defense when legal action is taken against nurses. Meticulous documentation of events enables the nurse to present a highly professional image and serves as one of the best defense resources during legal actions. When on the witness stand, the nurse must be able to formulate and present to others the theoretical and scientific bases for the judgment exercised while fulfilling professional responsibilities.

In addition to legal accountability, nurses must be able to formulate and present to others the ethical code or value system to which they refer when making judgments and using knowledge. They must answer consumers and others without becoming defensive when asked "Why did you do that?" "How did you come to that decision?" and "What makes you believe that was the most effective course of action?" Consumers have the right to know about all aspects of their nursing care, and nurses who are true professionals have the responsibility to know and provide the answers.

As knowledgeable professionals, nurses share accountability for the nation's health care delivery system with other health team members. When nurses blame others, such as physicians, administrators, or politicians, for the state of the health care delivery system or constantly look to others to improve the system, they weaken their position and power base. By accepting an appropriate degree of responsibility for the current situation and actively pursuing ways to improve it, nurses act on a more professional level and make their claim for a piece of the health care pie.

Nursing also is accountable to the public in guarding against any ill-prepared or apathetic UAP. During times of nurse shortages and cost containment, some hospitals provide brief (4- to 6-week) training programs for unlicensed workers to prepare them to assume complex nursing care tasks. In some cases, the quality of care is seriously compromised (see Concepts in Practice, "Accountability").

Concepts in Practice IDEA ──▶ PLAN ──▶ ACTION

Accountability

Rosetta has worked nights as a UAP for 20 years. She has heard the night nurses talks about how level of a patient's pain is really a fifth vital sign. One night, Rosetta finds herself working with Georgia, an RN. Rosetta volunteers to assess all the postoperative patients for pain. Georgia thanks Rosetta and teaches her how to assess patient pain using the 0 to 10 pain rating scale. By delegating this, Georgia is able to manage all the IV lines and perform dressing changes. Rosetta checks the pain level of all the patients who are not asleep at 2:00 AM and reports her findings to Georgia. Rosetta tells Georgia that no one needs pain medication (because Rosetta perceives that patients need pain medication when they report a pain level of more than 6. After all, it is a 0 to 10 pain scale).

Take a moment and jot down if you think that Georgia made a good decision and defend the reasons for your thoughts about this situation. Once you have completed your notes, continue reading.

Considering pain as a fifth vital sign and delegating its assessment to UAP deviates from judicious nursing practice. Effective pain management requires assessment by a professional nurse because UAP do not have the knowledge required to conduct a thorough pain assessment. In addition, a complaint of client pain needs to be managed by some form of independent or collaborative nursing intervention. Poor pain control may result in impaired healing, other potential physical complications, and client dissatisfaction with nursing care. If patients under Georgia's care complain about poor pain management and report that Rosetta was the one who asked about their pain levels and no action was taken, Georgia would have to provide answers to questions from the physicians, nurse manager, or other nurses on the unit for substandard pain management. Georgia is accountable to her patients for effective pain management based on her professional nursing pain assessment.

Take Note!

Nurses must work collectively and cohesively to protect the public against potential harm and protect aspects of health care delivery that belong to professional nursing.

Accountability to the Profession

The nursing profession exercises accountability toward itself in the performance of its duty to formulate its own policy and control its activities. Professional nurses determine standards for nursing licensure (the National Council of State Boards of Nursing and individual State Boards of Nursing) and entry into professional groups and associations (e.g., Association of Operating Room Nurses, American Association of Critical Care Nurses). When nurses determine and monitor compliance with professional nursing standards and guidelines, professional autonomy is preserved.

In connection with this aspect of accountability, individual nurses must understand the need to be aware of and accountable for not only their own actions but also those of their colleagues. For example, chemically addicted colleagues pose a danger to clients, themselves, and coworkers. Chemical abuse in nursing is a complex problem (Hastings & Burn, 2007; Lillibridge, Cox, & Cross, 2002). Nurses have a professional and legal responsibility to abide by the law and safeguard clients and other members of society, which means they need to report chemically impaired coworkers (U.S. Drug Enforcement Agency, 2005) (see Box 12.3, Learning, Knowing, and Growing, "Recognizing and Managing Possible Chemical Addiction in a Nursing Colleague").

Forty State Boards of Nursing offer alternatives to disciplinary actions that typically involve legally binding programs for detoxification, treatment, peer assistance, and recovery programs that include random monitoring for signs of chemical use (Maer-Brisen, 2007). When nurses police themselves, professional autonomy is enhanced.

Regular peer review programs provide another means for nurses to monitor their own profession. Benefits of peer review include increased self-awareness of practice, quality of client care, professionalism, and accountability. The Joint Commission recommends that nurses engage in peer review as part of professional practice (Roper & Russell, 1997). Peer review processes require that nurses look objectively at a colleague's performance, which sometimes can be difficult when the peer is a friend. Also, some nurses dislike pointing out deficiencies in another nurse's performance. Effective peer evaluations offer constructive suggestions to remedy identified performance deficiencies.

Finally, nurses are accountable for the survival of the profession. As members of a noble and well-respected profession, nurses need to recruit new members,

12.3 Learning, Knowing, and Growing

Recognizing and Managing Possible Chemical Addiction in a Nursing Colleague

Signs of Possible Chemical Addiction in a Nurse

- Arriving consistently early for work
- Departing late from work habitually
- Coming to work when not scheduled
- Wearing long-sleeved garments at all times
- Wasting controlled medications excessively
- Volunteering to administer controlled medications to unassigned patients
- Taking frequent breaks
- Spending excessive amount of time close to a controlled medication supply cart or computerized medication dispensing system
- Volunteering for overtime all of the time
- Keeping inaccurate records of controlled substances
- Failing to have another person with legal ability to witness wasting controlled medications during the time the drug is being prepared and administered
- Falsifying reasons for controlled medication variances in computerized dispensing systems
- Charting on electronic health records that seems incoherent

- Signing out medications for patients who have left the unit
- Increasing personal and/or professional isolation

Managing a Chemically Addicted Nursing Colleague

- Before confronting or reporting suspicions of illegal drug use, nurses should keep a written log (including time and date) of suspicious behaviors
- When confronting a colleague about suspected chemical impairment, the nurse should display genuine empathy and concern, be direct and open, share specific behaviors and incidents, and expect the colleague to deny allegations
- Experts in chemical impairment management advocate interventions involving the suspected nurse, colleagues who observed behaviors, the nurse's direct supervisor, and a chemical impairment counselor
- An intervention provides the suspected nurse with immediately available assistance should he or she want to seek professional help for the alleged problem

Maer-Brisen, P. (2007). Addiction: An occupational hazard in nursing. *American Journal of Nursing, 107*(8), 78–79; U.S. Drug Enforcement Agency (DEA). (2005). Drug addiction in health care professionals. Retrieved from http://www.deadiversion. usdoj.gov/pubs/brochures/drug_hc.htm. Accessed February 6, 2013.

support them through the education process, mentor them as they enter the workforce, and support them as experienced colleagues.

Accountability to Interprofessional and Unlicensed Health Care Team Members

As a professional in the interprofessional and multidisciplinary health care team, nurses are accountable for the unique contributions they make to client care. The nurse often spends more time with the client than any other health team member. Nurses who engage in holistic nursing care consider more than just client physiologic needs; they also identify psychological, sociocultural, and spiritual needs. Many times, nurses identify obstacles for client self-care by spending time in assessing, teaching, and evaluating client and family responses regarding what they need to know before discharge (see Concepts in Practice, "A Nurse's Contribution Makes a Big Difference").

Professional nurses also have accountability for informing UAP of potential hazards they might encounter when providing basic care to clients with

Concepts in Practice $\boxed{\text{IDEA}} \longrightarrow \boxed{\text{PLAN}} \longrightarrow \boxed{\text{ACTION}}$

A Nurse's Contribution Makes a Big Difference

Marian is a professional nurse who works on a rehabilitation unit. She is getting ready to dismiss Mrs. Garcia, an elderly woman who needs to learn how to perform glucose self-monitoring at home. The diabetes nurse educator who provided the basic instructions documented that the woman could effectively perform the required tasks. However, the evening before Mrs. Garcia's dismissal, Marian observes that Mrs. Garcia could not effectively use the glucose monitor because of limited manual dexterity and poor vision. Marian discovers that the woman lives alone and has no family members available for assistance. By documenting her assessment and informing the case manager, home health care is arranged, thereby preventing hospital readmission and reducing health care costs. Marian fulfills her obligation to the client, the organization, and interprofessional team members.

contagious diseases or to clients who have the potential for violence. UAP need to know what actions need to be taken to protect themselves. Likewise, UAP have the responsibility to inform professional nurses about changes in client status that indicate a potentially infectious disease or escalation of anger into physical violence. For example, UAP should inform the nurse of a new onset of frequent stools in a client (a possible sign of *Clostridium difficile* infection) and if a client (or family member) is disgruntled about received care. In situations such as the latter, the nurse can intervene through use of therapeutic communication techniques (see Chapter 4, "Establishing Helping and Healing Relationships") to discover and alleviate the issues and prevent escalation of anger into an episode of staff verbal abuse or physical assault.

Accountability to the Employing Agency

Nurses also are accountable to their employing agencies. Employees, even those with professional status, have responsibilities and must answer for job actions. The employing agency holds nurses accountable for the quality of nursing care they provide, including job preparation and fitness for duty. Optimal physical and mental status of nursing staff is essential for safe and effective client care. Nurses have the obligation to come to work well rested for peak performance. Nurses often work overtime to finish their daily jobs or take on extra shifts (scheduled or on-call) to support colleagues when care shortages arise (Bae, 2012; Olds & Clarke, 2010). Some nurses also work for more than one job to increase the income or to practice across nurse specialty areas.

The employing agency contracts with nurses for a specific job to be done at a specific time and place for a specific wage. Nurses must uphold their end of the agreement in all of these areas. They also have accountability for monitoring peer performance, providing effective supervision of UAP, and reporting safety issues (consumer or staff) when they arise.

Although not unimportant, accountability to the employing agency rightfully takes a back seat to accountability to the client, the public, the profession, and nurses themselves.

Accountability of Health Care Organizations to the Public and Employees: Quality and Safety

Nurse accountability to health care organizations requires that the employing agency creates working conditions that foster safety and quality in nursing care delivery. Just like nurses, health care organizations are accountable to the public for the quality and safety of care provided under its auspices. The agency is responsible for creating a culture of safety so that work processes and environments do not create care errors and staff can report issues without fear of reprisal.

The IOM report, *To Err Is Human*, identified gaps in health care delivery processes that sometimes resulted in death and permanent disability in patients (IOM, 2000). In 2001, the IOM followed up on safety issues by releasing *Crossing the Quality Chasm: A New Health System for the 21st Century*, which suggested actions that health care professionals can undertake to improve the quality and safety of health care delivery. In 2003, the IOM issued *Health Professions Education: A Bridge to Quality*, a report on how to completely transform the education of the interprofessional health care team so that team members would be effectively prepared to meet quality and safety issues encountered in daily practice. Nursing leaders acknowledge that the profession needed to address concerns raised by the IOM studies (IOM, 2011; Sherwood & Barnsteiner, 2012).

The Robert Wood Johnson Foundation provided a series of nursing grants to improve efforts for educating beginning and advanced practice nurses; these grants led to the development of the **Quality and Safety Education for Nurses (QSEN) Institute**. QSEN is an ongoing program that identifies core competencies and strategies to promote new health team members to develop essential competencies in knowledge, skills, and attitudes for patient-centered care, teamwork and collaboration, evidence-based practice, safety, quality improvement, and informatics. The QSEN Institute website offers detailed competencies and educational strategies for attainment (Sherwood & Barnsteiner, 2012).

In 2010, Sammer, Lykens, Singh, Mains, and Lackan conducted a comprehensive literature review to identify key elements that contribute to a hospital culture of patient safety. They concluded that communication, teamwork, learning, evidence-based practice, justice, leadership, and patient-centeredness are the hallmarks of a patient safety culture (Table 12.1). This text highlights many of these hallmarks (e.g., communication and teamwork in Chapters 4 and 21; evidence-based practice in Chapters 3, 4, 7, 8, 10, and 18; patient-centered care in Chapters 4, 7, 8, 11, 13, and 15; learning in Chapters 16 and 20; justice in Chapter 19; and leadership in Chapter 17).

TABLE 12.1   Factors Contributing to a Culture of Patient Safety

Element	Factors Involved
Communication	Transparency, structured techniques for intra- and interprofessional communication about patients and patient hand-offs, involvement in safety briefings and debriefings, effective feedback and conflict resolution, bottom-up approach, and clear, assertive communication patterns
Teamwork	Common mission, mission alignment among all members, referral to expert members when needed, flattened hierarchy, multidisciplinary meetings, mutual respect, intergenerational contributions valued, psychological safety, flexibility, adaptive ability, member support, and watching the backs of all members
Learning	Increased awareness and information transmission, success celebrations, data-driven actions, all members participate in educational endeavors, learning from mistakes, monitoring of outcomes using benchmarks, performance improvement programs, engagement in root cause analysis, proactive rather than reactive behaviors, and sharing of learned lessons
Evidence-based practice	Best practices followed, aim for zero-defect or high reliability, driven by outcomes, practice science of safety, standardized protocols, policies, checklists, and guidelines, effective use of technology and automation
Just Culture	Blame-free, open disclosure, non-punitive reporting processes and structures, awareness of at-risk behaviors, process, or systems rather than an individual as a source of errors, and high levels of trust
Leadership	Be accountable, manage change, display commitment, make administrative rounds, encourage participative governance, engage physicians, set priorities, supply material and human resources, role model desired attitudes and behaviors, be supportive, use vigilance and visibility, and determine and live values and mission
Patient-centeredness	Community involvement, grassroots efforts to change policies, patient and family empowerment, always focusing on the patient, formal patient participation in care, informed patients and families, and careful listening and paying attention to patient stories

Sammer, C., Lykens, K., Singh, K., Mains, D., & Lackan, N. (2010). What is patient safety culture? *Journal of Nursing Scholarship, 42*(2), 156–165; Sherwood, G., & Barnsteiner, J. (Eds.). (2012). *Quality and safety in nursing a competency approach to improving outcomes.* Oxford, UK: Wiley-Blackwell.

The employing agency administration is obligated to provide competent health care providers for the consumers of its services. Thus, the employing agency has the right to expect the nurse to be accountable to the agency. Dimensions of accountability include quality of work, unsafe practice situations, nurse attitudes toward the employing agency, and professional practice with outside agency staff. The agency must be open to suggestions from nurses to improve work processes and environment without being punitive to those who report unsafe or low-quality care situations.

Nurses also have the responsibility to inform their employers about situations that result in actual or potential unsafe nursing practice situations. Recent legislation has resulted in legal protection for nurses who report unsafe practice situations. Sometimes the employing organization may refuse to correct what the nurses perceive as an unsafe practice situation. Nurses must refuse to work in areas and situations they consider unsafe. This further fulfills accountability to the employer (as well as self) because such nurses are saying, in effect, "I will not put my employer in the position of giving unsafe care." Not taking action against unsafe practices places clients at risk, and clients will likely tell family members and acquaintances about the poor care received at the nurse's employing organization. However, refusal to provide client care as designated by terms of employment may result in reprimand, demotion, and even dismissal from the agency unless the nurse is employed in a state that offers whistleblower protection.

An additional aspect of the nurse's accountability to the employer involves the attitude toward that employer that the nurse projects to clients. The attitude should be one of objectivity and honesty. Nurses who find joy in working for a particular employer may appropriately and honestly promote the health care organization's strengths. However, if confronted with an employer's shortcoming, nurses must be honest in their responses. Sometimes, in the heat of the moment, when particularly taxed or following a disagreement, a nurse may denigrate a health care organization where he or she is employed. In this case, the nurse has not acted maturely and may not be aware of the impact of such statements on the client, visitors, or the health care organization.

Concerns have arisen recently regarding accountability to the employer because of a large and growing number of agency-employed nurses who are essentially "rented" to hospitals on a per diem basis. In most cases, agency nurses possess high levels of clinical competence. However, they may be unfamiliar with the employing institution's policies and procedures. A study by Pham and Papa (2011) revealed that emergency department temporary staff are twice as likely to be involved with harmful medication errors as permanent staff. Papa, a seasoned emergency room nurse manager, specifies that emergency rooms need to be properly staffed and believes that safety can be enhanced by providing adequate nurse orientation and pairing a temporary staff nurse with a seasoned full-time nurse employee so that questions regarding care protocols can be readily answered and guidance given for accessing agency information (Pham & Papa, 2011).

Agency nurses may have more accountability to the nursing agency, thus diminishing some of the support they might offer the hospital, or they may feel primarily accountable to the hospital's clients. When allegiance to the employing institution supersedes allegiance to the agency, nurses may run the risk of being dropped by the agency.

When nurses place their accountability to their employing agency above their accountability to all others, it detracts from a desirable image of nurses as working primarily in the public interest and instead fosters the impression of the nurse as being subservient to and under the control of the employing institution. Nurses must learn to balance their accountability to clients, society, the profession, and self with their accountability toward the employing agency; this may be more difficult in times of economic uncertainty.

■ QUESTIONS FOR REFLECTION

1. How do you define accountability to your employer or nursing program?
2. What would you do if you found yourself in a work/educational setting that required you to take care of more patients than you thought that you could safely handle?
3. Why do you think that some nurses fail to report unsafe patient situations to their managers?
4. What would you do if you heard a nursing colleague (professional nurse or nursing student) criticize where you work (or attend school)?

Accountability to Self

Professionals who are deeply committed to their careers sometimes can be exploited by the systems in which they work. In the early days of the nursing profession, hospitals and clients expected nurses to live on the premises in which they worked. Today, agencies no longer assume "ownership" of nurses and do not expect

them to work long hours without breaks. Employers and clients see nurses as free and independent individuals with multiple facets to their lives. In a recent study addressing nurse overtime, 10% of nurses reported working extra hours without being compensated (Bae, 2012).

When personal accountability is lacking, blaming, complaining, and procrastination are common. People who practice personal accountability experience healthier relationships, improved teamwork, and less stress while their employers enjoy increased productivity, greater teamwork, and improved customer service. Personal accountability begins with looking at oneself and seeing how things can be changed rather than pointing fingers at others. When things do not go smoothly, two key questions to ask are "What can I do?" and "How can I help?" These questions focus on action and include a role for the individual to make a difference (Miller, 2004).

However, some job situations may cause nurses and others to overlook these basic facts. Staff shortages may keep nurses from fulfilling their basic needs for nutrition and elimination. In addition, nurses' other life roles may affect professional performance. Therefore, nurses must be accountable to themselves for their actions both on and off the job because of the potential effects of their actions on themselves and others.

Fatigue, jet lag, minor illness, exhaustion, or the effects of alcohol or drugs can make the nurse a liability, rather than an asset, in the work situation (Fig. 12.1). Professional practice also may be hampered by nurses who put in too much overtime, allow themselves to be placed in a position far beyond their abilities and knowledge, and function in a constantly and highly stressed state. These nurses may find themselves too exhausted or unprepared to function effectively in professional and personal roles.

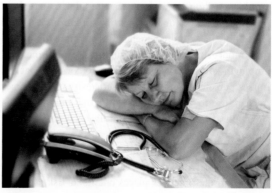

FIGURE 12.1 Nurses who come to work extremely fatigued remain accountable for clinical decisions that they make.

Significant others cannot always be expected to have lower priority than one's work, and work cannot always be expected to take second place to social and personal relationships. Nurses need to attain a certain balance. Overdoing the amount of time and energy expended on the job often leads to burnout, with the nurse becoming incapable of or unwilling to do adequate work. Burnout also may take a toll on nurses' personal and social lives (Chaska, 1983). Likewise, if the nurse ignores family needs, the family may disintegrate.

Nurses must assume responsibility for their own physical, mental, and spiritual health by maintaining a balanced lifestyle. They must decide when to give more energy to work and when to devote more energy to other life areas. When nurses sacrifice wholeness of life, they lose the capacity for optimal functioning as professionals and people. They must function at fullest capacity when on the job and yet set a pace to avoid despair and profound fatigue.

The nurse's accountability to self includes refusing to work in situations deemed unsafe. Each nurse defines unsafe situations individually. Some examples of unsafe practice situations include lack of knowledge or experience to work in an unfamiliar specialty area and insufficient staffing. Nurses must learn to see refusal to work in unsafe situations as the ultimate professional service to the consumer despite potential sanctions that may be applied as consequences for this action. Whistleblowing is the act of reporting unsafe or unethical situations or incompetence of another health care team member. Nurses must use professional judgment when deciding whether to report wrongdoing. Murray (2007) offered several suggestions for self-protection for nurses who opt to "blow the whistle" on unsafe client care situations (see Box 12.4, Professional Building Blocks, "Self-Protection Before Blowing the Whistle").

Accountability to self also involves acknowledging one's own limitations and knowing when additional education or assistance from another is needed for effective client care. Questioning physician orders requires confidence and sometimes courage, but it protects both client and nurse. Deciding when to assume a new nursing position (such as promotion to a nurse manager) should be based on each nurse's appraisal of his or her personal qualifications for the job rather than on opinions of other people. Completing an academic degree (such as a bachelor's degree in nursing) does not automatically prepare all nurses to assume a managerial role. Other factors such as personality, job description, and career goals should be considered before assuming an administrative position.

12.4 Professional Building Blocks

Self-Protection Before Blowing the Whistle

1. Hire an attorney for legal advice.
2. Verify the legalities of whistleblower protection at the federal and state levels.
3. Consult with the state nursing association for answers to or clarification of state laws and regulations.
4. Develop a written, accurate account of all observed events (including time, date, and incident).
5. Store all documents in a secure location and have multiple copies of each document.
6. Follow the facility's chain of command when reporting incidents.
7. Ask for help from experts, including the state attorney general, state and federal legislative bodies, and other agencies and organizations that have an interest in reducing unsafe health care delivery.
8. Forward all documents to outside agencies using certified mail for proper verification of receipt of records and materials.
9. Maintain professionalism at all times when presenting information to the employing and outside agencies.

Murray, J. (2007). Before blowing the whistle, learn to protect yourself. *American Nurse Today, 2*(3), 40–42.

Accountability to self involves protecting oneself against financial loss should an unforeseen incident occur. Many employing agencies carry insurance policies to protect themselves when client care errors and other accidents occur. Professional nurses who rely solely on the employing agency's insurance policy must remember that the agency will be looking out for its own best interests. On the other hand, when a nurse carries his or her own malpractice insurance, the legal counsel will focus on the nurse's interests and defend the nurse. When an error occurs resulting in patient harm, the nurse and the employing agency could very easily become adversaries (Anselmi, 2012). There have been incidents when professional nurses have been used as scapegoats to protect physicians and health care agencies, although there have also been cases in which agencies have supported professional nurses. With individual malpractice coverage the nurse knows that resources are available for legal consultation and defense. Some states require nurses to carry individual malpractice insurance policies as a condition for licensure application (Anselmi, 2012).

TABLE 12.2   Reasons for Nurse Malpractice Suits

Reason	Example
Failure to document	Failing to document procedures, medications, and physician interactions or not documenting events leading up to a situation resulting in patient harm as events occurred (charting after the fact)
Therapy error	Administering incorrect medication or treatment
Failure to follow standards of care	Using alternative treatments or procedures and/or failing to follow guidelines outlined by institutional policy and procedure manuals
Communication failure	Not listening intently to client concerns, providing inaccurate discharge instructions, not notifying a physician in a timely manner
Omitted assessment	Not performing routine assessments for various medical conditions or procedures, or neglecting to document a required assessment
Neglecting to be a client advocate	Not questioning physician orders when needed or not providing a safe environment for the client
Breach of confidentiality	Sharing of private information with others
Invasion of privacy	Failing to provide drapes for procedures requiring physical exposure
Release of medical information without permission	Failing to get written permission from clients when sharing medical information with others
Assault and battery	Performing invasive procedures without the client's informed consent
False imprisonment	Using of physical or chemical restraint inappropriately
Discrimination	Giving unequal treatment based on particular group membership or specific disease
Defamation	Harming the reputation of another person
Slander	Making false statements or misrepresentations that harm the reputation of another
Libel	Making written or oral statements or other representation published without just cause for the purpose of exposing another to public contempt
Impaired nursing practice	Working under the influence of controlled medications, illegal substances or alcohol OR being fatigued

Adapted from Helm, A., & Kihm, N. C. (2001). Is professional liability insurance for you? *Nursing, 31*(1), 48–49; Croke, E. M. (2003). Nurses, negligence and malpractice. *American Journal of Nursing, 103*, 54–64; and Watson, E. (2014). Nursing malpractice: Costs, trends & issues. *Journal of Legal Nurse Consulting, 25*(1), 26–31.

Table 12.2 presents reasons why lawsuits are filed against professional nurses. In the United States, client suits involving nurses rose from 307 in 1997 (Domrose, 2007) to 516 closed claims not including advanced practice nurses in 2011 (Watson, 2012). Between 1999 and 2011, 9,278 registered nurses actually were required to pay malpractice settlements (out of court and jury trial). One third of the claims were $50,000 or less and 195 claims were equal to or exceeded $2 million (Watson, 2014). Client suits against nurses fall into two main categories: failing to do what is expected and doing what is not expected (Aiken, 2003; Watson, 2012, 2014). Lawyers carefully examine client records for signs of breaches in nursing care standards and incidents of nurse failure to respond to, report, and follow-up on changes in client status (Domrose, 2007; Watson, 2012). Sometimes, a slight omission in documentation can precipitate legal action when harm comes to clients in a nurse's care.

As soon as money exchanges hands from a health care provider (including registered nurses), information regarding a settlement is entered into the National Practitioner Data Bank. Each State Board of Nursing where the nurse hold professional licensure status is also contacted (Watson, 2014).

Table 12.3 presents arguments for and against purchasing individual professional liability insurance. Professional liability insurance pays for individual nurse legal defense costs should a nurse be named in a malpractice suit or involved in an early settlement program. Liability coverage also pays damages to an injured party if the nurse is found negligent. As supervisors and coordinators of client care, nurses may be held accountable for actions of UAP, nursing assistants, other nurses, and clerical staff (Croke, 2003). According to direct online quotes from professional nurse liability providers, the annual cost for $1,000,000 in professional liability insurance coverage ranges from $102 to $450 for professional nurses not involved in advanced nursing practice. Advanced practice nurses (depending on their specialty) may pay up to $13,250

TABLE 12.3 Reasons for and Against Nurses Carrying Individual Liability Insurance

Reasons For	Reasons Against
Employer language may cover the facility but not individual employees	Attitude of being not at risk for malpractice
Employer policies may be insufficient to cover all claims, leaving the nurse responsible for the amount that exceeds the facility policy limits	Perceived adequate coverage from employer
Hospital insurer might seek indemnity from the nurse after lawsuit is settled	Clients may file malpractice claims several years after an incident, and the nurse may change jobs, or the facility could close or change its malpractice policy
Personal policies provide legal defense for the nurse, and some include costs for time off work and transportation during legal proceedings	Nurse could be caught in a facility's decision to side with a physician during legal proceedings, holding the nurse responsible for malpractice
Facility policy may have coverage gaps	Perception that carrying own insurance policy increases the likelihood of being sued
Most jurors assume nurses carry individual liability insurance	

Adapted from Helm, A., & Kihm, N. C. (2001). Is professional liability insurance for you? *Nursing, 31*(1), 48–49.

for liability coverage. Nurses who are self-employed and nurses working in some specialty areas (e.g., critical care, obstetrics) pay higher fees than nurses employed in medical-surgical units and extended-care facilities. In comparison, annual physician malpractice costs range from $10,836 to $45,550 (Gans, 2007).

Coverage terms vary according to the type of policy purchased. Claims-made policies cover the nurse for the time when the plaintiff files a court claim. In contrast, occurrence policies cover the nurse for the time in which the situation occurred that resulted in litigation. The nurse should know which type of policy he or she carries. When a nurse has claims-made coverage, the policy needs to be active until all chances of litigation have expired. Each state determines the time frame in which people can file legal claims for health care providers for undesirable care outcomes.

Some health care organizations have recently adopted early settlement programs to reduce litigation against physicians and hospitals when adverse client outcomes arise. Part of these programs includes established policies and procedures outlining exactly how appropriate disclosure is made to clients and families when an adverse event occurs. The process may include full apologies and early offers for compensation if deemed appropriate (Greenwald, 2008). However, no assurances have been made to professional nurses that the health care organization will not take punitive action against them should the adverse event occur because of a nursing error.

Finally, nurses are accountable to themselves to do their own personal best (Styles, 1985). Factors outside nursing can influence this aspect of accountability.

Federal and state governments can support or hinder the ability of professional nurses to be accountable. Government legislative efforts result in laws and regulations that facilitate or obstruct whistleblowing by professional nurses. Governments provide funding for health care services, research, and education. The federal government has established health care priorities for the United States by establishing and supporting *Healthy People 2020*. Most states also establish health care priorities. The IOM (2011) outlined a plan for advancing the nursing profession and outlined steps to alleviate the predicted professional nursing shortage. Managed care networks and third-party payers strive to provide health care services to subscribers at the lowest possible cost. The nurse must consider political activism as a means to the end of accountability to self, as a method of bringing public policy and the most expert care into congruence (see Chapter 19, "The Professional Nurse's Role in Public Policy").

QUESTIONS FOR REFLECTION

1. If a patient experiences a poor outcome and you were a part of the patient's care, who would be accountable?
2. What current resources are in place in your employing institution and your nursing program for employee or student defense should a medical malpractice suit be brought against you?
3. What actions can you take to prevent patient care errors in the health care setting where you practice (as a nursing student or professional nurse)?

THE GROUNDWORK FOR ACCOUNTABILITY

From this complex description of accountability, professional nurses must consciously prepare themselves to develop the skills and attributes that will enable its accomplishment. Nurses need to know the latest research, use theoretical bases, display competence in clinical practice, assume leadership, and engage in practice based on their personal ethical framework.

Research and the Establishment of a Theoretical Base for Nurse Accountability

One of the major factors in the movement of nursing toward professional status is the growth of its theoretical and conceptual base for practice. As the level of nursing education increases, nurses are incorporating theoretical, research-based, and other forms of evidence-based knowledge into daily practice. As evidence-based health care becomes commonplace, nurses are increasingly expected to use all forms of evidence, but especially research-based evidence, when providing nursing care services.

In practice, nurses use knowledge generated through research to substantiate their actions and develop clinical practice policies and procedures. Although most nurses have access to online and printed research findings, finding time to read and analyze nursing research results poses a dilemma for many. Some nurses (especially those educated in associate degree programs) have received no formal education on how to evaluate research findings for use in practice. In addition, the dissemination of nursing research results to practicing nurses occurs very slowly; sometimes it may be years before key findings are published.

With the advent of evidence-based practice and quality improvement initiatives, the use of research findings has become more desirable and acceptable. Nurses need help to access and understand available research reports and apply the findings to work situations. Some health care agencies have nursing research committees and offer resources to help nurses use research findings in practice. However, until nurses and all health care organizations value the use of nursing research, some nurses will continue to practice on the basis of tradition.

Clinical and Professional Competence

The public, consumers, health care agencies, and physicians expect nurses to have clinical competence.

Nurses in specialty areas of practice have specific knowledge and skills for competent practice. However, all areas of practice require that nurses understand and apply principles and techniques of asepsis, physical assessment, nursing process, pathophysiology, pharmacology, human growth and development, psychology, sociology, spirituality, and safety. Because all nurses hold their clients' lives in their hands, whatever a nurse does, it must be done well.

With many levels of nursing being reflected in the composition of today's health care teams, nurses at each level should have a clear idea of the scope of practice at their level, and should perform responsibly to the maximum limit of that level. A nurse's accountability may be called into question if he or she is functioning beyond the scope of practice at a particular level. It is no more appropriate for nurses who have been educated at the baccalaureate level to restrict professional activities to those they may have exercised at the associate degree level than it is for them to assume the role of the master's-prepared practitioner.

The key to expertise in practice lies in both knowledge and skill, a somewhat artificial distinction that nevertheless allows for more clarity in this discussion. Nursing has always had a strong manual skills component. To the extent that the nurse is in a role that calls for manual skills, gentleness, quickness, and accuracy remain hallmarks of excellence. Where the skills required are in the areas of communication, teaching, leadership, management, and research (the so-called hands-off skills), the need of expertise is no less pressing.

Underlying all skills is excellence in terms of command of "nursing knowledge." Nurses can never expect to contribute significantly to health care in its assessment, planning, implementation, and evaluation aspects if they do whatever they do in a mediocre manner.

Take Note!
Competence in nursing is an absolute prerequisite for accountability.

Leadership Skills

Leadership development frequently brings questions and puzzlement when first introduced to nursing students. A frequent response is "Not everyone can be a head nurse or a supervisor, or wants to be an instructor. I don't want to be a leader; I just want to be a nurse."

The fact is that the elements of leadership are inherent in any nurse role.

Leadership ability is one of the most important areas in laying the groundwork for accountability. The nurse's accountability extends into all areas of health care delivery, including health maintenance and promotion and promoting self-care. The nurse is a constant catalyst for change in health care quality and delivery, especially if he or she is "just" a nurse.

To fulfill the leadership role, nurses must be well versed in the theory and practice of change. Nurses are leaders because they influence others, provide others with desired health-related information, participate in the formation of health care and organizational policies, serve as role models of health, and coordinate client care. Accountable nurses cannot function without leadership skills.

Personal Ethical Framework

Nurses are accountable within a personal ethical framework. They cannot be accountable in a moral vacuum. They must have their guide standards and values in which they believe and to which they refer. To some extent, these are determined by the collective values of the profession, which, in turn, are partly determined by what the public expects of that profession and partly by what the profession demands of itself.

In nursing, these professional values are formalized by the *Code of Ethics for Nurses* (ANA, 2015a). However, in large measure, a nurse's ethical code is personal and highly individual, developed in the course and context of the individual's total life experience. It includes values learned in the home, in schools, from social groups, during religious training, in the work setting, and from the activities and contacts of daily life. It is influenced by the nurse's ethnic and religious background, the area of the country in which he or she lives, and his or her personality.

Often, a personal ethical code is something of which people are relatively unaware. It is unconsciously used in making decisions and running one's life but is rarely, if ever, pulled out and scrutinized or even acknowledged as existing. It is this code that is so essential in the professional nurse. A nurse must be aware of his or her code, how it affects decisions and actions, and where it is congruent with or departs from standard codes of the profession. Any conflicts must be worked through and compromise sought so that the nurse can feel comfortable with and confident in the ethical basis in which his or her practice is rooted.

■ QUESTIONS FOR REFLECTION

1. What do you truly value in life?
2. How do your values affect your nursing practice?

ACCOUNTABILITY IN AN ERA OF COST CONTAINMENT

As increases in health care costs continue to outpace inflation, public support for imposing controls on costs for health care increases. Prospective payment systems serve as the major reimbursement method for many health care services. In efforts to curb costs, Medicare no longer covers costs for hospital-acquired infections, complications, and errors. Thus, nurse accountability for the prevention of adverse effects of hospitalization increases.

For-profit and managed care providers consistently look for ways to provide cost-effective health care. Health care practices deemed to be effective will be increased and retained, while those determined to be ineffective will be decreased or discarded. Professional nurses must substantiate the benefits of the contributions they make to health care delivery.

All too often in health care, "effective" seems to mean "cost-effective." The idea of a universal right to top-quality care for all is being diluted to a standard of adequate care to those who meet specific criteria set by third-party payers. Nurses are now asked to be accountable for the care they give and for giving that care in the least expensive manner possible, often in a setting or time frame that severely limits the comprehensiveness of that care.

Disease-management programs offer a means to enhance the ability of clients to manage chronic health conditions (e.g., end-stage renal disease, diabetes, HIV/AIDS) by offering intensive client education and home support services to keep people with these conditions in their homes rather than in the hospital or an extended-care facility. As key providers of care in homes, professional nurses making home visits are held accountable for accurate client assessments, effective health education, and appropriate referrals. Because of the complexity of community interventions and algorithms present in the disease management programs, Goldstein (2006) recommends bachelor degree–level preparation as the minimum for nurses working in them.

Unlicensed Assistive Personnel

Increased use of UAP and LPN/LVNs adds layers of accountability for health care delivery. UAP and LPN/LVNs have always been accountable for proper performance of assigned duties and for knowing when other workers must be consulted for situations beyond the limits of the UAP's and LPN/LVN's knowledge and training. Unlicensed workers and LPN/LVNs must earn the trust of the professional nurse, and vice versa. Although the legal doctrine of respondeat superior (let the superior answer) applies, unlicensed and licensed practical/vocational workers do bear some accountability for their actions. Nevertheless, the principles that have guided nursing care for years apply: the professional nurse is still accountable for the client's overall care. Thus, the current situation requires that professional nurses broaden the scope of supervision and be more vigilant. They must be more aware of the abilities and activities of UAP and LPN/LVNs while increasing their own availability for consultation.

Managed Care and Third-Party Payers

Managed care, government health care plans, and private health insurance companies monitor access to services, strive to eliminate redundancy, look for ways to reduce overuse of services, and control health care costs. Unfortunately, in some managed care and insurance companies, people without health care experience or education make approval decisions for consumers needing or wanting specific health care services (including health insurance coverage).

With cost-containment efforts, the nurse's role as a client advocate becomes vital. The nurse advocate pays attention to and acts in instances in which clients are being denied access to essential care or seem to be short-changed by policies and actions directed primarily at cost containment (Aroskar, 1992; Stevens, 1992). The issue of access to care has been a legitimate one for nurses to address for years, as succinctly stated in the *Code of Ethics for Nurses* (ANA, 2015a):

The nurse assumes the responsibility and accountability for individual nursing judgments and actions.... The nurse collaborates with members of the health professions and other citizens in promoting community and national efforts to meet the health needs of the public (p. 1).

This notion has also been reiterated and emphasized by its inclusion in the ANA's *Nursing's Social Policy Statement* (2010). There can be no doubt that the nurse's accountability extends to exerting efforts to respond to the health care needs of the public in a collective sense.

Along with doing what is right for clients, nurses play a key role in reimbursement to the employing agency from managed care and other third-party payers. Meticulous documentation of all supplies and interventions provides evidence that consumers received care. Third-party payers frequently audit charts in efforts to disallow charges appearing on consumer bills.

ACCOUNTABILITY IN THE FUTURE

The future relies on current actions. The nursing profession has renewed its interest in accountability, and practice changes have occurred to increase nurse accountability.

Some nurses have assumed control of practice by adopting **shared governance** models that increase nurse participation in shaping professional practice. Nurses assume responsibility and accountability for developing unit-based and institution-wide procedures for clinical practice and quality improvement.

When adverse client events or failure of work processes arise, accountable nurses complete incident reports that are used to track reasons why errors occurred. Although incident reports are used internally to discover reasons for errors, nurses completing them admit that mistakes were made and examine the reasons why they occurred. A just culture approach to care errors uses incident reports as opportunities to identify flawed work processes and to help employees grow. Health care delivery (especially in hospitals) relies on many team members to execute physician orders. Each member of the health team makes a contribution, and all assume accountability for their actions. Nursing may have to learn to be accountable within a more ambiguous, multidisciplinary framework.

Advanced technology has provided the means for nursing to become more accountable. Technology can be used to clearly show what nurses do, including the care they deliver, the cost of that care, and its outcomes. Nursing must be rescued from burial in the category of "room and board" in budgets and on client bills. Once nursing services departments control their budgets, they will be empowered to make decisions and be accountable for them.

CHECKLIST FOR ACCOUNTABILITY

Preparation for accountability for action requires that nurses evaluate their actions periodically. Some nurses find it useful to use an **accountability checklist** that provides key questions to ask themselves that address their current behaviors, attitudes and resources required to protect everyone while engaging in clinical practice. Box 12.5, Professional Prototypes, "Accountability

12.5 Professional Prototypes

Accountability Checklists

Accountability to the Client

- Am I providing the best care of which I am capable?
- Is that care sufficient to meet the needs of the client in this situation?
- Is this client entitled to more than I can offer, and am I turning elsewhere to obtain the needed, additional dimension?
- Am I incorporating what I know of nursing theory and research into my practice in this situation?
- Am I using my leadership skills to encourage others to function to their optimal ability in the care of this patient?
- Am I acting in accordance with my own ethical code and that of the profession?
- If, by meeting the needs of this client, I am in conflict with my personal ethical code, am I seeking some alternative method or person to satisfy those needs?
- Have I given clients information they want or need about their health status, while considering the effect of that knowledge on them?

Accountability to the Public

- Am I seeking to improve health and nursing care?
- Am I speaking out against abuses I see in health and nursing care?
- Am I acting as a community resource in the areas of health and nursing?
- Am I remaining an active and contributing member of the profession and to society after using public funds to finance my education?
- Am I attempting to increase the knowledge of the public to enable people to make more informed choices about health and nursing care?
- Am I recruiting others to enter the profession to have future health care needs of clients met?
- Am I sharing my knowledge and expertise about health care with elected officials to shape public policy?

Accountability to the Profession

- Am I fulfilling my professional role in accordance with the requirements of the profession?
- Are other nurses in my setting doing the same?
- If I am not performing satisfactorily, or if others are not, am I taking steps to remedy that situation?

- Am I willing to help other nurses in my work setting?
- Am I a participant in professional meetings, organizations, seminars, conferences, and so forth, so that I may express my views on nursing to those in nursing?
- Am I working within the profession to improve practice, education, or research?
- Am I complying with the ethical code of the profession?

Accountability to the Agency

- Am I performing in accordance with the job description for the position for which I was employed?
- If I am not satisfied with that job description, am I seeking appropriate ways to change it?
- Am I seeking to ensure that I am practicing under safe, if not optimal, conditions?
- Am I giving the institution its money's worth in terms of my work?
- Am I working in accordance with the policies and procedures of the institution?
- If I am not satisfied with those policies and procedures, am I seeking to change those using principles of leadership and change with the total mission of the institution in mind?

Accountability to Self

- Am I satisfied in my chosen profession?
- Am I performing my professional role in the best way I can?
- Should I seek additional preparation for that role?
- Should I withdraw from that role until I receive additional preparation?
- In areas where I am dissatisfied, am I seeking alternative modes of action or thought?
- Am I comfortable, ethically, with the way in which I am performing my professional role?
- Am I shortchanging my patients, my significant others, or myself in the way I am performing my professional role?
- Do I have adequate financial protection for myself and family if I were to be involved in a professional litigation case?
- Am I satisfied with the position this role assumes within my total lifestyle?

Checklists," provides guidance for self-assessment of professional accountability by nurses. The list is not all-inclusive but offers a beginning tool for working the concept of accountability into one's life and work.

Because of the magnitude of the checklist provided in Professional Prototypes, most nurses could not confidently claim that they fulfill all criteria. Some activities are more appropriate than others for nurses in different settings and at different times. However, nurses who are to act in an accountable manner or increase the accountability of their decisions and actions must consider these and other questions. Those who wish to call themselves professional nurses must consider these questions to live a life of accountability.

Summary and Significance to Practice

Accountability in professional nursing is a complex phenomenon that requires nurses to look globally at how their actions affect clients, society, employing agencies, colleagues, and themselves. For a long time, nurses have assumed the responsibility of protecting clients and tending to their needs. Because of the nature of nursing practice, nurses have binding legal and ethical obligations to clients, the public, the employing agency, the profession, and themselves. Nurses need to have confidence in themselves and their cognitive skills if they are to tackle successfully situations with the potential to place clients in harm's way. Sometimes nurses have to make tough decisions such as reporting unsafe acts by a colleague or employer. In today's rapidly changing and chaotic health care environment, nurses become accountable for staying current with new treatments, research findings, cost containment issues, and clinical skills. Because of its breadth and depth, professional accountability takes time to develop. Professional accountability expands as nurses assume more autonomous and leadership career paths.

REAL-LIFE REFLECTIONS

Recall the scenario from the beginning of the chapter. In light of what you have learned in this chapter, revisit your list of who made mistakes in the care of Mr. Jones. Do you see the need for any changes to your answers? What mistakes did they make? Who is accountable for the actions of the people involved? How could this unfortunate incident have been avoided? What steps should be taken by everyone involved to avoid repeating the same errors with a future patient?

From Theory to Practice

1. Do you currently carry professional malpractice insurance? Why or why not?
2. How are student accountabilities addressed in your professional nursing program? How are they communicated to students? What are the consequences for a student breach of accountability?

Nurse as Author

Answer the questions contained in the accountability checklists provided in Professional Prototypes 12.5. Write an action plan to meet all areas for your future accountability in your personal and professional life.

Your Digital Classroom

Online Exploration

American Association of Colleges of Nursing: **www.aacn.nche.edu**

American Association of Legal Nurse Consultants: **www.aalnc.org**

American Nurses Association: **www.nursingworld.org**

Code for Nurses with Interpretive Statements: **www.nursingworld.org/codeofethics**

For a list of medical malpractice statutes and case outcomes including awards to plaintiffs visit **http://www.medicalmalpractice.com/lawsuit-and-award-limits/medical-malpractice-statutes.htm**

National Council of State Boards of Nursing: **www.ncsbn.org**

National League for Nursing: **www.nln.org**

Nurses Protection Group: **www.nursesprotectiongroup.com**

Nurses Service Organization: **www.nso.com**

Quality and Safety Education in Nursing (QSEN) Institute: **www.qsen.org**

Expanding Your Understanding

1. Visit the National Council of State Boards of Nursing website. Click on "About NCSBN" and read the organization's mission, vision, and purpose. Go back to the home page, and click on "Boards of Nursing" to access your state board of nursing. Find your state in the list and click on the website link to learn specific information related to professional nursing in your state.
2. View a sample nurse's malpractice insurance policy on the Nurses Service Organization website. Click on "Professional Liability Insurance" and "Individuals," and select either "Nurses" or "Student Nurses." Then select your state. Click on NSO's Professional Liability Insurance Program to get a sample of terms of liability coverage from this professional liability insurance provider.

Beyond the Book

Visit **thePoint®** **www.thePoint.lww.com** for activities and information to reinforce the concepts and content covered in this chapter.

REFERENCES

Aiken, T. M. (2003). Nursing malpractice: Understanding the risks. *Travel Nursing, 1*, 7–12.

American Nurses Association (ANA). (2010). *Nursing's social policy statement, the essence of the profession.* Silver Spring, MD: Author.

American Nurses Association. (2015a). *Code of ethics for nurses with interpretive statements.* Silver Springs, MD: Author.

American Nurses Association. (2015b). *Nursing scope and standards of practice* (3rd ed.). Silver Spring, MD: Author.

American Nurses Credentialing Center. (2011). Magnet Recognition Program(R) Program overview. Retrieved from http://nursecredentialing.org/Documents/Magnet/MagOverview-92011.pdf. Accessed April 8, 2017.

Anselmi, K. K. (2012). Nurses' personal liability vs. employer's vicarious liability. *Medsurg Nursing, 21*(1), 45–48.

Armstrong, A. (2011). Legal considerations for nurse prescribers. *Nurse Prescribing, 9*(12), 603–608.

Aroskar, M. A. (1992). Ethical foundations in nursing for broad health care access. *Scholarly Inquiry for Nursing Practice, 6*, 201–205.

Bae, S. H. (2012). Nursing overtime: Why, how much, and under what working conditions. *Nursing Economics, 30*(2), 60–72.

Batey, V. M., & Lewis, F. M. (1982). Clarifying autonomy and accountability in nursing service, Part 2. *Journal of Nursing Administration, 12*, 10–15.

Berwick, D. M. (2010). Campaign to save 5 million lives. Retrieved from http://www.ihi.org/offerings/Initiatives/PastStrategicInitiatives/5MillionLivesCampaign/Pages/default.aspx10. Accessed February 25, 2013.

Bixler, G. K., & Bixler, R. W. (1959). The professional status of nursing. *American Journal of Nursing, 59*, 1142–1147.

Chaska, N. L. (1983). *The nursing profession: A time to speak.* New York: McGraw-Hill.

Clifford, J. C. (1981). Managerial control versus professional autonomy: A paradox. *Journal of Nursing Administration, 11*, 19–21.

Copp, G. (1988). Professional accountability: The conflict. *Nursing Times, 84*(3), 42–44.

Croke, E. M. (2003). Nurses, negligence and malpractice. *American Journal of Nursing, 103*, 54–64.

Dachelet, C. Z., & Sullivan, J. A. (1979). Autonomy in practice. *Nursing Practice, 4*, 15–16, 18–19.

Dethmer, J. (2006a). Accountability: Part 1. Taking responsibility. In J. Ware, J. Dethmer, J. Ziegler, & F. Skinner (Eds.), *High performance investment teams.* Hoboken, NJ: John Wiley.

Dethmer, J. (2006b). Accountability: Part 2. Making and keeping agreements. In J. Ware, J. Dethmer, J. Ziegler, & F. Skinner (Eds.), *High performance investment teams.* Hoboken, NJ: John Wiley.

Domrose, C. (2007). Malpractice suits against nurses on the rise. *New Hampshire Nursing News,* 8–9.

Flexner, A. (1915). Is social work a profession? In Proceedings of the National Conference of Charities and Correction (pp. 576–590). Chicago: Heldman.

Fowler, M. D. M. (2015). *Guide to the code of ethics for nurses with interpretive statements* (2nd ed.). Silver Springs, MD: Nursebooks.com.

Gans, D. (2007). Malpractice insurance: A necessary but offensive cost. *MGMA Connexion, 7*(7), 20–21.

Goldstein, P. (2006). Impact of disease management programs on hospital and community nursing practice. *Nursing Economics, 24*(6), 308–314.

Greenwald, J. (2008), Stanford's medical center mulls expanding role of captive. *Business Insurance, 42*(17), 36–37.

Hastings, J., & Burn, J. (2007). Addiction: A nurse's story. Opioids became an obsession—until he was caught. *American Journal of Nursing, 107*(8), 75–77, 79.

Holden, R. J. (1991). Responsibility and autonomous nursing practice. *Journal of Advanced Nursing, 16*, 398–403.

Hylka, S. C., & Shugrue, D. (1991). Increasing staff nurse autonomy. *Nursing Management, 22*, 54–55.

Institute of Medicine (IOM). (2000). *To err is human: Building a safer health care system.* Washington, DC: National Academies Press.

Institute of Medicine. (2001). *Crossing the quality chasm: A new health system for the 21st century.* Washington, DC: National Academies Press.

Institute of Medicine. (2011). *The future of nursing: Leading change, advancing health.* Washington, DC: National Academies Press.

International Council of Nurses. (2012). *ICN code of ethics for nurses:* Retrieved from http://www.icn.ch/images/stories/documents/publications/free_publications/Code%20of%20Ethics%202012%20for%20web.pdf. Accessed February 25, 2013.

Joint Commission on Accreditation of Healthcare Organizations. (1991). *Nursing care accreditation manual for hospitals, 1991.* Chicago: Author.

Kopp, P. (2001). Fit for practice: Legal issues in accountability. *Nursing Times, 97*(5), 45–47.

Kramer, M., Schmalenberg, C., & Maguire, P. (2008). Essentials of a magnetic work environment. In *Nursing 2008 career directory* (pp. 36–37). Philadelphia, PA: Lippincott Williams & Wilkins.

Lillibridge, J., Cox, M., & Cross, W. (2002). Uncovering the secret: Giving voice to the experiences of nurses who misuse substances. *Journal of Advanced Nursing, 39*, 219–229.

Maer-Brisen, P. (2007). Addiction: An occupational hazard in nursing. *American Journal of Nursing, 107*(8), 78–79.

McCannon, C. J., Schall, M. W., Calkins, D. R., & Nazem, A. G. (2006). Saving 100,000 lives in US hospitals. *British Medical Journal, 332*(7553):1328–1330.

McGlothlin, W. J. (1961). The place of nursing among the professions. *Nursing Outlook, 9*, 214–216.

Merriam-Webster's Online Dictionary. (2015a). Accountable. Retrieved from http://www.merriam-webster.com/dictionary/accountable. Accessed October 10, 2016.

Merriam-Webster's Online Dictionary. (2015b). Responsibility. Retrieved from http://www.merriam-webster.com/dictionary/responsibility. Accessed October 10, 2016.

Merton, R. K. (1958). The functions of the professional association. *American Journal of Nursing, 58*, 50–54.

Miller, J. (2004). *QBQ! The question behind the question.* New York: G. P. Putnam's Sons.

Milstead, J. (2008). *Health policy and politics: A nurse's guide.* Sudbury, MA: Jones & Bartlett.

Murray, J. (2007). Before blowing the whistle, learn to protect yourself. *American Nurse Today, 2*(3), 40–42.

National Council of State Boards of Nursing. (2016). National guidelines for nursing delegation. *Journal of Nursing Regulation, 7*(1), 7–14.

Nightingale, F. (1946; originally published in 1859). *Notes on nursing: What it is and what it is not.* Philadelphia, PA: J. B. Lippincott.

Nolan, S., Burkard, J., Clark, M., Davidson, J., & Agan, D. (2010). Effect of morbidity and mortality peer review on nurse accountability and ventilator-associated pneumonia rates. *Journal of Nursing Administration, 40*(9), 374–383.

Olds, D., & Clarke, S. (2010). The effect of work hours on adverse events and errors in health care. *Journal of Safety Research, 41*(2), 153–162.

Pham, J., & Papa, A. (2011). Study: Temporary ED staff twice as likely to be associated with medication errors that cause harm to patients. *ED Management, 23*(12), 140–141.

Porter-O'Grady, T., & Malloch, K. (2015). *Quantum leadership: Building better partnerships for sustainable health (4th ed.).* Burlington, MA: Jones & Bartlett Learning.

Roper, K. A., & Russell, G. (1997). The effect of peer review on professionalism, autonomy and accountability. *Journal of Nursing Staff Development, 13*, 198–206.

Sammer, C., Lykens, K., Singh, K., Mains, D., & Lackan, N. (2010). What is patient safety culture? *Journal of Nursing Scholarship, 42*(2), 156–165.

Sherwood, G. (2012). Driving forces for quality and safety: Changing mindsets to improve health care. In G. Sherwood, & J. Barnsteiner (Eds.), *Quality and safety in nursing a competency approach to improving outcomes* (pp. 3–21). Oxford, UK: Wiley-Blackwell.

Sherwood, G., & Barnsteiner, J. (Eds.). (2012). *Quality and safety in nursing a competency approach to improving outcomes.* Oxford, UK: Wiley-Blackwell.

Stevens, P. E. (1992). Who gets care? Access to health care as an arena for nursing action. *Scholarly Inquiry for Nursing Practice, 6*, 185–200.

Styles, M. (1985). Accountable to whom? *Nursing Mirror, 160*, 36–37.

The QSEN Institute. (2013). *The new QSEN.* Retrieved from http://qsen.org/about-qsen/the-new-qsen/. Accessed February 25, 2013.

U.S. Drug Enforcement Agency. (2005). *Drug addiction in health care professionals.* Retrieved from http://www.deadiversion.usdoj.gov/pubs/brochures/drug_hc.htm. Accessed February 6, 2013.

Vaughn, B. (1989). Autonomy and accountability. *Nursing Times, 85*(3), 54–55.

Watson, E. (2014). Nursing malpractice: Costs, trends & issues. *Journal of Legal Nurse Consulting, 25*(1), 26–31.

Watson, S. (2012). New NSO study on nurse liability: Important implications for your practice. *Michigan Nurse, 41*(4), 15–19.

White, D. E., Jackson, K., Bessner, J., & Norris, J. M. (2015). The examination of nursing work through a role accountability framework. *Journal of Nursing Management, 23*(3), 604–612.

Chapter 13

Environmental and Global Health

KEY TERMS AND CONCEPTS

Environment
Global environment
Anthropocene era
Environmental health
Ecocentric
Pollution
Environmental surprises
Discontinuity
Extinct
Synergism
Unnoticed trend

Positive feedback
Cascading effects
Multiple chemical
 sensitivity
Community
 environment
Work environment
Home environment
Disaster
Disaster management
 cycle

LEARNING OUTCOMES

By the end of this chapter, the learner will be able to:

1. Explain how the global, community, work, and home environments affect human health.
2. Outline noxious environmental factors that may impair human health.
3. Identify elements within one's personal environment that are noxious to the global environment.
4. Identify factors within the environment that promote health.
5. Integrate personal behaviors that foster a health-promoting environment.
6. Relate environmental quality to the quality of human health.

REAL-LIFE REFLECTIONS

Arianna is a nursing student who lives next door to Elena, a registered nurse. Because of a blizzard, the electricity in their neighborhood stopped working. After checking with each other to verify that neither of them have power, they decide to spend the day clearing the sidewalks of snow with the help of Elena's two teenagers. At dusk, they notice that the porch light to the Garcias' house is lit. They also note that no one in the block appears to have electric service restored. Arianna asks Elena and her children if any of them recall seeing a gasoline or other-powered generator outside of the Garcias' home. None of them remember seeing any indications outside that a generator is being used. Because the Garcias rarely talk with the neighbors, they explore options of what to do.

- *What are the possible options for actions that Arianna and Elena might take?*
- *What are the potential health hazards for using a gas or other petroleum-fueled generator within the confines of a building?*
- *What would you do if you were in Arianna's or Elena's situation?*
- *How would you cope with the loss of electricity to your home?*

Objects, conditions, and circumstances create the environment. Living organisms depend on the environment for formation and survival. Not all environments have the capability of sustaining life. Multiple environmental systems must remain in balance to sustain life. For the purpose of this chapter, **environment** refers to "all the conditions and circumstances" that surround and influence life on Earth (Agnes, 2005, p. 476). The environment consists of physical domains (air, water, soil) and social domains (land use, industry, housing, transportation, agriculture). Depending on the context, environments may be miniscule or enormous. The **global environment** refers to the conditions of the entire Earth. **Environmental health** refers to conditions in the environment that preserve the balance of nature.

The current geologic era has been named the Anthropocene era, a term coined by Paul Crutzen, a Nobel Prize–winning atmospheric scientist from the Netherlands (Pearce, 2007). The **Anthropocene era** started approximately 200 years ago and encompasses the time during which humans appear to have dominated Earth. Some of the human-induced changes on Earth include the release of greenhouse gases and other environmental pollutants, deforestation, urban development, and pillaging of natural resources (Adeola, 2011; Fagan, 2008; Lynas, 2008; Pearce, 2007; Sachs, 2008).

Humans rely on the external environment for air, water, and food. Within a system's framework, interacting groups create a unitary whole. When the balance is altered, changes occur in the unitary whole experience. When those changes affect the quality of the external environment that supports life as we know it, they will affect human health status. Fagan (2008), Lynas (2008), Pearce (2007), and Sachs (2008) provide possible scenarios of the effects of global warming on Earth, some of which may result in marked population reductions and even the demise of the human race. This chapter examines the effects of the global, local, work, and home environments on human health and offers strategies for professional nurses to create a sustainable future.

THE GLOBAL ENVIRONMENT

In Victorian times, people tended to look at local, rather than global, environmental conditions. Florence Nightingale linked the quality of the environment to the health of soldiers during the Crimean War. Her writings documented reduced mortality of and infections in injured soldiers when pure air, pure water, efficient drainage, cleanliness, and light were provided

for them (Dock, 1912). After Nightingale's reforms, nurses paid close attention to the hospital environment to provide a healthy environment for patients. Nursing education textbooks provided detailed information on how to optimize the hospital environment to promote health and healing (Young & Lee, 1948).

When society became conscious of all the impact of pollution on human health and well-being, the nursing profession expanded its view of the environment. Instead of focusing on just the hospital home, or local community environments, nurses began to address issues related to the global environment (Kleffel, 1994). Because of the role that the environment plays in human health and its importance in professional nursing practice, Fawcett (1984) included environment in the metaparadigm for nursing.

Definitions of the environment depend on the philosophical stance of each theorist. Rogers (1990), Leddy (2004), and Newman (1994) defined the environment as an energy field, while Watson (1999), Neuman (2002), and Roy (1987) defined the environment as an open system. Neuman further separated the environment into internal and external domains that interact with each other.

With the development of the space program and advances in scientific technology, humans came to know much more about the environment. When the world saw pictures of Earth from outer space, many people understood the interconnectedness of nations and how global regulation (or its lack) could potentially affect everyone. As people realize the importance of the environment on human health, an **ecocentric** (the perspective of the environment as being whole, interconnected, and alive) approach to health care delivery becomes a societal priority (Kleffel, 1996).

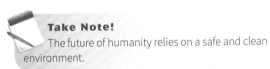

Take Note!
The future of humanity relies on a safe and clean environment.

Ecosystem Disturbance and Environmental Surprises

Earth is a delicate planet with balanced ecosystems that provide the resources to sustain many varieties of life. Humans upset this balance through environmental **pollution** (contamination with harmful chemicals) from waste products in manufacturing, energy production, and burning wood or petroleum products; chemicals used to control pests (animals, insects, plants); and widespread use of plastic products. When the balance becomes disturbed,

environmental surprises emerge. Bright (2000) identified three forms of environmental surprise:

1. **Discontinuity**: An abrupt shift in a trend or steady state. For example, forest habitat loss causes some animals to seek refuge elsewhere or travel to human-populated areas for food. The species (e.g., bears) becomes a menace to people by scouring human garbage cans for food; local governments spend money to control them; some people get harmed; and, in extreme cases, the species becomes endangered or **extinct** (ceases to exist).
2. **Synergism**: Simultaneous changes in several natural phenomena with greater-than-expected environmental effects. For example, a catastrophe with a high human death toll may result from the combined effects of a heavy rainstorm, cutting trees on a hillside, and people moving to an identified flood plain.
3. **Unnoticed trend**: An event that occurs undetected but does considerable damage to an ecosystem. For example, non-native weed invasion of fertile farm acreage in the United States displaced native plants that facilitated the balance of natural fire cycles. This resulted in the destruction of 9,884 acres of farmland during a 30-year period before it was detected (Bright, 2000).

To further complicate the maintenance of Earth's balance, synergisms can produce discontinuities. For example, ozone depletion combined with acid rain and other atmospheric contaminants (particles and gases) results in increased penetration of ultraviolet radiation in water, which leads to the destruction of microorganisms essential for the survival of coral reefs and fish. Alternatively, discontinuities can produce synergisms, such as the evolution of pesticide-resistant insects carrying plant viruses that destroy crops (Bright, 2000).

Positive feedback loops can also create discontinuities. In a positive feedback loop, the cycle of change continues to amplify itself. Global warming provides a prime example of a positive feedback loop. The Arctic ice cap is melting as the result of global warming. Although even a thick ice cap absorbs only 10% of the sunlight, with the oceans absorbing the rest, as the ice mass dwindles, the ocean becomes warmer, resulting in accelerated global warming (Adeola, 2011; Bright, 2000; Lynas, 2008; Pearce, 2007; Sachs, 2008).

Cascading effects can also lead to environmental changes. Cascading effects occur when a change in one component of a system results in a change in another component, which sets up a change in yet another component, with multiple changes occurring throughout various components. Cascading effects can produce discontinuities and synergisms. The Alaskan coastline provides an example of a cascading effect. When the Alaskan perch and herring populations declined, sea lions and seals starved. As the population of sea lions and seals declined, killer whales had to find new prey to survive. The sea otter was the ideal candidate. However, because sea otters feast on sea urchin, as the sea otter population declined, the sea urchin population exploded. The sea urchins then demolished the kelp forests. Many species of fish, marine invertebrates, marine mammals, and birds that rely on kelp for food are now at risk (Bright, 2000; Lynas, 2008; Pearce, 2007; Sachs, 2008).

Challenges of the 21st Century

Sachs (2008) identified the following six trends of the 21st century that are shaping the future of humankind.

1. The age of convergence (when the per capita income of poorer nations rises to, catches up with, and even exceeds that of rich nations).
2. Increased population growth of people with higher incomes (increased demands for goods, services, and energy).
3. Asian dominance of the world economy.
4. More people living in urban locales as a result of migration.
5. Environmental challenges (how to mitigate the effects of human environmental destruction).
6. The poverty trap (large income gaps between the rich and poor) with self-reinforcing and perpetual cycles of poverty.

Population Pressures

Pearce (2007) and Lynas (2008) shed more light on future environmental issues resulting from the exploding human population, such as rising global temperatures, falling water tables, declining croplands, diminishing fisheries, shrinking forests, and the loss of plant and animal species. When this chapter was prepared, the world population was 7.026 billion (U.S. Census Bureau, 2012); with current growth trends, the population is expected to reach 9.2 billion by 2050 (Sachs, 2008).

The growing population creates more demand for food, water, space, and goods. China, India, North Africa, and the United States pump more water than can be replenished through snow and rain. Farmers overpump water for crops, and many industries (e.g., paper, cotton) use enormous amounts of water for production. The processing of crops and livestock, and the production of consumer goods, result in an increased release of nitrogen and phosphorus into the atmosphere, triggering acid rain. Trees become more susceptible to disease and damage from extreme temperatures, effects of acid rain, and reduced rainfall. Deterioration of dead trees results in the release of more carbon dioxide and methane into the atmosphere, leading to increased global warming (Adeola, 2011; Lynas, 2008; Pearce, 2007).

Climate Change

Rising levels of carbon dioxide emissions (Fig. 13.1) since the advent of the Industrial Age have resulted in a rise in mean global from −0.19°C in 1880 to 0.87°C in 2015, according to 2016 data from National Aeronautics and Space Administration's Goddard Institute for Space Studies (NASA/GISS, 2016a). The year 2015 was the warmest on record and with the exception of 1998, the 10 warmest global temperatures were recorded within the last 10 years (NASA/GISS 2016a). Increased global temperature results in increased land ice melting. As of January 2016, the current sea level was measured to be 74.48 mm and sea levels are estimating to be rising at a rate of 3.42 mm annually because of melting land ice (increased water volume) and water molecular expansion in response to warmer temperatures (NASA/GISS, 2016b). Because of the uncertainty and complexity of Earth's ecosystem, projections for global warming by 2050 vary from 1°C to 12.7°C (1.7°F to 21°F).

Increases in global temperatures impact human health. As global temperatures increase, infectious diseases (especially those associated with insects) typically seen in tropical climates may be encountered in more temperate zones (Greer & Fisman, 2008; Lynas,

2008; Pearce, 2007). Additional human health effects of climate change also increased incidence and intensity of respiratory diseases from increased ozone levels and particulates in the air (allergic and air pollutant induced) (Albertine et al., 2014); adverse effects on pregnancy outcomes (preterm births, low birth weight, increased incidence of preeclampsia and eclampsia, and birth defects associated with infectious diseases) (Poursafa, Keitkha, & Kelishadi, 2015); massive migration of persons from coastal areas to higher ground form rising sea levels, mortality from extreme heat (Veenema, 2013; United States Environmental Protection Agency [US EPA], 2016), increased food and water-borne illnesses, altered density of nutrients of some plant life and potentially increasing mercury levels in seafood (US EPA, 2016).

Many unknowns exist among the climate change models, such as the long-term effects of manmade pollutants on the environment. Environmental research data and conclusions often appear to be in conflict. For example, ozone promotes the conversion of hydroxyl to a compound that oxidizes air pollutants such as sulfur dioxide, carbon monoxide, and methane so they can be washed away from the air by rain. However, when carbon dioxide does not oxidize out of the atmosphere, it diffuses into the oceans, with subsequent increases in ocean temperatures (Lynas, 2008; Pearce, 2007; Sachs, 2008). The U.S. Meteorological Society concluded that global climate change could increase the intensity level of storms, flooding, and drought conditions (Blunden & Arndt, 2012).

Urbanization

Urban sprawl impinges on available cropland and results in deforestation (Fig. 13.2). Burning harvested trees releases more carbon and methane into

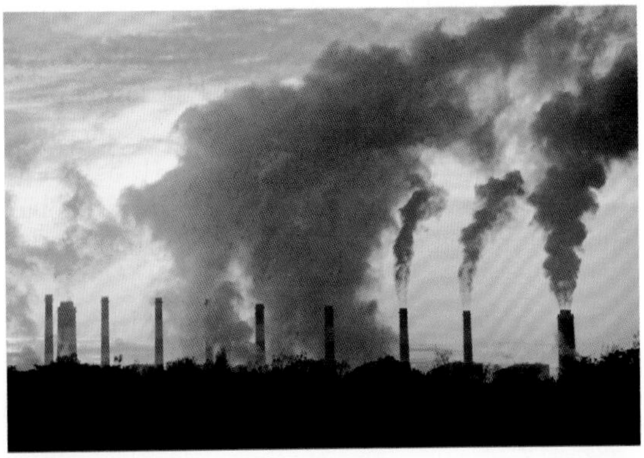

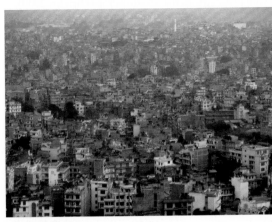

FIGURE 13.1 Air pollution contributes to global warming and human disease.

FIGURE 13.2 Urbanization results in deforestation, increased air pollution, and global warming.

the atmosphere, which increases global warming and reduces rainfall (Adeola, 2011; Lynas, 2008; Pearce, 2007; Sachs, 2008).

Urbanization increases the consumption of fossil fuels, which also contributes to global warming. Higher global temperatures and rising atmospheric carbon dioxide levels result in increased ocean temperatures and acidity, which destroy the plankton and coral that many fish rely on for survival (Lynas, 2008; Pearce, 2007; Sachs, 2008). From 1957 to 1997, the annual oceanic fish catch increased by 71 million tons (from 19 to 90 million tons). Many marine biologists theorize that the ocean cannot sustain an annual fish catch of more than 95 million tons (O'Meara, 2000). Recent research has demonstrated that some types of fish have resilience and have been able to reproduce at a rate fast enough to prevent extinction within the past 60 years, but many of these may be close to reaching a tipping point that will result in declining numbers (Vasailakopoulos & Marchall, 2015).

The Health Care Industry

American hospitals produce approximately 6,000 tons of medical waste per day. According to the Environmental Protection Agency (EPA, 2008), the health care industry is one of the major sources of mercury (found in medical equipment such as thermometers, sphygmomanometers, and endoscopes) and dioxin (from polyvinyl plastic materials) pollution. Other pollutants attributed to health care organizations include dead batteries, old computers, hazardous chemicals (cleaning products), chemotherapy agents, and radioactive isotopes (Shaner & Botter, 2003). Recent reports have identified various levels of human pharmaceuticals (analgesics, lipid regulators, beta-blockers, antidepressants, oral contraceptives, and antibiotics) being present in water treatment effluents, surface waters, groundwater, sea water, and even drinking waters (Adeola, 2011; Brausch, Connors, & Brooks, 2012; Fent, Weston, & Caminada, 2006; Hemminger, 2005).

Many developed countries, including the United States practice "toxic colonialism" or "toxic imperialism," a process by which wealthy nations pay poor, undeveloped nations to take waste. Much of American hospital waste (along with other dangerous chemical waste, discarded appliances, cell phones, MP3 players, and computer hardware) are sent to undeveloped, poor nations (Nigeria, South Africa, Ghana, Tanzania, India, Pakistan, and China) where children play among heavy metals (e.g., aluminum, arsenic, cadmium, barium, chromium, lithium, mercury) and low-level radioactive and transuranic waste (Adeola, 2011).

Efforts Toward Global Preservation

Environmental degradation demonstrates that Earth has undergone and is currently undergoing many changes as the result of human habitation. Ancient Greeks, Romans, Asians, and Native Americans viewed the world as a living organism. Traditional Native American and Eastern philosophies still espouse this belief. The Gaia hypothesis proposes that the difference between living and nonliving things is one of graded intensity and that Earth remains the sole provider of resources for humans. Many environmentalists profess a worldview of wholeness, in which each cell has equal value and is reflective of the entire cosmos. All cells within the environment interact and achieve a balance. Because everything is interconnected, all parts of the universe are equally important, and no organism should receive special status (Kleffel, 1994; Pearce, 2007). Unfortunately, humans have appropriated a special status for themselves, and the environment has become the casualty.

International efforts at global preservation have been formed by governmental, international, and private organizations (Fig. 13.3). Governmental agencies and nongovernmental organizations frequently exert pressure on companies to "clean up their acts."

- In 1992, the United Nations Framework Convention for Climate Change, an initiative to stabilize greenhouse gas emissions, was adopted. The U.S. Senate ratified the agreement in 1994.
- The Kyoto Protocol sought to reduce greenhouse emissions by 5% worldwide from 1997 to 2012. The protocol carried different guidelines for nations based on their wealth. Although adopted by the rest of the world, the United States has never accepted the Kyoto Protocol because of the perceived economic hardships it would cause.

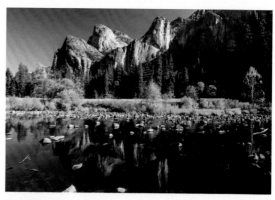

FIGURE 13.3 Efforts at preserving nature and natural habitats such as Yosemite Park provides a place for persons to enjoy the healthful benefits of being in an unspoiled natural environment.

TABLE 13.1 Global Environmental Organizations and Networks

Organization/Network	Purpose	Website
Good Guide	Monitors and communicates the status of the environment; creates an online data scorecard that ranks facilities, revealing the most offending polluters	www.scorecard.org
Association for Progressive Communications	Links nongovernmental organizations that promote human rights and environmental concerns	www.apc.org
OneWorld	Links many websites to provide information on economic development	www.oneworld.net
United Nations Environmental Programme (UNEP)	Links with partner institutions by satellite to improve the flow of environmental data	www.unep.org
Global Urban Observatory	Links researchers to a global network of data, statistics, and examples of best practices in urban management	ww2.unhabitat.org/programmes/guo/
Horizon Solutions (Horizon International)	Provides case studies on solutions related to water, waste, energy, transportation, toxic pollutants, public health, industrial manufacturing, biodiversity, air pollution, and agricultural issues	www.solutions-site.org
Intergovernmental Panel on Climate Change	Studies and reports on the current scientific and technologic knowledge about climate change while examining the sociocultural and economic effects of climate change; proposes ways to mitigate the effects of climate change.	www.ipcc.ch/
Environmental Defense Fund	Examines ways and strategies to promote environmental stewardship without compromising economic prosperity by informing the public of health hazards of chemical used in everyday life and working to pass environmental friendly legislation.	www.edf.og

Adapted from O'Meara, M. (2000). Harnessing information technologies for the environment. In L. R. Brown, C. Flavin, H. French, S. Postel, & L. Starke (Eds.), *State of the world 2000*. New York: W.W. Norton & Company. See also Environmental Defense Fund (2012) at www.edf.org, and the Intergovernmental Plane on Climate Change (2013) at www.ipcc.ch/.

- In 2005, the Earth Institute of Columbia University sponsored a Global Roundtable on Climate Change (GRTOCC) as a means to combat global warming on an international scale. A scientific consensus statement arising from the GRTOCC specified that "global warming is real and that it is caused by greenhouse gas emissions and primarily caused by our consumption of fossil fuels" (Sachs, 2008, p. 110). The GRTOCC outlined three methods to combat the issue of global warming: "mitigation, adaptation and research, development, and demonstration (RD&D) of new technologies" (Sachs, 2008, p. 110).
- In 2015, the UN held a Climate Change Conference in Paris, France. Participating countries agreed to limit global warming below 2°C for the entire century. The desired goal for global warming would be to keep less than 5°C above preindustrial global temperatures. Nations will need to begin serious efforts at reducing global warming within 30 days following ratification of the agreement by 55% of participating countries (United Nations, 2016).

In addition to formal governmental and international global efforts, nongovernmental organizations serve as environmental caretakers (Table 13.1). Global networking among environmentalists provides the opportunity for global solutions to global problems. Research universities such as the University of Michigan are also devoting resources to ecosystem toxicology. By exploring microscopic changes in the environment, such as measuring the content of specific pesticides in marine life and avian eggshells, damage to the environment can be discovered before deformed animals are found and freshwater sources become hazardous to drink (Scully, 2001).

Nurses can use information from established, reputable organizations to increase their awareness of global pollution, take steps to minimize pollution-promoting behaviors, and educate others about behaviors that may contribute to global pollution and destruction.

QUESTIONS FOR REFLECTION

1. What do you feel is the greatest threat to the global ecosystem and why?
2. What impact do you think changes in the global ecosystem will have on the nursing profession and clinical practice?

3. What impact does your personal life have on the environment?

4. What changes could you make to either your personal or professional life that would reduce your impact on the global environment?

Global Environmental Factors Threatening Health

Many global environmental factors threaten the health of people, plants, and animals. Professional nursing practice focuses on health promotion, as well as caring for the infirm. Nurses must be aware of environmental health risks.

- Many people drink chemical soups when they partake of water from local water supplies.
- People living in urban locales inhale chemical vapors, which results in an increased incidence of asthma, lung cancer, and other chronic pulmonary diseases.
- Agricultural workers have an increased incidence of lymphoma and other cancers that are linked to herbicide and pesticide exposure (McGinn, 2000).
- Persons remodeling or demolishing old buildings become exposed to asbestos and sometimes carry asbestos fibers home on their clothing.
- Miners inhale dust that results in the development of chronic lung diseases.

Infectious Disease

Environmental factors play a critical role in the rise and spread of infectious diseases. Many diseases have a higher prevalence in certain geographical locations. Others spread through animal migration, international travel, and the growth of a global economy.

- African mosquitoes have evolved to bite only humans, resulting in a high incidence of malaria. In areas without medication for treatment or chemically treated nets for sleeping places, malaria infects over a billion and kills over a million people (many of them are children) annually (Sachs, 2008). Some nations use pesticides to prevent malaria outbreaks, but this, in turn, raises concerns of land and water contamination.
- Human Ebola virus outbreaks in the early 2000s in the Republic of Congo, Sudan, and Gabon arose after hunters were infected by handling dead primates and subsequently spread the virus to other humans (LeRoy et al., 2004).
- West Nile virus originated in Africa but appeared in the United States when infected birds migrated

to the United States. The birds transmitted the virus to mosquitoes, which in turn passed the virus to humans. Documented cases of West Nile virus infection have since been linked to blood transfusions, organ donation, and breast milk (Bender & Thompson, 2003).

- Avian flu (H5N1) originated in China. Although not highly communicable, H5N1 spread rapidly across the globe, facilitated by the close contact of humans during air flights in 2003. Between 2003 and 2012, 605 laboratory-confirmed human cases of H5N1 were reported (World Health Organization [WHO], 2012). More than half of those infected died (WHO, 2012).
- Starting in 2013, another human ebola virus outbreak occurred in Guinea, Liberia, and Sierra Leone. It reached epidemic proportion in 2014. According to the Centers for Disease Control (CDC) (2016a), 28,616 confirmed cases resulting in 11,310 deaths were reported between March 2014 and February 2016. The United Nations declared the public health emergency was over in March, 2016.
- In 2015, the Pan American Health Organization issued a health alert regarding a Zika virus alert because of a confirmed case that occurred in Brazil. Zika viral illnesses have been confirmed occurred in Mexico, Central America, and South America. Confirmed cases of insect-borne cases have surfaced in some of the U.S. territories. Because the Zika virus caused mild symptoms, the virus would infect persons without being noticed. However, pregnant women infected with the Zika virus sometimes had babies with microencephaly and other congenital brain malformations. Zika viral infections have been associated with microcephaly and other severe congenital brain malformations. Zika virus is primarily transmitted to humans through a bite of an infected Aedes mosquito. The virus may also be spread through sexual transmission and to a fetus of an infected mother anytime during pregnancy. Because of unpredictable migration patterns of infected mosquitos, there are expected cases to occur in other parts of the western hemisphere including the United States (CDC, 2016b).

Human factors also play a major role in the rise of infectious diseases. In addition to diseases transmitted to humans by animals or insects, antibiotic-resistant bacteria (methicillin-resistant *Staphylococcus aureus* and vancomycin-resistant *Enterococcus* species) have become prevalent because of indiscriminate use of and client noncompliance with antibiotic therapy. *Clostridium difficile* sometimes causes serious outbreaks in acute and long-term care facilities. All health care workers bear the responsibility of containing the spread of infectious disease.

Along with infectious disease detection and containment, nurses and other health care providers must be aware of potential environmental health hazards (Table 13.2). Awareness of exposure to environmental toxins provides nurses with the ability to teach clients about ways to avoid long-term exposure to pollutants that sometimes result in devastating health consequences.

Multiple Chemical Sensitivity

No matter where they live, people may be exposed to a variety of chemicals. Some people experience severe reactions to such chemical exposures. Although many people may be somewhat sensitive to certain chemicals or environmental triggers, some people experience severe sensitivities to many chemicals, even at levels that would not trigger a reaction in the majority of the population, a condition known as **multiple chemical sensitivity** (MCS). MCS is a recognized form of physical disability (Cooper, 2007; Gibson, 2000; Heimlich, 2008). The National Institutes of Health describes MCS as a chronic, recurrent disorder resulting from a person's inability to tolerate a specific common environmental chemical or a class of foreign chemicals. A known cause for MCS has yet to be identified.

People with MCS often have sustained "systemic damage that causes them to react negatively to common chemicals in ambient air" (Gibson, 2000, p. 8) and typically have a heightened sense of smell (Cooper, 2007). Reactions range from slight drowsiness or nasal congestion to potentially fatal asthmatic attacks. Box 13.1, Professional Building Blocks, "Criteria for Multiple Chemical Sensitivity Diagnosis," outlines the criteria for MCS as determined by a consensus group of 34 researchers and clinicians who treat the condition. Reactions frequently result from exposure to solvents, pesticides, formaldehyde, fresh paint, new carpets, gas exhaust (diesel, car, propane, and natural gas appliances), perfumes, scented cleaners, air fresheners, aspirin, sugar, and food additives. Even processed lumber products used in new construction and electromagnetic fields from appliances can trigger reactions (Gibson, 2000; Heimlich, 2008). Gibson (2000) estimated that 11 million Americans have MCS and that 2% of these people have lost jobs as a result. Reports of MCS have been published in Denmark, Sweden, Norway, Finland, Germany, Holland, Belgium, Greece, and Great Britain (Gibson, 2000).

People with MCS frequently receive psychiatric diagnoses from health care providers (see Concepts in Practice, "Recognizing Multiple Chemical

13.1 Professional Building Blocks

Criteria for Multiple Chemical Sensitivity Diagnosis

- Identical symptoms are reproduced with repeated exposure to the same chemical.
- Reactions are chronic.
- Low levels of exposure to the offending chemical produce manifestations of the reactive symptoms.
- When the offending chemicals are removed, the symptoms lessen or resolve.
- Reactions occur to multiple, unrelated chemical substances.
- Symptoms affect multiple organ systems.

Adapted from Gibson, P. R. (2000). *Multiple chemical sensitivity: A survival guide* (p. 9). Oakland, CA: New Harbinger.

Sensitivity"). However, MCS appears to have a physiologic basis. For unknown reasons, the human body becomes damaged in response to repeated chemical exposures. The following physiologic theories related to the etiology of MCS have been proposed.

Concepts in Practice IDEA → PLAN → ACTION

Recognizing Multiple Chemical Sensitivity

Emily arrives at the emergency department of a teaching hospital with complaints of an intense headache, inability to concentrate, and slight dyspnea. Yolanda, the triage and charge nurse, asks Emily about her medical history. Emily provides a multipage list of allergies to medications, cleaning products, and foods. As the interview progresses, Emily begins to hyperventilate and can only whisper when answering questions. Yolanda becomes suspicious of Emily's many allergies and seemingly overdramatic behavior and concludes that Emily must be mentally ill. As Yolanda starts to page the psychiatric resident, Emily's allergist arrives, orders epinephrine, and states that Emily has a condition called chemical sensitivity, a rare disorder that the allergist says is becoming more prevalent in her practice. After receiving the epinephrine, Emily's symptoms subside.

- *How would you respond if you encountered a client like Emily in your clinical practice?*
- *What advice would you have given Yolanda if she consulted with you about Emily's case?*

TABLE 13.2 Environmental Health Hazards and Potential Remedies

Health Hazard	Geographical Locale(s)	Potential Remedy
Overpopulation	Pakistan, Sub-Saharan Africa, South and Central America	Education about and provision of birth control Governmental limits on number of children Voluntary sterilization
Shrinking croplands from soil erosion, persistent plant disease, and soil pollution	Worldwide	Environmentally sound agricultural practices
Deforestation	Brazil, Indonesia, Malaysia	Reduce demand for paper, lumber, and fuel wood
Increasing atmospheric carbon dioxide concentrations	Worldwide	Human population control Reduce demand for fossil fuels Reforestation
Global warming	Worldwide	Reduce demand for fossil fuels Reforestation Reduce demand for paper, lumber, and fuel wood
Declining/endangered fish population	Worldwide	Curb release of industrial waste chemicals into oceans, lakes, and waterways Judicious use of pesticides Reduce global warming Enforce catch limits
Falling water tables	Worldwide	Reduce use of water in industrial production Water conservation efforts Paper recycling Reduce agricultural crop irrigation
Ozone depletion	Worldwide	Limit demand for fossil fuels Replace appliances that use chlorofluorocarbons
Air pollution	Worldwide	Reduce use of coal, wood, and petroleum products for fuel sources Use hydrogen as an alternative fuel source Use solar and wind power plants Consider taxation for usage of polluting fuels
Malnutrition, undernourishment	Africa, Asia, Latin America, the Caribbean, and especially Bangladesh, India, Ethiopia, Vietnam, Nigeria, Indonesia	Promote breastfeeding efforts Improve prenatal care Alleviate poverty Examine and correct food distribution problems Use agricultural practice to prevent famine and improve yields.
Obesity, Overnourishment	United States, Russian Federation, United Kingdom, Germany, Columbia, Brazil (adults)	Educate about the health hazards of fast foods and highly processed foods Reduce food portion sizes Limit advertisements for food aimed at children Adopt a "junk food" tax
Persistent organic pollutants (dioxins, polychlorinated biphenyls, furans)	Russia, Japan, Holland, Belgium	Intensify recycling of batteries, electrical wiring, transformers, and computers Limit use of incinerators, and institute laws for business and agricultural use of these products Paper recycling Use autoclaves for sterilization Use of pesticide alternatives, such as barrier nets or steel mesh for control of insects, larvae-eating fish, and selected natural pests for agriculture Use environment-friendly pesticides
Chlorine (plastics, polyvinyl chloride)	Worldwide	Recycle products containing plastic and reduce demand for products made from plastic
DDT	Central Asia, India, China, Columbia, Ecuador	Rotate crops and use environment-friendly pesticides and herbicides

Adapted from Brown, L. R., Flavin, C., French, H., Postel, S., & Starke, L. (Eds.). (2000). *State of the world 2000.* New York: W.W. Norton & Company.

- Nervous system damage as a result of repeated exposures
- Limbic kindling through the olfactory-limbic system, resulting in triggered responses to repeated chemical exposure
- Depletion of or damage to enzymatic production within the body
- Repeated immunologic insults
- Airway and neurogenic inflammation
- Chronic candidiasis
- Carbon monoxide poisoning
- Altered brain chemistry, electrical activity, or neurotransmitter function

With the advent of positive emission tomography, evidence linking chemical brain changes with exposure to specific chemical substantiates that a physiologic phenomenon occurs in persons with MCS. Persons with MCS exhibit "different patterns of cortical and subcortical brain activation during olfactory stimulation" (Chiaravalloti et al., 2015, p. 734).

A physiologic process known as toxicant-induced loss of tolerance (TILT) may also be involved in the development of MCS. TILT is a two-stage process. The first step is initiation that occurs when person experiences exposure to chemicals below toxic levels (indoor or outdoor pollutants, pesticides, or other chemicals) that later become triggers for an MCS reaction. The second phase of TILT involves becoming hyperactive to the same or different chemicals upon exposure (Horowitz, 2014).

Along with the physiologic theories, the following psychological theories have surfaced.

- Psychological and behavioral conditioning
- Odor conditioning
- Increased vulnerability related to pre-existing anxiety and depression
- Amplification of symptoms
- Negative affectivity
- Personality disorders
- Somatization disorder
- Childhood trauma
- Excessively focused thought patterns and cognitions on chemicals

Practitioners who espouse a physiologic theory believe that avoidance of the offending chemicals is the only way to avoid continued health deterioration. Health care professionals who believe that MCS is a psychiatric disorder argue that chemical avoidance enables people with MCS to obsess more about their disorder. However, personality disturbances and panic attacks have been documented in workers exposed to organic solvents, and these problems may be the result of nervous system injury (Cooper, 2007; Gibson, 2000). Environmental Medical Units in which patients receive gradual exposures to one offending chemical at a time have been helpful in treating persons with MCS (Horowitz, 2014).

The Food Chain

Consumed food affects human health. Many chemicals are placed in foods to increase their visual appeal, enhance flavor, alter texture, and extend dates for safe consumption. How much do you know about the food that you eat? Do you know where it comes from and how it is produced? Consider the examples presented in Box 13.2, Learning, Knowing, and Growing, "The Food You Consume."

■ QUESTIONS FOR REFLECTION

1. Select a favorite packaged food and read its label to see how many chemicals or additives it contains.
2. After reading the label, are you going to think twice before consuming it again? Why or why not?

 13.2 Learning, Knowing, and Growing

The Food You Consume

Foods consumed by humans, especially those in developed countries, often contain an array of additives, contaminants, or modifications.

- To increase crop yields, many farmers use a variety of herbicides and pesticides; farmers also genetically manipulate crops.
- To improve meat production, some farmers use feed containing growth hormone and antibiotics.
- Many preservatives protect the consumer from foodborne infections.
- People trying to lose weight consume artificial sweeteners, such as aspartame and saccharin.
- To increase the visual appeal of food, some manufacturers use artificial dyes.
- Some foods contain flavor enhancers such as monosodium glutamate.
- Although some food chemicals reduce the risk for foodborne disease, others merely create another human chemical exposure (Gibson, 2000).

Consult your local food vendors and see how much they can tell you about the food that they sell. Informed consumers have the knowledge and power to make wise food choices for themselves.

The Nurse's Role in Promoting a Healthy Global Environment

Sachs (2008) and Papp (2007) identified nurses as key human resources to confront the future challenges of improving the health and well-being of all. Nurses possess communication and clinical skills to help people understand ways to promote a healthy global environment. Global leaders in the nursing profession have made key differences in the well-being of people around the world.

Kim, Woith, Otten, and McElmurry (2006) noted that to be successful, global nurse leaders must:

- remain open-minded and flexible, learn from others, and display cultural awareness, sensitivity, and interest.
- deal with complexity effectively, set high aspirations, and show resiliency, optimism, and energy.
- be honest and have integrity but be able to play politics.
- have patience and wait for others to assume responsibility.
- educate themselves formally and informally on global competencies.
- believe with conviction and passion about the importance of global nursing work.

Musker (1994) proposed a life of voluntary simplicity—a holistic, ecologically based lifestyle—to create a healing environment. In the voluntary simplicity outlook, "less is more," and people focus on the quality of life rather than the quantity of consumer products (contrary to Western culture, in which some think "more is better"). Voluntary simplicity consists of inner and outer processes.

- The inner process, "mindfulness," requires deep self-reflection to attend to personal needs and to separate them from personal desires. In this inner process, people discover their genuine, authentic self and discard the illusion of their preconceived self. Some people keep a journal to discover patterns of behavior.
- The outer or external process of "doing" results in responsible life behaviors that serve the world rather than pure self-interest.

As the inner and outer processes fuse, being becomes doing, and doing becomes being. Voluntary action involves making purposeful life choices by eliminating automatic choices. Simplification of life involves reducing overall consumption, purchasing durable and easily repaired products, consuming a more natural diet, pursuing work that contributes to the world while using more individual creativity and capacities, and changing transportation habits. Simplification also means releasing physical and mental clutter, emotional baggage, useless worries, and other concerns that distract from enjoying the present.

Take Note!

Through communication and education, nurses can play a key role in promoting a healthy global environment.

As individual global citizens, professional nurses can model environment-friendly behaviors for preventing pollution and conserving resources. When possible, nurses should look for ways to reduce energy consumption, recycle discarded products, and limit purchases to reusable items.

◼ QUESTIONS FOR REFLECTION

1. What actions in your workplace or school environment may be potentially harmful to the global environment?
2. What could you do differently to change those behaviors?

THE COMMUNITY ENVIRONMENT

Multiple environmental factors affect the health of the community. Community services that enhance health include public health departments, disease prevention services, and social support services. The individual health status of community residents relies on the quality of their physical and social community environments. For this discussion, the **community environment** refers to the geographical location where people live and work.

Community Environmental Factors Threatening Health

Although the local community provides services to promote health, most communities also have environmental factors that threaten the health of their citizens. Heavy traffic and industrial fumes pollute the air. Some municipalities and counties use pesticides to prevent the spread of insect-borne illnesses. High-tension power lines and power stations emit electromagnetic fields (Adeola, 2011; Gibson, 2000; Pearce, 2007; Sachs, 2008).

Along with business and industry, the level of affluence within a community affects the health of individuals and families. Taxes on the income of citizens enable communities to maintain infrastructure and provide services to enhance health. Persons with higher incomes typically have access to healthier food and better health care services.

However, affluence can also negatively affect health. Since 1980, Americans have increased the annual mileage on their cars by 80% (Adela, 2011; Gibson, 2000). Automobiles make it convenient to drive short distances, resulting in individuals getting less exercise from walking or cycling. Many people have long commutes from their homes to their workplaces. Traffic jams contribute to road rage and increased pollution.

Although obesity has multiple causes (genetics, metabolism, culture), for many Americans, the ease of obtaining high-calorie foods contributes to an unhealthy diet and an obesity epidemic. Between 2000 and 2011, the obesity rate among adult Americans rose 48%. The risk factors from an affluent lifestyle also contribute to the incidence of diabetes, cardiovascular disease, and stroke (U.S. Department of Health and Human Services, 2011).

Physical Threats to Community Health

The American Lung Association (2012) estimates that more than 127 million Americans live in areas where exposure to air particulate pollutants, including ozone, exceeded governmental health standards. The same report indicates that a disproportionate number of Hispanic and Pacific Islanders live in these areas. Air pollution results in shortness of breath, chest pain with inspiration, asthma attacks, increased susceptibility to respiratory infections, increased risk for pulmonary inflammation, and reduced lung capacity.

Although pesticides play a key role in preventing infectious disease epidemics, they can also cause systemic, long-lasting, environmental pollution. Many pesticides are persistent organic pollutants (POPs) that are fat soluble and resist being broken down by water. They rest in the soil for many years, and food grown in contaminated soil contains POPs. After consumption by animals, POPs accumulate in fat cells and enter the human food chain. The top 10 POP-contaminated foods are butter, cantaloupe, cucumbers/pickles, meatloaf, peanuts, popcorn, radishes, spinach, and summer and winter squash. Despite the potential negative effects of POPs, control of insect-borne illnesses justifies their use (Adeola, 2011). For example, West Nile virus has been linked to insects that infect birds, and Lyme disease has been linked to insects that infect deer. The proper application of pesticides limits environmental fallout from their use. Responsibility for the proper use of pesticides lies with homeowners and companies that secure community contracts. Professional nurses frequently participate in the development of community education programs or community service announcements to help citizens avoid contracting insect-borne infectious diseases.

To eliminate the risk for foodborne illness, local health departments license businesses and organizations that serve food. Poor handwashing by persons who handle food has led to outbreaks of hepatitis A, *Salmonella,* and *Escherichia coli* infections. Foodborne illnesses also occur when people fail to abide by guidelines for food storage and safe food preparation.

The potential for the spread of infectious illnesses, such as tuberculosis (TB), influenza, and viral or bacterial meningitis, is increased in people who are subjected to overcrowded conditions. College dormitories, schools, and day care centers also provide residence for a variety of disease-causing organisms.

Social Threats

In addition to threats to the physical integrity of communities, social problems also threaten human health. Poverty, substance abuse, incivility, and moral decay have led to a decline in communities. Violence occurs in urban, rural, and suburban settings. In urban areas, violence is the leading cause of death in young African American men. Among industrialized nations, the United States has the highest rate of childhood homicides (U.S. Department of Health and Human Services, 2000). In most instances, homicide victims know their killers. Domestic, child, and elder abuse occur in all socioeconomic groups but are more common when families struggle to meet basic human needs (food, water, and shelter).

In addition to economic factors, the media expose people to acts of violence in movies, fictional television programs, cartoons, and newscasts, and some computer and video games use violence as entertainment. As individuals are repeatedly exposed to images of violence, victims of violent crime become depersonalized, and violence becomes a part of life.

A number of mass shootings have occurred across the United States (Connecticut, Colorado, Oregon, Arkansas, Tennessee, Georgia, Kentucky, and Mississippi). Most of the shooters came from middle-class homes with two parents, and most used guns found in their homes. Preventive measures against teen violence focus on parents and include limiting teen exposure to violent movies, television programs, and video games.

Experts place emphasis on parents spending quality time with their children, serving as role models for them, and teaching them ethical and moral behavior (Steger, 2000).

Social interactions vary according to the type of communities in which people reside. People tend to socialize more with others who share similar life situations. In working-class neighborhoods (especially when both adults in a household are employed), relationships tend to be more casual. Time constraints present challenges for maintaining relationships with neighbors. Schools and places of worship provide opportunities for people with similar values to develop relationships.

The Professional Nurse's Role in Promoting a Healthy Community Environment

Professional nurses play key roles in promoting a healthy community environment. Nurses assess communities for actual and potential factors that are noxious to human health and well-being. When such factors are identified, nurses can inform community members, provide community education, and take action to eliminate the factors. Reporting local health hazards, such as deteriorating road conditions or dangerous thoroughfares that need traffic signs, signals, or speed controls, helps to prevent motor vehicle and pedestrian accidents. To avoid mosquito-borne illnesses, nurses can educate family, friends, and neighbors about the health hazards of standing water found in bird baths, fish ponds, and yard fountains.

Nurses can also inspire other community members to incorporate health promotion activities into their lives. For example, nurses who engage in a daily neighborhood walk or cycling trip serve as a role model for daily exercise. Nurses, like all citizens, have the freedom and obligation to attend local governmental meetings to express concerns related to community development projects. By participating in community cleanup programs, nurses reduce the community's risk for injury from exposure to broken glass, used needles, and sharp metal objects, as well as the risk for infectious illnesses from exposure to rotting food.

Nurses also can become active participants in local school, civic, and faith-based activities to foster mental health and offer safe recreation for people of all ages. To take a stance against societal violence, nurses can refuse to purchase products that promote violence as entertainment or from companies that advertise their products during violent television programs; they can also refuse to attend movies or plays that glorify violence. When working with teens, nurses should be alert to any precursors of imminent violent acts, including inappropriate angry outbursts, cruelty to animals, essays with violent themes, fascination with weapons (especially firearms), obsession with playing violent computer games, threats to harm self or others, vandalism (even of their own property), assumption of the victim role, involvement in fringe groups or gangs, behavior with the goal of getting suspended or expelled, and incidents of bringing weapons to show to other students.

Teaching violence awareness, stress management, self-esteem, gun safety, substance abuse prevention, and cultural diversity classes in the community serves as a means to help eliminate violence in society (Steger, 2000). In response to the December 2012 Sandy Hook Elementary School shooting incident in Newtown, Connecticut, the American Nurses Association and more than 40 other nursing organizations issued "A Call To Action" to improve access to mental health services for all Americans, increase student access to mental health professionals, and join together to ban assault weapons and to pass meaningful gun control legislation (American Nurses Association, 2013). Nurses also can serve as resources to local schools for violence prevention, violence recovery, and other health promotion programs. Finally, nurses can lobby local, state, and federal legislative bodies to protect environmental health.

> **Take Note!**
> Awareness, observation, participation, and education are key roles for nurses in promoting a healthy community environment.

▮ Questions for Reflection

1. How would you rate the health of your local community based on the information presented in this chapter?
2. What community resources are available to you as a citizen to improve the environment of your local community? As a professional nurse?
3. What strategies could you use to promote a healthy community environment?

THE WORK ENVIRONMENT

Many people spend more time in the workplace than they do at home. The quality of the **work environment** relies on physical and cultural factors. National, state, and local laws protect worker safety. Individual organizations have policies that guide worker behaviors and inform workers of potential health hazards.

Work Environmental Factors Threatening Health

Many offices and work settings contain factors that threaten the physiologic, psychological, and spiritual health of employees and consumers. Some industries and manufacturers rely on chemicals and solvents to produce products. Some jobs require workers to perform repetitive movements. According to the U.S. Occupational Safety and Health Administration (OSHA, 2007), each year 1.8 million U.S. workers experience disabling work-related musculoskeletal disorders, with close to 50,000 nurses or unlicensed assistive personnel sustaining a back injury that required being off work. According to the U.S. Bureau of Labor Statistics (2009), 23,000 licensed and unlicensed health care providers sustained work-related back injuries, tendonitis or carpal tunnel syndrome, and 46% decline in injuries among health care workers since the introduction of no direct lifting of patient work rules starting in 2005. Other common injuries sustained by nurses in clinical practice include overexertion, falls or slips, twisting injuries, bruises or lacerations (from bumping against or being struck by objects), injuries from violent acts, harmful substance exposure, transportation accidents, repetitive motion insults, and compression injuries. Health care professionals, including nurses, have a suicide rate 17.4 per 100,000 persons compared to an American suicide rate of 13 per 100,000 persons. More than half of the suicides of health care providers are women (McIntosh et al., 2016). In 2008, the American Society of Registered Nurses reported that female nurses were four times more likely to commit suicide than other American women.

Tasks required for patient care performed by nurses in hospitals create an "ergonomic nightmare" (Trossman, 2000, p. 1). Many nurses work 12-hour shifts and experience repetitive movement stress from lifting and turning patients, entering data into computers, drawing up parenteral medications, pumping sphygmomanometers, resetting monitor alarms, and moving heavy equipment.

The use of latex has been a source of concern for many years in health care settings, as allergies and sensitivities to it have increased among health care workers and clients. Currently, more than 40,000 medical and consumer products contain latex, including gloves, clothing, intravenous supplies, medication vials, urinary catheters, feeding tubes, endotracheal tubes, carpeting, furniture, blood pressure cuffs, tape, balloons, condoms, and chewing gum (Crippa, Belleri, Mistrello, Tedoldi, & Alessio, 2006; Dyck, 2000; Kellet, 1997; Kim, Graves, Safadi, Alhadeff, & Metcalfe, 1998; Lee & Kim, 1998). Since 1998, federal regulations specify that medical devices containing latex must be appropriately labeled to protect people who are sensitive to latex (Kim et al., 1998). Most health care workers report cutaneous allergic responses, but 1.3% of health care workers with latex allergy have allergic asthmatic responses with exposure. Since the federal mandate of removing powdered latex gloves from health care settings, the incidence of latex allergies among health care workers has decreased from a high of 17% to around 12% (Crippa et al., 2006). However, the vinyl gloves that have replaced latex tend to tear more readily, and vinyl gloves release toxic substances such as dioxin. Nitrile, neoprene, and thermoplastic gloves offer protection equal to that offered by latex gloves. However, like latex, these products may trigger allergic reactions because their chemical composition is similar (Worthington, 2000).

Depending on their practice area, nurses are at risk for exposure to a number of dangerous chemicals. OSHA has published standards for safe handling of all dangerous chemicals used in the workplace. In addition, nurse specialty organizations publish guidelines for safe practice use; these guidelines are usually covered in nurse specialty certification examinations. For example, antineoplastic agents may cause birth defects, allergic reactions, and skin, eye, and mucous membrane irritation. Radiation exposure can lead to birth defects, infertility, and increased risk of cancer in nurses. Chemicals used for sterilization and anesthesia have been associated with cancer development, birth defects, spontaneous abortion, respiratory tract irritation, central nervous system symptoms, dermatitis, eye irritation, liver dysfunction, and renal disorders (Papp, 2007).

In addition to chemical and radiation exposure, infectious diseases pose a workplace hazard to nurses and other health care workers. Nurses have the potential to contract hepatitis B and HIV from a percutaneous stick with a contaminated needle or other sharp implement. Strategies for preventing such an event include strict adherence to OSHA blood-borne pathogen standards and obtaining a hepatitis B vaccination. Nurses can encounter hepatitis A if they work in places where personal hygiene may be poor. Effective hand hygiene serves as the best method for preventing contraction of this virus. In recent years, nurse exposures to pulmonary illnesses such as SARS and TB have increased along with the incidence of those illnesses in clients. Contributing factors for resurgence in cases of TB include the acquired immunodeficiency syndrome (AIDS) epidemic, immigration, homelessness, and the evolution of drug-resistant strains. Diligent attention to isolation procedures and wearing special ventilation masks decrease the chance of contracting TB and SARS. Measles, rubella, mumps, and influenza also threaten the health of nurses as they engage in professional practice. Determination of immune status and offering appropriate immunizations eliminates the risk for nurses of contracting most of these diseases (Papp, 2007). Nevertheless, nurses bear the responsibility for protecting their own health by following specific isolation procedures and using protective devices when caring for clients with potentially contagious diseases.

Nurses may also come into contact with many organisms that cause nosocomial (hospital-acquired) infections. Vancomycin-resistant *Enterococcus* and methicillin-resistant *S. aureus* thrive in hospital environments. Frequently, nurses may be colonized with these organisms, but because of immunocompetence, not develop an infection. Other infections that threaten the health of nurses include herpes zoster and *C. difficile*. Diligent isolation practices, meticulous handwashing, and habits to promote immunocompetence protect nurses from contracting infectious diseases from clients or the work environment.

Table 13.3 presents strategies nurses can use to protect themselves from various potential physical dangers in the workplace. Box 13.3, Professional Building Blocks, "Nurses and Stress," outlines additional factors that can affect a nurse's physical and emotional well-being.

Violence in the Workplace

According to the International Council of Nurses (ICN, 2006), professional nurses worldwide have been victims of violence. Forms of workplace violence encountered by nurses include physical assault, verbal abuse, bullying, mobbing, and sexual harassment. Nurses can be assaulted physically or verbally by clients, clients' families and friends, physicians, administrators, and coworkers. On rare occasions, nurses and other health team members have been assaulted or shot by a client visitor when caring for an injured party from an act of gang violence (Carroll, 2004; Longo & Smith, 2011). According to the ICN (2006), the highest incidence of physical assault occurs in American emergency

13.3 Professional Building Blocks

Nurses and Stress

Stress is unavoidable, and nurses are no exception. Individuals perceive stress differently (Lazarus & Folkman, 1984), however, and those perceptions may affect physical and mental health (McLean, 1974). Nurses experience stress in the workplace as a result of the following workplace factors.

- Making decisions that may result in life or death
- Working with clients in pain
- Working with demanding clients
- Understaffing
- Rotating shifts
- Working long shifts (12 hours or more)
- Completing client documentation in a timely fashion
- Keeping current in the areas of pharmacology, technology, nursing standards, and procedural changes
- Dealing with authoritative managers
- Working with unlicensed personnel
- Being excluded from participating in decisions that affect nursing care delivery
- Coping with client deaths
- Feeling unappreciated by other health team members
- Practicing nursing without the time to establish meaningful and therapeutic client relationships
- Delegating tasks that serve as a source of accomplishment
- Dealing with reduced client length of stay (inpatient settings)
- Working in uncivil work settings

departments (36% of nurses reported being physically assaulted). Surveys of nurses reveal that incidences of psychological abuse and sexual harassment range from 24% to 91% (Bartholomew, 2006; ICN, 2006; Longo & Smith, 2011; Papp, 2007; Sutton, 2006). Of nurses who encounter violence in the workplace, 40% to 70% suffer posttraumatic stress disorder (Bartholomew, 2006; ICN, 2006; Papp, 2007). Although nurses once considered working with violent people to be part of the job, recent initiatives by health care administrators, nurses, and collective bargaining units have resulted in zero tolerance for workplace violence. In the United States, some states have passed legislation requiring health care facilities to provide a safe work environment, including provisions for rapid response teams to handle situations with a high potential to become violent. Efforts to promote a violence-free workplace include policies of zero tolerance for physical violence, sexual harassment, or verbal abuse. Staff education

TABLE 13.3   Strategies to Prevent Health Hazards in Nursing Work Environments

Health Hazard	Prevention Strategies
Needle stick injuries	Use needleless systems for IV therapy when possible. Use syringes with recapping devices for intramuscular, subcutaneous, and intradermal injections. Replace containers for used needles before they become more than two thirds full.
Back and shoulder injuries	Evaluate all clients for weight-bearing status and mobility before moving or lifting them. Use assistive devices (e.g., mechanical lifts, slide boards, sheets) and engineering controls properly. Verify that enough help is present before lifting, transferring, or ambulating clients. Take time to raise beds and equipment to a comfortable working level. Obtain training from physical therapy departments on proper body mechanics. Redesign workstations to provide ergonomically sound charting stations for standing and sitting. Provide supportive chairs for seated activities. Negotiate for ergonomically sound workplace practices. Lobby state legislators to enact ergonomic legislation.
Repetitive stress injuries	Increase worker and administrator awareness of how repetitive movements may result in musculoskeletal injury.
Carpal tunnel syndrome	Avoid long periods of computer data entry. Provide wrist support devices for computer mouse and keyboards. Teach employees wrist-stretching exercises.
Blood-borne infections	Use needleless and self-capping syringe devices.
Airborne infections	Use and change masks. Provide respirator masks for specific infections. Separate ventilation units for isolation rooms.
Other infections	Make soap and water accessible for handwashing. Make alcohol-based hand cleansers accessible.
Latex	Persuade employer to remove as many latex-containing supplies from the organization as possible. Use latex-free gloves exclusively. Follow extensive rinse procedures for any equipment rinsed with glutaraldehyde solutions. Encourage coworkers to refrain from touching telephone, intercom, keyboards, and other equipment buttons and light switches while wearing latex gloves.
Hazardous chemicals, antineoplastics	Follow OSHA and Oncology Nursing Society guidelines for safe handling of chemotherapeutic agents.
Ethylene oxide, formaldehyde, and glutaraldehyde (sterilization chemicals)	Follow OSHA guidelines.
Anesthetic gases (especially nitrous oxide)	Follow NIOSH recommendations for exposure limits.
Mercury	Do not touch mercury with hands. Request published standards for mercury disposal from environmental services or housekeeping departments.
Bleach and other disinfectant cleaners	Wear gloves when using bleach to clean surfaces and be sure the work location is well ventilated. Do not mix bleach with other cleaning ingredients
Radiation	Wear personal radiation safety equipment (such as lead aprons) and radiation safety badges (designed to measure radiation exposure). Limit exposure by using lead shields, keeping distance between self and radiation source, and limiting time spent in areas where radiation exposure may occur. Never touch a radioactive substance with your hands. The Nuclear Regulatory Commission (NRC) has set maximum exposure at 3 rem every 3 mo for safe exposure. If radiation dose exceeds exposure limit, workers are to be reassigned to work without radiation exposure risk. OSHA has guidelines for workers not covered by the NRC.
Suicide	Monitor self and others for addictive behaviors (including cigarettes). Talk to colleagues when intensely critical situations arise and after they are resolved. Be alert for colleagues who appear preoccupied with death or say they wish they were dead. Practice stress management and relaxation techniques. Do not be afraid to confront colleagues when suicidal warning signs occur and refer them to mental health professionals.

Adapted from American Nurses Association. (2011). 2011 Health and safety survey. Retrieved from http://nursingworld. org/2011HealthSurveyResults.aspx. Accessed January 23, 2013; Belanger, D. (2000). Nurses and suicide: The risk is real. RN, 63, 61–64; Kim, K. T., Graves, P. B., Safadi, G. S., Alhadeff, G., & Metcalfe, J. (1998). Implementation recommendations for making health care facilities latex safe. *AORN Journal, 67,* 615–632; Papp, E. (2007). *Occupational health and safety management programme for nurses.* Geneva, Switzerland: International Council of Nurses; and Shaner, H. (1994). Environmentally responsible clinical practice. In E. A. Schuster & C. L. Brown (Eds.), *Exploring our environmental connections practice. NLN Publication No. 14–2634.* New York: National League for Nursing.

may include the definition of what constitutes an act of violence, triggers of violent acts, causes of violent behaviors, assessment of potentially violent situations, signs and symptoms of anger, phases of the assault cycle, conflict resolution strategies, techniques to disrupt escalating violent behavior, strategies for effective intervention for potentially violent situations, procedures for reporting acts of violence, and techniques of medical and physical restraint (as a last resort). Some health care organizations have rapid response teams to deploy during situations when basic conflict management strategies fail and nurses (or other health care providers) feel threatened. These teams consist of people with advanced education in conflict management and resolution.

Prevention is the best protection against workplace violence. Studies indicate that there is no "reliable tool to predict the potential for violence" (ICN, 2006, p. 15). However, a history of violent behavior seems to be a predictor. Therefore, flagging the charts of clients with a history of assaultive or disruptive behavior alerts staff to the potential for violence should conflict arise. Clearly written policies and procedures offer staff actions to take to avoid and report acts of violence. Organization should keep records of actual and alleged acts of violence. Confidentiality of reports of violence must be ensured so that incidents involving supervisors and/or physicians will be reported. After an act of violence occurs, a debriefing session is useful to determine potential causes of the event, review steps taken, help victims cope with the effects, and determine if follow-up counseling or education is warranted (Bartholomew, 2006; ICN, 2006; Papp, 2007; Sutton, 2006).

The Nurse's Role in Promoting a Healthy Work Environment

Before a nurse can promote a healthy work environment, he or she must become cognizant of actual and potential hazards in the workplace. The nurse should assess the work setting systematically to identify the quality of the work environment, paying close attention to its impact on worker physical, mental, and spiritual health. When nurses identify actual or potential health hazards, they should educate staff about them and make referrals to people who can eliminate them. The nurse has an ethical obligation to protect the health of all health team members. The nurse should validate that governmental guidelines to protect workers and clients are followed and take risks to advocate for change when needed.

Along with protecting the physical health of coworkers, nurses play a key role in promoting the mental and spiritual health of colleagues and client care team members. Health care team members sometimes encounter ethical dilemmas, especially those who work in health care organizations that emphasize profits over client care quality, when they find themselves unable to provide services to all persons in need of health care, and have to make decisions on how best to use new technology in clinical practice. These conditions create an unhealthy work environment characterized by little or no commitment, worker rebellion, deflated morale, workplace anger, worker disengagement, inferior problem solving, and sloppy client care (Wilson & Porter-O'Grady, 1999).

Hierarchical relationships among health team members (physicians, nurses, administrators, and unlicensed personnel) compound the problem of unhealthy work environments (Bartholomew, 2006; Watkins & Mohr, 2001; Wesorick, Shiparski, Troseth, & Wyngarden, 1997; Wilson & Porter-O'Grady, 1999). Longo (2012) reports that bullying is a form of abusive behavior that occurs repeatedly in nursing and that 31% to 35% of nurses have been targets of bullying. Recognized forms of bullying include (1) personal attacks with the intent to isolate, intimidate or degrade another person; (2) behaviors aimed at eroding professional competence and reputation that result in deterioration of professional identity and limit career options (public criticism, unjustified blaming, gossip); and (3) personal attacks through work orders and tasks that obstruct work flow or deny due process. Factors increasing bullying include major organizational change, worker characteristics, poor workplace relationships, and undefined work systems.

When people connect deeply with each other to do important work, a healthy work environment emerges (Watkins & Mohr, 2001; Wesorick et al., 1997). Client care in any setting is important work. When nurses and other team members focus all efforts on what is best for clients, they become united in purpose. Finding meaning in one's existence nourishes the human spirit (Frankl, 1963). When coworkers share the same meaning in work, they connect on a spiritual level (Wesorick et al., 1997).

Efforts to create a healthy work environment require personal commitment, cooperation with others, and a courageous attitude to express genuine authenticity. Wesorick et al. (1997, p. 9) have identified three characteristics to connect souls and create healthy work cultures: (1) shared meaning and purpose in work, (2) healthy relationships, and (3) meaningful conversations. Identification of shared meaning and purpose in work requires that everyone working together is aware of and agrees to what matters most in their work. Wesorick and colleagues defined healthy relationships as partnerships and outlined the following six basic partnership principles.

1. **Intention:** A personal decision to connect with another at the deepest level of humanness
2. **Mission:** A calling to live out something that deeply matters or is meaningful
3. **Equal accountability:** Mutual ownership of the mission without one person having power over or instilling fear in another
4. **Potential:** The human capacity of all individuals (including oneself) to continuously learn, grow, and create
5. **Balance:** Harmonious relationships with self and others required to attain the mission
6. **Trust:** Synchronous sense on important things or issues that matter

Wesorick et al. (1997) outlined meaningful conversation as the vehicle for developing healthy and meaningful relationships in work settings. Participants engaging in dialogue feel welcomed and honored while they share ideas, thoughts, and feelings. In dialogue, messages are deeply listened to and not judged. The partnership approach to clinical practice has the potential to transform a toxic work setting for all health team members to one that promotes health in body, mind, and spirit.

Take Note!
A shared purpose, healthy relationships, and meaningful conversations all help to foster a healthy work environment.

The Magnet Hospital Model

In 1983, the American Academy of Nursing embarked on identifying "Magnet" hospitals that delivered excellent client care, recruited and retained professional nurses, and provided an empowering environment for nurses. Using descriptive research methods, the American Academy of Nursing derived eight essential elements that distinguished Magnet hospitals from other hospitals.

1. Support for education
2. Working with other nurses who are clinically competent

3. Positive nurse–physician relationships
4. Autonomous nursing practice
5. A culture that values concern for the patient
6. Control of and over nursing practice
7. Perceived adequacy of staffing
8. Nurse manager support (Kramer & Schmalenberg, 2004, p. 50)

In 2008, the American Nurses Credentialing Center (ANCC) revised the Magnet model, adding six new Magnet forces. The 14 forces of magnetism were then compressed into the following five model components:

1. Transformational leadership (quality of nursing leadership and management style)
2. Structural empowerment (organizational structure, personnel policies and programs, community and the health care organization, image of nursing, and professional development)
3. Exemplary professional practice (professional care models, consultation and resources, nurse autonomy, nurses as teachers, interdisciplinary relationships)
4. New knowledge, innovations, and improvements (quality improvement)
5. Empirical quality outcomes (quality of care)

Kramer and Schmalenberg (2002) and McClure and Hinshaw (2007) identified that health care organizations that held Magnet status had an increased ability to recruit and retain nurses.

At this writing, 433 health care organizations worldwide have earned Magnet status (ANCC, 2016). The majority of these are in the United States, but Magnet hospitals are also located in Australia, Lebanon, and Singapore. The ANCC outlines the following benefits of Magnet designation: ability to retain and attract the best possible nurses; improved patient satisfaction, safety, and care; attainment of a collaborative work culture; advanced nursing standards and practices; and increased business and financial success. Multiple studies have found that nurses working in Magnet hospitals have higher job satisfaction, more autonomy in practice, and better work environments (Goode, Blegen, Park, Vaughn, & Spetz, 2011). Some nurses apply only for positions in health care organizations that hold Magnet status because these organizations value nurse contributions to health care delivery. However, current nursing research studies demonstrate mixed results in Magnet hospitals in terms of better staffing patterns and patient outcomes (Focus on Research, "Magnet Status, Staffing, and Patient Outcome").

FOCUS ON RESEARCH

Magnet Status, Staffing, and Patient Outcome

The investigators set out to determine whether Magnet hospitals had better patient outcomes and staffing patterns compared with other hospitals within a university health systems consortium. The investigative team looked at patient outcomes from patient discharge data, patient safety indicators, and inpatient quality indicators published by the Agency for Healthcare Research and Quality as well as staffing patterns for 19 Magnet and 35 non-Magnet hospitals.

Study findings revealed that the percentage of RN staff was lower in Magnet hospitals (58% vs. 61% for general units and 75% vs. 77% for intensive care units). Patients in Magnet hospitals had fewer pressure ulcers, but patients in the non-Magnet hospitals had fewer incidences of health care–related infections, postoperative sepsis, and metabolic derangements.

The significance of this study is that there appears to be more mixed findings on the effects of Magnet designation on patient outcomes and RN staffing levels. Previous studies have shown some improvements in patient outcome when a larger percentage of the staff are RNs, especially when care is provided by baccalaureate-prepared nurses. This study failed to report the educational level of nurses. There also may be some Magnet characteristics of all hospitals in the consortium studies regardless of whether they had Magnet status. More research is needed at a national and international level to determine whether Magnet status improves patient outcome.

Goode, C., Blegen, M., Park, S., Vaughn, T., & Spetz, J. (2011). Comparison of patient outcomes in Magnet and non-Magnet hospitals. *Journal of Nursing Administration, 41*(12), 517–523. doi: 10.1097/NNA.0b013e3182378b7c

QUESTIONS FOR REFLECTION

1. How would you rate the health of your work or educational environment based on the information presented in this chapter?
2. In what ways have you promoted a healthy work or educational environment within the past month?
3. What factors in your work environment negatively affect the health of you and your coworkers?
4. What strategies can you take in the future to promote a healthy work or educational environment?

THE HOME ENVIRONMENT

The **home environment** plays a key role in health. A family's home creates a haven for individual autonomy and control. Some consider their home to be an extension of their personal identity. The quality of the physical structure, general cleanliness, storage of chemicals, and interpersonal relationships in the home affect the health of individual family members.

Home Environmental Factors Threatening Health

People seek safe living quarters. Even the homeless try to find some way to stay warm and dry. People with established residences live in single- or multiple-family dwellings. Homes may be purchased or rented. A home's arranged floor plan usually provides family members with space for privacy, sleeping, and interaction. In American culture, social status and self-esteem are linked to the home. Homeowners (or landlords) bear the responsibility for repairs to maintain environmental safety.

Accidents occur frequently in the home. The types of accidents vary according to the age and developmental level of family members. The structural integrity of stairs, railings, ceilings, walls, and furniture must be assessed periodically to prevent injury. Safe storage and proper labeling of cleaning products and medications are critical in homes with young children. Homes with throw rugs create hazards for falls, especially for the elderly. Fire safety relies on periodic inspection and maintenance of household appliances, functioning smoke detectors, storage of paper and flammable materials away from furnaces or other appliances that could generate sparks, and unobstructed access to home entrances and exits. Power sources such as natural gas and electricity can pose health hazards if basic rules for each are not followed.

Appliances provide another source for accidents, especially in households where children reside. Hot water may cause burns, especially if the hot water tank is set above 140°F. Stairs and throw rugs provide opportunities for falling. Fireplaces and improper storage of paper, rags, and combustible materials may create fire hazards.

In addition to accidents, the home can be a source of illness. Problems with cleanliness and personal hygiene result in outbreaks of infectious disease. An estimated 30 million cases of foodborne illnesses, resulting in 9,000 deaths, occur each year in the United States. *Salmonella, E. coli* (especially *E. coli* 0157:H7, found in raw ground beef), and *Pseudomonas aeruginosa* thrive on many kitchen counters (Rutala, Barbee, Aguiar, Sobsey, & Weber, 2000). Adequate water supply, plumbing, refrigeration, garbage disposal, and general household cleaning practices reduce infections in the home. Handwashing after using the toilet and before food preparation and eating remains the most effective measure for the prevention of infectious illness in the home. Proper kitchen counter cleaning using commercially prepared disinfectants or a 10% bleach solution effectively destroys bacteria when left on surfaces for at least 30 seconds. Note that vinegar and baking soda, a longstanding home cleaning "recipe," fail to provide effective disinfection (Rutala et al., 2000).

Indoor air pollution and allergens set the stage for the development of allergic disorders, especially asthma. Smoking has been named the main source of indoor air pollution. Sources of indoor allergens include dust mites, insect particles, pet dander, rodent dander, and mold. Limiting smoking to the outdoors and regular house cleaning help eliminate these factors that could potentially impair respiratory health.

Pets and insect infestation also may serve as vectors for infectious diseases. To control lawn and household infestations, people use pesticides. Organophosphate insecticides kill insects by inducing muscle paralysis. However, organophosphates can be easily absorbed by people and pets through inhalation, ingestion, and dermal and optical contact (Melum & Kearney, 2001). According to Cornell University's Pesticide Safety Education Program (2012), common symptoms associated with pesticide poisoning include increased saliva, abdominal cramps, excessive sweating, muscle weakness, muscle twitching, blurred vision, shortness of breath, and cough that can progress to respiratory distress, increased thirst, severe muscle twitching, convulsions, and loss of consciousness (Fig. 13.4). In addition to problems arising from direct contact, organophosphates contaminate freshwater supplies, especially if applied too heavily.

Many potentially noxious substances can be found in the home. Household chemicals, fixtures, construction materials containing organic compounds, and carbon monoxide may contaminate the indoor environment (Davis 2007; Gibson, 2000). Benzene, a known human carcinogen, is present in synthetic materials,

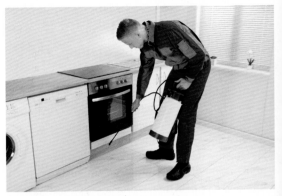

FIGURE 13.4 Sometimes making homes healthier, such as spraying for insects, results in indoor environmental pollution.

plastic, cleaning solutions, and tobacco smoke (Friedman & Morgan, 1992; Gibson, 2000). Construction materials such as particleboard and plywood emit formaldehyde, especially during the first year after construction. Most new carpeting contains a latex back, and latex carpet pads also are common. Newly poured concrete, fresh mortar, and paint emit gases (Davis, 2007; Gibson, 2000). Most commercial cleaners contain petrochemicals, fragrances, dyes, organophosphates, or bleach. Tap water contains pollutants such as bacterial colonies, nitrates, pesticides, particulates, and metals. Radon gas may seep into basements from rock foundations (Davis, 2007). Carbon monoxide is sometimes emitted from poorly maintained furnaces and when gasoline-powered generators are run inside or too close to a house.

In addition to indoor pollution, people are exposed to chemicals and vapors used by neighbors. Propane cookers, gas-powered lawn tools, gas appliances, and fresh paint emit fumes (Gibson, 2000). Many people apply dangerous herbicides and pesticides on lawns to make lawns look thicker and greener.

Psychological health requires privacy. People need to have a place for emotional release, to feel independent, and to express affection toward those they love. When people have time to recharge emotionally, the threat of domestic violence is reduced.

Factors contributing to domestic violence include the presence of weapons in the home, pregnancy, and drug or alcohol abuse. Many batterers have a history of violent behavior outside the home, depression, chemical dependency, and posttraumatic stress disorder. Children from homes where domestic violence occurs are at risk for becoming victims or perpetrators of violence. In addition, a history of head trauma has been associated with intense jealousy and violence (Gerard, 2000).

The Nurse's Role in Promoting a Healthy Home Environment

The professional nurse detects home health hazards by performing a comprehensive environmental assessment. When hazards are identified, the nurse provides education and support to help clients eliminate them. Sometimes, especially when nurses work with the disabled, community resources can be obtained to assist people with housekeeping and home maintenance.

Because of the high prevalence of domestic violence, health care providers, including nurses, routinely screen clients during outpatient visits and inpatient stays. Gerard (2000) reported that 35% of emergency department visits were linked to domestic violence. Many admission assessment forms contain direct questions to screen for physical and psychological abuse. Once violence has been confirmed, the nurse's priority is to ensure the safety of the victim and any dependents. Sometimes immediate referrals to social workers, police departments, or domestic shelters may be needed to protect the victim(s). If there is no threat of immediate danger, the nurse should outline a plan for safety if the violence escalates (Gerard, 2000). In some states, professional nurses are legally required to report incidents of child and elder abuse but not domestic violence between intimate partners.

Take Note!

Nurses can help promote a healthy home environment by screening for hazards, educating clients, and assisting clients with resources and referrals.

■ QUESTIONS FOR REFLECTION

1. How would you rate the environment of your home based on the information presented here?
2. What things could you change to promote a healthier home environment?

COMPREHENSIVE ENVIRONMENTAL HEALTH ASSESSMENT

Before professional nurses can take action to promote a healthy community environment, they must identify environmental factors that affect health. Shaner (1994) and Pope, Snyder, and Mood (1995) outlined various elements of an environmental health history (Table 13.4). The age of residences (lead paint was commonly used in home construction prior to the 1970s) and their proximity to military installations and industries provide clues to potential exposure to

substances and chemicals that impair health (Davis, 2007). Because people might be exposed to health hazards within work settings, information about occupations also provides clues to environmental health hazards. Workers in businesses that prepare foods for consumption (e.g., restaurants and grocery stores) may use latex gloves to prevent foodborne infections (Dyck, 2000; Kellet, 1997; Kim et al., 1999; Lee & Kim, 1998). Hobbies such as photography, furniture restoration, and gardening may result in exposure to hazardous chemicals. Household and lawn chemicals used on a regular basis also serve as a source of exposure to substances that may affect health. Nurses should also assess persons for being potential perpetrators or victims of violence and for potential disasters that might occur.

THE NURSE'S ROLE IN DISASTER PLANNING, MITIGATION AND RECOVERY

The education of professional nurses arms them with the knowledge and skills needed to help others in times of disaster. In addition, the public perceives nurses as people with knowledge and expertise with an obligation to provide care to them in times of distress. Nurses have a detailed understanding of first-aid principles, helping victims of trauma, and preventing the spread of contagious illnesses. Professional nurses also have well-refined teaching, organizational, and leadership skills that can be put to use in executing and coordinating care during all phases of a disaster. Finally, nurses have expertise in therapeutic communication skills to help provide psychological and spiritual support to people during times of uncertainty.

Take Note!

Professional nurses play a key role in helping people prepare for, survive during, cope with, and adapt to life after a disaster.

Veenema (2013, p. 3) defined a **disaster** as "any destructive event that disrupts the normal functioning of a community." Disasters may arise suddenly without warning (e.g., terrorist attack, plane crash, subway accident, earthquake), occur with warning (e.g., wildfire, hurricane, flood, tornado, blizzard), or evolve over an extended time (e.g., drought, famine). Disasters can be caused by nature (natural) or by humans. Disasters caused by humans fall into three broad categories: complex (e.g., multiple causation, such as a drought leading to a famine that stimulates political unrest and

TABLE 13.4 Elements of a Comprehensive Environmental Assessment

Location or Activity	Key Questions
Home	Where do you live?
	What is the distance from your home to a major thoroughfare, industrial complex, or military base?
	If your home is close to an industrial complex, what type of industrial plant is it?
	What is the drinking water source for your home?
	What types of cleaning agents do you use for housework and laundry?
	What types of chemicals do you use for yard care?
	What insecticides do you use inside the home?
	How old is your house/condo/apartment?
	How is your home heated?
	How is your home cooled?
	What is your fuel source for cooking?
	Have you tested your home for radon gas?
	Do you have a carbon monoxide alarm and smoke alarms in your home?
	Do you purify your home air or water?
	Have you recently acquired new furniture or carpeting?
	What type of paint is used on the exterior and interior of your home?
	Have you ever or recently refinished furniture or wood items in your home?
	What are the occupations of other household occupants?
	Do household occupants come into contact with chemicals as part of their employment or leisure activities?
	Does anyone living with you smoke inside the home?
Work	List your past jobs (including military experience) and whether you were exposed to any chemicals.
	Describe any work-related health problems or accidents.
	Did any of your coworkers have similar health problems or accidents?
	Where do you currently work?
	Are you employed full-time or part-time?
	How does your employer inform you of potentially hazardous chemicals, equipment, or procedures used in the workplace?
	Describe your work safety education programs (if applicable).
	What protective devices are available for your use?
	Do you use the protective devices?
	How old is the building in which you work?
	Do you have any symptoms associated with your work setting? If so, please describe them.
Hobbies	What hobbies do you have?
	Are any chemical agents used while engaging in the hobby?
Symptom assessment	What symptoms do you currently have?
	When did they start?
	When do they occur?
	Where do they occur?
	Does anyone who works with you or lives with or near you have the same symptoms?

Adapted from Shaner, H. (1994). Environmentally responsible clinical practice. In E. A. Schuster & C. L. Brown (Eds.), *Exploring our environmental connections practice.* NLN Publication No. 14–2634. New York: National League for Nursing; and Pope, A. M., Snyder, M. A., & Mood, L. H. (Eds.). (1995). *Nursing, health, and the environment.* Washington, DC: National Academy Press.

relocation of large numbers of people), technologic (e.g., destruction of community infrastructure, industrial accidents, massive power failure), or human settlement (e.g., migration of an entire ethnic group to avoid persecution).

The magnitude of a disaster depends on its location. Disasters in highly populated areas affect more people and strain more resources than those occurring in rural areas. In 2005, Hurricane Katrina paralyzed the city of New Orleans as well as much of the Louisiana coastal areas, and in 2012, Hurricane Sandy had a similar impact on the New Jersey coast/New York City area. Unfortunately, when disasters occur in remote areas, such as the 2008 earthquake in China, getting assistance

to the disaster site may be difficult. A medical disaster occurs when a catastrophic event creates more casualties than the health care resources within a community can effectively accommodate (Veenema, 2013).

In many developed nations, most communities have disaster plans in place (see Box 13.4, Professional Prototype, "Disaster Planning, Mitigation, and Recovery"). Disaster planning, mitigation, and recovery are the steps of the **disaster management cycle**. These plans address probable disasters that might occur within each community such as an earthquake along a fault line, hurricane in a coastal region, or a blizzard in temperate climate areas. Disaster preparedness,

13.4 Professional Prototype

Disaster Planning, Mitigation, and Recovery

Veenema (2013) and McGlown (2004) outlined a timeline for handling disasters that starts with preparation and ends with recovery.

- **Phase 1 (before the disaster):** In the first phase, which encompasses planning/preparedness, prevention, and warning, communities identify hazards and make attempts to remove them. If hazards cannot be removed (such as weather), then the community develops early warning systems, evacuates members at risk, institutes public awareness campaigns, performs disaster drills, develops nursing databases (mass casualty plans), and devises means to evaluate all components of the disaster response. During this phase, hospitals enact established disaster plans.

- **Phase 2 (during and 72 hours after the disaster):** The second phase consists of response, emergency management, and mitigation. In this phase, the disaster response plan is activated; potential and ongoing hazards are identified, and action is taken to relieve human suffering (mitigation); public health needs are anticipated; victims are triaged for effective use of available health care resources; emergency food and water distribution centers are established; and alternatives for sanitation and waste removal are established if the community infrastructure has been damaged. During this time, essential hospital personnel report to work per agency disaster policies so that enough personnel are available to provide care to anticipated victims (Adams & Berry, 2012).

- **Phase 3 (beginning 72 hours after the disaster):** The final phase focuses on recovery, rehabilitation, reconstruction, and evaluation. In this phase, victims receive medical and nursing care, disease surveillance continues, public health infrastructure is restored, family members are reunited, victims are monitored for long-term physical and psychological injuries, disaster responders attend debriefing and counseling sessions, and the disaster team evaluates the original disaster preparedness plan and revises it as needed (McGlown, 2004; Veenema, 2013).

Adams, L., & Berry, D. (2012). Who will show up? Estimating ability and willingness of essential hospital personnel to report to work in response to a disaster. *Online Journal of Issues in Nursing, 17*(2). Retrieved from www.nursingworld.org/MainMenuCategories/ANAMarketplace/ANAPeriodicals/OJIN/TableofContents/Vol-17-2012/No2-May-2012/Articles-Previous-Topics/Essential-Hospital-Personnel-and-Response-to-Disaster.html. Accessed February 24, 2013. doi: 10.3912/OJIN.Vol17No02PPT02; McGlown, K. (Ed.). (2004). *Terrorism and disaster management.* Chicago: Health Administration Press; and Veenema, T. (2013). *Disaster nursing and emergency preparedness for chemical, biological, radiological terrorism and other hazards.* New York: Springer.

mitigation, and recovery consume vast resources. Local and national governments pool resources to develop and maintain effective disaster plans. Note that plans remain intact only with stable governments.

Professional nurses play key roles in each phase of disaster response. Nurses who are uninjured at the disaster site offer basic first aid to victims. Some nurses, especially those working in emergency departments and as flight nurses, have special certification in trauma nursing and find themselves assisting in the rescue of victims in the field, triaging people for appropriate treatment, or treating victims in first-aid stations or emergency departments. Nurse administrators participate by assisting in communicating information about victims to families. Community health nurses and Red Cross volunteer nurses engage in setting up temporary shelters for people affected by the disaster. Some nurses may assume the responsibility of reuniting family members and friends who became separated during the disaster. Mental health nurses offer counseling to victims and relatives of victims. Acute care nurses may find themselves mobilizing supplies, adjusting staff assignments, and determining which patients can be discharged early to make room for other victims according to the facility's disaster plan. If the prospect of the spread of infectious disease surfaces, other nurses may participate in mass vaccination programs. Finally, nurses may become involved with shelter supervision.

In response to the terrorist attacks on September 11, 2001, the United States has developed the Emergency System for Advance Registration of Volunteer Health Professionals to rapidly mobilize required health care personnel. Using this system, individual states have created a nationwide database of 100,000 to 200,000 qualified volunteer health care professionals. Each state verifies its volunteers' credentials, offers access to disaster training and drilling, and develops a plan for requesting registration activation. Such a system is needed as People who volunteer spontaneously during disasters may get in the way or be denied participation in response efforts; even if used, a volunteer's skills may not be fully deployed because of lack of verification of professional status (Peterson, 2006). In the event of a disaster, an incident commander could use the system to identify and mobilize health care personnel with the skills to handle specific types of incidents (Association of Public Health Nurses [APH], Public Health Preparedness Committee, 2016).

Effective disaster planning for nurses involves personal and professional preparation (see Box 13.5, Learning, Knowing, and Growing, "Effective Disaster Planning for Nurses"). Nurses can access detailed checklists for emergency preparedness from the Red Cross or the

13.5 Learning, Knowing, and Growing

Effective Disaster Planning for Nurses

Personal Preparation	Professional Preparation
Be aware of possible or potential disasters.	Obtain disaster nursing certification through a local American Red Cross chapter or university.
Develop a personal household plan, including a 3-day to 3-week supply of food, medication, batteries, and water for all family members.	Provide community education about disaster preparedness, response, and recovery.
Drill the family on the emergency action plan, including what to do if separated.	Become involved in local disaster plan development.
Stay current on immunizations.	Participate in local disaster drills.
Keep first-aid supplies and skills up to date.	Make arrangements with employer for work relief if called to serve in a disaster.
Learn about wilderness survival, especially if power plants become disabled for prolonged periods.	
Become involved in community activities, and support leaders who want to pass ordinances that protect the community against floods, mudslides, or collapses.	

Gebbie, K., & Qureshi, K. (2006). A historical challenge: Nurses and emergencies. *Online Journal of Issues in Nursing, 11*(3), 6–8. Retrieved from www.nursingworld.org/MainMenuCategories/ANAMarketplace/ANAPeriodicals/OJIN/TableofContents/Volume112006/No3Sept06/NURSESANDEMERGENCIES.html. Accessed February 24, 2013; McGlown, K. (Ed.). (2004). *Terrorism and disaster management.* Chicago: Health Administration Press; Peterson, C. (2006). Be safe, be prepared: Emergency system for advance registration of volunteer health professionals in disaster response. *Online Journal of Issues in Nursing, 11*(3). Retrieved from www.nursingworld.org/MainMenuCategories/ANAMarketplace/ANAPeriodicals/OJIN/TableofContents/Volume112006/No3Sept06/tpc31_216083.html. Accessed February 24, 2013; Polivka, B., Stanley, S., Gorden, D., Taulbee, K., Kieffer, G., & McCorkle, S. M. (2008). Public health nursing competencies for public health surge events. *Public Health Nursing, 25*(5), 159–165; and Veenema, T. (2013). *Disaster nursing and emergency preparedness for chemical, biological, radiological terrorism and other hazards.* New York: Springer.

Department of Homeland Security. Many nurses realize that they must report to work in the event of a local disaster, but few have detailed disaster plans in place to care for family and pets (Nash, 2015). In 2015, Nash (2015) conducted a pilot study to learn about professional nurses personal preparation for a disaster following online education about personal disaster preparation planning. Her study is highlighted in the following research brief "Unveiling the Truth about Nurses' Personal Preparedness for Disaster Response: A Pilot Study."

FOCUS ON RESEARCH

Unveiling the Truth about Nurses' Personal Preparedness for Disaster Response: A Pilot Study

The investigator sought to determine the effectiveness of an online course on disaster preparedness on professional nurses intent to engage in personal disaster preparedness. A pre-test post-test research design was used to determine if intention to prepare oneself for a disaster would improve preparedness after participating in an online program for disaster preparedness.

Fifty-seven graduate nursing students (MSN or PhD levels of education) participated in the study and completed a 57-item investigator-developed survey addressing personal disaster preparedness before watching a 24-minute voice over PowerPoint presentation addressing the topic. Items in the survey addressed personal (27 items) and pet (4 items) preparation for a disaster should one occur. During the pre-education survey, more than 50% of the nurses reported not having the following things in place for a disaster: written evacuation plan, first-aid kit, 3-day water supply, bleach set for water purification, protective masks, battery-powered radio, matches or lighter, whistle, duct tape and plastic sheeting, document bag, extra prescription medication, copies of prescriptions, written medication list, alternative medical care provider, diabetic supplies (if they or family member were diabetic), electrical power backup system, pet first-aid kit and 3-day supply of pet medication.

The same survey minus demographic information items was given after the nurses viewed the disaster preparedness education program. Using paired t-tests, the investigator found statistical significant changes in general disaster and pet disaster preparedness ($p < 0.001$). Using correlation coefficients, the investigator discovered a large effect size for the educational program on both aspects of disaster preparedness (personal [$r = 0.83$] and pet [$r = 0.76$]).

The investigator identified the importance of disaster preparedness for professional nurses in order to provide direct care services to friends and families in the event of a local disaster when they are not working and to be able to report in a more timely fashion to their workplaces because they had plans in place to care for their loved ones. The results of this study should be exercised with caution because there was no validity or reliability testing on the survey used to collect study data. In addition, intention to act may differ from actually putting in place everything needed for nurses to have readily available for an impending disaster. Participants in the study were also graduate nursing students who may respond differently to education interventions than professional nurses not in school. The study also failed to collect information about individual nurse family obligation and how that might impact the nurse's response to disaster preparedness and reporting for duty. More research needs to be conducted to assess professional nurse disaster preparedness.

Nash, T. J. (2015). Unveiling the Truth about Nurses' Personal Preparedness for Disaster Response: A Pilot Study. *Med-Surg Nursing, 24*(6), 425–431.

Following a disaster, nurses play key roles in screening and assessing community members for symptoms associated with infectious illnesses and exposure to environmental toxins (APHN Public Health Preparedness Committee, 2016; Polivka et al., 2008; Veenema, 2013). Nurses also can offer valuable contributions to disaster debriefings to improve responses to future events (Polivka et al., 2008; Veenema, 2013).

Summary and Significance to Practice

The relationship of the environment to human health is highly complex. Professional nurses who have a solid knowledge about environmental factors affecting human health can effectively assess clients for injuries and diseases arising from various forms of exposure. Ecocentric professional nurses act to preserve the environment at the global, community, workplace, and home levels by practicing lives of voluntary simplicity. Nurses routinely assess factors that threaten health and provide education to promote environmental health for clients, each other, other health team members, and communities. Because professional nurses have specialized knowledge and skills to protect human health and promote healing, they be prepared to provide assistance in disaster preparedness, mitigation and recovery in the event of a natural or man-made disaster. When nurses become truly committed to improving the environment, they educate clients, coworkers, and community officials about potential hazards and advocate for change.

REAL-LIFE REFLECTIONS

Recall Arianna and Elena from the beginning of the chapter. Considering what you have learned, how would you handle the situation with Mr. and Mrs. Garcia? What would you say to them? What areas of their lives might you want to assess? Why is it important to perform a comprehensive environmental assessment, especially for older persons?

From Theory to Practice

1. What workplace environmental hazards can you identify in your clinical practice setting? What are the procedures for making changes in your health care organization? Why is it important to know the established policies and procedures for making changes in a workplace setting?

2. What individual behaviors could you change to promote a more healthy global, community, work, and home environment? What would be the consequences for making these changes?

Nurse as Author

1. Perform a home assessment using the questions related to "Home" found in Table 13.4. List areas for improvement or areas where you do not know the answers to the questions. Design a plan to improve the health of your home.
2. Write a short story of a personal or close encounter with a natural or man-made disaster. Include information about the disaster and your reaction to the disaster. Describe if you have any residual effects from the disaster. Relate how your experience with the personal or close encounter affects your ability to provide safe, effective nursing care.

Your Digital Classroom

Online Exploration

- Resources for global environmental health
  - Center for International Earth Science Information: **www.ciesin.org/data.html** (population distribution)
  - Centers for Disease Control and Prevention: **www.cdc.gov**
  - Environmental Protection Agency: **https://www3.epa.gov/**
  - Health Care Without Harm: **www.noharm.org/**
  - National Center for Environmental Health: **www.cdc.gov/nceh**
  - National Institute of Occupational Safety and Health: **www.cdc.gov/niosh**
  - Toxic Release Inventory Program: **https://www.epa.gov/toxics-release-inventory-tri-program**
  - Toxnet Toxicology Data Network: **https://toxnet.nlm.nih.gov/**
  - University of Wisconsin Space Science and Engineering Center: **www.ssec.wisc.edu/data/sst** (ocean and sea surface temperature)
- Resources for health in the home environment
  - Environmental Protection Agency: **https://www.epa.gov/indoor-air-quality-iaq** (Indoor Air Pollution: An Introduction for Health Professionals)
  - National Library of Medicine Household Products Database: **householdproducts.nlm.nih.gov/products.htm**

- University of Wisconsin-Extension: Resources for workplace health and safety
  - Elsevier Clinical Practice Model Resource Center: **http://www.elseviercpm.com/consortium/** (partnership, dialogue, and healthy workforce development)
  - Health Care Without Harm: **www.noharm.org** (safer cleaning products and pesticides in work settings)
  - OSHA Ergonomics: **https://www.osha.gov/SLTC/ergonomics/**
  - OSHA Workplace Violence: **https://www.osha.gov/SLTC/workplaceviolence/index.html**

Expanding Your Understanding

1. Visit the Good Guide website to learn about the environmental quality where you reside at **http://scorecard.goodguide.com/**. Type in your zip code and click "Get Report." Make a list of the top polluters in your county and the top chemicals released in your county. Learn about local lead hazards in houses and whether your area has a worst toxic site. Bring this information to share in class with your colleagues.
2. Visit the National Institute of Occupational Safety and Health (NIOSH) at www.cdc.gov/niosh/. In the search box at the top right hand of the page type in "Health Care Workers," and click to view the various topics covered. Select one of the 4,000+ documents that is a topic of interest. Pull the policies and procedures of your current clinical practice agency and compare these with those published by NIOSH. Observe health team members to see how well they comply with the agency and NIOSH guidelines. Note areas of compliance and noncompliance to the policy or guideline. Develop a report and action plan to improve compliance.
3. Visit the website of the nonprofit organization Bridging the Gap at **www.bridgingthegap.org**. Select one of the stories and then have a discussion with your family friends and colleagues to implement one of the selected strategies from one of the stories to improve your local environment (home, work, or community).

Beyond the Book

Visit thePoint® **www.thePoint.lww.com** for activities and information to reinforce the concepts and content covered in this chapter.

REFERENCES

Adams, L.M., & Berry, D. (2012). Who will show up? Estimating ability and willingness of essential hospital personnel to report to work in response to a disaster. *Online Journal of Issues in Nursing, 17*(2). Retrieved from www.nursingworld.org/MainMenuCategories/ANAMarketplace/ANAPeriodicals/OJIN/TableofContents/Vol-17-2012/No2-May-2012/Articles-Previous-Topics/Essential-Hospital-Personnel-and-Response-to-Disaster.html. Accessed February 24, 2013. doi: 10.3912/OJIN.Vol17No02PPT02

Adeola, F. (2011). *Hazardous waste, industrial disasters, and environmental health risk local and global environmental struggles.* New York: Palgrave MacMillan.

Agnes, M. (Ed.). (2005). *Webster's new world college dictionary* (4th ed.). Cleveland, OH: Wiley.

Albertine, J. M., Manning, W. J., DaCost, M., Stinson, K. A., Muilenberg, M. L., & Rogers, C. A. (2014). Projected carbon dioxide to increase grass pollen and allergen exposure despite higher ozone levels. *PLoS ONE, 9*(11), e111712. doi: 10.1371/

American Lung Association. (2012). State of the air 2012: Disparities in the impact of air pollution. Retrieved from www.stateoftheair.org/2012/health-risks/health-risks-disparities.html. Accessed December 27, 2012.

American Nurses Association. (2013). A call to action from the nation's nurses in the wake of Newtown. Retrieved from www.nursingworld.org/FunctionalMenuCategories/Media Resources/PressReleases/Call-to-Action-from-the-Nations-Nurses-in-the-Wake-of-Newtown.pdf. Accessed March 13, 2013.

American Nurses Credentialing Center. (2008). A new model for ANCC's Magnet Recognition Program. Retrieved from www.va.gov.nursing/docs/ANCC_NewMagnetModel.pdf. Accessed December 27, 2012.

American Nurses Credentialing Center. (2016). Frequently asked questions Magnet program. Retrieved from http://www.nursecredentialing.org/FindaMagnetFacility.aspx. Accessed May 15, 2016.

American Society of Registered Nurses. (2008). Nurses at risk. Retrieved from http://www.asrn.org/journal-nursing-to-day/291-nurses-at-risk.html. Accessed October 9, 2016.

Association of Public Health Nurses Public Health Preparedness Committee. (2016). The role of the public health nurse in disaster preparedness, response and recovery, a position paper. Retrieved from http://www.achne.org/files/public/APHN_RoleOfPHNinDisasterPRR_FINALJan14.pdf Accessed May 1, 2016.

Bartholomew, K. (2006). *Ending nurse-to-nurse hostility: Why nurses eat their young and each other.* Marblehead, MA: HCPro.

Belanger, D. (2000). Nurses and suicide: The risk is real. *RN, 63,* 61–64.

Bender, K., & Thompson, F. (2003). West Nile virus: A growing challenge. *American Journal of Nursing, 103,* 32–40.

Blunden, J., & Arndt, D. (2012). *State of the climate in 2011.* Washington, DC: American Metrological Society. Retrieved from www1.ncdc.noaa.gov/pub/data/cmb/bams-sotc/climate-assessment-2011-lo-rez.pdf. Accessed December 27, 2012.

Brausch, J., Connors, K., Brooks, B., & Rand, G. (2012). Human pharmaceutical in the aquatic environment: a review of recent toxicological studies and considerations for toxicity testing. *Review of Environmental Contamination & Toxicology, 218,* 1–99. doi: 10.1007/978–1–4614–3137–4_1.

Bright, C. (2000). Anticipating environmental "surprise." In L. R. Brown, C. Flavin, H. French, et al. (Eds.), *State of the world 2000.* New York: W. W. Norton.

Carroll, V. (2004). Preventing violence in the healthcare workplace. *The Missouri Nurse, 2,* 12–13, 31.

Centers for Disease Control. (2016a). 2014 Ebola Outbreak in West Africa -Case Count. Retrieved from http://www.cdc.gov/vhf/ebola/outbreaks/2014-west-africa/case-counts.html. Accessed May 15, 2016.

Centers for Disease Control. (2016b). About Zika virus disease. Retrieved from http://www.cdc.gov/zika/about/index.html. Accessed May 15, 2016.

Chiaravalloti, A., Pagani, M., Micarelli, A., Di Pietro, B., Genovesi, G., Alessandrini, M., et al. (2015). Cortical activity during olfactory stimulation in multiple chemical sensitivity: A 18F-FDG PET/CT study. *European Journal of Nuclear Medical Molecular Imaging, 42,* 733–740.

Cooper, C. (2007). Multiple chemical sensitivity in the clinical setting. *American Journal of Nursing, 107*(3), 40–48.

Cornell University Pesticide Safety Education Program. (2012). Symptoms of pesticide poisoning. Retrieved from http://psep.cce.cornell.edu/Tutorials/core-tutorial/module09/index.aspx. Accessed March 13, 2013.

Crippa, M., Belleri, L., Mistrello, G., Tedoldi, C., & Alessio, L. (2006). Prevention of latex allergy among health care workers and in the general population: latex protein content in devices commonly used in hospitals and general practice. *International Archive of Occupational Environmental Health, 79,* 550–557.

Davis, A. (2007). Home environmental health risks. *Online Journal of Issues in Nursing, 12*(2), 5.

Dock, L. L. (1912). *A history of nursing (Vol. 3).* New York: G. P. Putnam's Sons.

Dyck, R. J. (2000). Historical development of latex allergy. *AORN Journal, 72,* 27–29, 32–33, 35–40.

Environmental Protection Agency. (2008). Medical waste frequent questions. Retrieved from www.epa.gov/osw/nonhaz/industrial/medical/mwfaqs.htm. Accessed December 27, 2012.

Fagan, B. (2008). *The great warming.* New York: Bloomsbury.

Fawcett, J. (1984). *Analysis and evaluation of conceptual models of nursing.* Philadelphia, PA: F. A. Davis.

Fent, K., Weston, A., & Caminada, D. (2006). Ecotoxicology of human pharmaceuticals. *Aquatic Toxicology, 76,* 122–159.

Frankl, V. (1963). *Man's search for meaning.* New York: Washington Square Press.

Friedman, M., & Morgan, I. (1992). The health care function. In M. Friedman (Ed.), *Family nursing: Theory and practice* (3rd ed.). Norwalk, CT: Appleton & Lange.

Gebbie, K., & Qureshi, K. (2006). A historical challenge: Nurses and emergencies. *Online Journal of Issues in Nursing, 11*(3), 6–8. Retrieved from www.nursingworld.org/MainMenuCategories/ANAMarketplace/ANAPeriodicals/OJIN/TableofContents/Volume112006/No3Sept06/NURSESANDEMERGENCIES.html. Accessed February 24, 2013.

Gerard, M. (2000). Domestic violence: How to screen and intervene. *RN, 63,* 52–56, 58.

Gibson, P. R. (2000). *Multiple chemical sensitivity: A survival guide.* Oakland, CA: New Harbinger.

Goode, C., Blegen, M., Park, S., Vaughn, T., & Spetz, J. (2011). Comparison of patient outcomes in Magnet® and non-Magnet® Hospitals. *Journal of Nursing Administration, 41*(12), 517–523. doi: 10.1097/NNA.0b013e3182378b7c

Greer, A., & Fisman, D. (2008). Climate change and infectious diseases in North America: The road ahead. *The Canadian Medical Association Journal, 178*(6), 715–722.

Heimlich, J. (2008). The invisible environmental fact sheet series: Multiple chemical sensitivity. Retrieved from http://ohioline.osu.edu/cd-fact/pdf/0192.pdf. Accessed December 27, 2012.

Hemminger, P. (2005). Damming the flow of drugs into drinking water. *Environmental Health Perspectives, 13*, A678–A681.

Horowitz, S. (2014). Toxicant-induced loss of tolerance, a theory to account for multiple chemical sensitivity. *Alternative and Complementary Therapies, 20*(2), 96–100. doi: 10.1089/act.2014.20201

International Council of Nurses. (2006). *Guidelines on coping with violence in the workplace.* Geneva: Author.

Kellet, P. B. (1997). Latex allergy: A review. *Journal of Emergency Nursing, 23*, 27–36.

Kim, K. T., Graves, P. B., Safadi, G. S., Alhadeff, G., & Metcalfe, J. (1998). Implementation recommendations for making health care facilities latex safe. *AORN Journal, 67*, 615–618, 621–624, 626.

Kim, K. T., Wellmeyer, E. T., & Miller, K. V. (1999). Minimum prevalence of latex hypersensitivity in health care workers. *Allergy and Asthma Proceedings, 20*, 387–391.

Kim, J., Woith, W., Otten, K., & McElmurry, B. (2006). Global nurse leaders: Lessons from the sages. *Advances in Nursing Science, 29*(1), 27–42.

Kleffel, D. (1994). The environment: Alive, whole and interacting. In E. A. Schuster & C. L. Brown (Eds.), *Exploring our environmental connections (NLN Publication No. 14–2634).* New York: National League for Nursing.

Kleffel, D. (1996). Environmental paradigms: Moving toward an ecocentric perspective. *Advances in Nursing Science, 18*, 1–10.

Kramer, M., & Schmalenberg, C. (2002). Staff nurses identify essentials of magnetism. In M. McClure, & A. Hinshaw (Eds.), *Magnet hospitals revisited: Attraction and retention of professional nurses.* Kansas City, MO: American Nurses Publishing.

Kramer, M., & Schmalenberg, C. (2004). Essentials of a magnetic work environment: Part 1. *Nursing, 34*, 50–54.

Lazarus, R. S., & Folkman, S. (1984). *Stress, appraisal and coping.* New York: Springer.

Leddy, S. K. (2004). Human energy: A conceptual model of unitary nursing science. *Visions: The Journal of Rogerian Scholarship, 12*, 14–27.

Lee, M. H., & Kim, K. T. (1998). Latex allergy: A relevant issue in the general pediatric population. *Journal of Pediatric Health Care, 12*, 242–246.

Leroy, E., Rouquet, P., Formenty, P., Souquière, S., Kilbourne, A., Froment, J. M., et al. (2004). Multiple Ebola virus transmission events and rapid decline of central African wildlife. *Science, 303*, 387–390.

Longo, J. (2012). *Bulling in the workplace: Reversing a culture* (2012 Ed.). Silver Spring, MD: NurseBooks.

Longo, J., & Smith, M. (2011). A prescription for disruptions in care: Community building among nurses to address horizontal violence. *Advances in Nursing Science, 34*(4), 345–356.

Lynas, M. (2008). *Six degrees: Our future on a hotter planet.* Washington, DC: National Geographic.

McClure, M., & Hinshaw, A. (2007). The magnetic matrix: Building blocks of Magnet™ hospitals. *American Nurse Today, 2*(12), 22–24.

McGinn, A. P. (2000). Phasing out persistent organic pollutants. In L. R. Brown, C. Flavin, H. French, et al. (Eds.), *State of the world 2000.* New York: W. W. Norton.

McGlown, K. (Ed.). (2004). *Terrorism and disaster management.* Chicago: Health Administration Press,

McIntosh, W. L., Spies, E., Stone, D. M., Lokey, C. N., Trudeau, A. T., & Bartholow, B. (2016). Suicide Rates by Occupational Group — 17 States, 2012. *MMWR. Morbidity and Mortality Weekly Report, 65*, 641–645.

McLean, A. (1974). Concepts of occupational stress: A review. In A. McLean (Ed.), *Occupational stress.* Springfield, IL: Charles C. Thomas.

Melum, M. F., & Kearney, K. (2001). Organophosphate toxicity. *American Journal of Nursing, 101*, 57–58.

Musker, K. (1994). Voluntary simplicity: Nurses creating a healing environment. In E. A. Schuster & C. L. Brown (Eds.), *Exploring our environmental connections (NLN Publication No. 14–2634).* New York: National League for Nursing.

Nash, T. J. (2015). Unveiling the Truth about Nurses's Personal Preparedness for Disaster Response: A Pilot Study. *Med-Surg Nursing, 24*(6), 425–431.

National Aeronautics and Space Administration's Goddard Institute for Space Studies. (2016a). Global climate change-Vital signs of the planet: Global temperature. Retrieved from http://climate.nasa.gov/vital-signs/global-temperature/ Accessed May 14, 2016.

National Aeronautics and Space Administration's Goddard Institute for Space Studies. (2016b). Global climate change-Vital signs of the planet: Sea levels. Retrieved from http://climate.nasa.gov/vital-signs/sea-level/. Accessed May 14, 2016.

Neuman, B. (2002). The Neuman system model. In B. Neuman & J. Fawcett (Eds.), *The Neuman systems model* (4th ed.). Upper Saddle River, NJ: Prentice-Hall.

Newman, M. A. (1994). *Health as expanding consciousness* (2nd ed.). New York: National League for Nursing.

Occupational Safety and Health Administration. (2007). 2007 Industry injury and illness data. Retrieved from www.bls.gov/iif/oshwc/osh/os/ostab.pdf. Accessed November 12, 2008.

O'Meara, M. (2000). Harnessing information technologies for the environment. In L. R. Brown, C. Flavin, H. French, et al. (Eds.), *State of the world 2000.* New York: W. W. Norton.

Papp, E. (2007). *Occupational health and safety management programme for nurses.* Geneva: International Council of Nurses.

Pearce, F. (2007). *With speed and violence: Why scientist fear tipping points in climate change.* Boston, MA: Beacon.

Peterson, C. (2006). Be safe, be prepared: Emergency system for advance registration of volunteer health professionals in disaster response. *Online Journal of Issues in Nursing, 11*(3), 3. Retrieved from www.nursingworld.org/MainMenuCategories/ANAMarketplace/ANAPeriodicals/OJIN/TableofContents/Volume112006/No3Sept06/tpc31_216083.html. Accessed February 24, 2013.

Polivka, B., Stanley, S., Gorden, D., Taulbee, K., Kieffer, G., & McCorkle, S. M. (2008). Public health nursing competencies for public health surge events. *Public Health Nursing, 25*(5), 159–165.

Pope, A. M., Snyder, M. A., & Mood, L. H. (Eds.). (1995). *Nursing, health and the environment.* Washington, DC: National Academies Press.

Poursafa, P., Keitkha, M., & Kelishadi, R. (2015). Systematic review on adverse birth outcomes of climate change. *Journal of Research in Medical Sciences, 20*, 397–402.

Rogers, M. E. (1990). Nursing: Science of unitary, irreducible human beings: Update 1990. In E. A. M. Barrett (Ed.), *Visions of Rogers' science-based nursing.* New York: National League for Nursing.

Roy, C. (1987). Roy's adaptation model. In R. R. Parse (Ed.), *Nursing science; Major paradigms, theories and critiques.* Philadelphia, PA: W. B. Saunders.

Rutala, W. A., Barbee, S. L., Aguiar, N. C., Sobsey, M. D., & Weber, D. J. (2000). Antimicrobial activity of home disinfectants and natural products against potential human pathogens. *Infection Control and Hospital Epidemiology, 21,* 33–38.

Sachs, J. (2008). *Common wealth: Economics for a crowded planet.* New York: Penguin.

Scully, M. G. (2001). Taking the pulse of the Kalamazoo. *Chronicle of Higher Education, 47,* B16.

Shaner, H. (1994). Environmentally responsible clinical practice. In E. A. Schuster & C. L. Brown (Eds.), *Exploring our environmental connections practice (NLN Publication No. 14–2634).* New York: National League for Nursing.

Shaner, H., & Botter, M. (2003). Pollution: Health care's unintended legacy. *American Journal of Nursing, 103,* 79, 81, 83–84.

Steger, S. (2000). Killed in school! *RN, 63,* 36–38.

Sutton, R. (2006). *The no asshole rule: Building a civilized workplace and surviving one that isn't.* New York: Warner Business.

Trossman, S. (2000). Moving violations: Working to prevent on-the-job injuries. *The American Nurse, 32, 1,* 12–14.

United Nations. (2016). With Global Goals agreed, UN focuses on what it will take to achieve sustainability targets by 2030. Retrieved from http://www.un.org/sustainabledevelopment/blog/2016/04/with-global-goals-agreed-un-focuses-on-what-it-will-take-to-achieve-sustainability-targets-by-2030/. Accessed May 15, 2016.

U.S. Bureau of Labor Statistics. (2009). TABLE R1. Number of nonfatal occupational injuries and illnesses involving days away from work1 by industry and selected natures of injury or illness, private industry, 2009. Retrieved from www.bls.gov/iif/oshwc/osh/case/ostb2447.pdf. Accessed March 13, 2013.

U.S. Census Bureau. (2012). US & world population clocks. Retrieved from www.census.gov/main/www/popclock.html. Accessed December 27, 2012.

U.S. Department of Health and Human Services. (2000). *Healthy people 2010.* Boston, MA: Jones & Bartlett.

U.S. Department of Health and Human Services. (2011). HHS releases assessment of Healthy People 2010 objectives. Retrieved from www.healthypeople.gov/2020/about/HP2010PressReleaseOct5.doc. Accessed December 27, 2012.

United States Environmental Protection Agency. (2016). Climate impacts on human health. Retrieved from https://www3.epa.gov/climatechange/impacts/health.html. Accessed May 15, 2016.

Vasailakopoulos, P., & Marchall, C. T. (2015). Resilience and tipping points of an exploited fish population over six decades. *Global Change Biology, 21,* 1834–1847. doi: 10.1111/gcb.128

Veenema, T. (2013). *Disaster nursing and emergency preparedness for chemical, biological and radiological terrorism and other hazards* (3rd ed,). New York: Springer Publishing Co.

Watkins, J. M., & Mohr, B. J. (2001). *Appreciative inquiry.* San Francisco, CA: Jossey-Bass/Pfeiffer.

Watson, J. (1999). *Postmodern nursing and beyond.* Edinburgh: Churchill-Livingstone.

Wesorick, B., Shiparski, L., Troseth, M., & Wyngarden, K. (1997). *Partnership Council field book.* Grand Rapids, MI: Practice Field Publishing.

Wilson, C. K., & Porter-O'Grady, T. (1999). *Leading the revolution in health care* (2nd ed.). Gaithersburg, MD: Aspen.

World Health Organization. (2012). Influenza at the human-animal interface. Summary and assessment as of 4 June 2012. Retrieved from www.who.int/influenza/human_animal_interface/EN_GIP_20120706CumulativeNumberH5N-1cases.pdf. Accessed December 27, 2012.

Worthington, K. (2000). Seeking the perfect fit. *American Journal of Nursing, 100,* 88.

Young, H., & Lee, E. (Eds.) (1948). *Essential of nursing.* New York: G. P. Putnam's Sons.

Chapter 14

Informatics and Technology in Nursing Practice

LEARNING OUTCOMES

By the end of this chapter, the learner will be able to:

1. Discuss the roles and implications of informatics and technology in professional nursing practice.
2. Outline the educational preparation and roles of the informatics nurse specialist.
3. Identify current technologies used in clinical practice.
4. Debate the advantages and disadvantages of complex technology used in clinical practice.
5. Identify key ethical considerations as technologic advances become standard practice in professional nursing.
6. Outline ways to balance information and technology in personal and professional life.

REAL-LIFE REFLECTIONS

Jorge, Susan, and Amy graduated from the same nursing program several years ago. They now work at three different health care facilities. Jorge, who works at a large university medical center, has been documenting care using a computer for many years and has worked with two different computer documentation systems. Susan, a director of nursing at a rural hospital, just introduced a computerized client care documentation system at her facility. Amy works in a home health care agency that uses laptop computers to record home visits as well as computer technology for remote client monitoring. When they meet at a college alumni event, they compare notes about the strengths and weaknesses of the current computer systems and technology they use in practice. Susan poses the following questions during their discussion: "I know that computers are wonderful, but how can I get my older staff members to overcome their computer phobia? How can we ensure confidentiality of client information with computerized medical records? What key elements need to be included in an employee policy related to computer use and confidentiality of information? How much time is actually required of staff for computer documentation? What are the legal implications for nurses who use technology for remote client monitoring?

For optimal professional practice and client care, nurses must have well-refined computer skills. This chapter provides an overview of the informatics and technology used in today's nursing practice and explores the implications for professional nurses as technology plays an increasingly important role in health care delivery. Key computer competencies for professional nursing and advances in technology for clinical practice are presented. Finally, the chapter challenges students to consider the advantages, disadvantages, and ethical issues of technology use for client care.

Changes in technology occur quickly. In fact, by the time this chapter is published, some of the information presented will likely already be obsolete. Faster, improved models of computer equipment seem to be introduced just as soon as the latest model has been purchased. New materials superior to silicon continue to make computer chips smaller and faster. In fact, purchasing a hard copy of any book (including this one) may one day be a rarity, especially with the proliferation of e-readers capable of storing hundreds of books. Every day, more and more nurses access, record, and store clinically relevant information via computer.

INFORMATICS AND HEALTH CARE

The average person today has access to more information online than a single person could possibly comprehend in a lifetime. Information science deals with the discovery of "efficient collection, storage, and retrieval of information" (Agnes, 2005, p. 733). **Informatics**, or the science of information (Agnes, 2005), has emerged as the practical application of organizing information for a specific purpose. Because of the wide array of information available, devising effective methods for organizing and managing it is imperative. Essential information in one area of life may be irrelevant in another. For example, how informatics is used to generate, store, manage, and communicate information for computer gaming has little relevance to health care providers (unless a provider is working in the field of neuroscience and is studying the effects of computer gaming on memory).

Take Note!

In professional nursing, informatics plays a critical role in how nurses access, enter, manage, and store key knowledge essential for professional practice and client care.

Informatics and Professional Nursing

Nurses use a variety of computers in daily clinical practice. Nurses document various aspects of client care using computers, thereby creating an **electronic health record (EHR)** for each client. An EHR stores client health information digitally in a secure database (Fig 14.1). When consumers receive care from an integrated health system, EHRs can be accessed nearly seamlessly. Section 1461 of the 2010 Affordable Care Act sets regulations for EHR use across the care continuum and for the security of the protected health information contained in them, and sets specific dates for regulation implementation (HealthIT.gov, 2010). In the future, all health care providers across the continuum of care will be able to access EHRs when consumers receive care services.

The federal government recognized that for effective use of EHRs that they needed to be meaningful and so meaningful use was defined. Meaningful use means "the use of certified EHR technology to achieve health and efficiency goals" (HealthIT.gov, 2014, para 1). The government determined meaningful use objectives and classified them into the following patient-driven domains:

- Improve Quality, Safety, Efficiency
- Engage Patients & Families
- Improve Care Coordination
- Improve Public and Population Health
- Ensure Privacy and Security for Personal Health Information (HealthIT.gov, 2014, para 2)

The federal government set goals for meaningful use of EHRs. In order not to overwhelm health care organizations and providers, the government launched requirements in a series of stages. Stage one emphasized data capture and sharing and has been fully implemented

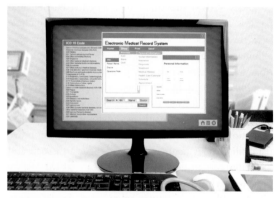

FIGURE 14.1 Electronic health records provide a seamless way to share client information across the continuum of care.

since 2013. Key components of stage one consisted of electronic health information entry using a standardized format, using this information to track common clinical conditions, communicating the information for care coordination, reporting quality measures (HealthIT.gov, 2013).

In 2013–2014, stage two was initiated. Stage two focused on advancing clinical processes. This phase was designed to enhance the rigor of health information exchange (between health care organizations and third-party payers), increased requirement for electronic prescriptions and including lab test results, transmission of patient care summaries across multiple care setting, and increased patient-controlled data (the right of a patient to request revisions to an EHR). Completion of this stage set the stage for stage three (HealthIT.gov, 2013).

The target date for complete implementation of stage three was 2015, but because of issues the date was delayed until the end of 2016. Stage three targets improved clinical outcomes. The goals for stage three include improving the quality, efficiency, and safety of health care interventions to improve health outcomes; implementing decision support systems for identified national high-priority health conditions, access to self-management of health computerized tools for all patients, seamless access to comprehensive patient data using patient-centered health information exchanges and improving the health of the entire American population (HeathIT.gov, 2013, 2015).

Most currently health care organizations used EHRs contain the following features: electronically stored health information in a standardized format, tracking key clinical conditions using the captured electronic health information, coordinating care using the data, reporting clinical quality measures and public health information, and engaging patients and families in their health care.

Duffy (2015) identified the benefits, barrier, and hazards to electronic documentation. Benefits include ease the health information documentation process, eliminated duplicate entries, permit automatic notifications to providers while giving care, provides standard terminology used by all providers, provide a consistent order and format to facilitate data retrieval, store data apart from the health record form enabling data extraction for quality reporting and research, improve readability (poor penmanship no longer an issue), and facilitates current documentation of care (if the facility provides each person involved in care access to a smart phone, tablet or computer where care is delivered). Barriers to EHR use include costs. Hazards identified

include inevitable system failures (computers go down, need updating, and power outages), overly simplified charting (checking boxes for health findings and loss of nurse ability to document detailed notes on abnormal assessment findings), and duplicate documentation on paper for later computer entry (increase chance for error or inconsistency of data).

Nurses frequently use paper to help organize their day. Many nurses find it useful to print and carry computerized reports. Privacy concerns arise if nurses accidently leave a report in a location with public access. Privacy issues also arise should a nurse forget to log off a computer following patient care documentation (Duffy, 2015).

However, when nurses realize that computerized systems provide them with messages about things that need to be done within a specific time frame, some nurses (including the text author) have abandoned the use of printed patient reports when providing inpatient care. Reduction in care errors is a key element of meaningful use of EHRs. Nurses who use nursing care reminders report having fewer misses or more near misses in care delivery (Piscotty, Kalisch, & Gracey-Thomas, 2015). The following Focus on Research, "How Health Care Information Technology Impacts on Nursing Practice" outlines how nurses perceive health care information technology assists them in providing the right care at the right time to patients in daily clinical practice.

Personal Electronic Health Records

Many people keep personal health records. Computer-savvy health care consumers typically keep a **personal electronic health record (PEHR)**. PEHRs emerged when people entered their personal health information into their home computers. Today, a number of insurance companies and primary care provider practices offer software or online tools for consumers to develop and maintain. Some PEHRs are stored in secure electronic databases; others can be accessed using smart phones. Benefits of a PEHR include error reduction and seamless health care delivery. A PEHR enables a new care provider to access specific health information about a client, including diagnostic tests (including viewing digitalized radiographic films if the PEHR is linked to an integrated health care delivery system), accurate lists of currently prescribed medications, and up-to-date third-party payment information (Nelson, 2007).

Unfortunately, there are no universal or standardized versions of PEHRs. The American Health Information Management Association keeps records

FOCUS ON RESEARCH

How Health Care Information Technology Impacts Nursing Practice

One hundred fourteen nurses working in a large teaching hospital participated in a descriptive study to identify the nurse perceived impact of health information technology on clinical practice mediated the relationship between nurse electronic reminder use and missed nursing care events.

Using online surveys, the participants completed three surveys, the Nursing Care Reminder Usage Survey (RCRS), the Impact of Health Information Technology Scale (I-HIT) and the Missed Nursing Care Survey (MISSCARE). Data were analyzed using multiple regression equations to identify any mediating effects among the variables.

The investigators found that nurses who perceived that health information technology affected their clinical practice reported fewer incidents of missed nursing care ($t = -4.12$, $p < 0.001$), and accounted for 9.8% variance in missed nursing care. When I-HIT was present, then the reminder use scores were no longer significant, but if I-HIT was not present the reminder use increased. Thus the investigators perceived that I-HIT mediated the relationship between reminder usage and missed nursing care.

The researchers concluded that nurses who recognize the impact of health care information technology tend to use electronic nurse messages and have fewer incidents of missed nursing care. Nurses who discount the impact of health information technology tended not to use electronic nurse messages and reported more incidents of missed care.

This study provides evidence that health care information technology improves the safety and efficiency of nursing care. However, sometimes nurses may tend to ignore key messages related to patient care if they discount the impact of technology over paper methods of keeping track of patient care in daily clinical practice.

These results should be interpreted with caution because there was no documentation on the validity and reliability of instruments used to collect data, no power analysis to determine sample size and the nurses who participated in the study 114 out of 169 nurses may differ from the nurse nonparticipants. The study is also limited to one hospital.

More research is needed to know what specific nurse reminders are useful to nurses in clinical practice, the effects of redundant nurse reminder messages and what nurses would prefer to have in the nursing component of EHRs software to facilitate organizing all the care activities required in a day of clinical practice.

Piscotty, R. J., Kalisch, B., & Gracey-Thomas, A. (2015). Impact of Healthcare Information Technology on Nursing Practice. *Journal of Nursing Scholarship, 47*(4), 287–293. doi: 10.1111/jnu.12138

---

of progress toward standardization and policy development about electronic health information on its website. The "Putting Patients First" initiative from the National Health Council was the first to specify that health information to be "portable, belong to the patient, and empower the patient to make informed decisions regarding care" (Nelson, 2007, p. 27). The National Health Council also emphasized the importance of standardization of electronic platforms used for PEHRs so that when a person changes insurance coverage or health care providers there is no loss of health information. The Affordable Care Act has also set regulations defining criteria for standardization of PEHRs (HealthIT.gov, 2010). Currently, more than 60 software programs are available for PEHRs; some offer the ability of transfer of data between software programs. Hospitals, outpatient facilities, physician offices, and integrated health care systems currently purchase computer platforms and software for keeping client EHRs and some offer clients access to PEHR software programs. Some physician offices send annual reminders to clients to update PEHRs.

Logue and Effken (2012, 2013) developed the Personal Health Records Adoption Model to explain why some people decide to use PEHRs. This model identifies four interactive factors that contribute to behavior required for PEHR adoption by health care consumers.

1. **Personal factors** encompass cognitive abilities, emotional attributes, and biologic characteristics that influence decisions for changing behaviors (intention to act and actual action).

2. **Environmental factors** include social and physical conditions that influence behavior.
3. **Technology factors** include resource availability, compatibility, and cost; perceived usefulness; perceptions of external control; ability to observe and try the system; complexity; and relative advantage.
4. **Chronic disease factors** are separated from personal factors based on the belief that self-management of and chronic diseases themselves create specific contexts and a variety of influencing factors, especially when people with chronic disease have specific care preferences, understand the complex nature of their disease, see multiple health care providers in various settings, engage in negotiated collaboration with health team members, and prefer to self-manage their condition.

Before people adopt PEHRs, they need to have some ability to understand and use computer technology, perceive that PEHRs would be useful and advantageous, and have the time to enter and update personal health data. Nurses can assist clients directly by helping them enter data or indirectly by providing education, support, and guidance as clients develop and maintain their PEHRs.

Many nurses currently use computer tablets, smartphones, and other electronic devices with software or apps for managing daily tasks, keeping calendars, calculating medication dosages or complex clinical calculations (e.g., body mass index, corrected serum calcium levels), and consulting clinical references (e.g., medication information and terminology, disease references, medical calculation software programs). Some health care organizations issue unit cell phones to nurses for use in the clinical setting to facilitate staff communications. Most health care organizations provide convenient ways for nurses to access and document information in client EHRs, such as having computers in every room, providing mobile, laptop, or tablet computers, or placing computers in strategic locations throughout the work setting.

> **Take Note!**
> Not only do EHRs eliminate the need for paper, they also allow instantaneous transfer of client information to all relevant health care personnel.

Information Beyond the EHR

Health care informatics encompasses more than EHRs. The **American Medical Informatics Association (AMIA)** identifies the following four categories of medical health care informatics (Kulikowski et al., 2012).

1. **Clinical research informatics** for new discoveries about health and illnesses
2. **Consumer health informatics** for patient/family use, especially in the areas of health literacy and education, with the aim of giving people valid and reliable information and resources, such as tools for identifying health risk assessments, maintaining PEHRs, and accessing all forms of health-related information in lay terminology
3. **Public health informatics** for disease surveillance and reporting, health promotion, electronic lab reporting, and coordination of outbreak responses
4. **Translational bioinformatics** for storage, analysis, and interpretation to optimize integration of new research and treatment strategies into predictive, preventive, and participatory health care, such as the use of molecular information (e.g., genomic data) into practical clinical applications

Nurses deal primarily with **clinical informatics**, which has been subdivided into specialty job positions of systems and support analysts, systems administrators, training managers, project managers and leaders, and chief information officers. To facilitate computer and information systems use for nurses, expert or nursing liaison positions have been developed. Informatics specialists design software programs and computer systems to manage information related to clients and health care. Specialists who focus on the health care delivery aspects design software and create integrated systems that facilitate health care delivery (American Nurses Association [ANA], 2008; **Alliance for Nursing Informatics [ANI]**, 2011).

The ANI is a collaboration of multiple organizations that provides a unified voice for **nursing informatics**, a subspecialty of health care informatics; it provides a nursing perspective on health care informatics, addresses issues surrounding nursing practice, and focuses on nursing phenomena and incorporating the values and beliefs of professional nursing (ANA, 2008; ANI, 2011). Professional nurses use nursing informatics as a means to integrate the vast amount of knowledge, information, and data required for effective clinical practice, education, and research (Carrington & Tiase, 2013; Shepard, 2013).

The ANI (2011) recognizes five subspecialties in the arena of nursing informatics. These are clinical informatics (used for direct and indirect client care), consumer-health informatics (used by clients to get health-related information), educational informatics (used for client, staff, and student education), public health informatics (used for tracking public health information), and research in nursing informatics (used to track client outcomes and the effectiveness of nursing interventions). ANI's vision is to "transform health and health care through nursing informatics and innovation" (ANI, 2011, para 1) by advancing "nursing informatics leadership, practice, education policy, and research through a unified voice of nursing informatics organizations" (ANI, 2011, para 2). ANI works closely with ANA to develop scope and standards of nursing informatics practice and to determine credentialing criteria for certification in the field of nursing informatics. ANA and ANI collaborate with the National League for Nursing and Technology Informatics Guiding Education Reform Collaborative Workgroup to determine informatics competencies across the nursing education spectrum. ANI also collaborates with AMIA and the Healthcare Information Management Systems Society so that nursing has a voice in the development of effective health care informatics and information systems (ANA, 2008).

> **Take Note!**
> For effective clinical practice, nurses must know how to use computers and manage enormous volumes of information.

QUESTIONS FOR REFLECTION

1. What are your current skills and abilities with computers and technology? How have you refined your skills and abilities to keep up with the pace of change in this area?
2. What additional skills would you like to acquire and why do you think they might be useful to you in your future nursing career?
3. What are the benefits and hazards of giving clients online access to their own EHRs from a provider's office? Why do you think that these are benefits and hazards?

Computer and Informatics Competencies for Professional Nurses

Computer use in health care delivery became prevalent in the early 21st century. In their pioneering efforts to determine professional nurse knowledge and skills in informatics, Staggers, Gassert, and Curan (2001, 2002) conducted a Delphi study that serves as the basis for today's competencies. The 2003 Institute of Medicine report, *Health Professions Education: A Bridge to Quality,* noted deficits in current education of all health professionals, including the following six core areas that needed vast improvement: patient-centered care, teamwork and collaboration, evidence-based practice, quality improvement, safety, and informatics (these are also the six key areas for Quality Safety Education for Nurses [QSEN] competencies). In 2004, President Bush issued a mandate that required all American health organizations providing direct client care to use EHRs by 2014. To meet this challenge, professional nurse leaders, educators, and informatics experts recognized the need to develop a vision for integrating informatics into practice, education, and research (Sherwood & Barnsteiner, 2012).

In 2006, the Technology Information Guiding Education Reform (TIGER) Initiative established seven "pillars" or key areas for nursing workforce development: management and leadership, education, communication and collaboration, informatics design, information technology, policy, and culture. The final report resulted in the TIGER Nursing Informatics Competencies Model, which addresses the basic computer competencies, information literacy, and information management skills nurses need. Listed competencies from the model have become part of most baccalaureate and higher-degree nursing programs (TIGER Summit, 2007).

In 2008, the American Association of Colleges of Nursing (AACN) revised its criteria for program accreditation to include informatics competences. The current AACN recommendations for professional nurse generalists outline the following informatics skills that nurses are expected to have.

- Use information and communication technology to document and evaluate patient care, advance patient education, and enhance the accessibility of care.
- Use appropriate technologies in the process of assessing and monitoring patients.
- Work in an interdisciplinary team to make ethical decisions regarding the application of technologies and the acquisition of data.
- Adapt the use of technologies to meet patient needs.
- Teach patients about health care technologies.
- Protect the safety and privacy of patients in relation to the use of health care and information technologies.
- Use information technologies to enhance one's own knowledge base.

In 2009, QSEN established specific knowledge, skills, and attitudes for all professional nurses to achieve competency in nursing informatics (and in the aforementioned key areas). Key knowledge for informatics outlined by QSEN competencies include: explaining the importance of information and technology skills that are essential for safe client care; identifying basic, essential information that must be contained within common databases for supporting client care; contrasting benefits and limitations of various communication technologies and their impact on the safety and quality of client care; providing examples of how technology and information management relate to client care quality and safety; and recognizing that time, effort, and skills are required for computers, databases, and other technologies before they can become effective, reliable instruments for client care delivery (Sherwood & Barnsteiner, 2012).

Knowledge is not enough for safe clinical practice. Professional nurses must also display skill in the application of knowledge in clinical setting. QSEN key pre-licensure nursing skills related to informatics include seeking education about health care information management before providing client care; applying technology and information management (computerized warning systems and resources) to promote safe client care; navigating the EHR documenting, planning client care using EHR programs, coordinating client care using communication technologies; responding effectively to clinical decision-making support systems and alerts (warning systems built into the EHR to prevent errors from occurring); using information generated from information management tools to track outcomes of nursing care delivered, and utilizing high-quality electronic sources of health care information for answering questions arising from practice and for client education (Sherwood & Barnsteiner, 2012).

Professional nurses are people who have attitudes, values, and beliefs about the use of technology, computers, and informatics when providing client care. The key QSEN Pre-licensure Competencies regarding informatics include appreciating the need for all health care professional to engage in lifelong, continuous learning of information and technology skills, valuing the technologies that support care coordination, error prevention, and clinical decision making (if they are valued, then they will be used); protecting the confidentiality of the client's protected health information contained within EHR, and valuing the involvement of professional nurses in the designing, selecting, implementing, and evaluating of information technologies used to support client care (Sherwood & Barnsteiner, 2012). Nurse experiences with health care informatics and technologies shape attitudes toward its use as well as identifying deficiencies within an adopted EHR

program, clinical decision support systems, and communication technologies.

The Nurse of the Future Nursing Core Competencies also addresses competencies related to computer and information technology in professional nursing. Professional nurses provide a bridge for the integration of informatics into health care. Nurses use computers to document patient care; find valid and relevant information for client education, access information to guide clinical actions and use technology and information to improve the health of the persons whom they serve (David, 2014).

The experienced nurse must be able to use applications for diagnostic coding, evaluate computer-assisted instruction as a teaching method, and integrate selected resources into a client file. The experienced professional should also be able to define how computerized information affects the nurse's role, assess the accuracy of health information posted on the internet, and serve as an advocate for client system users. Box 14.1, Professional Building Blocks "Checklist for Professional Nurse Competencies in the Use of Technology and Informatics" provides a tool for nurses to verify their level of competence with informatics and technology for general clinical practice. Nurses who specialize in nursing informatics have additional advanced competencies such as developing backup systems in the event of a computer systems failure, designing software programs applicable to clinical care settings, and troubleshooting software and computer system problems as they arise.

THE INFORMATICS NURSE SPECIALIST

The complex nature of designing, developing, implementing, and maintaining a health care clinical information system requires many experts. Therefore, numerous positions in the field of clinical informatics have emerged. Applied/professional roles focus on the design, development, execution, and maintenance of information systems (e.g., systems analyst, support analyst, systems administrator, software designer, project leader, chief information officer).

Sometimes, staff within a health care organization find themselves in the position of deciding what health care information system program would best fit their institutional needs. Informatics experts or liaisons focus on performing organizational needs assessments, helping organizations select particular hardware and software programs, implementing selected information systems, and training users on the selected programs.

Once an information system is designed and developed, nurses and other health care providers need to

14.1 Professional Building Blocks

Checklist for Professional Nurse Competencies in the Use of Technology and Informatics

Competency	Yes	No
Explain basic concepts of computer hardware, software, and networks.		
Use computer hardware, including a keyboard, screen, signing on, and turning on the computer.		
Use computer software, including basic word processing, spreadsheet, e-mail, and internet search programs.		
Use a computerized database to search professional nursing and other professional health care literature to access high-quality health care information.[a]		
Access dictated client reports such as histories and physicals, radiology and lab reports, surgery reports, pathology reports, and consultations.[a]		
Access telemetry, vital signs, and pulse oximetry data (all practice areas); access central venous pressure, cardiac output, pulmonary wedge pressure, and intracranial pressure (intensive care nursing areas); and access nursing and other health team members' electronic documentation (all areas of nursing practice).[a]		
Document client assessments electronically.[a]		
Document independent and collaborative nursing interventions electronically.[a]		
Document evaluation of independent and collaborative nursing interventions electronically.[a]		
Enter a basic care plan for clients electronically and update it as needed.[a]		
Take steps to ensure confidentiality of client personal health information.[b]		
Enter verbal and written orders (unless program requires physician direct entry).[a]		
Determine safe staffing needs for assigned unit.		
Perform basic maintenance and/or calibration of handheld computer devices.		
Enter and monitor client-ordered medication dosages on IV pumps with computer chips.		
Use telecommunication devices effectively (beepers or cell phones).		
Develop an attitude of confidence when using technologic devices in professional practice.		
Outline strategies for continued client care in the event of a situation during which computer systems may not be available.		
Specify the advantages of using computers and telecommunication device use in clinical practice.[c]		
List disadvantages of using computers and telecommunication devices in clinical practice.[c]		
Explain how and why information and technology skills enhance patient care safety.[c]		
Identify essential information that must be available in a common database for all health team members to use to support patient care.[c]		
Describe examples of how technology and information management are related to the quality and safety of patient care.[c]		
Recognize the time, effort, and skill required for computers, databases, and other technologies to become reliable and effective patient care tools.[c]		
Obtain education about how information is managed in care settings before working in them.[a]		
Use electronic technology and information management tools to enhance safe-care processes.[a]		

(continued on page 362)

14.1 Professional Building Blocks (continued)

Checklist for Professional Nurse Competencies in the Use of Technology and Informatics (continued)

Competency	Yes	No
Utilize communication technologies to coordinate patient care.[a]		
Respond effectively to clinical decision-making support tools and other clinical action alerts.[a]		
Appreciate the need for all health team members to participate in lifelong, continuous learning of new information technology skills.[b]		
Value technologies that facilitate clinical decision making, prevent errors, and foster care coordination.[b]		
Value the professional nursing involvement in designing, selecting, implementing, and evaluating all information technologies used to support patient care.[b]		

[a]Covered in QSEN skill competency.

[b]Covered in QSEN attitude competency.

[c]Covered in QSEN knowledge competency.

American Association of Colleges of Nursing. (2008). *The essentials of baccalaureate education for professional nursing practice.* Washington, DC: Author; American Nurses Association. (2008). *Nursing informatics: Scope and standards of practice.* Silver Spring, MD: Nursebooks.org; Barton, A., Armstrong, G., & Preheim, G. (2009). *Quality and safety education for nurses: Results of a national Delphi study of developmental level KSAs.* Denver, CO: University of Colorado; Ellerbee, S. (2007). Staffing through web-based open-shift bidding. *American Nurse Today, 2*(4), 32–34; Lin, J., Lin, K., Jiang, W., & Lee, T. (2007). An exploration of nursing informatics competency and satisfaction related to network education. *Journal of Nursing Research, 14*(1), 54–65; and Nelson, R. (2007). The personal health record. *American Journal of Nursing, 107*(9), 27–28.

learn how to use it. Organizations frequently employ nursing informatics specialists to educate staff on optimal use of the information system. Other expert/liaison positions include informatics coordinator, chief nursing informatics officer, and information technology nursing advocate. Professional nurses with specialization in computer applications are needed to develop nurse-friendly computer systems to support nurses working at the bedside (ANA, 2008).

The **informatics nurse specialist** has a graduate education, advanced levels of computer and information literacy, and professional development in leadership. The informatics nurse specialist can analyze information systems and work processes to apply knowledge to client care, health care administration, nursing research, and education. The **nursing informatics innovator** holds a doctorate degree and designs new technologic systems, techniques, and conceptual models for databases and information systems. He or she employs advanced knowledge and experience while formulating and developing unique methods to enhance current system or design new ones. The nurse informatics innovator also evaluates the safety, effectiveness, cost, and social impact of the technologic systems and researches theoretical foundations of the specialty itself (ANA, 2008; Staggers & Gassert, 2000).

Responsibilities of the Informatics Nurse Specialist

In 2008, the ANA revised its *Scope and Standards of Nursing Informatics Practice* to address the ever-increasing complexity of health care informatics. Informatics nurse specialists and nurse informatics innovators manage projects, offer specialized systems services, consult with information technology professionals and personnel, conduct quality improvement and research studies, educate nursing colleagues, and develop products and policies (ANA, 2008). Informatics nurse specialists and nurse informatics innovators work for health care organizations, for product vendors, and for themselves as entrepreneurs. Some informatics nurse specialists manage large databases specific to a specialty area of practice. Because of rapid advances in technology, all informatics nurse specialists must engage in lifelong learning. Knowledge of computers and information systems comes through formal education (collegiate and continuing education programs) as well as practical experience (ANA, 2008).

The perspective of the informatics nurse specialist gives the technologic development team a working knowledge of the nursing profession, so client care information can be better managed. Without input of nurses, health information systems may miss critical aspects of client care and may create procedures that reduce nursing effectiveness.

Education of the Informatics Nurse Specialist

Because nursing informatics is a new area of specialty practice, the educational preparation and role of informatics nurse specialists vary (Table 14.1). The informatics nurse specialist needs a thorough understanding of clinical practice in addition to detailed computer expertise.

Take Note!

Informatics nurse specialists have an integral role in the development of health information systems.

TABLE 14.1 Educational Requirements and Role Description of the Nursing Informatics Specialist

Educational Requirements	Role Description
At least 2 yrs of clinical nursing practice[a]	Thorough understanding of clinical practice to develop, implement, and maintain information systems that are relevant to clinical nursing practice
Successful completion of the ANA Certification Examination in Nursing Informatics[a]	Provides evidence for competence in the area of nursing informatics
Computer system design and analysis[b]	Develop novel system designs to meet nursing information needs Analyze available hardware and software to design a comprehensive nursing information system Recommend hardware and software to develop the information system Develop proposals for acquisition of resources needed for the system or system revisions Program computers to meet the needs of the health care organization
Information and support of systems[b]	Develop, plan, and implement education for nurses who use the information system Develop and implement policies and procedures for system use Develop documentation for staff education and support services Maintain collegial relationships with system users Outline strategies for system implementation Provide ongoing technical and clinical support for system users
Testing and evaluation of systems	Implement system testing to verify function Develop and implement system evaluation plan to detect strengths and weaknesses Assess current system and new products for potential updates
Managing information and databases[b]	Collect and analyze aggregate data Transform data into meaningful presentation format Plan future updates to system
Professional practice, issues, and trends[b]	Role components: nurse, information expert, computer expert, educator, and researcher Financial issues related to system development, utilization, and updates Future developments in technology Ethical issues, such as confidentiality of client information Federal regulations Interdisciplinary organizations for health informatics Professional standards for health and nursing informatics
Theoretical foundations for practice[b]	Concepts of nursing informatics Nursing taxonomy and nomenclature (e.g., North American Nursing Diagnosis Association, Nursing Interventions Classification System/Nursing Outcomes Classification System, Nursing Management Minimum Data Set, Omaha System, Patient Care Data Set, Nightingale Tracker) Mental models of data and information processing Nursing decision-making models and decision support systems

[a]Certification requirements from the American Nurses Credentialing Center (2016).

[b]Topics covered the American Nurses Credentialing Center Examination (2016).

Adapted from Thede, L. (1999). *Computers in nursing: Bridges to the future* (pp. 289–293). Philadelphia, PA: Lippincott Williams & Wilkins; Turley, J. P. (2000). Informatics and education: The start of a discussion. In B. Carty (Ed.), *Nursing informatics education for practice* (pp. 271–293). New York: Springer Publishing.

The ANA offers certification examinations to validate competence in nursing informatics. To stay abreast of changes, the ANA requires certified informatics nurse specialists to engage in clinical practice and complete continuing education. Hours of clinical practice vary. Eligibility requirements to take the American Nurses Credentialing Center (ANCC) exam in Nursing Informatics include a minimum of 2 years of full-time employment as a registered nurse and 30 continuing education contact hours in nursing informatics within 3 years along with one of the following criteria: 200 clock hours of practice in nursing informatics within the past 3 years; 1,000 hours of clinical practice in nursing informatics with 12 credit semester hours of graduate level courses in nursing informatics; or graduation with a master's degree in nursing informatics from a program that required a minimum of 200 clinical hours of a faculty-supervised clinical practicum in nursing informatics (ANCC, 2016). Certification in Nursing Informatics must be renewed every 5 years and the nurse renewing certification must document 75 contact hours in nursing informatics to qualify for renewal (ANCC, 2015).

Role of the Informatics Nurse

Software developers and computer programmers have expertise in computer systems but lack familiarity with clinical nursing practice and health care delivery. Thus, to develop software and computer systems that are compatible with nursing care delivery and facilitate, rather

TABLE 14.2 Components of Health Information Systems Used in Today's Health Care Institutions

Application	Function
Admission, discharge, and transfer	Tracks patient demographic data; insurance information; responsible parties; medical record number; care provider; and dates of admissions, transfer, and dismissals.
Financial	Keeps records related to billing information for medical supplies and services rendered, tracking of accounts receivable, general ledger, and institutional costs for care delivery.
Physician order entry	Provides computer order entry and almost instant notification of orders to ancillary departments. Sometimes, information related to specific test preparation is sent immediately to the unit.
Ancillary department	Shares information among various departments to facilitate scheduling of entered orders. These applications also provide information related to quality control.
Documentation	Consists of pop-up screens that enable care providers to select assessment parameters, document care delivered, and evaluate client response using checklists. These also have the capability of free text entry should the need arise. Most systems offer care alerts for nurses to see when ordered care has not been documented.
Care planning	Allows the nurse to select appropriate nursing diagnoses, expected care outcomes, and nursing interventions for any client.
Scheduling	Enables patient scheduling of radiographic, nuclear medicine, and other specialized diagnostic tests and surgery. Also provides a means to schedule staff. Both systems are integrated into the financial information system. Some systems allow scheduling of client appointments with care providers.
Acuity application	Provides a summary of client care needs based on the acuity of illness and, in some cases, the projected hours of nursing care in order to verify adequate staffing levels to fulfill client care needs.
Specialty practice	Provides health care providers within a specific specialty practice area to collect specific client data. Unfortunately, many of these systems fail to integrate data with other components of the health information system.
Decision support	Provides algorithmic decision making related to specific health problems, client demographics, and laboratory test results.
Communication	Provides e-mail and internet access. Some institutions publish policies and procedures in this system component.
Critical pathways	Streamlines the efforts of the interdisciplinary health team by focusing on specific care outcomes. Because all members document on the same form, a more coordinated approach to care results. When documentation is done by computer entry, comparisons of clinical data related to intervention, outcomes, and multidisciplinary approaches become possible.

American Nurses Association. (2008). *Nursing informatics: Scope & standards of practice.* Silver Spring, MD: Nursebooks. org; Hassert, M. (1999). Information systems. In L. Q. Thede (Ed.), *Computers in nursing: Bridges to the future* (pp. 237–247). Philadelphia, PA: Lippincott Williams & Wilkins.

than hinder, client care, health care systems and software companies seek nurse consultants or hire nurses with special education in nursing informatics. Nurses contribute critical information that affects client care. They also field-test software programs to determine the ease of use and feasibility of implementation in client care settings.

As computer technology and complex information systems permeate health care, more informatics nurse specialists will be needed to verify that systems address key nursing practice considerations and facilitate nursing care delivery. Table 14.2 and Box 14.2, Professional Prototypes, "Clinical Informatics in Practice," outline the complex nature of health information systems currently in use. Nearly every application has implications for professional nursing practice. As the need for automated systems to manage health care and document client health information increases, the need for computer analysts and computer support personnel is expected to rise. The U.S. Department of Labor Bureau of Labor Statistics (2012) projects that the need for professional nurses, health systems, computer analysts, and computer support specialists will grow by more than 36% between now and 2020. Nurses with advanced education in informatics will be able to design nurse-friendly systems, direct nurses effectively in their use, and provide support services to other nurses when they experience problems using computer and information systems.

14.2 Professional Prototypes

Clinical Informatics in Practice

Clinical informatics addresses the needs of nurses and other health care providers to streamline client care documentation, keep accurate client records, and integrate various aspects of client care to improve the quality of care. For example, a physician orders a diagnostic test by entering it directly into a computer. The request is received automatically by the department that performs the test. The nurse caring for the client receives a copy of routine client preparation orders and educational materials. When the client leaves the nursing unit for the test, a chip in the client's hospital identification bracelet monitors his or her location. After the test is completed, computerized postprocedure orders are generated and the client's hospital bill is updated to indicate that the test was performed and what supplies were used. In addition, the institution gathers data about the diagnostic procedure for quality improvement and electronically sends data to a registry collecting information about the procedure for research purposes. Finally, the updated bill is sent directly to the client's health insurance company.

QUESTIONS FOR REFLECTION

1. How do you currently use technology in your clinical or professional practice?
2. What are the benefits of using complex technology in professional nursing practice?
3. How does the use of technology affect the nurse–client relationship?
4. What is the impact of technology on the cost and quality of health care?

CONSUMER HEALTH INFORMATICS IN PRACTICE

Many people participate actively in health-related decision making by surfing the internet for information about health promotion, illness prevention, disease management, and specific symptoms. Consumers can watch video clips of surgical and other invasive procedures, subscribe to online health promotion newsletters, and receive checkup reminder text messages. Consumer health informatics focuses efforts on delivering health care services to people who need or want services. Consumer health informatics services include telemedicine, telehealth, and telemonitoring.

Telemedicine

Telemedicine provides medical care services to people who are physically distant from required medical services (Fig. 14.2). The term "telemedicine" first appeared in the literature in the 1960s, when telephone lines were used to transmit client information, such as test results sent via fax or electrocardiograph information sent using telephone lines. With advances in technology, telemedicine has expanded to a means to provide people residing in areas without specialized health

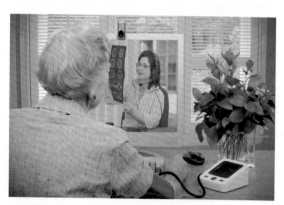

FIGURE 14.2 Online health visits with care providers enable homebound persons to receive health care services more conveniently and with reduced expenditures.

care services with access to those services using video technology (Institute of Medicine, 2012). For example, a victim of a motor vehicle accident who is seen in the emergency room of a rural hospital can receive consultation from a trauma team at a larger urban trauma center when both centers are equipped with video technology. Physicians at the trauma center can assess the victim, review all diagnostic tests, consult with the rural emergency physician, and make suggestions about how to deliver the best possible care. If needed, the victim may be transported to the trauma center or the trauma surgeon may walk the rural physician step-by-step through a life-saving procedure.

Besides delivering critical care services to remote locations, telemedicine is also used to expand the ability of physicians to work with clients though not physically present in their rooms. Some physicians have begun using robotic devices to make hospital rounds. Basic robotic equipment includes a two-way video feed, microphone, speaker, and bay that enables stethoscope use. The robot and the physician's laptop are connected to the internet using a secure wireless network. The physician uses a joystick to guide the robot to perform a physical assessment as if the physician were actually in the client's room. The physician can also use the robot to monitor critically ill clients several times daily. Using the robot's video and audio capabilities, clients and physicians can engage in conversation as if they were in the same room together (Wilke, 2007).

Telehealth

Telehealth, although sometimes used interchangeably with telemedicine, refers to the actual use of technology for disease diagnosis and treatment of a patient at a remote location by a physician. Telenursing refers to nursing care delivered to a client at a remote site. Today, a comprehensive telehealth system enables clients to interact in real time with health care providers using computer connections. In the process known as "store forward," images, photographs, and client records become digitized for transmission from one location to another (Thede, 1999). With telehealth, health care professionals working in remote locations can participate in continuing education programs that occur in large urban health centers. They also can receive step-by-step instructions from specialists in how to perform complex life-saving procedures.

Telemonitoring

Telemonitoring is another use of technology that allows for client data to be transmitted to health care providers. The earliest use of telemonitoring was when clients with pacemakers sent information to cardiology offices using the telephone.

Telemonitoring systems consist of a video camera, monitor, thermometer, blood pressure cuff, and stethoscope. The nurse calls the client to connect to the system and receives real-time images; data that can be stored electronically. This system provides client access to a home health nurse on a 24-hour basis (Institute of Medicine, 2012).

Telemonitoring also occurs in inpatient settings. The electronic intensive care unit (EICU) offers continuous remote monitoring and medical services for people in the intensive care unit (ICU). The EICU team is typically composed of a critical care physician and at least one critical care registered nurse who use telecommunication to provide additional monitoring of patients occupying ICU beds. The ICU staff can consult the EICU physician simply by picking up a special phone. In-room video cameras allow the nurse to send real-time video surveillance to the physician. The EICU team also contacts the critical care nurses when they notice a change in a monitored client and order early interventions. Remote monitoring improves critical care patient outcomes in addition to lengthening the career spans of ICU nurses and physicians (Loustau, 2007).

Some home health organizations offer clients the option of having a video or web camera along with monitoring devices (e.g., telemetry, blood pressure monitor, fetal heart monitor). Using a high-speed internet connection, the home health nurse and the client hold a video conference with each other. If the conference reveals no problems, the nurse does not have to make a home visit. However, if a client fails to contact the agency at the specified time or if the nurse determines during the conference that the client needs to be seen in person, the nurse makes arrangements to go see the client.

With consumer use of smart phones and computer tablets, telemonitoring using applications (apps) has emerged as a new way to manage chronic diseases. In an analysis of nine randomized control clinical trials, Whitehead and Seaton (2016) identified that some persons with chronic illnesses (diabetes mellitus, chronic lung disease, and coronary artery disease) had improved symptom control, fewer hospitalizations, reduced outpatient medical care visits and increased compliance to disease management regimens. Using Bluetooth© technology, patients could either manually record or use direct links for data to be uploaded and shared with health care providers using wireless technology. The studies reviewed also identified that patient compliance to data entry were improved for morning (70% to 75%) data transfer compared to evening data transfers (50% to 56%). Most study participants used the devices more readily when the apps were combined with either an instant message or phone call from a health care provider.

Advantages to using apps for managing health care conditions includes acceptance by persons who use either a smartphone or tablet on a daily basis, reducing consumer time for travel to and from provider office visits, and increased patient assurance that their data are constantly monitored. Costs for remote monitoring devices make the use of this technology prohibitive unless the costs are covered by a third-party payer (government or private health insurance provider). The cost for a wireless connection and fees for data transfer rest with the consumer. When this technology is used by consumers, then the health care provider incurs costs for personnel used to monitor incoming data, notifying clients as to what actions must be taken (should abnormal data be received), providing some form of acknowledgment of data receipt and sending messages or calling clients complimenting them on using the devices. Because the technology is new, more research is needed to discover the most appropriate use of this technology (Whitehead & Seaton, 2016).

Take Note!
Informatics nurses and clinical specialists develop and improve telemedicine, telehealth, and telemonitoring systems (Ozboltz et al., 2007).

EDUCATIONAL INFORMATICS

Educational informatics provides students, health care professionals, and clients with access to information. Health care professionals can earn continuing education credit by completing online courses. Nursing and other health care students have access to online collegiate courses. Students can choose from courses that are either synchronous (faculty and students meet online at the same time for classes) or asynchronous (students access course information at their own convenience).

Most programs use clinical simulations as a means to standardize student exposure to specific clinical situations without the fear of actually harming another person. The clinical simulation starts with the student preparation using media to learn about the client, the health issues being covered, and specific skills required to manage the case study that will occur in the simulation lab. The client may be a high fidelity mannequin loaded with software that makes it act like a real person, or an actor (or actress) may assume the role of the client. Simulations may be interdisciplinary in nature and offer students of all health professions opportunities to interact with each other or they may occur within the confines of the nursing program; students and/or faculty then assume the roles of other interprofessional team members. Documentation during the clinical scenario may occur on virtual client EHRs. The simulated experience may be simple or complex depending upon the level of the student. When a clinical simulation is used, all nursing students within a nursing program receive exposure to a common clinical practice situation (such as a birth or death), gain experience in clinical decision making (without harming anyone), and perform specific clinical nursing skills (Jeffries & Clochesy, 2012).

The use of high fidelity simulation may be used for formative (building student clinical skills, developing clinical decision making, and learning how to interact with others as a health care team) or evaluative (assessing student outcomes for skill attainment, clinical decision making, specific elements of the nurse–client relationship, and interprofessional team communication). Some health care facilities are using high fidelity simulations for orienting new graduate nurses, improving interprofessional team performance in client crisis situations (such as rapid responses and codes), skill building with newly acquired equipment for health care delivery, and facilitating team building among members of the interprofessional health care team.

Online Learning

Access to distance education is available to anyone with a high-speed connection to the internet—perhaps the course in which you are using this text is taught online. Each institution specifies required hardware and software for online courses, and many have vendor contracts for student discounts. Students can confirm with the program's information technology expert to verify that they have all required resources to access and run the learning platform, access student e-mail, and download required course resources. Many online education programs provide students with a list of all technologic resources required for optimal use of online learning platforms.

In addition to having the technologic resources needed (e.g., high-speed internet access, appropriate hardware and software), students must have the skills for success and verify the quality of education being offered before they enroll in an online course (see Box 14.3, Learning, Knowing, and Growing, "Is An Online Course the Best Choice?"). A self-assessment can reveal whether a student has the ability to connect to the class, engage in online class discussions, download complex documents, manage files, and access help. A student should ask questions related to available technical assistance and have a backup plan in place should technologic problems occur (Billings & Halstead, 2012; Mueller & Billings, 2000; Short, 2000). Some nursing programs may offer backup computers to students.

A key benefit of asynchronous online courses is the student's ability to develop an individually tailored class schedule, which is especially important to students juggling multiple roles. Access to 24/7 technical support

services enables students to meet program requirements based on their individual needs (Friesth, 2012; Short, 2000). Some programs offer hybrid courses that blend online learning with face-to-face classroom instruction.

Learning activities associated with online and hybrid courses include faculty-developed online lectures, podcasts, self-pace learning modules, online discussions, online exams and quizzes, and synchronous or asynchronous chats (Friesth, 2012; Halstead & Billings, 2012). The goal of online instruction is to promote student learning and professional growth. With effective faculty facilitation, learning communities can form and flourish (Halstead & Billings, 2012). Students can form online collegial relationships and friendships and engage in interactive problem-solving. In hybrid courses, students learn the key concepts and concepts surrounding a course topic and class time is spent in interactive learning activities such as solving a case study.

Educational informatics also enables practicing nurses to access continuing education programs at any time of the day. Some professional nursing associations offer online continuing education programs to nonmembers (for a fee) and their members (free or reduced cost). Some hospitals use online educational vendors (e.g., HealthStream®, eLeaP®) or their own educational platform to offer employees programs for meeting annual continuing education and competency requirements (privacy; infection control; fire, radiation, and electrical safety; age-related developmental care strategies; and domestic abuse).

Most colleges have a detailed website that contains useful student information. Students can obtain registration information and register online for courses, view student policies and faculty and staff information, and obtain financial aid information, class schedules, and a list of required textbooks for courses. Along with their websites, institutions that offer online and hybrid courses have an electronic learning management system. In the learning management system, faculty post course syllabi, online weekly lessons that outline required learning activities, course resources, and grades for exams and assignments. When learning management systems are used, there is 24-hour, 7-day a week help available to students. Students typically are required to have computer systems that have the hardware and software to use the learning management system effectively. Many colleges offer students the ability to purchase computers with all the required features. Some colleges even offer backup computers for student use in the event that a student computer ceases to function properly.

14.3 Learning, Knowing, and Growing

Is an Online Course the Best Choice?

Although online courses can offer many advantages over in-person learning, it is imperative for students to gauge the quality of the course and understand how they learn best *before* enrolling.

The Course

Asking questions about course content, the number of times the course has been offered online, and faculty experience with online education can provide clues about the quality of the instruction. In addition, the following five factors are usually good indicators of a high-quality online course: (1) reasonable faculty electronic office hours, (2) online library resources, (3) alternative ways to interact with student colleagues beyond e-mail, (4) secure online examinations, and (5) course content that balances passive lecture with interactive teaching techniques (Short, 2000).

The Student

Some students may not learn effectively in a virtual setting. The isolation of home study may impede learning for students who rely heavily on peer contact. Likewise, people who need structure and strict deadlines to complete course requirements do not fare well with online education (Short, 2000). Because most faculty–student and student–student interactions occur in written format in online courses, students with poorly developed writing skills may find such courses too burdensome (Mueller & Billings, 2000). Some students perceive that because they determine the time of instruction, online courses require less work than live courses, only to be surprised by the actual time commitment involved.

Through social networking, students can connect with other students in similar educational situations or with the same major. Students can check with other students to identify a tutor, participate in a study group, form a carpool, broadcast classes, serve as or find a student mentor, and establish social support groups (Skiba, 2007). Social networking can be done using online networking tools, accessing a professional nursing organization's website, or employing a discussion board feature found on many online learning platforms (e.g., Blackboard, Web CT, Angel). Faculty must set clear guidelines for online student discussion. For example, a faculty member may use the Oncology Nursing Society's networking feature for nursing students to share thoughts and feelings about working with oncology clients. In this case, a student from another nursing program may also enter into the discussion.

Although popular with young students, online discussions using Facebook, Twitter, or other social media have some disadvantages. It is almost impossible to remove information from the internet once it has appeared there, whether through a blog, Facebook, Twitter, or other means. Everything posted can likely be read by almost anyone, even future employers, and may "live" on in the electronic world long after you believe it has been deleted. Any person who posts things online may have to assume legal responsibility for the posting (Skiba, 2007). The National State Boards of Nursing (2011) have developed *Social Media Guidelines for Nurses*. The guidelines specify that nurses are legally accountable for any patient identifiable information posted on social media. Breaches of patient protected health information may result in formal actions by a state board of nursing against a nurse's professional license (warning, suspension, or revocation). The nurse may also be subject to legal action by a patient or patient's family for posting anything that can link a patient to a social media posting.

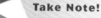

Take Note!

Social networking offers an opportunity for nursing students at all levels to connect with one other.

TECHNOLOGY IN THE ACUTE CARE CLINICAL SETTING

Effects of Technology on Direct Client Care

Technology has revolutionized client care delivery. Nurses use a variety of technologic tools in clinical

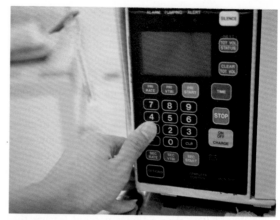

FIGURE 14.3 Nurses use technologic devices when providing patient care on a daily basis in clinical practice.

practice (Fig. 14.3). For client assessment, nurses use bedside and handheld monitors to collect a variety of information, including blood glucose level, clotting time, electrocardiograph rhythm, cardiac output, blood pressure, oxygen saturation of hemoglobin, and temperature. Some monitoring systems require that the client be physically connected to the device, and others require a drop or two of blood. Point-of-care testing enables nurses to receive instantaneous results for peripheral blood glucose levels for diabetics and activated clotting time for clients receiving anticoagulation therapy. Client monitoring systems that use wireless technology enable automatic nurse-paging capability when client measurements fall outside normal parameters. Pressure sensor monitors on beds also alert nurses when clients at risk for falling make maneuvers indicating that they may be getting out of bed.

Nurses also use technology for nursing interventions. Most intravenous pumps contain microprocessors for effective operation. Computerized pumps enable nurses to program administration rates for ordered medications without having to perform manual calculations. The pumps are also programmed for safe dosage limits over a specified time frame and have features for nurses to start infusions after hanging IV fluids or medications. Pumps with complex features enable nurses to program an infusion of multiple medications for specific timeframes and schedules. All pumps contain alarms to warn nurses that the pump needs attention.

Many other nursing care devices use computer technology as well. Even some air mattresses use computer components and software to regulate the amount of air inflation. Implantable subcutaneous pumps deliver local anesthetic along surgical incisions and have the technology to regulate the rate of subcutaneous drug administration. Some diabetics use computer-pro-grammed pumps for insulin administration.

Computerized documentation eliminates the need for nurses to shuffle through paper records. Nurses spend approximately 20% of their time documenting information on EHRs, which is about the same amount of time they spend in handwritten documentation systems (Yee et al., 2012). However, nearly instantaneous diagnostic test and assessment findings become available to the entire interprofessional team as soon as the data are entered into the computerized system. With wireless technology and highly integrated wired information systems, radiologists can access digital x-rays and then dictate their findings without leaving their homes.

Computers can also be used to plan client care. Many health care institutions provide software that enables nurses to enter care plans by selecting a specific nursing diagnosis. The software provides the nurse with appropriate expected outcomes and nursing interventions related to the identified nursing diagnosis. Software programs can also organize client care, store clinical forms, and house teaching protocol information. Some programs have the capability of translating client education materials into multiple languages.

Computerized medication-dispensing stations prevent nurses from making medication errors while automatically notifying the pharmacy when the stocked medications need to be replenished. These devices facilitate the work of nurses, especially when mounted on bases that enable mobility. Portable medication stations equipped with barcoding devices require that nurses scan client identification bracelets and medication prior to medication administration. This safety feature facilitates following the "5 rights": (right medication, right dose, right route, right patient, and right time) of medication administration, thereby reducing potentially costly errors. Successful implementation of computerized medication-dispensing stations relies on the system's ability to be user friendly, efficient, and well supplied. Some computerized stations offer information about the therapeutic action, pharmacokinetics, adverse effects, and incompatibilities of medications in device software. More sophisticated models offer features such as warning signs for potential drug interactions that require communication between physicians and pharmacists before dispensing medications (Hurley et al., 2007). Some even require biometric identification of users such as fingerprinting.

Nurses and other health care providers have access to computerized clinical decision-making support systems. Decision-making support systems help nurses define clinical problems, generate potential solutions, and select the best solution based on the likelihood of success. Many decision-making models use spreadsheets with formulae to predict the results of specific actions in a given client care situation (Thede, 2003). Nurses also have access to decision-making algorithms when clinical practice guidelines and procedures have been entered into computer systems.

Effects of Technology on Client Education

Going online enables consumers to use interactive educational materials and self-manage illnesses and health. Interactive websites may be sponsored by proprietary companies or nonprofit organizations. Some hospitals and integrated health care systems offer online educational materials to the public. For example, a woman diagnosed with early-stage breast cancer can visit the American Cancer Society to learn about her treatment options, view information about breast cancer from the National Institutes of Health and the National Library of Medicine, and view actual surgical procedures and radiation devices on the websites of medical centers, university-based cancer centers, and drug and device manufacturers. Sometimes clients may have more information about recent advances in the management of a particular disease than the health care provider, especially if the client has a rare medical condition. Access to comprehensive, detailed online information may result in client self-diagnosis and treatment based on information found online that may or may not be accurate or comprehensive.

Blogs and social networking sites such as Twitter and Facebook also offer consumers health-related information as well as links to others with a particular health problem. Often, health information accessed through blogs or other online resources has not been empirically tested and may even be harmful for consumers.

Effects of Technology on the Nursing Professional

Some nurses use computer tablets or handheld devices whose programs or apps enable the nurse to access current information, record self-reminders, set alarms, and perform clinical calculations without having to leave the bedside. The more sophisticated information systems enable nurses to record client care information onto the device and then place the device into a docking station or transmit the information wirelessly into the client's EHR. However, clients or families have reported incidents of nurses using handheld devices for personal use, such as checking e-mail or texting, while providing care.

When nurses connect their devices to a hospital's wireless system or use the hospital's internet network, the hospital can monitor and track all online activity. In some cases, nurses have been dismissed because they used their handheld devices for personal rather than professional reasons when on the job. Some hospitals have opted to ban nurse use of all personal handheld devices while in the clinical setting.

Some institutions make clinical practice guidelines and employee policies available on their intranets for ease of employee access.

Nurses frequently access institutional e-mail accounts to stay abreast of organizational news, receive policy updates, and access minutes of staff meetings. Most professional nursing organizations send e-mail messages to members routinely to inform them of new developments in clinical practice, organizational elections, and legislative issues.

Computer software is also used for staffing nursing units and making daily staff assignments. Programs can be used to determine the number of direct client care hours that are needed based on client acuity levels. Some staffing software allows nurses to look online for vacant shifts that fall outside their established schedules and then sign up to work those shifts. By allowing regular employees to sign up for extra shifts, overtime and the use of agency nurses have declined (Ellerbee, 2007).

Record Keeping and Documentation of Care Outcomes

Computer information systems enable nurses "to collect, process, store, retrieve, and display data and information" (Orlygsdottir, 2007, p. 283). When computer information systems include Nursing Minimum Data Set (NMDS) components, nursing care documentation encompasses all phases of the nursing process used by nurses in practice. As these phases are included in clinical documentation systems, the potential to report and merge client care information into a large multi-institutional database becomes possible. Thus, a large database may become available for use in nursing research studies and to compare the effects of nursing care across institutions and health care settings. In the United States, the NMDS includes information about patient demographics (personal identification, birth date, gender, ethnicity, and residence), nursing care elements (care intensity, nursing diagnoses, interventions, and outcomes), and service components (unique agency code, client health record, admission dismissal or termination dates, client disposition when leaving the facility, and expected bill payer). In contrast, the Nursing Management Minimum Data Set compiles data regarding nursing management decisions and actions across all settings. Establishment of a large database enables the nursing profession to develop best practices based on client outcomes.

Communication

The use of cell phones and smart phones reduces the time spent by health care professionals in trying to reach each other and decreases the need for overhead paging, which can disrupt client rest. Physicians can call nurses directly. Cell phones enable staff members to inform each other of specific events or assistance needs. Some nurses provide assigned clients with the cell phone number for direct communication.

E-mail also can be used to send messages about patients to physician's offices or inform staff of continuing education opportunities, special institutional events, and personal messages. Clients can be notified about health care appointments via e-mail and can e-mail questions to their health care providers. Because of the confidentiality of health-related information, e-mail message information about clients must be encrypted (digitally electronic coded). Encryption keeps personal health information private and accessible only to those directly involved in the client's care.

Protecting client identity in outpatient waiting rooms and hospital admission departments poses a challenge to health care providers. The use of technology fosters the protection of clients' personal identities in waiting rooms. Some facilities give clients a beeper, cell phone, or lighted handheld device that goes off when it is time to receive care. However, these devices can sometimes create confusion for elderly clients seeking health care services.

TECHNOLOGIC CHANGES AFFECTING NURSING PRACTICE AND HEALTH CARE

Robotics

In the future, some nursing tasks may be safely accomplished by machines. **Robotics** is the designing of machines to perform tasks usually done by humans. Pharmacy robots are currently used to perform mundane tasks associated with preparing and dispensing medications. As described earlier, robots equipped with video and audio capabilities allow nurses and physicians to see, hear, and talk to clients and staff even when not physically present. Some nursing tasks performed by robots (nursing bots) include meal tray delivery, filling water pitchers, making routine rounds, and taking vital signs (Jossi, 2004). Increasingly, surgery and other invasive procedures are being performed by robots because robots have better dexterity and eliminate human error when performing delicate procedures. Nevertheless, for the robots to perform, they must be controlled by an experienced physician. The use of robotics increases access to sophisticated procedures for people living in rural areas. Surgeons have the capability of controlling a robot in an urban medical center while the procedure is performed by the robot in a local hospital. The use of robots decreases surgical costs when clients who need specialized surgery no longer need to travel to a large metropolitan medical center to undergo the procedure (Jossi, 2004; Yuh, 2013). In some surgical cases, robotic surgery is less invasive, thereby resulting in less recovery time, reduced length of inpatient care, and smaller incisions.

Genomic Medicine

For many years, health care providers have relied on a client's family health history for understanding and predicting many disease processes. A **family health history** tracks incidences of illnesses that have occurred in people who share ancestors. Ideally, three generations worth of data should be collected.

Advances in genetics have transformed health care delivery. **Genomic medicine** applies knowledge generated from the human genome to develop new medical treatments and determine specific regimens for clients based on their particular human genetic sequence. Initial publicized findings of the Human Genome Project revealed that humans have approximately 34,000 genes and that the genetic makeup of all people is 99.5% identical. However, the 34,000 genes have the capability to make between 500,000 and 1 million proteins. This indicates that genes do not cause disease, but proteins do. Implications for disease screening and therapy most likely lie with the study of proteomics (human proteins). Diseases with verified or potential genetic links include some cancers (ovarian, breast, lung, and colon), mental illnesses (depression, schizophrenia, chemical addiction, and bipolar disease), birth defects (neural tube defects), preterm birth, obesity, type I and type II diabetes, cardiovascular disease, hypercholesterolemia, chronic sinusitis, immune deficiency disorders (X-linked combined immune deficiency), and neurologic diseases (Huntington chorea, Alzheimer disease,

multiple sclerosis) (Califano, Landi, & Cappuzzo, 2012; Calzone, Jenkins, Culp, Caskey, & Badzek, 2014; Check & Rodgers, 2001; Conley & Tinkle, 2007; Dolan, Biermann, & Damus 2007; Holden, 2003; Spiegel & Hawkins, 2012) (Genetic screening and genetic-based therapies have transformed many disease screening and treatment protocols) (Conley & Tinkle, 2007; Spiegel & Hawkins, 2012) (see Concepts in Practice, "It is in Your Genes").

Concepts in Practice [IDEA]──▸[PLAN]─▸[ACTION]

It is in Your Genes

Genetic differences in metabolism explain variations in therapeutic responses of medications based on ancestral heritage (Holden, 2003; Marshall, 2003b). Genetic differences have been identified to explain the lack of effectiveness of angiotensin-converting enzyme inhibitors in controlling blood pressure in some people of African descent. People from India have survived famines that resulted in a "thrifty gene" presentation in approximately one third of the Indian population. This gene is linked to the development of hypercholesterolemia when Indians westernize their diets (Holden, 2003). Risky genes have been identified in people who experience long QT syndrome after receiving specific medications (Marshall, 2003a). Twenty medications have warning labels specifying that fatal reactions may occur in people with inherited metabolism disorders (Conley & Tinkle, 2007; Calzone et al., 2014; Marshall, 2003b).

Genetic testing of malignant tumors is now commonplace and is used to help tailor treatment plans. Cancer is the disease where the most progress has been made for individualization of treatment plans. Progress on being able to develop individualized health promotion, disease prevention, and individualized therapies for all diseases is taking much longer than originally anticipated after sequencing of the human genome was completed (Califano et al., 2012; Calzone et al., 2014; Spiegel & Hawkins, 2012). Eventually, physicians may be able to send a genetic sample from a patient and receive a medication plan tailored to the patient's genotype, resulting in better disease management. Newborns may be genetically tested and receive a lifetime plan (including when to begin taking medications designed for their genotypes) to prevent illness (Spiegel & Hawkins, 2012; Stone, 2001).

Genetic testing may be offered to people at risk for a particular illness (Fig. 14.4). However, personal

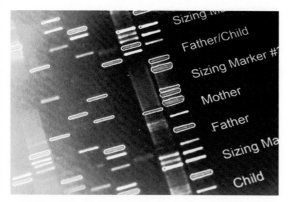

FIGURE 14.4 Genetic and genomic testing enable providers and consumers to make scientifically based decisions related to health promotion, early screenings, disease prevention, and tailored treatment plans for individuals.

behaviors and environmental factors also play a role in disease development. Once a genetic predisposition to an illness within a family is identified, the professional nurse sometimes becomes a resource for how to tell other family members they are at risk (Giarelli & Jacobs, 2001). In 2003 the cost of testing for a single gene that affects drug metabolism or identifying a person at risk for a particular disease ranges from $100 to $1,000 (Marshall, 2003b). Persons can now get genetic testing for ancestry for $99 (Ancestry.com, 2016) and a company known as "23 and Me Inc" provides genetic testing for individuals (23 and Me, 2016). Although clients can undergo genetic testing, they may not fully comprehend the meaning and implications of results and nurses play a key role in verifying client understanding of results, reinforcing information about treatment options and providing emotional support (Barnoy, Apel, Peretz, Meiraz, & Ehrenfeld, 2006; Calzone et al., 2014). Nurses who specialize in genetic counseling are frequently employed in health care facilities where genetic testing is frequently performed. In these settings, nurses provide clients with detailed information about the implications of positive and negative genetic tests.

In 2006, the National Coalition for Health Professional Education in Genetics established a list of essential professional nurse competencies in genetics. Jenkins and Calzone (2007, p. 13) presented the nurse's essential responsibilities with regard to genetic science.

1. Acknowledge when one's personal values and attitudes about genetics and genomic science could affect client care.
2. Advocate for client access to genetic/genomic services and support groups upon request.
3. Analyze personal competency with genomics and genetic science and seek additional education if needed.

4. Include genetics and genomic science as part of routine professional practice.
5. Tailor client education on genetics and genomic science to the client's culture, religious beliefs, literacy level, and preferred language.
6. Advocate for clients as they make autonomous, voluntary, and informed choices regarding genetic testing and genomic interventions.

Jenkins and Calzone (2007) also outlined the nurse's clinical practice competencies related to genetic science.

1. Displays an "understanding of the relationships of genetics and genomics to health prevention, screening, diagnostics, prognostics, selection of treatment, and monitoring of treatment effects" (p. 13).
2. Collects client family history for a minimum of three generations.
3. Uses standardized symbols and terms to construct a pedigree from a client's family history.
4. Assesses client's personal, health, and developmental histories inclusive of genetic, environmental, and genomic risks and influences on health status.
5. Analyzes health and physical assessment data for the presence of genetic, environmental, and genomic risks and influence on health status.
6. "Assesses clients' knowledge, perceptions, and responses to genetic and genomic in formation" (p. 13).
7. Creates a nursing care plan that considers genetic and genomic assessment findings.

Nurses can play a key role in shaping public policy regarding access to genetic testing and therapies for all people. Nurses also need to build knowledge for evidence-based practice so that effective public and client education about genomics and proteomics (the study of human proteins) can be implemented. Finally, nurses must collaborate with interprofessional team members to evaluate the effectiveness of advances in health care based on new genetic and protein information.

Take Note!

Technologic advances in health care diagnostics and treatment are changing the ways in which nurses will treat clients.

CHALLENGES IN MANAGING HEALTH-RELATED INFORMATICS AND TECHNOLOGY

The rapid introduction of **technology in clinical practice** provides a challenge to professional nurses. Just as a nurse becomes competent and confident with a new piece of patient care equipment, it seems the medical device manufacturers introduce a newer version. Although new generations of client care equipment usually contain features that increase accuracy or efficiency, some nurses find it challenging to adapt to constantly changing equipment.

The vast amount of available health-related information also creates challenges for health care professionals and consumers alike. The ever-increasing use of technology and computers in health care makes it imperative that professional nurses ensure ethical use of protected health information, determine the quality of health information for use in practice, maintain data security, and struggle to stay abreast of new developments.

Confidentiality

To protect people from discrimination based on genetic testing, the United States provided legal protection through the Genetic Confidentiality and Nondiscriminatory Act of 1997. When medical and pharmaceutical research centers use biologic material and data to develop new therapies for illnesses, the donors of human tissue and cells have a right to privacy. Nevertheless, pharmaceutical companies and research centers retain the right to ownership of discoveries from human-extracted materials (Lee, 2012).

The Health Insurance Portability and Accountability Act (HIPAA) mandates confidentiality of client medical records and certain information shared with insurance companies, physicians, hospitals, and other health care providers. Access to private health information (PHI) is limited either to people who are directly involved in the client's care or to people designated by the client (Huchenski, 2001). HIPAA requires health care organizations to offer education about PHI to all employees and that employees review PHI policies annually. Initial education about HIPAA occurs before employees (and nursing students) start working with clients in clinical setting. Content for HIPAA education includes a definition of PHI, strategies to protect PHI, legal use of PHI, and consequences for misuse of PHI.

Documented consent from the health care consumer is required before health care providers can disclose PHI to anyone not involved directly in the client's care (including family members). HIPAA provides health care consumers with the following four rights: (1) to receive written notice related to PHI storage and use changes before they are implemented, (2) to access and view one's health information, (3) to obtain an account of how PHI has been disclosed, and (4) to request a correction or amendment to PHI. Violators may be fined $25,000 to $250,000 and imprisoned for up to 10 years. Most health care providing organizations employ privacy officers to protect PHI (Huchenski, 2001). Some terminate employees for accessing the PHI of anyone who is not under their direct care.

Health care organizations take extreme care to ensure confidentiality of their client's PHI. Computer screens, fax machines, and even boards containing client names are placed in locations accessible only to health care providers. All e-mail messages containing PHI must be encrypted.

Health care institutions that use EHRs protect private data with passwords and firewalls. Many health care providers sign binding confidentiality agreements. Most health care organizations have departments devoted to information management that set policies for computer access and for managing violations of computer security policies.

Although telecommunication has greatly improved over the years, no connection offers complete security and information can be lost in cyberspace, or "broken into" by computer hackers. Computer hackers anywhere in the world have the capability of infiltrating any system containing private and personal information. Transmission of private medical data to an outside computer or server provides an opportunity for it to be viewed by unauthorized people (Foster, 2001; Thede, 2003).

Ethics and Technology

Ethical debates regarding new technology in health care are common. For example, stem cell therapy triggers debate about the definition of the beginning of human life (Does life begin at conception or when the fetus becomes viable?). Other ethical issues surround the cost of procedures and access to services. If insurance companies do not cover the cost (e.g., of storing umbilical cord stem cells or using genetically designed medications), then only people with adequate financial resources can reap the benefits of such technology (Korhonen, Nordman, & Eriksson, 2015). The Affordable Care Act will not be able to cover every complex, expensive medical, or surgical intervention. Health care consumers with ample resources will be able to pay for expensive therapies and may be able to access care services more readily. Thus, in the future, disparities over the quality of health care for the rich and poor may become more apparent (Korhonen et al., 2015).

Data Security

The potential loss of data (e.g., through hardware failures and system programming errors) is the biggest concern when using individual PEHRs. Data may be lost through the processes of acquisition, storage, and processing. PEHRs can be stored on personal computers, compact disks, on insurance company servers, or on private servers. Routine data backups and off-site storage protect information against natural disasters for health care institutions (Thede, 2003). Long-term storage of computerized data may be unstable. Recent observations indicate that data stored on CD-ROMs may begin to disintegrate after 5 years. Files and disks can become corrupt at any time (Korhonen et al., 2015; Thede, 2003).

Computer systems rely on quality information entry by humans. Bad information input results in poor use of technology. Computers cannot detect many of these errors, even though they are capable of performing complex mathematical operations and providing algorithms for complicated decision making (Thede, 2003). Finally, computers rely on a power source (electricity or battery) to work. When the power source is severed, the computer stops. During a power failure, most health care organizations have backup processes that use paper copies of documents so that client care can be seamlessly delivered. Once power is restored, paper documents are scanned and electronically stored.

The Struggle to Stay Abreast of New Technologies

The success of high-technology client care devices depends on the ability of the nurse (or consumer) to operate them. If a device is shown to promote client comfort or save time, nurses tend to adopt it readily. New devices are more readily accepted by nurses if nurses participate in making the decision to use them.

One of the disadvantages of high-tech care is the inclination of nurses to focus on the machinery rather than clients. Sometimes, nurses attend to machine alarms before observing clients. This practice may result in a nurse being perceived as cold or aloof.

Recent predictions suggest that information and technologic advancements will expand exponentially over the next 5 years (Kaku, 2011). With the vast amount of information required for effective client care, professional nurses frequently experience

information overload. To provide effective client care, nurses must stay abreast of new developments in health care information and technology, be willing to admit knowledge deficits, consult others when uncertain, and stay focused on the ever-increasing importance of authentic therapeutic relationships with clients and their significant others.

Take Note!
No machine can replace the warmth of a genuine, caring human interaction.

Accessing Information

The U.S. armed forces started the internet, which now has become the largest global computer network, in the late 1960s. The internet is a worldwide computer network that uses digitalized transmission of information. Information is shared by a network of collected websites that use the hypertext transfer protocol for communication. All web addresses use the same letters and symbols to begin their address (http://and https://), which is automatically inserted when a computer user enters a website address (Thede, 2003). To access the internet, people need an internet service provider that provides a server (a large computer linked to other computers to share information and provide services). E-mail is a mainstay of internet communication, while Facebook and Twitter enable anyone to share life events and personal views on current events and politics. Pinterest is another site that connects persons with common interests. However, internet users must be aware that absolutely anything can be posted on social media sites.

A website is a collection of pages posted on the internet (Akens, 1999). A home page is the beginning point of a website, where a browser enters the site and usually views content within the website. Most home pages contain text, graphics, sound, animation, and other interactive features (Akens, 1999). In the United States, the following six domains are commonly used to designate the type of server that hosts a website: (1) commercial = .com; (2) educational = .edu; (3) network = .net; (4) nonprofit organization = .org; (5) governmental = .gov; and (6) military = .mil (Thede, 2003). At this writing, the release of additional domains, including personalized domains, is planned.

Nurses can find internet sites through publishing guides, journal articles, and bibliographies. Millions of websites exist. Many have long lives, but some become obsolete when organizations merge or disband. Once a site has been found to be useful, the user can file it by using a bookmark or a list of favorites for easy access in the future.

Chat rooms and discussion boards connect people with similar interests. Information can be exchanged through synchronous or asynchronous postings. Many nursing programs use discussion boards for asynchronous communication and chat rooms for synchronous discussion. Some professional nursing organizations offer discussion boards and chat rooms, but require users to register and log in before posting entries. When posting information on a discussion board (or forum), a good rule to follow is not to post information that you would not want broadcasted on a televised news show.

Balancing Technology with Life

For some people, computers and smartphones can become an impediment to leading a balanced life. The purchase of each new device as soon as it becomes available serves as a status symbol for some people, but it may be a sign of an addiction to technology. Some people (including nurses) have become addicted to computer technology and spend hours on computers or handheld devices, participating in chat rooms, surfing the internet, shopping, tweeting, and playing games. Small handheld devices enable people to be constantly connected to the internet or to the job. Using technology may also serve as an excuse for not interacting personally with other people. Box 14.4, Professional Building Blocks, "Criteria for Internet Addiction," presents proposed criteria from Chinese and American researchers for identifying persons with **internet addiction**.

Some people rely heavily on cell phones. Having nearly instantaneous information related to medical emergencies and community health hazards enables nurses (especially those working in emergency departments or community health settings) to act swiftly, save lives, and prepare for victims of a disaster. However, the need to respond to them immediately sometimes impedes a person's ability to engage in deep, meaningful, face-to-face conversations. In addition, some people assume that because a nurse is issued a pager or an e-mail account in the workplace, he or she is available 24 hours a day, 7 days a week. Nurses need to have time away from their work setting and technology to cultivate personal relationships and outside interests.

Conversely, computers and other handheld technologic devices can enhance interpersonal relationships

14.4 Professional Building Blocks

Criteria for Internet Addiction

Current estimates of internet addiction range from 1% to 14% of the population (Tao et al., 2010). A person is considered to have an internet addiction if he or she meets criteria 1 and 2 plus one additional criterion.

1. **Preoccupation with the internet:** The internet becomes the dominant daily life activity. The user has a constant strong desire to use the internet, thinks about previous activity, and anxiously anticipates the next session.
2. **Withdrawal:** The user experiences dysphoric mood, anger, anxiety, irritability, or boredom if he or she does not use the internet for several days.
3. **Tolerance:** More internet use is required to achieve personal satisfaction.
4. **Use is difficult to control:** Efforts to cut back on use are futile.
5. **Disregard for harmful consequences of excessive use:** Internet users ignore personal, physical, or psychological needs, lose their job, or rack up high expenses online.
6. **Loss of social communications and interests**
7. **Emotional outlet:** Use of internet to alleviate negative emotions and a link is made that internet use results in feeling better emotionally.
8. **Deception:** The user lies about the actual time and costs of internet use to family members, therapist, or significant others.

Flisher, C. (2010). Getting plugged in: An overview of internet addiction. *Journal of Pediatrics and Child Health, 46,* 557–559. doi: 01.1111/j.1440–1754.2010.011879.x; Tao, R., Huang, Z., Wang, J., Zhang, H., Zhang, Y., & Li, M. (2010). Proposed diagnostic criteria for internet addiction. *Addiction, 105,* 556–564. doi:10.1111/j.1360–0443.2009.02828.x.

among professional colleagues, health team members, and families. Whitmore (2005) outlined etiquette for e-mail use and coined the term "netiquette" (Table 14.3).

▮ QUESTIONS FOR REFLECTION

1. How do you balance high tech with high touch in your personal life? In your professional life?
2. Why is it important to strike a balance between high tech and high touch in client care?
3. Why is it important to strike a balance between technology and other aspects of your personal life?

TABLE 14.3   E-mail "Netiquette"

Technique	Rationale
State the main reasons for the message in the subject line area.	Recipients can prioritize e-mail messages.
Consider e-mail messages as business letters.	E-mail has become a formal communication medium in business.
Use proper grammar and avoid using all uppercase letters.	E-mail is a means of professional communication, and using uppercase letters is known as "cyber shouting."
Avoid use of fancy or cute decorations.	This distracts the recipient's attention from message content.
Keep messages succinct but not abrupt.	Avoid being perceived as being rude when sending a message.
Treat e-mail as a public document.	Recipients can forward, print, or photocopy any message, and messages can be retrieved from computers.
Wait until anger passes before sending an e-mail message.	Strongly emotional messages can easily be misinterpreted because of the lack of body language and voice characteristics. Also, there is no opportunity to immediately clarify should a misunderstanding occur.
Praise people in person, or send them a handwritten note.	People usually cherish handwritten notes or greeting cards, and these forms of communication are more likely to be appreciated and saved.
Proof messages before sending them.	Use of automated correction devices for spelling or grammar may not always be accurate, especially when potential homonyms are used within a message.
Use the "Reply to All" feature only when everyone on the list requires a response.	This limits the number of e-mails sent and received, thereby increasing productivity.
Avoid sending multiple messages if the recipient fails to respond within your expected time frame.	If something is that urgent, contact people via phone or stop by their office. Some people check e-mail only once daily or less.
Respond as quickly as possible, especially to messages that are flagged as urgent.	Courtesy goes a long way in the work environment, especially when deadlines for responses are required.
Send attachments only when necessary.	Consider what is actually needed to get business done.
Less is more.	Sometimes an entire message can be sent using only the subject line, but end the line with the letters EOM to indicate "end of message."
Mark messages to denote whether they are urgent or just FYI (for your information).	Recipients can prioritize messages.
Think twice before sending unsolicited advertisements or humorous messages.	What you think might be humorous may not be humorous to others, and some organizations may enforce strict e-mail usage policies.
Inform others when you are unavailable by using an out-of-office feature, and provide contact information if something occurs during your absence that needs your immediate attention.	Senders of messages will know of your unavailability and contact you only if absolutely necessary.

Information adapted from Whitmore, J. (2005). *Business class etiquette: Essentials for success at work.* New York: St. Martin's Press.

Summary and Significance to Practice

Nurses must have competence in managing complex technology and must stay abreast of new advances in health care delivery. Increased technology and information have the ability to improve health care by providing early disease detection, reducing errors, and facilitating optimal use of limited resources. However, increased use of technology may threaten the therapeutic and effective relationships that nurses build with others because of the loss of face-to-face human interactions.

Effective use of informatics and technology has become a critical clinical skill for nurses practicing in today's complex and chaotic world of health care delivery. However, nurses must use their cognitive skills to determine how to best incorporate and evaluate the use of new information and technology in clinical practice.

Nurses need to strike a balance in providing high-tech and high-touch client care while taking time to lead satisfying personal lives.

REAL-LIFE REFLECTIONS

Recall the conversation among Jorge, Susan, and Amy from the beginning of the chapter. Based on your current use of computers and technology in clinical practice, what information would you share if you were part of the discussion?

From Theory to Practice

1. Take time and think about how you have used a computerized documentation system while giving client care during a clinical experience. What parts of the system were easy to use? What parts of the system were difficult for you to use? How would you go about learning how to better use the parts of the system that you had difficulty using?
2. What do you feel are the advantages of using computers and technology in clinical practice for nurses and consumers? Why are these advantages? What do you feel are the disadvantages of using them in clinical practice for nurses and consumers? Why are these disadvantages?

Nurse as Author

1. Look around your clinical unit and make a list of all the technology that you use in daily clinical practice. Select one technologic device and write a 5- to 6-paragraph essay on how it facilitates patient care quality and safety, and identify any ethical issues that could be encountered when using the device for daily patient care. In your final paragraph, summarize the benefits and hazards of using the device and indicate any identified areas to improve the device for patient care delivery.
2. Watch the National Council of State Boards of Nursing video "Social Media Guidelines for Nurses" (**https://www.ncsbn.org/347.htm**). Write an essay about how you use social media and what (if any) of your current practices regarding posting information related to school or work may need to change. Write your reactions to the student nurse's and professional nurse's actions as presented in the video, and discuss the penalties imposed by the nursing program or health care institution. Address what you would do if you found one of your colleagues either posting specific information about a patient for whom they provided care, or posting something derogatory about a health care agency or nursing program.

Your Digital Classroom

Online Exploration

Alliance for Nursing Informatics: **http://allianceni.org/about.asp**

American Health Information Management Association: **www.ahima.org**

American Nurses Association Health IT Position & Initiatives: **http://www.nursingworld.org/ MainMenuCategories/ThePracticeofProfessional Nursing/Health-IT**

American Nursing Informatics Association: **www.ania.org**

Cancer Genome Anatomy Project: **http://cgap.nci.nih.gov/**

Daniel Kraft: Medicine's Future? There's an app for that: **https://www.ted.com/talks/daniel_kraft_ medicine_s_future?language=en**

National Institute of Health Human Genome Project Fact Sheet: **https://report.nih.gov/ NIHfactsheets/ViewFactSheet.aspx?csid=45**

International Society of Nurses in Genetics: **www.isong.org**

National Human Genome Research Institute: **www.genome.gov**

Expanding Your Understanding

1. Select a topic that interests you as a professional nurse, and search for it online. Identify a number of potential websites to visit. Select two or three of these websites and compare and contrast them in terms of the type of website, the fees required (if any) to use the site, when the site was last updated, and whether the information presented is credible.
2. Visit the online source for the Institute of Medicine's 2012 report *The role of telehealth in an evolving health care environment: Workshop Summary* at rep **www.nap.edu/catalog.php?record_id=13466**. Click on "READ THIS BOOK ONLINE FOR FREE!" Scroll through the book and read Chapter 9, Technological Developments. After reading this chapter, answer the following questions:
   a. What do you perceive as advantages and disadvantages with the following aspects of telehealth: remote patient monitoring, increased social networking with patients and health care providers, and access to wireless health services?
   b. Do you think that there might be a time when a client might receive only telehealth services? Why or why not?

Beyond the Book

Visit thePoint® **www.thePoint.lww.com** for activities and information to reinforce the concepts and content covered in this chapter.

REFERENCES

23 and Me Inc. (2013). We bring the world of genetics to you. Retrieved from https://www.23andme.com/. Accessed May 22, 2016.

Agnes, M. (Ed.). (2005). *Webster's new world college dictionary* (4th ed.). Cleveland, OH: Wiley.

Akens, D. S. (1999). *Computers in plain English*. Huntsville, AL: PC Press.

Alliance for Nursing Informatics. (2011). *About ANI*. Retrieved from www.allianceni.org/about.asp. Accessed January 23, 2013.

American Association of Colleges of Nursing. (2008). *The essentials of baccalaureate education for professional nursing practice*. Washington, DC: Author.

American Nurses Association. (2008). *Nursing informatics: Scope and standards of practice*. Silver Spring, MD: Nursebooks.org.

American Nurses Credentialing Center (ANCC). (2015). *2015 Certification renewal requirements*. Retrieved from http://nursecredentialing.org/RenewalRequirements.aspx. Accessed May 21, 2016.

American Nurses Credentialing Center (ANCC). (2016). *Informatics certification catalog [Online]*. Washington, DC: American Nurses Credentialing Center. Retrieved from http://nursecredentialing.org/InformaticsNursing. Accessed May 21, 2016.

Ancestry.com. (2016). Discover the family story your DNA can tell. Retrieved from http://dna.ancestry.com/. Accessed May 22, 2016.

Barnoy, S., Apel, D., Peretz, C., Meiraz, H., & Ehrenfeld, M. (2006). Genetic testing, genetic information and the role of maternal-child health nurses in Israel. *Journal of Nursing Scholarship, 38*(3), 219–224.

Billings, D., & Halstead, J. (2012). *Teaching in nursing, a guide for faculty*. (4th ed.). St. Louis, MO: Elsevier Saunders.

Bureau of Labor Statistics. (2012). *Occupational outlook handbook*. Retrieved from www.bls.gov/oco. Accessed January 23, 2013.

Califano, R., Landi, L., & Cappuzzo, F. (2012). Prognostic and predictive value of K-RAS mutations in non-small cell lung cancer. *Drugs, 72*(Suppl. 1):28–36. doi: 0012–6667/12/0001–0028/$55.55/0

Calzone, K. A., Jenkins, J., Culp, S., Caskey, S., & Badzek, L. (2014). Introducing a new competency into nursing practice. *Journal of Nursing Regulation, 5*(1), 40–41.

Carrington, J., & Tiase, V. (2013). Nursing informatics year in review. *Nursing Administration Quarterly, 37*(2), 136–143. doi: 10.1097/NAQ.0b013e3182869deb

Check, E., & Rodgers, A. (2001). Solving the next genome puzzle. *Newsweek, 69*(46), 52–53.

Conley, Y., & Tinkle, M. (2007). The future of genomic nursing research. *Journal of Nursing Scholarship, 39*(1), 17–24.

David, D. (2014). Informatics and technology. *The Massachusetts nursing core competencies: A toolkit for implementation in education and practice settings*. Retrieved from http://www.mass.edu/nahi/documents/Toolkit-First%20Edition-May%202014-r1.pdf. Accessed May 21, 2016.

Dolan, S., Biermann, J., & Damus, K. (2007). Genomics for health in preconception and postnatal periods. *Journal of Nursing Scholarship, 39*(1), 4–9.

Duffy, M. (2015). Nurses and the migration to electronic health records. *American Journal of Nursing, 115*(12), 61–66. doi:10.1097/01.naj.0000475294.12738.83

Ellerbee, S. (2007). Staffing through web-based open-shift bidding. *American Nurse Today, 2*(4), 32–34.

Foster, A. L. (2001). The struggle to preserve privacy. *The Chronicle of Higher Education, 47*, A37–A39.

Friesth, B. (2012). Chapter 22: Teaching and learning at a distance. In D. M. Billings & J. A. Halstead (Eds.), *Teaching in nursing: A guide for faculty* (4th ed., pp. 386–400). St. Louis, MO: Elsevier Saunders.

Giarelli, E., & Jacobs, L. (2001). Issues related to the use of genetic material and information. *Oncology Nursing Forum, 27*, 459–467.

Halstead, J., & Billings, D. (2012). Chapter 23: Teaching and learning in on-line communities. In D. M. Billings & J. A. Halstead (Eds.), *Teaching in nursing: A guide for faculty* (4th ed., (pp. 401–421). St. Louis, MO: Elsevier Saunders.

HealthIT.gov. (2010). *Patient protection and Affordable Care Act Section 1461 recommendations*. Retrieved from www.healthit.gov/sites/default/files/rules-regulation/aca-1461-recommendations-final2.pdf. Accessed March 23, 2013.

HealthIT.gov. (2013). EHR incentives and certification: How to attain meaningful use. Retrieved from https://www.healthit.gov/providers-professionals/how-attain-meaningful-use. Accessed May 21, 2016.

HealthIT.gov. (2014). How to implement EHRs, Stage 5, Achieve meaningful use. Retrieved from https://www.healthit.gov/providers-professionals/ehr-implementation-steps/step-5-achieve-meaningful-use. Accessed May 22, 2016.

HealthIt.gov. (2015). EHR incentives & certifications, meaningful use: Definitions and objectives. Retrieved from https://www.healthit.gov/providers-professionals/meaningful-use-definition-objectives. Accessed May 21, 2016.

Holden, C. (2003). Race and medicine. *Science, 302*, 594–596.

Huchenski, J. (2001). New federal rule protects individual healthcare information privacy. *Computers in Nursing, 19*, 41, 43–44, 46.

Hurley, A. C., Lancaster, D., Hayes, J., Wilson-Chase, C., Bane, A., Griffin, M., et al. (2007). The medication administration system—nurses assessment of satisfaction (MAS-NAS) scale. *Journal of Nursing Scholarship, 38*(3), 298–300.

Institute of Medicine. (2003). *Health professions education: A bridge to quality*. Washington, DC: National Academies Press.

Institute of Medicine. (2012). *The role of telehealth in an evolving health care environment: Workshop Summary*. Retrieved from www.nap.edu/catalog.php?record_id = 13466, Accessed March 23, 2013.

Jeffries, P., & Clochesy, J. (2012). Chapter 20: Clinical simulation, an experiential student-centered pedagogical approach. In D. M. Billings & J. A. Halstead (Eds.), *Teaching in nursing: A guide for faculty* (4th ed., pp. 352–368). St. Louis, MO: Elsevier Saunders.

Jenkins, J., & Calzone, K. (2007). Establishing the essential nursing competencies for genetics and genomics. *Journal of Nursing Scholarship, 39*(1), 10–16.

Jossi, F. (2004). *Robostaff*. Healthcare informatics online. Retrieved from www.healthcare-informatics.com/issues/2004/04_04/jossi.htm. Accessed July 8, 2005.

Kaku, M. (2011). *The physics of the future*. New York: First Anchor Books.

Korhonen, E. S., Nordman, T., & Eriksson, K. (2015). Technology and its ethics in nursing and caring journals: An integrative literature review. *Nursing Ethics, 22*(5), 561–576. doi: 10.1177/0969733014549881

Kulikowski, C. A., Shortliffe, E. H., Curie, L. M., Elkin, P. L., Hunter, L. E., Johnson, T. R., et al. (2012). AMIA Board white paper: Definition of biomedical informatics and specification of core competencies for graduate education in the discipline. [Online.] *Journal of the American Medical Informatics Association, 19*(6), 931–938. doi:10.1136/amiajnl-2012–001053

Lee, T. (2012). Supreme Court to rule on patentability of human genes. Retrieved from http://arstechnica.com/tech-policy/2012/11/supreme-court-to-rule-on-patentability-of-human-genes/. Accessed March 29, 2013.

Logue, M., & Effken, J. (2012). Modeling factors that influence personal health records adoption. *CIN: Computers Informatics Nursing, 30*(7), 354–362. doi: 10.1097/NXN.0b013e3182510717

Logue, M., & Effken, J. (2013). Validating the personal health records adoption model using a modified e-Delphi. *Journal of Advanced Nursing, 69*(3), 685–696. doi: 10.1111/j.1365-2648.2012.06056.x

Loustau, L. (2007). Working to save lives—from a distance. *Kansas City Nursing News 2007 Guide to Nursing, 2*, 14.

Marshall, E. (2003a). First check my genome, doctor. *Science, 302*, 589.

Marshall, E. (2003b). Preventing toxicity with a gene test. *Science, 302*, 588–590.

Mueller, C. L., & Billings, D. M. (2000). Focus on the learner. In J. Novotny (Ed.), *Distance education in nursing*. New York: Springer.

National Council of State Boards of Nursing. (2011). Social media guidelines for nurses. Retrieved from https://www.ncsbn.org/347.htm. Accessed May 22, 2016.

Nelson, R. (2007). The personal health record. *American Journal of Nursing, 107*(9), 27–28.

Orlygsdottir, B. (2007). Use of NIDSEC-compliant CIS in community-based nursing-directed prenatal care to determine support of nursing minimum data set objectives. *CIN: Computers Informatics Nursing, 25*(5), 283–293.

Piscotty, R. J., Kalisch, B., & Gracey-Thomas, A. (2015). Impact of Healthcare Information Technology on Nursing Practice. *Journal of Nursing Scholarship, 47*(4), 287–293. doi: 10.1111/jnu.12138

Shepard, A. (2013). Clinical IT in a complex environment. *Nursing Administration Quarterly, 37*(2), 167–168. doi: 10.1097/NAQ.0b013e3182869e8c

Sherwood, G., & Barnsteiner, J. (2012). *Quality and safety in nursing, a competency approach to improving outcomes*. West Sussex, UK: Wiley-Blackwell.

Short, N. (2000). Online learning: Ready, set, click. *RN, 63*, 28–32.

Skiba, D. (2007). Nursing education 2.0: Poke me. Where's your face in space? *Nursing Education Perspectives, 28*(4), 214–216.

Spiegel, A., & Hawkins, M. (2012). 'Personalized Medicine' to identify genetic risks for type 2 diabetes and focus prevention: Can it fulfill its promise? *Health Affairs, 31*(1), 43–49. doi: 10.1377/hlthaff.2011.1054

Staggers, N., & Gassert, C. (2000). Competencies for nursing informatics. In B. Carty (Ed.), *Nursing informatics: Education for practice*. New York: Springer.

Staggers, N., Gassert, C., & Curan, C. (2001). Informatics competencies for nurses at four levels of practice. *Journal of Nursing Education, 40*(7), 303–316.

Staggers, N., Gassert, C., & Curan, C. (2002). A Delphi study to determine informatics competencies for nurses at four levels of practice. *Nursing Research, 51*(6), 383–390.

Stone, B. (2001). Wanted: Hot industry seeks supergeeks. *Newsweek, 137*, 54–55, 58.

Tao, R., Huang, Z., Wang, J., Zhang, H., Zhang, Y., & Li, M. (2010). Proposed diagnostic criteria for internet addiction. *Addiction, 105*, 556–564. doi:10.1111/j.1360-0443.2009.02828.x

Thede, L. (1999). *Computers in nursing: Bridges to the future*. Philadelphia, PA: Lippincott Williams & Wilkins.

Thede, L. (2003). *Informatics and nursing: Opportunities and challenges* (2nd ed.). Philadelphia, PA: Lippincott Williams & Wilkins.

TIGER Summit. (2007). *The TIGER initiative: Evidence and informatics transforming nursing: 3-year action steps toward a 10-year vision*. Retrieved from www.tigersummit.com/Downloads.html. Accessed January 23, 2013.

Whitehead, L., & Seaton, P. (2016). The effectiveness of self-management mobile phone and tablet apps in long-term condition management: A systematic review. *Journal of Medical Internet Research, 18*(5): e97. Retrieved from http://www.jmir.org/2016/5/e97/. Accessed May 15, 2016.

Whitmore, J. (2005). *Business class etiquette: Essentials for success at work*. New York: St. Martin's Press.

Wilke, A. (2007). With nurses' help REMi brings SMMC doctors to the bedside. *Kansas City Nursing News 2007 Guide to Nursing, 5*, 10.

Yee, T., Needleman, J., Pearson, M., Parkerton, P., Parkerton, M., & Wolstein, J. (2012). The influence of integrated electronic medical records and computerized nursing notes on nurses' time spent in documentation. *CIN: Computers Informatics Nursing, 30*(6), 287–292. doi: 10.1097/NXN.0b013e31824af835

Yuh, B. (2013). The bedside assistant in robotic surgery-keys to success. *Urologic Nursing, 33*(1), 29–32. doi: 10.7257/1053-816X.201333.1.29

PROFESSIONAL NURSING ROLES

Professional nurses assume a variety of roles—often simultaneously—as they engage in the complexities of clinical practice. Nurses consciously choose the roles they assume based on the nature of the client system, specific client needs, and the interprofessional team's efforts. Professional nurses aspire to provide the best quality health care by bringing a constellation of cognitive and clinical skills to empower clients while constantly assessing clinical practice environments for ways to improve the safety and quality of health care.

Nursing Approaches to Client Systems

KEY TERMS AND CONCEPTS

Human systems

Clients

Patient-centered care

Patient- and family-centered care

Change/growth view of change

Persistence view of change

Family functions

Community

Change/growth models

Change/stability models

Family

Family as client

Family system

Community as client

Health promotion

Risk

Disease prevention

Primary prevention

Secondary prevention

Tertiary prevention

LEARNING OUTCOMES

By the end of this chapter, the learner will be able to:

1. Define individual, family, and community as clients for professional nursing care.
2. Outline how various nursing conceptual models differentiate client systems in professional nursing.
3. Explain the concept and elements of patient-centered and patient–family-centered care.
4. Outline the differences in ethical issues when making decisions while delivering nursing care to an individual as client, family as client, and community as client.
5. Compare and contrast nursing approaches in the realms of family nursing using the change/growth view and the change/stability view.
6. Explain the differences in viewing communities as aggregates of people, human systems, and human field–environmental field process.
7. Outline the key differences in how nurses adapt their strategies based on their perceptions and theoretical approaches to the three-client systems.
8. Explain the concept of healthy community.
9. Articulate how nurses can define community in clinical practice settings.
10. Identify professional nursing career options in community health.

REAL-LIFE REFLECTIONS

Lisa is a teenager who prides herself on her skills in gymnastics, ballet, and academics. She strives for perfection in all her endeavors because she knows that her parents make great sacrifices so she can pursue her interests. Lisa's ballet teacher has been encouraging her to lose 9.07 kg (20 lb) because she carries 56.69 kg (125 lb) on her 170.18 cm (5 ft 7 in) frame. Today, Gina, a friend of Lisa who also takes ballet lessons, collapsed during physical

(continued on page 384)

education class. Gina had recently lost 9.07 kg (20 lb) as requested by the ballet teacher and secured a starring role in a local ballet production.

Upon hearing about Gina, Lisa has come to the health room complaining of dizziness. Her friend Cindy helps her to the health room. Nancy, an experienced school nurse, notices that both Cindy and Lisa have sunken eyes and appear to be extremely thin. Nancy gives both girls some orange juice. Nancy suspects that the girls have eating disorders. When she asks Cindy and Lisa about their eating habits, they both say they can eat anything they want without gaining weight. Both girls fail to make eye contact with Nancy when responding to her questions.

Nancy notices that both girls are wearing clothes similar to those worn by the cover model on a fashion magazine. Nancy, concerned for the health of both girls, recalls that families play a key role in eating disorders and that peer pressure sometimes makes teenagers do foolish things. Nancy realizes that she has an opportunity to help these individual clients, their families, and the school community.

Human systems are living systems open to interactions with other systems. Interacting systems are characterized by mutual change; that is, each human system can effect change in another and at the same time is influenced (changed) by that other system. Nurses involved in professional practice interact with client systems and the health care delivery system.

The nursing profession defines **clients** as the recipients of nursing care. In addition to being passive care recipients, clients assume the important role of active participants, or partners, with nurses when they seek the services of professional nurses. This chapter explores the professional nurse's role in client systems and differentiates between individuals, families, and communities as clients.

Recent efforts to improve quality and safety in nursing and health care emphasize the importance of **patient-centered care**, during which nurses use a holistic care approach considering each patient's/client's personal preferences, values, family situations, religious and cultural traditions, and specific lifestyle. In patient-centered care, nurses provide the knowledge, resources, and support that each client needs to be involved in informed decision-making processes, assume important aspects of total self-care (if capable), and change behaviors to promote health and a better quality of life. Patient-centered care cannot occur exclusively with an individual because most people are part of a family. Therefore, patient-centered care incorporates the family and becomes **patient- and family-centered care** (PFCC).

PFCC means that nurses consider the holistic needs of the family and the patient and the family works as a partner with the health and nursing care team (Fig. 15.1). Care coordination for smooth transitions across health delivery systems is a hallmark of PFCC. Care coordination promotes effective use of health care resources and results in reduced costs for patients, families, third-party payers, and governments. The Institute of Patient- and Family-Centered Care specifies that the following characteristics must be present in care coordination.

1. Dignity and respect occur for all people involved when receiving health care treatment.
2. Health care providers share complete and unbiased information with patients and families in a manner they can understand and use.
3. Care is focused on capitalizing and building on the strengths of patients and families by providing experiences that enhance independence and control.

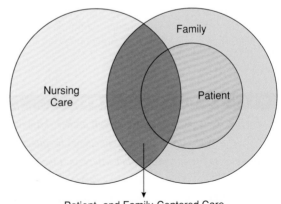

Patient- and Family-Centered Care

FIGURE 15.1 The patient- and family-centered care model.

4. Development of policies and programs, professional education, and care delivery occurs with effective collaboration among patient, family members, and health care providers.

Along with these characteristics, PFCC strives to provide physical comfort, emotional support, and involvement of family and friends (Moretz & Abraham, 2012; Walton & Barnsteiner, 2012).

Patients and families need and expect PFCC. National standards and regulations require that data regarding patient perceptions of a hospital experience be collected and reported. The Hospital Consumer Assessment of Healthcare Providers and Systems (HCAHPS) is a survey the federal government uses to collect, analyze, and report data about consumer experiences in hospitals. Hospital Compare (http://www.medicare.gov/hospitalcompare/) is a website that helps consumers compare local or national hospitals on communication, cleanliness, responsiveness, noise, and pain management. Many health care consumers visit the Hospital Compare website before selecting a hospital and physician for surgery or other invasive procedure. The Center for Medicare and Medicaid Services recently embarked on an incentive program to reward facilities for HCAHPS use, data reports, and actual results (Walton & Barnsteiner, 2012).

To be consistent with Fawcett's metaparadigm of nursing (see Chapter 5, Patterns of Knowing and Nursing Science), the conceptual models of nursing developed their views of "the person" (individual) even though nurses practice with families and communities (Fawcett & DeSanto-Madeya, 2012). In traditional practice, a person's family and community have actually been treated as a context of the client receiving nursing care. However, the person is integral to the family and vice versa. Families create communities when the family is incapable of providing for the family's entire needs. The major questions for the professional nurse are: How do I practice nursing with the individual client? With the whole family as client? With the community as client?

Take Note!

PFCC is not a new concept for professional nurses because nurses have for generations considered both the patient and the family when they provided nursing care services.

Change in human beings is lifelong, natural, and evolutionary. As people move through their lives, they establish themselves as integral elements of larger and more complex systems. The individual synthesizes the concept of "me" with "my family" and "my community." At times, nurses effectively and appropriately work with "me" in professional relationships (an independent adult receiving care). In other instances, the nurse must consider that working with "the family" may be more effective (child receiving care). Finally, nurses sometimes have to work with "the community," especially when the health of a large group of people may be affected.

According to the paradigm selected for application in this book—the growth or persistence view of change (Fawcett & DeSanto-Madeya, 2012)—it is the client–environment relationship that is most important. The way individual nurses think about change determines how they view clients. In the **change/growth view of change**, growth serves as the outcome of change. Nurses see clients with the ability for continuous growth, and nurses facilitate change by focusing clients on their strengths and abilities for potential growth. In the **persistence view of change**, the outcome is stability. Nurses see clients as potentially capable of stability and aim their efforts at solving problems to recapture a stable state.

When nursing conceptual models were originally developed, Fawcett's metaparadigm provided the foundation. Nursing scholars equated "person" with the individual client. The models have since been refined either by the model author or by other nursing scholars to explain how the models can be applied when the family and/or community becomes the client (or care recipient) (Anderson & McFarlane, 2015; Fawcett & DeSanto-Madeya, 2012; Kaakinen, Hanson, & Denham, 2010).

■ QUESTIONS FOR REFLECTION

1. As a health care consumer, have you ever been in a situation during which a family member or friend needed to have care? Describe the situation. How did the nurses handle the family member or friend of the person receiving health care services? Were the strategies used effective? Why or why not?

2. Have you ever encountered a nursing situation that required more than caring for the individual as client? Describe the situation. How did you handle the situation? Were your strategies effective? Why or why not?

3. Does consulting with family members breach client confidentiality? Why or why not?

4. How can you know when a health-related issue involves more than an individual or family system?

THE INDIVIDUAL AS CLIENT

As people progress through life and interact with their environment, unique patterns evolve. This philosophical assumption espouses that such patterns of interaction determine a person's health. In general, the changes that occur in the developing human being are characterized by higher abilities to organize and deal with more complex levels of interaction. The individual's patterns are unique and are continuously evolving from earlier life experiences, including biologic, genetic, cultural, interpersonal, and social influences, as well as current interactions and conceptions of the future.

Because the conceptual models of nursing were developed with people defined as the client, professional nurses derive directives for nursing practice from the discussion of nursing processes according to both the integration and interaction nursing models (see Chapter 6, Nursing Models and Theories). The following section reflects our efforts to differentiate the professional nursing care of families and communities from that of individuals.

THE FAMILY AS CLIENT

The question of what is a family evokes many definitions, from the conjugal or nuclear family (the family of marriage, parenthood, or procreation) to the extended family (the kinships of biologically related people—grandparents, aunts, uncles, and cousins). Such definitions have limited applicability in today's society. Families may be defined by legal, biologic, psychological, and social relationships (Kaakinen & Coehlo, 2015). Thus, the accepted definition of **family** is "two or more individuals who depend on one another for emotional, physical, and/or economic support. The members of the family are self-defined" (Hanson, 1996, p. 6; Kaakinen et al., 2010, p. 5).

Many terms are used to describe family nursing care, including family-centered care, family-based care, family-focused care, and most simply, family nursing. These different terms reflect confusion about whether the family is the client (the recipient of care) or the context of care (in which the individual family member is the care recipient). Family approaches to nursing care have been standard practice in the areas of maternal–child nursing, school nursing, and mental health nursing. In the era of cost containment in health care and early hospital dismissals, families frequently assume caregiver roles. Families also become the recipient of nursing care when they commit to caring for an aging family member in the home instead of sending the person to an extended-care facility (Bailey, 2007; Magnusson & Hanson, 2005; Stadnyk, 2006). The importance of

family as client emerges as a key component of cultural competence in professional practice (Andrews & Boyle, 2016; Knoerl, 2007) (see Chapter 11, Multicultural Issues in Professional Practice). When providing care to the terminally ill, nurses sometimes find themselves focusing more on families than on the individual who is dying (Schumacher, Stewart, & Archbold, 2007). In today's practice settings, nurses frequently view the family as the unit of care or clients.

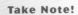

Take Note!

A family is any two or more people who depend on each other for support.

The **family as client** approach means that the entire family becomes the recipient of nursing services. Multiple approaches identify the indices and phenomena that represent the family as a holistic unit on which the professional nurse must focus. One approach is to view the family as a system interacting with subsystems and suprasystems. According to Artinian (1994), the following are some of the assumptions of the family systems perspective.

- A **family system** is an organized whole; individuals within the family are parts of the system and are interdependent.
- The family system is greater than and different from the sum of its parts.
- There are logical relationships (connectedness patterns) between the subsystems. In some families, the connectedness patterns may reflect rigid and fixed structures and relationships. In other families, the connectedness patterns may reflect highly flexible structures and relationships.
- Using feedback from the environment, the family system responds (adapts) to change in ways that reduce strain and maintain a dynamic balance.

REAL-LIFE REFLECTIONS

Recall Lisa from the beginning of the chapter, who is complaining of dizziness. If the nurse focuses on the unit of care as the individual, nursing interventions would address only specific interventions for Lisa. Because of Lisa's age and the nature of eating disorders, however, a more appropriate unit of care would be the family. Why do you think this is so? What could be achieved by considering the problem from a family-centered approach? Why would these things be important for providing care to Lisa and her family?

In the systems family approach, the phenomena of interest are wholeness, relationships, belief systems, family rules, family needs, roles, and tensions between individuation and togetherness. Two theories that are congruent with the family systems model are the Calgary family assessment model (Kaakinen & Hanson, 2010; Kaakinen & Coehlo, 2015; Wright & Leahey, 1988) and the framework of systemic organization (Friedmann, 1995). Box 15.1, Professional Building Blocks, "The Family Systems Model," summarizes key concepts.

Another approach to family as client focuses on the family as a structural–functional social system (Artinian, 1994). The focus is the family structure and its effectiveness in performing its functions. Friedman, Bowden, and Jones (2003) identified the following seven **family functions.**

1. **Affective support:** Meeting the emotional needs of family members

2. **Socialization and social placement:** Socializing children and making them productive members of society

3. **Reproduction:** Producing new members for society

4. **Family coping:** Maintaining order and stability

5. **Economic stability:** Providing sufficient economic resources and allocating resources effectively

6. **Providing physical necessities** (food, clothing, shelter)

7. **Maintaining health**

The Friedman family assessment model (Friedman, 1992; Friedman, Bowden, & Jones, 2003; Kaakinen & Hanson, 2010) appears congruent with a combination of the structural–functional model and the family systems model. Friedman stated that nurses must view the family in two ways when implementing family nursing: as each individual within the family context and the whole family as the unit of care. A summary of the structural–functional model presented in Box 15.2, Professional Building Blocks,

---

15.1 Professional Building Blocks

The Family Systems Model

Overview: Focuses on interaction between members of the family system and on the family system with other systems. A change in one member of the family system influences the entire system.

Concepts: Subsystems, boundaries, openness, energy, negentropy (energy that promotes order), entropy (energy promoting chaos), feedback, adaptation, homeostasis, input, output, internal system processes.

Assumptions: The family system is greater than the sum of its parts. Subsystems are related and interact with one another, and the whole family system interacts with other systems. Family systems have homeostatic features and strive to maintain a dynamic balance.

Clinical Application: Assess, diagnose, and intervene with family according to major concepts.

Sample Assessment Questions

- How did change caused by the critical illness event affect all members of the family?
- How are members of the family system relating with one another?
- How is the family system relating to the critical care environment?
- What is the "input" into the family system?
- Is the family system internally processing the input? What is the family system output?
- How open is the family system? Does the family system have homeostasis?
- How does behavior of all family members affect the patient?
- How does the patient's behavior affect the entire family?

Interventions

- Encourage nurse–family interactions by establishing trust and using communication skills to check for discrepancies between nurse and family expectations.
- Establish a mechanism for providing family with information about the patient on a regular basis.
- Foster the family's ability to get information.
- Listen to the family's feelings, concerns, and questions.
- Orient the family to the critical care environment.
- Answer family questions or assist the family in obtaining answers.
- Discuss with family members strategies for normalizing family life.
- Provide mechanisms for the patient and other family members to interact with one another through pictures, videos, audiotapes, or open visiting.
- Monitor family relationships.
- Facilitate open communication among family members.
- Collaborate with the family in problem solving.
- Provide necessary knowledge that will help the family make decisions.

Artinian, N. T. (1994). Selecting a model to guide family assessment. *Dimensions of Critical Care Nursing, 14,* 6. Used with permission of the publisher.

15.2 Professional Building Blocks

The Structural–Functional Model

Overview: Focuses on family structure and family function and how well the family performs its functions.

Concepts: Structural areas include family form, roles, values, communication patterns, power structure, and support network. Functional areas include affective, socialization, reproductive, coping, economic, physical care, and health care functions.

Assumptions: Family is a system and a small group that exists to perform certain functions.

Clinical Application: Assess, diagnose, and intervene with family according to major concepts.

Sample Assessment Questions

- What impact did the critical illness event have on family structure and function?
- How did the critical illness alter the family structure?
- What family roles were changed? What family functions have been affected?
- What are family members' physical responses to the illness event?

Interventions

- Assist the family to modify its organization so that role responsibilities can be redistributed.
- Respect and encourage adaptive coping skills used by the family.
- Counsel family members on additional effective coping skills for their own use.
- Identify typical family coping mechanisms.
- Tell the family it is safe and acceptable to use typical expressions of affection.
- Provide privacy for the family to allow for family expression of affection.
- Provide for family visitation.
- Encourage family members to recognize their own health needs.
- Help family members find ways to meet their health needs while helping them feel their concern for the patient has not diminished.
- Assist the family to use existing support structure.

Artinian, N. T. (1994). Selecting a model to guide family assessment. *Dimensions of Critical Care Nursing, 14,* 7. Used with permission of the publisher.

"The Structural–Functional Model," summarizes key concepts.

A third approach to family as client is the family stress model. Artinian (1994) outlined the following assumptions of this model.

1. The family is a system.
2. Unexpected or unplanned events are usually perceived as more stressful than expected events.
3. Events within the family that are defined as stressful are more disruptive than events outside the family.
4. Lack of experience with a stressor leads to greater perceived stressfulness.
5. Ambiguous stressor events are more stressful than unambiguous ones.

Artinian (1994) indicated that client assessment should include family resources, the meaning of the situation to the family (e.g., is it viewed as a threat or a challenge?), the level of crisis the family is experiencing, and coping mechanisms.

Patterson (1999) presented a postmodern view of a family and provided an ecologic perspective that requires nurses to think in layers. The smallest unit, the person, is in the center, with larger units extending outward from the person to include the family, social groups, the local community, and so on, until the

outermost layer comprises the entire cosmos. In this model, the family is an integral part of an ecosystem, and many variations in family form exist. Children receive support and protection from family members (parents, grandparents, siblings, and other relatives). The family serves as a unit of the **community** that encompasses schools, child care providers, faith-based groups, health care providers, workplaces, locally supportive services (police, fire, city, and county services), neighborhoods, and friends. The community is part of society, which is composed of the military, government, multinational corporations, online personal and professional networks, prisons, research institutions, courts, banks, insurers, transportation systems, media, and welfare systems. Patterson (1999) designated the following four family functions.

1. **Family formation and membership:** To provide a sense of belonging, personal and social identity, and meaning and direction for life
2. **Economic support:** To provide basic shelter, food, clothing, and other things to facilitate and enhance human development
3. **Nurturance and socialization:** To provide holistic development and support of members while instilling social values and norms

4. **Protection of vulnerable members:** To provide care for the young, disabled, ill, or aging family members incapable of self-care or at risk for harm

Patterson (1999) also proposed that each family develops specific functioning patterns that include consistent ways in which they display affection, show anger, cope with stress, deal with conflict, accomplish daily routines, discipline children, seek health care, and celebrate special occasions. The family alters these patterns as it experiences developmental transitions (birth, raising children, departing children, aging, and death). Because the familial experience is multidimensional, Patterson suggested that assessment using only family questionnaires limits the amount of data collected by health care providers. Health care professionals should consider observing family interactions when families enter the health care system. Because a family is a system, the conceptualization of family health requires consideration of the individual health status of each member and the health of the family's functioning patterns (Patterson, 1999). Alteration in the health of one member usually results in altered family functioning patterns.

Two theories that are congruent with a combination of the family stress model and the family systems model are the family assessment and intervention model (Kaakinen & Coehlo, 2015; Kaakinen & Hanson, 2010) and the resiliency model (McCubbin & McCubbin, 1993). Box 15.3, Professional Building Blocks, "The Family Stress Model," summarizes key concepts.

Anderson and Tomlinson (1992, p. 61) identified five realms of family experience that represent elements of the approaches identified and that direct professional practice.

1. **Interactive processes:** Family relationships, communication, nurturance, intimacy, and social support
2. **Developmental processes:** Family transitions and dynamic interactions between the stages of family development and individual developmental tasks
3. **Coping processes:** Management of resources, problem solving, and adaptation to stressors and crisis
4. **Integrity processes:** Shared meanings of experiences, family identity and commitment, family history, family values, boundary maintenance, and family rituals

---

15.3 Professional Building Blocks

The Family Stress Model

Overview: Focuses on stressors, resources, and perceptions to explain the amount of family disruption caused by a stressful event.

Concepts: "A"—stressful event with associated hardships; "B"—physical, psychological, material, social, spiritual, and informational resources of the family; "C"—the family's subjective definition of the stressful event; "X"—crisis, the amount of disruption or incapacitation within the family caused by the stressful event.

Assumptions: Family is a system. Unexpected and ambiguous illness events are more stressful. Stressful events within the family are more disruptive than stressor events outside the family. Lack of experience with a stressor event leads to increased perceptions of stressfulness.

Clinical Application: Assess, diagnose, and intervene with family according to major concepts.

Sample Assessment Questions

- Identify the family's understanding and beliefs about the situation.
- What family hardships are associated with the critical illness event?
- What are other situational stressors for the family?

- Did the family have time to prepare for the event?
- Has the family had experience with the event?
- What resources are available to the family?
- Are the resources sufficient to meet the demands of the event?
- What are the family's perceptions of the event?
- Do they perceive the event to be a threat or a challenge?
- Does the family blame themselves for the event?
- How incapacitated is family functioning?

Interventions

- Help the family to cope with imposed hardships.
- If appropriate, provide spiritual or informational resources for the family.
- Introduce the family to others undergoing similar experiences.
- Discuss existing social support resources for the family.
- Assist the family in capitalizing on its strengths.
- Assist the family to resolve feelings of guilt.
- Help the family visualize successfully handling all the hardships associated with the situation.
- If possible, encourage the family to focus on the positive aspects of the situation or cognitively reappraise the situation as positive.

Artinian, N. T. (1994). Selecting a model to guide family assessment. *Dimensions of Critical Care Nursing, 14,* 4–12. Used with permission of the publisher.

5. **Health processes:** Family health beliefs, health status, health responses and practices, lifestyle practices, and health care provision during wellness and illness

These realms remain applicable in the 21st century (Anderson, 2000; Bell, 2009). Therefore, nurses need to implement the nursing process in a way that facilitates exploration of all the family realms listed rather than focusing exclusively on health processes. In all of the conceptual nursing models, the client system is viewed holistically; thus, the nurse cannot extricate the health processes from the other processes (integrity, coping, development, and interaction).

Family nursing interventions depend on the clinical practice context. For example, early inpatient discharge planning requires that nurses teach and counsel families as they anticipate taking clients home. Nurses listen to families as they express concerns about the changes in the family's previous lifestyle. They give families knowledge and skills so that they can safely provide care, anticipate potential complications, and know what to do should complications occur. In inpatient

FOCUS ON RESEARCH

Maternal and Family Function and the Technology-Dependent Child

The investigators set out to explore the relationships of technology-dependent child functional status and Office of Technology Assistance group status on mother's depressive symptoms and normalization of familial functioning in families with a technology-dependent child over a 1-year time frame. They developed a conceptual model of family functioning for families with a technology-dependent child. The investigators used a descriptive, correlational, longitudinal study in which two interviews were conducted with mothers (defined as the primary female caregiver who could be a biologic, adoptive, or foster mother; or grandmother). The interviews consisted of completion of the following six instruments at 6-month intervals: Center for Epidemiological Studies Depression (CESD) Scale, Actual Effect of Chronic Physical Disorder on the Family Scale (AECPD), Feetham Family Functioning Survey (FFFS), Functional Status II—Revised (FS II-R), Level of Technology Dependency Questionnaire (LTDQ), and Demographic Characteristics Questionnaire (DCQ). Eighty-two mothers participated in the study. Data were analyzed using SPSS 15.0 and descriptive statistics; mean scores and repeated measures analyses of variance were calculated.

Results revealed that there were significantly reduced maternal depressive symptoms and improved normalization and family functions when the children in the study were no longer dependent on technology. Maternal depressive symptoms and poor normalization of family functions persisted as children continued to be dependent on technology. Normalization, caregiving duration, and required home nursing hours were found not to be directly related to family functioning. Baseline family functioning was found to predict future family functioning. Maternal depressive symptoms were positively related to reduced family functioning. There was no increase in maternal depressive symptoms or improvement in family functioning when the child remained technology-dependent for the year.

The clinical significance of this study is that maternal depressive symptoms remain relatively constant when caring for a technology-dependent child. Nurses should refer mothers to community mental health care professionals for assistance and support to screen for and prevent clinical depression. Nurses can also compliment primary caregivers on their performance in providing care and in dealing with technology-dependent children over time. The results of this study should be interpreted with caution because identified study limitations include limited geographical participation (midwestern United States), lack of cultural diversity of participants, small sample size, and sole focus on mothers. More research is needed to explore the effects of long-term technology-dependent children and adults on the entire family and primary caregiver, determine the effectiveness of nurse supportive and educational strategies, and examine the impact of the long-term technology-dependent lifestyle on the person with the disability.

Toly, V., Musil, C., & Carl, J. (2012). A longitudinal study of families with technology-dependent children. *Research in Nursing & Health, 35,* 40–54. doi: 10.1002/nur.21454 settings, families frequently find the ability to room-in with their loved one to be most beneficial. Nurses also assess family dynamics as families interact in all nursing care settings. Nurses collaborate with families in many nursing care settings to design family nursing care plans when needed (Ahmann & Dokken, 2012; Blanes, Carmagnani, & Ferreira, 2007; Gooding, Pierce, & Flaherty, 2012; Knoerl, 2007; Kwok, 2011; Li, Melnyk, & McCann, 2004; Stadnyk, 2006; Toly, Musil, & Carl, 2012). Sometimes nurses use creative arts as an innovation to reduce stress and lower anxiety in family caregivers (Walsh, Martin, & Schmidt, 2004). Focus on Research, "Maternal and Family Function and the Technology-Dependent Child," looks at the long-term effects on families of caring for technology-dependent children in the home setting and presents a nursing intervention to address maternal depressive symptoms.

Practice barriers may prevent nurses from addressing all relevant realms when the family is the client. Because of laws related to client privacy, nurses must exercise caution when disclosing protected health information about individuals to their family members. Some health care organizations limit the number of people who may receive client information, which sometimes creates friction among family members. Situations such as decreased length of stay in inpatient settings, inadequate staffing, poor coordination of services across the health care setting continuum, less-than-optimal communication among interprofessional health care providers, lack of nursing education regarding family structure and processes, and overwhelming complexity of family needs serve as the reasons for ineffective family nursing care. In addition, medical care supersedes nursing care in many health care settings (Rose, Mallinson, & Walton-Moss, 2004).

Nursing models presented in previous chapters explain how nursing care includes the concept of family as client and how nurses provide care to families. Following is a discussion of how the family may be understood in nursing models within the change/growth paradigm (Newman, 1983; Orem, 1983; Parse, 1996, 1998; Peplau, 1952; Rogers, 1983; Watson, 1996) and within the change/stability paradigm (King, 1983; Neuman & Fawcett, 2010; Roy, 1983).

▌ QUESTIONS FOR REFLECTION

1. How do you define family?
2. What ideas related to health and health care have you learned from your family?
3. Where and when did you seek health care services as a child?

4. Do you still use the same approach to health care services? Why or why not?
5. What obstacles to working with family as client have you experienced in your clinical practice setting? How can you create a clinical practice environment that supports family care?

The Family in the Change/Growth Models of Nursing

Nurses who use the **change/growth models** of nursing acknowledge that families experience growth when confronted with change. Like the individual, the family possesses great potential to develop in ways to maximize health for all members.

Orem's Self-Care Deficit Model

According to Taylor and Renpenning (1995, p. 356), Orem viewed family as a multiperson care system, defined as those courses and sequences of action which are performed by the people in multiperson units for the purpose of meeting the self-care requisites and the development and exercise of self-care agency of all members of the group and to maintain or establish the welfare of the unit. . . . The sub-systems of the multiperson system are the self-care systems of the individuals.

Whall and Fawcett (1991, p. 20) indicated that Orem's self-care conceptual framework primarily "views the family as only a backdrop for individuals." In her own words, Orem (1983, p. 368) directed the nurse to "first, accept the system of family living, the physical and social environment of the family, and the family's culture as basic conditioning factors for all the family members." She stressed that the family support system needs to be explored and "adjusted as needed and then incorporated into the system of family living" (Orem, 1983, p. 368).

Family is context in self-care, in which family members take actions to create conditions essential for human functioning and development, in dependent care, in situations in which family members need their care provided by others. Both self-care and dependent care are directed toward creating and maintaining conditions that support life and integrated functions and toward promoting human growth. Self-care and dependent care "are forms of deliberate action, learned behaviors, learned within the family and other social units within which individuals live and move" (Orem, 1983, p. 209). However, Orem also considered the family to be a unit, "a complex entity which can be regarded as a whole" (Taylor & Renpenning, 1995, p. 350). Thus, there is concern with the quality of interaction and the outcomes of those interactions on the family as a whole.

Two realms of family can be readily implemented in Orem's self-care model: the interactive processes, particularly the social support systems in the family, and the developmental processes, particularly in the understanding of dependent care needs at various life stages. "Conditions which justify identifying the multiperson unit include a need for protection and prevention, regulation of a hazard, need for environmental regulation, [and] need for resources" (Taylor & Renpenning, 1995, p. 366).

Lapp, Diemert, and Enestredt (1991) stressed the concept of the family as a partner in health care decision making. In keeping with the self-care perspective, they see "the primary responsibility for health and life choices as ultimately resting with the client family" (Lapp et al., 1991, p. 306). Lapp et al. further suggested that the main responsibility of the nurse is "ensuring that those choices were made on the basis of the most complete information possible while facilitating self-discovery of strengths and resources already existing for a family" (p. 306).

Chevannes (1997) specified that Orem's three levels of care enable nurses and family to develop a caring partnership. The nurse and family collaborate to determine the care level needed to fulfill the needs of the incapacitated member. In the wholly compensatory level of care, the nurse provides care to the incapacitated person while beginning to teach family members. The nurse assesses family needs for direct nursing care services and additional education as they assume a more active role in caring for the incapacitated family member. Eventually the nurse provides episodic care to the family (partially compensatory nursing care) when they no longer need continuous nursing care services. Finally, when families assume full care responsibilities, the nurse provides support and education as needs arise.

Watson's Human Science and Human Care Model

Watson's caring model lends itself to a view of the family as client if the nurse redefines the phenomenal field to be the family within the family system's environment. The nurse assesses family values by exploring the five realms of family experience (the integrity processes) (Anderson & Tomlinson, 1992; Bell 2009) through the following:

1. The family's shared meanings of experiences
2. The family's members' identity and commitment to that family identity
3. The family history
4. The family's members' shared values and rituals
5. The family's strategies for maintaining family boundaries

During actual caring occasions, nurses learn about the family and discover the needs for information and problem-solving abilities by identifying the family's past and current coping processes. Nurses and family members are "coparticipants in becoming in the now and the future and both are part of some larger, deeper, complex pattern of life" (Watson, 2007, p. 60). Together, nurses and family members analyze interaction processes, focus on familial relationships and communication patterns, explore the meanings of various transitions occurring within the family, identify support networks, and share feelings and meanings about family life. They also observe how the family members nurture each other and express intimacy, acting as coparticipants. In the human science and human care framework, nurses relate all familial processes to the health processes, clarifying with the family specific health beliefs, responses, and practices, and the patterns of caring for each other during times of wellness and illness.

REAL-LIFE REFLECTIONS

If Nancy practiced according to Orem's self-care deficit theory, she would assess Lisa and her family for their ability to access physical and mental health services independently and offer assistance if the family could not access services on their own, discuss treatment options for Lisa (and the family), and help them select specific services and treatment plans. Once the family obtained the help they needed, Nancy would offer education and support to them.

REAL-LIFE REFLECTIONS

If Nancy used Watson's approach to professional practice, she would offer education about eating disorders, help the family access required resources, and provide support during the treatment process. However, she would also pay more attention to the deep meaning of the experience for them, their family health beliefs, and their patterns of caring for each other.

Peplau's Interpersonal Relations Model

Peplau based her nursing model on the central concepts of growth and development facilitated by relationships with significant others. This model provides the foundation for the nurse to focus on the family as the unit of care if the patterns of interaction within the family and the family developmental processes replace individual needs as the central area of concern. Forchuk and Dorsay (1995, p. 114) stated that Peplau's model and family systems nursing "both share a common focus on interactions, patterns, and interpersonal relationships."

Perhaps Peplau's greatest contribution to the family nursing process is the enumeration of the stages of the nurse–client relationship. According to Friedman (1992, p. 42), "trust and rapport-building set the stage for and are the cornerstones of effective family nursing care." In the orientation stage, if the nurse and the family are to have an effective relationship, each member of the family must be able to share his or her concerns so that the nurse and other family members may more fully understand the whole family and the meaning of its experience together. In the planning stage, mutual goal setting—that is jointly formulated among family members and the nurse—and ways to meet commonly derived goals are directed toward reframing the need for help in the professional relationship to be a learning and growth experience.

It is proposed that, in the intervention stage (called the exploitation stage by Peplau) with families, Peplau's role behaviors originally designated as professional nursing roles could be developed as strategies for the entire family. Family needs replace individual needs, and the roles of resource person, teacher, leader, counselor, and surrogate may be played by both the nurse and various family members. Each role performance in the family should be fully explored in a way that the family learns about its interactive processes and the effect of those interactive processes on health processes.

REAL-LIFE REFLECTIONS

Using Peplau's model as a framework for professional practice, Nancy would work to build trust and rapport with the family unit, explore all family members' concerns, work with the family to understand the total experience, and collaborate with the family to set goals. Nancy would primarily assume the roles of teacher and counselor/teacher as the family learns about Lisa's eating disorder, what it means, and treatment options. She would emphasize how the disorder and treatment regimens would affect performance of family roles and how the overall interactive processes would affect the health of each family member and the family as a unit.

Rogers' Science of Unitary Human Beings Model

Various analysts agree that Rogers' conceptual model of nursing science lends itself readily to the family as the recipient of nursing care—the client system. As Friedman (1992, p. 62) said, "Rogers' legacy is clearly associated with general systems theory, and because of this orientation there is a good fit between Rogerian nursing theory and family nursing." Rogers herself said that the family system is an energy field that serves as the focus of study and interaction. She asserted that family fields and their respective environmental fields are engaged in a continuously evolving mutual process and that patterns identify this ongoing process (Rogers, 1983, p. 226). Some patterns may represent togetherness, others may represent activity/rest, and still others may represent rhythmicities in the family experience.

Whall and Fawcett (1991, p. 22) suggested that in the Rogerian model, the family is "viewed as an irreducible whole that is not understood by knowledge of individual family members." Newman, Sime, & Corcoran-Perry (1991, p. 4) pointed out that, from the unitary-transformative perspective (the perspective first described by Rogers), a phenomenon (any client system) is "viewed as a unitary, self-organizing field embedded in a larger self-organizing field . . . [and] identified by pattern and by interaction with the larger whole." Given this perspective, the family represents a unitary phenomenon embedded in the larger environmental field and a phenomenon that has patterns of energy exchange within its field and within its interactions with the larger environment.

Whall (1986) suggested that, despite Rogers not being completely clear about what assessment strategies are used in the unitary model, she deserves credit for the idea that the nurse providing care must assess the family as a whole. Other nurses have developed some of the tools needed for assessing the whole family. For example, Smoyak developed the idea of using genograms and the identification of family rules of organization as approaches in the nursing process (Whall, 1986). The genogram records information about family members and their relationships over at least three generations. It involves mapping the family structure, recording family information, and delineating family relationships. According to McGoldrick and Gerson (2008, p. 1), genograms "display family information graphically in a way that provides a quick gestalt of complex family patterns and a rich source of hypotheses about how a clinical problem may be connected to the family context and the evolution of problem and context over time."

The genogram is one of nursing's most useful tools for studying family patterns. By mapping relationships and patterns of functioning, it facilitates clinician systematic thinking about how events and relationships in client lives relate with patterns of health and illness (McGoldrick & Gerson, 2008). Using the historical data obtained by completing the genogram, the nurse assesses previous life cycle transitions. This assessment helps the nurse to identify important connections between the health of the family and the environment in which they arise (Jarvis, 2015). Readers are referred to McGoldrick and Gerson (2008) for additional details on constructing and interpreting the genogram as a tool for nursing assessment of the family. Genograms may also be generated by using online software programs.

All of the family realms described by Anderson and Tomlinson (1992) and discussed earlier in this chapter represent patterns of the family as a unitary phenomenon. Thus, these realms could be used as a basis for assessment, planning, intervention, and evaluation by nurses practicing on the basis of a Rogerian philosophy of nursing.

REAL-LIFE REFLECTIONS

If Nancy used Rogers' science of unitary human beings model to guide practice, she would see that the health status of both girls in her office was a manifestation of the pattern of the whole. She would focus on understanding all mechanisms that affect the life process of the girls, one of which is the family.

Parse's Human Becoming Model

The nursing models of Parse and Newman may be considered Rogerian-based. Thus, the nurse practicing within any of these models would incorporate Rogerian concepts in the caregiving process with the family.

In 2009, Parse published the human becoming family model in which she conceptualized the family as "an indivisible, unpredictable, ever-changing,

connectedness with close others" (Parse, 2009, p. 35). A family member is defined as any person who designates him- or herself as a family member, thereby transcending the need for a blood or legal relationship. Parse identified cocreated patterns of relating, involving, and being together and being alone while cotranscending with possibles. The ebb and flow of everyday life occurrences structures the deep personal meaning that results in seeing the familiar–unfamiliar differently. Parse (2009) identifies the following three key essences within the human becoming family model:

1. **Revering intentions** arise "with the wellspring of laughter and tears in honoring the personal significance of joy–sorrow" (Parse, 2009, p. 307).
2. **Shifting patterns** emerge when family members have opportunities and restrictions for being alone or together when they can either attend or distance themselves.
3. **Unfolding possibilities** occur as the result of family intentions and actions and lead to transcendence toward human becoming.

REAL-LIFE REFLECTIONS

Using Parse's human becoming model as a framework for professional practice, Nancy's approach would be similar to that of Rogers' science of unitary human beings model. However, Nancy would expend more energy to uncover the meaning that underlies the intentions and behaviors associated with eating disorders. To discover the true meanings, she would be truly present with the family as they expressed concerns that would ultimately reveal the meaning of thoughts, feelings, values, and changes that may have contributed to Lisa's problems. She would also provide a deep personal–professional relationship so that the family could express these things as they engaged in the treatment process and recover once treatment was completed.

Newman's Theory of Health as Expanding Consciousness

Newman, who views the individual as a center of energy, views the family the same way—a center of energy in constant interaction with the environment. Newman (1983) made five assumptions about families.

1. Health encompasses family situations in which one or more family members may be diagnosed as ill.
2. The illness of family members can be considered a manifestation of the pattern of the family interaction.
3. Elimination of the disease condition in the identified ill family member will not change the overall pattern of the family.
4. If one person's becoming ill is the only way the family can become conscious of its pattern, then that is health (in process) for that family.
5. Health is the expansion of consciousness of the family. Consciousness has been defined as the informational capacity of the system, a factor that can be observed in the quantity and quality of responses to stimuli.

The nature of nursing with the family would be the repatterning of partnerships between the family and the environment that promote higher levels of consciousness. Newman (1983) said that the purpose of nursing with the family is to facilitate the development of an increased range of responses of family members to each other and to the world outside the family and to facilitate the refinement of those responses (quality). She suggests that the first task is to assess the patterns of movement, time, space, and consciousness in the family. The nurse would consider the following factors to assess movement through observation: (1) the coordinated movement of language between speaker and listener, (2) other coordinated movements (such as dancing, lovemaking, and playing sports), (3) the freedom of individual movement within the family, and (4) movement outside the family.

Time is assessed for the quantity and quality of private time, coordinated time, and shared time. Space is assessed for territoriality, shared space, and distancing. Finally, consciousness is assessed by collecting data on the informational capacity of the family system, the quantity and quality of interaction within the family, and the quantity and quality of the interaction of the family with the community.

By completing these assessments, the nurse providing care for the family would be able to analyze the patterns of energy exchange between the family and the environment, and the transforming potential and life patterns of the family. These patterns will identify where the family energy is flowing and where it is blocked, depleted, or diffused, and will determine whether there is overload or buildup of energy in the

family. Newman (1983, p. 173) said that as these patterns emerge, the family's informational capacity will be increased in the nurse–client relationship. Assessment of these patterns also will reveal the family's evolving capacities, diversity, and complexity.

> **REAL-LIFE REFLECTIONS**
>
> *If Nancy used Newman's theory of health as expanding consciousness, she would intervene to facilitate repatterning the family into a higher level of consciousness.*

Consistent with the models of Rogers, Parse, and Newman is the fact that the family functions as a unitary, open system integrated with its environment. Family functions may be organized around Anderson and Tomlinson's (1992) five realms of family experience; thus the assessment, planning, implementation, and evaluation of the family as client by nurses practicing from any of the change/growth nursing models should reflect interactive, developmental, coping, integrity, and health processes and the relationship among all of these processes.

The Family in the Change/Stability Models of Nursing

When nurses use **change/stability models** of nursing, they acknowledge that nursing roles focus on assisting families in solving problems. This section presents a brief discussion of how the family may be viewed as the recipient of care in the nursing models in which the changes are directed toward restabilizing the client system.

King's Systems Interaction Model

King (1983, p. 179) viewed the family as "a social system that is seen as a group of interacting individuals." Thus, the family is an interpersonal system. In King's model, a theory of goal attainment in the family emphasizes interaction between family members.

The major concepts in this theory of goal attainment are self, role, perception, communication, transaction, stress, growth and development, time, space, and interaction. Each of these concepts is assessed in the nursing process between the nurse and the family. Communication is the interrelating factor among these concepts. Nurses and families make transactions to attain goals. King said that family movement through space and time may be social (called vertical movement) or physical (called geographic mobility). She also stated that family roles are related to growth and development and stress in the family.

According to King's perception of the family as client, the nurse assesses the family situation to identify real or potential problems. He or she "assist[s] family members in setting goals to resolve problems [and] provide[s] relevant information to help families make decisions about those factors that detract from or enhance healthy living" (King, 1983, p. 183).

REAL-LIFE REFLECTIONS

Using King's approach to professional practice, Nancy would assess the families to identify factors contributing to the suspected eating disorders, and help them to identify actual and potential issues and concerns regarding having a family member with an eating disorder.

Neuman's Health Care Systems Model

A stress/adaptation-based conceptual model for family nursing is Neuman's health care systems model. The nurse practicing with this model can modify assessment strategies to plan, implement, and evaluate primary, secondary, and tertiary interventions with families.

According to Neuman (1983, p. 241), "the concept of family as a system can be viewed as individual family members harmonious in their relationships—a cluster of related meanings and values that govern the family and keep it viable in a constantly changing environment." Stability is considered to represent the wellness state, instability the illness state, and transition the mixed wellness–illness state. The role of the nurse is "to control vigorously factors affecting the family, with special goal-directed activities toward facilitating stability within the system" (Neuman, p. 243). To understand influences on the stability of the family system, Neuman proposed the following points.

1. The nurse must deal with the needs of each family member in terms of his or her developmental age, developmental state, strengths and weaknesses, and environmental influences according to his or her perceptions of events.
2. The nurse must determine the structure and process of the family by studying the values and interaction patterns. The significant values and interaction patterns are the decision-making process (how power is distributed), coping style (how

differences are negotiated in relation to stress), role relationships (the controlling or facilitating effects of roles in meeting individual and family needs), communication styles and interaction patterns (congruence of verbal and nonverbal messages and the effects of situational or entrenched defense mechanisms in the family), goals (the sharing and supporting of concerns and feelings between members), boundaries (rules that define the type of behaviors that are acceptable or unacceptable to the family), socialization process (the adequacy of resources to support cultural and structural factors in meeting family needs), individuation (the quality of individuality of each family member that defines the wellness or stability of the unit), and sharing (an index for family stability).

3. The nurse must facilitate the meeting of family needs by intervening in the intra-family stressors (all things occurring within the family unit), inter-family stressors (all things occurring between the family and the immediate environment), and extra-family stressors (all things occurring between the family and the distal or indirect external environment). These interventions occur as primary prevention, secondary prevention, or tertiary prevention.

Tomlinson and Anderson (1995) described five areas of interface between Neuman's systems model and a general family health system paradigm.

1. **Complexity of the system:** The "need to consider not only the individual stressor response in relation to the family but also the family's response relative to lines of defense and resistance" (pp. 138–139).
2. **Conceptualization of the core of the family:** "The core of the family is composed of its individual members, and assessment of the family is done in relation to the dynamics of individual member contributions to the whole within their environmental interactive context . . . [in comparison] the core of the family systems is viewed as the interface of its members in interaction with the environment" (p. 139).
3. **Goal of family health:** "Neuman's central concern is to facilitate optimal client system stability or wellness in the face of change . . . [in comparison] from a family health system perspective, it is most desirable to facilitate family system wellness using strengths to reduce stressor effects and enhance family growth toward positive transformation" (p. 140).
4. **Entry point in caring for families:** The family becomes partners in health care. According to Neuman, "nursing functions to conserve system energy" (p. 140).

5. **Nursing interaction:** In the Neuman model, "the nurse role creates an explicit cooperative alliance with the client . . . [in comparison] based on a family systems perspective…in the family caregiving situation there may be considerable boundary ambiguity" (p. 141).

The nurse's prevention activities are the heart of Neuman's model of care. Primary preventions are the activities aimed at preventing stressors from invading the family. Secondary preventions are the protective activities that follow stressor invasion. Tertiary preventions are the activities during the family's reconstitution from stressors. All of these preventions are aimed at reestablishing stability within the family.

REAL-LIFE REFLECTIONS

If Nancy used Neuman's systems model as a foundation for practice, she would assess Lisa's family for stressors using five variables (physiologic, psychological, sociocultural, developmental, and spiritual). She would look for ways to minimize the impact of stressors associated with familial factors that may have contributed to the eating disorder, the stressors of living with a family member with an eating disorder, as well as the stressors associated with treatment.

Roy's Adaptation Model

Roy's adaptation model can be used by the nurse dealing with the family as client. Roy (1983) believed that the family as an adaptive system can be analyzed and that interventions can be organized around enhancing stimuli to the family.

Inputs for family include individual needs and changes within and among members as well as external changes in the environment. These inputs serve as focal stimuli for the family system. Processes handling the inputs are the control and feedback mechanisms. The control mechanisms—supporting, nurturing, and socializing—serve as contextual and residual stimuli to the family system. The feedback mechanisms are the transactional patterns and member control.

Outputs of the family system are the behaviors manifested. Roy (1983) has chosen three goals as the proposed output of the adaptive family system: (1) survival, (2) continuity (role function), and (3) growth (the system's self-concept). At the current stage of development, Roy (p. 275) simply said that "family behavior can be observed as it relates to the general family goals of survival, continuity, and growth."

The nurse observes for the outputs of survival, continuity, and growth and for the transactional and member controls that serve as feedback to the family to signal the need to adjust the behavior of a member or the group. Nursing practice emerges from the assessment of the previously described family factors. The nursing process continues to (1) identify and validate with family members the factor that is most immediately affecting their behavior, (2) identify individual family member needs as focal stimuli, (3) make nursing diagnoses and set goals, and (4) intervene to enhance stimuli configuration in the family.

Friedman (1992, p. 61) supported Roy's suggestion that "nursing problems involve ineffective coping mechanisms, which cause ineffective responses, disrupting the integrity of the person" and suggested that "this notion could easily be broadened to the family unit, where ineffective family coping patterns lead to family functioning problems." Whall and Fawcett (1991), p. 24) acknowledged the potential contribution of Roy's model of nursing care to the care of the family as an adaptive system but noted that "theories of family adaptation and nursing practice theories of family need to be generated and tested." Family adaptation theories need to be elaborated by identifying specific and concrete inputs, processes, and outputs of the family system.

It can be clearly seen that the family as client, rather than context, is a significant new conceptual basis for nursing. Although the attribution "of wellness and illness to the family unit is a recent phenomenon" (Gilliss, Highley, Roberts, & Martinson, 1988, p. 5), it is anticipated that an eclectic view of family incorporating both the nursing conceptual models and other social systems approaches will continue to be refined.

Nurses frequently integrate family approaches to clinical situations. Family theory and nursing models provide solid foundations for professional practice. Many family assessment tools exist. Most inpatient admission databases collect data surrounding family life. Although family models and theories are not specific to a particular nurse theorist, they complement many current nursing models and theories. Some cases, such as the structure provided by Anderson and Tomlinson (1992), provide an eclectic approach when working with families as clients. The family plays a key role in its own health and the health of individual members. Current family health practices evolve from previous health practices. When a family unit forms, the health practices of the new family frequently blend health patterns that the family heads learned as children. Women tend to assume primary responsibility for family health; family members have specific health routines; and community and cultural contexts affect family health (Andrews & Boyle, 2016; Blanes et al., 2007; Denham, 1999; Lundy & Janes, 2014; Schumacher et al., 2007).

> **Take Note!**
> Family models and theories are not specific to any specific nurse theorist; instead they complement many current nursing models and theories.

THE COMMUNITY AS CLIENT

This book philosophically defines community as a social system with open communication networks between structural and functional subsystems and the greater societal systems. Vertical bureaucratic relationships tie the community to the larger society. A community always has a sense of common identification, even if it does not exist as a common geographical location. Thus, the boundaries of a community can be determined in terms of role relationships as well as geography.

As with all open systems, the nurse influences change in the community. The change is directed toward higher levels of wellness in the system. Shuster and Geppinger (2004) specified that the community becomes the client when service providers aim to achieve what is best for the collective good of the population receiving care services instead of focusing on what is best for the individual. In addition, members of the community and nurses work collaboratively to identify community needs and develop programs to meet them.

Basic concepts from community health nursing apply to the care of **community as client**. Various community nursing scholars such as Neuman (1989), Pender, Murdaugh, and Parsons (2005) (see Chapter 8, The Health Process and Self-Care of the Nurse), and Canty-Mitchell, Little, Robinson, & Chandler (2008) have agreed that the following considerations are essential to professional nurses working with the community as client.

- **Health promotion**: Improving the well-being and quality of life of the community
- **Risk**: Identifying factors that increase the chance the community will either experience or be affected by a particular health problem
- **Disease prevention**: Protecting the population from diseases, disabilities, and their consequences

- **Primary prevention**: Preventing the occurrence of health problems or diseases
- **Secondary prevention**: Identifying and treating health problems and diseases
- **Tertiary prevention**: Preventing further deterioration following a health problem or restoring health and functioning after disease occurs

REAL-LIFE REFLECTIONS

Sometimes a social change may be needed to address the key considerations in community health nursing. For example, Nancy may find the need to confront the societal value that it is impossible to be too thin. In addition to educating the girls and their families, Nancy may find it necessary to consult with teachers, school administrators, the parent–teacher organization, other students, and the ballet teacher to inform them of the dangers and plan a community-wide program to alleviate malnutrition stemming from the desire to be thin.

Definitions of Community

Because community has been thought of primarily as a setting for care, nurses need to explore the various definitions of community to determine how they may view the community as a client for nursing services. Multiple definitions exist. Clark (1999, p. 6) defined a community as a "group of people who share some type of bond, who interact with each other, and who function collectively regarding common concerns." From a nursing perspective, Hanchett (1988, p. 7) said that community can be considered as an aggregate, a system, or a human–environment field. "As an aggregate, the individual is the basic unit of the community; that is, the community is a number of separate individuals." As a system, one must consider the "relationships among the individuals or groups who constitute the community" (Hanchett, 1988, p. 8). As a human–environment field, the community represents a human field integral with its environment and "manifesting correlates of the patterning of that field process" (Hanchett, 1988, p. 8).

If the nurse views the community as an aggregate, nursing truly is organized around the concept of the community serving as a context for individuals. Clark (1999, p. 56) defined community health nursing as a " synthesis of nursing knowledge and practice and the science and practice of public health, implemented via systematic use of the nursing process and other processes, designed to promote health and prevent illness in population groups. The focus of care is the aggregate." Clark indicated that community health nursing is characterized by the following attributes.

1. **Health orientation:** Health promotion and prevention of disease, rather than cure of illness
2. **Population focus:** Emphasis on aggregates, rather than individuals or families
3. **Autonomy:** Greater community control over health care decisions
4. **Continuity:** Providing continuing, comprehensive care rather than short-term, episodic care
5. **Collaboration:** Nurse and client interacting as equals
6. **Interactivity:** Awareness of interaction of a variety of factors with health
7. **Public accountability:** Accountability to society for public health
8. **Sphere of intimacy:** Greater awareness of the reality of client lives and situations

Nurses can select from a variety of community nursing and community health models to follow when working with the community as client. Christensen and Kenney (1990) proposed a comprehensive model for implementing the nursing process focusing on the aggregate within the context of a geopolitical environment.

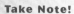

Take Note!
A community is a group of people who share a bond, interact with one another, and function as a unit.

Zotti, Brown, and Stotts (1996, p. 211) differentiated between community-based nursing and community health nursing (Table 15.1). Community-based nursing uses "a philosophy of nursing that guides nursing care provided for individuals, families, and groups wherever they are, including where they live, work, play, or go to school." In contrast, community health nursing is "a systematic process of delivering nursing care to improve the health of an entire community" (Zotti et al., 1996, p. 212).

When the community becomes the client, nurses may find themselves approaching ethical issues in a different manner. Many times ethical practice requires that nurses balance ethical considerations for the individual with those for the community. For example, protecting the community or collective becomes more important, especially when determining the allocation of scarce resources and when the need for community information supersedes the privacy and autonomy of an individual. Professional nurses must also look for ways to ensure social justice and equal access to offered care services while working with culturally diverse and marginalized groups within a designated community. When serving the community, professional nurses may encounter ethical conflicts arising from roles and responsibilities outlined by the profession and employing agency as well as conflicts arising among cultural

TABLE 15.1 Community-Based Nursing Versus Community Health Nursing		
Component	**Community-Based Nursing**	**Community Health Nursing**
Goals	Manage acute or chronic conditions Promote self-care	Preserve/protect health Promote self-care
Client	Individual and family	Community
Underlying philosophy	Human ecologic model	Primary health care
Autonomy	Individual and family autonomy Individual rights may be sacrificed for the good of the community	Community autonomy
Client character	Across the life span	Across the life span, with emphasis on high-risk aggregates
Cultural diversity	Culturally appropriate care of individual and families	Collaboration with and mobilization of diverse groups and communities
Type of service	Direct	Direct and indirect
Home visiting	Home visitor	Home visitor
Service focus	Local community	Local, state, federal, and international

From Zotti, M. E., Brown, P., & Stotts, R. C. (1996). Community-based nursing versus community health nursing: What does it all mean? *Nursing Outlook, 44*, 212. Used with permission of the publisher.

values and practices from different groups within the community. However, as with all clients, professional nurses serving the community must act with honesty, integrity, transparency, loyalty, and truthfulness (Allen & Easley, 2008; Kurtz & Burr, 2009).

If nurses view the community as a system, then they seek to introduce changes in the community systems and base interventions on their understanding of the impact of these changes on system functioning (Spradley, 1990). Christensen and Kenney (1990) also proposed a general systems assessment model for directing the nursing process with families. Considerable work on viewing the community as a system that is the recipient of nursing care has emerged from Neuman's conceptual model of nursing (discussed later in this chapter). Hanchett (1988) postulated that Roy's adaptation model of nursing and King's general system framework also offer nurses the opportunity to practice nursing with the community as a client system, in which the focus is on the pattern of relationships among the elements of the system.

Following are brief discussions of (1) a systems model of community as client based on Neuman's conceptual model, in which change is directed toward restoring stability to the system; and (2) a human field–environment model of community as client based on Rogerian nursing science, in which change is directed toward increasing capacities and evolving growth, and Parse's perception of community from a human becoming perspective. Despite their different approaches, these models tend to agree that community nursing interventions primarily address health promotion and interactions among the domains of space, human relationships, and the environment.

REAL-LIFE REFLECTIONS

If school nurse Nancy operates from a community as client perspective, her focus on eating disorders would shift. Instead of intervening with the individual students affected by the problem, she would consider how the problem affects the entire school community. She would plan and execute educational programs for students, faculty, staff, and administration on the detection and prevention of eating disorders. Along with education, Nancy would offer her time and attention to listen to concerns and counsel all people affected by the declining health of students with eating disorders.

A Systems Model of Viewing the Community as Client

Anderson and McFarlane (2015) adapted the Neuman health care systems model to provide a way for nurses to conceive of the community as the recipient of care. This effort synthesizes public health with nursing. In this systems approach, the community has eight subsystems: (1) recreation, (2) safety and transportation, (3) communication, (4) education, (5) health and social services, (6) economics, (7) politics and government, and (8) the physical environment.

The boundaries of a community are generally geopolitical. The interactive nature of these eight subsystems results in a whole that is more than the sum of its parts. Other nurse leaders have expanded views on this model in terms of the nursing process (Christensen & Kenney, 1990). For example, Beddome (1995) stressed the need to clearly define the client system that is the target of data collection and nursing intervention (geopolitical or aggregate).

The application of Neuman's model to the development of the nursing process with the community as the recipient of care is built around the redefinition of person, environment, health, and nursing. Community nursing scholars have described communities as groups of people who share common characteristics, such as language or culture, who may or may not live in a specific geographical area (Anderson & McFarlane, 2015; Lundy & Janes, 2014). They redefined the environment to include all conditions, circumstances, and influences that affect the development of the community. Health is equated with competence to function and "a definable state of equilibrium in which subsystems are in harmony so that the whole can perform at its maximum potential" (Saucier, 1991, p. 59).

Nurses participate in the care of the community by participating in community assessment, identifying and diagnosing problems amenable to nursing interventions, planning for and implementing interventions that enhance the interacting forces within the system, and evaluating the outcomes of the interventions on the community's health.

The systems model focuses on prevention.

- **Primary prevention strategies** for the professional nurse include (Saucier, 1991) (1) increasing the public's awareness of health problems, (2) increasing the public's knowledge of the available community resources and services to resolve the problems, (3) preparing the public to self-refer to appropriate resources, and (4) preparing the public to become involved in preventing the factors that lead to the problem.

- **Secondary prevention strategies** include facilitating self-screenings and referral to appropriate community resources.
- **Tertiary prevention strategies** include lobbying for adequate services and resources to meet the particular community health problems. An example is "health care reform by rethinking health policy and writing new health legislation at many levels of government" (Beddome, 1995, p. 571).

The systems model presents a comprehensive approach when nurses serve the community as client. The systems approach uses the change as stability perspective.

A Human Field–Environment Model of Viewing the Community as Client

The paradigm of nursing in which change is directed toward growth uses the Rogerian framework for viewing the community as client.

Hanchett (1988, p. 128) said that, in this view, the community is seen as an energy field in process with the environmental energy field, and health is viewed as the dynamic well-being of the community–environmental process. Manifestations of these energy fields in process may be reflected in visible expressions such as motion, rhythms of quiet and activity, and the togetherness of the community's members in participating in change.

For example, motion that is observable by the nurse is the speed of people and traffic in daily life. Rhythms of quiet and activity may be seen in the sleep–wake patterns of the community. Everyone has heard about how the streets are "rolled up at night" in some communities. Gatherings of people in community settings can be observed to analyze togetherness. Other pattern manifestations of this energy process include the "number of cultural and ethnic groups of the community, the variety of lifestyles and ideas that flourish, and pragmatic, imaginative, and visionary approaches to change evidenced by the community" (Hanchett, 1988, p. 129).

The goal of nursing is to help the community achieve maximum well-being. According to Hanchett (1988), this is done by the nurse participating in the process of change, assisting community groups to move toward well-being. Rogers' definition of health as "dynamic well-being" means that the community must become more aware of factors that maximize well-being and minimize conditions that limit actualization or realization of full potential.

This view of health as "dynamic well-being" directs the actions of the nurse in this model. His or her actions all center on facilitating for people the process of becoming more aware of their patterns of energy exchange with the environment and the evolving outcomes of these exchanges. Manifestations of field patterning include "diversity, rhythms, motion, the experience of time, sleep–wake and beyond-waking states, and pragmatic, imaginative, and visionary approaches to conscious participation in change" (Hanchett, 1988, p. 128). The nurse attempts to facilitate evolutionary change in the human field–environmental field process from lesser diversity to greater diversity; from longer rhythms and slower motion to seemingly continuous rhythms and motion; from experiencing time as slower, pragmatic foci to experiencing time as timelessness, visionary foci; and from longer sleeping to longer waking, perhaps even beyond waking (Hanchett, 1988).

The essence of this model for community nursing is that the community as a group–environmental field process determines the health of the community. In each community, the process unfolds at a unique pace and in unique patterns. The community's health is an expression of the mutually evolving process. Nursing's approaches to enhance the well-being of people-environment speak of community well-being. Influencing public policies to provide improved shelter, food, and clothing for all people is an example of approaches to improve community well-being (see Chapter 19, The Professional Nurse's Role in Public Policy). Nursing is "the science that the art of nursing uses in the conscious participation in the human–environmental field process toward the goal of maximum well-being" (Hanchett, 1988, p. 132).

In the Rogerian model of nursing, the community field–environmental field process integrates all other definitions of community; that is, it validates the community as a social system, as a place (space), and as people. The resultant health of the client system (community) is more than the sum of these identified parts. Well-being is an integral process in which human beings and the environment evolve toward greater awareness of their being. Respect for both diversity and sameness in patterns of energy exchange is essential for the professional nurse to operate out of this conceptual model of nursing.

It is evident from the general nature of the discussion of this model that much research is needed to assist further development of the Rogerian model. Determining manifestations of patterning of life, identifying patterns that maximize health, and developing strategies that focus on the community field–environmental field process are necessary for fuller implementation of this model in community nursing practice in which the community is the recipient of the care.

Similar to the Rogerian perspective of community, Parse (2003) espoused the interconnectedness of the community and the environment. Parse (2003) defined community as "a oneness of human-universe connectedness incarnating beliefs and values" (p. 1) that is "objective, measurable, and concerned with relationships, change, symbiosis, localism, cooperation, and the commonality of interests and goals" (p. 5). Parse (2003) further explained that the community is "an ever-changing incarnated interconnectedness correlated with all that is" (p. 21). Parse also envisioned a community that is more than just an acreage or a location. Using her consistent method of what seems to be nearly polar opposites, she identifies two key considerations for the ever-evolving community.

- **Anchoring–shifting** deals with the phenomenon of holding fast to some things while giving up others.
- **Pondering–shaping** refers to thoroughly thinking about how, dialoguing and listening to all community members, and considering all options before developing a means for change.

Parse also specified that when one barrier to change is removed, others typically appear. Parse specified that true presence serves as the core for nursing practice in the community and that nurses need courage and confidence along with the understanding of key community members in order to make changes. Cocreating rhythms occur within the community, thereby facilitating human interconnectedness that is ever-changing and creating new possibilities.

To learn how to care for communities as clients, nurses may benefit most from participating in service-learning projects or clinical experiences in community agencies. Community-based nursing experiences enable nurses to appreciate the value of being an engaged citizen in a community while learning how to provide nursing services to larger groups of people. Community-based experiences offer situations in which nurses give to the agency while they increase their repertoire of community nursing skills. When engaging in community nursing, nurses must expand their views to see how internal and external factors affect an agency while collaborating with community members to ensure that they offer relevant services (Narsavage, Batchelor, Lindell, & Chen, 2003). Nurses also work to build stronger communities as well as improve

community health. Through role modeling, nurses can inspire community members to participate actively in the political process, increase participation in community activities, develop community goals, manage conflicts effectively, attain consensus on goal priorities and how to reach them, use resources effectively, and obtain external resources for desired programs (Head et al., 2004). Finally, and most importantly, nurses advocate for underprivileged community members so that they gain access to health care and other basic services (McElmurry, Park, & Buseh, 2003).

From an idealist perspective, the goal of community health nursing would be to facilitate the development of healthy, healing communities. Nurses live and work with others in communities. If a community is defined as anyone who works together to attain a common goal, then nurses could view a community from a variety of perspectives. Provision of nursing services to any community begins with a community assessment.

Community Assessment

In a community assessment, community health care nurses assess the community in terms of status, structure, and process.

- *Status assessment* includes reported statistics related to birth, death, poverty, crime, and incidence of mental and physical illness.
- *Structure assessment* includes inpatient and outpatient health care facilities, local government structures, schools, law enforcement agencies, retailers, roads, and population demographics (socioeconomic status, gender, age).
- *Process assessment* includes factors such as member commitment, communication patterns, relationships of the community with the larger society, and how well the community voices its need for, accesses, and uses resources (Anderson & McFarlane, 2015; Clark, 2014; Hunt, 2008; Lundy & Janes, 2014; Maurer & Smith, 2013).

In the professional nursing work setting, the nurse would consider aspects of the building structure, actual and potential health hazards, employee demographics and incidences of work-related injuries and illnesses within the overall organization and at the nursing unit levels. For the academic setting, the nurse would look at the campus buildings, campus plan, demographics of students, faculty administration and staff; actual and potential health hazards, presence of academic support systems and instances of campus-related violence, injuries, and illnesses. In both settings, the nurse would examine current policies and procedures for getting the work done (patient care for a clinical setting or student education in an academic setting). The nurse would also look at how the institution communicates its mission and its commitments to local and global communities. Finally, the nurse would assess the frequency that the community accesses and uses the organizational (or institutional) services and resources.

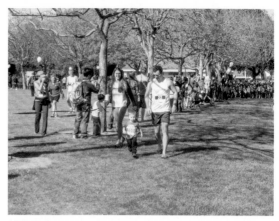

FIGURE 15.2 Communities play a key role in developing a local culture of wellness.

QUESTIONS FOR REFLECTION

1. What additional professional skills do nurses need when the community is the client?
2. What are current health concerns within your local community?
3. What are current health concerns within your academic community?
4. What health concerns can you identify in your clinical practice community?
5. Why are the health concerns you identify above important for each community?

HALLMARKS OF A HEALTHY COMMUNITY

The healthy city/community movement began in the mid-1980s in Europe. Hancock and Duhl (1986) specified that the following must be present for a community to be classified as healthy.

1. A clean, safe, and ecologically stable physical environment.
2. Resident access to resources that promote and maintain a healthy, diverse, vital, and innovative economy.
3. A strong, supportive, nonexploitative community.
4. Basic human needs (food, water, shelter, income, and safety) met for all members.
5. Access to a wide variety of experiences and resources (communications, cultural events, diverse contacts).
6. A connection to the community's heritage and past.
7. Equal access to public health and illness care services.
8. Good health status of citizens.
9. High levels of public participation in and control over decisions that affect individual citizens' lives, health, and well-being.

Morse (2004) denoted characteristics of successful communities that plan for and adapt to change. Healthy communities have members who understand their relationship and responsibility to others rather than focusing solely on individual pursuits (Fig. 15.2).

By strategically planning for change, communities ensure their survival and enable brighter futures for members following in their footsteps. Morse identified the following seven key points that result in successful community adaptation to change.

1. Making the right investments/decisions the first time
2. Working together instead of as individuals or special interest groups with specific agendas
3. Building on current community strengths
4. Using a democratic process
5. Preserving the community's history
6. Growing their own leaders
7. Inventing a better and brighter future

COMMUNITY-LEVEL NURSING INTERVENTIONS

Health promotion within a community encompasses collective efforts. Community nursing interventions work best when the community assumes ownership of the plan, responsibility for community health program maintenance, and control for planning future programs. Nurses use multiple strategies to help communities improve their health. They empower, collaborate with, build capacity for, and advocate for individual members and the entire community (Leddy, 2003; Lind & Smith, 2008).

Nurses empower communities by investing time and resources to enable communities to assume control over their destinies. Some community members view the nurse as a health expert who has much knowledge and expertise in developing programs and supporting others to attain better health, while others see the nurse as someone who plans to force sometimes culturally incompatible ways on them (Andrews & Boyle, 2016; Leininger & McFarland, 2006; Lind & Smith, 2008). Poverty-stricken communities perceive a lack of control over their destinies and feel powerless because they may not be valued by others, have few (or no) resources, lack economic and political power, have no experience in making decisions, and have learned helplessness. Sometimes, community members have a history of fighting with each other. Nurses can serve as mediators to settle long-standing disputes so community members can determine which programs are needed. Nurses also serve as consultants, coaches, and cheerleaders as community members plan, implement, and evaluate community health programs.

Collaboration with the community requires that the nurse and community members share information and resources with each other, but above all, trust each other. Lind and Smith (2008) proposed the use of appreciative inquiry as a means to connect with the community and identify community strengths. Appreciative inquiry provides opportunities for people to share their stories and to perceive that they have been heard and that their ideas are valued. Everyone involved shares ideas and listens intently. Through the use of appreciative inquiry, the community health nurse becomes familiar with traditional folk medicine, key community concerns, and community leaders. Appreciative inquiry fosters deep personal connections while encouraging the participation of everyone engaged in the development, planning, and implementation of community nursing interventions. The community and nurse work in partnership to promote health rather than merely identify health problems.

Capacity building occurs with individual members, small groups, and the entire community. Capacity building involves building on the current strengths, resources, and abilities already present in the community. Individual capacity building involves changing personal values for health-enhancing outcomes, having a positive attitude toward collaboration, making decisions using consensus, sharing power and information, showing respect, giving support, participating in egalitarian relationships, perceiving self-efficacy, setting future goals, feeling a sense of coherence, identifying with others who have similar problems, feeling able to help others, and understanding community member roles and responsibilities. Small-group capacity building includes interacting with others to help them assume control, fostering a sense of connectedness, establishing trust, and creating positive interactions. Capacity in building communities involves helping

members and the community to articulate health problems and potential solutions, providing them with access to information, supporting current community leadership, and assisting them to overcome obstacles to action. While building capacity within a community, the nurse may act as a strategist, coach, meeting facilitator, mediator, and developer of community leadership (Leddy, 2003).

Once the community has mobilized its internal human and physical resources, the community shares a group consciousness. With a united purpose, the community becomes capable of taking social and political action to obtain additional resources for use in community building and improvement. Disenfranchised people may not have the ability to develop independently as a community. The nurse helps these people achieve community-building skills through role modeling, providing support, and listening to them share their problems and concerns. Nurses have the ability to service communities in multiple ways and there are many opportunities for nurses to pursue a career in community health nursing.

CAREER OPPORTUNITIES IN COMMUNITY HEALTH NURSING

Nurses have many opportunities to engage in community nursing, including in public health departments, factories, businesses, camps, homes, homeless shelters, prisons, schools, parishes, and the armed forces. Some nurses engage in volunteer nursing. Community members who know professional nurses sometimes ask them for health advice and information outside the work setting. Nurses who give health-related advice to friends and acquaintances are practicing nursing and should assume accountability for their actions. Thus, the professional nurse should keep a record of nursing actions (including consultations with neighbors) and evaluate outcomes of health education, advice, recommended consultations, and nursing procedures.

In an examination of state health rankings and the 2004 National Survey of Registered Nurses, Bigbee (2008) reported that an increased nurse-to-population ratio resulted in higher state health rankings in terms of reduced motor vehicle deaths, crime rates, incidence of infectious diseases, childhood poverty, uninsured people, premature deaths, and time off work for poor physical and mental health. In addition, the higher nurse ratio resulted in increases in high school graduation rates, recommended immunizations, and prenatal care. The study also revealed that higher nurse-to-population ratios resulted in an increased level of healthiness and general well-being in the community, whereas higher physician-to-population ratios resulted in improved physical health of individuals. Therefore, the study findings "suggest that more RNs per capita may be associated with healthier populations" (Bigbee, 2008, p. 250), substantiating the need for effective strategies to alleviate the current and projected future nursing shortage (see Chapter 3, "Contextual, Philosophical, and Ethical Elements of Professional Nursing").

The following section briefly describes selected practice areas for community health nursing. More detailed information regarding community nursing opportunities may be found by consulting website resources or references at the end of this chapter.

Public Health Nursing

Public health nurses have been serving individuals, groups, communities, and populations since 1893. The Institute of Medicine (2003) defined public health as what a society does collectively to guarantee that conditions occur so that people can be healthy. Public health nurses respond to societal health needs by focusing on promoting and protecting the health of populations. Public health nurses do not work in isolation; rather, they collaborate with interprofessional health care team members, typically within a local government agency (city or county health department). When health issues arise that concern more than the local community, public health nurses find themselves consulting and working with national governments (e.g., U.S. Public Health Service) and even world organizations (e.g., United Nations). Health promotion and protection are the top priorities for public health nurses (American Nurses Association [ANA], 2013b; Lind & Smith, 2008; Quad Council of Public Health Nursing Organizations, 1999).

Since 1999, the Quad Council of Public Health Nursing Organizations has stipulated the baccalaureate degree as the entry level for public health nursing practice. The ANA offers certification in community/public health nursing. Bekemeier (2007) noted that the certification has intrinsic value for nurses (personal satisfaction, sign of professional growth, evidence of professional accomplishment and specialized knowledge, increased confidence, and professional credibility). However, many nurses report the certification has little extrinsic value such as employer and public recognition. Very few nurses report receiving salary increases by earning community/public health nursing certification (Bekemeier, 2007).

Currently, advanced practice public health nursing requires graduate-level education with a master's degree in either nursing or public health. Most state nurse practice acts fail to recognize advanced nursing practice in the realm of public health nursing (Levin et al., 2008). In many states, when practice focuses on health and illnesses of individuals residing in a community, less highly educated nurses may engage in public health nursing practice.

Public health nurses aim to promote and protect the health of populations through the creation of situations and provision of services to help people optimize their health. Along with using foundational nursing knowledge, public health nurses incorporate knowledge from the social and public health science into practice (ANA, 2013b). Public health nurses provide services to meet government-specified health objectives as outlined in *Healthy People 2020* (USDHHS, 2010). Essential services offered by public health service nurses include (1) monitoring the health status of a particular population, (2) diagnosing community health problems, (3) identifying community health hazards, (4) investigating community health problems when they arise, (5) developing partnerships with those they serve, (6) solving community health problems, (7) developing policies and action plans to support community health, (8) enforcing laws and regulations to ensure public safety and health, (9) linking people to appropriate health care services, (10) educating current and future public health personnel, (11) evaluating the effectiveness and quality of public health services, (12) identifying future health threats, and (13) researching innovative solutions to maximize the health and safety of the public (Bekemeier, 2007; Bender & Salmon, 2009; Clark, 2014; Levin et al., 2008; Quad Council of Public Health Nursing Organizations, 1999; Smith & Maurer, 2013).

QUESTIONS FOR REFLECTION

1. Do you know how to contact your local public health department?
2. What services does your local public health department offer? Have you or a member of your family ever made use of those services?

Community Mental Health Nursing

Promoting the mental health of citizens is extremely important for the quality of life in a community. Many countries, including the United States, provide a full array of mental health services (from acute and long-term residential programs to home health care) for citizens who need them. In 1963, the passage of the Community Mental Health Centers Act provided federal funding for community mental health centers, resulting in the deinstitutionalization of mentally ill people who were once confined to psychiatric inpatient facilities. These individuals became part of local communities and were no longer required to conform to the restrictions required by hospitals, shelters, and group homes.

Because of the lack of residential programs, many people with severe mental illness may live at home. In addition, many people with mental disorders cannot hold a job, which means they frequently have no health care insurance. Many homeless people suffer from mental illness. When left to fend for themselves, some mentally ill people have no access to mental health services to receive the psychotropic medications necessary to function effectively as citizens. Some communities have civil ordinances against people living on the streets, some provide homeless shelters, and others rely on private agencies or faith-based organizations to provide shelter for the homeless. Some homeless shelters provide mental health services for their clients.

Community mental health nurses may find themselves working with people who may have a history of violent behavior or have been victims of violence. Some people living in high-crime areas become isolated because of their fear for their safety or the safety of their property. Community mental health nurses work in a variety of settings, such as mental health clinics, public health departments, chemical abuse programs, homeless shelters, group residential homes, prisons, and home health, to address the needs of these populations.

When working in community settings, community mental health nurses assume the following client care activities: assessing client condition and progress, managing medication, promoting health, supporting clients and families, and intervening to prevent (hopefully), and manage psychiatric emergencies. When signs of mental deterioration occur, community mental health nurses collaborate with physicians for emergency management and make referrals for emergency or immediate care. In life-threatening situations, community mental health nurses activate the emergency response system. Advanced practice mental health nurses may have prescriptive privileges for psychotropic medications and frequently have education and credentials to offer counseling services (ANA, 2014b; Elsom, Happell, & Manias, 2007).

Community mental health nurses collaborate with and support community members as they make autonomous decisions. They also work with other health care professionals to maximize use of available resources for health promotion, such as using a social worker to help secure food stamps or vouchers (ANA, 2014b). Many people with mental disorders receive mental health services from home health nurses who specialize in psychiatric-mental health care.

Not all public health departments provide mental health services for their communities. When they do, community health nurses provide mental health services to clients who seek care in public health clinics. If the public health department fails to provide mental health services, community members receive mental health services from free-standing, government-supported, nonprofit, or for-profit mental health centers. To access mental health services, community members must be informed of the location and nature of the mental health services offered by each center. They receive such information from nurses or other health care providers.

If a major event occurs within a community that has the potential to affect the mental health of its members, coordinated efforts from all facilities offering mental health services are required. For example, community mental health nurses from various mental health facilities may be consulted to support students and teachers in schools after an act of violence or student loss of life has occurred.

In *Healthy People 2020,* the U.S. government specified goals to improve and increase access to quality mental health services (USDHHS, 2010). Mental health services targeted for improvement include preventive services for suicide, adolescent suicide attempts, and eating disorders. An increased effort aimed at providing employment for people with serious mental illnesses is another goal. The initiative also hopes to improve services for homeless adults with serious mental illnesses. Areas for treatment expansion for mental health and illness include (1) primary care, including screening and assessment; (2) pediatric mental health services, including screening for mental disorders in juvenile justice facilities; and (3) improving treatment services for adults, especially the elderly (USDHHS, 2010). More community mental health nurses are and will be needed to attain these goals.

Healthy People 2020 also provides mechanisms to track consumer satisfaction with offered mental health services, determine cultural competence, and develop plans to address the mental health needs of the burgeoning elderly population (USDHHS, 2010).

Electronic Community Health Nursing

Online chat rooms, blogs, and social media create a "virtual" gathering place for people with similar interests or conditions. When a chat, blog, Facebook page, or other social media message is formed for a specific purpose, such as providing support, education, and resource information for people with a similar health condition or life situation, the purpose is consistent with the ANA's *Scope and Standards of Public Health Nursing Practice* (2013). When nurses participate in these online interactions with the aim of promoting and protecting the health of their community members, they could be considered to be providing community nursing services. In such forums, nurses may provide social support to other members, model therapeutic communication techniques, reinforce positive behaviors among group members, offer self-care or health-promoting advice, provide health-related information, and monitor group dynamics (Copeland, 2002).

Before electronic community health nursing can be recognized, current international, national, and state laws require changes. The following questions about professional nursing practice must also be addressed.

1. How will professional nurses receive compensation for their services (or will they)?
2. What accountability will the nurse have to the members of the electronic community?
3. What are the roles of the professional nurse providing e-community health nursing services?
4. If the nurse shares a similar condition as other chat room participants, how will professional and personal boundaries be delineated?
5. How will states and/or the federal government regulate online professional nursing practice?

Camp Nursing

Camps are temporary, small communities. "Like all communities, camps provide basic services for their members, including food, shelter, socialization, protection from harm, meaningful activity, and the other necessities of life" (Lishner & Bruya, 1994, p. 7). Although seen primarily as a form of recreation, camps offer opportunities for nurses to practice first-aid skills and care for the injured and infirmed in more rustic settings, thereby providing practice in skills that might be required when responding to disaster situations and caring for disaster victims (Erceg & Pravda, 2009).

Camp nurses work toward attaining a healthy camp community. Depending on the type of camp, camping allows individuals of all ages to experience nature; escape the stress of a fast-paced, highly technologic society; and learn self-reliance while learning skills for survival and recreation. Camp enables people to live with others unlike themselves and shows them how to establish a community for a prescribed time. Skills learned at camp transfer to other settings.

Professional nurses have opportunities to participate in a variety of camping experiences. Day camps provide sessions of varying lengths, with participants and staff returning home at night. Residential camps require participants and staff to live on site for a few days or up to 2 months. Residential camps assume great responsibility to ensure the safety and health of participants and staff. Travel camps typically involve some form of motorized transportation so that participants can move from site to site. Trip camps use individually guided vehicles or animals (such as horses, bicycles, or canoes). Special-needs camps offer people with special physical, cognitive, or emotional needs, an opportunity to reap the benefits of camp life. Special-needs camps include the various members of the interdisciplinary health care team on staff to ensure that the participants' special health needs are met (Erceg & Pravda, 2009).

Camp nurses confront a variety of health care needs in professional practice. Generally speaking, camp nurses provide the following.

- Emergency care for accidents and acute care for minor illness and injuries (e.g., insect bites, sore throats, cuts).
- Plans to avoid spread of contagious illnesses (foodborne illness, athlete's foot, plantar warts).
- Health education for campers and staff.
- Screening for and elimination of health hazards in the camp environment (insects, snakes, mice, and poison ivy, oak, and sumac).
- Verification of healthy nutritional offerings and daily camp schedules.
- Supervision to ensure that campers abide by health-related rules.

Nurses working or volunteering in special-needs camps find themselves providing direct care to campers by administering medications, performing specialized procedures and therapies, and monitoring the effects of interventions and the camping experience on those with special needs. Camp nurses also must be aware of, develop relationships with, and secure camp contracts for emergency care with health care providers located in the camp's vicinity (Erceg & Pravda, 2009).

Occupational Health Nursing

Because employers and employees in work settings share a common goal and spend time together, workplaces fit the definition of community. Occupational health nurses provide primary, secondary, and tertiary care to people in the work setting. Occupational health nurses ensure employee safety by collaborating with agencies that set standards for safe and healthy working environments. Federal guidelines for worker safety specify that employers bear responsibility for deleterious effects encountered by workers for occupational and environmental hazards (Clark, 2014; Rogers, 2001). Large businesses may have an occupational health department that employs many nurses; small businesses may employ only one nurse or contract with health care providers to provide occupational health services for employees.

In addition to direct care services, occupational health nurses may provide health education to employees. They also compile statistical reports summarizing the annual incidence of employee occupational illness and injuries. By law, these reports are submitted to federal, state, and local agencies and made available to employees. Commonly occurring occupational illnesses include repetitive stress injuries, allergic and contact dermatitis, respiratory disorders caused by inhalation of toxic agents, poisoning, hearing loss, low back disorders, traumatic injuries, fertility problems, and pregnancy abnormalities (Clark, 2014; Rogers, 2001).

In 2004, the American Association of Occupational Health Nurses (AAOHN) developed 11 standards for occupational and environmental health nursing practice (the entire document is available from AAOHN) which were revised in 2015.

1. Assess the health status of clients, workforce, and work environment using a systematic approach.
2. Analyze the health data from the assessment and develop nursing diagnoses that need to be addressed.
3. Develop specific expected client outcomes to address identified nursing diagnoses.
4. Create a goal-directed plan with comprehensive interventions and therapies to achieve care outcomes.
5. Implement identified interventions to achieve desired care plan outcomes.
6. Evaluate the developed care plan systematically and continuously in response to client responses.
7. Manage and use corporate resources to support occupational health and safety programs.
8. Assume responsibility for professional self-development for enhancement of professional growth and competency.
9. Collaborate with clients and other health team members to prevent health issues while promoting and restoring health in the work environment.
10. Use research findings in and contribute to the scientific knowledge base for occupational and environmental health nursing for improving practice and advancing the profession.
11. Use an ethical framework when making practice decisions.

AAOHN (2007) identified core competencies based on the results of a Delphi process using Benner's (1984) "novice to expert" framework for ranking professional nurse competency levels in the following areas: clinical practice; case management; efforts at keeping the workforce healthy and safe while promoting a safe and healthy workplace and environment; regulatory and legislative efforts (abiding by current regulations and impacting future public policies); management, business, and leadership skills; health promotion and disease prevention; health and safety education and training; occupational and environmental health research; and professionalism. The AAOHN competencies were revised in 2015 and added competencies to address provision of culturally appropriate services to a diverse workforce, independent management of employee health issues by an advanced practice nurse and application of principles of the current business climate when providing employee health services (AAOHN, 2015b).

Occupational health nursing provides nurses with an opportunity to improve the health of employees and the work environment. By screening employees for various health problems related to their work before symptoms occur, occupational health nurses not only improve the health of workers but also reduce long-term health care costs for employers (AAOHN, 2007, 2015a).

▌ QUESTIONS FOR REFLECTION

1. What occupational health hazards are present in your current work setting?
2. What health hazards are present in your position as a student and in the building where you attend classes?
3. How can you reduce health hazards that you find in your work or school setting?
4. Does your school or workplace offer opportunities to better your health?

Home Health Nursing

Home health nurses provide nursing services to clients within the confines of each client's residence (Fig. 15.3). Although home health nursing practice focuses primarily on individuals, the home health care nurse also considers the needs of the family and designated caregivers. Home health nursing is considered a form of community nursing because the care occurs within the community and numerous community resources are used. Home health nurses view the client, family, and designated caregivers as partners when planning and implementing nursing care. The nurse performs a detailed home assessment to determine the safety of the home for the client (ANA, 2014a; Bailey, 2007). The home health nurse performs an assessment of the community in which the client's home is located to determine access to services and availability of resources for client support. The home health nurse provides direct care; educates the client, family, and caregivers about how to independently meet health care needs; counsels the client and family; and coordinates community resources and benefits. Home health

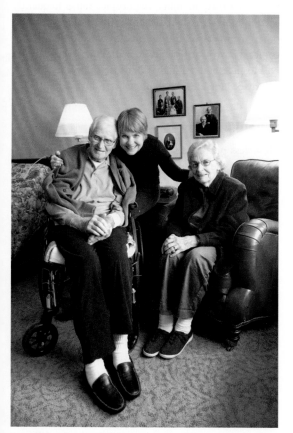

FIGURE 15.3 Home health nursing enables clients to stay in their own homes, and may be a rewarding nursing career.

nurses continually evaluate the effectiveness of planned interventions and community resources as nursing care is delivered (ANA, 2014a; Bailey, 2007).

The nurse–client relationship differs in home health nursing because the client (and family) considers the nurse a guest (ANA, 2014a). This perception sets up vastly different dynamics for the nurse–client relationship. The nurse must work diligently to ensure that he or she is welcome while helping the client and family assume responsibility for meeting individualized health needs. The nurse exercises special care not to offend the host or disaffirm client and family self-determination. Sometimes, the nurse must politely refuse client requests when they fall outside the arena of professional nursing practice (Clark, 2014). When such requests are made, the nurse might consider referring the client to appropriate community resources or set up visits by a homemaker or unlicensed care provider.

Home health nurses frequently supervise visits by unlicensed care providers and coordinate the schedules of other members of the health care team and home care services so that the client has someone visiting each day of the week. Home health care nurses frequently take calls on weekends and holidays so that homebound clients have access to a nurse should health care problems arise.

Advances in technology now enable home health nurses to have daily contact with clients. Telehealth and satellite home monitoring systems enable home health nurses to check client weight, blood pressure, pulse, peripheral blood glucose, and prothrombin times remotely. Some home monitoring systems set alarms and verbally prompt clients when it is time to get connected and send physical assessment data to the home health care agency. Certain systems offer direct video monitoring and/or wireless technology to obtain results of client home monitoring. With computer technology, the home health agency can create printed records of client data using tables or graphs to detect trends toward meeting expected outcomes or to indicate deteriorating parameters. Some systems even have the capability to ask a client specific questions to assess for potential disease complications.

Home health nurses use these systems for planning the sequence of daily visits or determining if an additional, unscheduled visit should be made. They also can call clients when they fail to perform required, daily monitoring tasks. Medicare covers home monitoring systems as long as clients have been certified for home health nurse visits. Once clients no longer need home health care, the monitoring system may be removed from the home. Some clients with financial resources elect to keep the monitoring system in their home using private funds. Home health nurses need to stress to clients that home monitoring systems do not replace calling 911 or an ambulance when an emergency arises.

For home health agencies to be reimbursed for services, the professional nurse maintains detailed records of home health visits. Complete, accurate documentation of the visit serves as data for third-party payer reimbursement, validation of services rendered, and data for nursing research. The professional nurse completes approval and recertification forms to validate the need for nursing services.

Hospice and Palliative Care Nursing

Hospice and palliative care nurses visit clients where they live and assist care providers with end-of-life care issues (Fig. 15.4). This may include the home or extended-care or residential facilities. The goal of hospice and palliative care is to promote the best possible quality of life for terminally ill persons and their significant others by alleviating suffering, promoting comfort, providing support services, and recognizing that the terminally ill are living until they die. According to the Hospice and Palliative Nurses Credentialing Center *CHPN® Candidate Handbook* (2016), over 16,000 nurses have attained certification in hospice and palliative care nursing (CHPN).

The nurse generalist provides direct care to patients and families and coordinates hospice and palliative care agencies. Nurse practitioners and clinical nurse specialists also offer advanced practice nursing care (including prescriptive services) in accordance with state laws (ANA & Hospice and Palliative Nurses Association, 2014 Since 1983, Medicare has covered home health services for the terminally ill (Lundy, Utterback, Lance, & Bloxsom, 2009; Lundy & Janes, 2014; Stanhope & Lancaster, 2014).

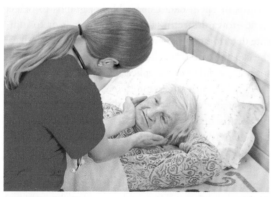

FIGURE 15.4 Hospice nursing helps terminally ill clients to achieve a peaceful, dignified death.

Nurses have a long history of caring for the dying. In 1950, Dr. Cicely Saunders founded the hospice movement at St. Christopher's Hospital in London. Hospice aims to add more life to each day when medical science cannot add additional time to a person's life. Hospice uses a team approach to maximize quality of life for the terminally ill client and caregivers by providing the following: (1) intermittent nursing services; (2) physician services aimed at alleviating human suffering; (3) medications for relieving pain, nausea, and other discomforts associated with the dying process; (4) home health aides; (5) medical equipment and supplies; (6) pastoral services for spiritual support; (7) continuous care when crises arise; and (8) follow-up bereavement services for the family for as long as a year after the client has died.

Hospice nurses receive special education on the dying process, grief, and bereavement management. To effectively care for terminally ill clients and their caregivers, hospice nurses must have confidence in their clinical skills and spiritual beliefs. Much of the nursing care focuses on helping the terminally ill and their families find meaning in their past, present, and future lives. As a team member, the hospice nurse frequently spends more time with clients and families than do other members of the hospice care team and shares comprehensive information with the team (ANA & Hospice and Palliative Nurses Association, 2014; Lundy & Janes, 2014; Stanhope & Lancaster, 2014).

Nursing the Homeless

Homeless people lack a fixed, regular night-time residence, or use a shelter, mission, or transient hotel, or who live in some other physical place not designed for human slumber or occupation (e.g., under a bridge, in a subway tunnel). For some people, homelessness may be temporary (the person has no home, but community membership remains), episodic (several bouts of having no home), or chronic (no home as a way of life). Homelessness is not confined to single adults; children appear among the ranks of the homeless as well. During times of economic recession, the number of homeless families increases. Reasons for homelessness include poverty, lack of affordable housing, unemployment, lack or inadequacy of government financial support, crime, violence, lack of kin support, mental illness, substance abuse, mental illness (addressed above), and socially stigmatizing infectious diseases (Anderson & Riley, 2008; Butts & Lundy, 2009; Clark, 2014).

In American life, securing a job, societal privileges, or government-sponsored social services requires a permanent address. Accessing health care services can be difficult if not impossible for the homeless. Frequently, homeless people use emergency rooms for the treatment of illnesses or enter the health care system as victims of crime. They receive emergency and acute care for sustained injuries in acute-care facilities. Once they recover, placing them in a safe situation where they can meet the demands of follow-up care poses a challenge to social workers and case managers.

Because of their inability to pay for services rendered, homeless people rarely have a consistent primary care provider. When health care is needed, some homeless people rely on free community health clinics or homeless shelters. Unfortunately, some of these organizations depend solely on volunteer health care providers, and the consistency of seeing the same client over time becomes problematic. Nurses also see homeless clients in soup kitchens and on urban streets.

Homelessness is not confined to urban settings. Migrant workers also fit the definition of homelessness. Rural county health departments frequently serve as the vehicle for health care for transient farm workers and homeless people seeking refuge in rural areas.

For effective nursing practice with the homeless, the community health or volunteer professional nurse must develop and maintain a realistic understanding of the world of homelessness. Many times, homeless people lack knowledge of available local programs and services to which they are entitled. Sometimes, homeless people become so overwhelmed in securing food and shelter that they lose hope. To survive, some homeless individuals develop street-smart behaviors that include manipulation, lying, and panhandling.

Professional nurses may play a variety of roles when working with and for the homeless. Nurses can work with clients to prevent the factors contributing to homelessness. Nurses also can lobby for legislation that increases services to homeless people and provide government officials with information about the plight of the homeless (see Chapter 19, The Professional Nurse's Role in Public Policy). Nurses can provide direct care and health screening to people who seek help at public health departments, free health clinics, homeless shelters, places of religious worship, or soup kitchens. Finally, nurses can refer the homeless to mobile treatment centers, mental health facilities, and drug and alcohol rehabilitation programs.

Nursing the Incarcerated

Nurses who work in prisons and detention centers provide physical and mental health care to persons who have committed crimes. Professional nurses engage in primary, secondary and tertiary interventions for those who are incarcerated. Professional nurses do not participate in procedures exclusively for correctional purposes; professional nursing practice in correctional facilities emphasizes disease prevention, promotes health enhancement activities, and recognizes and treats physical and mental illnesses and injuries from accident or act of violence. Nurses frequently administer medications for the purpose of controlling behavior and diagnosed mental illnesses. They also evaluate the effectiveness of care and look for ways to improve health services for those incarcerated (ANA, 2010). In prison settings, nurses make most health care decisions. They work with medically approved care protocols for the use of physical and chemical restraints when persons are in danger or harming themselves or others (Stringer, 2001).

Watson, Stimpson, and Hostick (2004) reported that as many as 90% of incarcerated people may have mental health problems, 80% smoke, 12% may be infected with HIV, and 8% may have hepatitis. As prison sentences lengthen, nurses encounter older inmates, as many as 85% of whom may have more than one chronic major illness. Although not common, some terminally ill prisoners may be seen by prison hospice workers or volunteers (Watson et al., 2004).

Security systems at correctional facilities apply to health care professionals and other staff members. Security systems protect staff, volunteers, and visitors from acts of violence. Prison officials have corrections officers stand outside examination rooms and accompany nurses to cells as they deliver health care to inmates who have a history of violence (Stringer, 2001). Some inmates receive outpatient care in prison clinics and, if 24-hour nursing care is needed, most prisons have an infirmary. Prisons frequently develop partnerships with university health care centers and the private sector to obtain medical staff coverage for clinics. However, prisons staff infirmaries with nurses and with unlicensed care providers who are employed by the prison system (ANA, 2013a; Watson et al., 2004).

Nurses who work in correctional institutions must display self-confidence and strength. They must avoid performing favors for inmates because inmates frequently try to take advantage of anyone who displays kindness toward them (ANA, 2013a; Stringer, 2001).

Forensic Nursing

The scientific study of forensics is a vital arm of law enforcement. In recent years, the application of forensic science to investigate trauma in emergency departments has created the need to secure reliable evidence and support victims of violent crime. The practice of forensic nursing includes forensic nursing sexual assault examiners, forensic nursing educators/consultants, nurse coroners, nurse death investigators, legal nurse consultants, nurse attorneys, correctional nurses, clinical nurse specialists, forensic pediatric nurses, forensic gerontology nurses, and forensic psychiatric nurses. Forensic nurses use the nursing process to determine the occurrence of sexual assault, homicide, physical assault, spouse abuse, and child abuse (International Association of Forensic Nurses & ANA, 2009).

Forensic nurses identify injuries with forensic implication. Using strict protocols, they collect evidence when a crime has occurred. Nurses who collect evidence frequently provide expert witness testimony as to the integrity of the evidence. They also meticulously document client interactions and evidence collection because the documentation will be used in legal proceedings as evidence. Forensic nurses also interact with the victims of crime and their grieving families. Finally, forensic nurses may consult with other agencies and law enforcement personnel when forensic information is shared (International Association of Forensic Nurses & ANA, 2009).

Armed Forces Nursing

The branches of the U.S. armed forces work and live together for a common purpose: to protect the country. Because each branch of the military has a specific area of expertise, each branch fits the definition of community. Armed forces nursing provides nurses with the opportunity to work with military personnel and their families, as well as civilians affected by warfare. The U.S. Army, Navy (whose nurses serve the Marines as well), and Air Force each have a nursing corps. Nurses serve the military by enlisting for active duty, for reserve status, or in the National Guard. Military nurses have the opportunity to practice with clients of all ages in ambulatory clinics, community hospitals, large medical centers, hospital ships, field hospitals, and aircraft. Military nurses receive comparable compensation to nurses in civilian practice settings. Branches of the armed services offer generous signing bonuses, a full array of benefits, and the option to retire with full benefits after 20 years of service. Nurses in all branches of the armed forces have great potential for upward mobility (Marquand, 2004). Professional practice responsibilities vary according to assignment.

Military nurses confront special personal and professional challenges when deployed into a combat zone.

Some of the challenges include long separations from family (up to a year or longer), language and cultural differences, climate issues (temperature extremes, dust, or tropical storms), supply shortages, severe trauma exposure, violent threats from enemy combatants or insurgents, and posttraumatic stress disorder. When serving in a combat zone, military nurses, like soldiers, receive increased pay (Spencer, 2006).

Armed forces nursing provides professional nurses with opportunities for advanced education. Nurses can earn graduate degrees in nursing, receive specialty education, and pursue graduate degrees outside the discipline of nursing. Military nurses have opportunities for teaching patient care skills to corps members and leadership classes to future officers (Marquand, 2004). The branches of the armed forces also conduct nursing research related to issues of deployment, the needs of military personnel and their beneficiaries in times of war and peace, and cultural aspects of military nursing (Committee on Military Nursing Research, Institute of Medicine, 1996; Marquand, 2004).

Military nursing provides the opportunity for nurses to work with other health team members as equal partners. Camaraderie among health team members is high because everyone focuses on what is best for the service member receiving care. Physicians and nurses have weapons training together. In some circumstances, nurses may outrank physicians. When armed forces deploy active duty and reserve nurses during times of war, they expend energy and resources to recruit civilian nurses to fill vacancies left in stateside hospitals and clinics (Marquand, 2004).

School Nursing

Within a school, many people work together to attain the goal of imparting cognitive, affective, or psychomotor knowledge and skills to others. Thus, all levels of schools meet the definition of a community. Many people tend to view school nursing as confined to the kindergarten through high school levels, but many colleges and universities also provide health services to students, and some nurses work with college students (Fig. 15.5).

Regardless of student age group, school nurses use the nursing process to guide client care activities and bear a number of responsibilities (see Box 15.4, Professional Building Blocks, "Responsibilities of the Professional School Nurse"). They also systematically evaluate the effectiveness of nursing practice and health care services. School nurses must abide by various regulations in the state in which they practice.

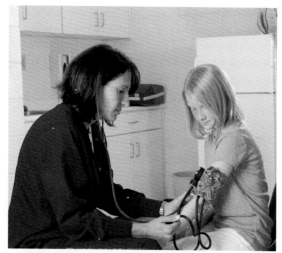

FIGURE 15.5 School nursing helps detect health issues early as well as teaching students healthy habits that may last a lifetime.

Elementary and High School Settings

The role of the school nurse remains consistent across all levels of education. However, when nurses work with children and minors, they also spend much time working with the parents of these younger clients. As a nursing specialty, school nursing aims to advance student well-being, academic success, lifelong achievement, and health. School nurses work to facilitate positive student responses to normal growth and development, promote safety and health, intervene when health problems arise or are anticipated, and provide community referrals and other case management services (National Association of School Nurses [NASN], 2011).

School nurses have various roles. They provide direct health care to students who have bouts of acute physical or chronic illness, as well as to students with special health care needs resulting from a disability. Professional school nurse generalists also provide first aid; administer medications; screen students for health problems, general fitness, and signs of abuse; monitor vital signs; participate in case management activities; change dressings; and perform urinary catheterizations. School nurses develop individualized nursing care and health educational plans for students with chronic illness or those who need to learn complex self-care skills to cope with a disability. School nurses also engage in enhancing the wellness of teachers, administrators, counselors, and nutritional, janitorial, and clerical staff. School nurses perform periodic environmental assessments to ensure a safe and health-promoting school environment. They also may review the daily menu for

15.4 Professional Building Blocks

Responsibilities of the Professional School Nurse

- Maintain competence.
- Assess, diagnose, identify outcomes, plan, implement, and evaluate student health care services.
- Coordinate student health care services.
- Provide health teaching.
- Promote student health.
- Consult with other health professionals.
- Abide by state and federal laws when using prescriptive authority, treatments, and therapies (advanced practice nurses only) in regard to knowledge and issues affecting their student populations.
- Provide ethical care.
- Use research findings and best evidence in practice.
- Conduct research studies when gaps in practice are identified.
- Engage in quality improvement processes.
- Use school resources judiciously.
- Collaborate with others to develop relevant health care services.
- Communicate effectively in all areas of professional nursing.
- Demonstrate leadership in practice setting and the profession.
- Collaborate with health care consumers, families, and others.
- Evaluate one's practice against practice standards.
- Maintain environmental safety.
- Manage student health programs.

National Association of School Nurses. (2011). *School nursing: Scope and standards of practice* (2nd ed.). Silver Spring, MD: Nursebooks.org.

school cafeterias to verify that healthy meals are being served. When specific health care needs arise, school nurses make referrals to local health care providers (Martin, 2009; NASN, 2011).

In some school systems, nurses frequently develop the health education program in collaboration with the school administration, teachers, and parents. Health education programs may be tailored to an individual school's needs or be developed to meet the needs and concerns of a school district. Many times, the school nurse teaches health education classes to students, parents, school staff, or community groups (Martin, 2009; NASN, 2011).

School nurses spend much time maintaining student health records. They verify that all students have received required immunizations and that students have received screening for visual, hearing, and skeletal deformities. When students visit the school nurse, the nurse documents the reason for the visit, interventions performed, parental contact (if needed), and referrals made (if required). Most school health programs have protocols indicating actions that can be taken by nurses without parental consent. Many schools have parents sign forms specifying particular over-the-counter medications (such as acetaminophen, antibiotic or steroid ointments, antihistamines, and decongestants) the nurse may administer to their children. School nurses also receive detailed information about routinely prescribed medications that students may require. Because of the prevalence of drug abuse and zero-tolerance laws in many school districts, students taking prescription medications must visit the school nurse to receive their scheduled doses (Martin, 2009).

The school nurse serves as a resource for health information for students, faculty, and staff. Sometimes, faculty and staff consult the school nurse when they suspect a potential health-related problem among students. The nurse may develop several approaches to the problem and consult with school administration before activating a plan. Sometimes nurses work collaboratively with teachers and administrators to develop plans for students with learning disabilities and mental health problems. In some cases, the school nurse assumes responsibility for monitoring school compliance with specific portions of student disability regulations (Martin, 2009; NASN, 2011).

School nursing is a specialized area of nursing practice, and additional education beyond the baccalaureate degree is recommended for optimal clinical effectiveness. School nurses may become certified through the NASN or ANA. Many states also have certification requirements for school nursing. The Rehabilitation Act in 1973 required that public schools provide appropriate and free education for disabled children; this required that nurses be readily available to attend to needs of "medically fragile children" (Martin, 2009, p. 1009). In 1990, the Americans with Disabilities Act specified that all children with any form of cognitive, physical, or social disability had equal rights to educational opportunities. The school nurse has the responsibility to develop and monitor student individualized health plans with other health team members to address identified student health needs. The school nurse is legally bound to write emergency individualized health plans for students with potentially life-threatening health issues (seizures, insulin-dependent diabetes, asthma, or anaphylactic reactions to peanut exposure) (Martin, 2009). Some school districts offer school-based clinics that are staffed by a school nurse practitioner who provides primary health care services to students (including prescriptions for contraceptives and treatment for sexually transmitted infections). School-based clinics have been credited with reducing the number of school absences for students with chronic diseases, especially asthma (Martin, 2009; NASN, 2011).

In addition to providing nursing services and health education, the school nurse participates in research, investigates cases, and delegates health-related tasks to unlicensed personnel. Unfortunately, not every school has a nurse on campus, and certain tasks must be delegated to school staff members. When this happens, the nurse must provide the staff members with education to safely accomplish health-related tasks (Martin, 2009; NASN, 2011).

College Campus Setting

College health nursing focuses primarily on the health care needs and concerns of people between the ages of 17 and 24 years. Nurses working with college students emphasize self-care and wellness. College nursing services vary in size and scope. Some college health programs offer ambulatory care services with scheduled office hours exclusively, whereas others provide an infirmary for acute care staffed by a multidisciplinary health team. The American College Health Association Review Group, in collaboration with the ANA, has published guidelines for collegiate nursing practice. Many colleges and universities provide clinics that have an advanced practice nurse on staff to deliver required health services to students (ANA, 1997).

▮ Questions for Reflection

1. What are the health care services offered at the college you attend?
2. What health-promoting factors are present within the college you attend?
3. What are your major health-related concerns as a nursing student? Why are these important to you?

Faith Community Nursing

Faith community nursing provides nurses with an opportunity to practice within faith communities. Faith communities are groups of people who share a common faith tradition and meet in a place of worship (church, mosque, synagogue, etc.) (ANA & Health Ministries Association Inc. [HMAI], 2012). In 1984, Granger Westberg started a parish nursing program at Lutheran General Hospital in Chicago. The International Parish Nursing Resource Center offered the first continuing education program in parish nursing in 1987 (Solari-Twadell & McDermott, 2006). In 1998, the ANA published *Scope and Standards of Parish Nursing Practice,* thereby acknowledging parish nursing as a distinct specialized area of professional practice. These guidelines were revised in 2012 and renamed *Faith Community Nursing: Scope and Standards of Parish Practice* (ANA & HMAI, 2012).

Two models for faith community nursing exist: the congregational model and the institutional model. In the congregational model, the nurse acts autonomously and nursing and health programs arise from the community in which the nurse serves. The nurse is held accountable to the congregation and the governing body. In the institutional model, the nurse collaborates more closely with local hospitals, medical centers, extended-care facilities, and educational institutions. Sometimes the faith community nurse holds contracts with the collaborating agencies. The nurse works in partnership with the local health care and educational institutions to meet the needs of faith community members (Solari-Twadell & McDermott, 2006).

Nurses holding membership in a faith-based community frequently serve as first responders when a congregation member has a health-related problem during a service or activity. Parish nurses also engage in health ministry activities, such as visiting homebound congregation members, arranging for meals for families in times of crises, forming prayer circles or chains, serving healthy meals and refreshments at congregational activities, and volunteering for local community care groups. In some faith communities nurses provide volunteer service. Other faith communities have formalized programs staffed by paid directors, coordinators, and nurses. Some faith community nursing programs allow the nurse to run clinics to serve poor or marginalized congregations. These clinics may be staffed by nurse practitioners (Solari-Twadell & McDermott, 2006).

As a specialized area of professional practice, the following factors distinguish faith community nursing from other practice areas.

1. The client spiritual dimension is the core and central dimension of faith community nursing practice.
2. The faith community nurse balances knowledge of nursing science, humanities, and theology as nursing services are delivered.
3. The faith community and its ministry become the focus of practice.

4. The faith community nurse emphasizes individual, family, and faith community strengths.
5. Spiritual health, physical health, and healing are viewed as dynamic ongoing processes (Solari-Twadell & McDermott, 2006).

Nursing skills used when providing care to faith-based communities vary across programs. No two faith community nursing programs are identical, and the nursing services offered in them cannot fully meet all health needs of the community. The eight key functions of the faith community nurse have been identified as health education, personal health counseling, health care referral services, support group development, volunteer facilitation, volunteer training, faith and health integration, and health care advocacy. Westberg envisioned the faith community nurse as a part-time paid position assumed by a baccalaureate-prepared nurse (Solari-Twadell & McDermott, 2006).

Education preparation for faith community nurses has evolved from a 1- or 2-day continuing education seminar into more formalized programs. Nurses can attend a 1-day continuing education program or take a formal course of study lasting several years to earn a master's degree in nursing or a graduate degree in divinity. In 1996, 50 parish nurse coordinators identified key elements of a standardized curriculum for parish nursing. Curricular content addresses the church's role in health; health theology; the history and philosophy of parish nursing; models of parish nursing practice; the teaching, counseling, referring, and educating functions of the parish nurse; the integration of faith and health; parish community assessment; health promotion and maintenance; families and faith communities as client; parish nurse self-care; working with churches and within a ministerial team; legal and ethical issues; accountability and documentation techniques; prayer and worship leadership; and how to start a faith community nursing program. Additional content for faith community nurse coordinators includes budgeting, writing grants, managing human and fiscal resources, developing spiritually, and planning continuing education for parish nurses. Advanced practice and health ministry specialty practice education along with practical experience in community health nursing enrich faith community nursing services (ANA & HMAI, 2012).

Faith community nursing offers an avenue for the development of new spiritual (or religious), community, and interpersonal nursing diagnoses and interventions. Proposed new nursing diagnoses include the potential for enhanced acceptance, spiritual concern, altered spiritual development, spiritual isolation, altered spiritual ritual patterns, risk for cultural incongruity, ineffective boundaries, ineffective meditation skills, and communication enhancement. Spiritual nursing interventions focus on enhancing health through strengthening faith and hope while preventing religious addiction. Faith community nurses empower faith communities to engage in unified political actions on health-related legislation, support and teach each other to provide volunteer assistance to ill and frail members, and promote health by enhancing the spiritual dimensions of congregation members (Solari-Twadell & McDermott, 2006).

Volunteer Nursing

Many nurses volunteer to provide nursing services in community settings. Some nurses routinely schedule volunteer activities into life routines, such as serving on organizational or institutional boards, monthly or weekly duties at a free health clinic, and regularly scheduled community health screening activities. Other nurses may provide volunteer service for episodic events such as health fairs, camps, community service projects (e.g., Habitat for Humanity), faith-community activities, and community events. When volunteering, nurses have an obligation to have adequate knowledge about actual and potential situations that may arise. For example, when volunteering in a foreign country, nurses must be knowledgeable about any specific laws that govern clinical practice as well as laws that may govern personal behaviors (Leffers & Plotnik, 2011).

When providing services, the nurse assumes responsibility for providing accurate health information and ensuring that those served receive the care they require. In the case of blood pressure screening, the nurse must establish guidelines for people who require emergency treatment, those with dangerously high or low blood pressure measurements, those who need medical referral for abnormal measurements, and those with borderline measurements. While engaging in blood pressure screening, nurses can teach people about blood pressure and ways to avoid hypertension. Sometimes, nurses provide clients with a form containing the client's blood pressure reading and recommended actions for various readings. The professional nurse cannot force anyone to seek immediate treatment for blood pressure problems or verify that clients participating in the screening follow through with referral recommendations.

Summary and Significance to Practice

Conceptual models of the client–environment relationship provide frameworks to guide practice with family and community clients as well as individual clients. Views of change reflected by the models underlie strategies to promote growth of the family or community or to facilitate return to stability. When working with the family or community as clients, nurses must develop an ability to think in multiple dimensions because more than one person becomes the client system. In most cases, the impact of an individual's health-related change affects a family system. The impact of a health change also may have implications for the entire community. As health care professionals, nurses must look beyond individual clients and develop strategies to provide relevant care for families and communities. There are many opportunities for nursing wanting to pursue a career in community health. Nursing models provide a theoretical foundation for guiding professional nursing actions as nurses work with individuals, families, and communities.

REAL-LIFE REFLECTIONS

Recalling what you have learned in this chapter, consider the following questions about school nurse Nancy, and Lisa, the student she suspects of having an eating disorder.

- *List the individual as client, family as client, and community as client in this school nursing scenario.*
- *Why is it important in this situation to expand the definition of client to include the family and community?*
- *What do you think is Nancy's top priority? Why do you think this issue should be addressed first?*
- *What other issues need to be addressed? Why are these important?*

From Theory to Practice

1. After reading this chapter, do you think it is possible to provide nursing care services only to individuals? Why or why not?
2. Which definition of family appeals most to you? How will you incorporate PFCC concepts into your current or future professional practice? What potential obstacles might occur when trying to

include the family unit when caring for an individual client?

3. Which of the nursing models presented in the chapter would you consider using if you were providing nursing services to a community? Why do you prefer this model over the other nursing theoretical approaches to caring for communities?

Nurse as Author

1. Think of areas where the health of your current educational community or professional practice community could be improved, and list several strategies you might use to address them. Select one of these strategies and search peer-reviewed literature, such as journal articles and books, for four to six references to support it. Develop a nursing care plan for the community or a concept map for your chosen strategy. After completing this exercise, write a 4- to 5-paragraph essay about your experience, what you learned about the specific health issue, and what you learned about your community's openness toward tackling the health issue.

2. Most states identify professional nurses as mandatory reporters for identified instances of child abuse or neglect. Write 2- to 3-paragraphs about how you feel about becoming a mandatory reporter, and what future issues you might encounter should you directly witness an incident of child abuse or neglect. Include a list of persons who might be of help should you find yourself in such a position.

Your Digital Classroom

Online Exploration

For Family as Client

American Academy of Pediatrics: **www.aap.org**
Children Now: **www.childrennow.org**
Children's Institute: **www.childrensinstitute.org**
Center for Health Care Strategies: **www.chcs.org**
Centers for Medicare and Medicaid Services: **https://cms.hhs.gov**
Hospital Compare: **www.hospitalcompare.hhs.gov**
March of Dimes: **www.marchofdimes.org**
Child Welfare Information Gateway: **https://www.childwelfare.gov/**

For Community as Client

Centers for Disease Control and Prevention National Immunization Program: **www.cdc.gov**

Healthy People 2020: **www.healthypeople.gov**
National Highway Traffic Safety Administration: **www.nhtsa.gov**
Substance Abuse and Mental Health Services Administration: **www.samhsa.gov**

Expanding Your Understanding

1. Visit the Child Welfare Information Gateway at **www.childwelfare.gov**. Under the TOPICS menu on the left side of the page click on "Child Abuse & Neglect." Find Tools on the next screen. Underneath "Tools" find "State Statutes Search." On the State Statutes page, click on the name of your state of residence from the drop down menu (for number one) and select all topics under child abuse and neglect for number two. After selecting the state and topics, read your state laws for topics including: Immunity for Reporters of Child Abuse and Neglect, Mandatory Reporters of Child Abuse and Neglect, and Penalties for Failure to Report and False Reporting of Child Abuse and Neglect.

2. Visit the Centers for Disease Control and Prevention website. Under POPULAR TOPICS, click on "Seasonal Flu" to read information about this year's influenza season and "Vaccines and Immunization" to access national immunization guidelines. Check to see if you and your family are protected according to CDC guidelines for infectious diseases and this year's influenza.

3. Visit the Healthy People 2020 website, and click on "Leading Health Indicators." On the next screen, click "What Are the Leading Health Indicators?" Assess your family, academic community, clinical practice community, and neighborhood to see where improvements to health could be made. Outline a plan to assist family and community members to make improvements in one of the identified areas.

Beyond the Book

Visit **thePoint®** **www.thePoint.lww.com** for activities and information to reinforce the concepts and content covered in this chapter.

REFERENCES

Ahmann, E., & Dokken, D. (2012). Strategies for encouraging patient/family member partnerships with the health care team. *Pediatric Nursing, 38*(4), 232–235.

Allen, C., & Easley, C. (2008). Ethics and human rights. In L. Ivanov & C. Blude (Eds.), *Public health nursing: Leadership, policy and practice.* Clifton Park, NY: Delmar Cengage Learning.

American Association of Occupational Health Nurses. (2004). Standards of occupational and environmental health nursing. *American Association of Occupational Health Nurses Journal, 52*(7), 270–274.

American Association of Occupational Health Nurses. (2007). Competencies in occupational and environmental health nursing: By the American Association of Occupational Nurses, Inc. *American Association of Occupational Health Nurses Journal, 55*(11), 442–447.

American Association of Occupational Health Nurses. (2015a). *Competencies in occupational and environmental health nursing.* Retrieved from http://www.aaohn.org/practice/ohn-practice/competencies.html. Accessed May 28, 2016.

American Association of Occupational Health Nurses. (2015b). *Occupational health nursing practice standards.* Retrieved from http://www.aaohn.org/practice/ohn-practice/standards.html. Accessed May 28, 2016.

American Nurses Association. (1997). *Scope and standards of college health nursing practice.* Washington, DC: Nursebooks.org.

American Nurses Association. (1998). *Scope and Standards of parish nursing practice.* Washington, DC: Author.

American Nurses Association. (2010). *Nursing social policy statement, the essence of the profession* (2010 ed.). Silver Spring MD: Author.

American Nurses Association. (2013a). *Correctional nursing: Scope and standard of practice* (2nd ed.). Silver Spring MD: Author.

American Nurses Association. (2013b). *Scope and standards of public health nursing practice* (2nd ed.). Silver Springs, MD: Author.

American Nurses Association. (2014a). *Home health nursing: Scope and standards practice* (2nd ed.). Silver Springs MD: Author.

American Nurses Association. (2014b). *Psychiatric-mental health nursing: Scope and standards of practice* (2nd ed.). Silver Spring, MD: Author.

American Nurses Association, & Health Ministries Association Inc. (2012). *Faith community nursing: Scope and standards of practice* (2nd ed.). Silver Spring, MD: Nursebooks.org.

American Nurses Association, & Hospice & Palliative Care Nurses Association. (2014). *Palliative nursing: Scope and standards of practice.* Silver Spring, MD: ANA.

Anderson, K. H. (2000). The family health system approach to family systems nursing. *Journal of Family Nursing, 6*(2), 113–119.

Anderson, E. T., & McFarlane, J. (2015). *Community as partner, theory and practice in nursing* (7th ed.). Philadelphia, PA: Wolters Kluwer Health.

Anderson, D., & Riley, P. (2008). The homeless population. In L. L. Ivanov & C. L. Blue (Eds.), *Public health nursing leadership, policy & practice.* Clifton Park, NY: Delmar Cengage Learning.

Anderson, K. H., & Tomlinson, P. S. (1992). The family health system as an emerging paradigmatic view for nursing. *Image, 24,* 57–63.

Andrews, M., & Boyle, J. (2016). *Transcultural concepts in nursing care* (7th ed.). Philadelphia, PA: Wolters Kluwer.

Artinian, N. T. (1994). Selecting a model to guide family assessment. *Dimensions of Critical Care Nursing, 14,* 4–12.

Bailey, V. (2007). Satisfaction levels with a community night nursing service. *Nursing Standard, 22*(5), 35–42.

Beddome, G. (1995). Community-as-client assessment. A Neuman-based guide for education and practice. In B. Neuman (Ed.), *The Neuman systems model* (3rd ed.). East Norwalk, CT: Appleton & Lange.

Bekemeier, B. (2007). Credentialing for public health nurses: Personally valued . . . but not well recognized. *Public Health Nursing, 24*(5), 439–448.

Bell, J. (2009). Family systems nursing: Re-examined. *Journal of Family Nursing, 15*(2), 123–129.

Bender, K. W., & Salmon, M. E. (2009). Public health nursing: Pioneers of health care reform. In B. S. Lundy & S. Janes (Eds.), *Community health nursing: Caring for the public's health* (2nd ed.). Sudbury, MA: Jones & Bartlett.

Benner, P. (1984). *From novice to expert.* Menlo Park, CA: Addison-Wesley.

Bigbee, J. (2008). Relationships between nurse-and physician-to-population ratios and state health rankings. *Public Health Nursing, (3),* 244–252.

Blanes, L., Carmagnani, M., & Ferreira, L. (2007). Health-related quality of life in primary caregivers of persons with quadriplegia. *Spinal Cord, 45,* 399–403.

Butts, J. B., & Lundy, K. S. (2009). Urban and homeless populations. In K. S. Lundy & S. Janes (Eds.), *Community health nursing: Caring for the public's health* (2nd ed.). Sudbury, MA: Jones & Bartlett.

Canty-Mitchell, J., Little, B., Robinson, S., & Chandler, R. (2008). Racial and ethnic health disparities. In L. Ivanov & C. Blude (Eds.), *Public health nursing: Leadership, policy and practice.* Clifton Park, NY: Delmar Cengage Learning.

Chevannes, M. (1997). Nursing caring for families: Issues in a multiracial society. *Journal of Clinical Nursing, 6,* 151–157.

Christensen, P. J., & Kenney, J. W. (1990). *Nursing process: Application of conceptual models* (3rd ed.). St. Louis, MO: Mosby.

Clark, M. J. (1999). *Nursing in the community* (3rd ed.). Stamford, CT: Appleton & Lange.

Clark, M. J. (2014). *Population and community health nursing* (6th ed.). Upper Saddle River, NJ: Pearson Education.

Committee on Military Nursing Research, Institute of Medicine. (1996). The program for research in military nursing: Progress and future direction. Retrieved from www.nap.edu/catalog/5257.html. Accessed February 23, 2013.

Copeland, M. (2002). e-community health nursing. *Journal of Holistic Nursing, 20,* 152–165.

Denham, S. A. (1999). Part I: The definition and practice of family health. *Journal of Family Nursing, 5,* 133–159.

Elsom, S., Happell, B., & Manias, E. (2007). Exploring the expanded practice roles of community mental health nurses. *Issues in Mental Health Nursing, 28,* 413–429.

Erceg, L., & Pravda, M. (2009). *The basics of camp nursing* (2nd ed.). Martinsville, IN: American Camping Association.

Fawcett, J., & DeSanto-Madeya, S. A. (2012). *Contemporary nursing knowledge: Analysis and evaluation of nursing models and theories* (3rd ed.). Philadelphia, PA: F. A. Davis.

Forchuk, C., & Dorsay, J. P. (1995). Hildegard Peplau meets family systems nursing: Innovation in theory-based practice. *Journal of Advanced Nursing, 21:*110–115.

Friedman, M. M. (1992). *Family nursing: Theory and practice* (3rd ed.). East Norwalk, CT: Appleton & Lange.

Friedmann, M. L. (1995). *The framework of systemic organization.* Thousand Oaks, CA: Sage.

Friedman, M., Bowden V., & Jones, E. (2003). *Family nursing: Research theory & practice* (5th ed.). East Norwalk, CT: Prentice-Hall.

Gilliss, C. L., Highley, B. L., Roberts, B. M., & Martinson, I. M. (1988). *Toward a science of family nursing.* Reading, MA: Addison-Wesley.

Gooding, T., Pierce, B., & Flaherty, K. (2012). Partnering with family members to improve the intensive care unit experience. *Critical Care Nursing Quarterly, 35*(3), 215–222. doi: 10.1097/CNQ.0b013e31826066a

Hanchett, E. S. (1988). *Nursing frameworks and community as client.* East Norwalk, CT: Appleton & Lange.

Hancock, T., & Duhl, L. (1986). *Healthy cities: Promoting health in the urban context (Healthy Cities Paper No 1.).* Copenhagen: World Health Organization Europe.

Hanson, S. (1996). Family assessment and interventions. In S. Hanson & S. Boyd (Eds.), *Family care nursing: Theory, practice and research.* Philadelphia, PA: F. A. Davis.

Head, B., Aquilino, M., Johnson, M., Reed, D., Mass, M., & Moorehead, S. (2004). Content validity and nursing sensitive community-level outcomes from the nursing outcomes classification (NOC). *Journal of Nursing Scholarship, 36,* 251–259.

Hospice and Palliative Nursing Credentialing Center. (2016). *CHPN® Candidate Handbook.* Retrieved from http://documents.goamp.com/Publications/candidateHandbooks/HPCC-CHPN-Handbook.pdf. Accessed October 31, 2016.

Hunt, R. (2008). *Introduction to community-based nursing* (4th ed.). Philadelphia, PA: Lippincott Williams & Wilkins.

Institute of Medicine (2003). *Health professions education: A bridge to quality.* Washington DC: National Academies Press.

International Association of Forensic Nurses & American Nurses Association. (2009). *Forensic nursing: Scope and standards of forensic nursing practice.* Silver Spring, MD: Nursebooks.org.

Jarvis, C. (2015). *Physical examination and health assessment* (7th ed.). St. Louis, MO: Elsevier.

Kaakinen, J. R., & Coehlo, D. P. (2015). *Family health care nursing: Theory, practice and research.* Philadelphia, PA: F.A. Davis.

Kaakinen, J., & Hanson, S. (2010). Theoretical foundations for the nursing of families. In J. Kaakinen, V. Gedaly-Duff, D. Coehlo, & S. Hanson (Eds.), *Family health care nursing, theory, practice and research* (4th ed.). Philadelphia, PA: F.A. Davis.

Kaakinen, J., Hanson, S., & Denham, S. (2010). Family health care nursing: An introduction. In J. Kaakinen, V. Gedaly-Duff, D. Coehlo, & S. Hanson (Eds.), *Family health care nursing, theory, practice and research* (4th ed.). Philadelphia, PA: F.A. Davis.

King, I. M. (1983). King's theory of nursing. In I. W. Clements & F. B. Roberts (Eds.), *Family health: A theoretical approach to nursing care.* New York: Wiley.

Knoerl, A. (2007). Cultural considerations and the Hispanic cardiac client. *Home Health Care, 25*(2), 82–86.

Kurtz, P., & Burr, R. (2009). Ethics and health. In B. Lundy & S. Janes (Eds.), *Community health nursing caring for the public's health* (2nd ed.). Sudbury, MA: Jones & Bartlett.

Kwok, S. (2011). Perceived family functioning and suicidal ideation, hopelessness as a mediator or moderator. *Nursing Research, 60*(6), 422–429. doi: 10.1097/NNR.0b013e31823585d6

Lapp, C. A., Diemert, C. A., & Enestredt, R. (1991). Family-based practice. In K. A. Saucier (Ed.), *Perspectives in family and community health.* St. Louis, MO: Mosby-Year Book.

Leddy, S. (2003). *Integrative health promotion.* Thorofare, NJ: Slack.

Leffers, J., & Plotnik, J. (2011). *Volunteering home and abroad: The essential guide for nurses.* Indianapolis: Sigma Theta Tau International.

Leininger, M. & McFarland, M. (2006). *Culture care diversity and universality: A worldwide theory for nursing* (2nd ed.) Sudbury, MA: Jones & Bartlett.

Levin, P., Cary, A., Kulbok, P., Leffers, J., Molle, M., & Polivka, B.J. Association of Community Health Nursing Educators. (2008). Graduate education for advanced practice public health nursing: At the crossroads. *Public Health Nursing, 25,* 176–193.

Li, H., Melnyk, B., & McCann, R. (2004). Review of intervention studies of families with hospitalized elderly relatives. *Journal of Nursing Scholarship, 36,* 54–59.

Lind, C., & Smith, D. (2008). Analyzing the state of community health nursing: advancing from deficit to strengths-based practice using appreciative inquiry. *Advances in Nursing Science, 31*(1), 28–41.

Lishner, K. M., & Bruya, M. A. (Eds.). (1994). *Creating a healthy camp community: A nurse's role.* Martinsville, IN: American Camping Association.

Lundy, K., & Janes, S. (2014). *Community health nursing: Caring for the public's health* (3rd ed.). Burlington, MA: Jones & Bartlett.

Lundy, K., Utterback, K., Lance, D., & Bloxsom, I. (2009). Home health and hospice nursing. In S. Lundy & S. Janes (Eds.), *Community health nursing: Caring for the public's health.* Sudbury, MA: Jones & Bartlett.

Magnusson, L., & Hanson, E. (2005). Supporting frail older people and their family careers at home using information and communication technology: Cost analysis. *Journal of Advanced Nursing, 51*(6), 654–657.

Marquand, B. (2004, Spring). An army (and navy and air force) of opportunities. *Minority Nurse, 26*–30.

Martin, F. (2009). School health nursing. In S. Lundy & S. Janes, (Eds.), *Community health nursing: Caring for the public's health.* Sudbury MA: Jones & Bartlett.

Maurer, F. A., & Smith, C. M. (2013). *Community/public health nursing practice: Health for families & populations* (5th ed.). Philadelphia, PA: Elsevier-Saunders.

McCubbin, M. A., & McCubbin, H. I. (1993). Families coping with illness: The resiliency model of family stress, adjustment, and adaptation. In C. B. Danielson, B. Hamel-Bissell, & P. Winstead-Fry (Eds.), *Families, health, and illness: Perspectives on coping and intervention.* St. Louis, MO: Mosby.

McElmurry, B., Park, C., & Buseh, A. (2003). The nurse-community health advocate team for urban immigrant primary health care. *Journal of Nursing Scholarship, 35,* 275–281.

McGoldrick, M., & Gerson, R. (2008). *Genograms: Assessment & intervention* (3rd ed.). New York: WW Norton & Co.

Moretz, J., & Abraham, M. (2012). Implementing patient-and family-centered care: Part II. Strategies and resources for success. *Pediatric Nursing, 38*(2), 106–109, 71.

Morse, S. (2004). *Smart communities.* San Francisco, CA: Jossey-Bass.

Narsavage, G., Batchelor, H., Lindell, D., & Chen, Y. (2003). Developing personal and community learning in graduate nursing education through community engagement. *Nursing Education Perspectives, 24,* 300–305.

National Association of School Nurses. (2011). *School nursing: Scope and standards of practice* (2nd ed.). Silver Spring, MD: Nursebooks.org.

Neuman, B. (1983). Family interventions using the Betty Neuman health care systems model. In I. W. Clements & F. B. Roberts (Eds.), *Family health: A theoretical approach to nursing care.* New York: Wiley.

Neuman, B. (1989). *The Neuman systems model.* (2nd ed.) Norwalk, CT: Appleton & Lange.

Neuman, B., & Fawcett J. (2010). *The Neuman systems model* (5th ed.). Upper Saddle River, NJ: Pearson Education Inc.

Newman, M. A. (1983). Newman's health theory. In I. W. Clements & F. B. Roberts (Eds.), *Family health: A theoretical approach to nursing care.* New York: Wiley.

Newman, M. A., Sime, A. M., & Corcoran-Perry, S. A. (1991). The focus of the discipline of nursing. *Advances in Nursing Science, 14,* 1–6.

Orem, D. E. (1983). The self-care deficit theory of nursing: A general theory. In I. W. Clements & F. B. Roberts (Eds.), *Family health: A theoretical approach to nursing care.* New York: Wiley.

Parse, R. R. (1996). The human becoming theory: Challenges in practice and research. *Nursing Science Quarterly, 9,* 55–60.

Parse, R. R. (1998). *The human becoming school of thought.* Thousand Oaks, CA: Sage.

Parse, R. (2003). *Community: A human becoming perspective.* Sudbury, MA: Jones & Bartlett.

Parse, R. (2009). The human becoming family model. *Nursing Science Quarterly, 22,* 305–309.

Patterson, J. M. (1999). Healthy American families in a postmodern society: An ecological perspective. In H. M. Wallace, G. Green, K. J. Jaros, L. L. Paine, & M. Story (Eds.), *Health and welfare for families in the 21st century.* Sudbury, MA: Jones & Bartlett.

Pender, N., Murdaugh, C., & Parsons, M. (2005). *Health promotion in nursing practice* (5th ed.). Upper Saddle River, NJ: Pearson/Prentice Hall.

Peplau, H. (1952). *Interpersonal relations in nursing.* New York: G. P. Putnam's Sons.

Quad Council of Public Health Nursing Organizations. (1999). *Scope and standards of public health nursing practice.* Washington, DC: American Nurses Publishing.

Rogers, B. (2001). Occupational health nursing. In K. S. Lundy & S. Janes (Eds.), *Community health nursing: Caring for the public's health.* Sudbury, MA: Jones & Bartlett.

Rogers, M. E. (1983). Science of unitary human beings: A paradigm for nursing. In I. W. Clements & F. B. Roberts (Eds.), *Family health: A theoretical approach to nursing care.* New York: Wiley.

Rose, L., Mallinson, K., & Walton-Moss, B. (2004). Barriers to family care in psychiatric settings. *Journal of Nursing Scholarship, 36,* 39–47.

Roy, C. (1983). Roy adaptation model. In I. W. Clements & F. B. Roberts (Eds.), *Family health: A theoretical approach to nursing care.* New York: Wiley.

Saucier, K. A. (Ed.). (1991). *Perspectives in family and community health.* St. Louis, MO: Mosby-Year Book.

Schumacher, K., Stewart, B., & Archbold, P. (2007). Mutuality and preparedness moderate the effects of caregiving demand on cancer family caregiver outcomes. *Nursing Research, 56*(6), 425–433.

Shuster, G., & Geppinger, J. (2004). Community as client: Assessment and analysis. In M. Stanhope & J. Lancaster (Eds.), *Community and public health nursing.* St. Louis, MO: Mosby.

Smith, C. M. & Maurer, F. F. (2013). *Community health nursing theory and Practice* (5th ed). Philadelphia: Elsevier Saunders.

Solari-Twadell, P. A., & McDermott M. A. (Eds.) (2006). *Parish nursing: Promoting whole person health within faith communities* (2nd ed.). Thousand Oaks, CA: Sage.

Spencer, B. (2006). Nursing care on the battlefield, how the war in Iraq is changing critical care. *American Nurse Today, 1*(2), 24–26.

Spradley, B. W. (1990). *Community health nursing: Concepts and practice* (3rd ed.). Glenview, IL: Scott, Foresman/Little Brown Higher Education.

Stadnyk, R. (2006). Community-dwelling spouses of nursing home residents: Activities that sustain identities in times of transition. *Topics in Geriatric Rehabilitation, 22*(4), 283–293.

Stanhope, M., & Lancaster, J. (2014). *Foundations of nursing in the community, community-oriented practice* (4th ed.) St. Louis, MO: Mosby-Elsevier.

Stringer, H. (2001). Prison break. *Nurse Week, 2,* 24–25.

Taylor, S. G., & Renpenning, K. M. (1995). The practice of nursing in multiperson situations, family and community. In D. E. Orem (Ed.), *Nursing: Concepts of practice.* St. Louis, MO: Mosby.

Toly, V., Musil, C., & Carl, J. (2012). A longitudinal study of families with technology-dependent children. *Research in Nursing & Health, 35,* 40–54. doi: 10.1002/nur.21454

Tomlinson, P. S., & Anderson, K. H. (1995). Family health and the Neuman systems model. In B. Neuman (Ed.), *The Neuman systems model* (3rd ed.). East Norwalk, CT: Appleton & Lange.

U.S. Department of Health and Human Services. (2010). *Healthy People 2020.* Retrieved from www.healthypeople.gov/2020/topicsobjectives2020/pdfs/hp2020_brochure.pdf. Accessed March 23, 2013.

Walsh, S., Martin, S., & Schmidt, L. (2004). Testing the efficacy of a creative-arts intervention with family caregivers of patients with cancer. *Journal of Nursing Scholarship, 36,* 214–219.

Walton, M., & Barnsteiner, J. (2012). Patient-centered care. In G. Sherwood & J. Barnsteiner (Eds.), *Quality and safety in nursing, a competency approach to improving outcomes.* West Sussex, UK: Wiley-Blackwell.

Watson, J. (1996). Watson's theory of transpersonal caring. In P. H. Walker & B. Neuman (Eds.), *Blueprint for use of nursing models: Education, research, practice and administration.* New York: National League for Nursing.

Watson, J. (2007). *Nursing human science and human care, a theory of nursing.* Sudbury, MA: Jones & Bartlett.

Watson, R., Stimpson, A., & Hostick, T. (2004). Prison health care: A review of the literature. *International Journal of Nursing Studies, 41,* 119–128.

Whall, A. L. (1986). *Family therapy theory for nursing: Four approaches.* East Norwalk, CT: Appleton-Century-Crofts.

Whall, A. L., & Fawcett, J. (1991). *Family theory development in nursing: State of the science and art.* Philadelphia, PA: F. A. Davis.

Wright, L. M., & Leahey, M. (1988). Family nursing trends in academic and clinical settings. *Paper presented at the International Family Nursing Conference,* Convention Centre, Calgary, Alberta, Canada, May 24–27, pp. 29–37.

Zotti, M. E., Brown, P., & Stotts, R. C. (1996). Community-based nursing versus community health nursing: What does it all mean? *Nursing Outlook, 44,* 211–217.

The Professional Nurse's Role in Teaching and Learning

LEARNING OUTCOMES

By the end of this chapter, the learner will be able to:

1. Provide the rationale for identifying clients and nurses as "experts" in the client education process.
2. Specify key client assessment data to collect before developing and implementing client education.
3. Explain the concept of health literacy and how it affects client education.
4. Explain how mutuality enhances client learning.
5. Describe each step of the traditional teaching–learning process.
6. Outline key strategies for effective client education.
7. Specify ways to validate client learning.

REAL-LIFE REFLECTIONS

Lillian works as a staff nurse in a rural community hospital. She often cares for people with poorly controlled diabetes, cancer, and other chronic illnesses. During her recent performance evaluation, the nurse manager suggested that Lillian improve her patient teaching. Although Lillian agrees with the nurse manager, she also feels that client education is very time consuming. She knows that improved client education will likely prevent recurrent hospital admissions and promote the general health and well-being of dismissed clients, but her heavy workload prevents Lillian from spending much time teaching clients and families. She wonders how she can deliver effective education to clients and families while frequently being the only registered nurse on her unit.

Patient- and family-centered care focuses on developing partnerships with individuals, families, and communities to empower them with knowledge, skills, and attitudes that promote health, safety, and well-being. The American value of independence means that most Americans prefer to meet their own physical, psychological, and spiritual needs. When knowledge is viewed as power, teaching becomes a key element of professional nursing practice.

Teaching is the process of imparting or sharing knowledge and skills with another. Teaching involves instructing, coaching, and guiding another through unfamiliar content or procedures. Without proper education, health care treatments—especially medications—could be very dangerous.

Professional nurses have been teaching clients for decades, well before the nursing conceptual models on

421

which many nurses base their practice were developed. In 1918, the National League for Nursing Education issued a statement that expressed the need to educate professional nurses to assume teaching responsibilities. In all health care settings, clients and families need the knowledge and skills surrounding encountered health care issues. Historically, compliance with treatment plans has served as the main reason for client education (Falvo, 2004). Current views of client education focus on empowering clients by providing them with knowledge and skills to manage their own health.

In daily practice, nurses share a lot of information with clients. Some nurses have discovered that clients learn more effectively when health education emerges from a mutually determined process between the nurse and the client. Each client encounter provides an opportunity for sharing health-related information rather than simply following standardized teaching outlines from standardized clinical paths or computer programs. Clients must have information about their health problems, potential complications, treatment options, and prevention strategies to make informed choices regarding treatment and health promotion. In some cases, clients must make behavioral changes to avoid and manage certain diseases. As health care professionals, nurses serve as role models of good health for their clients and communities. Optimal education for lifestyle changes improves when clients see that nurses and other health care providers follow healthy lifestyle habits (Joos & Hickam, 1990).

Take Note!
Nurses provide clients with educative experiences that increase the integration of knowledge, skills, behaviors, and attitudes that improve health.

Teaching–learning is considered a public duty of most professions. Lawyers inform clients about the law, physicians teach clients about diseases, physical therapists teach clients how to ambulate safely, social workers educate clients about available community resources, and pharmacists teach clients about medications. As part of the interprofessional health team, nurses have an obligation to educate clients so that the clients can safely and effectively manage their own health and well-being. Professional nurses extend educational efforts beyond individuals and families by providing community-based health education programs, leading support groups, and steering public discussions about needed public health policy changes. By listening to and learning from all clients (individuals, families, and communities), nurses become capable of

providing relevant information that promotes health and improves well-being.

The health education needs and wants of consumers vary. Some clients want to learn how to best promote personal health and avoid illnesses, while others do not see the value of health information until they find themselves ill and in need of health care services (Rankin, Stallings, & London, 2005). Many clients use the internet to access health information, but they may not be able to evaluate the quality of the information they obtain. Clients need to be aware of methods to prevent illness and treatment options for diagnosed health issues so they can make informed choices and comply with complex treatment regimens (Bosek & Savage, 2007; Falvo, 2004; Herzlinger, 2004; Rankin et al., 2005). Topics of interest to health care consumers include the following.

- Complex health care delivery systems
- Health insurance options
- Available community resources
- How to ask questions of health care providers to get desired information
- Medication safety, including how to avoid potential complications of prescribed therapies
- Finding valid and reliable health information using the internet
- When to consult health care providers
- Safe use of assistive devices and other technology

Some clients have multiple health care providers. Nurses play a pivotal role in ensuring client safety across the continuum of care. Nurses carefully gather current client information regarding medications and complementary therapies being used, document this information, and look for any potential harmful interactions with new treatment orders. When clients and families are informed of prescribed medications and treatments, fewer errors occur (The Joint Commission, 2008, 2016b). Shorter hospital stays coupled with ineffective client education have been linked to increased hospital readmission rates (Herzlinger, 2004).

HEALTH LITERACY

The Institute of Medicine (2004) defined health literacy as "the degree to which individuals have the capacity to obtain, process, and understand basic health information needed to make appropriate health decisions" (p. 2). Factors associated with high levels of health literacy include high reading comprehension, well-refined vocabulary, membership in the dominant cultural group, higher income, previous knowledge and experience with health care situations, intact cognitive status, and the ability to communicate orally and understand oral health information. Women tend to have higher health literacy than men because they typically manage the health care needs of the family (Ingram & Kautz, 2012). Limited or low health literacy levels have been associated with limited knowledge about encountered illnesses and disease management, difficulty completing health care forms and surveys, decreased access to high-quality health care information, incorrect use of prescription medication, increased health care expenses, higher use of emergency rooms, and problems keeping appointments and scheduling follow-up visits (Hersh, Salzman, & Snyderman, 2015; Ingram & Kautz, 2012; Morris, Grant, Repp, MacLean, & Littenberg, 2011; Mulder, Tzeng, & Vecchioni, 2012; Remshardt, 2011; Roett & Wessel, 2012; Ward-Smith, 2012).

According to the U.S. Department of Education, an estimated 90 million Americans have low health literacy levels; that is, they experience problems comprehending and acting on health information (Beagley, 2011; Hersch et al., 2015). Low health literacy levels seem to increase as a person ages which may be the result of cognitive, memory and executive function declines associated with old age (Hersch et al., 2015; Ingram & Kautz, 2012; Kabayashi, Wordle, Wolf, & von Wagner, 2015; Morris et al., 2011). Hersch, Salzman, and Snyderman (2015) report 80 million Americans or 36% of American adults have a basic or below level of health literacy. Low levels of health literacy are associated with reduced reading ability. The average reading level of American adults is 8th grade level, but 75% health information and educational materials are written at the high school or college reading levels (Hersh et al., 2015). Low health literacy has been linked to readmissions to the hospital. Reports estimate that between 13% and 24% of hospitalized Medicare patients re-enter the hospital within 30 days of dismissal and cost taxpayers an additional $2 to $5 billion annually (Mulder et al., 2012). Ingram and Kautz describe low health literacy as a "silent epidemic" (p. 22). Teaching health care consumers health literacy basics is a challenge for all health care professionals. Information regarding how to plan and carry out client education in this chapter includes specific strategies to address low health literacy.

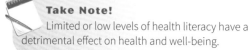

Take Note!
Limited or low levels of health literacy have a detrimental effect on health and well-being.

PHILOSOPHICAL ASSUMPTIONS ABOUT TEACHING AND LEARNING

Education can be defined as a product or as a process. As a product, education can be perceived as a commodity for purchase that yields intended results. As a **process**, the focus becomes how education is planned and implemented; the teaching–learning process considers the relationships among **experts**, thereby emphasizing the essential nature of communication. Clients are experts in how health issues affect them, and nurses are experts in the health issues encountered.

Process—Not Product

Interpersonal relationships with others deeply affect human health and well-being. Through relationships, growth can occur when a person integrates new knowledge, attitudes, and skills that lead to a more healthful and satisfying life. Teaching–learning in the nurse–client relationship is aimed toward such growth.

Education involves personal growth and development. In professional nursing, nurse–client relationships facilitate the educational process. Agnes (2005, p. 816) defined **learning** as "the acquiring of knowledge and skill." In recent years, neuroscientists have identified physiologic processes that alter the brain to develop different types of memory for knowledge and skill acquisition. Lupien and McEwen (1997), as cited in Collins (2007), described the process of memory in the following three phases: acquisition (exposure to knowledge to be remembered), consolidation (transformation of short-term to long-term memory), and retrieval (recall of knowledge or skill). Without long-term memory, learning cannot be recalled. Because of the neurophysiologic processes required for learning, nurses must recognize that a patient's physical health may affect the ability to learn. If the patient possesses impaired cognition, then the nurse needs to delay patient education efforts until full cognition returns.

Nurses who view education as a product ignore the physiologic and psychological processes required for long-lasting learning. When education is viewed as a process, the nurse offers clients information and experiences to reinforce the necessary knowledge, skills, and attitudes required for self-care and personal growth. The nurse also assesses the client for high stress levels and fatigue, which might impair the learning process. In addition, the nurse can offer information in small chunks to facilitate knowledge acquisition and consolidation (Collins, 2007). Client education culminates with the client receiving validation from the nurse that mastery of new knowledge, ideas, or skills has occurred.

Teaching–learning is an interpersonal process in which both the teacher and the learner acquire and consolidate new information, experience new relatedness, and behave in new ways.

Current health care seeks to empower consumers to make informed, autonomous decisions. Many facilities strive to become centers of excellence for a particular disease, health condition, or procedure. Effective client education is a hallmark of a center of excellence. Typically, effective education facilitates learning by engaging clients in purposeful, sequenced learning activities while providing them with support and guidance for mastering required knowledge and skills. The final outcome of learning becomes apparent when clients can recall key information and independently perform skills required for self-care. Nurses can assess recall and comprehension of client education by engaging in a variety of methods. Nurses can ask direct questions about information shared, provide computerized or pencil and paper quizzes for completion, or have the patient participate in a return demonstration of skills or "teachback" (which is simply asking clients to explain what was taught and state what they plan to do when they are at home) (Roett & Wessel, 2012).

When nurses believe that clients have the required abilities for self-care management, they view learning as far more than discovery by their clients. Their educator role becomes focused on "learning that leads to new action and new problem-solving, which enable individuals and systems to continue to learn" (Argyris, 1982, p. 160). Thus, teaching–learning becomes an ongoing dynamic process.

If learning is to be more than the passive acceptance by the learner of information from the teacher, then nurses must commit themselves to collaborative relationships with clients to fulfill the responsibility for providing optimal client education. The nurse invites and expects clients to participate in the process, define their own strengths and problems, share information about personal preferences for teaching strategies, and construct their own meanings. Thus, teaching–learning is a collaborative process that is most effective when nurses fully engage clients as participatory learners.

Relationship Between Experts

Teaching–learning can be viewed as a relationship between experts. Experts are people who have special knowledge and skills about a particular subject (Agnes, 2005). In the professional nursing process, nurses are the experts on health and clients are the experts on their health experiences and life circumstances (ANA,

2015). In the teaching–learning process, clients and nurses view nurses as the experts on knowledge about health and the information that enables people to achieve health, and clients as experts on the context of their life and the need for information and experiences to achieve their intentions to maximize health.

The Nurse: Information and Knowledge Expert

Teaching–learning may be viewed as a part of the healing process. Nurses who have reported that they believed their interventions made a difference in their clients' progress de-scribed several steps in that healing relationship (Benner, 2000, p. 49): mobilizing hope for the nurse as well as for the client; finding an acceptable interpretation or understanding of the illness, pain, fear, anxiety, or other stressful emotion; and assisting the client to use social, emotional, or spiritual support.

Viewing teaching as a coaching function, Benner (2000) proposed that "nurses become experts in coaching a patient through an illness. They take what is foreign and fearful to the patient and make it familiar and thus less frightening" (p. 77). The teacher also needs to have expertise in helping. Helping the learner become aware of learning and thinking processes and helping the person understand the nature of the problems may be equally as important as providing information.

To be an expert in the teaching–learning process, the nurse also must enable the person to feel free to express opinions; react honestly to how content is presented; and assume responsibility for mastering knowledge, skills, and attitudes to change behavior to maximize potential for optimal health and well-being. Learning is facilitated when teachers treat learners as responsible people. In addition, learning empowers clients to take action and assume responsibility for their health (Rankin et al., 2005).

In addition to coach and enabler, several other roles have been proposed for the nurse–teacher (Forbes, 1995, p. 99).

1. **Learning facilitator:** Breaks down barriers to learning by listening, probing, and being aware of feelings
2. **Authority:** Sets up a teaching structure and rules
3. **Ego ideal:** Serves as a role model for the client's "altered existence"
4. **Socializing agent:** Acknowledges concerns and fears for the future
5. **Person:** Relates to clients as people rather than just a disease diagnosis

Which roles should be assumed and outlining the teaching–learning situations during which they would be most effective needs to be validated through qualitative and quantitative research methods?

Take Note!

For the teaching and learning process to be successful, the nurse may need to assume multiple roles.

▌ QUESTIONS FOR REFLECTION

1. How do you prefer to learn new things? What teaching strategies enhance your learning? How might you employ your preferred teaching strategies in the future when teaching clients, families, and communities?
2. How do you involve your clients and their families during health teaching?
3. How frequently do you teach clients/families/communities about things that promote health?
4. What education strategies do you tend to use when providing client/family/community education?
5. What factors in your current practice environment support your role as a client teacher?
6. What factors in your current practice environment prevent you from providing effective client education?

The Client: Context and Need Expert

No one knows better the meaning of his or her life, individual health status, and full circumstances integral to life experiences than the client (ANA, 2015). Thus, clients serve as the experts on the context in which they will be attempting to implement new health behaviors. They are the experts on their own individualized needs for information, support, and relatedness. When nurses appreciate their professional expertise and the personal expertise of the client, the teaching–learning process can truly be implemented as a mutual responsibility.

The Joint Commission, formerly the Joint Commission on Accreditation of Healthcare Organizations (JCAHO), has developed standards for client and family education as an essential element of nursing. According to the Joint Commission (JCAHO, 2006a), **patient education** should convey knowledge and understanding, create a different perspective or attitude, build self-care skills, and change behavior. The Joint Commission's educational standards (2006b) include the following elements for effective client education.

1. Facilitate, plan, support, and provide client education
2. Comprehensive learner assessment before education occurs (ability, readiness, literacy, learning style preferences, cultural or language obstacles, physical or mental limitations)
3. Age and educational level; appropriate teaching methods and materials
4. Consideration of client-preferred learning style
5. Education on safe and effective use of medications, medical equipment, potential food–drug medication interactions, therapeutic diets, and rehabilitation techniques performed by the best qualified member of the interprofessional health care team
6. Information on available community resources and how to obtain additional treatment (if needed)
7. Education on client and family responsibilities for ongoing health care needs and the knowledge and skills on how to fulfill these responsibilities (e.g., ways to promote personal privacy and demonstrating respect when providing basic personal hygiene on incapacitated persons; knowing specific signs and symptoms that require immediate medical attention)
8. Educational strategies that are interactive, provide detailed instructions, and present available and reliable resources for future use
9. Use of a medical translator when needed
10. Evidence that intended learning outcomes for education have been achieved

The Joint Commission standards provide a framework for nurses to follow as they plan and execute client educational activities. In 2006, the Joint Commission (JCAHO, 2006b) developed a client information brochure, *Patient 101* that steers health care consumers to a variety of valid and reliable online sites for health education; the list includes governmental organizations, disease-specific nonprofit organizations, and academic organizations.

Because the Joint Commission accreditation is required for federal reimbursement to organizations for delivered health care, documentation of client education is critical. During accreditation visits, the Joint Commission surveyors examine client care documentation for evidence of client education. Ninety percent of client charts (paper or electronic) should contain this evidence to avoid a citation for improvement. In addition to facilitating reimbursement and accreditation, documenting client education provides solid evidence of nursing's contributions to the interdisciplinary client care efforts. Documentation of education also may provide useful information regarding specific communication strategies that work well with individual clients and families.

Federal- and state-funded reimbursement programs for health care services also require proof of client education in documentation. The Centers for Medicare and Medicaid Services (CMS) identify core measures (evidence-based practice interventions) that indicate that high-quality health care services have been rendered. Currently, CMS requires documentation of core measures for smoking cessation education (if applicable), detailed education on the management of congestive heart failure (HF), and dismissal education regarding home medications (with special attention on informing clients about possible side effects), follow-up care, and other special treatments before reimbursing health care facilities for services.

Along with external agency requirements for patient education, the ANA Scope and Standards of Practice for Nursing (2015) specify that professional nurses are responsible to assess patients and families for anticipated or actual health education needs. They also recognize that nurses can identify gaps in knowledge in patients for effective management of health conditions and for health promotion. The standards also expect nurses to develop health education plans for patients, families, and other caregivers. Nurses bear responsibility and accountability for implementing and evaluating individualized educational plans to determine patient mastery of knowledge and skills for effective self-management of health.

Communication: The Condition for Teaching–Learning

Nurses who display empathy, respect, mutuality, and genuineness while teaching are likely to create effective teaching–learning environments. By using empathy, nurses are more apt to understand client global situations and take full advantage of client expertise. Likewise, clients need to perceive that nurses are sensitive to their needs and will generate effective educational plans that include measurement of the cognitive, affective, and psychomotor (if needed) domains of learning.

Some clients perceive that nurses and other health care professionals have a superior status and, therefore, may be reluctant to ask questions. To combat this issue, the National Patient Safety Foundation developed the "Ask Me 3" campaign. This program outlines three key questions consumers should ask during each visit to a health care provider: (1) What is my main problem? (2) What do I need to do? (3) Why is it important for me to do this?

An effective teaching–learning process occurs when both nurses and clients share a mutual responsibility for the education process and experience respectful communication. Feelings of self-worth facilitate teaching

and learning because teachers and learners need to see themselves as capable of effectively fulfilling their roles. Teachers believe and know they can create and execute meaningful learning experiences, and learners believe and know they have the capabilities to master the content and skills being taught.

Full exploration and analysis of the health concerns and information needed to change behaviors cannot occur unless nurses and clients perceive each other as real, as genuinely human, open, honest, and caring in their responses to each other. Nurses must provide clients with accurate health-related information, and clients must perceive that nurses have information to facilitate health promotion, maintenance, or restoration. Although clients may display an authentic interest in the information being shared with them, the client makes the final determination of what, if, and when received information will be used.

When providing clients with printed or web-based materials, nurses should consider the client's ability to read, reading level, language preferences, and access to the internet. Published, printed, and posted internet educational materials are often written above the average fifth-grade reading level of Americans (Remshardt, 2011; Taylor-Clarke et al., 2012). The Centers for Medicare and Medicaid services have a toolkit for health care professionals to develop clearly and effectively written materials that can be printed or posted online (https://www.cms.gov/Outreach-and-Education/Outreach/WrittenMaterialsToolkit/index.html) (Centers for Medicare & Medicaid Services, 2016). Some facilities offer client educational software programs that can provide printed materials in a variety of foreign languages to meet the educational needs of clients who do not have fluency in English.

Nurses empower clients to have control over their lives when they give them information or teach them skills to care for themselves. Rankin et al. (2005, p. 75) outlined the following four-step counseling model for empowering individual clients.

1. Identify the problem or issue (past)
2. Explore feelings and meanings (present)
3. Identify goals and choices (plan for the future)
4. Commit to action (future)

To identify the problem or issue and its impact on the client, the nurse uses holistic assessment skills. Once the issue or problem has been identified, the nurse uses the nursing process step of planning to specify goals and strategies to resolve the problem or issue in collaboration with the client. Once the client has committed to action, the change process begins.

TEACHING–LEARNING PROCESS APPROACHES

The Traditional Approach

Nurses can choose from a variety of approaches when providing client education. The traditional process has been used with success by many nurses and provides a structured approach. Similar to nursing process, the steps of the traditional teaching–learning process are assessment, identification of learning needs, planning (including the development of learning objectives and selection of educational materials), implementation, evaluation, and documentation (Rankin et al., 2005; Redman, 1993).

Assessment and Identification of Learning Needs

The first activity on the part of the nurse–teacher is assessment: gathering facts and information that will help the nurse meet the client's or the family's learning needs. Rankin et al. (2005) indicated the following four steps in the assessment process: (1) selecting the areas to be assessed, (2) gathering the data, (3) sorting and categorizing the data, and (4) writing a summary statement (nursing diagnosis). Box 16.1, Professional Building Blocks, "Purposes of Client Assessment for Education," outlines the purposes of client assessment (Rankin et al., 2005; Redman, 1993).

Assessment may be conducted by listening and questioning, observing, reviewing records, collaborating with the health care team, and integrating the client's verbal description with the nurse's observation. Nurses can also use formalized tools to assess learners to determine preferred learning styles and levels of health literacy. The Agency for Healthcare Research and Quality offers a Health Literacy Universal Precautions Tool Kit (available at http://www.ahrq.gov/professionals/quality-patient-safety/quality-resources/tools/literacy-toolkit/index.html) that helps nurses identify clients at risk for not being able to understand and use health care information. Of all these assessments, the client's perceptions of what is needed serve as the most important factor in determining educational needs. Therefore, the nurse must engage in active listening and validate professional perceptions with the client.

Nurses must consider reading ability of the persons for whom they provide education. A recent study released by the United States Department of Education, National Institute of Literacy revealed that the reading level of Americans has remained consistent over the past decade. Data from this study revealed that only 13% of Americans read a proficient level, 44% read

16.1 Professional Building Blocks

Purposes of Client Assessment for Education

1. Identify what the client wants to learn.
2. Identify what the client needs to know.
3. Establish a point of reference for learning (relate new information to pre-existing knowledge).
4. Identify incorrect information and assumptions.
5. Determine what environmental factors may pose barriers.
6. Identify potential client barriers to learning (language, culture, education level, cognitive skills, reading ability, health literacy level, physical limitations).
7. Identify what will need to be evaluated.
8. Build trust and rapport.
9. Provide for involvement of family.
10. Set priorities for the needs and problems to be addressed by education.

Beagley, L. (2011). Educating patients: Understanding barriers, learning styles, and teaching techniques. *Journal of Perianesthesia Nursing, 26*(5), 331–337. doi: 10.1016/j.opan.2011.06.002; Ingram, R., & Kautz, D. (2012). Overcoming low health literacy. *Nursing 2013 Critical Care, 7*(4), 22–27; Rankin, S., Stallings, K., & London, F. (2005). *Patient education in health and illness* (5th ed.). Philadelphia, PA: Lippincott Williams & Wilkins; Redman, B. K. (1993). *The process of patient education* (7th ed.). St. Louis, MO: Mosby Year Book; and Roett, M., & Wessel, L. (2012). Help your patient "get" what you just said: A health literacy guide. *The Journal of Family Practice, 61*(4), 190–196.

at an intermediate level, 29% read at a basic level, and 14% read at below a basic level. Nineteen percent of high school graduates read below a basic level. Demographics reveal that 44% Hispanic, 24% African Americans, 9% Caucasian, and 13% other ethnic groups read below a basic level (Statistic Brain, 2015).

Planning and Implementation

After determining the learning needs in the assessment stage, the nurse and the client collaboratively develop a plan that contains objectives/outcomes for the client's learning. These objectives/outcomes clarify what is to be taught, what is to be learned, what and how to evaluate, and what to document. An objective/outcome must be singular to be specific, inclusive of all elements of content necessary to be understood, measurable, and realistic to the extent that it can be attained by the client.

After objectives/outcomes are clarified and validated, the nurse continues planning by determining and analyzing the information to be presented. The nurse validates the knowledge, skills, and attitudes (competencies) to be incorporated into health education, then selects presentation modalities based on the client's learning styles and preferred learning methods. Using physiology of learning principles, the nurse also strives to use presentation methods that involve the client, stimulate as many human senses as possible, and link new ideas to previous learning. Often, the nurse complements the presentation of information by using supplemental materials, such as audiovisual aids or printed materials. To verify that the client is absorbing new material, developing new skills, and changing personal attitudes during educational sessions, the nurse should frequently observe the client's reaction to the teaching–learning activities. Unfortunately, many health educational materials do not meet the level of client health literacy.

Two instruments are available for measuring the suitability and readability of health care consumer educational materials: The Fry Reading Formula (FRF) and the Suitability Assessment of Materials (SAM). The FRF determines reading grade level by plotting on a graph the syllable and sentence counts from three 100-word passages. Longer sentences and larger word syllable counts are plotted onto a graph. Reading level increases with longer sentences and more words with three or more syllables. The SAM analyzes patient education materials for message content, text appearance, visual displays, layout, and design. For example, text font size should be at least 12 points; key points should be summarized at the end of each section; strategically placed learner evaluations for success should be present; visual displays should be age appropriate, relevant, culturally sensitive, and easy for readers to follow and comprehend; key messages should be organized; no dense text blocks or large amounts of white space should be present; and the text formatting should be easy for the eye to follow. A SAM score of more than 70% indicates superior suitability; scores ranging from 40% to 69% indicate average suitability. Some research studies have revealed that only 10% to 36% of free, health care consumer educational materials (print or internet) meet readability and suitability standards for use. Some of these health resources may also contain factual errors about ways to prevent and manage disease (Taylor-Clarke et al., 2012; Wiener & Weiner-Pla, 2014).

Evaluation and Documentation

As the final activity in the teaching–learning process, the nurse and client determine whether the client has achieved the identified learning objectives/outcomes. Criteria for evaluation include specifications of what the client will do and the particular behavior that the client will demonstrate, which were previously stated in each objective/outcome. To provide proof of client learning, the nurse documents what was taught and whether the client met the desired educational objectives/outcomes. A way to assess attainment of desired objectives/outcomes is to have the client teach back the information to the nurse. If learning objectives/outcomes are not met, then the nurse needs to either provide additional teaching or report to other interprofessional health team members that additional education is needed (see Concepts in Practice, "Client Education—A Collaborative Process").

The Holistic Approach

The holistic approach to the teaching–learning process offers another avenue for nurses to use for client education. Holistic teaching–learning espouses the use of active learning principles. Holistic active learning links the concepts of experiences (doing, seeing, simulating), information and ideas (formal or informal acquisition of knowledge, learning on your own or from others, original ideas or ideas from others or resources), and reflection (taking time to think about what is being learned, either alone or with others) (Fink, 2003). The holistic approach addresses the cognitive, affective, and psychomotor domains of learning simultaneously and facilitates clients finding personal meaning in information that is needed for self-care and health promotion.

The holistic approach provides foundational knowledge for clients while paying attention to human interactions, caring, and learning how to learn while learners work toward meeting intended learning goals (Fink, 2003). Self-assessment by clients toward achieving health education–related goals instills confidence in their ability to do what is needed to care optimally for themselves or their loved ones. Taking time to reflect on what is learned facilitates the development of the implicit memory that recalls sensory, emotional, and skeletal responses along with procedural skills (Collins, 2007). However, little research is available to validate whether the holistic approach to client health education is better than the traditional teaching–learning process.

TEACHING–LEARNING AS A RESPONSIBILITY OF THE ADVOCATE

As nurses engage in the teaching–learning process with clients, they assist clients to become better informed about how to manage their own health. Thus, clients are able to make informed choices about the type of health care that they receive. By eliminating the

Concepts in Practice

IDEA ——→ PLAN —→ ACTION

Client Education—A Collaborative Process

Mr. H is a 75-year-old man who has been admitted to the hospital for slurred speech, right arm weakness, and right leg weakness. His wife has accompanied him and is very concerned and worried. Within 18 hours of admission, his symptoms subside completely. The neurologist sends him home on clopidogrel 75 mg and aspirin 325 mg daily.

When planning dismissal instructions, Juliana, the nurse caring for Mr. H, sets the following learning objectives for the client educational encounter.

1. Accurately describe the signs and symptoms of a stroke.
2. Explain the emergency measures to take if signs and symptoms occur (activate the Emergency Medical System [EMS] and get to a hospital as soon as possible).
3. List the side effects of clopidogrel and aspirin.
4. Outline ways to reduce the gastrointestinal irritation that may arise from the dismissal medication.
5. Specify when to contact the physician for adverse effects of the dismissal medication.
6. Explain the reasons for newly ordered medication, dietary and activity restrictions, and follow-up care with their primary care physician and neurologist.

Juliana provides Mr. and Mrs. H with instructions about the side effects of the medications, signs and symptoms of a stroke, and what to do if any should occur. Along with verbal instructions, Juliana provides them with a booklet about transient ischemic attacks and brain attacks (cerebral vascular accidents or strokes).

Mr. and Mrs. H tell Juliana all of the required information correctly with the exception of what they will do if either one of them has the signs and symptoms of brain attacks. They insist that their first action would be to contact their closest family member for a ride to the hospital rather than activating the Emergency Medical Response System.

Recognizing that transporting family members using a family member's care as a patient preference, Juliana can try to Figure out how to motivate them to call 911 first. However, if unsuccessful, additional teaching will be needed and this educational need should be shared with a home health nurses (if one was ordered) and/or someone in an outpatient setting where Mr. and Mrs. H will be receiving follow-up care. Juliana could also refer the couple and their family members to a community-based stroke education program.

Juliana notifies the neurologist about the need for further education. The neurologist states that this information will be re-taught during the follow-up office visit. Based on the results of the response from the neurologist, Juliana provides the couple with information about the local stroke educational program and support group. Mrs. H expresses intense interest in attending these programs.

"mysteries" behind navigating the health care system, medical interventions, and complementary therapies, nurses assume the role of client advocate.

The belief in advocacy as an appropriate role of the nurse has evolved in harmony with the current societal characteristics and values of consumerism, self-care, justice and human rights, equal opportunity for all, and individual accountability for health. Many people no longer believe that illness is an event over which they have control. One of the most significant activities of the nurse advocate is to provide informational support to assist the client to make the wisest possible decisions in the pursuit of well-being.

The Purpose of Teaching–Learning

The search for meaning in professional nursing should be focused on the client's perceptions of his or her health situation. The phenomenologic model of curriculum proposed by Diekelmann (1988) fits the role conception of the nurse as an advocate for the client. In this model, "the central concern is the communicative understandings of meanings given by people who live within the situation" (Diekelmann, 1988, p. 142). Thus, the purpose of teaching–learning is to provide the opportunity for the nurse and the client to explore together the importance and meaning of the client's experience.

Applying Diekelmann's proposition, the essential aspect of the process is not transmitting or acquiring facts; rather, it is "making meaning and giving meaning ... through the initiation and maintenance of dialogue" (Diekelmann, 1988, p. 143). In addition, Diekelmann (p. 143) proposed that the teacher's role is to "link the contextual and conceptual worlds of students," who are, in this discussion, clients participating in the nursing process. In this kind of dialogue, clients retain the authority and responsibility for their decisions and health behaviors.

According to Babcock and Miller (1994), if nurses expect clients to take interdependent and independent responsibilities for decision making, clients need nurses who can identify central issues, recognize underlying assumptions, recognize evidence of bias and emotion, solve problems, and think creatively. The development of these abilities appears in definitions of critical thinking, a key cognitive skill for effective professional nursing practice. In client education situations, nurses guide the client to master the knowledge and skills that are needed to make decisions.

Take Note!
As clients begin to make informed choices for health and health care–related decisions, they look to professional nurses for support.

Functions of the Advocate in the Teaching-Learning Process

Providing the opportunity for dialogue to fully explore health concerns is the major function of the nurse acting as an advocate for clients, regardless of whether those clients are experiencing high or low levels of wellness. Within this exploration, nurses use their expertise to "not only offer information [but also] offer ways of being, ways of coping, and even new possibilities" for the clients (Benner, 2000, p. 78).

Benner (2000) proposed that teaching–learning transactions take on new dimensions when the learner (client) is ill. She cited the following competencies necessary for the nurse to assume the teaching–coaching function with a client who is ill.

1. Carefully time the interventions to capture the client's readiness to learn.
2. Help the client integrate the implications of the illness and recovery into his or her lifestyle.
3. Elicit and respect the client's interpretation of the illness.
4. Respond fully and cogently to the client's request for an explanation of what is happening (within the limits of both the client's and the nurse's own understanding).
5. Make approachable and understandable any culturally avoided or uncharted aspects of an illness by exploring ways of being and coping for the client and the family and by identifying new possibilities.

Growth through learning is maximized if the nurse fulfills these functions with the client.

Mutuality in the Teaching-Learning Process

One of the primary characteristics of an advocate–client relationship is mutuality. Watson (2007) stressed that nurses must strive to develop with client interactions that are liberating and empowering. Teachers and learners should learn from each other. Learning should be mutual, characterized by anticipatory–participatory behaviors, shared power, and knowing, doing, and being to become one. Watson's model of nursing is cited as one that mandates mutuality in the nursing process and places high priority on teaching–learning as a significant intervention mode in a reciprocal nurse–client relationship.

Mutuality can be defined as "a connection with or understanding of another that facilitates a dynamic process of joint exchange between people. The process of being mutual is characterized by a sense of unfolding action that is shared in common, a sense of moving toward a common goal, and a sense of satisfaction for all involved" (Henson, 1997, p. 80). Mutuality balances power and respect, encourages accountability, and "facilitates active involvement of both nurses and clients in effectively working toward mutually identified goals" (Henson, 1997, p. 77). Mutuality is consistent with any learning theory used to guide the teaching-learning process.

QUESTIONS FOR REFLECTION

1. Have you ever learned anything from a client, client's family, or community? If so, what did you learn?
2. Have you ever received health education from a nurse? How effective was the education? What key things do you remember from your experience that you might want to incorporate into your future professional practice when educating clients, families, or communities?
3. How do you feel when clients or their family members learn a new skill or grasp key information regarding self-care for the first time?
4. How do you promote active participation by clients, families, and communities in the client education process?
5. Why is active participation important in the teaching-learning process?

LEARNING THEORIES

The process by which learning occurs has been described in multiple ways. Learning theories and models explain how people learn. When nurses use models and theories to guide the client education process, they can use principles to structure meaningful client educational experiences, prevent overloading clients with information, and understand the reasons for unsuccessful client education encounters. Educational effort should be focused on learners (individuals, families, significant others, and communities). Because the vast amounts of information available on learning theories is too broad to cover in this text, the following section outlines Bruner's perspective, which encompasses five different learning models.

Bruner's Learning Models

Bruner (1986) cited five popular models of how the learner learns: empiricism, hypothesis generator, nativism, constructivism, and novice-to-expert. Empiricism is considered the oldest model. It is based on the premise that "one learns from experience" and that "such order as there is in the mind is a reflection of the order that exists in the world" (Bruner, 1986, p. 199). People need life experience for success in educational situations based on empiricism.

Unlike the rather passive view of the empiricism model, the hypothesis generator mode includes a major premise of intentionality. "The learner, rather than being the creature of experience, selects that which is to enter" and possesses an active curiosity guided by self-directed projects" (Bruner, 1986, p. 199). A person is a successful learner in this model if he or she has a good theory from which hypotheses are generated. This perspective of learning supports the use of active learning educational strategies.

The nativism model proposes that the mind is innately shaped by "a set of underlying categories, hypotheses," both forms of organizing experiences (Bruner, 1986, p. 199). The task of the learner in this model is to develop a way of organizing perceived reality. Using the innate powers of the mind is the formula for successful learning in this model. Concept mapping facilitates the organization of concepts to be learned under the nativism model.

The constructivism model was developed primarily by Piaget, who, according to Bruner (1986, p. 199), stated that "the world is not found, but made, and according to a set of structural rules that are imposed on the flow of experience." These structural rules provide boundaries for learning. The learner goes through stage-like progressions characterized by tension between previously assimilated structural rules and changes in the rules that come in later stage development. In accommodating these new rules, the learner is successful if his or her learning structure changes by

moving to higher systems that subsume earlier structures. Thus, the constructivism model supports a holistic approach to teaching–learning.

The novice-to-expert model "begins with the premise that if you want to find out about learning, ask first about what is to be learned, find an expert who does it well, and then look at the novice and figure out how he or she can get there" (Bruner, 1986, p. 199). In this model, the formula for success is to be specific and explicit in taking the steps to attain expertise. The novice-to-expert model substantiates the use of collaborative partnerships in the teaching–learning process.

Bruner (1986, p. 200) suggested that there is not just one kind of learning and that we would be better served if we understood that "the model of the learner is not fixed but various." In many health care organizations, nurses use standardized teaching guides; documentation frequently consists of checking off items on a list. Nurses who use Bruner's learner models individualize client education, thereby maximizing client mastery of desired outcomes.

Types of Learning

Bevis (1988, p. 40) outlined six types of learning that may be useful in the teaching–learning process (see Box 16.2, Professional Building Blocks, "Bevis's Six Types of Learning"). She suggested that different educational approaches work best for different types of learning, but noted that syntactic, contextual, and inquiry learning are necessary for change that can truly maximize the client's abilities to gain the best control of his or her health. Item learning, directive learning, and rational learning typically are needed for safe performance of a skill. For example, item learning generates lists or outlines procedures (think about gathering all supplies for preparing an injection and then learning the skill of how to give an injection). Directive learning involves rules, injunctions, and exceptions to rules (do not give an injection where there is a break in the skin). Rational learning involves the use of theory and other information to make logical judgments (If an injection is given where the skin is broken, there will be an increase chance of causing an injection site infection.).

In contrast, syntactic, contextual, and inquiry learning incorporate personal meaning, cultural considerations, and discovery in the client education process rather than approaching learning as an exercise in mastery of relationships, rules, and logic. For example, syntactic learning would result when a person with a newly diagnosed case of diabetes links improved cognitive abilities based on optimal blood glucose control or

16.2 Professional Building Blocks

Bevis' Six Types of Learning

1. **Item learning:** Simple relationships between separate pieces of information, as seen in mechanistic and ritualistic lists and procedures
2. **Directive learning:** Rules, injunctions, and exceptions, as seen in safety requirements
3. **Rational learning:** Use of theory to buttress action, enabling logical decision making, and logical judgments
4. **Syntactic learning:** Seeing meaningful wholes, relationships, and patterns that enables the learner to develop insights and find meaning
5. **Contextual learning:** Acceptance of culture, mores, folkways, rites, and rituals as ways of being; these learning transactions are "caring, compassionate, and positive"
6. **Inquiry learning:** Investigating, categorizing, and theorizing in a way to generate ideas and develop a vision

Bevis, E. O. (1988). *New directions for a new age. In National League for Nursing. Curriculum revolution: Mandate for change.* New York: National League for Nursing; p. 40.

excessive urination with poor glucose control. Contextual and inquiry learning might occur simultaneously while finding ways how to participate fully in family celebrations centered on special holiday foods without disrupting optimal glucose control.

Principles of Learning

Principles identified by Babcock and Miller (1994) are considered useful in any of these learner models or types of learning (see Box 16.3, Professional Building Blocks, "Babcock and Miller's Guiding Principles in the Teaching–Learning Process"). In addition, because individual learning preferences of clients vary, the professional nurse needs to understand the multiple models and types of learning to personalize the teaching–learning process effectively. Effectiveness is measured by the success of the nurse and the client in changing the client's health behaviors in a positive direction.

▌ QUESTIONS FOR REFLECTION

1. How do you assess clients for preferred learning styles?
2. How do you learn best? Why is it important for you to know your preferred learning style?

IMPLICATIONS OF CHANGE THEORY ON TEACHING–LEARNING

Growth is inherent in the definition of learning. Growth implies that change occurs. Because change is about the only thing that occurs constantly, change, growth, and learning happen continuously throughout life. Desired outcomes of education are changes in behavior, attitude, and psychomotor abilities (Bloom, 1974). However, in the process of learning, the human brain also experiences long-lasting changes (Collins, 2007).

Change as a Goal of Teaching: Growth

The mutually determined goal of the nurse and the client who are participating in the teaching–learning process is "becoming different than before" (Douglass, 1988, p. 226). Douglass noted that forces that influence change can be external or internal. The nurse is an intentional external force assisting the client to demonstrate different and better health behaviors.

The nurse in the teaching–learning relationship needs to follow a series of sequential steps that

16.3 Professional Building Blocks

Babcock and Miller's Guiding Principles in the Teaching–Learning Process

1. Focusing intensifies learning.
2. Repetition enhances learning.
3. Learner control increases learning.
4. Active participation is necessary for learning.
5. Learning styles vary.
6. Organization promotes learning.
7. Association is necessary to learning.
8. Imitation is a method of learning.
9. Motivation strengthens learning.
10. Spacing new material facilitates learning.
11. Recency influences retention.
12. Primacy affects retention.
13. Arousal influences attention.
14. Accurate and prompt feedback enhances learning.
15. Application of new learning in a variety of contexts broadens the generalization of that learning.
16. The learner's biologic, psychological, sociologic, and cultural realities shape the learner's perception of the learning experience.

Babcock, D. E., & Miller, M. A. (1994). *Client education: Theory and practice.* St. Louis, MO: Mosby Year Book; pp 45–48.

are consistent with planned change theory. Planned change is a deliberate process to make a desired change in a situation, knowledge, skill, or attitude (such as redecorating a room, learning to play a musical instrument, searching for information on an unfamiliar topic, or adjusting one's attitude and approach when working with a person different from oneself). Unplanned change is unanticipated and may arise from an unexpected situation such as a sudden illness, motor vehicle accident, falling and injuring oneself, or house fire (see Box 16.4, Professional Building Blocks, "Sequential Steps Consistent with Planned Change Theory") (Douglass, 1988). The steps mirror nursing process: exploring and identifying factors for the change (assessment), determining specific knowledge gaps (diagnosis), selecting an educational strategy (planning), executing the strategy (implementation), and determining the overall results (evaluation).

Outcomes of Knowledge Acquisition

The outcome of knowledge acquisition in the teaching–learning process may not always be satisfying to the nurse and the client. Harmony within the human system results when the newly acquired information is congruent with previously integrated functions. However, if the new information is incompatible with the previously integrated functions, clients and nurses may perceive disharmony. Feelings of being unsettled, restless, and uncertain frequently accompany periods of growth. Nurses often need to help clients understand that change may not be a painless process.

To reduce the discomfort that sometimes occurs in the teaching–learning process, nurses and clients can analyze the current situation using a holistic perspective. The holistic approach would consider all aspects of the client's life, including how the change would affect the client as an individual, impact all people involved in the client's life, and alter social structures along with the client's motivation for change. Both the situational context and the motivational aspects of planned change play a significant role in the client's ability to integrate information and develop new behaviors.

Readiness for Learning

A central issue for nurses in implementing the teaching–learning process as a strategy for changing behaviors is the client's **readiness for learning** (Fig. 16.1). Benner (2000, p. 79) noted that teaching–learning interventions often are dictated by schedules in the health care delivery environment: "Assessing where a patient is, how open he is to information, deciding when to go ahead even when the patient does

---

16.4 Professional Building Blocks

Sequential Steps Consistent with Planned Change Theory

1. Explore the client's perceived need for change.
2. Identify the forces for change with the client.
3. Help the client state his or her health concerns.
4. Identify constraints and opportunities in the situation.
5. Provide the information needed to analyze both the change needs and the potential strategies to achieve the desired change.
6. Critique each of the possible change strategies on the basis of both the information understood and the situational factors.
7. Select the change strategy to be attempted in the effort to achieve a different and better health behavior.
8. Plan the implementation, filling in all of the informational gaps perceived by the nurse and the client.
9. Design an evaluation process to determine success in changing health behavior.
10. *Client:* Implement the planned behavioral activities. *Nurse:* Offer feedback and facilitate opportunities in the delivery system environment to promote success of the client.
11. Evaluate the overall results of the teaching–learning interaction and the specific health behavior changes on the part of the client.

Douglass, L. M. (1988). *The effective nurse: Leader and manager* (3rd ed., pp. 226–232). St. Louis, MO: Mosby Year Book.

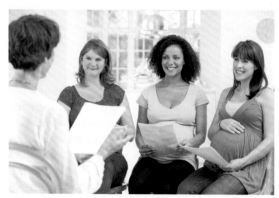

FIGURE 16.1 Anticipated future labor enhances readiness for learning in prenatal classes.

Concepts in Practice

Complex Client Education

IDEA ──→ PLAN ──→ ACTION

A newly diagnosed diabetic has multiple learning needs. In today's fast-paced society, effective control of blood sugar is very challenging.

Such would be the case for a single, working mother who has just found out that she has insulin-dependent diabetes while in the hospital.

1. The nurse would teach the woman how to perform blood glucose checks using a handheld glucometer. Effective use of the meter involves turning on the meter, calibrating it, checking glucose strips for expiration dates and calibrating them to the meter, acquiring blood safely for accurate testing, reading, and understanding meter testing results, turning off the meter, and caring for the meter.

2. In order to affirm understanding of how and when the insulin would be prepared and administered, the nurse would share information about proper storage of insulin, when insulin would become outdated and how to safely prepare and administer insulin injections.

3. While observing the client performing all the required skills for safe home management of diabetes, the nurse would note any visual (inability to see syringe markings), literacy (inability to read or understand printed directions), psychomotor (poor/fine motor hand coordination), and psychological (extreme anxiety or denial) barriers in performing any required skills.

4. In addition to glucose testing and insulin injection administration, the nurse would review the signs and symptoms of hypoglycemia and its management. The nurse would also provide education about signs and symptoms of hyperglycemia, the importance of managing strict glucose control, and the complications of poorly managed glucose levels.

5. The nurse would stress the importance of daily inspection of feet, daily foot hygiene, and proper toenail care and actions to take if foot problems are identified.

6. The nurse would verify that the woman received effective education about current diabetic dietary needs. Typically, newly diagnosed persons with diabetes receive special nutritional education from a dietitian. However, the nurse needs to validate client understanding of nutritional strategies to promote optimal glucose control (testing blood glucose levels before meals, eating regularly scheduled meals, counting carbohydrates consumed, and knowing how to follow a sliding scale insulin regimen).

7. For identified gaps in education, the nurse would make referrals to a specialized diabetic educator for further education. The nurse would consult a social worker to facilitate acquisition of diabetes testing and management supplies if problems securing them arose.

Unless the client understands the benefits of controlling glucose levels, she may put taking care of herself behind caring for her children.

---

not appear ready, are key aspects of effective patient teaching."

Nurses frequently find themselves pressured to implement client teaching quickly, especially when clients want to go home immediately, physicians write discharge from the hospital orders, or the dismissal from the hospital is unanticipated. Unless a preferred learning style assessment has been performed sometime during the hospital stay (many institutions include this as part of the nursing admission database), the nurse must quickly ask clients and significant others how they learn best. Nurses quickly assess clients for learning readiness and most of the time, clients are ready to learn because they want to go home and many clients want to assume responsibility for their own health (see Concepts in Practice, "Client Education—A Collaborative Process," earlier in this chapter).

For commonly encountered surgical procedures and disease processes, many health care organizations have standardized teaching plans for nurses to follow when providing client education. Because many clients use computers and mobile phones daily, if the health care facility's policies permit, nurses can provide photos or videos for client education, especially if the client identifies video technology as the preferred teaching–learning strategy (Holt, Flint, & Bowers, 2011).

Most people experiencing a newly diagnosed disease, illness, or surgical procedure experience some anxiety (see Concepts in Practice, "Client Education—A Collaborative Process," earlier in this chapter). Thus, learning readiness must be evaluated in terms of the degree of anxiety the client expresses. Minimal anxiety serves as a positive force for attention, alertness, or awareness, all of which are necessary for learning and integration of functions to occur. Moderate anxiety usually is associated with selective inattention and decreasing awareness; extreme anxiety is associated with lack of attention and loss of awareness. Moderate or extreme anxiety usually is an indicator of the client's lack of readiness for learning. In these two anxiety states, the nurse's focus needs to be on reducing anxiety to enable the client to regain a sense of security and repossess the energy required for attention and awareness, which are prerequisites for learning (Collins, 2007; Rankin et al., 2005).

Validating Learning: Feedback

Validation, a process of confirmation, is a necessary element of teaching–learning. In client education, validation means that the client understands the educational material, has mastered a particular health care skill, or uses the new information or skill effectively. For a behavioral change to become well integrated, it must be validated by people significant to the client. Nurses frequently play a significant role in clients' lives.

As teachers, nurses share their knowledge and expertise with clients. Learners appreciate feedback from teachers. **Feedback** is the transmission of information regarding how well learning outcomes are being met by learners. Frequently, constructive feedback stimulates learners to want to learn more. In client education, nurse feedback provides clients (and families) with specific information on how well they have absorbed the knowledge and skills needed to care for themselves (Rankin et al., 2005).

Take Note!
Throughout life, a person requires validation through feedback from significant others to maintain the integrity of his or her self-system.

STRATEGIES FOR EFFECTIVE TEACHING AND LEARNING

Patient-Focused Teaching

Although nurses often use standardized teaching plans, **patient-focused teaching** hones in on individual client learning needs and preferences. Client education works better when nurses and clients involved in the teaching–learning process know about each other (Rankin et al., 2015; Redman, 1993). As they use their repertoire of therapeutic communication skills and as they conduct their assessments, nurses get to know their clients. However, clients may know very little

about their nurses other than the information found on the nurse's employer name badge. Some health care facilities include professional licensure, earned academic degrees, and nurse specialty certifications on name badges. Some nurses carry business cards that they give to clients specifying their academic degrees, certification, and scope of practice. In addition to providing their credentials, nurses should communicate clearly their intentions in the teaching–learning process, share a clear plan of the time commitments to clients, and offer information about how a contract can be established if clients desire one.

For instructions to be effective, the nurse should know the following information about clients involved in the education process: (1) how the client perceives the health situation; (2) physical, cultural, linguistic, or psychological limitations that may impede learning (including anxiety or cognitive impairment); (3) intended learning outcomes; (4) interprofessional team members' plans for the client; (5) what the client's conscious intentions and desires are regarding health behaviors; and (6) what information the client perceives is needed to achieve his or her health goals. With this basic information, nurses and clients should be able to engage fully in the teaching–learning process (Rankin et al., 2005; Redman, 1993).

Motivational Strategies

Many teaching strategies are available to enhance client **motivation** (stimulus) to participate in learning but only a few are mentioned in this chapter. Additional motivational teaching strategies may be found in books devoted to teaching strategies (see the reference list at the end of the chapter).

Theis and Johnson (1995) synthesized the existing research examining teaching strategies and found "66% of subjects receiving planned teaching had better outcomes than did control group subjects receiving routine care" (p. 100). Current literature also supports the effectiveness of structured approaches, reinforcement, independent study, and multiple strategies (Allen, Iezzoni, Huang, Huang, & Leveille, 2008; Budin et al., 2008; Chang & Kelly, 2007; Edwardson, 2007). Box 16.5, Professional Building Blocks, "Effective Teaching Strategies," suggests additional approaches (Babcock & Miller, 1994; Rankin et al., 2005; Redman, 1993).

Motivation for learning is enhanced if the student and the teacher trust and respect each other, the teacher assumes and expects that the student can learn, the teacher is sensitive to the student's individual needs, and both the student and the teacher feel free to learn

16.5 Professional Building Blocks

Effective Teaching Strategies

- Computer-based instruction
- Observation and assessment scales
- Demonstration
- Lecture/discussion
- Modeling
- Programmed instruction
- Role playing
- Group activities
- Use of media (posters, flip charts, overhead projections, videotapes, audiotapes, films)
- Games and simulations
- Concept maps

Babcock, D. E., & Miller, M. A. (1994). *Client education: Theory and practice.* St. Louis, MO: Mosby Year Book; Fink, L. (2003). *Creating significant learning experiences.* San Francisco: Jossey-Bass; Rankin, S., Stallings, K., & London, F. (2005). *Patient education in health and illness* (5th ed.). Philadelphia, PA: Lippincott Williams & Wilkins; and Redman, B. K. (1993). *The process of patient education* (7th ed.). St. Louis, MO: Mosby Year Book.

and make mistakes in their own unique styles. Boswell, Pichert, Lorenz, and Schlundt (1990) reinforced the idea that active participation in learning is a strong motivator. Box 16.6, Professional Building Blocks, "Effective Motivational Strategies for Learning," suggests additional motivational approaches (Bevis, 1988).

16.6 Professional Building Blocks

Effective Motivational Strategies for Learning

- Engaging the learner in active analysis
- Raising questions
- Nurturing
- Finding ways to make the learning meaningful and significant for the learner
- Following the ethical ideal in giving clients all the information they need to make sound choices
- Displaying a caring attitude
- Using and encouraging creativity in the teaching–learning process
- Encouraging curiosity and the search for satisfying ideas
- Being assertive
- Desiring to engage in and to seek dialogue

Bevis, E. O. (1988). *New directions for a new age. In National League for Nursing. Curriculum revolution: Mandate for change.* New York: National League for Nursing; p. 45.

▥ QUESTIONS FOR REFLECTION

1. Look back at the teaching struggles and motivational strategies presented here. Which have you experienced in your nursing education program? Were they helpful to you? Why or why not? Which have you used in clinical practice? Do you think that they were helpful when providing client education? Why or why not?

2. Can you identify additional teaching and motivational strategies for working with clients? Make a list and indicate why you think they would be effective.

Take Note!

Teaching is more effective when nurses tailor the education strategy to fit client-preferred learning styles.

Contextual Constraints and Opportunities

Some contextual constraints, such as the dilemma of insufficient time and great need on the part of the client, have been mentioned. To attempt to control environmental constraints that might be imposed on the teaching–learning process, the nurse should keep the following teaching strategies in mind.

- Try to arrange learning experiences when the learner feels relatively healthy.
- Provide time for learning at a comfortable pace.
- Have sufficient grasp of the subject matter to translate concepts into different terms for different learners.
- Make sure expectations and standards are clear.

Certain clients, such as the elderly, require a slower pace of instruction to allow for increased time for mental processing. The Hartford Foundation offers a vast array of resources for nurses working with elderly clients, including tips for effective teaching and learning (Fulmer, 2007).

Bruner (1986, p. 198) suggested that educators need to assist learners to perceive the value of the rich diversity in the world. He encouraged educators to view the learner as "equipped to discriminate and deal differentially with a wide variety of possible worlds exhibiting different conditions, yet worlds in which one can cope." The nurse should perhaps heed this advice and have confidence in the client's ability to mutually participate in teaching–learning and to succeed in a diverse world, rather than trying to control all the contextual constraints that might interfere with learning.

Power sharing would be more likely by nurses with this confidence in clients. Perceived abilities and learning are more likely in such relationships.

SPECIFIC CLIENT EDUCATION ACTIVITIES

Many routine nursing activities involve client (and family) education. When clients enter a health care institution, they frequently need instructions related to their expected role responsibilities. Health care professionals cannot deliver effective care unless clients are willing to provide them with information related to health problems and educational needs. During an initial client encounter, the nurse may learn more about the client needs and concerns, and the client actually assumes the role of teacher. To plan effective nursing care, the nurse needs to understand the client's perspective of the health problem or illness. Usually additional information related to specific care needs (special adaptive devices, cultural concerns) also surface during the initial encounter.

Nurses assume the role of educator when they inform clients and families of the purposes behind nursing interventions and rationales for administered medications. Educational efforts such as these enable clients to understand the reasons behind care activities and learn why they must comply with the ordered medical regimen. Most teaching related to medication administration reinforces information clients have received from physicians. However, sometimes, as in the case of a client with newly diagnosed diabetes, the physician delegates the task of teaching insulin administration to a nurse or certified diabetic educator (who usually is a professional nurse).

The Joint Commission has a consumer education campaign for clients and families known as "Speak Up™". The campaign emphasizes the importance of health care consumers to ask questions in home, inpatient, and outpatient settings about their care. The campaign emphasizes the importance of consumes to ask questions if something does not seem correct to prevent errors (right treatment and right identification), insist the health care providers follow infection control guidelines, learn about their disease processes and treatment (to avoid rehospitalization), know what they need to do before having surgery, understand risks for falling, know how to take medications safely, acknowledge principles of safe antibiotic use, know their rights, select a personal advocate for health care, advocate for children, and report pain and feelings of depression to health care providers. In 2015, the Joint Commission surveyed users of the program and results revealed that 83% of respondents perceived that the campaign was easy to use and understand, increased health care consumer empowerment and perceptions as an equal partner in their health care, adds value to health care organizations, and perceive that the Joint Commission is an authoritative source of information related to health care (The Joint Commission, 2016b). Sixty-nine percent of the respondents reported that they would recommend the use of the campaign to others seeking health care services (The Joint Commission, 2016a). However, some patients must feel comfortable with their health care providers before asking questions or reminding them of proper infection control or identification strategies.

Sometimes the roles of educator and client advocate become intertwined. As a client advocate, the nurse frequently verifies that patients understand procedures that are about to happen. Nurses commonly obtain signatures on informed consent forms before clients undergo invasive procedures. Informed consent requires that the client is competent, has had other treatment options explained to him or her, understands the treatment/test and its potential adverse effects, agrees to the procedure without coercion, and consents to having the procedure performed (Bosek & Savage, 2007; Rankin et al., 2005). Nursing process is used to determine the multiple elements of informed consent. When assessing for the elements required for informed consent, questions related to the procedure may arise. The nurse who answers them engages in the process of client education. However, if the nurse discovers that the client does not fully understand the anticipated procedure, the role of educator is put aside and the nurse assumes the role of advocate, informing the physician of an inability to obtain a signature on a consent form because the client fails to understand the procedure's risks and benefits.

Nurses also participate in community health education. Successful community education starts with the participation of community members. Nurses secure community input when planning community education programs by performing a needs assessment. In a manner similar to that used to identify individual client learning needs, the nurse asks community members to identify community learning needs. Methods for performing a needs assessment include individual interviews, informal polls, focus groups, or written surveys. Key community leaders must also be asked to identify group learning needs to ensure successful program development and implementation. Once a learning need has been identified, professional nurses secure credible resources and financial support for the program. Financial support may be secured in the form of grants or corporate sponsorships, or from the community. Involvement of community members during the program-planning process increases the chance that the program will appeal to community members.

Teaching strategies that appeal to individual clients (videos, slides, and flip charts) may be highly effective for community education. However, the teaching strategies must consider the projected number of people who will attend the program (Rankin et al., 2005). Within

FOCUS ON RESEARCH

Examining Associations between Health Information Seeking Behavior and Adult Education Status in the United States: An Analysis of the 2012 PIAAC Data

The investigators wanted to discover if there was a difference in health information seeking behaviors (HISB) for Americans with and without a high school diploma and if there were any relationships among HISB, health status, and use of preventive health measures.

They analyzed data from the Program for International Assessment of Adult Competencies (PIAAC), an international household survey that assesses adult competencies. The survey is given under the guidance of the Organization of Economic Cooperation and Development in 26 nations. Frequency of source use for health information data (books, health care providers, internet, magazines, newspapers, radio, or television) were generated using a Likert scale and boxes to check yes or no were used to assess preventive service use (flus vaccines, mammography, pap smear, screening for colon cancer, prostate cancer and osteoporosis, dental care visit and vision examinations). The United States was the only nation that added five items to address health information seeking behaviors.

Five thousand adults between the ages of 16 and 65 years completed the survey. Of the adults surveyed, 4,256 had high school diplomas (85%) and 629 did not (15%). Seventy-nine percent of respondents reported having health insurance. Health was rated as excellent by 4%, very good by 11%, good by 28%, fair by 33%, and poor by 24% of the adults.

The researchers found that younger adults and adults with high school diplomas tended to use the internet as their main source of health care information. Persons with high school diplomas reported also using newspapers, television, books, and magazines. Persons without high school diplomas

reported using magazines, radio, and television more for health information. Both groups used health care professionals for health care information. However, health care professionals were used less frequently as the main source of health information. Most adults used the internet, magazines, television more frequently. Persons without high school diplomas also used information from the radio more frequently than information from a health care provider.

Persons without a high school diploma reported their health status as lower than persons with a high school diploma. Adults with a high school diploma reported using health preventive services more frequently than adults without a high school diploma.

The clinical significance of this study is that the internet is the fastest growing source of health information and educated people are consulting internet resources for health information. In addition, persons without internet access may soon become disadvantaged in access to health information. Health care professionals must ascertain that available internet health resources contain valid, reliable information and need to review internet resources that health consumers are accessing for health information. Weaknesses of this study include the use of ordinal and nominal level of measurement for statistical analyses, the cross-sectional design, and that not all screening tests (mammography, colon, prostate, and osteoporosis) applied to the age of each respondent and that these tests may not be performed on an annual basis. More research is needed to determine where access health information, the accuracy and quality of online health information materials, and how to help persons decipher valid health information from health information linked to a product advertisement.

Feinberg, I., Frijters, J., Johnson-Lawrence, V., Greenberg, D., Nightingale, E., & Moodie, C. (2016). Examining associations between health information seeking behavior and adult education status in the U.S.: An analysis of the 2012 PIAAC data. *PLoS ONE 11*(2): e0148751. doi: 10.1371/journal.pone.0148751 recent years, health care consumers are using technology to access health care information. Computer, tablet, and cell phone applications help consumers keep records regarding health promotion efforts (dietary intake and exercise) and disease management strategies (blood pressure, blood sugar readings). Americans are increasingly using the internet for health information according to Feinberg et al. (2016). Their study appears in the following Focus on Research, "Examining Associations between Health Information Seeking Behavior and Adult Education Status in the United States: An Analysis of the 2012 PIAAC Data."

Not all client education occurs in a formalized setting, such as a health care organization or community agency. Nurses reside in neighborhoods and are members of families. Family members, neighbors, and friends frequently consult nurses they are acquainted with or related to when health care concerns or questions about a health condition arise. Sometimes, the questions fall within the realm of the professional nurse's area of expertise; at other times, they do not. Directing family, friends, and acquaintances to credible resources sometimes poses a great challenge for the professional nurse. As more people use the internet as a source of health information, the professional nurse should become aware of the quality of information posted on various popular websites. Nurses have an obligation to share accurate health-related information or refer the question or concern to another health team member when unable to provide the requested information.

Rankin et al. (2005) and Smeltzer (2005) outlined several factors that distinguish credible from less reputable information for client education and care (see Box 16.7, Learning, Knowing, and Growing, "Assessing the Suitability of Sources"). The process of peer review increases the credibility of information because the information has been appraised by experts in the field. Before suggesting materials for client education,

---

16.7 Learning, Knowing, and Growing

Assessing the Suitability of Sources

How do you know if an information source is credible and suitable for health education for clients? Certain defining characteristics can help you identify suitable sources for use in your studies or with your clients. Other characteristics should be considered based on client needs.

Suitable Source Characteristics

- Peer reviewed
- Primary source of information
- Written or developed by known experts in a field
- Editorial ideas clearly documented as such
- Governmental or higher educational sources
- Professional nursing organization
- Recognized nonprofit organizations for a disease process (e.g., American Cancer Society, American Diabetes Association, Multiple Sclerosis Society)
- Websites from government, higher education, and nonprofit organizations that are updated on a regular schedule
- Clearly delineate editorials and advertisement from objective information
- Display biographic information of all content authors (academic and professional credentials) as well as their relationship to the organization
- Disclaimer present that sends clients to physicians or other health care providers for specific use of content provided

- Open disclosures if funds from companies were used to develop the study or website
- Hyperlinks to reports of original studies or primary sources of information
- Website design easy to navigate in order to reach desired information

Unsuitable Source Characteristics

- Use of secondary sources of information
- Use of editorial ideas as facts
- Product advertisements or information for sale
- Websites that are not updated on a regular basis
- No content review by medical experts
- For-profit organizations
- Nonprofit organizations displaying narrow viewpoints
- Poorly designed websites
- Websites linked directly to advertisements (automatic pop-up ads come when site accessed)
- No disclaimer statement to warn clients of the need to consult with a health care provider to meet specific needs

Additional Considerations Based on Client Needs

- High level of literacy required to read and/or understand content
- Print or font less than 12 points in size (for the visually impaired or elderly)
- Only the English language option (for persons who have limited fluency in English)

Rankin, S., Stallings, K., & London, F. (2005). *Patient education in health and illness* (5th ed., pp. 280–282). Philadelphia, PA: Lippincott Williams & Wilkins; Smeltzer, S. (2005). Is that information safe for patient care? *Nursing, 35,* 54–55.

nurses must review them to verify accuracy, readability, and ease of use.

QUESTIONS FOR REFLECTION

1. How do you currently evaluate the educational information that you give to clients? That you use in your own studies?
2. Why is it important for nurses to determine the suitability of client educational materials before using them with clients?

CLIENT EDUCATION AS AN INTERDISCIPLINARY PROCESS

Along with nurses, other members of the health care team make significant contributions to client education. Because nurses tend to spend more time with clients than other providers, nurses have the opportunity to assess client learning needs and responses to health teaching implemented by other team members (Fig. 16.2). The nurse also has the ability to determine whether the client has the capability to absorb teaching from other disciplines. Thus, the nurse may suggest that other health team members (e.g., dietitians, physical therapists, social workers, pharmacists) refrain from educational activities until clients are physically stable and emotionally ready to benefit from detailed self-care education.

In addition to determining the best times for client education, the nurse has the responsibility to coordinate educational activities and verify that clients receive the same information from all health care team members. Documentation of teaching by all disciplines (including nursing) is key so that instructions from one discipline can be effectively reinforced. Documented teaching content also may eliminate duplicate teaching efforts, ensure continuity of content, and

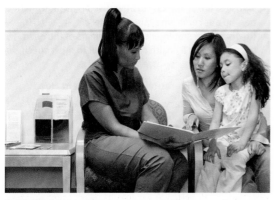

FIGURE 16.2 Explaining test results is one way that nurses engage in patient education.

provide a detailed record to meet the Joint Commission standards for client education and for third-party reimbursement.

For decades, nurses have participated in the development of client care paths. Most of these care paths are integrated into client electronic health records. Care paths designate specific client educational activities so that client education does not occur haphazardly or at the last minute when the physician writes a dismissal order. Some institutions have formed multidisciplinary educational committees to develop guidelines for client education and identify continuing educational needs for the entire health care team.

Summary and Significance to Practice

Teaching–learning is presented as a complex process among experts, the teacher, and the learner, in which all acquire new information, experience new relatedness, and change behavior as a result of the interaction. The nurse–teacher is an expert on health, and the client–learner is an expert on the client's experience of health and life circumstances. As the person who bears responsibility for developing and implementing effective client education, the nurse uses communication skills to assess and collaborate with learners to develop relevant learning experiences. Cognitive skills prove useful when determining priorities, materials, and specific strategies to use during the teaching–learning process. When clients need to learn procedural skills, the nurse shares clinical skills with them. Effective teaching and learning result in increased confidence and competence for nurses and clients.

REAL-LIFE REFLECTIONS

Recall Lillian, the nurse from the beginning of the chapter. What barriers does Lillian encounter in providing effective client education? What suggestions could Lillian make to the hospital to improve client education? What potential barriers might prevent her suggestions from being implemented? How could these suggestions be financed?

From Theory to Practice

1. After reading this chapter, what ideas will you incorporate into your client education in clinical practice? Why are these ideas important?

2. What are the consequences when clients are dismissed without receiving detailed education about medications, diet, activity, and follow-up health care?

Nurse as Author

Using ideas presented in this chapter, write a 3- to 4-paragraph essay about key considerations that need to be made for health care consumer education. Include ideas related to assessment of learning needs, identification of educational outcomes, development of an individualized educational plan, facilitators and barriers to plan implementation, and evaluation of educational outcomes.

Your Digital Classroom

Online Exploration

American Academy of Family Practitioners: **www.aafp.org**
American Cancer Society: **www.cancer.org**
American Heart Association: **www.heart.org**
American Medical Association: **www.ama-assn.org**
National Patient Safety Foundation: **www.npsf.org**
Cancer Control P.L.A.N.E.T.:
http://cancercontrolplanet.cancer.gov
Centers for Disease Control and Prevention:
www.cdc.gov
The John A. Hartford Foundation:
www.johnhartfound.org
The National Library of Medicine MedLine Plus Program for Evaluating Health Information:
www.nlm.nih.gov/medlineplus/evaluatinghealthinformation.html
National Institutes of Health: **www.nih.gov**
The Joint Commission: **www.jointcommission.org**
Centers for Medicare & Medicaid Services Toolkit for Making Written Material Clear and Effective:
https://www.cms.gov/Outreach-and-Education/Outreach/WrittenMaterialsToolkit/index.html

Expanding Your Understanding

1. Search online for a health topic of interest to you. Scan the first 10 websites in your search results. How many of these sites are trying to sell a product? How many are nonprofit organizations? How many are sponsored by a national or local government agency? Compare the quality of each website. Which sites would you recommend to a potential client for health information? Why or why not? Which sites would you use for personal health information? Why or why not?

2. Visit one of the websites listed above in Online Exploration. Print out information that you would like to use for client teaching and bring it to class. Analyze the information according to the following criteria:
   ▪ Readability
   ▪ Visual appeal
   ▪ Accuracy of information
   ▪ Use of more than one language
   ▪ Ability to sustain interest and actively engage the learner

3. What types of policies does your current work setting have related to distribution of internet resources for client education? Describe the materials available for client education in your current work setting. Search the internet to find teaching materials on the same topic. Compare and contrast the two resources.

Beyond the Book

Visit **thePoint® www.thePoint.lww.com** for activities and information to reinforce the concepts and content covered in this chapter.

REFERENCES

Agnes, M. (2005). *Webster's new world college dictionary* (4th ed.). Cleveland, OH: Wiley.

Allen, M., Iezzoni, L., Huang, A., Huang, L., & Leveille, S. (2008). Improving patient-clinician communication about chronic conditions: Description of an internet-based nurse E-coach intervention. *Nursing Research, 57*(2), 107–112.

American Nurses Association. (2015). *Nursing: Scope and standards of practice* (3rd ed.). Silver Spring, MD: ANA.

Argyris, C. (1982). *Reasoning, learning, and action: Individual and organizational.* San Francisco, CA: Jossey-Bass.

Babcock, D. E., & Miller, M. A. (1994). *Client education: Theory and practice.* St. Louis, MO: Mosby Year Book.

Beagley, L. (2011). Educating patients: Understanding barriers, learning styles, and teaching techniques. *Journal of Perianesthesia Nursing, 26*(5), 331–337. doi: 10.1016/j.opan.2011.06.002.

Benner, P. (2000). *From novice to expert: Excellence in power and clinical nursing (Commemorative edition).* Menlo Park, CA: Addison-Wesley.

Bevis, E. O. (1988). New directions for a new age. In *National League for Nursing. Curriculum revolution: Mandate for change.* New York: National League for Nursing.

Bloom, B. (Ed.). (1974). *Taxonomy of educational objectives.* New York: D. McKay.

Bosek, M., & Savage, T. (2007). *The ethical component of nursing education.* Philadelphia, PA: Lippincott Williams & Wilkins.

Boswell, E. J., Pichert, J. W., Lorenz, R. A., & Schlundt, D. G. (1990). Training health care professionals to enhance their patient teaching skills. *Journal of Nursing Staff Development,* 6, 233–239.

Bruner, J. (1986). Models of the learner. *Education Horizons, 64,* 197–200.

Budin, W., Hoskins, C. N., Haber, J., Sherman, D. W., Maislin, G., Cater, J. R., et al. (2008). Breast cancer: Education, counseling, and adjustment among patients and partners: A randomized clinical trial. *Nursing Research, 57*(3), 199–213.

Centers for Medicare & Medicare Services. (2016). Toolkit for making written material clear and effective. Retrieved from https://www.cms.gov/Outreach-and-Education/Outreach/WrittenMaterialsToolkit/index.html. Accessed May 30, 2016.

Chang, M., & Kelly, A. (2007). Patient education: Addressing cultural diversity and health literacy issues. *Urology Nursing,* 27(5), 411–416.

Collins, J. (2007). The neuroscience of learning. *Journal of Neuroscience Nursing, 39*(5), 305–315.

Diekelmann, N. (1988). Curriculum revolution: A theoretical and philosophical mandate for change. In *National League for Nursing. Curriculum revolution: Mandate for change.* New York: National League for Nursing.

Douglass, L. M. (1988). *The effective nurse: Leader and manager* (3rd ed.). St. Louis, MO: Mosby Year Book.

Edwardson, S. (2007). Patient education in heart failure. *Heart & Lung, 36*(4), 244–252.

Falvo, D. (2004). *Effective patient education, a guide to increased compliance* (3rd ed.). Sudbury, MA: Jones & Bartlett.

Feinberg, I., Frijters, J., Johnson-Lawrence, V., Greenberg, D., Nightingale, E., & Moodie, C. (2016) Examining Associations between Health Information Seeking Behavior and Adult Education Status in the U.S.: An Analysis of the 2012 PIAAC Data. *PLoS ONE, 11*(2): e0148751. doi:10.1371/journal.pone.0148751

Fink, L. (2003). *Creating significant learning experiences.* San Francisco, CA: Jossey-Bass.

Forbes, K. E. (1995). Please, more than just the facts. *Clinical Nurse Specialist, 9,* 99.

Fulmer, T. (2007). How to try this: Fulmer SPICES. *American Journal of Nursing, 107*(10), 40–49.

Henson, R. H. (1997). Analysis of the concept of mutuality. *Image, 29,* 77–81.

Hersh, L., Salzman, B., & Snyderman, D. (2015). Health literacy in primary care practice. *American Family Physician, 92*(2), 119–124.

Herzlinger, R. (2004). *Consumer-driven health care.* San Francisco, CA: Jossey-Bass.

Holt, J., Flint, E., & Bowers, M. (2011). Got the picture? Using mobile phone technology to reinforce discharge instructions. *American Journal of Nursing, 111*(8), 47–51.

Ingram, R., & Kautz, D. (2012). Overcoming low health literacy. *Nursing2013 Critical Care, 7*(4), 22–27.

Institute of Medicine. (2004). *Health literacy: A prescription to end confusion.* Washington, DC: National Academies Press.

Joint Commission on Accreditation of Healthcare Organizations. (2006a). 2006 hospital requirements related to the provision of culturally and linguistically appropriate health care. Retrieved from www.jointcommission.org/NR/rdonlyres/A2B030A3-7BE-4981-A064-309865BBA6720/hl_standards.pdf. Accessed July 5, 2008.

Joint Commission on Accreditation of Healthcare Organizations. (2006b). Patient 101: How to find reliable health information. Retrieved from www.jointcommission.org/assets/1/18/patient_101.pdf. Accessed February 10, 2013.

Joint Commission on Accreditation of Healthcare Organizations. (2016a). *Facts about Speak-Up™.* Retrieved from https://www.jointcommission.org/facts_about_speak_up/. Accessed May 30, 2016.

Joint Commission on Accreditation of Healthcare Organizations. (2016b). *Speak Up Initiatives,* Retrieved from https://www.jointcommission.org/speakup.aspx. Accessed May 30, 2016.

Joos, S. K., & Hickam, D. H. (1990). *How health professional influence health behavior: Patient-provider interactions and health care outcomes.* San Francisco, CA: Jossey-Bass.

Kabayashi, L. C., Wordle, J., Wolf, M. S., & von Wagner, C. (2015). Cognitive function and health literacy decline in a cohort of aging English adults. *Journal of General Internal Medicine, 30*(7):958–64. doi: 10.1007/s11606–015–3206–9.

Lupien, S. J., & McEwen, B. S. (1997). The acute effects of corticosteroids on cognition: Integration of animal and human model studies. *Brain Research Reviews, 24,* 1–27.

Morris, N., Grant, S., Repp, A., MacLean, C., & Littenberg, B. (2011). Prevalence of limited health literacy and compensatory strategies used by hospitalized patients. *Nursing Research, 60*(5), 361–366. doi: 10.1097/NNR.0b013e31822c68a6.

Mulder, B., Tzeng, H., & Vecchioni, N. (2012). Preventing avoidable rehospitalizations by understanding the characteristics of "frequent fliers." *Journal of Nursing Care Quality, 27*(1), 77–82. doi: 10.1097/NCQ.0b013e318229fddc.

Rankin, S., Stallings, K., & London, F. (2005). *Patient education in health and illness* (5th ed.). Philadelphia, PA: Lippincott Williams & Wilkins.

Redman, B. K. (1993). *The process of patient education* (7th ed.). St. Louis, MO: Mosby Year Book.

Remshardt, M. (2011). The impact of patient literacy on healthcare practices. *Nursing Management, 42*(11), 25–29. doi: 101097/01/01.NUMA.0000406576.26956.53.

Roett, M., & Wessel, L. (2012). Help your patient "get" what you just said: A health literacy guide. *The Journal of Family Practice, 61*(4), 190–196.

Smeltzer, S. (2005). Is that information safe for patient care? *Nursing, 35,* 54–55.

Statistic Brain. (2015). Illiteracy statistics. Retrieved from http://www.statisticbrain.com/number-of-american-adults-who-cant-read/. Accessed May 30, 2016.

Taylor-Clarke, K., Henry-Okafor, Q., Murphy, C., Keyes, M., Rothman, R., Churchwell, A., et al. (2012). Assessment of commonly available education materials in heart failure clinics. *Journal of Cardiovascular Nursing, 27*(6), 485–494. doi: 10.1097/JCN.0b013e318220720c.

The Joint Commission. (2008). The Joint Commission hospital accreditation program 2009 chapter: National patient safety goal (prepub. version). Retrieved from www.jointcommission.org/NR/rdonlyres/3:23E-9BE8-F05BDICBOAA8/09_NPSG_HAP.pdf. Accessed July 5, 2008.

Theis, S. L., & Johnson, J. H. (1995). Strategies for teaching patients: A meta-analysis. *Clinical Nurse Specialist, 9,* 100–105.

Ward-Smith, P. (2012). Health literacy. *Urologic Nursing, 32*(3), 168–170, 167.

Watson, J. (2007). *Nursing human science and human care: A theory for nursing.* Sudbury, MA: Jones & Bartlett.

Wiener, R. C., & Winer-Pla, R. (2014). Literacy, pregnancy and potential oral health changes: The internet and readability levels. *Maternal Child Health Journal, 18*(3), 657–662. doi: 10.1007/s10995–013–1290–1

Leadership and Management in Professional Nursing

LEARNING OUTCOMES

By the end of this chapter, the learner will be able to:

1. Explain contemporary thoughts about the concepts of leadership and management.
2. Compare and contrast the concepts of leadership and management.
3. Identify the essential habits of effective leaders.
4. Outline the strengths of a feminine approach to leadership.
5. Specify the value of empowering others and oneself in professional nursing relationships.
6. Outline criteria to evaluate leadership effectiveness.

REAL-LIFE REFLECTIONS

Elena is a registered nurse (RN) who graduated from school a year ago. While attending a parent–teacher association (PTA) meeting at her son's school, Elena learns that the school does not have a full-time nurse. At the previous meeting, many parents voiced complaints related to the school's current health education and health care services. The PTA forms a task force and elects Elena to chair it because she is an RN. Uncomfortable with her new leadership position, Elena decides that she needs to read about principles of leadership and finds her nursing leadership textbook.

- *Do you think the PTA made a wise decision in selecting Elena as their leader?*
- *How would you feel if you were in Elena's position?*
- *What would be the first things you would do as the task force chair? Why?*

Distinguishing leadership and **management** is difficult because the concepts overlap and business literature often uses the terms interchangeably. **Leaders** are people who influence others. Leaders view issues globally, create visions of what might be, inspire others, tolerate chaos and ambiguity, do not fear taking risks, and work with others in a more connected way. **Managers** usually receive their title because of an appointment to a position within an organization. Managers tend to focus energy and efforts to ensure a smooth workflow and the efficient use of resources to meet the objectives of the organization. Effective managers and leaders both possess expertise in working with people, understand organizations as being authentic, and pursue their work with passion (Covey, 2004).

Formal leaders are people who hold a position of power via appointments or elections in groups, organizations, or workplaces. In contrast, **informal leaders** are not formally appointed to their position; rather, they emerge when members of a group recognize that a person has special knowledge, expertise, communication skills, or other personality traits they respect and admire (Donnelly, 2003; Videback, 2008).

Nurses influence clients and other members of the health care team as they fulfill professional roles and responsibilities. A strong knowledge base of **leadership and management skills** enables nurses to influence others (including clients) to make optimal health care decisions. As leaders of the interprofessional health care team, nurses coordinate efforts and inspire others to provide the best possible client care.

Take Note!

Because they influence clients and the health care team in performing their everyday duties, all nurses are leaders.

CONCEPTUAL AND THEORETICAL APPROACHES TO NURSING LEADERSHIP AND MANAGEMENT

Leadership is a complex term with multiple definitions but is typically defined as a process of influencing others or guiding or directing others to attain mutual goals (Agnes, 2005). Leadership can be transactional (relationships based on the exchange of effort or something valued by followers) or transformational (empowering others to create and work toward achieving anything that is possible). Transactional leaders typically use strategies that exercise power over others, whereas transformational leaders use strategies that empower others (Bass & Riggio, 2005; Burns, 2003).

Perceptions of Power and Empowerment

The ideas of mutuality, empowerment, and transformation as key elements of leadership surfaced in the late 1970s (Burns, 1978). These ideas comprise a

feminine approach to leadership because they emphasize "power with" rather than "power over," which is the more masculine approach toward the world (Noddings, 1984). Table 17.1 presents some current leadership theories classified according to gender approaches the use of power, focus on tasks and emphasis on relationships. Leaders choose how they use power based on their philosophical beliefs while considering specific situations.

Mutuality, empowerment, and transformation serve as hallmarks of contemporary leadership. In health care, the interprofessional team and unlicensed assistive personnel (UAP) work collectively toward attaining optimal client outcomes. Professional nurses assume leadership roles when coordinating care and making recommendations to interprofessional team members. In an ideal world, all members of the health care team assume leadership roles when needed because of their special expertise. Author and motivational speaker Covey (1996) proposed that today's leaders must combine personal values and visions to develop a strategic pathway, and align organizational resources and processes to fulfill visions and missions while empowering others. Leaders create a vision that inspires commitment and empowers people by sharing authority. Empowering leaders prefer to be transformational, thereby changing individuals, organizations, and societies.

According to Covey (1989, p. 222), the real test of interpersonal leadership is the leader's ability to permit others to validate themselves and realize that they will benefit more by working toward accomplishing goals that are shared by the leader and team members. In **transformational leadership**, there is "mutual learning, mutual influence, and mutual benefits" (Covey, 1989, p. 216). Donnelly (2003) noted that all definitions of leadership contain the following elements: "relationship, context, purpose, and accountability" (p. 40).

TABLE 17.1 Gender Approaches to Leadership and Management

Theory Name	Theory Creator(s)	Key Principles	Gender Approach to Leadership/Management
Leadership styles	White and Lippitt (1960)	The leader's style affects worker performance. Identifies three basic leadership styles. *Authoritarian:* Leader exercises great control to get the work done. *Democratic:* Leader and group work together to get things accomplished. *Laissez-faire:* Leader abstains from leading and lets subordinates lead themselves.	Masculine More feminine than masculine Feminine to empower workers, but no attention paid to relationships
Theory X	McGregor (1960)	The manager must control, direct, and motivate workers by offering rewards or threatening punishment. Workers avoid responsibility and seek security. Workers cannot be trusted.	Masculine
Theory Y	McGregor (1960)	Managers can trust workers to do the best possible job. Workers value their work, are motivated by rewards, contribute to the organization, and derive satisfaction from meeting goals. Workers can solve work-related problems with their own initiative and creativity. Managers can create an environment to increase worker commitment and self-direction.	Feminine
Managerial grid model	Blake and Morton (1964)	Identifies five basic leadership styles based on balancing concern for task and concern for people. *Impoverished:* Low concern for task and people. *Produce or Perish:* High concern for tasks with low concern for people. *Country club:* High concern for people with low concern for tasks. *Middle of the road:* Balanced, but not high concern for people or tasks. *Team:* High concern for people and tasks.	Neither Masculine nor Feminine Poor use of both masculine and feminine Feminine Balance of feminine and masculine
Be–know–do	U.S. Army (2004)	Leaders influence other people by providing them with purpose, direction, and motivation while operating to achieve the mission and improve the organization. Effective performance is the result of transforming human potential. To be a leader means to have values and attributes of a leader (loyalty, duty, respect, selfless service, honor, integrity, and personal courage). To know involves knowledge and mastery of interpersonal, conceptual, technical, and tactical skills. To do means to live out the values, use knowledge and skills to influence others to achieve the mission, and improve the organization by providing everyone with purpose, meaning, and motivation. There is a high level of trust among soldiers and officers. Officers have a duty to protect their subordinates, and subordinates have a duty to follow orders issued by officers.	Masculine
Theory Z	Ouchi (1981)	Leaders share responsibility with workers. Leaders match work with employee strengths. Work processes are designed and work problems are solved by using quality circles in which workers and managers have equal status. Decisions are made by democracy and consensus building. However, leaders consider the long-term effects to evaluate management decisions.	Feminine

(continued on page 446)

TABLE 17.1 Gender Approaches to Leadership and Management *(continued)*

Theory Name	Theory Creator(s)	Key Principles	Gender Approach to Leadership/Management
Contingency leadership	Fieldler (1967)	A leader selects a particular leadership style to best fit a given situation that includes the nature of staff–leader relationships, formal position of the leader, and the nature of the task.	Masculine or feminine depending of the style of leadership selected by the leader to fit the specific situation
Leader participation model	Vroom and Yetton (1973)	Leaders choose from autocratic, consultative, or participative styles when making decisions. The leader uses a list of questions to analyze the environmental contingencies that may affect the quality of the decision made.	Autocratic: masculine Consultative: primarily masculine Participative: primarily feminine
Transformational leadership	Burns (2003)	Identifies two types of leaders. *Transactional leaders* maintain daily operations using rewards to motivate subordinates. *Transformational leaders* inspire and empower everyone with the vision of what could be possible. The transformational leader has a high level of trust, gets others to share common values and mission, shows a committed work ethic, defines reality, keeps the dream alive, examines effects of actions, and makes adjustments as needed.	Masculine Feminine
Path–goal theory	House and Mitchell (1974)	Leaders coach, guide, and reward staff to select the best paths to meet organizational goals using one of four leadership styles. *Achievement-oriented:* Used to set challenging goals for competent followers. *Directive:* Used to set expectations and operational methods for followers. *Participative:* Used when the leader wants follower suggestions. *Supportive:* Used to build follower trust and confidence.	Masculine Masculine Feminine Masculine and feminine
Situational theory	Hershey and Blanchard (1977)	The leader selects from four leadership styles while considering the amount of direction required, specific factors about the situation, and the maturity of followers. *Telling:* High task/low relationship (leader needs to be in command in a situation with one correct response). *Selling:* High task/high relationship (leader has most of the controls but assists followers to boost confidence).	Masculine Masculine
		Participating: High relationship/low task (leader and followers share decision making). *Delegating:* Low task/low relationship (leaders assume the followers are competent and capable of assuming full responsibility for the decision or task).	Primarily feminine Feminine and Masculine
Transforming leadership	Anderson (1998)	"Transforming leadership is vision, planning, communication, and creative action that has a positive unifying effect on a group of people around a set of clear values and beliefs to accomplish a clear set of measurable goals. This transforming approach simultaneously impacts the personal development and corporate productivity of all involved" (p. 270). Transforming leadership anticipates future trends; develops new leaders; assesses, plans, and implements organization-wide leadership and self-leadership development programs; and creates a community within the organization. The leader uses communication, counseling, and consulting to create the organizational community.	Primarily feminine

Theory Name	Theory Creator(s)	Key Principles	Gender Approach to Leadership/Management
Authentic leadership	George (2003)	Leadership is not about style but rather authenticity. Five qualities of authentic leaders are "understanding their purpose, practicing solid values, leading with heart, establishing connected relationship, and demonstrating self-discipline" (p. 17). Leadership is more effective when the leader leads a balanced life with authenticity in each of life aspects.	Feminine
Servant leadership	Greenleaf (1977)	Leaders use their values to empower workers by providing them with all the needed resources and an environment that enables each one to achieve their maximum potential. The top priority for the leader is to serve others (employees, customers, and the community).	Feminine
Quantum leadership	Porter-O'Grady first presented the idea in 1997; Porter-O'Grady and Malloch (2015)	"Leadership emerges from the combined active engagement of all members in the organization" (p. 261) because the group has a deep commitment to a shared mission. Effective leaders possess technical capabilities (having knowledge of service, skills, and abilities), relational skills (connecting interpersonally with others while remaining connected to the technical aspects), and intentional aspirations (possessing goals that are based on values and skills). Typically various group members assume leadership to achieve a group or organizational mission (or goal) based on their areas of expertise and skill. Leadership is shared among group members, who use systems thinking to thrive in a complex, chaotic, and constantly changing world.	Feminine
Trait theories	Evolved in the early history of man	Leaders are born. They inherit characteristics that make them suitable as leaders.	Masculine or feminine, depending on how the leader uses power

Anderson, T. (1998). *Transforming leadership* (2nd ed.). Boston, MA: St. Lucie Press; Blake, R., & Morton, J. (1964). *The managerial grid: Key orientations for achieving production through people.* Houston, TX: Gulf Publishing; Burns, J. (2003). *Transformational leadership.* New York: Grove/Atlantic; Fieldler, F. (1967). *A theory of leadership effectiveness.* New York: McGraw-Hill; George, B. (2003). *Authentic leadership.* San Francisco, CA: Jossey-Bass; Greenleaf, R. (1977). *Servant leadership: A journey into the nature of legitimate power and greatness.* Mahwah, NJ: Paulist Press; Hershey, P., & Blanchard, K. (1977). *Management of organizational behavior: Leading human resources* (3rd ed.). Upper Saddle River, NJ: Prentice Hall; House, R., & Mitchell, T. (1974). Path–goal theory of leadership. *Journal of Contemporary Business, 3,* 81–97; McGregor, D. (1960). *The human side of enterprise.* New York: McGraw-Hill; Ouchi, W. (1981). *Theory Z: How American business can meet the Japanese challenge.* Reading, MA: Addison-Wesley-Longman; Porter-O'Grady, T., & Malloch, K. (2015). *Quantum leadership: A resource for health care innovation* (2nd ed.). Sudbury, MA: Jones & Bartlett; U.S. Army. (2004). *Be-know-do: Leadership the Army way.* San Francisco, CA: Jossey-Bass; White, R., & Lippitt, R. (1960). *Autocracy and democracy: An experimental inquiry.* New York: Harper & Row; and Vroom, V., & Yetton, P. (1973). *Leadership and decision making.* Pittsburgh, PA: University of Pittsburgh Press.

REAL-LIFE REFLECTIONS

Elena's leadership position means that she needs to spend time building and cultivating relationships to enhance teamwork and influence people who make decisions about student health services and education. If you were in Elena's position, what persons in the decision-making process would you consult? Why would the input of these persons be important? What key topics should Elena cover when talking to these key persons?

QUESTIONS FOR REFLECTION

1. Think of your current manager or a faculty member. Which of the leadership theories do you see that person using to motivate employees or students? Why do you think they use this theory?
2. List the pros and cons of masculine and feminine approaches to the use of power.
3. Identify separate clinical practice situations and whether a masculine or feminist approach to leadership would best fit each identified situation. Explain your choices.

Leadership as a Process of Empowerment

Perceptions of power and power relationships have changed markedly in recent years. In the past, physicians were viewed as all powerful and dominated health care because they held a monopoly on key medical information and refused to share it with others. Today, many people have access to state-of-the-art information about health care advances. Health care professionals and consumers have easy access to videos about health conditions and how to manage them. Online electronic databases can be readily accessed on the National Library of Medicine website. Anyone with internet access can read information available on a variety of health care professional association and academic medical websites. If knowledge is perceived as a power source, power becomes redistributed as more people gain access to it.

Porter-O'Grady and Malloch (2015) proposed that power has conflicting connotations. People can think of power in terms of either coercion and domination or influence and strength. All people have power and the right to exercise that power legitimately. Instead of centralizing power to people in administrative positions or to an elite group, Porter-O'Grady and Malloch suggested that power should be shared by all (decentralized) so that all people can use their expertise in delivering client care. By sharing knowledge and expertise with others, nurses empower clients, families, each other, health team members, and communities.

Blanchard, Carlos, and Randolph (1996) perceived **empowerment** as a releasing of the knowledge, experience, and motivation that people already possess. They identified the following three keys to empower people within organizations.

1. **Share information:** Trust people with information, and they will act responsibly.
2. **Create autonomy through boundaries:** Clearly delineate purposes, values, images, goals, roles, structure, and systems; thus everyone within an organization understands and executes his or her own role to meet the mission.
3. **Replace the traditional organizational hierarchy with self-directed teams:** Workers assume full responsibility for entire work processes and products.

> **Take Note!**
> When knowledge is perceived as a power source, power becomes redistributed as more people gain access to it.

Empowering leadership gives energy to the work of nursing and provides leaders and followers to maximize personal areas of strength. Empowered persons make decisions about the work that they pursue and feel valued by the organization and leaders. Empowerment becomes an outcome of leadership. Bennis (1989, p. 23) said that empowerment is evident in the four themes (adapted for nursing) shown in Box 17.1, Professional Building Blocks, "Empowerment Themes Related to Nursing Leadership."

Empowered nurses make each person with whom they interact feel important. Nurse leaders also value the knowledge and skills that each person brings to a health care situation. Finally, clients, nurses, and health care team members collaborate to determine a preferred vision for the future, and all work together to attain optimal client care.

LEADERSHIP DEVELOPMENT

When nurses envision themselves as leaders, they embark on the journey of **leadership development**.

17.1 Professional Building Blocks

Empowerment Themes Related to Nursing Leadership

1. **People feel significant:** All feel that they make a difference and that what they do has meaning and significance. In the nursing process, the nurse and the client are equal in significance; both have meaning, and what they do together is mutually significant.

2. **Learning and competence matter:** The nurse and the client value learning and mastery. The nurse makes it clear that there is no failure, only mistakes that provide feedback and tell us what to do next.

3. **People are part of a community:** The nurse, other health care providers, and the client are experienced as a team, a family, a unit. A person does not have to like another to feel a sense of community (striving for a common goal).

4. **Work is exciting:** The nursing process is stimulating, challenging, and fun. The nurse "pulls," rather than "pushes," a client toward a goal. This pull style of influence energizes the client to "enroll in an exciting vision of the future.... It motivates through identification, rather than through rewards and punishments" (Bennis, 1989, p. 23). The nurse articulates and embodies the ideals of health toward which both the nurse and the client strive.

Adapted from Bennis, W. (1989). *Why leaders can't lead: The unconscious conspiracy continues.* San Francisco, CA: Jossey-Bass.

Aspiring leaders need to realize that leadership does not automatically occur with position appointment, but rather must be learned and developed (Barrett, 1998; Donnelly, 2003; Dotlich, Noel, & Walker, 2004; Kouzes & Posner, 2010, 2012; Porter-O'Grady & Malloch, 2015; Van Velsor, Moxley, & Bunker, 2004). Table 17.2 outlines two different approaches for leadership development and includes examples of how a nurse might experience it. Most of the approaches begin with establishing a personal leadership mission followed by self-analysis. Once aspiring leaders envision the type of leader they want to become, they engage in a process of mastering key leadership skills that fit with the desired leadership approach.

Take Note!

Leadership must be learned and developed; it is not automatically acquired when one is appointed to a leadership position.

Leaders learn from challenging assignments, education, significant people, hardship, and other unidentified situations. McCauley and Van Velsor (2004) specified that leadership development occurs from a variety of experiences. They proposed that through leadership development programs, aspiring leaders learn self-management capabilities (increasing self-awareness, balancing conflicting demands, learning new skills and ideas, and developing a personal set of values for leadership). Along with personal capacity for development, novice leaders learn social capabilities (building and maintaining relationships, developing effective work groups, enhancing interpersonal communication skills, and learning how to develop other people). Finally, leaders develop work facilitation capacities by learning management skills, learning how to engage in strategic thought and action, increasing their ability for creative thinking, and learning how to imitate and implement change (McCauley & Van Velsor, 2004). Porter-O'Grady and Malloch (2015) concurred with this leadership development framework, but also added that leaders must learn how to take risks.

Nurses embark on a career in nursing leadership for a variety of reasons. Some nurse leaders assume leadership positions because they displayed leadership qualities throughout life. Others view an administrative position as being less physically taxing. Some find daytime hours and salaries attractive. Nurses may find themselves in a leadership position because no other nurse in the organization would assume it, whereas others enter

TABLE 17.2 Three Approaches to Leadership Development

Barrett (1998)	Leadership Passages (Dotlich et al., 2004)	Professional Nurse Experience
Becoming a facilitator by focusing on physical, emotional, mental, and spiritual balance and aligning personal mission, vision, and values with those of an organization	Joining an organization or company and learning the organizational culture	Finding a first nursing job, learning work expectations and the culture of the particular nursing department as well as the larger organization
	Moving into a leadership role that results in losing one's personal identity, losing one's status as the upcoming star, and learning how to balance tasks and people	Realizing that some enjoyable client care tasks must now be delegated to other people in order to provide efficient client care
	Moving into a leadership role that results in losing one's personal identity, losing one's status as the upcoming star, and learning how to balance tasks and people	Realizing that some enjoyable client care tasks must now be delegated to other people in order to provide efficient client care
Becoming a collaborator by developing one's emotional intelligence; learning effective interpersonal skills; building collaboration and team spirit; accessing the intuition and creativity of others; empathizing with others; and giving and receiving effective feedback	Accepting the stretch assignment resulting in the need for overcoming feeling like a victim, coping with skepticism and hostility from others, and realizing what is not known and when to seek out other trustful team members	Accepting the position of "charge nurse"
	Assuming responsibility for actions by valuing the unfamiliar, displaying resiliency despite setbacks, and accepting the paradoxical characteristics of the work	Taking responsibility when the nursing unit fails to run smoothly, realizing that more tasks need to be delegated, deciding that more knowledge and practice are needed for managing coworkers effectively, and doing what is needed to improve job performance

(continued on page 450)

TABLE 17.2   Three Approaches to Leadership Development *(continued)*

Barrett (1998)	Leadership Passages (Dotlich et al., 2004)	Professional Nurse Experience
Becoming a servant/partner or wisdom/visionary by increasing individual role awareness, understanding the role of the organization, creating a sustainable future, partnering, forming strategic alliances to attain long-lasting success, and deepening and strengthening personal and professional growth as a leader	Dealing with significant failures one has caused or is responsible for by examining decisions that resulted in the failure; sharing experience with a trusted boss, coach, or advisor; reflecting on the failure and devising different actions for future situations; and rallying the energy needed for perseverance	Sharing personal frustrations with a trusted nurse who has more experience; developing a mentoring relationship; generating alternative actions if similar situations are encountered in the future; and keeping oneself physically, emotionally, and spiritually healthy to remain in professional nursing practice
	Coping with a bad boss or competitive coworkers by developing a strategy to manage the ineffective relationship; analyzing your reaction to the boss or peer regarding what it tells you about yourself; and defining personal values	Finding effective strategies to manage an ineffective manager or jealous coworkers and engaging in a process of clarifying one's personal values and identifying own personal weaknesses
	Dealing with losing a job or not getting an expected promotion by using the following strategies: not letting a job or event define you as a person, trying to understand what occurred by contemplation, using a support network, and devising a strategy to address "what next"	Engaging in conversations with other nurses who have survived similar circumstances, recognizing that professional nursing does not need to consume one's total being, and perhaps changing to a new area of professional practice (or leaving the profession)
	Being part of an acquisition or merger	Learning new ways of working and learning a new organizational culture (this is true especially when a nonprofit health care organization becomes part of a larger for-profit network)
	Living in a different country or culture	Learning alternative ways of living and working (some nurses may go on medical missions, travel abroad, relocate to a different area, or go to a different location to further their education)
	Finding and maintaining a meaningful balance between family and work	Achieving an effective balance between one's personal and professional lives
	Letting go of ambition by realizing that you do not have to be "the best" or "first," accepting that all people cannot be the best forever, redirecting energy to other things, and redefining a personal definition of achievement	Acknowledging that "perfection" in nursing is impossible, developing a meaningful professional practice, becoming more involved in things outside nursing, and realizing that others need to be educated to fill nursing positions as you and some of your colleagues consider retirement
	Facing personal upheaval by accepting tragedy as a means for humanization by revealing personal vulnerabilities to others, being authentic, and accepting fate and carrying on	Using personal losses and challenges to connect more effectively with clients, colleagues, and other health team members
	Losing faith in the system by finding meaning in one's life and current work, sponsoring a protégé for a leadership position, finding fulfillment with a current project, achieving new skills, reconnecting with what originally led you to your area of expertise	Being a mentor to a younger professional nurse, clarifying personal values, and finding joy and meaning with current professional work

the profession with the intention of becoming a nurse administrator. In a qualitative research study, Bondas (2006) identified several paths to nursing leadership.

- The *path of ideals* was followed by nurses who had a desire to seek knowledge and education. These nurses engaged in self-reflection and dreamed about making a professional difference. Previous positive and negative experiences with nurse leaders also influenced their career decision.
- The *career path* was selected by nurses who used personal power in making the decision to assume a leadership position because they perceived themselves to have personality traits, skills, and previous experiences to offer. They also perceived themselves as being very self-directed, wanting desirable daytime hours, and needing to have a less physically demanding job.
- The *path of chance* occurred when the nurses found that a leadership position was the only available nursing job when they were seeking employment.
- The *temporary path* resulted when nurses substituted for other nurse leaders, and viewed the experience as a trial to see if a leadership position worked for them.
- The *path of choice* happened when the nurses developed a career plan to assume a nursing leadership position.

Nurses following the temporary path or path of chance often had no formal leadership education. The path of chance was a more passive approach in which the nurses felt that the choices were made by others.

Business scholars Kouzes and Posner have spent over 30 years studying people globally in leadership positions in a variety of fields, including professional nursing. Their research revealed that characteristics of admired leaders appear to be consistent regardless of age and geographic location; the top descriptors include honest, forward-looking, inspiring, competent, intelligent, broad-minded, dependable, supportive, fair-minded, and straightforward. They also identified the importance of clarity in personal values for exemplary leadership and organizational commitment.

Exemplary leaders accomplish extraordinary things by empowering others. Kouzes and Posner (2010, 2011, 2012) identified the following five practices of exemplary leadership.

1. *Modeling the way* starts with clarifying personal values and asserting shared ideals and values. Once values and ideals are affirmed, exemplary leaders role model by living out the values and ideals.
2. *Inspiring a shared vision* involves envisioning the future, imagining all possible exciting and ennobling future states, and enlisting others to refine and subscribe to the shared visions.
3. *Challenging processes* consist of looking externally for innovative ways for improvement and taking risks to try new ways.
4. *Enabling others to act* necessitates building trust among others, facilitating relationships, fostering collaboration to strengthen others to promote self-determination, and developing increased competence.
5. *Encouraging the heart* affirms the importance of recognizing the contributions of others and expressing appreciation to them for individual excellence through meaningful celebrations that foster creation of a spirit of community.

Take Note!

Exemplary leaders are credible because they display consistency between words and actions (they do what they say they will do).

QUESTIONS FOR REFLECTION

1. What steps have you taken to develop leadership in yourself or others?
2. Have you encountered any obstacles toward developing leadership? If yes, what were they and how did you handle them?
3. What areas do you need to develop to improve your leadership abilities? Why are these areas important to develop?

KEY LEADERSHIP AND MANAGEMENT SKILLS FOR NURSES

The nature of professional practice dictates that all nurses need to develop leadership skills. Nurses use many leadership and management skills when engaged in their multiple professional nursing roles (Table 17.3).

The professional nursing roles of critical thinker, caregiver, client advocate, change agent, counselor–teacher, coordinator, and colleague require use of many leadership and management skills. Nurses must believe they have personal power to execute each role effectively. Hagberg (1994) proposed that the first step in establishing personal power is to perceive oneself as being powerless. Feelings of powerlessness sometimes occur when people encounter new situations. However, as time progresses, all people (including nurses) will develop some power as they succeed in a particular arena. Box 17.2, Learning, Knowing, and Growing, "Strategies for Professional Nurses to Develop a Personal Power Base," provides ideas for accomplishing this.

TABLE 17.3 Key Leadership and Management Skills for Nurses

Leadership Skills	Management Skills	Skills for Leadership and Management
Maintain a focused and intense approach to work.	Clarify organizational goals and expectations.	Expand one's self-awareness.
Challenge others to expand thinking and actions.	Use established relationships to influence others in the organization.	Maintain composure and a high energy level when encountering multiple competing demands (stress management).
Deliver compelling messages.	Create a strong organizational culture.	Learn from experience.
Take risks.	Use all incentives available to motivate others.	Seek feedback from a variety of sources.
Set personal goals.	See that day-to-day operations are executed effectively.	Find common ground with others.
Have a deep, connected, and emotional involvement with subordinates/followers.	Set organizational goals.	Demonstrate sincere empathy toward others.
Keep a strong concern and investment with ideas.	Remain fair by keeping a low level of emotional involvement with employees.	Make self available to others.
See the gestalt of situations.	Be concerned with results.	Listen effectively.
Inspire others.	Make a strong investment in the organization.	Express appreciation for the contributions of others toward goals.
Tolerate ambiguity.	Staff inpatient and outpatient departments.	Abide consistently and constantly with ethics and principles.
Tolerate diverse perspectives.	Enhance productivity.	Establish trust with all people.
	Budget to meet operations.	Establish and agree on goals using collaboration.
	Market the organization.	Use facts or evidence to clarify expectations rather than assumptions or rumors.
	Reduce risks in the organization.	Identify rumors, clarify their truth, and dispel them if false.
	Write and deliver employee performance appraisals.	Display optimism in all situations.
	Follow organizational guidelines and procedures.	Analyze situations from multiple perspectives to identify issues and concerns.
		Network with others to identify issues and concerns that need to be addressed.
		Monitor the impact of change.
		Learn new things quickly.
		Set effective priorities.
		Generate multiple courses of action.
		Take decisive action but know when to change to a different course of action.
		Commit self to effective action plans.
		Attract others to assume leadership or management positions.
		Share power with subordinates/followers.
		Form alliances with key players in any given situation.
		Communicate precisely and consistently.
		Communicate in ways that are acceptable and clear to others.
		Manage resistance.
		Clarify roles of others and encourage them to assume a leadership role.
		Resolve conflicts.
		Motivate others to be their best.
		Manage the vast sea of information.

Leadership Skills	Management Skills	Skills for Leadership and Management
		Master computers and other high-tech equipment.
		Meet standards of professional nursing practice.
		Work to attain optimal client outcomes.
		Delegate tasks to others.
		Deconstruct 20th century barriers and structures.
		Recognize future trends that will point to a need to change to meet the needs of the future.
		Celebrate all progress toward change to meet 21st century health care demands.

Adapted from Blank, W. (2001). *The 108 skills of natural born leaders.* New York: AMACOM; Donnelly, G. (2003). How leaders work: Myths and theories. In T. Steltzer (Ed.), *Five keys to successful nursing management* (pp. 31–60). Philadelphia, PA: Lippincott; Porter-O'Grady, T., & Malloch, K. (2015). *Quantum leadership: A resource for health care innovation* (2nd ed.). Sudbury, MA: Jones & Bartlett; and McCauley, C., & Van Velsor, E. (2004). *The Center for Creative Leadership handbook of leadership development* (2nd ed.). San Francisco, CA: Jossey-Bass.

17.2 Learning, Knowing, and Growing

Strategies for Professional Nurses to Develop a Personal Power Base

- Develop and nurture a high personal energy.
- Display a powerful image to others.
- Work hard and diligently to become accepted by members of the nursing and interprofessional health team.
- Identify the powerful people within the organization, remembering that those with informal power are sometimes more influential than those with formal power.
- Study, learn, and master the language, symbols, and entire organizational culture.
- Use the organization's priorities to meet professional and personal goals.
- Increase expertise by expanding professional skills and knowledge.
- Envision broadly by looking upward and outward to expand organizational influence.
- Seek and use counsel from expert role models.
- Be flexible and open to others and change.
- Become a visible voice within the organization.
- Inform others of personal talents and professional accomplishments without bragging, and compliment others on their talents and accomplishments.
- Laugh at yourself, and do not take yourself too seriously.
- Empower others by sharing knowledge and experience while building a cohesive team.
- Support others whenever possible.

Adapted from Marquis, B., & Huston, C. (2012). *Leadership roles and management functions in nursing, theory and application* (7th ed., pp. 291–294). Philadelphia, PA: Wolters Kluwer/Lippincott Williams & Wilkins.

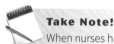

Take Note!

When nurses have personal power, the likelihood of professional power increases.

Like Kouzes and Posner (2010, 2011, 2012) and Marquis and Huston (2014), Hagberg (1994) stressed the importance of self-awareness and the value of teamwork when establishing personal power. However, Hagberg proposed that true empowerment does not occur until people no longer use power by association (hoping the power of strong people or superiors will be transferred to you) or power by symbols (displaying signs of success such as having an extravagant lifestyle, the newest gadget, or the need to impress others). True empowerment occurs when people have the freedom to be their true authentic selves (power by reflection), live out their life purposes (power by purpose), or have power by gestalt (turning to higher powers without the need for social prominence). Truly empowered people give power to others by fostering in others their ability to share special gifts and make meaningful contributions to the world (Bass & Riggio, 2005; Hagberg, 1994).

Empowerment is a key factor in the practice of nursing leadership. In order to empower others, nurse leaders and managers must feel empowered themselves. The following research brief "Factors that influence the approach to leadership: directors of nursing working in rural health services" by Bish, Kenny, and Nay (2015) identify key factors to the development of empowered nurse leaders.

Leadership in the Role of Critical Thinker

Most nurses engage in critical thinking as they perform all aspects of clinical practice. Critical thinking

FOCUS ON RESEARCH

Factors Influencing Nursing Leadership in Rural Australia

The investigators sought to identify factors that determined how rural director of nurses approached leadership in rural and regional, Victoria, in Australia. Using semi-structured audio-taped interviews the research team asked questions focused upon discovering the insights of directors of nursing into their perceptions about nursing leadership and the circumstances in which they practiced leadership. Five nursing leaders participated in the study and answered open-ended questions regarding their current position, nursing philosophy evolution, career path, leadership style, nursing, general ideas on leadership, and main issues related to nursing leadership in rural Australia. After transcribing and coding the audiotapes, the investigators sent the transcripts to the participants for review and response.

Using thematic analysis, the investigators found that empowerment was the key theme that was the most important to the nursing directors. They identified three factors contributing to empowerment (capital, influence, and contextual understanding). Under the theme of capital, they identified that information, support and resources as key contributing elements. They identified that self-knowledge and formal and informal power contributed to influence. Contextual understanding factors identified were situational factors, career trajectory and connectedness. The nursing directors all identified the desire to empower staff.

This study provides evidence of the complexity and demanding nature of nursing leadership. In addition, the study provides how important it is for nurses to have the knowledge, resources and support to be effective in their roles as well as understanding themselves and sources of power. Contextual understanding such as understanding all situational factors before making decisions, realizing the impact of their career path and connectedness to the community, profession and organization makes a key difference in how nurse leaders and managers implement their roles. Many of the contributing factors of empowerment are being presented in this chapter.

The authors address elements of trustworthiness and credibility in this study and also mention that the sample size was small and that only nursing directors practicing in rural settings in Victoria, Australia participated in the study so more research is needed to see if empowerment is the key theme for other nursing directors and if the same contributing factors apply.

Bish, M., Kenny, A., & Nay, R. (2015). Factors that influence the approach to leadership: directors of nursing working in rural health services. *Journal of Nursing Management 23*, 380–389. doi: 10.1111/jonm.12146

---

prevents nurses from blindly following physician orders and jumping to conclusions about client care situations. Nurses use critical thinking to analyze situations, identify problems, set priorities, develop multiple possible approaches to a specific situation, and consider the consequences of a strategy before taking action. Nurse leaders also use critical thinking when clarifying personal values, envisioning missions, challenging processes, and enabling others to act independently.

Leadership in the Role of Caregiver

When driven to do what is in the client's best interest, nurses use power to ensure that client care needs are met. Empowered nurses share power with others, thereby empowering clients to manage their own health. When nurses understand levels of power, they use power more effectively. Rafael (1996) described the following three levels of power as it is exercised in caring.

1. **Power in ordered caring** uses a patriarchal (male supremacy) ideology; fosters separation, strength, and control (esteemed properties of masculinity); relates to having control over others and nature; sustains organizational hierarchies; and is "vested in certain positions and legitimized as authority over nurses" (p. 8). Examples of ordered caring include physician dominance in health care settings or nurses using autocratic methods to delegate tasks to UAP (Standing & Anthony, 2008).

2. **Power in assimilated caring** is gained through "access to male power through assimilation of male characteristics, practices, and values" (Rafael, 1996, p. 12). Assimilated caring is ethically based on "maelstrom ethics," with its emphasis on application

of universal principles, such as self-determination, beneficence, and rights-based justice. As client advocates and caregivers, nurses use this power level when manipulating the health care system to help clients access needed services.

3. **Empowered caring** is distinguished by equal power and knowledge distribution among all people regardless of gender, position, social status, or education. People act with a commitment to resolve social problems as equal colleagues. All participants in health care situations participate equally in determining goal setting and become transformed in the relational way of becoming within the therapeutic relationship. Relational ethics drive decision making for each situation within its specific context. With empowered caring, nurses share their knowledge and skills freely with others while valuing the contributions all persons bring to nursing care situations. Changes arising from empowering situations tend to become, realistic, genuine, long-lasting habits.

Nurses use a range of power sources while engaging with clients and others in a variety of clinical practice settings. Expert power is used when nurses bring their specialized knowledge and skills to any practice. Nurses use power based on legitimate right and authority (position power) in daily practice situations. Nurses use referent power (based on identification with the personal qualities of the nurse) to mobilize others to facilitate desired outcomes.

The professional nurse must be an activist in the work setting and in the community while setting an example of what it means to live a healthy lifestyle and be a health advocate for all people. When assuming the activist role, the professional nurse exercises all power bases to improve the quality of and access to health care.

Leadership in the Role of Client Advocate

The concept of client advocacy has many meanings. An advocate "supports or defends someone or something and recommends or pleads in another's behalf … [and] works to change the power structure so that a situation will be improved" (Douglass, 1988, p. 259). Box 17.3, Professional Building Blocks, "What Is Advocacy?" outlines beliefs of the nurse advocate.

Nurses cannot be effective advocates unless they believe fully in their strengths. Power is shared among nurses and the people they serve. Frequently, nurses serve as resources for clients, subordinates, or colleagues. Because advocacy requires conviction, it is

17.3 Professional Building Blocks

What is Advocacy?

Nurses who believe in advocacy share the following beliefs.

1. Clients have the right to a nurse–client relationship based on mutuality, shared respect, consideration of information and feelings, and full participation when solving problems regarding their health and health care needs.

2. Nurses have the responsibility to ensure that clients have access to appropriate services to meet their health care needs.

3. Clients are responsible for their own health.

4. Nurses are responsible for mobilizing and facilitating client strengths in achieving the highest possible level of health.

important for the nurse to overcome personal feelings and beliefs about nurses' "powerless-ness" to take the first step in the process of empowerment (Richardson, 1992, p. 38).

Key Attribute: Mutuality

Evidence shows that decisions made when all involved people are actively engaged in the process have an increased chance of success. Nurses have expertise to facilitate health and healing. Clients are the experts of their bodies, minds, spirits, and life situations, and possess the knowledge of how to best control them. Decisions affecting clients must be made by the clients, with full informational support, empathy, and respect from nurses.

Mutuality means that the nurse and client collaborate to fully identify the client's health situation (strengths and weaknesses), agree on needed changes, set goals, explore alternative ways to achieve those goals, and work together to meet those goals. At this stage, the advocate verifies that technical and informational resources are available to the client. If needed, the nurse assists the client in gaining access to the needed health care services and additional resources.

Two essential elements of mutuality are respect and sharing. Respect means that the client has the right to make decisions and find meaning in them. Sharing means that the client openly communicates information, needs, and expectations while the nurse freely provides information and services in an empathetic manner. It is important to understand empathy in the advocate role because "empathy involves feelings of mutuality with another" (Olsen, 1991, p. 67). Olsen also said that "empathy can exist simply because both parties share humanity" and that "justification of another's humanity would make little sense in the way that justifications of another's actions or feelings do" (p. 70). Thus, empathized humanity is the crux of the nurse–client relationship and the advocate's role.

The most important factor in mutuality is that the nurse and the client are seen as equally able and responsible for outcomes. Their areas of expertise vary, but their authority and significance in the relationship are equal. Each person's potential can be more fully realized in a relationship characterized by mutuality.

Key Attribute: Facilitation

Facilitation in the advocacy process requires that the advocate take responsibility to ensure the client has all the necessary information to make informed decisions and to support clients in the decisions they make (Snowball, 1996). King (1984, p. 17) suggested that an effective way for the nurse to facilitate growth in self and others is through values clarification; that is, to help the client think through issues and develop a personal value system that aids decision making. Hames and Joseph (1980) suggested that facilitation is enhanced by helping clients understand the tasks before them, ensuring that they experience some success when they are trying to accomplish something, providing an environment that is conducive to learning (one of trust and respect), and offering information and emotional supports.

Key Attribute: Protection

Client advocacy has been associated with an assumption that nurses have a responsibility to protect their clients. Since the time of Florence Nightingale, nurses have been called on to protect clients from harm. Bandman and Bandman (1995) reported that nurses often are caught in ethical dilemmas when working with people who are terminally ill or hopelessly disabled, especially when physicians or family members want to force treatments on clients or withhold life-saving measures. Bandman and Bandman concluded that morality tends to support a client's right to live over letting others decide that the client's life should be terminated. In addition, there may be cases in which the nurse can legitimately protect a client's wish to end life.

Perhaps the greatest need for nurses to act as protectors occurs when nurses identify threats to client safety such as situations in which care is inadequate or environmental hazards surface. As client advocates, nurses assume leadership roles in promoting access to health care for all, preserving the rights of people to make health care decisions, keeping clients safe, monitoring care quality, and intervening in a nonadversarial manner when harmful (or potentially harmful) situations arise. The nurse may have to take risks to protect clients. When nurses defend patient rights, they act as client advocates even if they must engage in an adversarial struggle against the forces of institutional oppression, including those arising from cost containment or discrimination.

Challenges and Rewards of the Client Advocate Role

For nurses to effectively carry out the role of client advocate, the health care delivery system must be restructured, especially in terms of professional nurse positions within health care organizations. In many health care delivery systems, nurse advocacy efforts are hampered by the lack of nurse equality with administrators or physicians. A recent trend toward interprofessional education of health care team members has resulted in improved collaboration, equality, and responsibility in practice settings. Each discipline assumes full responsibility and accountability for its own practice.

Until health care organizations eliminate hierarchical approaches to authority, nurses advocating for clients will continue to start from a position of disadvantage. Thus, nurses attempting to operate as client advocates in a hierarchical system need to learn how to negotiate such situations and develop strategies that promote the significance of advocacy work. If nurses believe that equal authority to fulfill the advocate's role is important, then they must demonstrate the effectiveness of the advocacy work (such as improved client outcomes, improved service, and affordable cost). Because many nurses entered the profession because they possess compassion, they become satisfied with their careers when they effectively execute the role of client advocate.

Emphasis should be placed on the knowledge and skills needed to assist clients to increase competence in assuming responsibility for their health. In such a restructured system, nurses and other health team members need to be supported as they engage in practical applications to promote client self-care (see Box 17.4, Professional Building Blocks, "Six Ways to Promote Self-care in Clients").

The challenge to professional nursing is to restructure the work to facilitate the role of client advocate (see Box 17.5, Professional Building Blocks, "Duties of Nurses Serving as Client Advocates"). By gaining acceptance of, demonstrating the effectiveness of, and

17.4 Professional Building Blocks

Six Ways to Promote Self-Care in Clients

1. Develop an understanding of clients' responses to various threats to health as well as strategies to respond effectively to these responses.

2. Refine and further develop health promotion and illness prevention abilities, as well as restorative abilities.

3. Re-evaluate belief systems about the independent versus dependent role of clients and self.

4. Assume collaborative responsibility for monitoring the effectiveness of the delivery system, as well as independent responsibility for evaluating the effectiveness of the nursing interventions in responding to the client's health needs.

5. Implement interdisciplinary dialogue, with all professional workers sharing equal responsibility and authority for meeting clients' health needs.

6. Provide an opportunity for all members of the team to evaluate effectiveness in collaboration, thereby avoiding the establishment of adversarial relationships.

placing emphasis on key behaviors and duties of professional nurses, the role of client advocate for professional nurses becomes legitimate and solidified.

To restructure their working conditions, nurses must be advocates for professional colleagues and for themselves. Chapter 7 ("Professional Nursing Processes") and Chapter 10 ("Developing and Using Nursing Knowledge Through Research") suggest that an effective method for gaining control over practice is to develop and use evidence as a basis for recommending changes. Evidence, rather than opinion, strengthens the need for change. Advocacy for anyone is more effective if the advocate is working from a position of strength, is armed with solid evidence, and holds the steadfast belief that what one proposes will improve the safety and quality of client care.

Leadership in the Role of Counselor–Teacher

Professional nurses provide emotional support and education to clients (see Chapter 4, "Establishing Helping and Healing Relationships," and Chapter 16, "The Professional Nurse's Role in Teaching and Learning"). Nurse leaders also teach and counsel colleagues.

17.5 Professional Building Blocks

Duties of Nurses Serving as Client Advocates

1. Interact with the client in a manner and quantity that permits the following.
   - Exploration of the client's personal responses to health or threats to health.
   - Evaluation of the environmental circumstances in which the client exists.
   - Identification of client strengths and limitations.
   - Identification of resources perceived to be needed.
   - Clear allocation of responsibilities of client and nurse, which ensures the client's assumption of responsibility for health and the nurse's assumption of responsibility for the informational and interactional supports needed.

2. Prepare for and implement teaching programs needed by the client.

3. Update technical skills as new therapeutic techniques and equipment become available.

4. Discuss beliefs about the client's abilities with professional peers in an effort to evaluate own values about independence and dependence in various states of health.

5. Update nursing care plans in an effort to evaluate outcomes of nursing care.

6. Participate in nursing research as a consumer and assist in nursing studies conducted in the health care setting.

7. Identify all units of the delivery system that need to be involved in the client's care.

8. Coordinate efforts of the multiple health care workers involved in the client's care.

9. Assess the adequacy of efforts of all workers involved in care, according to the client's stated needs.

10. Resolve conflicts that might occur in relation to advocacy efforts for the client by the following.
    - Respecting the position of all involved.
    - Gathering data that describe the whole system of client–environment.
    - Promoting expression of conflicts.
    - Participating in the problem-solving process.
    - Allowing the client to make decisions based on data, rather than on advice from others.

11. Recognize and show appreciation for the contributions of team members to the client's health care.

12. Periodically discuss and evaluate the quality of the interactions among health care team members and evaluate own interpersonal effectiveness with the client and team members.

Most nurse practice acts contain a clause that states that RNs teach others in any nursing care activities. Most institutions set basic standards for educating UAP in collaboration with nurses. As direct supervisors, professional nurses assess the educational needs of staff and design educational programs. When nurses keep the client and family at the center of health care, they serve as role models for all health team members regarding the provision of patient- and family-centered care. Nurses teach UAP daily when different approaches are required to meet individual client care needs and preferences. Many times, nurses teach other professional team members about new work processes (e.g., electronic documentation changes), potential client safety issues (e.g., reminding physicians to comply with hand hygiene or posted isolation procedures), and specific client home care needs (e.g., imparting information from client stories about home life).

Professional nurses frequently find other members of the health care team experiencing distress. Nurses who spend time listening to the concerns of team members can offer support and guidance. Through this informal counsel, nurses may refer coworkers to community health resources as indicated (see Concepts in Practice, "The Colleague–Counselor Role in Action"). When nurses counsel team members and each other, they acknowledge the humanness of all colleagues, care enough to listen to personal stories and issues, provide needed emotional support, and display an ability to lead from the heart. Helping colleagues through difficult times and issues builds trust and fosters the development of meaningful team relationships.

Concepts in Practice IDEA → PLAN → ACTION

The Colleague–Counselor Role in Action

The following scenario demonstrates how a nurse leader might teach and counsel a colleague.

Luisa, an RN, finds Sara, a UAP, crying in the nurse's lounge instead of performing her delegated tasks. Luisa takes time to listen as Sara shares that she discovered a breast lump during her morning shower and just knows that it must be cancer. Luisa shares her knowledge about various breast tumors and available treatment centers, and helps Sara make an appointment for diagnosis. Later that week, Luisa accompanies Sara to a breast care center, where a needle biopsy is performed and the tumor is found to be benign.

Leadership in the Role of Coordinator

Nurses often find themselves in the role of coordinator. Nurses assume responsibility for delivering basic client care, carrying out physician orders, and promoting optimal client outcomes. When competing demands are placed on the nurse's time, he or she must frequently prioritize activities.

The role of coordinator becomes more apparent when professional nurses assume administrative positions. Managers assume responsibility for using people, supplies, money, and systems effectively to provide high-quality, cost-effective care. They coordinate the efforts of others so that the job is performed efficiently. To meet the challenges of management, nurse managers use a variety of skills, including interpersonal ("people") skills, budgeting and finance skills, information technology skills (see Chapter 14, "Informatics and Technology in Nursing Practice"), and quality management skills (see Chapter 18, "Quality Improvement: Enhancing Patient Safety and Health Care Quality").

Interpersonal Skills for Nursing Management and Supervision

Effective managers strive to bring out the best in their employees while providing them with required resources and support to provide effective client care. Nurse managers need to set and effectively communicate expectations for their departments. Nurse managers must also interact with administrators, other department managers, physicians, and other interprofessional team members. Strategies for developing helpful and healing relationships (outlined in Chapter 4, "Establishing Helping and Healing Relationships") serve as the basis for developing effective communication with staff and all members of the interdisciplinary health care team.

Empowering Team Members: Decisions by Consensus

Decisions related to problems or changes in practice tend to work better when made by consensus rather than by an individual. A major tenet of transformational leadership is to inspire and empower others to achieve the best possible future state (Burns, 1978, 2003). In any given clinical situation, everyone involved has a unique perspective and a specific skill set that must be used to facilitate optimal outcomes. Sharing power and responsibility for outcomes is facilitated when all stakeholders (those affected by the decision) participate in the process.

Consensus provides an avenue for participatory decision making because it relies on all parties sharing key information, generating alternatives, listening with respect to the views of others, and taking time to explore all options and their consequences. In most situations, generating several options for action may be more effective than generating an exhaustive list. Singular solutions are rare in human health concerns or in work situations. Although reaching consensus takes more time than other decision-making processes, the people making the decision will have a commitment to execute it (Burns, 1978; McCauley & Van Velsor, 2004; Porter-O'Grady & Malloch, 2015).

Connectedness underlies the process of consensus. When a team works together toward a common goal (e.g., optimal client outcomes), team cohesion is enhanced when decisions are made by consensus. Consensus means that everyone will try to implement the decision even though each person may not agree fully with it. All people participating in the process feel that they played a significant role in decision making, especially if participants engaged in meaningful dialogue (Wesorick & Shiparski, 1997). See Concepts in Practice, "Nursing in Action: Making Decisions by Consensus" for an example of consensus decision making.

Concepts in Practice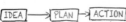

Nursing in Action: Making Decisions by Consensus

The following scenario demonstrates how nurses can work together to attain a common goal that benefits all parties.

Because of low client census on a hospital unit, nurses have been sent home on a rotating basis as a cost-saving measure. Nurses who have accrued vacation time may use it. The policy states that each nurse must take a turn being sent home. A group of older nurses with more seniority (and more vacation time) collaborate with younger nurses who have recently been hired. The nurses reach a consensus that those with more vacation time will go home twice for every one time that a new nurse is sent home. With their revised plan fully designed, all the nurses meet with the nurse manager, who agrees to its implementation. In the process of working together, these nurses developed more meaningful working relationships and feel more connected to each other.

All people in consensus share equal accountability and responsibility for the quality of the decisions made. However, when hierarchical relationships are established in the health care setting, health care providers

TABLE 17.4 Transformational Leadership and Constructed Knower Attributes	
Transformational Leader Attributes	**Constructed Knower Attributes**
Relationships engaged	Relationships networked
Individual consideration	Caring
Leader as moral agent: values and needs	Moral responsibility
Mutual dependence/trust	Reciprocity and cooperation
Communication	Integration of voices
Builder of self-esteem	Positive self-esteem
Listens to intuition, balances with analysis	Use of intuition and logic
Empowerment	Empowerment

Adapted from Barker, A. M., & Young, C. E. (1994). Transformational leadership: The feminist connection in postmodern organizations. *Holistic Nursing Practice, 9,* 20. Used with permission of the publisher.

(including some nurses) tend to use command styles rather than participatory styles when coordinating efforts of the health team (Porter-O'Grady & Malloch, 2015; Standing & Anthony, 2008) or attempting to influence client decision making (Taylor, Pickens, & Geden, 1989). Participatory decision making is a hallmark of transformational leadership (Burns, 2003; Porter-O'Grady & Malloch, 2015).

Common themes and meaning between the characteristics of transformational leaders and the attributes of women who are constructed knowers are described in Table 17.4. Barker and Young (1994) indicated that constructed knowers participate in a network or web that includes caring, moral responsibility, positive self-esteem, and use of intuition and logic. Transformational leaders seek to establish an environment that generates empowerment in self and/or others (Barker & Young, 1994, p. 20). As a change agent, the professional nurse collaborates with clients and team members to identify when and what changes are needed for better health and positive work environments.

Team-Building Skills

Positive work environments are enhanced when all workers display commitment to the work and work together as a cohesive team (Porter-O'Grady & Malloch, 2015; Wesorick & Shiparski, 1997). Effective teamwork enables all team members to use their skills. Effective teams have members who collaborate to set visions and goals while identifying how they will work together to attain them.

Effective teamwork balances unity with diversity. If a group is too unified, new ideas and divergent thinking may become stifled, resulting in groupthink. Groupthink occurs when group members' drive for unanimity supersedes their motivation to consider alternative actions. Antecedents to groupthink include decision-maker cohesiveness, group insulation, leadership responsibilities assigned to a select few members, deeply shared norms, homogeneity of members, high levels of external stress, low member self-esteem, reduced acceptance for individualism, and time constraints. Symptoms of groupthink are closed-mindedness, overestimation of group abilities, and peer pressure toward uniformity. Groupthink results in defective decision-making stemming from incomplete information (failure to consider things external to the group) and poor outcomes (Shirey, 2012).

Divergent opinions allow the team to remain open to alternative processes and new possibilities (McCauley & Van Velsor, 2004). When teams express openness to new ideas, they are better equipped to adapt to the continual change that is so prevalent in today's health care organizations (Kouzes & Posner, 2012). If a group has too much diversity, however, conflicts may impede progress toward attaining mutually agreed goals.

Strategic Planning

A **strategic plan** provides a long-term roadmap for ensuring the future and sustainability of an organization. Organizations must continually adapt to keep pace with the ever-changing world. Strategic plan development requires a detailed analysis of internal and external factors affecting offered services. Strategic plan time frames typically range from 3 to 10 years (Calhoun, 2006; Marquis & Huston, 2014).

The strategic planning process typically begins with a thorough analysis of the current situation followed by identification of an ideal future state. Organizational vision, mission, and philosophy are reviewed and revised as needed. Next, the organization identifies goals to fulfill its vision and mission. To ensure organizational sustainability, strategic planning should include goals for the organization's environmental impact (carbon footprint and pollution from health care services waste), sociocultural relevance (how well services meet the demographics and cultural idiosyncrasies of the targeted service areas), financial stability (feasibility of acquiring monetary and other requisite resources), political commitment (internal governance and external legal and governmental issues), and organizational development capacity (new operational systems, current and new facilities, human resources plan,

assessment of current and new technology, creation of a strong organizational culture, continuous quality improvement and safety programs, and effective management of knowledge and information) (Ramirez, Oetjen, & Malvey, 2011). Some organizations identify current strengths (S), weaknesses (W), opportunities (O), and threats (T) (SWOT) during the organizational analysis phase (Marquis & Huston, 2014; Porter-O'Grady & Malloch, 2015). After the strategic goals have been finalized, the organization outlines a deployment plan, which includes providing a culture, structures, and resources for plan implementation. Some organizations manage the plan using a strategic planning matrix that includes departmental goals (broadly written statement depicting a desired state), objectives (things to complete within a specific time frame), measurements or benchmarks (targeted dates and data collection to verify objective attainment), target date (deadline), and people responsible for achievement of each goal (Calhoun, 2006). Table 17.5 outlines considerations for strategic plan development and deployment.

Strategic plans work best when organizations hold individuals accountable for successful implementation. To track progress toward meeting objectives outlined in a strategic plan, a means to evaluate progress must be devised. Some organizations opt for the use of balanced scorecards to ensure that strategic objectives are accomplished by all departments. Balanced scorecards collect and analyze data regarding four aspects of organizational performance: (1) financial, (2) customers, (3) processes, and (4) learning and growth. Balanced scorecards may be completed at the organizational, departmental, and individual employee levels. Balanced scorecards typically contain the measurement methods and action steps outlined by the strategic plan. When the annual action steps do not happen as outlined by the strategic plan, a detailed analysis takes place to determine why. If results indicate that step failure was a result of unpredictable events (such as a major economic downturn), the organization reviews and revises the strategic plan appropriately. However, if the analysis reveals that the action steps were not executed because of managerial inaction, the organization may demote or terminate the manager (Calhoun, 2006; Marquis & Huston, 2014).

Budgeting Skills

To implement a personal or organizational mission, resources must be acquired, mobilized, and used. Human and material resources are required to provide health care services. Viability of a health care

TABLE 17.5 Key Elements of a Strategic Plan

Direction Statement	Strategic Objectives	Strategic Priority Issues
Mission statement: purpose and why	Measures performance on the direction statements	Broad issues that should be addressed to meet a desired future state
Vision statement: desired future state	Measures success in meeting intentions	Internal changes to continue to hold a competitive advantage over competitors
Business definition: clear and concise presentation of products, offered services, target consumers, technology, distribution of products and services, and geographic area served	Frequently addresses performance on profitability, shareholder value (if a for-profit), market position, services, quality, and innovations	Target areas in which to develop measurable action plans
Competitive advantage: what makes you better than other organizations offering the same or similar services		
Core competencies: key systems, assets, intellectual prowess, programs, and special skills to enhance the competitive advantage		
Values/beliefs: philosophy and values that guide organizational behavior and processes		

Adapted from Fogg, C. D. (1999). *Implementing your strategic plan.* New York: AMACOM; Marquis, B., & Huston, C. (2012). *Leadership roles and management functions in nursing: Theory and application* (7th ed.). Philadelphia, PA: Wolters Kluwer/Lippincott Williams & Wilkins.

organization (from a large medical center to the smallest office or clinic) relies on effective use of human and material resources.

Budgeting serves as a process to plan for attaining the required material and human resources to accomplish an organizational (or personal) mission. Budgets outline the costs of organizational operations. For example, acquiring the resources needed to go to school requires planning, determining the amount of money needed to finance educational costs, and developing a plan to verify that all personal responsibilities can be met. Likewise, an organization must be certain that it has the capital, equipment, and people to meet its mission effectively. The planning phase of the budgeting process is not an exact science, but rather is a process in which nurse managers look at the current direction of health care, anticipate what future services may be needed, and make decisions based on sound business principles and education. For example, the staffing budget projects the amount of money and the number of nursing personnel needed to provide safe, effective client care.

Nurse managers use critical thinking skills when developing departmental budgets. Budgets are typically determined for a 12-month time frame and include costs for staff (staff salaries and fringe benefits), client care (supplies and equipment), and environmental maintenance. Some nurse managers also submit budgets for capital expenditures along with expected revenue (Marquette, Dunham-Taylor, & Pinczuk, 2006; Marquis & Huston, 2014). Capital expenditures include material resources that are expensive and have a projected lifespan (e.g., cardiac monitors, computers). In contrast, the supply budget consists of inexpensive or disposable items that are used for a short time (e.g., syringes, dressings, office supplies).

Once the budget is approved by a governing body (e.g., board of directors), nurse managers compare actual spending with the projected amounts outlined in budget reports. Periodic review of reports enables nurse managers to monitor resource utilization and control excessive spending. Nurse managers must account for budgeting variances. Simply, a budget variance occurs when there is a difference between estimated and actual costs, revenue, or activity. For example, if more money was spent on nurses' salaries than projected on a cardiac unit, the nurse manager must discover why this occurred and then justify the reason for the variance. Sometimes reasons may be beyond the manager's control (Marquette et al., 2006; Marquis & Huston, 2014). In the above example, a nurse manager discovered that unit census was above projections due to increased numbers of invasive cardiac procedures resulting from the addition of a new staff cardiologist. If the overtime was the result of ineffective delegation of tasks to UAP, then the manager must submit an action plan to remedy the situation.

Staffing

Ensuring that enough nurses are available to deliver client care seems to be one of the most challenging tasks for nurse managers. The **staffing** process involves proving to the finance department how many people are needed to provide quality nursing care and then finding qualified people to those fill positions. Many staffing plans use the full-time equivalent (FTE) model to develop staffing plans. An FTE is defined as a person who would work 2,080 hours annually if no vacations, holidays, or sick days were taken. The following formula is used to calculate the number of FTEs to staff a nursing department in a hospital.

$$\frac{\text{Number of hours worked per shift}}{40 \text{ hours}} \times \text{Number of shifts worked per week}$$

When nurses work less than 40 hours per week, the nurse manager must hire additional nurses to fill the gap in settings that provide services 24 hours a day, 7 days a week. Along with productive employee hours (hours actually spent working), managers must budget for nonproductive hours such as paid time off (e.g., vacation, sick leave), jury duty, holidays, education time, and other benefits (Marquette et al., 2006; Marquis & Huston, 2014).

To determine daily staffing requirements, the nurse manager must consider client census, client acuity, and the number of nursing care hours needed for each client. To accomplish staffing projections, nurses calculate the nursing hours per patient day. The number of nursing hours per patient day varies across nursing units, with intensive care nursing units having more required hours of nursing care than short-stay surgical units. To determine daily staffing needs, the unit manager multiplies the average daily census times the nursing hours per patient day. With daily census fluctuations, some nurse managers prefer to use a staffing matrix, which is a staffing plan based on the number of clients needing nursing care. The matrix also presents a ratio of RNs, licensed practical/vocational nurses, UAP, and unit secretaries/clerks for each shift (Marquette et al., 2006; Marquis & Huston, 2014).

Eighty percent of workload on a nursing unit can be predicted (Porter-O'Grady & Malloch, 2015). Prudent nurse managers realize that in health care settings, staff workloads and the timing of essential nursing tasks cannot be predicted accurately. Therefore, they build overtime expenses into the staffing budget. For example in acute-care nursing, the following situations might result in unplanned overtime: (1) a client may have a medical emergency as nurses are changing shifts, (2) a nursing unit could receive unexpected multiple admissions within a short time, (3) a family emergency may require a staff member to leave work, or (4) a staff member may experience exposure to a health hazard or sustain a work-related injury.

When staff nurses have input into staffing plans, they are more apt to understand the process, feel capable of making decisions about unit staffing, and have increased job satisfaction. Dent (2015) suggests that the following dimensions should be considered when formulating staffing plans for nursing unit: using evidence-based staffing guidelines determined by the National Nursing Database of Quality Indicators, include planning for staff turnover (increasing staffing during the orientation of newly hired nurses), using acuity-based patient classification systems for making staff assignments, accommodating for travel nurse use, and considering nurse fatigue management. Nurses should not be permitted to work more than 12.5 hours in a given day, 36 hours in any 3-day period and 602 hours within a 7-day time frame because working more produces fatigue and increases the chance or care errors (Dent).

Marketing Skills

When nurse leaders engage in promotional activities to bring someone to something, they are using **marketing** skills. Many nurses find themselves marketing the facility (engaging in promotional activities to bring clients or employees to a facility in which they work) and/or marketing the nursing profession. Marketing goals might include increasing volume, maximizing client and staff satisfaction, and improving quality of life for the community. The steps of the marketing process mirror the steps of nursing process, starting with assessing the current situation. Considerations for a marketing assessment include listing services offered and assessing the community served by the facility. The next step is selecting strategies to inform potential clients about the organization and its services. Sometimes, health care organizations have marketing budgets that nurses can use. Marketing strategies used in nursing are outlined in Table 17.6. Of all the strategies outlined, personal recommendation tends to be the most effective (Hunt, 2003).

Leadership in the Role of Change Agent

One constant throughout the world is **change**. When people are actively involved in designing and implementing change, the change is usually sustained. Henriksen, Keyes, Steens, and Clancy (2006) defined transformational change as the process of reinventing

TABLE 17.6 Marketing Strategies for Nurses

Strategy	Description	Expense
Personal recommendation	Word-of-mouth compliment	None
Newspaper advertisement	Print ad	Rates depend on circulation of the newspaper
Radio or television advertisement	Broadcast message	Free for a public service announcement; charge rates vary
Printed materials	Brochures, fact sheets, catalogs	Printing costs Free distribution if volunteer time Mailing costs Fee for distribution racks housed in hotels, restaurants, or businesses
Community outreach	Speaking engagements, health screenings at health fairs, or contacting agencies where potential customers may be	Free if services volunteered Work release time for employees Cost for health screening supplies, props, and printed materials
Introductory offers	Health promotion classes on a trial basis Reduced cost for a new service	Costs of running program and delivering services
Traditional sales call	Sell health-related services to other companies	Salesperson salary, supplies, and fringe benefits

Adapted from Hunt, P. (2003). Marketing your facility. In T. Stelzer (Ed.), *Five keys to successful nursing management* (pp. 276–286). Philadelphia, PA: Lippincott Williams & Wilkins.

an organization or a single work unit to improve performance, thereby enabling it to respond more effectively to external environmental changes and forces. As health care organizations look for ways to continually improve the quality and safety of health care, they seek ways to streamline work processes and use resources more efficiently. Some people find moving from a current, comfortable state (or process) distressing, whereas others find it exciting. The professional nurse confronts change on a daily basis. As change agents, nurses steer change while helping themselves and others cope with it.

Organizational change requires resources and energy (Perlman & Takacs, 1990). Change has an emotional meaning for people and often is associated with feelings of loss or pain (Davis, 1991). Based on the Kübler-Ross model of death and dying, Perlman and Takacs (1990) proposed a 10-stage model to explain the psychological issues associated with change, the signs and symptoms of each stage, and nursing interventions to help others grow during the change process (Table 17.7).

In another model, Carnall (1990, pp. 141–146) proposed the following five stages in coping with change.

- **Stage 1:** Denial of the validity of new ideas
- **Stage 2:** Defense (experiencing depression and frustration)
- **Stage 3:** Discarding (acknowledging change as inevitable or necessary)
- **Stage 4:** Adaptation (feeling anger)
- **Stage 5:** Internalization

Bridges (2003) approached change from the perspective of psychological adaptation. Unlike other approaches to change, he proposed that transitions start with endings and end with beginnings. He acknowledged that during any change, people enter a period of uncertainty (the neutral zone) when they fail to understand fully the meaning of and their role in implementing the change.

Table 17.8 compares the Perlman and Takacs model, Carnall model, and Bridges model of change. The models address various psychological responses experienced by people when confronted with change. Before change can be internalized, people tend to progress through various stages of acceptance. Pritchett and Pound (1995) suggested pitfalls that frequently arise when coping with organizational change (see Box 17.6, Learning, Knowing, and Growing, "Common Mistakes When Coping With Organizational Change").

Team Roles in the Change Process

Roles of the Professional Nurse Change Agent

Based on a comparative analysis of the literature, Wooten and White (1989) identified five basic change roles: (1) educator/trainer, (2) model, (3) researcher/theoretician, (4) technical expert, and (5) resource linker. The **change agent** (the person who brings about a change) must model appropriate behaviors in an atmosphere of trust and openness, accept responsibility for getting data in an appropriate manner, provide skills and

TABLE 17.7	Growing with Change: The Emotional Voyage of the Change Process	
Stage	**Characteristics/Symptoms**	**Interventions for Successful Change**
1. Equilibrium	High energy level, state of emotional and intellectual balance, sense of inner peace with personal and professional goals in sync.	Make employees aware of changes in the environment that will impact the status quo.
2. Denial	Energy is drained by the defense mechanism of rationalizing a denial of the reality of the change. Employees experience negative changes in physical health, emotional balance, logical thinking patterns, and normal behavior patterns.	Employ active listening skills (e.g., being empathic, nonjudgmental, using reflective listening techniques). Nurturing behavior, avoiding isolation, and offering stress management workshops also will help.
3. Anger	Energy is used to ward off and actively resist the change by blaming others. Frustration, anger, rage, envy, and resentment become visible.	Recognize the symptoms; legitimize employees' feelings and verbal expressions of anger, rage, envy, and resentment. Active listening, assertiveness, and problem-solving skills are needed by managers. Employees need to probe within for the source of their anger.
4. Bargaining	Energy is used in an attempt to eliminate the change. Talk is about "if only." Others try to solve the problem. "Bargains" are unrealistic and designed to compromise the change out of existence.	Search for real needs/problems and bring them into the open. Explore ways to achieve desired changes through conflict management skills and win–win negotiation skills.
5. Chaos	Diffused energy, feeling of powerlessness, insecurity, sense of disorientation, loss of identity and direction, no sense of grounding or meaning, breakdown of value system and belief, defense mechanisms begin to lose usefulness and meaning.	Quiet time for reflection, listening skills, inner search for both employee and organization identity and meaning, approval for being in state of flux.
6. Depression	No energy left to produce results. Former defense mechanisms no longer operable. Self-pity, remembering past, expressions of sorrow, feeling nothingness, and emptiness.	Provide necessary information in a timely fashion. Allow sorrow and pain to be expressed openly. Exhibit long-term patience, take one step at a time as employees learn to let go.
7. Resignation	Energy expended in passively accepting change; lack of enthusiasm.	Expect employees to be accountable for reactions to behavior. Allow them to move at their own pace.
8. Openness	Availability to renewed energy, willingness to expend energy on what has been assigned to individual.	Patiently explain again, in detail, the desired change.
9. Readiness	Willingness to expend energy in exploring new events, reunification of intellect and emotions begins.	Assume a direct management style: assign tasks, monitor tasks and results so as to provide direction and guidelines.
10. Re-emergence	Re-channeled energy produces feelings of empowerment, and employees become more proactive. Growth and commitment are reborn. Employee initiates projects and ideas. Career questions are answered.	Mutual answering of questions; redefinition of career, mission, and culture; mutual understanding of role and identity; employee's action based on own decisions.

Adapted from Perlman, D., & Takacs, G. J. (1990). The ten stages of change. *Nursing Management, 21,* 33–38. Used with permission of the publisher.

expertise, and link needed resources in ways that make the intervention effective. The selection and timing of particular roles depend on the specific needs of the situation.

Roles of the Client System

Effective change depends on the client system assuming various roles. Wooten and White (1989) also described four basic roles of the client system: (1) resource provider, (2) supporter/advocate, (3) information supplier, and (4) participant. The client system provides effort, time, and money resources; advocates the change; provides information involving self and others; and participates in the change process. It is crucial that the change agent and the client collaborate to promote effective change.

TABLE 17.8 Comparison of Theoretical Stages in Coping with Change

Perlman and Takacs (1990)	Carnall (1990)	Bridges (2003)
Equilibrium		*Endings*
		Disengagement
		Dis-identification
		Disenchantment
Denial	Denial	*The Neutral Zone*
		Disequilibrium
Anger	Defense	Dis-identification
Bargaining		
Chaos		
Depression		
Resignation	Discarding	
Openness	Adaptation	*New Beginnings*
		Re-engagement
Readiness		Realignment
Re-emergence	Internalization	Re-identification

Mutual Roles

Wooten and White (1989, p. 657) indicated that "mutual role enactment is at the heart of the change process." The mutual roles include (1) problem solver, (2) diagnostician, (3) learner, and (4) monitor. Instead of relegating full responsibility for the entire change process to the change agents, this model focuses on joint responsibility and action.

Problem solving involves identifying a problem, generating alternatives, and testing assumptions. Diagnosis necessitates sensitivity to issues in the relationship. Learning includes knowledge, skills, or new attitudes, and monitoring involves "remain [ing] aware

17.6 Learning, Knowing, and Growing

Common Mistakes When Coping with Organizational Change

- Assuming that the role of management is to keep you comfortable
- Expecting another or others to reduce your stress
- Aiming for a low-stress work setting
- Attempting to control uncontrollable factors
- Refusing to abandon the expendable
- Facing the future with fear
- Choosing the wrong battles to fight
- Unplugging psychologically from your job
- Avoiding acceptance of new assignments

of alternatives, ascertain [ing] the consequences of action, [and] gaug[ing] the effectiveness of the change effort and relationship at each stage of the intervention" (Wooten & White, 1989, p. 657). Each role can be adopted independently or simultaneously.

Selecting a Change Strategy

As change agents, professional nurses select specific change strategies to use in practice situations. The strategy selected depends on the type of change involved. Change strategies are classified into the following six categories: empirical–rational, normative–re-educative, power–coercive, facilitative, re-educative, and persuasive and power. The following discussion defines each major category and provides examples of how they are used in professional nursing practice.

Empirical–Rational Strategies

The empirical–rational category assumes that people will act in a way that is rational and in their own self-interest. These strategies focus on educating a person about the available options and assuming that the individual will change behavior because he or she knows that the new behavior will be beneficial and desirable.

For example, in-service education may include a demonstration of the latest techniques available for a particular task, with the expectation that nurses will apply that knowledge to improve their care of clients. Another example is nurses who do not take breaks during work hours and have an increased chance of making an error in client care. Nurses who attend a staff in-service on the need to take breaks during their shifts may incorporate this idea into practice. However, if the nurses have the deep personal value that clients come first, they may not take breaks. Thus, sometimes the empirical–rational strategy may be ineffective in establishing and maintaining a desired change, especially if the change encompasses shifting personal values and beliefs (Cummings & McLennan, 2005).

Normative–Re-Educative Strategies

The normative–re-educative category assumes that sociocultural norms are fundamental to a person's behavior. In addition to rationality and intelligence, change must involve modification of attitudes, values, skills, and significant relationships. Thus, when working with clients and colleagues, the change process must be based on mutuality and collaboration. This allows for the problem solving and personal growth believed necessary to promote effective change.

For example, a young woman who needs to have surgery for ovarian cancer refuses to have it because of her firm belief that the purpose of a woman's life is to bear children. When listening to the client, the RN discovers that the client had a childless aunt who received the undivided attention of her husband, had a lavish lifestyle, and was considered by the family to be spoiled and selfish. Once widowed, the aunt became very demanding of other family members. The client expresses fear that she will become like her childless aunt. The nurse acknowledges the fear, and the two of them engage in meaningful dialogue about the purpose of life. The young woman's attitude changes, and she consents to having the surgery.

Power–Coercive Strategies

Power–coercive strategies are based on the use of power. It is believed that despite the need for knowledge and for modification of attitudes and values, change will occur only when it is supported by power that is based on potential punishment and rewards. This rationale is the basis for much political action, and it may imply the use of legitimate channels of authority or violent, non-sanctioned methods (Chin, 1976). This strategy effects change more quickly than do other strategies, but the change that results usually is not lasting (Haffer, 1986).

For example, a professional nurse working with a particular UAP notices that every time they work together, the UAP fails to complete delegated tasks in a timely manner. Because the nurse supervises the UAP, the nurse initiates the first step of a progressive discipline process, which is documenting the conversation held with the UAP about not fulfilling job responsibilities. For a month, the UAP completes delegated tasks quickly, but returns to previous habits thereafter.

Facilitative Strategies

Facilitative strategies are used to make clients and others aware of the availability of help in sufficient detail and clarity so that they know exactly how to access and use assistance. Facilitative strategies are appropriate when there is openness to change. This type of strategy can include (1) simplifying data, providing feedback, and providing other necessary tools to help others recognize a problem; (2) providing multiple potential solutions to a problem; and (3) involving others in the decision-making process. These strategies produce greater commitment to change, but the change agent must be sure that there are sufficient resources, commitment, and capability to maintain the change after leaving the situation.

For example, a nursing research consultant is hired to help staff nurses develop and implement evidence-based practice or nursing research on hospital nursing units. The consultant meets with interested nurses every other month, helps them develop research projects, and coaches them on project implementation. When the consulting contract ends, the nurse researcher contacts doctoral-prepared nursing faculty from a local nursing program to continue helping the nurses execute and publish their research projects. The unit nurses select the faculty with whom they will work to finish their projects.

Re-Educative Strategies

Re-educative strategies are based on empirical–rational theory but are different because the person needs to acquire new skills and knowledge. They also facilitate change when resistance is prevalent, when people have inaccurate information, when the change involved is a radical departure from past practices, and when the person lacks confidence about the ability to implement the new practices. However, re-educative strategies work to bring about change only when there is a strongly felt need and a strong motivation to change.

Re-educative strategies work slowly, so they are feasible only when time is not a pressing factor. Examples of re-educative strategies include creating awareness that a problem exists by indicating how much better things could be when symptoms can be connected with causes, and outlining the benefits of new practices. Re-educative strategies work well when people receive a new diagnosis of a chronic illness, such as diabetes or renal disease that requires special self-monitoring and compliance with strict regimens for optimal outcomes. Re-educative strategies heighten awareness of a problem and possible solutions, but they fail to increase the motivation to change.

Persuasive and Power Strategies

Persuasive and power strategies involve active participation of all persons involved and consume much time. Research findings and other forms of evidence serve as useful tools when presenting a case to move from one way of doing things to another (see Chapter 10, "Developing and Using Nursing Knowledge Through Research").

Persuasive and power strategies involve active discussion and debate. Process participants each bring an idea of what should be done and how the change should be implemented. They also outline the consequences if change does not occur.

For example, persuasive and power strategies permeate the federal and state legislative process (see Chapter 19, "The Professional Nurses Role in Public Policy"). As a result of the Affordable Care Act (see Chapter 9, "Health Care Delivery Systems"), many health care organizations are preparing for reductions in federal and state reimbursement for services rendered to the elderly and poor. Hospital administrators (including nursing administrators) possess a global perspective of the implications of reduced income to provide safe, effective health services. Nurses and other care providers have undertaken the challenge to look for ways to reduce costs for patient care services. If costs cannot be contained, then many health care organizations may have to close, resulting in reduced access to care and increased unemployment of health care providers. Motivation for change is driven by aversion to potentially undesired consequences rather than the need for improved processes or relationships.

Benefits of Change Strategies

Professional nurses who understand the basic types of change strategies may select the best way to proceed when confronted with situations where change is indicated. People vary in their responses to the many change strategies. For example, sometimes the power–coercive strategy may be met with much resistance, while at other times it may be very successful.

The professional nurse also must assess the ability of individuals to cope with change and how many changes are occurring simultaneously. When one strategy fails, the nurse can try another one to bring about the desired change. At times, the professional nurse must prioritize changes for clients, health care team members, or organizations to avoid extreme psychological distress arising from too much change in too little time.

Leadership in the Role of Colleague

Whether working with individual clients, client groups, other health care team members, or an entire organization, nurses must establish collegial partnerships with others. Collegial partnerships enable equality among all people involved in an interaction. Over time, health care team members develop collegial partnerships with each other in which each person acknowledges the contributions and skills that the other members bring to client service.

A collegial partnership is a relationship in which all people view each other as providing equal contributions to a mutually defined outcome. Collaboration begins when individuals realize that they need others to attain an envisioned goal (Porter-O'Grady & Malloch, 2015; Wesorick & Shiparski, 1997; Wilson & Porter-O'Grady, 1999). Collegial partnerships may occur between nurses and clients, nurses and UAP, nurses and other nurses, nurses and physicians, nurses and other health team members, and even nurses and a community group. Partnerships may be short lived or

last for an extended time. When working in partnership with others, various partners assume leadership when an issue arises that falls within the realm of his or her expertise. The development of clinical paths or client care maps within health care organizations represents one outcome of interdisciplinary collegial partnerships.

Various barriers can undermine the development of effective collaboration among health care partners (Wilson & Porter-O'Grady, 1999).

- Old animosities, such as perceived physician superiority, sometimes prevent the nurse from trusting and relating effectively with physicians.
- Incongruence of philosophy related to the partnership may create tension. However, when these philosophical differences are acknowledged and a new common ground is found, professional partnerships may flourish.
- Competitive behavior may limit the ability to form effective collegial partnerships.
- Social status and inequality in educational levels may interfere with the development of partnerships. Information sharing is critical, and systems must be designed so all partners have access to the same information and responsible decisions and behaviors can occur.
- Partners sometimes equate collaboration with total agreement on every issue, and processes must be in place for negotiating differences between and among partners when disagreements arise.

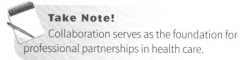

Take Note!
Collaboration serves as the foundation for professional partnerships in health care.

LEADERSHIP EFFECTIVENESS

Professional nurses serve as experts on health issues, care coordinators, client advocates, counselors, educators, and change agents. Box 17.7, Professional Building Blocks, "Forms of Influence Within the Nurse–Client Relationship," outlines different forms of nurse influence in the nurse–client relationship. These forms of influence may also apply when the nurse works with UAP. For example, nurses make legitimate requests to UAP when delegating tasks to them. At times, nurses may use coercion or rational persuasion to get them to perform the delegated tasks. With time, UAP may recognize nurses as experts, internalize some of the values of nurses they respect, relinquish control of independence to comply with nurse requests, participate actively

17.7 Professional Building Blocks

Forms of Influence within the Nurse–Client Relationship

1. **Legitimate request:** Responding to legitimate power, the client complies with the nurse's request because the client recognizes the nurse's right to make such a request. The client's compliance represents internalized values of obedience, cooperation, courtesy, respect for tradition, and loyalty to the organization.

2. **Instrumental compliance:** Responding to reward power, the client complies because the nurse has made an explicit or implicit promise to ensure some tangible outcome that the client desires.

3. **Coercion:** Responding to the threat of adverse outcomes, such as economic loss, embarrassment, or expulsion. Because the influence is motivated by fear, it is most effective when it is credible.

4. **Rational persuasion:** Responding to a logical argument, the client is convinced that the nurse's suggested behavior is the best way to satisfy needs or attain objectives.

5. **Rational faith:** Acting out of faith in the nurse's expertise and credibility. Such a response is based on expert power.

6. **Inspirational appeal:** Responding to expressions of values and ideals without any tangible reward, the client acts from obedience to authority figures, reverence for tradition, self-sacrifice, and so forth.

7. **Situational engineering:** Responding to manipulation of relevant aspects of the physical and social situation. The nurse must have control, and the client must accept the situation.

8. **Personal identification:** Responding to referent power. The client imitates the behavior of an admired nurse.

9. **Decision identification:** Responding to involvement in decision making.

in client care decisions, and begin to imitate nurses whom they admire. Likewise, some professional nurses acknowledge the valuable and unique contributions UAP make to client care (Standing & Anthony, 2008).

In transformational leadership, rational persuasion and shared decision making serve as the most valid forms of influence because they promote empowerment. Research findings and the literature suggest that transformational leadership promotes staff empowerment, increased job satisfaction for staff and managers, improved client satisfaction with care, supportive work environments, the development of mutual team

goals, and an optimal mix of nursing skill and expertise (Marquis & Huston, 2014; Porter-O'Grady & Malloch, 2015). Increased staff nurse retention saves money because recruitment and replacement costs for new professional nurse employees range from $37,000 to $58,400 (Nursing Solutions Inc., 2016). The areas of high turnover in hospitals occur in the specialty practice areas of behavior health (25.5%) and the emergency department (21.7%). Lower rates of turnover occur in critical care nursing (17.7%) women's health (14.5%) and pediatrics (11.7%). More than a quarter of newly hired nurses (28.9%) leave a position within a year (Nursing Solutions Inc. 2016). Arnold (2012) reported that $1,700 was spent on pre-employment costs for all nurses being hired (application process, job interviews, drug testing, criminal background check, and pre-employment physical) and $5,000 could be added to cover costs of a facility's mandatory week-long orientation. For new graduate nurses being employed in acute-care settings, an additional $77,145 can be spent on clinical educator, preceptor and new graduate salaries, and time spent in classroom and skill-building activities for mandatory clinical competencies over an additional 5-month orientation period (Arnold, 2012). Thus, effective development of transformational leadership competencies in nurse managers can reduce the costs for acute-care health care delivery from increased nurse retention rates.

> **Take Note!**
> The sharing of power—rather than the wielding of power—characterizes the transformational relationship of the nurse with all members of the health care team, including the client.

Transformational Leadership Competencies

Gurka (1995, p. 170) identified the following qualities of transformational leaders.

1. **Individual consideration:** Promoting others' growth, recognizing and supporting others' needs and feelings, and giving positive feedback and recognition

2. **Charisma:** Inspiring and motivating, demonstrating enthusiasm, and communicating in a positive manner

3. **Intellectual stimulation:** Creating a questioning environment, acting as a mentor, and challenging others to grow and learn

4. **Vulnerability:** Communicating authentically and openly, expressing emotions as well as ideas, and sharing the self with others

5. **Knowledge, concern, and courage:** Seeking knowledge through study and experience, showing concern and caring for others, and being willing to take risks

6. **Feminine attributes:** Maintaining accessibility, paying attention to process as well as outcomes, and practicing balance in lifestyle

Based on these and other transformational leadership concepts (Bennis & Nanus, 1985), Box 17.8, Learning, Knowing, and Growing, "Leadership Competencies," suggests way to foster your personal and professional growth. When these actions become part of the nurse's character, they are called habits. Leadership habits of the nurse also determine the nurse's effectiveness in practice.

17.8 Learning, Knowing, and Growing

Leadership Competencies

- Acknowledging and using the inner wisdom of self and others
- Setting goals and working to achieve them
- Working with others to achieve a common vision and mission
- Recognizing the interconnection of everyone on everything
- Abandoning the hierarchical approach to leadership
- Recognizing that people performing the work are specialists
- Engaging in systems thinking
- Recognizing patterns
- Synthesizing new ideas and processes
- Committing to lifelong continuous learning
- Adapting to and accepting chaos
- Facilitating each team member's involvement and accountability
- Empowering others
- Being receptive to new ideas and the ideas of others
- Facilitating group meetings and participation of everyone in organizational processes (especially decision making)
- Coaching
- Acting with immediacy and equality
- Displaying technical expertise (organizational culture and design, financial management, economics, business ethics, evaluation methods, health care jurisprudence, information technology, and strategic planning for the long term)
- Practicing knowledge of relationship dynamics
- Sharing administrative functions
- Favoring collaboration over competition
- Mentoring others for leadership

Covey's Habits of the Effective Leader

Covey (1989, p. 47) defined a habit as "the intersection of knowledge, skill, and desire that has great power in a person's life." Covey has described knowledge as the "what to do and why," skills as the "how to do," and desire as the motivation or the "want to do" (p. 47). He emphasized that without desire or motivation, essential, effective leaderships skills such as sharing knowledge confidently and listening intently to others will never become ingrained habits.

Habits of effective leaders are the internalized principles and patterns of behavior that reflect the three inter-related factors of knowledge, skills, and desire. Seven habits that Covey (1989) designated for effective leadership are based on the theoretical premise of sequential growth—moving people from dependence to independence and finally to interdependence, the phase in which true mutuality can occur.

In 2004, Covey added another habit of great leaders: The eighth habit involves hearing one's own voice and inspiring others to find theirs. Finding one's own voice means periodic analysis of values and beliefs and finding quiet time to listen to oneself. Once found, the voice must be expressed by developing a personal vision, practicing discipline, showing passion in action, and not doing anything against one's conscience. Inspiring others means being a "trim-tab" (a small rudder that turns the large rudder of a ship), modeling character and competence, instilling trust, and blending voices to develop shared vision. Once others have discovered their voices, the great leader aligns goals and systems to achieve desired results (the shared vision) while empowering others to use their talents and live out passions.

Covey identified the four roles of leadership as modeling (inspiring trust), path finding (creating order), aligning (nourishing vision and empowerment), and empowering (getting others to internally unleash their human potential). Great leaders use their influence to serve others. Box 17.9, Learning, Knowing, and Growing, "Covey's Eight Habits, Adapted for the Nurse," outlines the eight habits identified by Covey (1989, 2004) in terms of nursing leadership and enhanced personal and professional growth. Habits represent the integrated principles of the professional nurse while providing consistency in action.

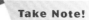

Take Note!
When leaders use effective habits, they earn the trust of their followers.

17.9 Learning, Knowing, and Growing

Covey's Eight Habits, Adapted for the Nurse

1. **Be proactive:** Nurses need to set a goal and work to achieve it. They commit themselves to the client's perceptions and serve as a model for health, not a critic of those with expressed concerns. They accept their own ability to be "response-able" in dealing with clients' whole human responses to their health concerns. They believe that "it's not what happens to us, but our response to what happens to us that hurts us" (Covey, 1989, p. 73).

2. **Begin with the end in mind:** The nurse should identify what is really important and try to do what really matters the most every day. The nurse also must differentiate management from leadership. Management, representing the bottom line, focuses on how the nurse can best accomplish certain things with the client, whereas leadership, representing the top line, focuses on what the nurse wants to accomplish. "Management is efficiency in climbing the ladder of success; leadership determines whether the ladder is leaning against the right wall" (Covey, 1989, p. 101).

3. **Put first things first:** The formula for the nurse who wants to stay focused on the important business of nursing and give less energy to the unimportant is to set priorities, organize and, finally, perform. The challenge for the nurse is to manage time in such a way that most of the time is used for urgent activities, such as crises, pressing problems, and deadline-driven projects, as well as the not urgent but important projects, such as health promotion/illness prevention, relationship building, recognizing new opportunities, planning, and recreation.

4. **Think win–win or no deal:** Interdependence is the most mature goal for any relationship; thus, in professional relationships, interdependence would emphasize mutual benefits. Activities would reflect a commitment to both parties' growth, development, and satisfaction. For example, a client benefits from being empowered by the professional nurse providing informational support, and the nurse benefits by having the interventions validated and the sense of presence with the client valued. When such mutuality is experienced, neither person in the relationship loses or feels powerless.

5. **Seek first to understand, then to be understood:** Empathy is the habit reflected in this principle. The ability to focus on the client's reality as he or she experiences it is vital to positive communication. (Empathy is discussed in detail in Chapter 18, Quality Improvement: Enhancing Patient Safety and Health Care Quality). "Credibility problems, such as the client's feeling that "you just don't understand," are prevented to the extent that the nurse empathizes with the client.

6. **Value differences and bring all perspectives together:** Respect is the characteristic that enables the nurse to develop this habit. (Respect is discussed further in Chapter 15, Informatics and Technology in Nursing Practice). To the extent that the nurse facilitates respect for differing perspectives, the client is likely to feel freer to seek the best possible alternative. If the nurse also experiences respect for his or her perspectives, synergistic relationships are enhanced. Using the principle of synergy, the nurse and client multiply their individual talents and abilities, and the outcome of their efforts is greater than the sum of the parts.

7. **Have a balanced, systematic program for self-renewal:** Consistency in having a regularly planned and balanced program for self-renewal prevents weakening of the body, mechanization of the mind, exposure of raw emotions, and desensitization of the spirit. Clearly, nurses' leadership ability is enhanced if they consistently participate in activities that renew four aspects of the self: physical, mental, emotional–social, and moral. Renewal energizes capabilities that are necessary for productive helping relationships in nursing.

8. **Find your own voice and inspire others to find theirs:** Being truly authentic toward one's personal life mission, and helping others find themselves, fosters the development of new leaders and promotes deep satisfaction with life and work. Others quickly detect lack of authenticity in a relationship, especially when nurses establish helping and healing relationships with clients and health team members.

Adapted from Covey, S. R. (1989). *The 7 habits of highly effective people.* New York: Simon & Schuster, and Covey, S. R. (2004). *The 8th habit.* New York: Free Press.

EVALUATING LEADERSHIP EFFECTIVENESS

As professionals, nurses engage in the process of self-evaluation and look for ways to improve their leadership performance. Unfortunately, not all leaders are effective. Competing demands force leaders (especially managers) to make difficult decisions, which may result in win–lose situations. Ineffective leadership takes many forms, including the person who assumes a leadership position without proper qualification, the person who bides his or her time until retirement, or the person who received a leadership appointment because of success in a previous appointment. Frequently, the personal insecurities of people in charge results in dysfunctional leadership (Fitzpatrick, 2004). Poor nursing leadership also may occur when the well-respected, competent, professional nurse is forced into accepting a leadership position. The quality of leadership suffers when the person assuming the leadership position would rather be doing something different. Nurses who know themselves as people and have a clear idea of their life passions can thwart the influences of others before assuming a leadership position that they really do not want.

McCauley and Van Velsor (2004) proposed that people who assume a leadership position should conduct periodic self-evaluations of their performance. They suggest self-reflection and eliciting information from followers to provide a complete, accurate picture of one's leadership. Box 17.10, Professional Prototypes, "Nursing Leadership Self-Evaluation Criteria," provides pertinent questions to use.

17.10 Professional Prototypes

Nursing Leadership
Self-Evaluation Criteria

1. Can I be trusted?
2. Do I use effective verbal and nonverbal communication skills?
3. Am I accessible to the persons whom I serve as a leader?
4. Am I aware of all the issues encountered by nurses engaged in client care activities?
5. Do I provide support to staff when problems arise?
6. Can I initiate, maintain, and terminate effective professional relationships?
7. Do I understand the impact of self on others, leading to effective use of self?
8. Can I effectively modify my behavior and that of others?
9. Do I effectively delegate tasks to others, or do I try to micromanage everything?
10. Do I provide the needed resources to provide quality nursing services?
11. Do I set high standards and hold others and accountable for them?
12. Am I willing to help others grow as professional nurses?

Adapted from McCauley, C., & Van Velsor, E. (2004). *The Center for Creative Leadership handbook of leadership development* (2nd ed.). San Francisco, CA: Jossey-Bass.

Summary and Significance to Practice

Effective nursing leadership is critical in today's complex, chaotic health care environment. Because all professional nurses are leaders, they need to use cognitive and communication skills to empower others to make decisions, facilitate access to needed care services, share knowledge, coordinate care delivery, plan for the future, use resources judiciously, and facilitate adaptation to change. Effective leaders in nursing display caring, compassion, commitment, confidence, and competence in their roles and periodically conduct self-evaluations to discover additional areas for lifelong learning.

REAL-LIFE REFLECTIONS

Recall Elena from earlier in the chapter. Which of the leadership theories would be most useful to Elena as she leads the group of parent volunteers to determine how to get an RN in every school? Why do you think the selected theory would work best? What are the potential outcomes for having an RN in every school for students, faculty, school administration, the local school board, and school district taxpayers? What obstacles do you think Elena and the task force might encounter in achieving the goal of a nurse in every school?

From Theory to Practice

1. How do you rate your effectiveness as a nurse leader? What are your strengths? Your weaknesses?
2. What are your opportunities for future growth as a leader? Outline an action plan to facilitate your growth as a nursing leader.

Nurse as Author

Think about the best leader/manager/teacher/coach that you have encountered in your working career or as a student. Think about the worst leader/manager/ teacher/coach that you have encountered in your working career or as a student. Write a 2- to 3-page essay comparing the traits and practices of these two persons. In one paragraph, include each person's strengths and weaknesses. In another paragraph, specify what you learned from both persons. Please do not identify either person by name. In your concluding paragraph, specify what you plan to do in a future leadership role based upon your experiences with both persons.

Your Digital Classroom

Online Exploration

American Academy of Nursing: **www.aannet.org**
American Organization of Nurse Executives:
   www.aone.org
American Nurses Association:
   www.nursingworld.org
Changing Minds—Transformational Leadership:
   http://changingminds.org/disciplines/leadership/ styles/transformational_leadership.htm
Center for Servant Leadership: **www.greenleaf.org/**
Sigma Theta Tau International:
   www.nursingsociety.org
The Center for Innovative Leadership: **www.cfil.com**

Expanding Your Understanding

1. Visit the International Council of Nurses website and access the Leadership for Change™ **http:// leadership.icn.ch/lfc/**. Read the following information about the program (Background, LFC Vision, Mission and Key Strategic Aims; Outcomes and Benefits, Planning and Methodology, LFC Activities, Evaluation, and the most recent Leadership-Bulletin) and answer the following questions.
   a. What perceptions about nurses held by others prevent nurses from assuming leadership roles?
   b. How can the nursing profession dispel the negative perceptions of others?
   c. What do you think about the vision and mission statements for the leadership for change initiative?
   d. How would you like to change health care delivery in your locale?

Beyond the Book

Visit thePoint® **www.thePoint.lww.com** for activities and information to reinforce the concepts and content covered in this chapter.

REFERENCES

Agnes, M. (Ed.). (2005). *Webster's new world college dictionary* (4th ed.). Cleveland, OH: Wiley.

Anderson, T. (1998). *Transforming leadership* (2nd ed.). Boston, MA: St. Lucie Press.

Arnold, J. (2012). Cost of hiring new nurses. Advanced Healthcare Network for Nurses Retrieved from http://nursing.advanceweb.com/Features/Articles/Cost-of-Hiring-New-Nurses.aspx. Accessed May 31, 2016.

Bandman, E. L., & Bandman, B. (1995). *Nursing ethics through the life span* (3rd ed.). East Norwalk, CT: Appleton & Lange.

Barker, A. M., & Young, C. E. (1994). Transformational leadership: The feminist connection in postmodern organizations. *Holistic Nursing Practice, 9*, 16–25.

Barrett, R. (1998). *Liberating the corporate soul: Building a visionary organization.* Boston, MA: Butterworth-Heinemann.

Bass, B., & Riggio, R. (2005). *Transformational leadership* (2nd ed.). Mahwah, NJ: Erlbaum.

Bennis, W. (1989). *Why leaders can't lead: The unconscious conspiracy continues.* San Francisco, CA: Jossey-Bass.

Bennis, W., & Nanus, B. (1985). *Leaders: The strategies for taking charge.* New York: Harper & Row.

Bish, M., Kenny, A., & Nay, R. (2015). Factors that influence the approach to leadership: directors of nursing working in rural health services. *Journal of Nursing Management, 23*, 380–389. doi: 10.1111/jonm.12146

Blake, R., & Morton, J. (1964). *The managerial grid: Key orientations for achieving production through people.* Houston, TX: Gulf Publishing.

Blanchard, K., Carlos, J. P., & Randolph, A. (1996). *Empowerment takes more than a minute.* San Francisco, CA: Berrett-Koehler.

Bondas, T. (2006). Paths to nursing leadership. *Journal of Nursing Management, 14*(5), 332–339.

Bridges, W. (2003). *Managing transitions* (2nd ed.). Cambridge, MA: Perseus.

Burns, J. (1978). *Leadership.* New York: Harper & Row.

Burns, J. (2003). *Transformational leadership.* New York: Grove/Atlantic.

Calhoun, S. K. (2006). Strategic management: Facing the future with confidence. In J. Dunham-Taylor & J. Pinczuk (Eds.), *Health care financial management for nurse managers: Merging the heart with the dollar* (pp. 607–645). Sudbury, MA: Jones & Bartlett.

Carnall, C. A. (1990). *Managing change in organizations.* Upper Saddle River, NJ: Prentice Hall.

Chin, R. (1976). The utility of systems models and developmental models for practitioners. In W. G. Bennis, K. D. Benne, & R. Chin (Eds.), *The planning of change* (3rd ed.). New York: Holt, Rinehart & Winston.

Covey, S. R. (1989). *The 7 habits of highly effective people.* New York: Simon & Schuster.

Covey, S. R. (1996). Three roles of the leader in the new paradigm. In F. Hesselbein, M. Goldsmith, & R. Beckhard (Eds.), *The leader of the future: New visions, strategies, and practices for the next era.* San Francisco, CA: Jossey-Bass.

Covey, S. R. (2004). *The 8th habit.* New York: Free Press.

Cummings, G., & McLennan, M. (2005). Advanced practice nursing: Leadership to effect policy change. *Journal of Nursing Administration, 35*(2), 61–66.

Davis, P. S. (1991). The meaning of change to individuals within a college of nurse education. *Journal of Advanced Nursing, 16*, 108–115.

Dent, B. (2015). Nine principles for improved nurse staffing. *Nursing Economic$, 35*(1), 44–44, 66.

Donnelly, G. (2003). Why leadership is important to nursing. In T. Stelzer (Ed.), *Five keys to successful nursing management*. Philadelphia, PA: Lippincott Williams & Wilkins.

Dotlich, D., Noel, J., & Walker, N. (2004). *Leadership passages*. San Francisco, CA: Jossey-Bass.

Douglass, L. M. (1988). *The effective nurse: Leader and manager* (3rd ed.). St. Louis, MO: Mosby.

Fieldler, F. (1967). *A theory of leadership effectiveness*. New York: McGraw-Hill.

Fitzpatrick, M. (2004). Facing challenges. In N. Holmes (Ed.), *Five keys to successful nursing management*. Philadelphia, PA: Lippincott Williams & Wilkins.

George, B. (2003). *Authentic leadership*. San Francisco, CA: Jossey-Bass.

Greenleaf, R. (1977). *Servant leadership: A journey into the nature of legitimate power and greatness*. Mahwah, NJ: Paulist Press.

Gurka, A. M. (1995). Transformational leadership: Qualities and strategies for the CNS. *Clinical Nurse Specialist, 9*, 169–174.

Haffer, A. (1986). Facilitating change: Choosing the appropriate strategy. *Journal of Nursing Administration, 16*, 17–22.

Hagberg, J. (1994). *Real power: Stages of personal power in organizations* (2nd ed.). Salem, WI: Sheffield.

Hames, C. C., & Joseph, D. H. (1980). *Basic concepts of helping: A holistic approach*. New York: Appleton-Century-Crofts.

Henriksen, K., Keyes, M., Steens, D., & Clancy, C. (2006). Initiating transformational change to enhance patient safety. *Journal of Patient Safety, 2*(19), 20–24.

Hershey, P., & Blanchard, K. (1977). *Management of organizational behavior: Leading human resources* (3rd ed.). Upper Saddle River, NJ: Prentice Hall.

House, R., & Mitchell, T. (1974). Path–goal theory of leadership. *Journal of Contemporary Business, 3*, 81–97.

Hunt, P. (2003). Marketing your facility. In T. Stelzer (Ed.), *Five keys to successful nursing management*. Philadelphia, PA: Lippincott Williams & Wilkins.

King, E. C. (1984). *Affective education in nursing*. Rockville, MD: Aspen Systems.

Kouzes, J., & Posner, B. (2010). *The truth about leadership, the no-fads, heart-of-the-matter facts you need to know*. San Francisco, CA: Jossey-Bass.

Kouzes, J., & Posner, B. (2011). *The five practices of exemplary leadership*. San Francisco, CA: Pfeiffer.

Kouzes J, & Posner B. (2012). *The leadership challenge* (5th ed.). San Francisco, CA: Jossey-Bass.

Marquette, R., Dunham-Taylor, J., & Pinczuk, J. (2006). Budgeting. In J. Dunham-Taylor & J. Pinczuk (Eds.), *Health care financial management for nurse managers: Merging the heart with the dollar*. Sudbury, MA: Jones & Bartlett.

Marquis, B., & Huston, C. (2014). *Leadership roles and management functions in nursing: Theory and application* (8th ed.). Philadelphia, PA: Wolters Kluwer Health.

McCauley, C., & Van Velsor, E. (2004). *The Center for Creative Leadership handbook of leadership development* (2nd ed.). San Francisco, CA: Jossey-Bass.

McGregor, D. (1960). *The human side of enterprise*. New York: McGraw-Hill.

Noddings, N. (1984). *Caring: A feminine approach to ethics and moral education*. Berkeley: University of California Press.

Nursing Solutions Inc. (2016). *2016 National healthcare retention & RN staffing report*. Retrieved from http://www.nsinursingsolutions.com/Files/assets/library/retention-institute/NationalHealthcareRNRetentionReport2016.pdf. Accessed November 3, 2016.

Olsen, D. P. (1991). Empathy as an ethical and philosophical basis for nursing. *Advances in Nursing Science, 14*, 62–75.

Ouchi, W. (1981). *Theory Z: How American business can meet the Japanese challenge*. Reading, MA: Addison-Wesley-Longman.

Perlman, D., & Takacs, G. J. (1990). The 10 stages of change. *Nursing Management, 21*, 33–38.

Porter-O'Grady, T., & Malloch, K. (2015). *Quantum leadership: Building better partnerships for sustainable health* (4th ed.). Burlington, MA: Jones & Bartlett Learning.

Pritchett, R., & Pound, R. (1995). *A survival guide to the stress of organizational change*. Dallas, TX: Pritchett & Associates.

Rafael, A. R. (1996). Power and caring: A dialectic in nursing. *Advances in Nursing Science, 19*, 3–17.

Ramirez, B., Oetjen, R., & Malvey, D. (2011). Sustainability and the health care manager. *The Health Care Manager, 30*(2), 13–138. doi: 10.1097.HCM.0b013e317216f4e5.

Richardson, P. (1992). Hospital practices that erode nursing power by promoting job dissatisfaction. *Revolution: The Journal of Nurse Empowerment, 2*, 34–39.

Shirey, M. (2012). Group think, organizational strategy and change. *Journal of Nursing Administration, 42*(2), 67–71. doi: 10.1097/NNA.0b013e3172433510.

Snowball, J. (1996). Asking nurses about advocating for patients: "Reactive" and "proactive" accounts. *Journal of Advanced Nursing, 24*, 67–75.

Standing, T., & Anthony, M. (2008). Delegation: What it means to acute care nurses. *Applied Nursing Research, 21*(1), 8–14.

Taylor, S. G., Pickens, J. M., & Geden, E. A. (1989). Interactional styles of nurse practitioners and physicians regarding patient decision making. *Nursing Research, 38*, 50–55.

U.S. Army. (2004). *Be-know-do: Leadership the Army way*. San Francisco, CA: Jossey-Bass.

Van Velsor, E., Moxley, R., & Bunker, K. (2004). The leadership development process. In C. McCauley, & E. Van Velsor (Eds.), *The Center for Creative Leadership handbook of leadership development* (2nd ed.). San Francisco, CA: Jossey-Bass.

Videback, S. (2008). *Psychiatric-mental health nursing* (4th ed.). Philadelphia, PA: Wolters Kluwer Health/Lippincott Williams & Wilkins.

Vroom, V., & Yetton, P. (1973). *Leadership and decision making*. Pittsburgh, PA: University of Pittsburgh Press.

Wesorick, B., & Shiparski, L. (1997). *Can the human being thrive in the workplace? Dialogue as a strategy of hope*. Grand Rapids, MI: Practice Field Publishing.

White, R., & Lippitt, R. (1960). *Autocracy and democracy: An experimental inquiry*. New York: Harper & Row.

Wilson, C. K., & Porter-O'Grady, T. (1999). *Leading the revolution in health care* (2nd ed.). Gaithersburg, MD: Aspen.

Wooten, K. C., & White, L. P. (1989). Toward a theory of change role efficacy. *Human Relations, 42*, 651–669.

Quality Improvement: Enhancing Patient Safety and Health Care Quality

LEARNING OUTCOMES

By the end of this chapter, the learner will be able to:

1. Define the term *quality*.
2. Outline the hallmarks of quality health care.
3. Compare and contrast quality assurance, total quality management, and continuous quality improvement.
4. Explain the plan, do, check, act (PDCA) cycle used in quality improvement programs.
5. Identify internal and external customers in health care settings.
6. Explain Six Sigma and how it could be used to improve health care quality.
7. Describe the process of benchmarking.
8. Specify core measures and nursing-sensitive outcomes for patient care delivery.
9. Explain how recent quality and safety initiatives improve the quality of health care services.

REAL-LIFE REFLECTIONS

Laura is a nurse working on a busy cardiac care unit. This evening, she has admitted two people with chest pain and transferred another of her assigned patients to the intensive care unit. Upon returning to the unit, Laura notices that one of her other patients did not receive ordered medications per the scheduled time. Laura missed giving an ordered antibiotic on time by 2 hours. She notifies the attending physician who yells at her. Laura completes an incident report on herself. Because she is new to the unit, Laura wonders how the nurse manager and her colleagues will react to her mistake.

This chapter was co-authored with Karen Wiegman, PhD, RN.

QUESTIONS FOR REFLECTION

1. How does the organization in which you practice nursing handle medication errors? How does your nursing program handle medication and other care errors made by students?
2. What steps could you take to prevent the medication error that happened to Laura?
3. Are you afraid to complete incident reports? Why or why not?
4. Who is at fault when a nurse makes an error?

The term **quality** means "a degree of excellence which something possesses" (Agnes, 2005, p. 1173). Quality in health care means different things depending on individual perspectives.

- The Institute of Medicine (IOM) stated that **quality health care** is safe, timely, efficient, equitable, effective, and patient centered (IOM, 2001; IOM, 2011).
- Consumers look for caring providers, timely services, technical competence, error-free care, accurate bills, and improved health status as indicators of quality.
- Nurses consider nurse–patient ratios, adequate time to spend with patients, availability of supplies, quality of ancillary staff, easy access to resources for procedures, and educational information and assistance as quality indicators (IOM, 2011).

Most health care consumers assume that health care providers and organizations will keep them safe. However, according to a 2016 study from John Hopkins University, safety experts have estimated that more than 250,000 Americans died as a result of medical care errors in 2013. Thus, medical care errors across care settings has become the third highest cause of death in the United States (Makary & Daniel, 2016). Deaths from medical errors, however, are extremely hard to track as they never appear on death certificates as the cause of death. "Medical error has been defined as an unintended act (either of omission or commission) or one that does not achieve its intended outcome" (Makary & Daniel, 2016, p. 1). Medical errors have been defined as situations in which health care providers failed to complete planned actions as intended, used an incorrect care plan to manage care or prescribed or administered medications for an unapproved reason. Omitted and unintended interventions may result in no adverse patient outcomes, in reversible patient harm, in temporary or permanent disability, or even in death (IOM, 2004; Makary & Daniel, 2016). Manufacturing companies would be out of business if they had as many errors as occur in the health care arena.

Hospital nurses today care for more acutely ill patients than in the past, requiring nurses to be able to change their thinking rapidly, keep a mental list of multiple tasks to accomplish, document all care activities, and supervise unlicensed care providers. According to a poll conducted by the American Nurses Association (ANA, 2013) with 16,295 nurse participants, 118,130 nurses believed that inadequate staffing compromised the quality of nursing care services.

Take Note!
The hallmarks of quality health care are safety, timeliness, efficiency, equitability, effectiveness, and patient-centeredness.

QUESTIONS FOR REFLECTION

1. As a consumer, what do you consider elements of quality care when you receive health care services? Why are these important?
2. As a professional nurse, what do you consider the elements of quality care? Why are they important?
3. How well do your lists of quality care match?

HISTORY OF QUALITY IMPROVEMENT IN HEALTH CARE

Quality management became popular in business and industry after American manufacturers lost market share to Japanese competitors in the late 1970s (Ouchi, 1981). As American businesses began incorporating quality management principles in the 1980s, they noticed improved sales. American workers also became involved in shaping work processes and a new sense of pride emerged.

Florence Nightingale can be considered the first nurse who engaged in quality improvement (QI) activities. During the Crimean War, Nightingale's work at the Barrack Hospital demonstrated the effects of quality nursing care on wounded and infirm soldiers. The mortality rate at the Barrack Hospital was 60% when Nightingale arrived. By the time she departed, it had fallen to just a fraction over 1%. Nightingale kept detailed records that included statistics about the effects of cleanliness, good nutrition, and fresh air on the survival of the soldiers (Kalisch & Kalisch, 2004). Her diligent attention to detailed records and continuous analysis of the data provided evidence that nursing care could reduce mortality. In 1855, Nightingale's interventions resulted in a reduction of mortality from 33% in January through March to just 2% by July through September of the same year (Gill & Gill, 2005). She reported her success to the British government and documented her work in three books: *Notes on Matters Affecting the Health, Efficiency and Hospital Administration of the British Army*

(1858); *Notes on Hospitals* (1858); and *Notes on Nursing* (1859) (Kalisch & Kalisch, 2004).

In 1913, a group of surgeons concerned about the quality of care in American hospitals formed the American College of Surgeons. By 1918, their work led to the implementation of the Hospital Standardization Program (HSP), which evolved into an accreditation process for hospitals. The HSP developed minimum standards for physician credentialing, hospital privileges, and methods to evaluate physician care and medical equipment. To create a standardized system for record keeping, the HSP established the first known standards for health care recipient medical records (DesHarnais & McLaughlin, 1999; Koch & Fairly, 1993).

The Evolution of the Joint Commission and Hospital Accreditation

In 1951, the HSP evolved into the Joint Commission on Accreditation of Hospitals (JCAH), a private, nonprofit, voluntary agency that ascertained that a hospital met American College of Surgeons Standards. Concerned about the quality of care received by subscribers during hospitalizations, the insurer Blue Cross required that participating hospitals be accredited by the JCAH by the early 1970s. Eventually, JCAH accreditation became a way for hospitals to prove that they met quality care requirements to receive Medicare program payments. By the mid-1970s, JCAH accreditation automatically guaranteed Medicare reimbursement (the other option for hospitals was to design their own system for meeting all Medicare program quality of care requirements) (DesHarnais & McLaughlin, 1999; Koch & Fairly, 1993; Sultz & Young, 2004; The Joint Commission 2013b).

Hospitals began to develop health care systems that also included primary care services for consumers in the mid-1980s. Accreditation by JCAH meant that each health care–providing organization demonstrated effective, high-quality services to persons. JCAH accreditation became a requirement for many health care organizations to qualify for insurance company reimbursement (Sultz & Young, 2004). In 1987, JCAH changed its name to the Joint Commission on Accreditation of Healthcare Organizations (JCAHO) (Koch & Fairly, 1993). In addition to assuring health care quality, JCAHO accreditation standards addressed efficacy of health care interventions and appropriateness of services delivered. Aspects for quality services include the following (DesHarnais & McLaughlin, 1999; Sultz & Young, 2004; The Joint Commission 2013b).

1. Availability of the needed health care intervention.
2. Timeliness of services.
3. Effectiveness of health care interventions.
4. Continuity of health care services across various health care settings.
5. Safety of patients and others.
6. Efficiencies of provided care and services.
7. Respect given to consumers and caring with which services are rendered.

In 2003, JCAHO recognized the impact of nursing care on patient quality outcomes and established a Nursing Advisory Council to address evolving nursing and patient care issues (The Joint Commission 2013d). Today, the Nursing Advisory Council has nursing organization, chief nursing officer, staff nurse, magnet hospital, research, academic, and nurse leader representation (The Joint Commission, 2016a).

JCAHO, known as **the Joint Commission** since 2007, accredits approximately 21,000 health care organizations which include general pediatric, long-term acute, rehabilitation, and specialty hospitals, home health agencies, laboratories, and extended-care and outpatient facilities. The Joint Commission uses standards, performance outcomes, and consumer perception of rendered services as criteria for accreditation (The Joint Commission, 2016b). In 2006, the World Health Organization (WHO) acknowledged the Joint Commission's contributions to ensuring quality health services, and today the Joint Commission accredits health care organizations internationally.

The Joint Commission and the Centers for Medicare and Medicaid Services (CMS) set annual national patient safety goals aimed at averting errors that compromise patient safety in hospitals, home care agencies, outpatient facilities, and laboratories (see Box 18.1, Professional Prototypes). The Joint Commission's 2016 National Patient Safety Goals for Hospitals included correct identification of patients, improved health team communication, safe use of medications, infection prevention, patient safety risk identification (patients at increased risk for suicide), and surgical mistake prevention (The Joint Commission, 2016c). The annual safety goals are broadly written. For most of the goals, the Joint Commission outlines elements of performance that typically include patient and health provider education along with a series of critical steps to follow. For example, 17 performance elements are identified for preventing central line bloodstream infections. The Joint Commission accreditation process requires that health care organizations compile data on the safety goals, communicate findings to staff, and develop plans to address each of the safety goals (The Joint Commission, 2016c).

Along with the development of national patient safety goals, the Joint Commission has collaborated

18.1 Professional Prototypes

The Joint Commission's 2016 Hospital National Patient Safety Goals

2016 Hospital National Patient Safety Goals

The purpose of the National Patient Safety Goals is to improve patient safety. The goals focus on problems in health care safety and how to solve them.

Identify patients correctly

NPSG.01.01.01

Use at least two ways to identify patients. For example, use the patient's name *and* date of birth. This is done to make sure that each patient gets the correct medicine and treatment.

NPSG.01.03.01

Make sure that the correct patient gets the correct blood when they get a blood transfusion.

Improve staff communication

NPSG.02.03.01

Get important test results to the right staff person on time.

Use medicines safely

NPSG.03.04.01

Before a procedure, label medicines that are not labeled. For example, medicines in syringes, cups and basins. Do this in the area where medicines and supplies are set up.

NPSG.03.05.01

Take extra care with patients who take medicines to thin their blood.

NPSG.03.06.01

Record and pass along correct information about a patient's medicines. Find out what medicines the patient is taking. Compare those medicines to new medicines given to the patient. Make sure the patient knows which medicines to take when they are at home. Tell the patient it is important to bring their up-to-date list of medicines every time they visit a doctor.

Use alarms safely

NPSG.06.01.01

Make improvements to ensure that alarms on medical equipment are heard and responded to on time.

Prevent infection

NPSG.07.01.01

Use the hand cleaning guidelines from the Centers for Disease Control and Prevention or the World Health Organization. Set goals for improving hand cleaning. Use the goals to improve hand cleaning.

NPSG.07.03.01

Use proven guidelines to prevent infections that are difficult to treat.

NPSG.07.04.01

Use proven guidelines to prevent infection of the blood from central lines.

NPSG.07.05.01

Use proven guidelines to prevent infection after surgery.

NPSG.07.06.01

Use proven guidelines to prevent infections of the urinary tract that are caused by catheters.

Identify patient safety risks

NPSG.15.01.01

Find out which patients are most likely to try to commit suicide.

Prevent mistakes in surgery

UP.01.01.01

Make sure that the correct surgery is done on the correct patient and at the correct place on the patient's body.

UP.01.02.01

Mark the correct place on the patient's body where the surgery is to be done.

UP.01.03.01

Pause before the surgery to make sure that a mistake is not being made.

The Joint Commission
Accreditation
Hospital

This is an easy-to-read document. It has been created for the public. The exact language of the goals can be found at www.jointcommission.org.

2016 Hospital National Patient Safety Goals. Retrieved from https://www.jointcommission.org/assets/1/6/2016_NPSG_HAP_ ER.pdf © The Joint Commission, 2016. Reprinted with permission.

with the CMS since 2003 to align specific core measures for the management of disease processes such as acute myocardial infarction and heart failure. The CMS is in the process of determining graduated levels of reimbursement to health care organizations based on performance on core measures, thereby creating Accountable Care Organizations (ACOs) are voluntary provider partnerships who integrate and align providers to provide coordinated care services to a specifically defined group of patients (e.g., older adults with congestive heart failure). The long-term goal is to pay organizations with higher levels of performance more and establish a competitive reimbursement structure in which the best performers attain the highest reimbursement. ACOs constantly look for ways to improve the quality of health care delivered to the defined patient group (IOM, 2011; Joshi, Ransom, Nash, & Ransom, 2014; The Joint Commission, 2013a and 2015a).

The Joint Commission (2015) identifies accountability measures as quality measures that meet the following four criteria: (a) research (performance of evidence-based care processes that have been supported by research to influence desired patient outcomes), (b) proximity (performance of direct care process most closely linked to a desired outcome), (c) accuracy (that measure accurately the care process associated with a positive outcome, and (d) adverse effects (implementation of a measure is unlikely to produce undesired, negative outcomes). The Joint Commission uses these measures for evaluating organization for accreditation, reporting comparative results of organizations, and determining pay-for-performance (The Joint Commission, 2015; CMS, 2016). Accountability measures provide the basis for QI processes for many hospitals.

Quality Assurance Programs

Quality assurance (QA) programs became part of the hospital accreditation process in the 1970s. The Joint Commission standards require that health care organizations (especially hospitals) regularly review the following data as part of their QA programs: (1) mortality rates by department or service, (2) hospital-acquired infections, (3) patient falls, (4) adverse drug reactions, (5) unplanned returns to surgery, and (6) hospital-incurred trauma (Sultz & Young, 2004, p. 108). QA programs examine patient outcomes retrospectively. QA also includes planning operational and strategic plans for an organization to compare past performance with current performance including communication of standards, identifying key indicators for mentoring compliance to

standards as well and assessing compliance to standards. Because of its punitive nature toward individual health care providers and reactive approach to errors, QA has been losing popularity (Joshi et al., 2014).

Total Quality Management and Continuous Quality Improvement

The terms **total quality management** (TQM) and **continuous quality improvement** (CQI) are used synonymously in the business and health care–related literature. The Joint Commission standards (2013a and 2016b) emphasize the importance of CQI or TQM. Success in CQI and TQM is based on the premise that if staff members who are closest to the point of service delivery are empowered and educated on the process of incremental change, the quality and efficiency of patient care will improve (Sultz & Young, 2004). QI differs from QA in that QA programs tend to be reactive in nature and focus on the correction of specific identified causes of problems with limited responsibility using authoritative problem solving. In contrast, QI is a proactive program aimed at correcting common system problems; QI holds everyone involved in a process responsible, has leaders who actively lead, and actual and potential problems are identified and solved by all employees (Koch & Fairly, 1993). Table 18.1 outlines the differences between QA and QI programs.

> **Take Note!**
> QI, CQI, and TQM all basically mean the same thing—processes used constantly and continuously to improve all aspects of goods and services that are offered to consumers.

TABLE 18.1   Comparison of Quality Assurance (QA) and Quality Improvement (QI) Programs

Quality Assurance Program	Quality Improvement Program
Conformance focused	Improvement focused
Reactive in nature	Proactive in nature
Looks for special sources of variation within a system	Focuses on internal variations within a system
Variation results from actions of specific people or work groups	Variation results from increased complexity of work processes or may be random in nature

Adapted from McLaughlin, C., & Kaluzny, A. (1999). *Continuous quality improvement in healthcare.* Gaithersburg, MD: Aspen.

THE NEED FOR IMPROVED PATIENT SAFETY AND CARE QUALITY

The Institute of Medicine's Quality Chasm Series

In light of issues with patient safety and health care quality, the IOM conducted a series of quality studies known as the **Institute of Medicine Quality Chasm Series.** The findings of the first study, *To Err Is Human: Building a Safer Health System* (2000), shocked many health care consumers and providers. This landmark study, with findings derived from the analysis of aggregate data, estimated that between 44,000 and 98,000 people die annually as a result of preventable medical errors. The report also concluded that medical errors in health care settings were the leading cause of unexpected deaths in the United States, more than any other form of sudden, unexpected death (including motor vehicle accidents). The report identified ineffective communication as the root cause of 65% of errors that resulted in death or permanent disability. As a result of the report, Congress appropriated funds starting in the fiscal year 2001–2002, to establish a Patient Safety Network within the Agency for Healthcare Research and Quality that would also establish national safety goals, track progress in safety improvement, and fund research to learn how to prevent health care–related errors.

The second IOM (2001) study, *Crossing the Quality Chasm: A New Health System for the 21st Century,* proposed radical reforms for the American health care system. The report determined a set of performance expectations to ensure that patient care is safe, timely, effective, efficient, equitable, and patient-centered. The goal of the reforms was to align payment and accountability with QI initiatives. The report identified the complexity of current health care organizations that resulted in increased risk for errors and higher care delivery costs. Complicated work processes and ineffective communication were cited as two key factors interfering with health care safety and quality.

Results from the 2001 IOM study led to additional recommendations for education of the health care professions outlined in *Health Professions Education: A Bridge to Quality* (IOM, 2003). The report called for education based on five competencies: (1) patient-centered care, (2) teamwork and collaboration, (3) evidence-based practice, (4) QI (and safety), and (5) informatics. Key recommendations included the development of a common language for interdisciplinary team members, educational experiences including all members of the interprofessional health care team, creating evidence-based health professions curricula, providing evidence-based teaching and learning methods, initiating faculty development programs for effective role modeling of desired competencies, and developing and implementing plans for monitoring student, graduate, and faculty proficiency in the five competencies.

The 2004 IOM report, *Keeping Patients Safe: Transforming the Work Environment of Nurses,* linked the work environment of nurses with the quality and safety of patient care. The report acknowledged the high-stress, complex work processes; inadequate resources (human and material); and environmental barriers nurses face in providing safe, effective patient care. Key recommendations included the creation and maintenance of a satisfying and rewarding work environment for nurses, adequate nurse staffing levels, increased focus on patient safety at the bedside *and* by governing boards, use of evidence-based nursing management strategies, determination of ways to build and maintain trust between nurses and facility administration, participative decision making, development of ways to support and promote learning for all nurses, establishment of interdisciplinary collaboration, work environment redesign for improving patient care processes, and creation of a patient safety culture.

Aspen, Walcott, Bootman, and Cronenwett (2007) conducted a study aimed at discovering the prevalence and reasons for medication errors by nurses. This final study in the IOM Quality Chasm series, *Identifying and Preventing Medication Errors,* found that over 7,000 patients died as a result of medication errors each year and that most inpatients are subjected to at least one medication error per day on average. The authors projected that 1.5 million preventable adverse drug events occur annually, adverse drug events account for 2% of hospital admissions, and the annual cost for these events is $2 billion in national health care expenditures.

The federal government examined societal trends and noted increasing diversity of citizenship, numbers of elderly, and demands for high-quality health care services. Analysis of data and literature revealed the important roles that nurses fill. To plan for the future of health care delivery, the IOM formed an ad hoc committee to explore how to maximize the use of professional nurses in reshaping the American health care delivery system. In 2011, the IOM published the findings of the committee, *The future of nursing: Leading change, advancing health.* The report identifies four key messages that resulted from a thorough examination of the literature, nursing workforce data, interview transcripts, and research studies.

- **Message 1:** "Nurses should practice to the full extent of their education and training" (IOM, 2011, p. 4)

The first message addresses legal and regulatory restrictions encountered by APRNs and the national and state levels of government. Scope of practice barriers must be removed for APRN practice in order to practice to their full capability and receive reimbursement for rendered services. Some states restrict the ability for APRN practice and removal of these barriers has the potential for increasing health care access for all while reducing costs.

- **Message 2:** "Nurses should achieve higher levels of education and training through an improved education system that promotes seamless academic progression" (IOM, 2011, p. 4).

The IOM (2011) recommends "increasing the proportion of practicing nurses with a baccalaureate degree to 80% by 2020" (p. 12) and doubling "the number of nurses with a doctorate by 2010" (p. 13). As diversity of health care consumers and complexity of care increases, a more highly educated nurse workforce is needed. Health care organizations and nursing faculty must collaborate with each other and form partnerships so that the newly educated nurses have the required knowledge, skills, and attitudes required for effective clinical practice. Higher education levels also enable professional nurses to lead changes to improve the quality of health care delivery in complex health organizations collaboratively with other professional health team members.

- **Message 3:** "Nurses should be full partners, with physicians and other health professionals, in redesigning health care in the United States" (IOM, 2011, p. 4).

Currently, the multiple educational level of practicing registered nurses creates barriers to recognition as a full partner when providing patient care. Some physicians view APRNs as competitors rather than collaborators. Unfortunately, some nurses perceive that they are not treated as equal partners in the interprofessional health care team. Redesigning the current mechanisms of health care delivery must include all members of the health team to avoid duplication of services, to improve quality, to reduce costs and to meet holistic needs of health care consumers (IOM, 2011).

- **Message 4:** "Effective workforce planning and policy making require better data collection and

an improved information infrastructure" (IOM, 2011, p. 4).

To meet the future health care needs of American society (increased diversity of the population and numbers of the elderly), the National Health Workforce Commission and the Health Resources and Service Administration must improve the way that nursing workforce data are collected. Current predictions are made from the National Registered Nurses Sample Survey (NRNSS) conducted every 4 years and from reports from state licensing boards. Suggested ways to improve data include conduction of the NRNSS biannually and developing state nursing workforce centers to determine regional health care workforce needs, set regional health care workforce targets, and plan appropriately to expand the supply of health professionals to meet future needs (IOM, 2011). Once these programs are in place, then efforts to improve their quality will be needed.

In response to the IOM *Future of Nursing Report,* the Robert Wood Johnson Foundation and the American Association of Retired Persons collaborated with the nursing profession to develop a Nursing Campaign for Action to design and implement programs to attain the four key messages in the report. In the action campaign, each of the 50 states formed a State Nursing Coalition in order to prevent duplicative efforts for each key message. The Future of Nursing Campaign for Action (2016) reported the following progress on the four key messages:

- Message 1: In 2010, only five states permitted independent practice for APRNs. In 2015, eight states now permit full scope of independent practice for RNs. In 2010, 16 states allowed APRNs to have full prescriptive authority. In 2016, APRNs enjoy full prescriptive authority in 42 states.
- Message 2: The number of practicing RNs with a BSN rose from 49% to 51% from 2010 to 2014 and the number of RNs with earned doctorates increased from 11,589 to 21,280 from 2010 to 2016.
- Message 3: At the top-ranked nursing schools by *US News and World,* the number of graduate clinical nursing courses that required collaboration with other graduate student health team members rose from 6 to 23 from 2010 to 2016.
- Message 4: Thirty-one states collected data related to nursing education program enrollment, current nurse supply and projected demand for nurses in 2010. In 2016, 47 states collect some data related to nursing workforce supply and demand.

Improving the Quality and Safety of Health Care Delivery

Progress toward meeting the recommendations of the IOM Quality Chasm reports has been slow. Brady (2015) reported that from 2010 to 2013 that with the implementation of Comprehensive Unit-Based Safety Programs and TEAMSTEPPS©, there were 1.3 million fewer hospital-associated complications (a 17% decline), 50,000 lives saved and $12 billion in health care expenditure avoidance. Patient safety has also improved because of tougher accreditation standards and mandatory error reporting requirements. National and international campaigns aimed at improving patient safety and care quality include the "5 Million Lives Campaign" by the Institute for Healthcare Improvement (IHI), evidence-based care protocols from the Agency for Healthcare Research and Quality, the national patient safety goals from the Joint Commission, and the Millennium Development Goals from WHO.

The National Quality Forum (NQF) is a private, non-partisan, nonprofit group of individuals and group interested in improving the quality (effectiveness and efficiency) of health care delivery in the United States. The NQF was formed following a 199 Presidential Advisory Commission on Consumer Protection & Quality in the Healthcare Industry. The NQF sets performance standards for health care and establishes routine measures of quality outcomes that have been determined by consensus of all persons involved in health care delivery represented by specialty councils (consumers, health care plans, health professionals, public/community health providers, suppliers, and industries). Participating members have access to a dashboard that displays collected data on key performance indicators of delivery of high-quality health care. The NQF also engages in CQI/TQM and constantly updates data reports and uses the best possible evidence to set quality performance standards. Nursing sensitive outcomes measures are included in NQF performance standards (National Quality Forum, 2016).

Many health care organizations have adopted a "just culture" for managing errors when they occur; such a culture emphasizes that work processes rather than people are usually the cause of mistakes in health care delivery. According to the just culture approach, there are four main categories of failures and the levels have differing remedies. The first failure level is that of unintentional harm when an unintended result occurs typically as a result of ambiguous work processes or systems. In this case, focus is placed on the system and how it might be improved. The second failure level is provider carelessness or at-risk behavior such as inattentiveness to details that resulted in an error. When this happens, the provider receives counseling and education about how to avoid repeating the same mistake. The next two levels require some form of punishment because of the severity of their nature. A level three situation involves recklessness with complete disregard for established work processes or norms resulting in a care error (such as a health care provider coming to work under the influence of alcohol). The fourth level arises when providers simply refuse to follow standards and procedures or show flagrant disregard at organizational authorities. The last two levels typically result in either a suspension from duty or cessation of employment (Joshi et al., 2014).

The CMS has moved to value-based purchasing (VBP). VBP represents a shift from reimbursement based on fee-for-service and high volume to reimbursement for predictions of achieving optimal patient outcomes (Aroh, Colella, Douglas, & Eddings, 2015). The movement toward VBP started when industry was looking for ways to provide the best possible health insurance coverage for employees. Using data from national quality organizations, companies could compare outcomes for disease processes for hospitals, individual health care providers and how services were organized and delivered across the continuum of care. In response to the rising costs of health care and prevalence of potentially avoidable complications, the United States initiated the Provider Payment Reform for Outcomes, Margins, Evidence, Transparency, Hassle-Reduction, Excellence, Understandability, and Sustainability (PROMETHEUS) (Joshi et al., 2014, p. 533). By instituting the PROMETHEUS model, the National Quality Forum was able to collect detailed data and compare outcomes for health care providers and settings. The NQF discovered that 27% of health care costs were the result of potentially avoidable complications arising from health care interventions. Therefore, CMS had evidence to move to a payment for performance reimbursement structure (Joshi et al., 2014).

■ QUESTIONS FOR REFLECTION

1. How does VBP change care delivery using a fee-for-service approach?
2. What problems do you see for different health care organizations when receiving reimbursement for patient outcome attainment?
3. How do nurses contribute to optimal patient outcomes across the continuum of care?

The Joint Commission sets annual National Patient Safety Goals and requires accredited organization to educate patients and families on how to stay safe in the hospital (see Box 18.1, Professional Prototypes). Along with the National Patient Safety Goals, the Joint Commission has developed the SPEAK UP™ initiative that educates patients and their significant other to do the following things when receiving health care services.

Speak up if you have questions or concerns.
Pay attention to the care you get.
Educate yourself about your illness.
Ask a trusted family member or friend to be your advocate (advisor or supporter).
Know what medicines you take and why you take them.
Use a health care organization that has been carefully checked out.
Participate in all decisions about your treatment.

This initiative emphasizes the importance of all individuals to participate actively and to be knowledgeable about personal health and health issues (The Joint Commission, 2016d).

The QI/TQM/CQI process offers approaches to meet recommendations to improve the quality and safety of health care delivery. To understand variances in QI/TQM/CQI process encountered in practice, several approaches are presented in the following section.

Quality and Safety Education for Nurses (QSEN)

Starting in 1995, several annual invitational Dartmouth Summer Symposia were held, led by Paul Batalden, a pediatrician who was concerned about the quality of health care in the United States. Meeting participants included physicians, nurses, hospital administrators, and educators who referred to themselves as "an interprofessional community of educators devoted to building knowledge for leading improvement in health care" (Cronenwett, 2012, p. 6). Using basic principles of QI (identification of ways to improve, developing an action plan, implementing the plan, measuring plan results, comparing results with baseline data, and determining the effectiveness of the plan), the participants designed a program to improve the safety and quality education for the health professions, especially the nursing profession. The Robert Wood Johnson Foundation agreed to fund the project, which would start by educating faculty on the quality and safety goals outlined in *Transforming Care at the Bedside* and became known as **Quality and Safety Education for Nurses (QSEN)**.

Phase I of the project (2005 to 2007) identified the following areas for nurses to display competence in providing safe, effective, high-quality care: "patient-centered care, teamwork and collaboration, evidence-based practice, QI, safety, and informatics" (Cronenwett, 2012, p. 52) which are known as the **QSEN competencies**. The work group established the knowledge, skills, and attitudes for each of the identified areas to be used in nursing pre-licensure programs. Along with the identified competency areas, the work group advocated open sharing of information, keeping the work open for exploring other ideas, practicing trustworthiness, sharing generously (no stealing of others' ideas) to protect the future of all colleagues, engaging in dialogue and listening, and using the gift of silence for time of reflection. The name Quality and Safety Education for Nurses (QSEN) was created in 2005, along with a website to share teaching strategies for QSEN competencies.

Phase II of QSEN (2007 to 2008) involved generating and sharing ideas. The QSEN faculty/advisory board developed educational materials to train faculty trainers. Faculty in pre-licensure programs were invited to develop, implement, test, and disseminate various teaching strategies for QSEN competencies. The IHI model for learning collaboration was implemented so that faculty could easily access educational materials related to QSEN. Workshops were held and 13 professional nursing organizations generated knowledge, skills, and attitudes for graduate education. By the end of phase II in 2008, 40 nurse educators had joined the expert QSEN faculty and provided consultation to all types of nursing pre-licensure programs across the nation. Nursing programs and clinical agencies formed partnerships in which the agencies freely shared with students and faculty current QI and safety initiatives (Cronenwett, 2012).

Phase III (2008 to 2011) of QSEN involved promoting innovations in evaluation and assessment of student learning of knowledge, skills, and attitudes in the six competency areas. Further development of faculty expertise was needed to assist learning and assess attainment of QSEN competencies in all types of nursing education programs, as well as to create ways to change nursing programs to embrace QSEN by including QSEN competencies in textbooks, adding them to standards for accreditation and certification standards for advanced practice nursing, incorporating them into professional nursing licensing exams, and developing program outcomes based on QSEN knowledge, skills, and attitudes. Nine faculty workshops were held in 2011 across the United States for faculty innovating with QSEN competencies and new teaching strategies.

Phase IV of QSEN (2010 to present) will include increased interprofessional collaboration in the education of all future health care professionals. Goals include determining strategies for developing knowledge, skills, and attitudes for interprofessional practice, including "values/ethics for interprofessional practice, role/responsibilities for collaborative practice, interprofessional communication, and interprofessional teamwork and team-based care" (Cronenwett, 2012, p. 62). If QSEN meets its lofty goals, then the goals of all members of the interprofessional health care team will be attuned to safety issues in health care and use QI strategies to improve the quality and safety of health care delivery.

QUALITY IMPROVEMENT APPROACHES

QI education appears as a QSEN competency for nursing undergraduate and graduate programs. The American Association of Colleges of Nursing also list QI education as an essential element of undergraduate (AACN, 2008) and graduate nursing education (AACN, 2011). The expectation is that nurses will be capable of using data to monitor care process outcomes and utilizing methods outlined in the QI process to identify targeted areas for improvement, design ways to change current work systems and processes, test the new way of care delivery, and determine whether the tested innovations enhance the quality and safety of health care. If the innovations are shown to improve health care systems, then they will become the new standard practices.

In health care, providers have traditionally rated quality in terms of mortality and morbidity, and many institutions hold "mortality and morbidity conferences" on a regular basis. Others hold regularly scheduled conferences to analyze precipitating factors and outcomes of rescue efforts following cases of respiratory and cardiac arrest and other deaths that occur in the hospital. Some health care professionals consider death as a failure of the health care system and believe detailed analyses of the reasons for a death should be thoroughly investigated so that measures can be taken to avoid similar deaths in the future.

QI/TQM/CQI offers an alternative way to measure, analyze, and control quality in health care.

W. Edwards Deming

W. Edwards Deming (a physicist, mathematician, and engineer) was responsible for postwar construction in Japan. In 1950, he presented a quality management workshop that emphasized the importance of statistical control for managers. To maintain a competitive edge, Deming proposed that dedication to quality and productivity was essential. Deming suggested that errors increased and productivity declined as a result of flawed work processes rather than individual actions. He also believed that productivity and quality would improve when workers became empowered to make decisions about work processes (Walton, 1986).

Deming developed a cycle, today known as the Deming cycle, to improve quality (Fig. 18.1). The cycle is a continuous loop consisting of the following steps: **plan, do, check, and act (PDCA).** Using the Deming cycle, organizations *plan* what improvements need to be made, *do* by implementing the plan, *check* results of plan implementation using statistical data, and *act* by correcting work processes to improve the quality of services or products. The IHI uses a variation of the PDCA cycle (Walton, 1986).

Deming also emphasized that a successful QI program requires total commitment and accountability from all workers (including management). He created 14 points that must be applied for successful QI processes (see Box 18.2, Professional Prototypes).

Along with proposals for successful QI programs, Deming warned of the following seven "deadly diseases" and obstacles that could derail the process.

1. Lack of constancy of purpose (everyone working toward different goals without a single strategic plan to ensure organizational survival).

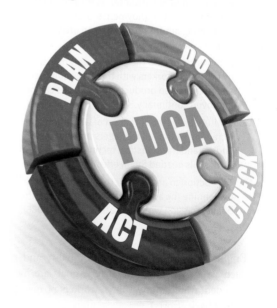

FIGURE 18.1 Deming's Plan-Do-Check-Act Cycle, the first quality improvement method.

18.2 Professional Prototypes

Deming's 14 Points for Successful Quality Improvement Processes

1. Create a constancy of purpose for improvement of products and services.

2. Adopt the philosophy that poor workmanship and services must not be tolerated.

3. Cease dependence on mass inspection by entrusting and expecting workers to develop ways to improve production processes and have them make decisions during the production process whether to discard or rework a product.

4. End the practice of awarding business based solely on the lowest cost.

5. Work constantly and endlessly to improve the systems of production and service.

6. Institute training for all workers.

7. Reconfigure leadership so that supervisors help workers perform better.

8. Drive out fear in the workplace because fear prevents people from asking questions or expressing ideas and perpetuates errors in performance.

9. Remove all barriers between staff areas by bringing various departments together to work toward the common purpose and find more opportunities for improvement.

10. Eliminate slogans, exhortations, and targets for the workforce by having the workers write their own slogans and specify production targets.

11. Eliminate numerical quotas as they create the perception that employment status is based only on meeting quotas rather than on producing high-quality goods and services.

12. Remove barriers to the pride of workmanship by providing workers with the best equipment and materials so products and services can be improved continually.

13. Institute a vigorous program of education and retraining so that all managers and workers understand the statistical techniques and teamwork skills needed for an effective QI program.

14. Take action to accomplish the transformation by defining the action plan required to lead the quality mission with dedication (Walton, 1986).

2. Emphasis on short-term profits (quality and productivity may decline if quarterly goals are met or exceeded, which may result in workers or managers scaling back efforts).

3. Evaluation by performance, merit rating, or annual performance reviews (sets up a competitive environment with the potential for destroying teamwork, instilling rivalry, creating despondency, and encouraging management upward mobility).

4. Mobility of management away from production or service (management must understand the work and complete changes for improved productivity and quality, which means managers must be on the job long enough to accomplish these tasks).

5. Running a company solely on visible figures (the effects of a satisfied or dissatisfied customer remain unknown).

6. Excessive medical costs (reveal potential problems within the work environment or no time for employees to engage in health promotion activities).

7. Excessive costs of warranty, fueled by lawyers working for contingency fees (high losses reveal that inferior goods or services are being provided to customers) (Walton, 1986).

Deming provided businesses with an innovative approach. He outlined strategies for success that empowered workers. In addition, his obstacles warned about potentially catastrophic effects arising from failure to develop strategic plans, relying on technology rather than people to solve problems, and generating excuses for less-than-optimal performance (Walton, 1986).

If Deming's principles are applied to clinical nursing practice; QI efforts would be made to streamline work processes related to direct patient care. For example, nurses would not be blamed if errors occurred while taking care of patients. Each error that occurred would be analyzed fully to determine all contributing factors. Work processes would be changed to prevent the error's recurrence. Nurses would be empowered to make changes in clinical policies and procedures as well as assume control over their clinical practice environments.

Joseph Juran

Like Deming, management consultant and engineer Joseph Juran stressed the importance of careful planning to generate product quality. In 1945, Juran took his concepts to Japan, where he used statistical quality control as a management tool. He created the Juran Trilogy, consisting of quality planning, quality control, and QI.

- Quality planning consists of identifying specific customers and their needs, developing products to meet customer needs, developing processes to produce product features, and transferring production plans and product features to operating forces.

- Quality control consists of evaluating actual performance, comparing it with product goals, and acting on the difference.
- QI consists of establishing an infrastructure, identifying specific improvement projects, establishing project teams, and providing the improvement teams with resources, training, education, and motivation. The QI team works to diagnose causes of less-than-desired quality, propose and simulate remedies to identified causes, and establish control systems to maintain the gains (Juran, 1989).

Juran (1989) also differentiated quality circles from QI project teams. Quality circles serve primarily to improve human relationships and secondarily to improve quality. Quality circles usually occur within a single department where members volunteer to tackle many QI projects. Managers and workers hold equal status in quality circles. In contrast, QI project team membership crosses departmental boundaries, has a primary mission of improving quality, is run by a manager (or professional), and disbands once the project ends.

Juran (1989) outlined the following eight factors to distinguish institutions that have improved quality and reduced quality-related costs.

1. Upper managers lead the quality process and serve on quality councils (QI teams) as guides.
2. **Internal customers** (people working within the organization) and **external customers** (people outside the organization but receiving products or services) needs are considered as QI processes are applied to businesses and usual operating processes.
3. Senior managers are given clear responsibility to adopt mandated, annual QI with a defined infrastructure that identifies opportunities for improvement, and are held accountable for making the improvements.
4. Managers involve everyone who affects the plan in the QI process.
5. Managers use modern quality methodology rather than empiric methods in quality planning.
6. Senior managers train all management team members in quality planning, quality control, and QI.
7. Managers train all workers in how to participate actively in QI.
8. QI becomes a major feature in the strategic planning process.

Philip Crosby

Businessman Philip Crosby (1979) proposed that quality is free but specified that time, manpower, and resources cost money. Crosby advocated for doing things right

the first time, stating that quality saves money, thereby increasing profits. He defined quality as "conformance to requirements" (Crosby, 1979, p. 8). Crosby's emphasis on doing things right the first time particularly resonates in health care delivery because health care professionals usually get only one chance to deliver effective, safe patient care (e.g., the nurse has only one chance to administer the right medication to a patient). He proposed that organizations needed to create climates in which attitudes and controls make error prevention possible.

Like Deming, Crosby saw the need for all within an organization to be committed to the QI process. However, Crosby believed that "management needs to understand their personal roles in implanting quality and engaging employees in the vision of the company" (Crosby, 1979, p. 78). Crosby identified 14 essential elements of a quality management program.

1. Management commitment to the QI process
2. QI teams to oversee actions
3. Measurement tools appropriate to specific activities going through the QI process
4. Consideration of the costs of quality evaluation (using estimates as needed)
5. Quality awareness promotion from all involved
6. Corrective action as needed to correct measurement tools and reduce costs associated with the QI process
7. Planning for zero deficits
8. Supervisory education and training for management at all levels
9. Holding a zero defects day to celebrate the new standard of performance
10. Goal determination for individual workers and work teams
11. Worker rather than management removal of causes of error after notification
12. Recognition of all involved once performance goals are attained
13. Quality circle sharing of ideas, experiences, and problems
14. Constant repetition of all steps (after all, QI is a continuous, never-ending process)

Crosby's thesis of the importance of doing things right the first time has been recently expanded by Toyota's Lean operations and Chowdhury's Six Sigma Design approach to quality management.

Lean

Since the 1980s, Toyota automobiles have been known for their quality construction and performance. The

Toyota Production System involves creation of a learning environment that uses the following four key practices.

1. **How people work:** Workers follow strict production specifications, are encouraged to identify changes in work processes, and then perform controlled trials of new work processes.
2. **How workers connect:** Workers across all levels of the organization interact directly following standardized methods. These practices reduce ambiguity, prevent key issues from losing attention, encourage requests for help (to which assistance is provided immediately), set deadlines for problem resolution, and foster trust among everyone in the organization.
3. **How work is constructed:** Work processes are designed to attain maximum reliability, eliminate repetition, and follow principles to promote worker health and well-being.
4. **How work is improved and errors are reduced:** All workers are trained in how to effect change, assume responsibility for making errors, and use the scientific method to identify and propose changes to improve productivity and product quality, and reduce errors (Joshi et al., 2014).

Toyota also uses **Lean** operation techniques that advocate the use of desired, value-added activities while eliminating undesirable activities and waste in all work processes. Lean techniques eliminate waste by using visual controls, streamlined physical plant layouts, standardized work processes, and point-of-use storage. If a health care organization operated using Lean principles, operations flowcharts outlining steps for delivering various services would be posted in departments (Joshi et al., 2014). Nursing units and other ancillary departments would be designed to promote the flow of activities required for patient care. Routine work processes would be standardized (many institutions already use standardized clinical care pathways for commonly encountered diseases, surgeries, and invasive diagnostic and intervention procedures). Finally, supplies, equipment, information, and procedures would be housed in convenient locations where patient services are delivered (IOM, 2004).

The Lean system outlines seven categories of waste: (1) poor utilization of resources, (2) excess motion, (3) unnecessary waiting, (4) transportation, (5) process inefficiency, (6) excess inventory, and (7) defects/quality control. Often, waste is identified by asking a series of why questions as in the case of nurses not finding the equipment on a hypothetical clinical unit (see Concepts in Practice).

Concepts in Practice IDEA ──→ PLAN ──→ ACTION

Using Root Cause Analysis and Learning to Discover Quality Defects Leading to Reduced Nursing Productivity

Location: A medical-surgical nursing unit

Problem: The nurses cannot find basic patient care equipment such as a bedpan, toothbrushes, and soap. This results in wasted time searching for patient care supplies.

- *Why do the nurses have difficulty finding a bedpan?* Because a new bedpan is not available in the supply room.
- *Why is the equipment not in the supply room?* Because the bedpan was not specified on the list of supplies that should be restocked.
- *Why are the supplies not on the list?* Because the nursing staff did not scan the computer-based bar code and charge the patient for the bedpan when one was taken from the supply room.
- *Why did the nursing staff not scan the bedpan?* Because the nurse was in a hurry to get the patient a bedpan.
- *Why was the nurse in such a hurry?* Because the nurse did not want the patient to eliminate in the bed because the patient was ordered on complete bed rest.

Possible Resolutions

- Stock a bedpan in each patient room (excess inventory possible).
- Position the computer-based bar coding device in a strategic location to make bar scanning quick and easy (may be a process inefficiency or excessive motion by staff).
- Educate the nursing staff about how the bar scanning device is used for supply inventory control (correct a quality defect).
- Install cameras to videotape staff as supplies are removed from the supply room and then generate reports for specific staff members who fail to comply with bar scanning supplies when removing them from a supply room (correct a process inefficiency, however, this process is incongruent with QI philosophy).

When nurses go searching for equipment needed for patient care, hospitals practice poor utilization of resources, excess motion, unnecessary waiting, and process inefficiency. Many times patients wait for long periods after undergoing diagnostic tests because of the unavailability of someone to return them to their rooms (waste from transportation, unnecessary waiting, and process inefficiency). Nurses may make medication errors because they engage in multitasking to meet patient care needs (waste in terms of process inefficiency). Hospitals frequently buy supplies in bulk to reduce cost per unit, resulting in a higher inventory of supplies than actually needed; some supplies may become outdated and have to be discarded (excess inventory) (IOM, 2004).

However, health care organizations constantly look for ways to reduce delivery costs. Some health care organizations have identified that by removing waste and improving work flow processes (e.g., the use of interprofessional team developed client care paths), better patient outcomes occur.

Six Sigma

In the late 1980s, Motorola developed the Six Sigma strategy as a means to sharpen its focus on QI and help accelerate the pace of change in a highly competitive technologic and telecommunications market (Pande, Neuman, & Cavanagh, 2000). The concept was expanded by other companies, including General Electric, Allied Signal, and Honeywell (Pande et al., 2000). Six Sigma has its basis in the quality principles outlined by Deming, Juran, and Crosby, and in the Lean model, but takes quality to a new level. "In a nutshell, **Six Sigma** is a management philosophy focused on eliminating mistakes, waste, and rework" (Chowdhury, 2002, p. 4).

Sigma (the Greek letter for deviation) measures variation within a process. The standard deviation of a process quantifies how far a process functions from its ideal. Instead of using percentages (based on a system of 100 performances), Six Sigma looks at "defects per million opportunities" (Chowdhury, 2002; Pande et al., 2000). Table 18.2 summarizes the levels of Six Sigma, translates the levels in terms of performance accuracy, and presents health care–based scenarios using Six Sigma.

Six Sigma methodology strives to improve products and work processes during the design rather than the

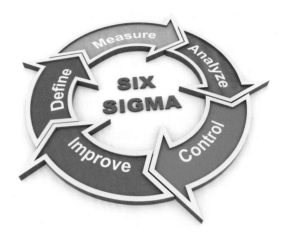

FIGURE 18.2 The Six Sigma process: Define, Measure, Analyze, Improve, and Control incorporates customer focus and wise use of facts to improve and manage work processes.

quality control stage. Like TQM, Six Sigma processes emphasize providing the highest possible quality of goods and services to consumers. Pande et al. (2000, p. 68) identified a Six Sigma Roadmap consisting of the following five sequential steps: (1) identify core processes and key customers; (2) define customer requirements; (3) measure current performance; (4) prioritize, analyze, and implement improvements; and (5) expand and integrate the Six Sigma system.

The steps apply to situations related to business transformation, strategic improvement, and problem solving. When transforming business, Pande and colleagues suggested limiting the scope of change to one or two core processes. However, in health care, Six Sigma (Fig. 18.2) may best be used for strategic improvement (finding out what patients and families need and want, followed by implementation of initiatives to fulfill

TABLE 18.2 Six Sigma Levels, Performance Accuracy, and Implications for Nursing Practice			
Sigma Level	Performance Accuracy/Million	Defective Performance/Million	Implication for Nursing Practice
1	310,000 (30.9% accuracy)	690,000	309 of 1,000 patient interactions make patients feel that the nurse truly understood their concerns.
2	692,000 (69.2% accuracy)	308,000	692 of 1,000 IVs are inserted successfully on the first attempt.
3	933,200 (93.3% accuracy)	66,800	933 of 1,000 postoperative complications are detected and treated effectively.
4	993,790 (99.4% accuracy)	6,210	994 of 1,000 medications are administered accurately.
5	999,680 (99.98% accuracy)	320	4,999 of 5,000 physician orders are transcribed accurately.
6	999,996.6 (99.9997% accuracy)	3.4	Between three and four errors are made per million patient care documentation entries in medical records.

Adapted from Pande, P., Neuman, R., & Cavanagh, R. (2000). *The Six Sigma way.* New York: McGraw-Hill.

patient and family expectations) and for problem solving (looking for ways to improve effective health care delivery while reducing costs).

Six Sigma uses a cyclical process similar to the PDCA cycle.

1. **Define:** Identify the problem, determine requirements, and set goals.
2. **Measure:** Validate the problem or flawed process, refine problems or goals, and measure key steps and inputs.

3. **Analyze:** Develop causal hypotheses, identify the "vital few" root causes, and validate a causal hypothesis.
4. **Improve:** Develop ideas to eliminate root causes, test solutions, standardize to a single solution, and measure results.
5. **Control:** Establish standard measurements to maintain performance and correct problems as needed.

Six Sigma has one definition: "a business system for achieving and sustaining success through customer focus, process management and improvement, and the

FOCUS ON RESEARCH

Interruptions During Medication Administration: A Descriptive Study

The investigators want to determine what and how many interruptions occur with nurses while they administered medications and the length of time the interruptions consumed during the medication administration process. The investigators employed a descriptive design that collected data using direct observation of nurses while they administered medications using a checklist of commonly encountered interruptions. The investigators watched nurses as they administered medications to 30 patients in 4 different units (2 medical telemetry, 1 medical, and 1 combined medical–oncology unit) at a Magnet© suburban Midwestern hospital. They observed and timed the process of medication administration from when the nurses obtained the medication until the medication administration was documented.

The investigators found that the nurses in the study were interrupted 63% of the time when administering medications. One to two interruptions occurred 33% of the time. Three to five interruptions happened 30% of the time. A single interruption resulted in an increase of an average time increase of 7 minutes. Two interruptions increased the average time to 10.5 minutes. A 16-minute time increase was noted to occur if more than three interruptions occurred. The maximum interruptions were observed during data collection. The most common interruption was the need to retrieve needed supplies for medication administration (43%). Other observed interruptions included

telephone calls, other staff, physicians, families, and other procedures. The day shift nurses experienced all the interruption. The highest number of two or more interruptions occurred during the night shift. In the evening, the only interruptions observed were other staff and telephone calls. Telephone calls were classified as emergent patient care needs, routed to others to address the concern and other (personal phone calls or follow-up calls with extended-care facilities).

Clinical implications of this study reveal the need for nurses to gather all required supplies for medication administration before entering the patient's room, assuring the availability of unlicensed assistive personnel when nurses are scheduled to administer medications, limiting the number of telephone calls during times when nurses are administering medications (phone calls for emergent needs, but text messaging for other needs), and checking the patient schedules to know if patients will be going to other departments before starting medication administration. Interruptions while administering medication prolong the process and increase task complexity thereby increasing the chance of process errors. Results of this study should be exercised with caution because of the small sample size, limitation of observations to one hospital, and the nurses knew that they were being observed. More research is needed to determine what are the major barriers encountered by acute care nurses to complete medication administration in a timely fashion.

Cooper, C. H., Tupper, R., & Holm. L. (2016) Interruptions during medication administration: A descriptive study. *MEDSURG Nursing,* *25*(3), 186–191.

wise use of facts and data" (Pande et al., 2000, p. 3). Six Sigma is tied to the bottom line of the organization because funding efforts for it are based more on the fact than TQM funding, which is based on faith (Chowdhury, 2002; Pande et al., 2000). Six Sigma sets a no-nonsense but ambitious goal of 3.4 defective parts per million opportunities (Chowdhury, 2002; Pande et al., 2000) rather than using **benchmarking** (comparing outcomes or results with those of other similar organizations) systems as indicators for improvement. Six Sigma has the capability to detect incremental and exponential change. TQM/CQI initiatives focus on product quality, whereas Six Sigma solutions attend to all business processes. Six Sigma may hold the key to delighting both patients and nurses in health care environments as Morgan and Cooper (2004) used the process to change the methods for making staff assignments and to increase the availability of patient care supplies. Results of improved work processes included higher consumer satisfaction score, less overtime, and increased job satisfaction (Morgan & Cooper, 2004).

However, the professional nurse's job in the hospital environment remains highly complex. Complex work processes increase the likelihood of errors, especially when nurses experience multiple interruptions when performing essential patient care tasks (see Focus on Research).

▌ QUESTIONS FOR REFLECTION

1. Which of the QI approaches seems the best to you? Why do you think it is superior to the others presented in the chapter?
2. What is the QI approach used in your current clinical practice setting? What QI approaches are used in your nursing program?
3. How have you participated in the QI process in your current clinical practice setting or nursing program?
4. Is it important for nurses or students to participate in the QI process? Why or why not?

IMPLEMENTING CONTINUOUS QUALITY IMPROVEMENT AND TOTAL QUALITY MANAGEMENT

Celebrating Successes

One of Deming's 14 principles for QI is to recognize participants when performance goals are attained (Walton, 1986). Responding to the perception in the 1980s that the American manufacturing industry was trailing the Japanese manufacturing industry,

Congress enacted the "Malcolm Baldrige National Quality Improvement Act" (Public Law 100–107), with the "objective of encouraging American business and other organizations to practice effective quality control in the provision of their goods and services." The law was named after the Secretary of Commerce, who had been killed in a rodeo accident that year and provided funding for recognizing organization who excel in QI implementation. Only two **Malcolm Baldrige National Quality Awards** per category (manufacturing, small business, service, education health care, and nonprofit) can be given in any year (National Institute of Standards & Technology, 2015; Hart & Bogan, 1992).

The National Institute of Standards and Technology (2011) developed the criteria for the award and presents it annually. Criteria for the award are known as the "seven pillars"; they are (1) leadership, (2) strategic planning, (3) customer focus, (4) measurement, analysis and knowledge management, (5) workforce focus, (6) operations focus, and (7) results. Several integrated health care systems and hospitals have won this prestigious award (National Institute of Standards and Technology, 2011).

In addition to the Baldrige National Quality Award, health care systems in most states are eligible for state-sponsored quality award programs. Winning a state or a national quality award serves as a valuable marketing strategy in a health care system increasingly driven by competition and the need to reduce costs (Sultz & Young, 2004).

To showcase the accomplishment of QI goals, some institutions prominently post baseline and improvement data for health care team members and consumers to see. Posters highlighting goal attainment frequently recognize members of process improvement teams. Sometimes, intra-agency publications express appreciation to workers for gains in quality. Ceremonies for nurses and other team members who achieve performance improvement goals provide recognition of those achievements (Sultz & Young, 2004). To inform staff of progress and needed improvements, some units limit their posting of QI data to exclusively staff areas.

Key Concepts of Total Quality Improvement and Other Quality Management Approaches

Total quality improvement (TQI) may be viewed as an organizational value and process to deliver the best possible goods and services to consumers. TQI works to improve constancy in actions while meeting (and exceeding) product and service standards.

TABLE 18.3   Key Principles and Health Care Examples of TQI Based on ISO 9000

TQM/ISO Principle	Goal/Purpose	Examples
Customer focus	Delight external and internal customers.	■ Provide external customers (recipients of health care services) with "the little" extras that make big differences, such as customized menus, backrubs, esthetically appealing rooms. ■ Create and open, trusting work environment for internal customers (physicians, interdisciplinary health care professionals, nursing staff members, and other supportive patient services staff) that encourages collaboration and suggestions to improve work-related processes that are studied and, if feasible, implemented.
Leadership	Provide vision, direction, and understanding of the constancy of purpose among all members of the organization.	■ Empower all workers by inviting them to participate in departmental strategic planning. ■ Provide education about the mission, values, goals, and objectives of the organization to all workers.
Involvement of people	All people within the organization should feel ownership in the TQM values and processes.	■ Form a nursing unit and other departmental-based quality circles. ■ Form interdepartmental and interdisciplinary QI teams to improve work processes that involve more than one department or discipline. ■ Institute interdisciplinary shared governance systems for nursing and other professional disciplines.
Process approach	Desired results are more effectively accomplished when related resources and activities are defined and managed as a process.	■ Constantly monitor organizational performance, comparing results with similar organizations (benchmarking), and share results on a regular basis with all organizational members. ■ Consistently use patient care pathways.
Systems approach to management	Leaders and people in the organization must look outside the organization to plan how best to use physical, monetary, and human resources.	■ Analyze local, regional, and global trends to plan future services. ■ Review and analyze current work processes to determine how to improve health care and health education services. ■ Stay abreast of the latest scientific advancements in disease management, illness prevention, health promotion, and health care delivery.
Continual improvement	Constant improvement becomes a permanent organizational objective.	■ Always look for ways to improve delivery of health care services. ■ Continually reinforce with staff the importance of improving quality via education, informing staff of performance results. ■ Share data with all organizational members who deliver specific services.
Factual approach to decision making	Actual data, current trends, and other forms of objective information serve as the basis for decision making within the organization.	■ Stay informed of current trends and advances in health care. ■ Use data generated by QI processes to guide actions, changes, and plans. ■ Pilot new equipment before making purchases.
Mutually beneficial supplier relationships	The organization forms partnerships with external contractors based on the quality of goods and services they can provide.	■ Identify vendors that provide high-quality products. ■ Secure exclusive purchasing contracts with identified vendors.

Adapted from Institute of Medicine. (2004). *Keeping patients safe: Transforming the work environment of nurses.* Washington, DC: National Academies Press; St. Luke's Hospital of Kansas City Organizational Manual. (2012). Kansas City, MO: Saint Luke's Health System.

All TQI programs focus efforts in the following four areas: (1) customer service (both internal and external customers); (2) ways to improve the quality of key work processes; (3) development and use of quality tools and statistics; and (4) involvement of all people and organizational departments that provide service to the consumer.

Benchmarking

Effectiveness of QI initiatives relies on institutional benchmarking, a process that uses standardized performance evaluation tools and compares results within the institution (to track gains in quality) or with similar institutions (to determine how well the organization is performing against others). One tool used to evaluate quality is a balanced scorecard system that examines performance in the four following areas: consumer satisfaction, financial performance and stability, use of clinical services and outcomes, and change and system integration (Hall, Peterson, Baker, 2007; Sultz & Young, 2004). When performance fails to reach the benchmark, all people within the organization work together to fix the work process rather than blaming individuals or each other.

ISO 9000

The International Organization for Standardization (ISO) is a nongovernmental organization composed of a network of national standards institutes from 146 countries. Its goal is to set international standards for all businesses and for the broader needs of the global human society. ISO standards benefit society by prompting fair trade; compatibility of technology; conformity of consumer products in terms of safety, quality, and reliability; and scientific knowledge and technology for health; and provide guidelines to prevent global environmental contamination (ISO, 2017). The ISO outlines eight key principles for TQM known as ISO 9000, which ensures consistency among all international efforts aimed at TQM, CQI, and TQI (Table 18.3).

TQM/CQI Processes in Health Care

Key principles of TQI consider people who receive services and attend to people providing services. Therefore, TQI enhances the health care delivery experience for everyone.

TQM/CQI places consumers first. People providing services seek to find ways to streamline work processes. Deming proposed that more complex work processes have a greater chance for error. Consistency of action reduces error rates (Sultz & Young, 2004; Walton, 1986). TQM/CQI programs use a variety of instruments to identify variations in work processes (Table 18.4). With the exception of regression analysis, most of the instruments diagram the steps of a given process, thereby providing QI team members with a picture and facilitating identification of variations along with potential sources for error.

Once the work process has been fully described, participants in the TQM/CQI process can proceed to implement the Deming PDCA cycle. Note that the process starts with planning, requires implementation of plans, and concludes with the final step that restarts the cycle by looking for ways to improve the process. Concepts in Practice provides an example of the TQM/CQI process in action.

Concepts in Practice IDEA ⟶ PLAN ⟶ ACTION

Use of the TQM/CQI Process to Reduce Medication Errors

The following example shows how Laura, the nurse presented at the beginning of the chapter, and the nursing department where she works could use TQM/CQI to avoid the problem of medication errors.

- Step 1: Identify a work process to be improved—Accuracy of antibiotic administration.
- Step 2: Organize a CQI/TQM team—Select health team members to serve on the CQI/TQM team who are involved in this work process. In this case, members would include a physician who writes antibiotic orders, a unit secretary who transcribes the physician order, a pharmacist who fills the order, a courier who delivers daily doses to the nursing units, two nurses who verify the physician order and administers the antibiotics to patients.
- Step 3: Clarify the current work process—The team meets and diagrams the current process from the time the order is written until the patient receives the ordered medication.
- Step 4: Identify and understand all variation sources—The team notices that six people are involved in the process of antibiotic administration (physician, unit secretary, pharmacist [who reviews the patient data, validates that it is safe for the patient to receive the medication, and enters it into the patient electronic medication administration record], another pharmacist [who mixes and prepares the IV antibiotic and places it in the box for delivery to the nursing unit], the pharmacy courier [who delivers the medication to the unit] and the nurse who administers the antibiotic dose to the patient). The team also notes that antibiotic orders may be written at any time during the day, leading to scheduling issues. The team analyzes all the medication incident reports filed related to antibiotic administration to confirm the information generated from the brainstorming session. In addition, the team creates a checklist for collecting data regarding administration of intravenous antibiotics in the 2 weeks before the next meeting.
- Step 5: Select the improvement—The team discovers after its data collection that delay in administration was a prevalent quality problem. Therefore, the team decides that perhaps commonly administered dosages could be placed in the computerized medication-dispensing station so that the nurse can access it more readily and not have to wait for unit delivery. Another suggestion is that nurses on the unit should notify at least two nursing colleagues when they leave the unit for more than 5 minutes and inform their colleagues of any patient care needs, especially antibiotic administration.

- Step 6: Implement the improvement—The nurses obtain ordered antibiotic doses from the computerized medication-dispensing system and comply with the recommended notification of other nurses when leaving the unit for longer than 5 minutes.
- Step 7: Check and compare results with desired outcome—Within a month of implementing step 6, the number of incident reports filed related to antibiotic administration decreases by 80%.
- Step 8: Take steps to maintain improved performance and suggest ways to further improve the process—Proposals are made for hospital-wide implementation. The first proposal is that all nurses will contact a minimum of two other nurses on the unit when leaving the unit for more than 5 minutes and provide them with the status of medication administration and other patient care needs. The second proposal is that commonly ordered antibiotics will be placed in all hospital-computerized medication dispensing systems.

Using a TQM/CQI approach, Laura does not receive a reprimand for missing the ordered dose of antibiotics; rather, work processes are found that contributed to her error. In health care, the professional nurse plays a pivotal role in TQM/CQI.

To recognize their success in implementing the TQM/CQI project, the hospital acknowledges contributions of the QI team in the organizational newsletter. The team also posts graphs indicating reduction in warfarin administration errors in the staff lounge of the cardiac unit.

▌ QUESTIONS FOR REFLECTION

1. What do you like about using a CQI/TQM process when quality issues arise in health care delivery?
2. What are the benefits of the process?
3. What barriers might interfere with the process?
4. Would you be willing to participate as a CQI/TQM team member? Why or why not?

EFFORTS TO IMPROVE THE QUALITY OF HEALTH CARE

In 1986, a group of health care providers saw the gap between ideal and actual health care safety and quality. Their efforts to improve health care for all people worldwide led to the formation of the IHI a nonprofit organization that works collaboratively with professional health care teams to establish a scientific foundation for improving the quality and safety of health care delivery (IHI, 2016). Using the goals outlined by the IOM, the IHI developed a "Always Events" list that capture what is vitally essential to patients and families when they receive health care to a "Never Event: list that is an event that results in a patient death, permanent disability or severe, intense suffering of any nature" (Balik, 2016). The IHI also addresses helplessness in health care consumers and providers, undesirable waiting for services, wasteful expenditure of health care resources and denial of access to care (IHI, 2016). The IHI strives to re-instill the passion that health care professionals have toward their work.

Some of the key IHI contributions to health care that have become practice standards include the Ventilator Bundle (specific care protocols for people on respirators), Applying Operations Research to Healthcare, Transitions Home Program (a program that reduces hospital readmission rates and improves patient outcomes), Rapid Response Teams, and Medication Reconciliation Process (IHI, 2010). The IHI offers free information and education for health care professionals and students about how to improve quality and safety in health care, and coordinates interprofessional QI teams.

Many agencies and organizations have developed indicators of quality health care in terms of processes and outcomes. The NQF was established in 1999 in response to the President's Advisory Commission on Consumer Protection and Quality in the Healthcare Industry; its mission is to standardize health quality measurement and reporting. The NQF tabulates data from multiple databases and publishes reports on the quality of health care services at a national and local level. The organization provides consumers with online information regarding the quality of institutions, organizations, and agencies that provide health care services.

In 2003, JCAHO (now the Joint Commission) and the CMS collaborated to identify and deliver core measures for use by both agencies for measuring quality of health care services. The 2012 core measure sets address improvements in surgical care (Surgical Care Improvement Project), substance use and prevention, tobacco cessation education and treatment, prevention of venous thromboembolism, prevention of nosocomial pneumonia, management of acute myocardial infarction, immunization compliance, management of heart failure, asthma care in children, hospital-based inpatient psychiatric services, perinatal care, management of stroke, and hospital outpatient department care (The Joint Commission, 2013a). Each core measures set identifies multiple key interventions (a range of 5 to 24 interventions per core measure) that must occur based on evidence from the Agency for Healthcare

TABLE 18.4 Instruments Used in TQM/CQI Programs

Instrument	Description	Advantages
Check sheet	Generic instrument to collect data over time to identify "patterns, trends, defects, or causes of defects" (Joshi, Ransom, Nash, et al. 2014, p. 94).	Excellent for tracking progress over time and captured data easily converted to visual tool such as a histogram or Pareto chart.
Five Whys	Asking repetitive why questions helps to drill down to identify the flaws in a process or design failure to identify the root care. Caution is needed to cease prematurely which may result in failure or misidentification of a root cause.	Provides a structured process to identify a root cause.
Flowchart	Graphic representation of a sequence of events required to attain a specific outcome. Specific symbols depict steps of a process (e.g., rectangle, activity; diamond-shaped polygon, decision; triangle, wait; large circle, file; small circle, go to another point); arrows indicate the direction of the overall process. Symbols may vary according to organizational practices.	Easily identifies sources of variation and easily updated to remain current.
Fishbone diagram	A horizontal line depicts the work process with the desired outcome appearing at the far left side of the diagram. Inputs into the work process are represented as lines (or spines) that intersect the horizontal line drawn obliquely from the baseline in upward or downward directions. The diagram looks like a fish skeleton.	Great for depicting work processes during brainstorming sessions, readily stratified to show details. Easy to identify causes and effects in a work process.
Run chart	Displays the frequency of events or a particular observation over time. Frequency counts are connected by a line.	Wonderful way to depict data alterations arising from changes and key for determining whether improvements have resulted from changes.
Pareto chart	Displays data using a rank order. Factors with the most frequent observation appear first, followed by less frequent observations.	Offers the ability to stratify causes and identify the top causes, helpful to prioritize changes and useful to show results of changes.
Histogram	Bar-type graph that displays the frequency of something occurring.	Offers the ability to detect the frequency of root causes in a process and useful for tracking results of changes.
Control chart	Depicted as a run chart, but with statistically determined upper and lower limits of variation above and below the average performance.	Essential to see if the process remains under control.
Scatter diagram	A point is placed across a vertical and horizontal axis to demonstrate the relationship between two variables.	Useful to see if any relationships between two variables are occurring to detect causes and monitor the effects of changes.
Regression analysis	Statistical testing of correlational models.	Tests hypothesis used by organizations for decision making.

Adapted from Joshi, M. S., Ransom, E. R., Nash, D. B, & Ransom, S. B. (2014). *The healthcare quality book, vision strategy and tools* (3rd ed.). Chicago: Health Administration Press & Arlington, VA: Association of University Programs in Health Administration; Koch, M., & Fairly, T. (1993). *Integrated quality management, the key to improving nursing care quality.* St. Louis: Mosby; and McLaughlin, C., & Kaluzny, A. (1999). *Continuous quality improvement in healthcare* (2nd ed.). Gaithersburg, MD: Aspen.

Research and Quality that constitutes "best practices"; these, in turn, are based on meta-analyses of research studies including outcomes-based research. Nurses meticulously document key assessments and interventions on patient electronic health records following requirements of core measure sets, thereby increasing the number of required documentation entries. Hospitals collect data on each core measure in the electronic health records of patients and submit reports to the NQF, which compiles all the data.

The Joint Commission (2013c) issues an annual report on efforts to improve American hospitals that lists the top performers among accredited hospitals by using a program called ORYX® that integrates patient outcomes and other performance measures with the accreditation process. The results of hospital outcomes are published by the Joint Commission online in Quality Check® and help health care consumers to compare the quality of accredited hospitals and other health care facilities online (www.qualitycheck.org). The

Joint Commission also certifies health care organization according to specific diseases such as stroke, heart failure, acute myocardial infarction, chronic obstructive pulmonary disease, and inpatient diabetes management (The Joint Commission, 2017). The Joint Commission also lists certified specialty disease centers on its website.

In 2005, the NQF endorsed the Hospital Consumer Assessment of Healthcare Providers and Systems (HCAHPS) Survey to collect data regarding the quality of health care received by consumers in hospitals. The HCAHPS survey was developed by the Center for Medicare and Medicaid Services (CMS) in 2005 to collect information about the hospital experiences of program recipients. The survey includes 27 items, 18 of which request patient perspectives of care in the following 8 areas: communication with physicians, communication with nurses, hospital staff responsiveness, pain management, communication about prescribed medications, discharge information, environmental cleanliness, and hospital environmental quietness. The survey also collects four screener questions and five patient demographic items (CMS, 2012). Under the implementation of the Patient Protection and Affordable Care Act, Medicare and Medicaid reimbursement rates to hospitals will be adjusted based on HCAHPS survey scores. Higher scores mean higher rates of reimbursement. Hospital administrators and nurse managers have begun directing staff to use key phrases when communicating with patients, families, and visitors so that they will be able to answer HCAHPS items correctly. For example, when a nurse provides dismissal instructions to a patient (or family member), the nurse needs to use the term "side effect" when discussing prescribed medications at home.

PROFESSIONAL NURSING ROLES IN QUALITY IMPROVEMENT

TQM/CQI provides professional nurses with an opportunity to showcase the unique contributions they make to interdisciplinary health care delivery. Because nurses have always been concerned with patient safety and quality of care, they can assume leadership roles in TQM/CQI processes. Data collection by nurses as part of routine care delivery sometimes identifies a quality initiative (an area for improvement). In addition, the professional nurse serves as a key player in developing work processes and strategies to improve care quality. The following discussion outlines how nurses might use professional nursing roles to promote QI.

Role of Caregiver

Professional nursing continues to study the effects of nursing care on patient outcomes. Patient outcomes that arise directly from nursing assessment and intervention are known as **nursing-sensitive outcomes**. Box 18.3, Professional Building Blocks, displays nursing-sensitive

18.3 Professional Building Blocks

Patient-Related Nursing-Sensitive Outcomes

- Safety from medication and other treatment-related errors
- Functional status
- Self-care
- Effective symptom management
- Effective pain management
- Satisfaction with received health care services
- Effective management of fatigue
- Effective management of nausea and vomiting
- Effective management of dyspnea
- Early detection and effective management of postoperative complications
- Reduced incidence of urinary tract infections
- Reduced incidence of pneumonia
- Increased incidence of successful rescue following cardiac or respiratory arrest
- Reduced rate of injury from falling
- Reduced rates of institutionally acquired pressure ulcers
- Reduced use of physical or chemical restraints
- Reduced incidence of bloodstream infections from central line use
- Failure to rescue

National Quality Forum Nursing-Sensitive Measures
- Hospital-acquired pressure ulcers
- Nursing staff skill mix
- Nursing hours per patient day
- RN Survey: Practice Environment Scale
- Restraint use prevalence
- Nurse turnover
- Ventilator-associated pneumonia
- Central line–associated bloodstream infection
- Catheter-associated urinary tract infections

Adapted from Doran, D. (Ed.). (2003). *Nursing-sensitive outcomes: The state of the science.* Sudbury, MA: Jones & Bartlett; Dunton, N. (2008). Take a cue from the NDNQI. *Nursing Management, 39*(4), 20, 22, 23; Institute of Medicine. (2004). *Keeping patients safe.* Washington, DC: National Academies Press; and Dunton, J. Montalvo, I. & Dunton, N. (2011). *NDNQI Case studies in nursing quality improvement.* Silver Spring, MD: American Nurses Association; National Quality Forum (2016) Reports. Retrieved from http://www.qualityforum.org/Publications.aspx. Accessed June 26, 2016.

outcomes that have been identified to date. Most of these outcomes have been identified through nursing research or comprehensive literature reviews of nursing research studies examining the impact of professional nursing care on patient outcomes (Doran, 2003; Dunton, 2008; Dunton, Montalvo, & Dunton, 2011). Research suggests that the increased presence of RNs and RNs with specialty certification improves patient outcomes, reduces hospital-acquired complications, and decreases health care costs (Boltz, Capezuti, Fulmer, & Zwicker, 2012; Park, Blegen, Spetz, Chapman, & De Groot, 2012; Roche, Duffield, Aisbett, Diers, & Stasa, 2012; Twigg, Duffield, Bremmer, Rapley, & Finn, 2012).

The ANA (2015) incorporates nurse participation in QI programs as a required professional practice standard (Standard 14, Quality of Practice). Required QI competencies include identifying areas of practice for quality monitoring; using indicators to monitor the quality, safety, and effectiveness of practice; collecting, analyzing, and interpreting data to improve practice; developing, implementing, and evaluating policies, procedures, and guidelines to improve quality of practice; and analyzing factors, systems, and processes to remove barriers to safety and quality. To practice ethically, nurses must assert themselves when needed to question practices that may endanger patient safety, jeopardize the best interests of consumers, or affect QI (Standard 7, Ethics).

To facilitate nurse attainment of Standard 14, the ANA has compiled the National Database of Nursing Quality Indicators (NDNQI), which addresses the structures, processes, and outcomes of nursing care. The database collects information and reports some findings to the NQF. Specific data collected by the NDNQI include information on patient falls, fall injuries, pressure ulcers, physical/sexual assault, all aspects of pain assessment and management, peripheral IV infiltration, use of physical restraints, health care–associated infections (central line, ventilator-associated pneumonia, catheter-associated urinary tract infections); nursing staff mix; nursing care hours provided per patient day, nurse turnover, RN education/certification, and RN practice environment scales and job satisfaction (ANA, 2010). In 2014, Press Ganey acquired the NDNQI from the ANA (Press Ganey, 2015).

In daily practice, nurses collect data that substantiate adherence to Centers for Disease Control and Prevention (CDC) and institutional standards for care when they document routine care processes. Some institutions have a quality council that determines what work processes need evaluation to determine QI opportunities. For example, for hospitals to receive third-party reimbursement for IV tubing and supplies, the information must be documented in patient medical records. If a hospital is interested in determining how well nurses are following CDC and institutional standards for IV therapy, the nurse working at the bedside is the best qualified person to perform electronic health record audits (a review of records) to identify when nurses are changing IV sites and tubing. After audit data are tabulated, nurses receive the results. If results reveal that standards are not being followed, a QI team analyzes the work processes for changing IV sites and tubing. Depending on the outcome of the analysis, the team then determines how to change work processes and provides staff education to ensure that all nurses follow outlined processes rather than taking shortcuts. However, if the chart audits reveal that the performance meets or exceeds the desired performance, some form of recognition is given to the staff responsible for effective IV management.

Because cost-effectiveness has been identified as an indicator of quality health care, nurses in clinical practice look for ways to use human and material resources judiciously. Professional nurses use cost-effective strategies when they take time to attend to the little details associated with care delivery that, if ignored, could result in poor patient outcomes.

Role of Critical Thinker

Critical thinking is an essential cognitive skill used by nurses in clinical decision making. To ensure safe and quality nursing care delivery, professional nurses engage in multiple activities requiring critical thinking, from determining what assessments are appropriate for a clinical situation to evaluating how well patients have met desired care outcomes.

The process of safe administration of medication provides a key example of how nurses use critical thinking to promote high-quality care and identify areas for QI. Medication administration, an activity frequently performed by nurses, poses great risks to patients. More than 770,000 people die or suffer irreversible injury annually because of adverse drug events (including medication errors) (IOM, 2004). Causes of medication errors include prescription errors; increased nurse responsibility for knowing medication dosages, action, and potential adverse effects; errors in calculated dosages; and nurse interruptions (Cohen, Robinson, & Mandrack, 2003;

IOM, 2004). Work-related processes identified by nurses as contributing to medication errors included being distracted or interrupted when administering medication, having inadequate staff, caring for high numbers of patients, reading illegible medication orders, working with medications with similar names and packaging, and having incorrect dosage calculations. The IOM (2004) also identified problems with miscommunication, lack of patient information, infusion pump malfunctions, and IV delivery (extravasations, incompatibility of medications, diluents, and ordered fluids).

Nurses use critical thinking to develop theoretical approaches to evaluate and improve the quality of nursing care (Sidani, Doran, & Mitchell, 2004). Five key characteristics produce direct effects on patient outcomes, thereby accounting for individual and variable responses to nursing and health care interventions.

1. **Patient characteristics:** Personal, sociocultural, and health-related factors
2. **Professional characteristics:** Personal factors (dedication, commitment, and finding meaning in work), educational preparation, keeping current with new practice advances, and sociocultural factors
3. **Health care setting:** Physical layout, availability of supplies, and organizational culture
4. **Health care interventions for patient:** Invasiveness, risks, type, and if individualized to specific patient
5. **Nature and timing or attainment of expected outcomes for health care interventions**

Sidani et al. (2004) also identified two forms of indirect effects: "moderating and mediating" (p. 61). Moderating effects address the effectiveness of care to produce desired outcomes according to different levels of the five factors. An example of this would be how soon a patient admitted to the hospital for a severe infection receives the first dose of an antibiotic. Mediating effects explain variance based on all factor effects on the intervention provided to the patient (see Concepts in Practice).

A nursing-specific theoretical approach to evaluate nursing care is more valuable to nurses than relying on approaches used by medicine or business. As critical thinkers, nurses who use a theoretical approach can generate questions to gather data for a holistic approach to nursing care concerns and choose instruments to consistently measure the effects of nursing care. A theoretical approach also fosters an understanding of the unique contributions nurses make in the health care

Concepts in Practice [IDEA]→[PLAN]→[ACTION]

Mediating Variables in a Patient Case

Mr. Jones is a patient with a pre-existing condition of diabetes and knows that recovering from an infection is a complex process. He notices that his right leg has become very warm, red and swollen after his beloved cat scratched him 3 days ago. He opts to seek care for the infection in a large teaching hospital where there will be multiple specialty physicians available to attend to the complex needs, especially an endocrinologist who will manage his blood sugar.

Mr. Jones knows that in patients with limited veins in which to start an IV for antibiotics, the hospital uses an IV team to initiate IV lines. He anticipates being on antibiotics for a long time and will request the insertion of a peripherally inserted central catheter (PICC) so that the number of sticks to maintain an IV line will be limited.

Mr. Jones is admitted to the hospital and his antibiotics are not started until 6 hours after admission because of the need for the IV team to insert a PICC. Knowing the risks of bloodstream infections with central catheter use, Eugenia the nurse recognizes that Mr. Jones will be at higher risk for a blood stream infection because of his diabetes. She also realizes that the delay in starting the antibiotic means that Mr. Jones also has an increased risk of systemic complication from his right leg cellulitis.

setting. A consistent approach to evaluating nursing care fosters QI initiatives because comparisons can be tracked over time.

Role of Patient Advocate

Nurses work endlessly to consider the patient's best interests. When participating in QI activities, nurses advocate for all patients. Improvements in work processes reduce care errors.

For example, nurses who acknowledge the effects of physical and mental fatigue advocate for patients when they refuse to work overtime. Nurses who provide direct patient care services for 12.5 hours or longer triple the chance for making errors (Rogers, Hwang, Scott, Aiken, & Dinges, 2004). Working extra shifts also increases the chance for committing nursing care errors (IOM, 2004; Rogers et al., 2004). However, despite the research evidence linking long shifts and overtime to nursing errors, some nurses volunteer for overtime shifts to fill staffing shortages. Some institutions require nurses to work overtime. Many nurses consider long hours and overtime acceptable and agree to work them despite the effects of fatigue on judgment (Leighty, 2004). Nurses who refuse extra shifts may be perceived as not being good members of the nursing care team. Nevertheless, refusing to work long hours and overtime may be the best way to prevent nursing care errors, increasing the quality of health care services while ultimately looking out for the patient's best interest.

Role of Change Agent

Professional nurses act as change agents when they identify needed changes in work processes to improve the quality of nursing care. Change occurs rapidly in the health care arena. As new health care devices, medications, and treatment advances become available, nurses need to change practice procedures. Because they are stakeholders in the delivery of health care services, nurses must continuously determine which rituals and routines remain applicable and which should be discarded (Porter-O'Grady & Malloch, 2015).

As leaders of a nursing care team, professional nurses must clearly communicate changes in practice procedures to all team members. Some staff members (especially those who have worked in nursing for a long time) need to learn new approaches, new skills, and new equipment procedures. Replacing traditional practice may create distress for some older nurses. Successful integration of change requires that the innovation fits well with the practice setting, has congruence with staff roles, improves patient outcomes, and complements values and beliefs. Empowering staff to make work-related decisions and empowering patients to assume responsibility for their own health increases the chance of successful change (Porter-O'Grady & Malloch, 2015). Because change requires unlearning old ways and learning new ones, the role of counselor/teacher becomes critical.

Role of Counselor/Teacher

Before adopting an innovation, the staff must be educated about the reasons for the innovation, changes in practice policies, and how to operate new equipment (if applicable). Staff educational programs may be planned using the teaching/learning principles outlined in Chapter 17, Leadership and Management in Professional Nursing. Interdepartmental educational programs provide staff with the opportunity

to network, share successes with change, and support each other.

Along with education, nurses and other care providers need emotional support during times of nonstop change. Psychological effects of change have been delineated in Chapter 17, Leadership and Management in Professional Nursing.

Staff need time to grieve for the way things have been done traditionally before they can fully embrace innovations. When the innovation process becomes tough or stuck, staff relationships may be the only glue holding the nursing care team together. Taking time to listen to peers and team members fosters capturing the messages and the meanings that surround continual change processes associated with TQM/CQI programs (Porter-O'Grady & Malloch, 2015).

Role of Coordinator

As coordinators of care, professional nurses must seek ways to provide quality of care while using resources effectively. Nursing unit characteristics directly affect patient outcomes. Increased nurse perception of autonomy/collaboration has been instrumental in reducing incidences of urinary tract infections and failure-to-rescue events. When specialized nurses provide care with continuity, lower rates of pneumonia and cardiac arrests are reported along with shorter length of hospital stays. Likewise, high levels of nurse manager support have been associated with reduced levels of pressure ulcer prevalence in patients and patient mortality (Aiken, Smith, & Lake, 1994, 2000; Boyle, 2004; Haven & Aiken, 1999; Twigg, Duffield, Bremmer, et al., 2012).

Role of Colleague

The American way of life values independence and self-sufficiency. Nurses frequently have a strong sense of responsibility for individual vigilance that accentuates independence and self-sufficiency. Some nurses believe that asking for help with patient assignments might be viewed as a sign of incompetence, while others are afraid of being perceived as being weak if they need to ask for assistance with a problem (Tucker & Edmondson, 2003). The QI process discourages this form of thinking, instead giving all health team members the responsibility to point out work process flaws.

As a colleague on an interdisciplinary (multidisciplinary or interprofessional) health care team, nurses have an equal responsibility to engage in collaboration with team members to promote safe, effective health care delivery. Nurses have the responsibility to share concerns about patients when they arise with other members of the health care team.

Establishment of a culture of safety in health care organizations requires trust among nurses, physicians, hospital administration, and all health team members. A culture of safety uses errors as an opportunity for learning rather than blaming. Team training for patient emergencies using simulated experiences helps team members identify each other's roles, learn how to best execute their roles confidently, create a venue to dispel stereotypes associated with each team member, and provide an opportunity for collegial networking (Barnsteiner, Disch, Hall, Mayer, & Moore, 2007; Finkleman & Kenner, 2007; Grey & Connolly, 2008; Weaver, 2008).

When flaws are identified with work processes, multidisciplinary QI teams are formed. Participation in the QI project team provides opportunities for nurses to network with other members of the health care team, thereby strengthening working relationships with them. During team deliberations, members of the QI team have opportunities to see and value the unique skills and approaches they bring to patient health care delivery.

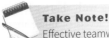

Take Note!
Effective teamwork facilitates safety and quality in health care.

▍ Questions for Reflection

1. Can you think of other roles held by nurses that might affect QI efforts?
2. Which of the nursing roles discussed above do you believe is most critical to QI? Why?

AN INTEGRATED APPROACH TO QUALITY IMPROVEMENT AND SAFETY IN HEALTH CARE

Since the inception of their profession, nurses have assumed the obligation of keeping patients safe. Improving the quality and safety of health care requires a fully integrated approach from all stakeholders. QI initiatives from various stakeholders tend to overlap. Table 18.5 compares and contrasts QI and safety programs from the IOM, reports (primarily physician-based), QSEN competencies, and the

Joint Commission accreditation standards and safety goals. QSEN opted to separate safety from quality because nurses traditionally have assumed the role of patient advocate. Nurse educators establish desired knowledge, skills, and attitudes associated with each QSEN competency to provide guidance for basic and continuing nursing education. The competencies, standards, and safety goals of these organizations cross the entire health care continuum; although they differ slightly, improving the quality and safety of health care delivery is the ultimate goal of each group.

Effectiveness and safety serve as two hallmarks of quality health care (Finkleman & Kenner, 2007). To ensure fiscally responsible tax expenditures, the federal government no longer covers expenses incurred from hospital-acquired injuries and illnesses. The government also bestows awards (e.g., the Baldrige National Quality Award) and recognizes health care organizations by publishing lists for consumer use to facilitate decision making about where to access quality health care. The Joint Commission also publishes and posts online lists of fully accredited providers, along with deficiencies found in others. For-profit health care insurance companies sometimes follow the lead of the federal government in cutting health care costs.

Consumers play a key role in QI and safety in health care. When they enter the health care system, consumers must communicate their needs to providers. Consumers also need to freely share all information (such as a complete list of all medications, including those obtained over the counter, herbal supplements, and other home remedies) that could impact the health care provider's decisions for a safe treatment plan. Consumers are more apt to share detailed information when providers develop helping and healing relationships with them (see Chapter 4, Establishing Helping and Healing Relationships). Along with freely shared information about themselves, consumers provide valuable input into health care delivery processes when they complete satisfaction questionnaires for rendered services.

The development of a culture of safety and quality may mean that some stakeholders might have to change behaviors and attitudes. When all have access to knowledge and take time to listen to each other, health care safety and quality improve. Everyone involved in health care delivery becomes capable of making evidence-based decisions. Evidence ranges from individual patient values and preferences to a

TABLE 18.5 Improving the Quality of Health Care: Comparing and Contrasting Recommendations of the Institute of Medicine (IOM), Quality and Safety in Nursing Education (QSEN), and The Joint Commission

Key Consideration	IOM	QSEN Competencies	Selected Joint Commission Standards and Goals
Keeping health care services focused on consumers/ patients	*Provide patient-centered care* Pros and cons of decentralized care Fragmentation of care Self-management support Health care literacy Effective use of interpreters Patient health information Family and/or caregiver preparation Consumer perceptions of health care needs Care coordination	*Patient-centered care* Acknowledgment of the patient (or designated other) is the course of control Compassionate, coordinated care is delivered in full partnership with the patient (or designee) Care is planned and delivered considering patient values, preferences, and needs	Standards address the need for care, treatment, and services based on assessment of patient needs, individualizing the treatment or care plan based on identified patient strengths and weaknesses along with relevant health education for patient self-care based on patient ability, educational level, reading ability, and language National standards for culturally and linguistically appropriate services in health care Reconciliation of all medications across the care continuum Facilitate patients' active involvement in their care as a strategy to promote patient safety Required screening for patient and family complaints
Use special expertise to foster the best possible care across the care continuum for consumers of health care services	*Work on interdisciplinary teams* Creation of a culture of safety Development of an environment of learning rather than blaming Team learning, education, and training Adaptation to constant change	*Teamwork and collaboration* Team efforts are aimed at attaining high-quality patient care Nurses communicate and function as effective teams with each other Nurses function effectively in interprofessional teams Effective teamwork is characterized by open communication, mutual respect, and shared decision making	A nurse executive serves as a senior leader and provides effective leadership to coordinate nursing care treatment and services Nurse executives are licensed professional nurses, have advanced education (graduate or postgraduate degree in nursing or a related field), and have managerial experience A nurse executive directs and establishes guidelines for nursing care, treatment, and services, while directing nursing standards, policies, procedures, and staffing plans Improve communication among caregivers, including written or computer-entered physician orders, read-back-order verification for telephone orders, and test results along with mechanisms to document the read-back procedure Standardized hand-off communication procedures that include time for asking and responding to questions Emergency department guidelines for nutritional screening, immunization status, and repeated visits Required screening for facility selection of human resource indicators (e.g., overtime, staffing plan, staff injury, and nursing care hours per patient day)

(continued on page 500)

TABLE 18.5 Improving the Quality of Health Care: Comparing and Contrasting Recommendations of the Institute of Medicine (IOM), Quality, and Safety in Nursing Education (QSEN), and The Joint Commission *(continued)*

Key Consideration	IOM	QSEN Competencies	Selected Joint Commission Standards and Goals
Decision making by using all possible forms of evidence to provide the best possible outcomes for recipients of health care services	*Employ evidence-based practice* Use of evidence-based practice resources Involvement in quality and safety research projects Evaluating evidence (systematic literature reviews and research studies)	*Evidence-based practice* Integration of best current evidence, nurse clinical expertise, and patient preferences and values to deliver optimal health care	Implement best practices or evidence-based guidelines to manage central lines and prevent surgical site infections Health professional access to the latest developments in health care delivery and methods to facilitate optimal patient outcomes Evidence of multidisciplinary approaches to manage complex patient situations
Provide the safest and best quality care possible	*Apply quality improvement* Error management (analysis of actual errors, human factors, generation of solutions, and legal issues) The Joint Commission and QI (informed about latest standards) Medication administration (increased use of drugs, multiple-drug use in a single patient, medication administration processes, preventing adverse drug events, collaborative approaches to medication management, and effective medication management) Safety in Care Plan (avoiding wrong-site surgeries, preventing falls, setting safety standards, containing infections, attending mortality and morbidity conferences, participating in risk management programs, accessing standards of care and clinical guidelines, and making safety an essential staff competency)	*Quality improvement* Use data to assess outcomes of care delivery processes Use QI method cycles (plan, do, check, act) to test proposed changes before making them standard practices for improving the safety and quality of health care systems *Safety (set as a separate competency because of longstanding nurse professional responsibility to keep patients safe)* Analyze individual effectiveness strategies to keep patients and providers safe Analyze system process to keep patients and providers safe	Use of a minimum of two patient identifiers when giving medication, blood, or blood components; acquiring lab specimens; and providing treatments or procedures Use of a standardized list of abbreviations that do not contain dangerous abbreviations, symbols, and designations for medication dosages Procedures for reporting critical results and values along with processes for measuring desired outcomes Limit the use of look-alike–sound-alike medications to a total of 10 Labeling of all medications, medication cups, syringes, and solutions (on and off sterile fields) Standardized protocols for anticoagulation therapy Compliance with CDC or WHO hand hygiene and infection control practice guidelines Root cause analysis of sentinel events Fall reduction risk program Programs for improved early recognition and response to patient condition changes Preprocedure verification process following a universal protocol prior to invasive procedures that include a "time out" before a procedure is started
Integration of available technology to provide optimal safe health care services across the health care continuum	*Utilize informatics* Clinical computer information systems that share patient information across the care continuum Use computer-based reminder systems Use computers as a means to access comprehensive patient information. Clinical decision-making support programs	*Informatics* Utilize information systems to facilitate knowledge communication and management Use technology and information systems to prevent and mitigate errors Use technology and information systems as resources to support clinical decisions	ORYX™ is an outcome and performance measurement system for monitoring patient outcomes with an emphasis on optimal outcome attainment Computerized system required to track errors and near misses that occur in care delivery Ownership or access to knowledge-based information using systems, resources, and services for health care professionals to access the latest information, produce optimal patient outcomes, avoid adverse events in the facility, provide needed education and information to patients (and significant others) and satisfy professional research-related needs

Key Consideration	IOM	QSEN Competencies	Selected Joint Commission Standards and Goals
Ethical care delivery	*No competency outlined by IOM; however, one of the 10 rules that apply to the core IOM competencies, need for transparency* Collaborative teamwork Privacy of protected health information Transformational leadership Maximal use of workforce capability, including safe staffing levels, knowledge and skill acquisition, collaborative skills, verbal abuse management, interdisciplinary team forums, and work process and workspace designs (work hours, medication delivery systems, transfers, paperwork, physical layout of workspaces, use of contingent workers, development of learning organizations, and revival of nurse internships and residencies)	*No competency identified*	Accreditation standards address ethical behavior in the delivery of care services, patient decision making, patient rights, and need for effective communication Hospital standards for frequent repeated emergency visits by a single patient and readmissions to confront access to and use of health care services Short-term and long-term planning for meeting the needs of consumer base such as continued service programs, plans to expand services, and/or considerations for and actual discontinuation of provided services

Adapted from Cronenwett, L., Sherwood, G., Barnsteiner, J., et al. (2007). *Teaching IOM: Implications of the Institute of Medicine reports for nursing education.* Silver Spring, MD: American Nurses Association; The Joint Commission (2016). 2016 National Patient Safety Goals (2016). Retrieved from https://www.jointcommission.org/assets/1/6/2016_NPSG_HAP_ER.pdf. Accessed June 26, 2016.; The Joint Commission. (2015a). Joint Commission Measure Sets Effective January 1, 2016. Retrieved from https://www.jointcommission.org/joint_commission_measure_sets_effective_january_1_2016/3. Accessed June 26, 2016.

meta-analysis of research studies and/or clinical trials to determine best practices.

Take Note!

Many people play key roles in developing and maintaining a culture of safety and quality for health care.

Summary and Significance to Practice

The process of delivering high-quality and safe health care is highly complex. Professional nurses use cognitive, communication, and clinical skills when working as partners with patients and in multidisciplinary teams. TQM/CQI programs look for opportunities to change the processes of health care delivery in order to improve safety, effectiveness, patient focus, and efficiency. When nurses and health team members subscribe to a TQM/CQI approach, they constantly look for ways to improve care delivery. Professional nurses bring a unique perspective and offer valuable skills to enhance health care quality. All health team members must be invested in developing and maintaining a culture of safety and QI.

REAL-LIFE REFLECTIONS

Recall Laura from the beginning of the chapter, who was unable to administer the patient antibiotic as ordered. What advice would you give her based on the information presented in this chapter? Do you feel that writing a care variance report is a sign of professional weakness? Why or why not? What suggestions would you make to improve unit practices to prevent a similar error from occurring again?

From Theory to Practice

1. Do you think the health care industry should be held to the same quality standards as those in big business and industry? Why or why not?
2. How would you have to change your practice and practice environment to strive toward attaining the same level of quality that is required of the business and manufacturing industries?

3. How does your clinical practice setting view incident reports? What are the advantages of having staff complete incident reports for quality monitoring purposes? Are you afraid to complete incident reports? Why or why not?

4. How would you change your nursing program to improve its quality? What steps would you take to present these ideas to nursing program administration? Would you be afraid to share your ideas with program administration? Why or why not?

Nurse as Author

In four to six paragraphs, report on how you have seen QI used in a clinical setting among an interprofessional health care team. How did this collaboration enhance the quality of patient care? In what ways did the collaboration fall short? Using one of the QI processes outlined in this chapter, briefly describe a way to improve such interprofessional collaboration in a clinical practice setting.

Your Digital Classroom

Online Exploration

Baldrige Performance Excellence Program:
  https://www.nist.gov/baldrige
GE—Six Sigma: **http://www.ge.com/en/company/ companyinfo/quality/whatis.htm**
Institute for Healthcare Improvement: **www.ihi.org**
Juran Institute: **www.juran.com**
National Quality Forum: **www.qualityforum.org**
Philip Crosby Associates: **www.philipcrosby.com**
The Joint Commission: **www.jointcommission.org**
The W. Edwards Deming Institute: **www.deming.org**

Expanding Your Understanding

1. Visit the NQF and the Joint Commission websites, and compare the information you find. Which site do you think offers the best information for nurses? Why? Which site offers the best health-related information for consumers? Why?

2. Visit GE's Six Sigma web page to learn more about the concept of Six Sigma and how GE uses Six Sigma to ensure quality products and services.

3. Make a list of reasons for going to a specific hospital if you would need inpatient care. Visit the Quality Check® **http://www.qualitycheck.org**. Perform a search of hospitals within a 25-mile radius of your home. View the information. After reading this information, would you change your mind about seeking care at the hospital you originally selected?

Beyond the Book

Visit **the Point®** **www.thePoint.lww.com** for activities and information to reinforce the concepts and content covered in this chapter.

REFERENCES

Agnes, M. (Ed.). (2005). *Webster's new world college dictionary* (4th ed.). Cleveland, OH: Wiley.

Aiken, L., Clarke, P., & Sloane, D. (2000). Hospital restructuring: Does it adversely affect care and outcomes? *Journal of Nursing Administration, 30,* 457–465.

Aiken, L., Smith, H., & Lake, E. (1994). Lower Medicare mortality among a set of hospitals known for good nursing care. *Medical Care, 32,* 771–787.

American Association of Colleges of Nursing. (2008). The essentials of baccalaureate education for professional nursing practice. Retrieved from http://www.aacn.nche.edu/education-resources/baccessentials08.pdf. Accessed March 10, 2013.

American Association of Colleges of Nursing. (2011). The essentials of master's education in nursing. Retrieved from http://www.aacn.nche.edu/education-resources/MastersEssentials11.pdf. Accessed March 10, 2013.

American Nurses Association. (2010). NDNQI: Transforming data into quality care. Retrieved from https://www.nursingquality.org/discover.aspx. Accessed March 10, 2013.

American Nurses Association. (2013). Safe staffing saves lives: Safe nursing staffing poll results. Retrieved from http://www.safestaffingsaveslives.org/WhatisANADoing/PollResults.aspx. Accessed February 6, 2013.

American Nurses Association. (2015). *Nursing: Scope and standards of practice* (3rd ed.). Silver Spring, MD: Author.

Aroh, D., Colella, J., Douglas, C., & Eddings, A. (2015). An example of translating value-based purchasing into value-based care. *Urologic Nursing, 35*(2), 61–74. doi:10.7257/1053-816X.2015.35.2.61

Aspen, P., Walcott, J., Bootman, L., & Cronenwett, L. (Eds.), and the Committee on Identifying and Preventing Medication Errors. (2007). *Identifying and preventing medication errors.* Washington, DC: National Academies Press.

Balik, B. (2016). What is an 'Always Event'? Retrieved from http://www.ihi.org/education/IHIOpenSchool/resources/Pages/Activities/Balik-WhatIsAnAlwaysEvent.aspx. Accessed July 1, 2016.

Barnsteiner, J., Disch, J., Hall, L., Mayer, D., & Moore, S. (2007). Promoting interprofessional education. *Nursing Outlook, 55*(3), 144–150.

Boltz, M., Capezuti, E., Fulmer, T., & Zwicker, D. (2012). *Evidence-based geriatric nursing protocols for best practice* (4th ed.). New York: Springer Publishing.

Boyle, S. (2004). Nursing unit characteristics and patient outcomes. *Nursing Economic$, 22,* 111–123.

Brady, J. (2015). *Health care safety: Progress & Opportunities.* Presentation given at the NIH Inter-Society Coordinating Committee to Practitioner Educators in Genomic, Porter

Neuroscience Research Center, NIH, May 21, 2015. Retrieved from https://www.genome.gov/pages/research/researchfunding/dgm/healthcare_safety_052115.pdf. Accessed June 26, 2016.

Centers for Medicare & Medicaid Services (CMS). (2012). *HCAHPS online.* Baltimore, MD: Centers for Medicare & Medicaid Services. Retrieved from http://www.hcahpsonline.org. Accessed August 18, 2012 (citation format required by CMS).

Centers for Medicare & Medicaid Services. (2016). Quality measures. Retrieved from https://www.cms.gov/Medicare/Quality-Initiatives-Patient-Assessment-Instruments/QualityMeasures/index.html. Accessed June 26, 2016.

Chowdhury, S. (2002). *The power of Six Sigma.* Chicago: Dearborn Trade.

Cohen, H., Robinson, E., & Mandrack, M. (2003). Getting to the root of medication errors: Survey results. *Nursing, 33,* 36–46.

Cronenwett, L. (2012). A national initiative: Quality and safety education for nurses (QSEN). In G. Sherwood, & J. Barnsteiner (Eds.), *Quality and safety in nursing, a competency approach to improving outcomes.* Chichester, UK: John Wiley and Sons, Inc.

Crosby, P. (1979). *Quality is free: The art of making quality certain.* New York: Mentor.

DesHarnais, S., & McLaughlin, C. (1999). *Continuous quality improvement in healthcare* (2nd ed.). Gaithersburg, MD: Aspen.

Doran, D. (Ed.). (2003). *Nursing-sensitive outcomes: State of the science.* Sudbury, MA: Jones & Bartlett.

Dunton, N. (2008). Take a cue from the NDNQI. *Nursing Management, 39*(4), 20, 22, 23.

Dunton, J., Montalvo, I., & Dunton, N. (2011). *NDNQI case studies in nursing quality improvement.* Silver Spring MD: American Nurses Association.

Finkleman, A., & Kenner, C. (2007). *Teaching IOM: Implications of the Institute of Medicine reports for nursing education.* Silver Spring, MD: American Nurses Association.

Future of Nursing Campaign for Action. (2016). Welcome to the Future of Nursing: *Campaign for Action Dashboard.* Retrieved from http://campaignforaction.org/resource/dashboard-indicators/. Accessed May 1, 2016.

Gill, J. C., & Gill, G. C. (2005) Nightingale in Scutari: Her legacy reexamined. *Clinical Infectious Diseases, 40*(12), 1799–1905. Retrieved from http://cid.oxfordjournals.org/content/40/12/1799.full Accessed November 1, 2016.

Grey, M., & Connolly, C. (2008). "Coming together, keeping together, working together": Interdisciplinary to transdisciplinary research and nursing. *Nursing Outlook, 56*(5), 102–107.

Hall, L., Peterson, J., Baker, G., et al. (2008). Nursing staffing and system integration and change indicators in acute care hospitals: evidence from a balanced scorecard. *Journal of Nursing Care Quality, 23*(3), 24–52.

Hart, C., & Bogan, C. (1992). *The Baldrige.* New York: McGraw-Hill.

Haven, D., & Aiken, L. (1999). Shaping systems to promote desired outcomes. *Journal of Nursing Administration, 29,* 14–20.

Institute for Healthcare Improvement. (2010). Closing the quality gap. Retrieved from http://www.ihi.org/about/Documents/IntroductiontoIHIBrochureDec10.pdf. Accessed February 6, 2013.

Institute for Healthcare Improvement. (2016). About IHI. Retrieved from http://www.ihi.org/about/Pages/default.aspx. Accessed July 1, 2016.

Institute of Medicine. (2000). *To err is human: Building a safer health system.* Washington, DC: National Academies Press.

Institute of Medicine. (2001). *Crossing the quality chasm: A new health system for the 21st century.* Washington, DC: National Academies Press.

Institute of Medicine. (2003). *Health professions education: A bridge to quality.* Washington, DC: National Academies Press.

Institute of Medicine. (2004). *Keeping patients safe: Transforming the work environment of nurses.* Washington, DC: National Academies Press.

Institute of Medicine. (2011). *The future of nursing, leading change, advancing health.* Washington, DC: National Academies Press.

International Organizations for Standardization (ISO) (2017). About ISO. Retrieved from https://www.iso.org/about-us.html Accessed April 14, 2017.

Joshi, M. S., Ransom, E. R., Nash, D. B., & Ransom, S. B. (2014). *The healthcare quality book, vision strategy and tools* (3rd ed.). Chicago: Health Administration Press & Arlington, VA: Association of University Programs in Health Administration.

Juran, J. (1989). *Juran on leadership for quality.* New York: Free Press.

Kalisch, P. A., & Kalisch, B. J. (2004). *The advance of American nursing* (4th ed.). Philadelphia, PA: Lippincott Williams & Wilkins.

Koch, M., & Fairly, T. (1993). *Integrated quality management: The key to improving nursing care quality.* St. Louis, MO: Mosby.

Leighty, J. (2004, August 23). Test pilots. *Nurseweek* (Heartland ed.), pp. 15–16.

Makary, M. A., & Daniel, M. (2016). Medical error: The third leading cause of death in the U.S. *British Medical Journal, 353,* i2139.

Morgan, S., & Cooper, C. (2004). Shoulder work intensity with Six Sigma. *Nursing Management, 35,* 28–32.

National Institute of Standards and Technology. (2011). Baldridge 20/20, An executive's guide to performance excellence. Retrieved from http://www.nist.gov/baldrige/publications/upload/Baldrige_20_20.pdf. Accessed July 1, 2016.

National Institute of Standards & Technology. (2015) How Baldrige works. Retrieved from https://www.nist.gov/baldrige/how-baldrige-works. Accessed April 14, 2017.

National Quality Forum. (2016). NQF's History. Retrieved from http://www.qualityforum.org/about_nqf/history/. Accessed June 26, 2016.

Ouchi, W. (1981). *Theory Z: How American business can meet the Japanese challenge.* Reading, MA: Addison Wesley.

Pande, P., Neuman, R., & Cavanagh, R. (2000). *The Six Sigma way: How GE, Motorola and other top companies are honing their performance.* New York: McGraw-Hill.

Park, S., Blegen, M., Spetz, J., Chapman, S, & De Groot, H. (2012). Patient turnover and the relationship between nurse staffing and patient outcomes. *Research in Nursing & Health, 35,* 277–288. doi: 10.1002/nur.21474.

Porter-O'Grady, T., & Malloch, K. (2015). *Quantum leadership: Building better partnerships for sustainable health* (4th ed.). Burlington, MA: Jones & Bartlett Learning.

Press Ganey. (2015). *Press Ganey acquires national database of nursing quality indicators NDNQI®.* Retrieved from http://pressganey.com/resources/reports/press-ganey-acquires-national-database-of-nursing-quality-indicators-(ndnqi-). Accessed July 1, 2016.

Roche, M., Duffield, C., Aisbett, C., Diers, D., & Stasa, H. (2012). Nursing work directions in Australia: Does evidence drive the policy? *Collegian, 18*(4), 231–238.

Rogers, A., Hwang, W., Scott, L., Aiken, L., & Dinges, D. (2004). The working hours of hospital staff nurses and patient safety. *Health Affairs, 23*, 202–212.

Sidani, S., Doran, D., & Mitchell, P. (2004). A theory-driven approach to evaluating quality of nursing care. *Journal of Nursing Scholarship, 36*, 60–65.

Sultz, H., & Young, K. (2004). *Healthcare USA: Understanding its organization and delivery* (4th ed.). Sudbury, MA: Jones & Bartlett.

The Joint Commission. (2013a). Core measure sets. Retrieved from http://www.jointcommission.org/core_measure_sets.aspx. Accessed March 10, 2013.

The Joint Commission. (2013b). Facts about the Joint Commission. Retrieved from http://www.jointcommission.org/about_us/fact_sheets.aspx. Accessed February 6, 2013.

The Joint Commission. (2013c). Fact about ORYX® for hospitals. Retrieved from http://www.jointcommission.org/facts_about_oryx_for_hospitals. Accessed March 10, 2013.

The Joint Commission. (2013d). Nursing Advisory Council Fact Sheet. Retrieved from http://www.jointcommission.org/assets/1/18/Nursing_Advisory_Council2.PDF. Accessed March 10, 2013.

The Joint Commission. (2015a). Facts about accountability measures. Retrieved from https://www.jointcommission.org/facts_about_accountability_measures/. Accessed June 26, 2016.

The Joint Commission. (2015b). Joint Commission Measure Sets Effective January 1, 2016. Retrieved from https://www.jointcommission.org/joint_commission_measure_sets_effective_january_1_2016/. Accessed June 26, 2016.

The Joint Commission. (2016a). Facts about the Nursing Advisory Council. Retrieved from https://www.jointcommission.org/facts_about_the_nursing_advisory_council/. Accessed April 11, 2016.

The Joint Commission. (2016b). Facts about hospital accreditation. Retrieved from https://www.jointcommission.org/accreditation/accreditation_main.aspx. Accessed January 29, 2016.

The Joint Commission. (2016c). 2016 National Patient Safety Goals. Retrieved from https://www.jointcommission.org/assets/1/6/2016_NPSG_HAP_ER.pdf. Accessed June 25, 2016.

The Joint Commission. (2016d). Facts about SPEAK UP™. Retrieved from https://www.jointcommission.org/facts_about_speak_up/. Accessed June 26, 2016.

The Joint Commission (2017). Disease-Specific Care Certification. Retrieved from https://www.jointcommission.org/certification/dsc_home.aspx. Accessed April 14, 2017.

Tucker, A., & Edmondson, A. (2003). When problem solving prevents organizational learning. *Journal of Organizational Change Management, 15*, 122–137.

Twigg, D., Duffield, C., Bremmer, A., Rapley, P., & Finn, J. (2012). Impact of skill mix variations on patient outcomes following implementation of nursing hours per patient day staffing: a retrospective study. *Journal of Advanced Nursing, 68*(12), 2710–2718. doi: http://dx.doi.org/10.1111/j.1365-2648.2012.05971.x

Walton, M. (1986). *The Deming management method.* New York: Putman.

Weaver, T. (2008). Enhancing multiple disciplinary teamwork. *Nursing Outlook, 56*(3), 108–114.

The Professional Nurse's Role in Public Policy

LEARNING OUTCOMES

By the end of this chapter, the learner will be able to:

1. Define the terms public policy, politics, political competence lobbyist, and political action committee.
2. Explain the key concepts and relationships of the Kingdon model for agenda development and policy formation.
3. Differentiate between the roles of lobbyists and political action committees.
4. List the strategies used to lobby elected officials.
5. Discuss the key elements of effectively written letters to elected officials.
6. Outline a plan for a personal visit with an elected official.
7. Specify strategies to stay abreast of current legislative and public policy issues.

REAL-LIFE REFLECTIONS

As a result of budget cuts and loss of grant funding, school districts in Florida no longer have the resources to provide registered nurses (RNs) for student health services. Some counties in the state have a licensed practical nurse (LPN) in every school who keep records of specific health issues encountered with students. In other schools, students, health issues, and concerns are managed by health aides, teachers, or school staff members resulting in many children automatically being sent home for complaints of physical illness (Roth, 2011). Without RNs to manage complex chronic student illnesses, provide preventive health care services, and develop and implement health promotion education, there has been an increase in several adolescent health problems, including alcohol abuse, drug abuse, sexually transmitted infections, teenage pregnancy, obesity, and immunization noncompliance.

Several nurses with school-aged children band together to work to overturn state policy. Assuming the roles of client advocate and change agent, these nurses approach the members of the state legislature and the governor to see if they would propose legislation mandating "an RN in every school." After all, the state of Delaware requires an RN in every school (Roth, 2011).

Working to lower the speed limits on public roads, petitioning the city to install stoplights at a busy intersection, visiting an elected official to support legislation regarding unlicensed assistive personnel in acute health care settings, organizing a group of nurses to develop a legislative agenda, and lobbying for a bill aimed at increasing governmental funding for nursing education are some examples of how professional nurses can influence public policy. Governmental and institutional policies greatly affect nursing practice and health care delivery.

This chapter provides an overview of public policies, including the various levels of governmental influence on the development and implementation of public policies and how nurses influence public policies. It offers strategies for nurses to use when working with people in charge of public policy development and implementation. Finally, it highlights nurses who have influenced public policy development and outlines strategies to help other nurses learn the art and science of political action.

Politics plays a key role in policy development. *Merriam-Webster's Collegiate Dictionary* defines politics as "the science and art of political government" (Agnes, 2005, p. 1114). Being political means "taking sides or prudently crafting a plan." People use political activities to influence policy development, revision, and implementation. Most laws are public policies, but not all public policies are laws. Some policies may evolve into law. **Laws** are a set of established rules that create a system of privileges and a process for people to solve problems with minimal force. Laws outline and govern the relationships between citizens, between citizens and organizations, and between citizens and their government. In democratic societies, citizens use political action to influence the legislative process required for law enactment.

Once laws become established, policies must be developed to ensure their uniform enforcement. **Policies** are the formalized procedures followed by people responsible for delivering governmental or institutional services (Mason, Gardner, Hopkins-Outlaw, & O'Grady, 2016). In most cases, the government acts as the ultimate authority within the society for policy enforcement.

THE KINGDON MODEL FOR POLITICAL PROCESSES

The processes of law passage and policy development are highly complex. Political action that results in policy changes requires the cooperation of legislators, special interest groups, and administrative agencies (Mason et al., 2016; Milstead, 2016). To bolster their policymaking efforts, nursing experts in political processes identify and use models from political science. The research-based **Kingdon model for political processes** attempts to make sense of the complex American political process by offering a conceptual approach that can be used by nurses to aid in the development of legislative agendas and public policies.

Kingdon's model addresses how issues become part of the political agenda and how alternative approaches for resolving them are developed. Kingdon (1995) specified that people within and outside the government play key roles in the processes of agenda development and policy formation. These processes are dynamic and fluid rather than linear and sequential, and include three key streams: (1) problem streams, (2) policy streams, and (3) political streams. A window of opportunity affects each of the three streams, thereby influencing the development of an agenda.

The problem stream starts with the recognition of conditions (issues that ought to be solved). Conditions become problems when people believe that something ought to be done about them. Triggers for conditions to transform into problems might be a key study report, an unexpected crisis, media attention to an issue, or a thoughtful, well-executed plan from a special interest group (Kingdon, 1995). For example, if the unemployment rates were to rise sharply, many Americans would lose health care insurance benefits. Conditions affecting disenfranchised members of society or those without resources to grant political favors, however, are sometimes ignored (Kingdon, 1995). Sometimes, a group of people interested in publicizing an issue can develop a media campaign to illuminate the issue for the public (Abood, 2007).

The policy stream involves determining viable approaches to solving an identified problem. Stakeholders (people who have an interest in how the issue is addressed) present their views on how to best resolve it. During this phase, multiple approaches are generated and studied. Experts from the governmental, private, and academic arenas provide testimony about the issues. Kingdon (1995) called these experts actors. The actors know each other's views because they are aware of each other's publications and are involved in professional organizations and networking activities. Before addressing the problem in the formal agenda, ideas must be "softened up," which is the process of getting people accustomed to new approaches, building support for new ideas, and gaining acceptance for new proposals (Kingdon, 1995). For example, if too many people lose health care coverage, health care providers, insurance companies, public health officials, and special interest groups might collaborate to generate alternative solutions.

The political stream aims at creating a political culture in elected bodies that support tackling the problem. This stream involves changing the public mood, using pressure group campaigns, influencing election results, and changing the partisan composition of the legislature and administration. During this phase, coalitions are built based on negotiation and persuasion. Political parties reach consensus on campaign platforms. Frequently, trading favors becomes a key way to build coalitions (Kingdon, 1995). For example, if there were to be a spike in gun violence in schools then the political climate would indicate the need for more restrictive gun control laws and regulations. Public pressure and media advertisements might change the attitude of many citizens who believe that the right to bear arm is a basic fundamental right for all Americans and that perhaps there may be real benefits toward tighter restrictions of gun ownership. Thus, the outcomes of the next election might put into office, officials who espouse to work diligently to passing strict gun control laws.

Agenda formation occurs when streams couple together during a window of opportunity. A formal agenda is developed when a group of persons sharing similar interests (such as a professional nursing organization) band together and decide upon what issues that they would like to see resolved. Members of the group agree to work toward achieving desired action on agenda issues. In the United States during general elections, each major political party develops a platform. A party's platform is basically a formal agenda that outlines key positions on issues confronting American society that may be solved by changing laws or regulations (Kingdon, 1995).

According to Kingdon (1995), windows of opportunity rapidly open and close. Kingdon specified that the problem and political streams drive agenda formation, whereas alternative solutions tend to be driven by the policy stream.

Kingdon (1995) acknowledged the contributions that elected officials bring to the processes of agenda development and policy formation. Elected officials bring issues to legislative bodies that are merged to become the formal agenda. The ability of the elected official to influence formal agenda development depends on his or her position as a member of the body. A legislative committee chairperson determines which issues are brought before a committee, a ranking member of the minority party on a committee has the power to influence committee proceedings, and a committee member with long tenure as an elected official may be viewed as being more powerful than his or her colleagues. Each elected official wants to serve constituent interests to ensure reelection, enhance his or her reputation, and pass sound public policy legislation.

> **Take Note!**
> A political model such as Kingdon's provides a framework to understand the complex art and science of influencing public policy and guide nurses as they engage in that process.

THE NURSE'S ROLE IN INFLUENCING PUBLIC POLICY

Nurses have a great deal of knowledge about health and the delivery of health care. Practicing nurses frequently identify flaws in the health care delivery system. Although nurses represent the largest health care professional group in the United States, they have historically failed to play a proportionate role in shaping health policies for Americans at all levels of government (Abood, 2007; Bissonnette, 2004; Mason et al., 2016; Milstead, 2016). According to Wakefield (2004), nursing lacks the financial resources prevalent in more highly influential groups such as organized medicine, insurance corporations, and pharmaceutical firms. In the United States (and elsewhere), money determines how much political power and influence a group possesses.

The Nurse's Role as a Responsible Citizen

The U.S. Constitution ensures the right of American citizens to have a voice in the government. Americans have the freedom to ask questions, offer suggestions, and debate the effects of public policies.

Nurses have a history of political activism. During the women's suffrage movement of the early 2000s, the American Federation of Nursing (now the American Nurses Association [ANA]) joined forces with other women's groups to win women the right to vote. Nurses quickly discovered that they could affect public policy by working independently and with other women's organizations to exert pressure on elected officials to develop policies that support health promotion and disease prevention (Feldman & Lewenson, 2000).

The degree of political action varies among nurses. In 1996, Cohen et al. (1996) outlined four stages of political activism in nursing that still apply.

1. **Buying in:** Nurses become aware of the importance of political activism to attain professional goals, and use the political system to provide input into public policy development.
2. **Self-interest:** Nurses use the political system exclusively to advance their own agenda.
3. **Political sophistication:** Nurses engage in complex political activity such as building coalitions and running for political office.
4. **Leading the way:** Nurses influence other people by holding key governmental positions and in the process select the course for public policy changes.

Nurses participate in public policy formation in a variety of ways; most nurses, however, tend to be in the first stage of political activism. Casting an informed vote during an election is the first level of responsible citizenship in a democracy (Fig. 19.1). **Responsible citizenship** consists of being an active participant in the governing process. The second level of responsible citizenship is engaging in the process of affecting governmental policies. Once they are successful in affecting public policy by providing input, some nurses progress to higher levels of political activism.

Political activism by nurses started with Florence Nightingale's efforts during the Crimean War (Abood, 2007) and fits with professional nursing goals of enhancing health and improving the quality of life for all. The public perceives nurses as being trustworthy and credible. Nurses advocate for large groups of clients when they use their specialized knowledge to influence policy makers to create and fund public health programs. Nurses also have well-refined communication and assessment skills that enhance their ability to determine what types of health programs are needed (and wanted). Because they understand nursing and health-related research, nurses can present strong cases based on solid evidence to document the need for new programs and to continue existing ones. Politically active nurses frequently use the nursing process to guide their thinking for public policy development and evaluation (Abood, 2007; Mason et al., 2016; Milstead, 2016).

Feldman and Lewenson (2000) noted that some nurses begin political careers because of grassroots efforts to accomplish a particular public policy goal. **Grassroots efforts** start at the basic unit of society (local community or special interest group) and expand to reach more centralized areas of influence. Grassroots efforts frequently start as an action to improve a local community that snowballs into a larger action. Grassroots activities involve building coalitions, contacting and visiting elected officials, and testifying before governmental committees. When nurses successfully attain political action goals, they directly affect public policy (Abood, 2007; Feldman & Lewenson, 2000; Mason et al., 2016; Milstead, 2016). Successful action in grassroots efforts builds the nurse's self-confidence and reputation that he or she can be trusted to get the job done (Milstead, 2016).

The second stage of political activism is that of self-interest. An analysis of the current American government reveals that many times, small groups of people expend great resources and much energy to have their agendas approved (especially when competing for a piece of the federal budget). During the third stage of political activism, individuals and groups collaborate and reach consensus about how to best use available resources to better society. Running for office or receiving a political appointment to a key governmental agency are key elements of the fourth stage of political involvement (Abood, 2007; Feldman & Lewenson, 2000; Mason et al., 2016; Milstead, 2016). Examples of nurses serving in legislative bodies and governmental posts are presented later in this chapter. There is little research that has been done to address political activity of nurses and none has been published in the last decade in peer-reviewed journals. Focus on Research, "Empowerment Skills and Values Among Nurses and Social Workers," describes and compares the political activity levels of nurses and social workers.

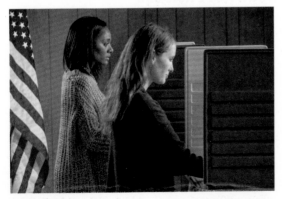

FIGURE 19.1 Voting is a right and responsibility that nurses need to exercise.

FOCUS ON RESEARCH

Empowerment Skills and Values Among Nurses and Social Workers

The investigators sought to discover the differences between nurses' and social workers' perceptions and reported actions using the skills and values of the concept of empowerment. Participants in this cross-sectional survey study included 213 social workers and 152 RNs in Israel. Participants completed Frans' Social Worker Empowerment Scale, Alperin and Richie's Social Service Skills Scale, and Schwartz's Human Values Survey.

Using multiple analysis of variance techniques, the investigators identified the following differences.

1. The nurses scored higher than social workers in knowledge, self-concept, critical awareness, and propensity to act; social workers scored higher on the scale measuring collective identity.
2. Nurses scored higher than social workers in therapeutic communication skills.
3. Social workers ranked higher than nurses in social action skills (including finding government resources, lobbying, and contacting elected officials).

4. Nurses reported having more emphasis on spiritual and material values than social workers.
5. Social workers had higher levels of political activity than nurses.

These findings reveal that nurses and social workers, although both employed in helping professions, have distinct differences. The investigators suggested that the differences could have arisen because nurses use therapeutic communication daily. Results also reveal that nurses tended to think of themselves as individuals rather than as a collective group. Results of this study must be interpreted with caution because the study was conducted in Israel. However, the study points to the need to increase nurses' awareness of the political process and how they could influence public policy. More research is needed to see how all members of the interdisciplinary health team perceive empowerment and how they use their influence in helping to shape public policy and health care delivery.

Itzhaky, H., Gerber, P., & Dekel, R. (2004). Empowerment skills and values: A comparative study of nurses and social workers. *International Journal of Nursing Studies, 41*, 447–456.

Governments and institutions create policies to achieve their missions. However, policy development and implementation are not limited to governments and institutions. Any health care–providing agency, professional organization, nonprofit organization, or family may make policies for its members to follow. Professional nurses bring special expertise to the process of developing and revising health care policies.

> **Take Note!**
> Being part of a successful grassroots effort builds the nurse's confidence and enhances the nurse's reputation.

▌ QUESTIONS FOR REFLECTION

1. In which stage of political activism do you fit?
2. What are the current barriers to your participation in the political process?

3. Do you want to be more politically active? Why or why not?
4. What current behaviors do you need to change to become more politically active?

The Role of Government in Public Policy Development

The federal government and most state governments are organized into three branches: legislative, executive, and judicial. The legislative branch develops and approves legislation for executive branch consideration. The executive branch approves legislative acts and administers and regulates governmental policies. Once laws are passed, the administrative and executive branches of government develop policies to enact them. The judicial branch interprets laws and their application, and the meaning of approved policies.

Legal bases for legislative action in health care are found in Article I, Section 8 of the U.S. Constitution, which states that the government bears the

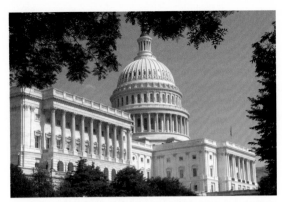

FIGURE 19.2 The US Congress where elected officials draft and approve health care acts that result in national health care laws and policies.

responsibility to provide for the general welfare of its citizens, regulate interstate commerce, fund the military, and provide funds for governmental operations (Fig. 19.2). Each state bears the responsibility to enforce national policies while protecting the safety, health, and welfare of its citizens. Local governments implement national programs and develop laws, regulations, and policies to ensure public health.

The Role of Nurses in Public Policy Development

Nurses have a dual stake in public policy legislation and enforcement: laws not only govern professional nursing practice, but they also impact research, professional education, and the scope of and access to health care by citizens. Nurses shape legislative proposals by contacting their elected officials to influence actions during the legislative process. Some nurses engage in proactive political action by proposing legislation, persuading an elected official in the legislature to introduce a bill, devising public relations campaigns around their proposal, **lobbying** (attempting to sway an elected official to take a desired action) to get the bill passed by legislative bodies, and influencing the head of the executive branch to sign it. A national or statewide effort to pass legislation requires the participation of many for success. Once legislation becomes law, some nurses continue to work with the state or federal agencies responsible for devising the regulations and/or policies to implement the law.

Nursing's Legislative Priorities

Every 2 years, the ANA develops and publishes a list of legislative and regulatory priorities for each session of the U.S. Congress. The identified priorities help to shape the goals of an organization and the actions it will take to influence the passage of legislative proposals

and the development of governmental policies. ANA's legislative goals are developed by its Governmental Affairs Committee, approved by its Board of Governors and accepted by the House of Delegates (ANA, 2013). Once finalized, the ANA publicizes its **legislative and regulatory agendas**. Its membership bears the responsibility for supporting the agenda, whereas the ANA staff advances it. State nursing associations (SNAs) follow a similar process.

The ANA and SNAs also hire professional lobbyists to help draft and promote legislation that favorably affects professional nursing practice (Abood, 2007; Mason et al., 2016; Milstead, 2016). The ANA's Legislative Priorities are developed collaboratively by the ANA Membership Assembly and the ANA Board of Directors. Frequently, priorities are carried over from one Congressional session to another. The legislative and regulatory initiatives for the 114th Congressional session that will likely be applied to the 115th session of Congress (meeting from January 3rd 2017 to January 3rd 2019) are listed below (ANA, 2016c).

1. Work for promoting safe, ethical work environments to protect patient safety and health and wellness of nurses in all practice settings that includes legislative initiatives for acute and nursing home staffing as well as safe patient handling and mobility. Regulatory initiatives include working to include specific staffing patterns on the Centers for Medicare and Medicate Hospital Compare website.

2. Work for enhancing patient care safety and quality during the transformation of the health care system. Legislative initiatives include supporting incentives for Advanced Practice Registered Nurse (APRN) aim toward inclusion and parity for nurses in telehealth legislation, oppose efforts to redefine fulltime work, improve health care benefits, practices in meaningful use, include APRNs as providers of service in telehealth with payment parity, and support new models for payment of RNs and APRNs in medical homes and accountable care organizations. Regulatory initiatives include supporting standardization, attribution and interoperability of nursing information in electronic health records, improve health care benefits in subsidized health insurance plans, aim for patient and provider nondiscrimination in health insurance exchanges, and include RNs and APRNs for leadership in new payment models.

3. Ensure the full use of RN and APRN leadership abilities, knowledge and skills to optimize nursing practice and quality of health care. Legislative efforts include continued support and reauthorization of

Title VIII Nursing Workforce Development Programs; removing barriers to APRN full scope of practice in all ability to certify patients for home health services, durable medical equipment (national acts passed and signed into law in 2015), perform and be reimbursed fully for monthly resident assessments in skilled nursing facilities, and eliminate unnecessary physician supervision requirements; and to seek a permanent fix to the spiraling costs of health care.

Unmet legislative priorities for one Congressional session usually become key initiatives for the next session of Congress.

The first step in publicizing action toward achieving legislative goals and priorities is to develop position papers for each of the identified legislative goals. A position paper is a brief (usually one page) paper that specifies a goal, and clearly and concisely communicates the rationale behind the agenda based on solid facts and persuasive arguments. Supportive evidence such as research findings, statistics, and published articles are used to solidify the position. Typically, nursing organizations print the paper using their official logo, thereby adding credibility to the publication.

The Art of Lobbying

The world of politics moves quickly—sometimes a piece of legislation changes in less than an hour. To stay abreast of the proposed legislation and its changes, nursing organizations hire lobbyists. The ANA has lobbyists for federal legislation. Most SNAs hire a lobbyist for state legislation. Lobbyists visit with elected officials in the hopes of influencing action on a piece of pending legislation. In addition, lobbyists are responsible for keeping their organizational membership informed of the proposed changes to a piece of legislation. At the local level, nurses directly engage in lobbying activities by attending city council and other community organizational meetings.

In addition to hiring lobbyists, the ANA and SNAs offer the Nurses Strategic Action Team (N-STAT), a grassroots lobbying group organized to ensure that nurses' voices are heard at the federal and state governmental levels.

When presenting information on a legislative or local issue, nurses and lobbyists must do their homework to develop expertise on the impending issue. Before briefing an elected official on an issue, it is mandatory to develop expertise on it. Having the facts and statistics related to an issue provides a solid foundation for the art of persuasion. Effective use of statistics involves (1) putting the numbers in human terms; (2)

reporting the statistics in simple terms while avoiding the use of percentages; (3) including practical and statistical significance when reporting numbers; (4) using national, state, and local statistics (elected representatives are most concerned with the local impact of an issue on the constituents whose votes will affect their electability); and (5) citing the source of information (Abood, 2007; Mason et al., 2016; Milstead, 2016).

In addition to statistics, the use of personal stories may be effective in influencing elected officials. Effective use of personal stories involves (1) telling a personal story about a citizen who resides in the elected official's district; (2) telling the story in clear, concise, declarative, strong, and simple terms; (3) requesting a specific action by the legislator; and (4) emphasizing the importance of the issue (Abood, 2007; Mason et al., 2016; Milstead, 2016).

Take Note!

Because elected officials deal with multiple issues every day, they appreciate a clear, concise, precise, and persuasive presentation of the individual's or the organization's goal.

Before effective lobbying can occur, nurses must be aware of current changes in the proposed legislation. To stay aware of current and proposed legislation and policies, nurses must have access to information. Information on legislative issues may be found in newspapers and news magazines (print and online), television and radio, nursing and professional publications, and websites. Along with these sources, legislative bodies offer their own websites to inform constituents of pending legislation and the legislator's position on that legislation. The U.S. Library of Congress has a website that links to federal legislative information. This site posts the status of pending legislation and committee hearing transcripts, which may be studied, downloaded, and printed. In addition, legislative body websites have features for citizens to find the legislators representing them.

Professional nursing associations post legislative issue information on their websites. The ANA and the Canadian Nurses Association websites also contain information about pending national legislation affecting health care and professional nursing practice. The ANA offers an online *Capitol Update* newsletter as well as opportunities for its membership to participate in N-STAT. RN Action (Facebook© and Twitter© accounts) is the ANA's efforts to publicize key political issues affecting the professional nursing practice, access to care, and patient care quality and safety.

Availability of information regarding state issues depends on the state or provincial nursing association. Several SNAs reserve access to information on current state legislative issues for their members (Abood, 2007), whereas others post key information on the public pages of their website. Some SNAs also have Facebook© and Twitter© accounts.

Elected legislators frequently provide their constituents with periodic reports during the legislative session, such as weekly electronic updates and annual reports from state representatives and state senators. Reports may be delivered to constituents via email or the postal service. Reports sent to constituents before the end of the legislative session usually ask for voter opinions on pending legislative issues. When nurses return questionnaires addressing pending legislation, they are participating in the legislative process.

Because of the complex process set forth in the constitution, the path of legislation provides ample opportunity for citizen input. Box 19.1, Learning, Knowing, and Growing, "**The Federal Legislative Path**," outlines the complicated process by which an idea becomes law, and how nurses can influence that process.

Lobbying Strategies

Lobbying strategies are techniques that are used by citizens to influence others to take a desired action. Lobbying strategies are classified into two types: direct and indirect (Table 19.1). Direct lobbying involves personal contact with elected officials. Indirect lobbying involves influencing public opinion on a particular issue.

Before implementing lobbying strategies, nurses should outline a plan that contains a timeline for recording lobbying activities and their results. By keeping records of reactions and responses from elected officials,

---

19.1 Learning, Knowing, and Growing

The Federal Legislative Path

When you step into the voting booth on election day, you set in motion the legislative process. Your elected representatives are charged with taking your ideas and beliefs and carrying them forward to their ultimate enactment into law.

A member of the House of Representatives or the Senate must introduce a bill before it can be considered. They may do so based on their perception of a public need, in support of their elected colleagues, or on the urging of their constituents or of professional associations such as the ANA. Once a bill is introduced, it goes to a committee, where it may be referred (passed to another committee), become the topic of a hearing, be marked up (rewritten and amended), or be reported out (sent to the House or Senate for floor action).

The chair of the committee considering the bill decides on its action. This person possesses much power because he or she may delay the presentation of the bill to the committee (Kingdon, 1995; Mason et al., 2016; Milstead, 2016). During this phase of the legislative process, interested individuals and groups, including nurses, may brief the committee chair to attempt to influence the scheduling of the bill for committee discussion or action on the floor.

Bills that make it out of committee go to the legislative chamber for debate. Once either chamber passes a bill, it goes to the other chamber and is subjected to the entire legislative process again. After the second chamber approves the bill, it is submitted to a conference committee that consists of members from both chambers. The conference committee negotiates differences between the two versions of the bill, adopts the bill, and submits

(reports) it to both chambers for adoption or rejection. If both chambers adopt the conference bill, it becomes an Act of Congress (or of the state legislature). At each of the stages through which a bill moves, constituent input, including that of nurses, can be critical to the outcome.

Each adopted act (also known as an enrolled bill at the federal level) is referred to the president (or governor in state legislatures), who signs or vetoes it. The influence of the public is key at this stage as well—likely, you have seen stories in the news of individuals and groups demonstrating to have the president sign/veto a bill. If the bill is signed, it becomes law. If the bill is vetoed, the House and Senate may override the veto by a two thirds majority vote, and the bill becomes public law. If the veto is sustained, the bill dies (Mason et al., 2016; Milstead, 2016).

The U.S. Constitution gives the president 10 days (excluding Sundays) to act on an enrolled bill. The president has four possible options. The bill may be approved by signature, approved by inaction (i.e., the president takes no action within 10 days, an option used when it is considered unnecessary or politically unwise to sign a bill, or if there are questions regarding its constitutionality), pocket vetoed (used at the end of a legislative session when the Congress adjourns before the 10-day expiration date), or vetoed (the president refuses to sign the bill and presents both bodies of the Congress with a message stating his or her objections to it) (Mason et al., 2016; Milstead, 2016). When the enrolled bill is submitted for executive approval, nurses should contact the president or governor via phone, fax, or email to voice the desired action.

TABLE 19.1 Lobbying Strategies

Direct Lobbying: Through a Legislative Body	Indirect Lobbying: Through Public Opinion
Participate in party platform development.	Publicize nursing organizational agendas.
Contribute time and money to political campaigns.	Use traditional media (especially television) and social media (such as Facebook and Twitter) to further the agenda.
Influence the legislative committee members by personally visiting, writing, or emailing them preferably using the legislator's published form.	Write editorial pieces for print and electronic media, such as newspapers or news magazines, ezines, and blogs, and/or establish a website or Facebook page that promotes the cause.
Influence the agency regulators by personally visiting, writing, or emailing them preferably using the legislator's published form	Seek public opinion by polling the public and publishing the results.
Engage in direct lobbying by visiting or writing to elected officials or hiring a professional lobbyist.	Use paid media advertisements (television, radio, print, online).
Attend social events at which elected officials appear.	Print and distribute books or pamphlets, or set up a website or Facebook page.
Develop an understanding of elected officials' key positions on issues.	Develop and execute educational campaigns.

de Vries, C., & Vanderbilt, M. (1992). *The grassroots lobbying handbook: Empowering nurses through legislative and political action.* Washington, DC: American Nurses Association; Glassman, M. E., Straus, J. R., & Shogan, C. J. (2010). Social networking and constituent communications: Member use of Twitter during a two-month period in the 111th Congress. *Congressional Research Service 7-5700* www.crs/gpv R41066. Retrieved from http://assets.opencrs.com/rpts/R41066_20100193.pdf. Accessed April 19, 2013; Mason, D. J., Gardner, D. S., Hopkins outlaw, F. & O'Grady, E. T. (Eds.). (2016). *Policy and politics in nursing and health care* (7th ed.). St. Louis, MO: Elsevier; Milstead, J. (2016). *Health policy and politics: A nurse's guide* (5thd ed.) Burlington, MA: Jones & Bartlett Learning; and The Partnership for A More Perfect Union (2011). Communicating with Congress, perceptions of citizen advocacy on Capitol Hill. Retrieved from www.congressfoundation.org/storage/documents/CMF_Pubs/cwc-perceptions-of-citizen-advocacy.pdf. Accessed April 19, 2013.

nurses may use this information in future interactions. Appointment of a spokesperson can help to maintain a consistent lobbying approach and enhance public recognition of a particular issue viewpoint.

Constituent pressure is perhaps the most effective weapon for the lobbyist, and mobilization of a group of individuals for collective action provides numbers that influence action. Letter-writing and email campaigns are effective when a bill is pending in the Congress or in a state legislative body. Communicating by form letter or form email is superior to sending nothing. If a specific piece of legislation is supported by a nursing organization, the organization may have a sample letter or email message drafted for membership use. However, according to a survey of 280 Congressional staff members conducted in 2010, the *content* of the communication is more important than its form. Communications are most effective when the constituents share a personal story related to the issue or bill, specific reasons to support or oppose a particular bill or issue, and key information about the impact pending legislation would have on the legislator's district or state (The Partnership for A More Perfect Union, 2011).

Since 2009, email has made possible for elected officials to receive a flood of messages from persons other than their constituents. An elected official may receive thousands of messages in one day and only a fraction of them may have been sent by his or her constituents. Most elected officials now post a contact form for constituent use that requires detailed identification about who is sending the message, thereby facilitating the separation of messages sent to an official from a constituent (Congress.org, 2016).

Electronic media and technology have become essential vehicles for elected officials to communicate with constituents. Along with traditional face-to-face town hall meetings, personal visits, telephone calls, and mailed letters, elected officials use email updates, websites, teleconference town hall meetings, online videos, social networking sites, and other forms of technology to connect with the constituents. Between 1995 and 2008, postal mailings to Congressional members declined 50%. In 2008, members of the United States House of Representatives received close to 190 million email messages. Twitter has become a relatively inexpensive way for members of the Congress and several legislative branches of the federal government (e.g., U.S. Government Accountability Office, Library of Congress, the Government Printing Office, and the Law Library of Congress) to inform interested persons of events, views, and new products or services (Glassman, Straus, & Shogan, 2010).

Because elected officials rely on voter support for reelection, each letter, email, tweet, and personal contact counts. Follow-up messages of appreciation for action on an issue enhance relationships among elected officials and their constituents. Box 19.2, Learning, Knowing, and Growing, "Characteristics of Effective Written Communication to an Official," provides strategies to enhance the impact of your communication with your elected officials.

Using email to lobby an elected official has advantages and disadvantages. It is economical and quick and enables users to send messages at any time. The message is not dependent on postal delivery, and delivery is instantaneous, which can be particularly crucial when a critical vote is only minutes or hours away. In the light of recent security issues with chemically and infectious-agent tainted letters, some elected officials prefer email messages over handwritten letters for their personal safety (Roll Call CQ, 2013; Roll Call CQ Staff, 2009). Many members of the Congress also use software to tabulate constituent views and positions on pieces of pending legislation (Roll Call CQ Staff, 2009).

However, email also has some disadvantages. The ease of email also means that its impact may be watered down by sheer numbers especially when form email messages are sent. Some special interest groups bombard legislators with emails, many of which may be identical, as group members simply forward the messages without bothering to personalize them. If an individual tries to send multiple messages on a subject to one representative, the messages may get trapped as spam or flagged as such by staffers. Messages from individuals who fail to identify themselves clearly as a constituent may not be given as much attention (with mailed letters, postmarks help identify the writer's location). As is the case with traditional letters, many elected officials receive large volumes of email and must rely on staff to read and sort it, and to relay crucial information (Roll Call CQ, 2013). Because legislators tend to hear exclusively from dissatisfied constituents, they may be led to believe falsely that large numbers of their constituents disagree with a pending issue when a large volume of email is received.

A bill may be introduced years before it is passed, and in multiple sessions of the Congress or state

---

19.2 Learning, Knowing, and Growing

Characteristics of Effective Written Communication to an Official

1. Limit letters or emails to one page (approximately 250 words) if possible, but no longer than two pages.

2. Focus on one issue for each email or letter.

3. Identify the issue in the subject heading if using email.

4. Correctly address the person to whom you are writing, referring to an elected official as The Honorable (first name followed by surname).

5. Greet the official according to the title (e.g., Dear Senator _____, Dear Representative _____, Dear Congressman/Congresswoman _____, Dear Mr. Chairman or Madam Chairwoman _____, or Dear Mr./Madam Speaker _____), using a colon for punctuation after the greeting.

6. Identify yourself as a constituent, a health care expert, a member of a large organization, and a credible source on the issue within the first paragraph.

7. Refer to the specific piece of legislation by title (H.R. [number] for a House bill; S. [number] for a Senate

bill) in the first paragraph if the letter pertains to a specific legislative proposal.

8. Emphasize the local importance of the proposed issue.

9. Be brief and specific when presenting key information.

10. Add personal experiences and views, thus eliminating the tone of a form letter.

11. If you are sending your message on paper, handwrite letters, and use professional but personalized letterhead.

12. Verify that the email or letter is neat and free of spelling, grammatical, or typographical errors, and is neat (if handwritten or typewritten).

13. Be specific about the desired action on the part of the elected official.

14. Offer personal assistance or the organization's assistance in the closing.

15. Thank the official for his or her anticipated action.

16. Provide your contact information.

Mason, D. J., Gardner, D. S., Hopkins outlaw, F., & O'Grady, E. T. (Eds.). (2016). *Policy and politics in nursing and health care* (7th ed.). St. Louis, MO: Elsevier; Milstead, J. A. (2016). *Health policy and politics: A nurse's guide* (5th ed.). Burlington, MA: Jones & Bartlett Learning; and Congress.org (2016). Advocacy 101: A new age of online advocacy. Retrieved http://congress. org/advocacy-101//. Accessed June 5, 2016.

legislatures. "Persistence and patience are two key factors in lobbying" (deVries & Vanderbilt, 1992, p. 59). When nurses stay in regular contact with elected officials, the officials are more likely to remember them and work to help support nursing's agenda.

A telephone call offers a way to deliver a brief and quick message to an elected official. A legislator's staff members frequently keep a tally of how many calls support and how many calls disapprove of pending legislation. Many nurses find it beneficial to have the desired message scripted for reading to an elected official. A phone call, like an email, is superior to traditional written and mailed media because it best communicates the urgency of an issue.

All national elected officials have offices in Washington, DC as well as in the state or district where they reside. When legislators return home during breaks, nurses can arrange to meet with them to share their views, eliminating time, and travel barriers to this personal communication. Email messages are effective tools to send quick messages requesting prompt action. Petitions containing large numbers of signatures usually are effective only for public relations because it is difficult for the staff to verify whether all signatures on the document represent the constituents.

In addition to written communication, a personal visit is an effective method of lobbying. Constituents are often invited to meet with elected officials in the local or governmental office. A personal visit lays the foundation for future contacts. A scheduled appointment usually ensures a personal meeting with an elected official. Frequently, visits are limited to 15 to 30 minutes. Because of legislative emergencies, appointments may be canceled, especially if a floor vote is scheduled during the planned meeting. Box 19.3, Learning, Knowing, and Growing, "Steps for Facilitating a Personal Visit with an Elected Official," provides suggestions for how you can effectively visit with your elected official.

When lobbying for specific action on an issue, inviting an elected official for a personal tour of a local hospital, or to participate in a local community service event may assist in advancing the cause. These activities increase the official's visibility and provide an opportunity for interaction with constituents. Because this may be viewed as an opportunity for press coverage, special attention to the press secretary at this time may increase the likelihood of future access to the elected official (deVries & Vanderbilt, 1992; Mason et al., 2016).

Once reliable relationships are established with elected officials, nurses may be invited to testify at legislative committee hearings. When this happens, careful preparation is required, and a technical expert

---

 ## 19.3 Learning, Knowing, and Growing

Steps for Facilitating a Personal Visit with an Elected Official

1. Confirm the appointment and arrive several minutes early, using this time to establish relationships with the official's staff members.

2. Provide the official with a business card after greeting him or her with a firm handshake and confident personal introduction.

3. Start the meeting by establishing a tie between you (such as where you live) so that the official knows you are a constituent who may be responsible for his or her reelection.

4. Inform the official of your mission and clearly identify the issue. If there is pending legislation, refer to it by the bill number and the title.

5. Present statistics and personal stories when appropriate, while emphasizing the issue's importance to the local community.

6. Request the name of the staff member who handles the issue, and request follow-up.

7. Be concise and focus solely on the issue of the meeting.

8. Leave a one- or two-page fact sheet summarizing the issue and your position on it.

9. Conclude the meeting by thanking the official for spending time with you.

10. Send a thank you note or email several days after the meeting.

11. If the legislator requests more information about the bill and the issue, provide all requested information within 1 or 2 weeks of the visit.

de Vries, C., & Vanderbilt, M. (1992). *The grassroots lobbying handbook: Empowering nurses through legislative and political action.* Washington, DC: American Nurses Association; Mason, D. J., Gardner, D. S., Hopkins outlaw, F., & O'Grady, E. T. (Eds.). (2016). *Policy and politics in nursing and health care* (7th ed.). St. Louis, MO: Elsevier; and Milstead, J. A. (2016). *Health policy and politics: A nurse's guide* (5th ed.). Burlington, MA: Jones & Bartlett Learning.

or attorney may accompany a witness. ANA's president frequently testifies at committee hearings when issues regarding professional nursing practice are debated. Karen Daley, PhD, MPH, RN, FAAN, a former ANA president, provided testimony regarding the 2013 Fiscal Year appropriations for the Title VIII Nursing Workforce Development Programs and in support of nurse-managed health clinics. Rich sources of evidence for testimony include the Agency for Health Care Research and Quality (AHRQ; formerly the Agency for Health Care Policy and Research), the Center for Telehealth and e-Health

Law, the National Council of State Boards of Nursing (NCSBN), and the U.S. Department of Health and Human Services.

Sending emails or letters and visiting the legislators are the best lobbying techniques. Traditionally, people lobby the officials they have elected into office while ignoring powerful legislators, such as party leaders and committee chairpeople. Different lobbying strategies work more effectively during different phases of the legislative process. Table 19.2 outlines specific lobbying strategies recommended for use during each phase of the legislative and regulatory processes.

TABLE 19.2 The Legislative Process: Steps and Suggested Lobbying Strategies

Steps in the Legislative Process	Suggested Lobbying Strategy
Legislation introduction	Hold a technical expert meeting to map out a strategy. Form a coalition of people and organizations with the same goal. Identify a legislator in each legislative chamber (House and Senate) who would be likely to introduce the proposal. Schedule a meeting with the legislator's staff members. Initiate a letter-writing campaign to other legislative members who may wish to cosponsor the bill.
Immediately following introduction of legislation before committee assignment	Meet with interest groups to map out additional lobbying strategies. Create a one-page fact sheet to distribute to interested parties. Initiate a letter-writing campaign to elected officials to urge bill cosponsorship. Draft proposed amendments to bill.
Committee consideration	Write letters to all committee members to emphasize the need for a public hearing. Enlist a letter-writing campaign by members of other interested organizations. Submit written information about oral or written testimony if a hearing is to occur. Have someone monitor the mark-up session and share information with letter writers. Conduct a letter-writing campaign to committee members either supporting or disagreeing with the bill amendments added in the committee. Conduct a letter-writing campaign to elected officials from the local district outlining support or disapproval of the revised bill, or to enlist their support by contacting committee members or testifying at a committee meeting. Call a meeting of interested people to verify whether new amendments are tolerable. Work with committee staff in drafting the final draft of the bill. Notify the press about the bill.
Rules Committee action	Work with Rules Committee members to determine whether amendments can be made while the bill is debated on the floor of either chamber.
Legislation on the floor of a chamber	Send short messages to all members of the chamber in great quantities (email messages, phone calls, postcards). Develop a swing list of officials. Initiate personal visits to officials on undecided, leaning no, and leaning yes lists.
Conference Committee action	Meet with other interested people to verify which version (House or Senate) is to be supported. Email, write, visit, or call district officials and members of the Conference Committee.
Return to both chambers for approval	No lobbying strategies are needed if work has been consistent. Email, write, or call elected officials from district.
Presidential or gubernatorial signature	Call the White House or governor's staff, leaving a message for veto or signature.
Veto override	Email, write, or call locally elected official. Intensify lobbying efforts at those who appeared on the leaning yes list.

de Vries, C., & Vanderbilt, M. (1992). *The grassroots lobbying handbook: Empowering nurses through legislative and political action.* Washington, DC: American Nurses Association; Mason, D. J., Gardner, D. S., Hopkins outlaw, F, & O'Grady, E. T. (Eds.). (2016). *Policy and politics in nursing and health care* (7th ed.). St. Louis, MO: Elsevier.

Obstacles to Effective Lobbying

Major obstacles encountered by nurses include not knowing whom to lobby, where to contact officials, or the best time for contact. Some do not know the names of their elected officials. Before contacting an elected official, nurses should find out about the official's personal biography, committee memberships, voting record, and introduced or cosponsored legislative activity. Knowledge of the official's personal causes or pet projects may also be useful.

The Importance of Legislative Staff Members

Because of their enormous responsibilities, all elected officials have staff. (Elected officials may work with thousands of pieces of legislation during one legislative session.) Staff members routinely handle much of the elected official's work. Good relationships with legislative staff at the national and local offices provide invaluable contacts and advantages when engaging in lobbying activities.

An elected official's personal staff may include an administrative assistant, a legislative director, legislative assistants, legislative correspondents, a press secretary, caseworkers, a secretary, an office manager, and a receptionist. Staff members are responsible for scheduling appointments and activities. More importantly, officials fill staff posts with highly qualified people who assist them in making decisions, including members of the nursing profession. For example, Sheila Burke, RN, MPA, FAAN, served as chief of staff for Senator Robert Dole when he was the Senate majority leader (Goldwater & Zusy, 1990). Mary Wakefield, PhD, RN, was a member of Senator Tom Daschle's staff. Both of these nurses advised the respective senators on issues related to health care delivery and workforce development. Dr. Wakefield currently serves as the head administrator for the U.S. Health Resources and Services Administration, a key department of the U.S. Department of Health and Human Services.

Nurses who serve as staff members bring their expertise on health and safety issues to the team. To become a staff member, nurses should get to know political candidates, join political parties, donate time to work for election campaigns, contribute funds to campaigns, and market their nursing expertise on issues related to health care and health promotion.

Maintaining a Working Relationship

Expressing appreciation is a frequently overlooked step in the lobbying process. Elected officials should be acknowledged for introducing and supporting legislation that enhances professional nursing practice. Some SNAs bestow honors on elected officials who have developed records for supporting "nursing-friendly" legislation. A thank you note that includes a statement about informing other nurses living in the district about an official's action in supporting legislation increases the support for an official running for reelection.

Honesty is perhaps the most important factor contributing to effective lobbying. When lobbying, nurses must be willing to spend the time to explore the issues and collect valid and reliable data surrounding them. When encountering questions that cannot be answered accurately with complete certainty, nurses should refer the question to another expert or offer to find the desired information and present it to the official at a later date. Attempts to "wing it" or inadvertently sharing untrue information could sabotage the personal relationships established with officials (deVries & Vanderbilt, 1992; Mason et al., 2016).

There are multiple ways to cultivate a working relationship with an elected official. Wakefield (2004) suggested that working for an election (or reelection) campaign and becoming a member of a political party foster networking with elected officials. Attendance at events where legislators are scheduled to speak or fundraise serves as an additional opportunity for access. Some SNAs offer programs to meet political candidates at district meetings or during special programs held in state capitols. A political campaign contribution offers a token of appreciation (Wakefield, 2004). Taking time to listen to candidates running for office when they canvass neighborhoods enables nurses to meet the candidates.

In the United States, public policy development and implementation are affected by money, power, and societal position. To maintain their position and power, elected officials must work for reelection. Because officials acknowledge the importance of pleasing their constituents, their actions are aimed at protecting and serving their voters. Politically astute people acknowledge the importance of building **coalitions** (forming a larger group from smaller groups of people with similar goals and interests) and contributing resources to a political campaign to get their candidate elected to office.

Take Note!

Without nurses' active participation in the legislative and election processes, public policy may not remain friendly to the nursing profession or health care consumers.

▌ Questions for Reflection

1. Do you know the number of the congressional district in which you reside?
2. Who are the senators serving your state in the Congress?
3. Who is your congressional district's House of Representatives member?
4. Who are your representatives in the state legislature?
5. Which of the lobbying strategies is most appealing to you? Why?

Coalition Building

Although difficult to establish and maintain, coalitions unite diverse groups, organizations, and people for a common specific purpose. Coalitions operate under the assumption that "there is strength in numbers." Many coalitions begin with an informal structure that formalizes as the coalition evolves and becomes more active. Before extending an invitation for membership, a background check verifies any strengths or weaknesses individuals or organizations bring to the coalition. The goal of building a coalition is to capitalize on all members' strengths (Skaggs, 1997). Usually, the organization that started the coalition becomes its leader. When the ANA and American Medical Association (AMA) work together to support a piece of legislation, they build a coalition of health care providers. Once a formal structure has been established, a coalition may need to hire employees to accomplish its goals.

The ANA (2016b) has built coalitions with a variety of groups in order to advance efforts for improving health care funding, protecting the environment, enhancing public safety, seeking funding to advance health care delivery, and protecting patient rights. Current coalitions in place include 50 States United for a Healthy Air, Alliance of Nurses for Healthy Environments, Coalition for Health Funding, Coalition for Patient Rights, NDD United (a group aimed at securing funding for nondefense discretionary spending at all government levels), Get Covered America, Friends of the National Institute of Occupational Health & Safety, Nursing Community, the Public Affairs Council, Smart Disposal and Safe Chemicals, Healthy Families.

Political Action Committees

Political action committees (PACs) are created by existing organizations for the purpose of financing campaigns for political office. Federal election guidelines prohibit nonprofit groups from contributing to political campaigns. Funding for a PAC is independent of the founding organization's funding.

Federal election guidelines mandate that PAC donations may be solicited from an organization's membership only for candidates of public office. However, general organizational funds may finance a political education program for members of the PAC's founding organization. Sometimes candidates for office receive political contributions from the PAC. However, some candidates may request only a public endorsement of their campaigns.

The ANA-PAC, founded in 1972, supports political candidates with "nursing-friendly" agendas (Flanagan, 1976). "The ANA-PAC is an unincorporated committee of the ANA Board of Directors" (Conant & Jackson, 2007, p. 24). Conant and Jackson reported that the ANA-PAC has a separate fund dedicated for the sole use of supporting candidates running for federal office. The ANA-PAC report to the Federal Election Commission for March 2016 revealed a total of close to $99,568 in available funds with no disbursements for the calendar year (Federal Election Commission, 2016). Typical disbursements to have been between $250 and $2,000 to support candidates for federal Senate or House of Representatives (Federal Election Commission, 2013). Before supporting candidates, the ANA offers them the opportunity to complete a questionnaire about their positions on issues important to nurses. The ANA-PAC Board sets concrete endorsement criteria and then forwards information to the ANA-PAC Board of Trustees to review relevant information addressing the criteria. The ANA-PAC Board votes to endorse candidates for federal office. However, each constituent State Nurses Association may agree or disagree with endorsements for federal political offices. Once a candidate is endorsed, ANA staff members notify the candidate. Once the candidate agrees to the endorsement, the ANA-PAC contributes funds to their campaigns and receives ANA candidate endorsement (ANA, 2016a). The ANA-PAC supports a political candidate for president and frequently the candidate wins the election as Barak Obama did in the 2008 and 2012 presidential elections. Many SNAs also have PACs, and each designates specific criteria for endorsing a candidate running for office and contributing to state candidate political campaigns.

Currently, the AMA PAC is ranked as the second largest health-related PAC in the country, the American Hospital Association ranks fourth, and the American Association of Retired Persons (AARP) ranks fifth. The American Association of Nurse Anesthetists PAC is the top nursing PAC (Twedell & Webb, 2007).

CURRENT POLITICAL AND LEGISLATIVE ISSUES AFFECTING PROFESSIONAL NURSING PRACTICE AND HEALTH CARE

Laws regulate nursing practice and health care delivery. Each state regulates nursing practice through its nurse practice act. Federal and state governments regulate health care access and indigent health care service reimbursement. Many issues confronting legislators affect citizen safety, health care policy, and the control of nursing practice.

Hundreds of bills addressing health care are introduced into the Congress and state legislatures annually. If a bill is not passed during the session of Congress in which it is introduced, it dies. However, the bill may be reintroduced during each successive session of Congress until it passes. Issues that are current today may become history tomorrow.

In the recent past, nurses have been successful in influencing the passage of legislation related to patient safety, nursing and health care research funding, human immunodeficiency virus programs, family leave, tobacco settlements, abuse programs, direct Medicare reimbursement to APRNs, Medicare prescription coverage, expanded scope of practice for APRNs, and nursing education funding. Often, a particular issue surfaces over several legislative sessions before legislative action occurs. For example, health care reform has remained on the legislative table for decades. The following section discusses pending legislative issues that may be of interest to professional nurses.

Annually, the federal government develops a budget for all expenditures, including a number of longstanding programs related to public health, nursing education, and nursing research. Nurses need to be aware of the funding proposals made for such programs (Wakefield, 2004). Nurses can become aware of proposed program cuts or increases through the efforts of the ANA and other specialty nurse organizations.

The American Nurses Association's 114th Congress Federal Legislative Agenda

When the Institute of Medicine (IOM) released the report *To err is human: Building a safer health system* in 1999, health care consumers and providers began questioning the general safety of health care delivery. An IOM follow-up report issued in 2011, *The future of nursing: Leading change, advancing health*, offered suggestions to improve the quality of health care by increasing the educational level and optimizing the use of professional nurses (RNs and APRNs) to create a more efficient, patient-centered health care system (see Chapter 9, "Health Care Delivery Systems," and Chapter 18, "Quality Improvement: Enhancing Patient Safety and Health Care Quality"). Nurses seized the opportunity to validate their contributions to quality health care by conducting studies and sharing results that demonstrated improvements in hospitalized patient outcomes with increased RN hours per patient day (Agency for Healthcare Research and Quality [AHRQ], 2007; Buerhaus et al., 2007; Institute of Medicine, 2011). The American Nurses Association's *114th Congress Federal Legislative Priorities* outlines ways to implement recommendations from the 2011 Institute of Medicine's study and to promote the overall health for all Americans. The ANA develops a new legislative agenda for each new session of the Congress and state nurses associations also create legislative agendas for each state legislative session (see Box 19.4, Professional Prototypes, "Items from the ANA 113th Congress Federal Legislative Agenda & 114th Congress Legislative Priorities"). The ANA will develop a list of new legislative priorities for the 115th Congressional Session and for all future sessions.

The federal government spends billions of dollars to monitor and improve the quality of health care services. It funds the AHRQ, the National Institutes of Health, the Centers for Disease Control and Prevention, the Food and Drug Administration, the Health Care Financing Administration, and the Health Resources and Services Administration. Without adequate federal funding, the quality of health and health care in the United States would suffer.

Safe Nursing and Patient Legislation and Nursing's Legislative Efforts

Legislative initiatives on safe nursing and patient care have been introduced with each session of the Congress since 2003. All of the legislative proposals on this issue have had provisions that would prohibit mandatory overtime for RNs and other licensed members of the interdisciplinary care team, but would not set limits on voluntary overtime (IOM, 2004; McKeon, 2008). Despite IOM (1999) evidence-based findings denoting increased errors made by nurses when they work for more than 96 hours per week or longer than 12 hours at a time, no federal legislation has been enacted to reduce the number of hours that RNs can work within a week's time frame. Passage of any law limiting the amount of overtime

19.4 Professional Prototypes

Items From the ANA 113th Congress Federal Legislative Agenda & 114th Legislative Priorities

Scope of Practice for Advanced Practice Registered Nurses

- **Barriers to the Practice of Advanced Practice Registered Nurses.** Need to enact laws, rules, and regulations that remove barriers and discriminatory practices that interfere with APRNs from being able to participate to their full scope of abilities and educational background in the health care system.
- **Home Health: Plan of Care Designation.** Need to enact laws, rules, and regulations that enable APRNs to certify the need for home health care services without the need for physician approval and to reimburse APRNs for conducting in-home visits for primary care and chronic disease management. Currently this requires a physician's signature. Projected savings for this practice for a 10-year time frame are estimated at $273.1 million.
- **Medical Coverage of Advanced Practice Nurses.** Medicare and Medicaid should cover all services that APRNs provide according to state laws. The Children's Health Insurance Program should also cover all APRN services.

Health Care Innovation and Quality

- **Provider Neutral Language:** All future health care rules, laws, and regulations should be written containing the words "primary health care provider" that would include physicians, physician assistants, and APRNs.
- **Care Coordination:** All future health care laws, rules, and regulations regarding the coordination of health care services should include APRNs in the list of persons eligible for reimbursement of services for coordinating a patient's care.

- **Health Care Quality Measures:** Development of a federal system to measure health care quality to provide consistency of measuring quality of care to fairly implement health care accountable organization guidelines.

Safe Health Care Environment

- **Appropriate Staffing for Acute Care:** National standards for direct care RN-to-patient ratios need to be set in accordance with nursing research study findings. (S. 1132 & H.R. 20852 for the 114th Congressional Legislative Session).
- **Safe Patient Handling:** Laws need to be passed to make physical lifting by nurses and other care providers illegal and require agencies that require lifting of patients to provide mechanical lifting equipment for staff to use (S. 2408 & H.R. 4266 Nurse and Health Worker Protection Act of 2015 in the 114th Congressional Legislative Session).

Other Nursing Legislative Issues

- Patient safety/advocacy
- Appropriations
- Rules and regulations
- State exchange implementation
- Medical malpractice liability/tort reform
- Social security
- Protection of Medicare and Medicaid
- Gun violence
- Mental health care

Nursing Shortage

- **Title VIII Funding for Nursing Workforce Development Programs:** Each year the Congress allocates funding for this program that supports all levels of nursing education.
- **Immigration and Nursing Workforce**

American Nurses Association. (2013). 113th Congress Federal Legislative Agenda Retrieved from www.nursingworld.org/MainMenuCategories/Policy-Advocacy/Federal/113th-Congress-Federal-Legislative-Agenda. Accessed April 19, 2013; Library of Congress. (2013). Thomas. Retrieved from http://thomas.loc.gov/home/thomas.php. Accessed April 19, 2013. American Nurses Association. (2016b). Legislative and regulatory priories for the 114th Congress. Retrieved on from http://nursingworld.org/MainMenuCategories/Policy-Advocacy/Federal/114-Congress-Federal-Legislative-Agenda. Accessed June 11, 2016.

or hours nurses work might create a financial hardship for some nurses.

At this writing, the 115th session of Congress has not addressed the issue of mandatory nurse overtime. However, several states have enacted laws prohibiting health care organizations from requiring nurses to work mandatory overtime, although some states have provisions requiring nurses to work overtime in the event of a natural or man-made disaster.

The Registered Nurse Safe Staffing Act of 2015 (S. 1132 and H.R. 2083) have been introduced in the 114th Congress. This legislative proposal would hold hospitals accountable for developing and implementing staff plans for each nursing unit, utilizing collaborative efforts with nurses providing direct care services and incorporating each unit's specific, unique needs. Justification for the passage of a safe staffing act incorporates research findings on the increased incidence of patient complications and mortality when a nurse's daily workload in acute care settings exceeds four patients. In addition, many nurses have left the profession because the stress of high patient care assignments makes the delivery of safe, effective patient care impossible. This piece of legislation seems to get stuck in committee hearings (Library of Congress, 2013; Congress.gov 2016b).

The Nurse and Health Worker Protection Act of 2015 (S. 2408 and H.R. 4266) was introduced in both bodies on Congress to promote safe patient handling in response to the high injury rate sustained by nurses and other health care workers (Congress.gov, 2016a). As of 2013, 12 states have enacted "Safe Patient Handling" legislation (California, Hawaii, Illinois, Maryland, Minnesota, Missouri, New Jersey, New York, Ohio, Rhode Island, Texas, and West Virginia). In these states it is illegal for health care providers to directly lift patients; the legislation requires the use of assistive lifting device for patient handling (ANA, 2016e). Musculoskeletal disorders, especially back injuries, have resulted in the most lost work time, need for prolonged medical care, and permanent disabilities for people involved in direct patient care activities. Each shift, the average nurse lifts 1.8 tons, and 38% of all nurses have sustained a back injury as a direct result of their employment. Permanent disability from a back injury shortens a nurse's career and contributes to the current and future nursing workforce shortage (ANA, 2017).

Nursing Workforce

The U.S. Bureau of Labor Statistics (2015) projects an RN demand of approximately 493,300 by 2024. To keep RNs active in the workforce, the federal and state governments have introduced health care workforce legislation. Each year, Congress approves funding for Title VIII the Nursing Workforce Development program. For the 2016 fiscal year final budget signed by President Obama, $229.5 million was approved to cover grant funding for all levels nursing education (nursing students, advanced practice nursing students, and nursing faculty pursuing doctoral studies) (ANA, 2016d). At the time of final manuscript preparation, there are no legislative initiatives to entice currently employed nurses to remain in the workforce.

State Legislative Initiatives

States frequently address similar health care issues in their legislative bodies. To track state legislative initiatives, SNAs monitor pending legislation that affects health care and professional practice. Some of the issues that are active in various state legislatures include the prohibition of mandatory overtime, safe patient handling, minimum nurse–patient ratios, malpractice tort reform, whistleblower protection for nurses, mandatory development of valid nursing staffing systems for acute and long-term care, state funding for nursing education, and passage of mutual state compacts for nursing licensure.

Mutual Recognition State Compact Legislation

Within the past few years, NCSBN developed a system in which professional nurses wishing to practice across state lines would not have to secure individual state licenses; this system is known as the **Nurse Licensure Compact (NLC)**. Under this provision, the RN holds a professional nursing license in the state of his or her primary residence but would not have to hold another professional nursing license in states abiding by the NLC in order to practice. However, the RN is held accountable to the nurse practice act of the state in which nursing practice occurs. The compact is quite attractive to nurses who live close to state lines and to those employed by traveling nurse agencies (NCSBN, 2001, 2015).

Each state regulates professional nursing practice within its borders. For a state to participate in the mutual recognition program, the state legislature must adopt the NLC. In some states, such as Kansas, participation in a multistate compact violates the state constitution and requires a constitutional change (NCSBN, 2001). Currently, 25 states have approved NLC (NCSBN, 2015).

■ QUESTIONS FOR REFLECTION

1. What are your views on some of the current nursing legislative issues at the federal level? Which of these do you feel is the most important to you as a student or a practicing nurse?
2. Do your views match those of the professional nursing organizations to which you belong?
3. Do the legislative goals of the professional nursing organizations make you more or less likely to joint those organizations? Why?

EXAMPLES OF NURSES INFLUENCING PUBLIC POLICY

Although politics frequently is equated with corruption and abuse of power, the combination of political activity and professional nursing does not create cognitive dissonance. Nurses bring a caring perspective to the political process. Health care delivery and access are greatly affected by the political process. Nurses can fulfill the roles of client advocates and change agents by becoming politically active.

In addition to influencing legislation, as noted earlier in this chapter, nurses have assumed responsibility in the legislative process by becoming members of legislative bodies. In 2016, 60 nurses held seats in state legislatures. Minnesota had the highest number of RNs serving in the State Legislature (3 RNs as State Senators & 3 RNs as State Representatives). Sixteen states do not have an RN in their legislative bodies. (ANA, 2015a). Currently, three nurses serve in the U.S. Congress (see Box 19.5, Professional Prototypes, "Nurses in Congress"). The number of RNs serving in the U.S. Congress fell from five to three following the November 2016 General Election. They are scheduled for re-election in 2018.

Many nurses, officers of nursing organizations (ANA, SNA, specialty nursing), and nursing education program deans and directors testify before congressional committees when issues regarding health care and nursing arise. The president of the ANA frequently shares nursing expertise before the Congress. ANA President Karen Daley, PhD, MPH, RN, FAAN, testified before the House Ways and Means Committee as committee members engaged in federal budget fiscal year 2013 deliberations. Mary Wakefield, PhD, RN, frequently provides Congressional Testimony as the Director of the Health Services Resource Administration regarding the current and future health care workforce needs. Nurses at the state level also provide committee testimony.

Persons are asked to provide testimony because of their position of special expertise. Persons receive a letter requesting participation in the hearing from the committee chair conducting the hearing (Congressional Activities Office, n.d.). If called upon to provide testimony related to a committee or governmental agency, it is best to prepare a written document according to the guidelines presented in Box 19.6, Learning, Knowing, and Growing, "Guidelines for Preparing Testimony to a Committee or Governmental Agency."

Take Note!
Nurses fulfill the roles of client advocate and change agent when they become politically active.

19.5 Professional Prototypes

Nurses in Congress

Membership of the 115th congressional session in the U.S. House of Representatives includes the following nurses (ANA, 2017a; Govtrack, 2017):

- Eddie Bernice Johnson, RN (D-TX), was the first nurse elected to the Congress (in 1992) and won her most recent election with more than 65% of the popular vote (ANA, 2017a). Representative Johnson current services as the Democratic Deputy Whip of the House and as a ranking member of the Transportation & Infrastructure and Science, Space & Technology Committees. She also serves as the Secretary of the Congressional Black Caucus (Johnson, n.d.).
- Karen Bass, RN, is the Democratic representative from the 37th congressional district of California and was first elected to serve in 2010. Representative Bass serves on the Committee on Foreign Affairs and the Steering and Policy Committee. She has served

as the Whip of the Congressional Black Caucus. Her legislative interests include reforming the American foster care system and strengthening the relationships of United States with African nations. Prior to her election, she worked as a physician's assistant and clinical instructor for the University of Southern California School of Medicine Physician's Assistant Program (Bass, n.d.).
- Diane Black, RN, is the Republican representative from the sixth congressional district of Tennessee starting in 2011 after winning the 2010 election. Black serves on the Committee of the Ways and Means and chairs the Committee on the Budget. She also serves on the Subcommittee on Health. She was a primary sponsor of the American Health Care Act of 2017. Prior to election, Black practiced nursing for 40 years in the areas of emergency room nursing, long-term care, and outpatient surgery (Black, n.d.).

19.6 Learning, Knowing, and Growing

Guidelines for Preparing Testimony to a Committee or Governmental Agency

- Study and review material related to the issue for which the testimony is to be given.
- Learn about the congressional committee members (chair, ranking members) and committee staff.
- Prepare three versions of your statement—an official written statement, a shorter version consisting of opening remarks and verbal statements, and abbreviated opening remarks.
- Make certain that all versions are consistent and free of grammatical and spelling errors as the official statement will be entered into the record; the other versions are given to expedite committee proceedings.
- Memorize the shorter version and have all materials printed with large font and on the top half of the sheet (this prevents head bobbing).
- Limit the opening remarks to three key points.
- Write each version using concise sentences.
- In the document, provide the following:
    - Your name, the issue being addressed, and the group receiving the testimony (provide this in the heading).

- Salutation of persons receiving the testimony and group name.
- Identification of self and professional credentials and any persons whom you represent.
- Background information of the group if you are representing one.
- Personal request for desired action.
- Evidence for desired action (cite relevant research findings, societal trends).
- Describe the specifics of the program to resolve or help the issue being presented including potential negative results if the program is not developed, funded, or continued.
- State the desired action again.
- Express appreciation for the committee's time and attention and then offer to answer questions (Anticipate possible questions and prepare answers to them).
- Rehearse aloud all three versions of documents with one or more persons.

U.S. Congressional Activities Office. (n.d.). So you've been asked to testify before Congress. Retrieved from http://www.tradoc.army.mil/tpubs/misc/handbooktestifyingbeforecongress.pdf

OPPORTUNITIES TO LEARN THE ART OF INFLUENCING PUBLIC POLICY

There are many ways nurses can learn the art of influencing public policy development and legislative activity. ANA membership and involvement provide an avenue to learn how to play the political game. The ANA employs political action specialists who educate nurses about the political process, communicate directly with elected officials about pending legislation, collect information about elected officials' voting records, identify politicians who are friends of nursing, and advise the ANA-PAC Board on potential candidates for ANA endorsement. In addition to active involvement in national politics, some SNAs offer daylong or weeklong internships in the art and science of influencing public policies.

Fellowships and internships also offer the nurses an opportunity to learn the process of public policy development through actual experience. Fellowships and internships inform participants about the complexities of health care policy and legislative priorities and provide knowledge and skills to function in the public policy arena. Nurses may participate in formal fellowships

and internships or create their own internship in the nation's capital. Some colleges and university graduate programs offer college credit to students who complete a Capitol Hill practicum. Internships offer nurses the ability to network professionally with members of the Congress and their staff. An internship may start a long-term relationship with a legislator or an influential staff member and increase political passion within the nurse.

Informal internships can be set up by sending a brief cover letter and résumé (by email or post office) to an elected official. The information should be sent to the member's administrative assistant or chief of staff. A number of groups offer formal public policy fellowships (see Box 19.7, Professional Building Blocks, "Groups Offering Formal Public Policy Fellowships").

Take Note!

Through advocacy and lobbying efforts and by serving as elected officials, nurses influence the future of health care delivery, public safety, and nursing practice.

19.7 Professional Building Blocks

Groups Offering Formal Public Policy Fellowships

- The Robert Wood Johnson Foundation
- David A. Winston
- The W.K. Kellogg Foundation
- The Congressional Black Caucus Foundation
- The White House Commission
- The Women's Research and Education Institute
- The Coro Foundation
- The American Association of University Women Educational Foundation
- The Business and Professional Women's Foundation
- The Everett McKinley Dirksen Congressional Leadership Research Center
- The U.S. Supreme Court
- The Woodrow Wilson National Fellowship Foundation
- The Employee Benefit Research Institute
- The Office of Technology Assessment of the United States Congress
- The U.S. Department of Health and Human Services Office of the General Counsel
- IOM
- AHRQ
- The American Public Health Association
- The Centers for Disease Control and Prevention Health & Aging Policy Fellows Program
- SNAs

Mason, D. J., Gardner, D. S., Hopkins outlaw, F. & O'Grady, E. T. (Eds.). (2016). *Policy and politics in nursing and health care* (7th ed.). St. Louis, MO: Elsevier; and Sharp, N., Biggs, S., & Wakefield, M. (1999). Public policy: New opportunities for nurses. *Nursing & Health Care, 12*(1), 16–22.

Summary and Significance to Practice

In these chaotic times, change is needed to provide safe, effective, patient-centered, timely, and efficient health care. By virtue of their training, nurses possess the cognitive and communication skills necessary to successfully navigate the complex political processes required to influence public policy. To change the health care system, nurses can use critical thinking to analyze issues and communication skills to illuminate elected officials, policy makers, and the public about pressing health care issues. A model for political processes such as Kingdon's provides nurses with an evidence-based framework to guide political action efforts. Developing expertise in influencing public policy requires dedication, time, practice, and a willingness to work with others. When nurses succeed with political action, they become confident in their ability to improve health care for all.

Issues affecting personal and public health are too important to be left to politicians. They and their constituents need nurses to ensure that future public health care policies are based on solid evidence and improve access to health care for all.

REAL-LIFE REFLECTIONS

Recall the scenario presented at the beginning of the chapter, in which state school districts no longer have the resources to provide RNs for student health services. Do you think that all schools within a state should have an RN on the premises at all times during school hours? Why or why not? What impact would having an RN on school premises during school hours have on students? Faculty? School staff and administration? Parents? Taxpayers? Does your state provide resources for RNs in its schools? What actions might you take to change your state's policies?

From Theory to Practice

1. Identify a legislative proposal at either the federal or state level that you think may affect your future as a nurse, or your current nursing practice or client care delivery. Write a one- to two-page position paper on the pending legislation using research and other evidence to support your position. Give the paper to a colleague to critique it in terms of clarity, conciseness, and strength of your position argument. Revise the paper based on your colleague's critique.

Nurse as Author

Identify a currently introduced bill in the national or your state legislature. Using information from the ANA or your State Nurses' Association, write an email message that conveys the importance of the issue to professional nursing practice and/or patient safety. You will find that Position Papers or White Papers on the topic will provide substantial information and data related to the issue that should be included in your message. Once your message has been approved by your faculty member, send it using the form designated by your legislator found on your legislator's website.

Your Digital Classroom

Online Exploration

Agency for Healthcare Research and Quality:
www.ahrq.gov

American Academy of Nursing Health Policy Issues:
http://www.aannet.org/health-policy

American Hospital Association (Advocacy Issues):
http://www.aha.org/advocacy-issues/index.shtml

American Nurses Association:
http://www.nursingworld.org/
MainMenuCategories/Policy-Advocacy

Canadian Nurses Association:
http://www.cna-aiic.ca/en/

Congress.org: http://www.congress.org

Center for Telehealth and e-Health Law:
http://ctel.org/

Centers for Medicare and Medicaid Services:
www.cms.hhs.gov

Department of Health and Human Services:
www.hhs.gov

Government Made Easy (database of more than
1.5 million U.S. government web pages):
www.usa.gov

Institute of Medicine:
http://www.nationalacademies.org/hmd/

Library of Congress (U.S. government legislative
website): https://www.congress.gov/

National Council of State Boards of Nursing:
www.ncsbn.org

Occupational Safety and Health Administration:
www.osha.gov

RN Action: http://www.rnaction.org

U.S. House of Representatives: www.house.gov

U.S. Senate: www.senate.gov

Expanding Your Understanding

1. Visit the websites of the U.S. Congress (www.senate.gov and www.house.gov) and complete the following exercises:
   a. Visit the home pages of your two state Senators and your Representative to the U.S. House of Representatives. If you do not know their names, you can find them by entering your home zip code, clicking your home location on a map, or typing in the number of your legislative district found on your voter registration card in the information request section.
   b. Search for the current legislation affecting nursing and health care delivery by performing a topic search or typing in key words. Read the full bill text or its summary.
   c. Send an email to your Senators and Representative using the strategies for composing letters and messages found in this chapter.
   d. Find your state legislature by conducting a search for "(your state's name) legislature." On your state's legislative site, search for "nursing" and "health care delivery" as key words to find information about the current legislative efforts affecting professional nursing in your state.

2. Visit the ANA website (www.nursingworld.org) and complete the following exercises:
   a. Find on the menu bar the words "Policy & Advocacy" at the top of the page.
   b. On the next screen click on "Take Action" either by using the drop down menu or clicking on the link in the list of choices under "Policy & Advocacy" on the left.
   c. Click on all of the "Alerts" and select one and take the requested action on it.
   d. When you come to class or participate in a course online discussion board, report on the action you took. Include the reasons why you selected to act on one alert over another, state the action that you took and if you received any follow-up communication from your Representative or Senator. How did it feel to take political action? Would you take action on another issue? Why or why not?

3. Visit the NCSBN website (www.ncsbn.org) and complete the following exercises:
   a. At the top of the page, click on "Licensure Compacts." On the next page click on "Find out more" under the tab "About the NLC." On this page, scroll down until you see a map of the United States that identifies current states that have enacted the NLC. You will see a map of the United States with certain states highlighted in blue. These are the states that participate in the Nurse Licensure Compact. What states participate in the compact? Does your state participate in the interstate nursing licensure compact?
   b. Scroll down and continue reading information that appears below the map of the United States that specify NLC compact states. On a piece of paper write down information to explain the NLC to a nurse who does not live in a participating state and to a nurse who lives in a participating state, but is considering a move to a non-participating state.
   c. Once you have read all the information posted to answer questions for learning exercise b, scroll

to the top of the page. On the left side of the screen, click on NLC FAQs and read answers to frequently asked questions about the NLC. In addition, download the NLC Toolkit that contains Fact Sheets and Flow Charts. Click on the Flow Charts for" Licensure by Examination" and "Licensure by Endorsement". Compare and contrast this information. Consult with a nursing faculty member from your program if you have any questions. Click on the following Fact Sheets: "What Nurses Need to Know" and "Fact Sheet for New Graduates". What did you find important and interesting? Why did you find this information important and interesting?

Beyond the Book

Visit thePoint® **www.thePoint.lww.com** for activities and information to reinforce the concepts and content covered in this chapter.

REFERENCES

Abood, S. (2007). Influencing health care in the legislative arena. *The Online Journal of Issues in Nursing, 12*(10), 3. Retrieved from www.nursingworld.org/MainMenuCategories/ANA-Marketplace/ANAPeriodicals/OJIN/TableofContents/Volume122007/No1Jan07/tpc32_216091.aspx. Accessed February 26, 2013.

Agency for Healthcare Research and Quality. (2007). *Nursing staffing and quality of patient care (AHRQ Publication No. 07-E005).* Rockville, MD: Author. Retrieved from www.ahrq.gov/clinic/tp/nursesttp.htm. Accessed July 2008.

Agnes, M. (Ed.). (2005). *Webster's new world college dictionary* (4th ed.). Cleveland, OH: Wiley.

American Nurses Association (ANA). (2013). *113th Congress federal legislative agenda.* Retrieved from http://nursingworld.org/MainMenuCategories/Policy-Advocacy/Federal/113th-Congress-Federal-Legislative-Agenda. Accessed April 19, 2013.

ANA. (2015a). *Nurse state legislators and administrative leaders directory.* Retrieved from http://nursingworld.org/NurseLegislatorDirectory.aspx#mo. Accessed June 5, 2016.

ANA. (2015b). *Nurses currently serving in Congress.* Retrieved from http://nursingworld.org/MainMenuCategories/Policy-Advocacy/Federal/Nurses-in-Congress. Accessed June 5, 2016.

ANA. (2016a). ANA-PAC Endorsement Process. Retrieved from http://www.rnaction.org/site/PageNavigator/nstat_pac_endorsement_process.htmll. Accessed June 11, 2016.

ANA. (2016b). Coalitions. Retrieved from http://www.rnaction.org/site/PageNavigator/nstat_ana_coalitions.html. Accessed June 11, 2016.

ANA. (2016c). Legislative and regulatory priories for the 114th Congress. Retrieved from http://nursingworld.org/MainMenuCategories/Policy-Advocacy/Federal/114-Congress-Federal-Legislative-Agenda. Accessed June 11, 2016.

ANA. (2016d). President Obama's final budget prompts praise and pause from the American Nurses Association. Retrieved from http://www.rnaction.org/site/PageNavigator/nstat_take_action_title_viii_issues.html. Accessed June 11, 2016.

ANA. (2017). *Safe patient handling and mobility (SPHM).* Retrieved from http://www.nursingworld.org/MainMenu-Categories/Policy-Advocacy/State/Legislative-Agenda-Reports/State-SafePatientHandling Accessed April 15, 2017.

ANA (2017a). Nurses Currently Serving in Congress. Retrieved from http://www.nursingworld.org/MainMenuCategories/Policy-Advocacy/Federal/Nurses-in-Congress. Accessed April 15, 2017.

Bass, K. (n.d.). *About me: Full biography.* Retrieved from http://bass.house.gov/about-me/full-biography. Accessed June 5, 2016.

Bissonnette, T. (2004). Passion, engagement, and political action. *Michigan Nurse, 77*, 1.

Black, D. (n.d.). *About me: Biography.* Retrieved from http://black.house.gov/about-me/full-biography. Accessed June 5, 2016.

Buerhaus, P. I., Donelan, K., Ulrich, B. T, Norman, L., DesRoches, C., & Dittus, R. (2007). Impact of the nurse shortage on hospital patient care: Comparative perspectives. *Health Affairs, 26*, 853–862.

Bureau of Labor Statistics. (2015). *Occupational outlook handbook, Registered nurses.* Retrieved from http://www.bls.gov/ooh/healthcare/registered-nurses.htm. Accessed June 11, 2016.

Capps, L. (n.d.). *Congresswoman Lois Capps' full biography.* Retrieved from http://capps.house.gov/about-me/full-biography. Accessed June 5, 2016.

Cohen, S. S., Mason, D. J., Kovner, C., Leavitt, J. K., Pulcini, J., & Sochalski, J. (1996). Stages of nursing's political development: Where we've been and where we ought to go. *Nursing Outlook, 44*, 259–266.

Conant, R., & Jackson, C. (2007). Brief overview of ANA political action committee. *American Nurse Today, 2*(3), 24.

Congress.gov. (2016a) Legislative search results. Retrieved from https://www.congress.gov/search?q=%7B%22source%22%3A%22legislation%22%2C%22search%22%3A%22safe%20patient%20handling%22%7D. Accessed June 11, 2016.

Congress.gov. (2016b). Legislative search results. Retrieved from https://www.congress.gov/search?q=%7B%22source%22%3A%22legislation%22%2C%22search%22%3A%22RN+safe+staffing%22%7D. Accessed June 11, 2016.

Congress.org. (2016). Advocacy 101: A new age of online advocacy. Retrieved http://congress.org/advocacy-101//. Accessed June 5, 2016.

Congressional Activities Office. (n.d.). *So, you've been asked to testify before Congress.* Retrieved from http://www.tradoc.army.mil/tpubs/misc/handbooktestifyingbeforecongress.pdf. Accessed June 19, 2013.

deVries, C., & Vanderbilt, M. (1992). *The grassroots lobbying handbook: Empowering nurses through legislative and political action.* Washington, DC: American Nurses Association.

Ellmers, R. (n.d.). *Congresswoman Renee Ellmers biography.* Retrieved from http://ellmers.house.gov/biography/. Accessed June 5, 2016.

Federal Election Commission. (2013). *American Nurses Association PAC, FEC Form 3X.* Retrieved from http://query.nictusa.com/pdf/313/13940555313/13940555313.pdf#navpanes=0. Accessed April 19, 2013.

Federal Election Commission. (2016). *Detail for Committee ID: C00559229.* Retrieved from http://www.fec.gov/fecviewer/CandidateCommitteeDetail.do?candidateCommitteeId=C00559229&tabIndex=1. Accessed June 11, 2016.

Feldman, J. R., & Lewenson, S. B. (Eds.). (2000). *Nurses in the political arena.* New York: Springer.

Flanagan, L. (1976). *One strong voice: the story of the American Nurses Association.* Kansas City MO: ANA.

Glassman, M. E., Straus, J. R., & Shogan, C. J. (2010). *Social networking and constituent communications: Member use of Twitter during a two-month period in the 111th Congress* (Research Report No. 7-5700 www/crs/gpv R41066). Retrieved from Congressional Research Service website: http://assets.opencrs.com/rpts/R41066_20100193.pdf. Accessed April 19, 2013.

Goldwater, M., & Zusy, M. (1990). *Prescription for nurses: Effective political action.* St. Louis, MO: Mosby.

Govtrack (2017). Members of Congress. Retrieved from https://www.govtrack.us/congress/members/current. Accessed April 15, 2017.

Institute of Medicine. (1999). *To err is human: Building a safer health system.* Washington, DC: National Academies Press.

Institute of Medicine. (2004). *Keeping patients safe: Transforming the work environment of nurses.* Washington, DC: National Academies Press.

Institute of Medicine. (2011). *The future of nursing: Leading change, advancing health.* Washington, DC: National Academies Press.

Itzhaky, H., Gerber, P., & Dekel, R. (2004). Empowerment skills and values: A comparative study of nurses and social workers. *International Journal of Nursing Studies, 41,* 447–456.

Johnson, E. (n.d.). *About Eddie Bernice Johnson.* Retrieved from http://ebjohnson.house.gov/about/full-biography. Accessed June 5, 2016.

Kingdon, J. (1995). *Agendas, alternatives and public policy.* New York: Harper Collins College.

Library of Congress. (2013). *Thomas.* Retrieved from http://thomas.loc.gov/home/thomas.php. Accessed April 19, 2013.

Mason, D. J., Gardner, D. S., Hopkins Outlaw, F., & O'Grady, E. T. (Eds.). (2016). *Policy and politics in nursing and health care* (7th ed.). St. Louis, MO: Elsevier.

McKeon, E. (2008). Legislative updates: 110th Congress wrap-up. *Capitol Update, 6*(9). Retrieved from www.capitolupdate.org/Newsletter/index.asp?nlid=199&nlid=1054. Accessed January 3, 2009.

Milstead, J. A. (Ed.). (2016). *Health policy and politics: A nurse's guide* (5thd ed.). Burlington, MA: Jones & Bartlett Learning.

National Council of State Boards of Nursing. (2001). *Mutual recognition information.* Retrieved from www.ncsbn.org/mutual_compact.pdf. Accessed January 12, 2002.

National Council of State Boards of Nursing. (2015). *25 Nurse Licensure Compact States.* Retrieved from https://www.ncsbn.org/NLC_Implementation_2015.pdf. Accessed June 11, 2016.

Roth, L. (2011). A nurse in every school?—not in Florida—not even close. *The Orlando Sentinel.* Retrieved from http://articles.orlandosentinel.com/2011-09-26/business/os-fewer-school-nurses-florida-20110925_1_school-nurses-practical-nurses-students-with-chronic-illnesses. Accessed April 19, 2012.

Roll Call CQ. (2013). *Communicating with Congress.* Retrieved from www.congress.org/ Roll Call news/communicating-with-congress/. Accessed April 19, 2013.

Roll Call CQ Staff. (2009). *Why Congress prefers email.* Retrieved from www.congress.org/news/why-congress-prefers-e-mail/. Accessed April 19, 2013.

Sharp, N., Biggs, S., & Wakefield, M. (1999). Public policy: New opportunities for nurses. *Nursing & Health Care, 12*(1), 16–22.

Skaggs, B. (1997). Political action in nursing. In J. Zerwekh, & J. Claborn (Eds.), *Nursing today: Transitions and trends* (2nd ed.). Philadelphia, PA: WB Saunders.

The Partnership for A More Perfect Union. (2011). *Communicating with Congress, perceptions of citizen advocacy on Capitol Hill.* Retrieved from www.congressfoundation.org/storage/documents/CMF_Pubs/cwc-perceptions-of-citizen-advocacy.pdf. Accessed April 19, 2014.

Twedell, D., & Webb, J. (2007). The value of the political action committee: Dollars and influence for nurse leaders. *Nursing Administration Quarterly, 31*(4), 279–283.

Wakefield, M. (2004). A call to political arms. *Nursing Economic$, 33,* 166–167.

Envisioning and Creating the Future of Professional Nursing

As a profession, nursing can count on change. Nurses have many career options. A rewarding and satisfying career depends on the interests and passions of each individual nurse. Once nurses discover what they want to do, they can use specific career development strategies to ensure success. Many nurses move from one area of professional practice to another throughout their professional nursing career. To meet the future needs for professional nursing and to secure a future for the profession, nurses need to examine current trends, develop future scenarios, and envision a preferred future. Once a preferred future is envisioned, professional nurses can develop plans to create a future that optimizes the contributions that nurses make in enhancing the health and well-being of all people.

Chapter 20

Career Options for Professional Nurses

KEY TERMS AND CONCEPTS

Universal job skills
Licensure
Registration
Certification
Advanced nursing
   practice
Graduate nursing
   education

Nurse practitioners
General nursing practice
Specialized nursing
   practice
Clinical ladders
Nursing administration
Nursing academia
Nurse entrepreneur

LEARNING OUTCOMES

By the end of this chapter, the learner will be able to:

1. Outline universal job skills.
2. Specify which universal job skills nurses possess.
3. Identify career options for nurses educated at the generalist level.
4. Explain the differences between general and advanced nursing practice.
5. Distinguish certification from advanced nursing practice.
6. Describe advanced nursing practice roles and responsibilities.

REAL-LIFE REFLECTIONS

Laura is thinking about entering the nursing profession. As she explores professional nursing, Laura interviews three nurses and finds that there are many career options within the profession. One nurse Laura interviewed remained employed for over 20 years as a staff nurse at the same clinical site where she had her capstone nursing experience as an undergraduate student. Another nurse shared her experiences with a nursing career that began as a nursing assistant, followed by several years each of hospital staff nursing, school nursing, and outpatient clinic nursing that resulted in more education to work as a nurse practitioner (NP) in a small rural clinic. The third nurse Laura interviewed was a nurse faculty member who held a nursing doctorate and enjoyed researching and teaching. After learning about the diverse career options in nursing, Laura realizes that she does not have to decide on a specialized area of practice and will keep her options open until she finds her niche.

Setting career goals begins with self-assessment. Ideally, career goals should match personal values and acquired skills. This chapter explores many of the possible career options in professional nursing.

UNIVERSAL JOB SKILLS

In 1992, the *Occupational Outlook Handbook* published by the Federal Bureau of Labor Statistics delineated the following **universal job skills** for all types of work: (1) leadership/persuasion, (2) problem solving/creativity, (3) working as part of a team, (4) manual dexterity, (5) helping or instructing others, (6) initiative, (7) frequent contact with the public, and (8) physical stamina. These skills remain relevant today. Yee-Litzenberg (2011) identified similar universal job skills, but expanded the skill set to include media use and technical skills (including computer software

TABLE 20.1 Universal Job Skills and How Professional Nurses Use Them

Occupational Outlook Handbook (Bureau of Labor Statistics, 1992)	Yee-Litzenberg (2011) (University of Michigan)	Professional Nurse Example
Leadership/persuasion	Management	Supervising unlicensed assistive personnel
Problem solving/creativity	Analytical/problem-solving skills	Utilizing nursing process
Working as part of a team	Multidisciplinary team experience/interpersonal skills	Working in partnership with patients, families, and other health care providers
Manual dexterity	Technical skills	Executing complex clinical nursing and computer skills (e.g., starting IVs and accessing and entering information from computers)
Helping or instructing others	Interpersonal skills	Establishing and maintaining therapeutic relationships Teaching
Initiative	Leadership/initiative	Performing surveillance activities to detect complications before they arise Providing optimal, high-quality patient care services
Frequent contact with the public	Interpersonal skills	Working with patients, families, visitors, and communities
Physical stamina		Meeting physical demands of patient care activities Working long hours
	Communication/media	Developing patient, family, and community education materials Giving public presentations

abilities); physical stamina does not appear in her list. Table 20.1 compares these two sets of universal job skills and provides examples of how professional nurses use them. The comprehensive skill set required by professional nurses may be one reason for the diversity of nursing career opportunities.

Individuals rank the importance of job skills differently, thereby providing clues to how nurses perceive what is important to them. For example, a nursing position that limits direct communication with patients and families would be a less than optimal choice for a nurse who values establishing and maintaining therapeutic relationships with others. By taking time to rank each job skill, nurses discover what type of a nursing career fits with their personal values.

Take Note!

The job skills mastered by nurses readily transfer to multiple fields within and outside the nursing profession.

QUESTIONS FOR REFLECTION

1. How might you use each of the eight universal job skills in your daily professional nursing practice?
2. How do people with non-nursing jobs use the skills differently than nurses?

3. Why does nursing require mastery of all eight universal job skills?

LEVELS OF NURSING PRACTICE

In the United States, state legislatures and state boards of nursing regulate practice. In most of Canada (except Ontario and Quebec), provincial/territorial professional nursing associations regulate practice. In Ontario, diploma nursing programs are approved and monitored by the Ministry of Training Colleges and the Council of Ontario University Programs in Nursing (COUPN). All university nursing programs in Ontario are also approved by each university senate or governing council. In 2008, COUPN delegated its authorship for approving university-based nursing programs to the Canadian Association of Schools of Nursing (CASN). CASN accreditation constitutes nursing program approval. In Quebec, diploma nursing programs are approved and monitored in the Collège d'Enseignement Général et Professionnel, and university programs are monitored by the particular university in which they reside (Ross-Kerr, 2011). In both countries, regulation of practice involves determining educational qualifications, setting standards of professional practice, limiting the use of the title "registered nurse (RN)," approving nursing education programs, determining the extent of continuing education and competency, disciplining professional members who endanger the public, and specifying the scope of nursing practice (Ross-Kerr, 2011; National Council of State Boards of Nursing [NCSBN], 2012).

When nurses complete a preparatory nursing education program (associate degree, diploma, or baccalaureate degree), successfully pass the National Council Licensure Examination for Registered Nurses (NCLEX-RN), and pay nursing licensure fees, they begin professional practice as RNs. **Licensure** is a process of legal authorization for nursing practice. **Registration** encompasses a listing of qualified, licensed nurses in good standing that is available to the public. Newly licensed nurses practice as generalists initially. However, with increased experience in a particular area of practice, many nurses become specialized.

Professional nurse associations recognize competence in a particular nursing field through certification. **Certification** means that an individual meets specified requirements, which usually include specialized knowledge and skills in a particular area of nursing practice. Most certifications in professional nursing practice require a specified number of years of experience within a specialty along with successful completion of a competency examination. Each nursing organization sets criteria for nurses to maintain specialty certification. Most organizations require a combination of clinical practice hours along with a determined number of continuing education contact hours. Some nursing regulatory agencies recognize certification from professional nursing associations as credentials for an advanced nursing practice licensure.

Advanced nursing practice extends the scope and responsibilities beyond what is typically expected of an RN. According to the American Nurses Association's *Nursing: Scope and Standards of Practice, 3rd ed* (American Nurses Association [ANA], 2015), advanced practice registered nurses (APRNs) are defined as nurses who have "completed an accredited graduate-level education program" that prepares them for one of the following roles: "certified nurse practitioner, certified registered nurse anesthetist, certified nurse-midwife or clinical nurse specialist" (p. 2). Along with earning a graduate nursing degree, APRNs pass "a national certification exam that measures the APRN role and population-focused competencies" (ANA, 2015, p. 3). APRNs are also licensed for advanced practice by the state in which they practice and must undergo periodic recertification (ANA, 2015), which typically includes a minimum number of clinical practice hours in their area of practice. Hallmarks of advanced nursing

practice include **graduate nursing education** (master's degree or doctorate in nursing), national certification for the role and focused population for whom they will be providing services.

Early in the profession's history, graduate nursing education was not required for entry into advanced nursing practice. Today, depending on the nature of advanced practice, additional state nursing licensure is required. Most states require that **nurse practitioners** (who deliver primary, secondary, and tertiary health care services in collaboration with a physician) enter into collaborative practice agreements with physicians licensed in their state of practice (Jansen & Zwygart-Stauffacher, 2010).

GENERAL NURSING CAREER OPPORTUNITIES

The nursing profession offers a wide array of opportunities. Nurses have the flexibility to focus on one area of practice or work in several practice areas. In addition, nurses may work for an organization or for themselves. **General nursing practice** encompasses areas of practice in which no additional or specialized formal education is required. **Specialized nursing practice** occurs when nurses work in a specific clinical area (e.g., obstetrics, oncology, intensive care) in which additional education and training are needed to meet specific client concerns or master unique clinical nursing skills. In many specialty areas of nursing practice, nurses become certified in the area of practice, which means they have mastered specific skills and possess a unique knowledge to deliver client care.

When a nurse identifies a problem in practice, a potential opportunity arises for a new area of nursing practice. An identified problem sometimes leads to the development of a personal business or an entirely new health service to be offered by a large medical center.

This section briefly summarizes the more common areas of nursing practice. Detailed information about specific nursing careers can be found in this and other chapters, including advanced practice nursing (later in this chapter), nursing informatics (Chapter 14, "Informatics and Technology in Nursing Practice"), lobbying as a nurse (Chapter 19, "The Professional Nurse's Role in Public Policy"), and nursing careers in community health nursing (Chapter 15, "Nursing Approaches to Client Systems").

Acute Care or Hospital Nursing Options

When asked about professional nursing, persons not involved in health care tend to describe a nurse as someone who provides direct care to patients in inpatient settings. According to the U.S. Bureau of Labor Statistics (2016a), 61% of the employed RNs worked in hospitals in 2014, with most of them being engaged in direct client care. Recent changes in the health care delivery system have resulted in a variety of career options for nurses working in acute care.

Staff Nursing

Nurses engaging in direct client care find themselves in a fast-paced and challenging position. Within the past decade, the acuity of hospitalized clients has increased dramatically. Nurses today often care for clients who once would have been admitted only to intensive care units. As complex specialized skills become requirements for various types of staff nursing (such as oncology and cardiac specialties), many nurses become certified in specialty practice areas. Experience and certification in specialty areas of practice result in highly trained experts delivering client care. As nurses develop more technical expertise in specific areas, they cannot be expected to provide expert nursing care to clients outside those areas of clinical specialties. However, because basic nursing education effectively prepares nurses to assume safe care responsibilities as nurse generalists, hospitals sometimes assign nurses to work outside their clinical specialty areas.

In all practice settings, professional nurses must become experts at juggling multiple tasks simultaneously as they fulfill numerous obligations. Nurses confront competing client care priorities such as balancing the quality of care with cost containment. They use leadership skills for effective delegation and supervision of unlicensed assistive personnel (UAP) and licensed practical/vocational nurses (LPN/LVNs) rather than performing direct care activities themselves. They serve as the primary coordinators of client care when consumers receive care in health care organizations. In order to remain in control of and have a voice in daily practice, some nurses assume shared governance responsibilities. When getting patients the services that they need, nurses coordinate care activities. They also use therapeutic communication skills to effectively soothe disgruntled clients, families, and physicians. Sometimes they use humor judiciously for optimal management of emotionally charged situations (especially when work colleagues are involved). Above all, professional nurses keep health care consumers safe and look for ways to enhance environmental safety for all involved in health care delivery.

Keeping nurse experts at the client bedside poses challenges for acute care organizations. Some hospitals have designed nursing **clinical ladders** as a means to keep highly qualified and experienced nurses at the bedside. Clinical ladders reward experienced bedside staff nurses for ongoing professional development activities. Rewards include increased income and job titles that denote professional accomplishments and experience. Frequently, nurses who climb clinical ladders have the opportunity to serve as mentors or preceptors to novice nurses. Many employers use educational status, specialty professional nurse certification, integration of nursing research in clinical practice, and participation in shared governance activities as criteria for promotion.

Forensic Nursing

Forensic nurses provide care to victims of violent crime. Many hospital emergency departments have a nurse who has special education in working with victims of violent crimes. Nursing care provided by forensic nurses includes caring for the victim's injuries, identifying and documenting injuries (including taking photographs), determining wound patterns, collecting evidence (samples of hair, tissue, and body fluids) for future trials, and testifying in court to present and explain evidence and examination findings.

Victims of violent crime benefit from having forensic nurses because these nurses know how to approach and counsel the victims of violent crime while collecting evidence (Fig. 20.1). Some emergency departments have special rape crisis or abuse crisis programs in which victims receive care in specially designated rooms from RNs educated as sexual assault nurse examiners (SANEs). The International Association offers two certifications for SANEs, SANE-A (for

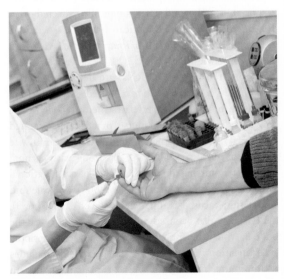

FIGURE 20.1 Forensic nurses collect evidence from victims.

adolescent and adult victims) and SANE-P (for pediatric victims). SANEs preform physical, psychological, developmental and safety patient assessments; collect and document evidence; manage the care of sexually assaulted patients from a holistic perspective; respond to subpoenas and court orders; provide factual or expert witness testimony during trials. Initial management of victims of sexual assaults postevidence collection involves referrals to social workers (International Association of Forensic Nurses, 2016; International Association of Forensic Nurses & ANA, 2009; Stevens, 2004).

Certification in advanced forensic nursing is available through the American Nurses Credentialing Center (ANCC). There is no current certification examination to pass. Credentialing is attained by submitting a portfolio that documents 2 years of experience as a registered nurse, academic qualifications (earned MSN, post-masters certificate or doctoral degree in nursing or forensic nursing), 2,000 practice hours in forensic nursing within the past 3 years, 30 continuing education hours in forensic nursing within the last 3 years, and evidence of fulfilling two of the following professional development criteria: academic credit, professional presentations, publications/research, preceptor to nursing student or other nurses in the field, and professional nursing service (ANCC, 2014).

Take Note!

Due to changes in the health care delivery system, a variety of career options have recently arisen for all professional nurses.

■ QUESTIONS FOR REFLECTION

1. What are the benefits for nurses of having nursing clinical ladders? For hospitals?
2. Would a clinical nursing ladder keep you at the bedside? Why or why not?

Staff Development

Concerns related to staff competency and improving the quality of care have provided impetus for hospitals to maintain nursing staff education and training departments (sometimes called staff development). Staff development roles vary from organization to organization. Typically, staff development personnel provide organizational orientation and continuing education programs. Sometimes, the staff development educator has the responsibility for maintaining American Nursing Credentialing Center (ANCC) certification for the department in order to provide continuing education credit for all offered continuing education programs (an essential part of the job in states that have continuing education requirements for nursing license renewals).

Staff development departments typically manage professional nurse competencies that must be verified on a regular basis (e.g., annual reviews for infection control and safety or biannual cardiopulmonary resuscitation [CPR]). Staff development departments also become involved in offering education for professional nurses on new equipment and new nursing protocols that may arise from quality improvement or initiatives. Verification of professional nurse competence to perform specific clinical skills may be centralized through this department or may occur within individual nursing units. Staff development educators also develop, plan and execute transition programs for new graduate nurses as they assume their first professional nurse position (Association for Nursing Professional Development [ANPD], 2016).

When a facility trains its own UAP the staff development department offers and coordinates training efforts to ensure consistency in UAP preparation. The staff development educator may also manage UAP competencies and provide additional education and training for new equipment, policies, and procedures.

Some hospitals require graduate degrees in nursing or education for staff development positions. ANCC offers certification for nursing staff development educators (ANPD, 2016). Titles for nurses working in this field include staff educator, clinical education specialist, in-service educator, and educational specialist. Some institutions (usually smaller ones) also use staff development personnel to plan community education programs. When a hospital is used as a clinical site for multiple nursing programs, staff educators frequently coordinate clinical day availability, set up programs to verify clinical faculty competence, develop student clinical orientation programs, and keep records related to nursing program satisfaction with the agency as a clinical site.

Utilization Review

In response to Medicare regulations, many hospitals have utilization review programs. To verify the effective use of hospital services, many hospitals and insurance companies use nurses to streamline inpatient care. Because they have the education and experience to understand the effective use of resources, some nurses obtain employment as utilization reviewers. Some managed care organizations employ nurses as preadmission coordinators who prepare the clients for hospital admission by coordinating preadmission testing and providing clients with education related to the usual hospital course (especially for surgical procedures). In addition, some managed care organizations use nurses as case managers who act as the client care advocate to make care-related decisions, recommend medical treatments, certify insurance coverage, and listen to customer expectations and problems.

Working as a utilization reviewer requires a strong clinical background, refined communication skills, good research skills, and well-developed analytical skills. Nurses in these positions often serve as liaisons among the provider, physician, and consumer.

Risk/Quality Management

Most hospitals have departments to monitor care quality, track unusual reported incidents, identify potential liability areas, provide the staff education on the documentation and reporting of incidents, and assist the staff when legal actions or malpractice suits arise. Risk management focuses on reducing institutional financial losses because of care errors and accidents. Nurses employed in risk management departments sometimes hold law degrees.

Although all nurses play a role in managing the quality of health care provided within their institutions, some larger organizations may have a centralized quality management department to assess the quality of services provided. Some quality management departments employ nurses who have earned graduate degrees or doctorates in quality management. Because a large portion of the services offered by hospitals is nursing care, nurses may be members of the quality department. However, some organizations opt for a decentralized approach to quality management. In these cases, staff nurses assume a larger role in monitoring the quality of nursing care and may be required to perform periodic review of client care documentation to verify that quality indicators have been met. As pay for performance and Accountable Care Organizations become more prominent in today's health care delivery system, there may be an increased need for nurses to assume leadership positions in quality management departments.

Travel Nursing

With regional and seasonal RN shortages, some nurses (especially those who like variety, taking risks, and traveling) elect to travel to different inpatient institutions to practice bedside client care. Travel nurses accept staff nurse assignments in all areas of the hospital. Travel nurses may contract with a travel nurse agency or work as independent contractors. Most traveling agencies require that a nurse has 1 to 2 years of acute care experience before a contract is offered.

Travel nurse agencies may contract with hospitals to fill vacant staff nurse positions. The agency offers nurses positions from which to choose as well as assistance with housing, moving, and professional licensure expenses; some agencies may offer benefits (health insurance, life insurance, and retirement plans). Terms of contracts with travel nurse agencies vary greatly. Most temporary agencies require nurses to fulfill their current contract and then wait for a period of time before accepting a position once held as a travel nurse (Morrison, 2014). For example, conditions of a contract may specify that the nurse may not accept employment at a hospital where the agency sent the nurse for 2 years after severing ties with the nursing agency.

Extended-Care Facility Nursing

The Bureau of Labor Statistics (2016a) estimated that close to 196,600 RNs worked in extended-care facilities in 2014. Most of these nurses were educated in diploma or associate degree programs.

Elderly Long-Term Care

For nurses who wish to escape the fast pace of acute care nursing and establish long-term relationships with clients, LTC nursing provides these opportunities. In most LTC facilities, professional nurses assume supervisory roles and delegate tasks to LPN/LVNs, certified medication technicians, and other UAP. With the push for earlier hospital dismissals, complex care needs (e.g., mechanical ventilation, tracheotomy, hyperalimentation, tube feeding) have become common among clients in LTC facilities. Some LTC clients are residents only long enough to complete postoperative therapy or to regain strength after a hospital stay. Thus, the professional nurse can maintain some acute care clinical skills when working in LTC.

Some LTC facilities offer assisted living services. Professional nurses conduct initial periodic client assessments, screen clients for health problems, see clients when health-related problems arise, develop the client care plan, manage client medications, supervise licensed and unlicensed personnel as they provide client care, and determine staff in-service educational needs (Mitty, 2003). Instead of providing an institutional approach to client care, most LTC facilities view themselves as the client's home.

Some nurses find great rewards in working with the elderly. Unfortunately, some elderly clients have no families or support systems, and members of the LTC staff become their only link to the outside world. Many elderly clients develop strong personal relationships with LTC staff. Because death is viewed as a normal part of life in LTC facilities, residents may not be subjected to many invasive procedures or become tethered to technologic equipment that is used only to preserve life. Most LTC facilities permit visits by hospice when death is imminent, enabling comfortable, dignified, and peaceful deaths. Some nurses find a sense of personal and professional satisfaction by easing discomfort in the dying process for the person who is dying and for their significant others.

With the projected increases in the elderly population needing assisted living, LTC nursing represents one of the fastest-growing careers. LTC offers professional nurses the chance to make a significant difference in individual lives.

Rehabilitation Nursing

Advances in trauma care and increases in chemical dependency have resulted in an explosion in the number of rehabilitation facilities. Insurance companies have identified that transferring clients to rehabilitation facilities after bouts of acute illness or surgery saves money. Rehabilitation units have opened as part of acute care and LTC facilities as well as freestanding rehabilitation centers. Some centers specialize in specific rehabilitation needs for a particular health problem such as stroke, head injury, spinal cord trauma, chemical dependency, chronic respiratory illness, amputation, cancer survival, or blindness.

In contrast to nurses working in acute care, rehabilitation nurses participate as equal partners of an interdisciplinary health team. Rehabilitation nurses need to be cooperative team players and have excellent organizational and communication skills. In rehabilitation, there is a strong focus on client education because the goal of rehabilitation is to get the clients to care for themselves or coach someone on how to care for them. Rehabilitation nurses may become very involved with clients and families and experience great satisfaction from being part of the client's journey toward mastering an independent lifestyle. The Association of Rehabilitation Nurses offers special certification in rehabilitation nursing.

Outpatient Nursing Opportunities

Many nursing opportunities occur in outpatient settings. Some outpatient nursing opportunities demand specialized education and training.

Outpatient Clinics and Physician Offices

Nurses working in outpatient clinics and physician offices usually work with clients who have less acute conditions. In 2014, ambulatory care centers employed close to 200,000 RNs (Bureau of Labor Statistics, U.S. Department of Labor, 2016a). Many nurses choose these settings because of better hours (usually daytime hours with no weekend shifts) and less stressful working conditions. Depending on the clinic or office, the professional nurse may be a specialist or a generalist. Some nurses work in clinic settings, where a specialized clinic may be held on a specific day of the week. Clinics and offices may be located close to a hospital, in professional office buildings, shopping malls, pharmaceutical retail establishments, or even department stores. Some urgent care clinics offer services 24 hours a day, 7 days a week for illnesses and injuries not requiring emergency services.

Outpatient Surgery Centers

The number of outpatient or ambulatory surgical centers has exploded within the past 20 years. Many surgical procedures do not require a postoperative hospital stay. Although outpatient centers do not have all the resources available in an acute care setting, they do have emergency equipment available and policies to guide staff should life-threatening emergencies arise. Many nurses working in outpatient surgery centers have operating room experience. In this setting, some nurses admit clients, assist with surgical procedures, provide care after anesthesia administration, give clients discharge instructions, and accompany them to vehicles for the ride home. Some outpatient surgery centers have nurses call to check on client progress the day after a procedure.

> **Take Note!**
> There are myriad nursing opportunities in outpatient settings, some of which require specialized education and training.

Special Care Centers

In addition to outpatient clinics and surgery centers, disease-focused centers provide expert care to people with health problems such as diabetes, heart disease, renal failure, and cancer. Some large urban medical centers have opened breast care centers that provide a comprehensive approach to breast health. Services include screening mammography, breast self-examination education, a comprehensive library related to breast cancer, ultrasound testing, and breast biopsy. In these settings, nurses work as interdisciplinary team members to provide holistic, comprehensive client care.

Community Nursing Centers

Community nursing centers offer primary health care services to middle- and low-income clients at a lower cost than traditional clinics and physician offices. Nurse-run centers usually have an NP and nurses with specialized skills in health education, stress reduction, weight issues, lifestyle management, and other wellness-focused health topics to deliver services. According to a literature review by Coddington and Sands (2008), nurse-managed clinics provide an important safety net for delivering health care services to the underinsured and uninsured. Along with removing barriers to care, nurse-managed centers encourage meaningful, therapeutic relationships between clients and NPs; reduce the incidence of emergency use for primary care and minor illnesses; reduce hospitalizations; promote health; improve patient compliance with treatment plans; and have the same level of consumer satisfaction compared to the care received from a physician's office. Bicki et al. (2013) reported serving 256 patients in a nurse-run community-based clinic and reported saving an estimated $1.28 million in future health care expenditures for these persons by providing vaccinations, screening and effective management of chronic illnesses such as hypertension, diabetes, asthma, and arthritis. Community nursing centers may be located in schools or places of worship. Some communities even offer mobile clinics in converted buses or recreational vehicles. Many nursing centers are affiliated with a collegiate nursing program. If the required care is not available at the community nursing center, nurses make referrals and sometimes arrange for services. Depending on funding, the nursing center may pay for services arranged within a provider network.

Outreach and Education

As consumers seek wellness education, professional nurses frequently find themselves volunteering for various community education groups to teach a variety of health classes (see Chapter 15, "Nursing Approaches to Client Systems"). Local businesses, civic organizations, and faith-based organizations frequently want to offer their staff and members information regarding CPR, first aid, cancer self-examinations, parenting skills, babysitting, and healthy lifestyles. Some organizations request health screenings and may sponsor health fairs.

Cardiac Rehabilitation

Within the past 20 years, most cardiac clients have received offers to participate in cardiac rehabilitation programs after undergoing cardiac catheterization, pacemaker implantation, or open heart surgery. People recovering from myocardial infarctions also qualify for cardiac rehabilitation. Cardiac rehabilitation centers can be found in hospital settings, physician offices, or fitness centers. These programs rely on the expertise of professional nurses and exercise physiologists to develop and supervise a physical workout for patients with cardiac disease.

Most cardiac rehabilitation nurses have a background in critical care nursing and have Advanced Cardiac Life Support (ACLS) certification. Many also have certification in critical care and/or cardiovascular nursing. Cardiac rehabilitation nursing responsibilities include observing cardiac monitors as clients exercise, performing periodic pulse and blood pressure measurements, assessing for signs of overexertion, and teaching relaxation and stress reduction techniques. Some cardiac rehabilitation programs use the nurse for nutritional lifestyle counseling and mental health counseling when nutritionists (or dietitians) and psychologists are not part of the program.

Hospice and Palliative Care Nursing: Outpatient and Inpatient Settings

As the number of elderly increases, so does the incidence of life-limiting diseases. Palliative care occurs across a continuum in which nurses provide care and support to patients and families who experience a serious or potentially life-limiting progressive illness. The goal of hospice and palliative care nursing is to help patient and families live full and comfortable lives as much as possible when encountering serious, life-altering illnesses. In recent years, palliative care has become an option for persons undergoing medical treatments that have profound adverse effects (such as cancer chemotherapy). When an illness is diagnosed as terminal, hospice care is initiated. Hospice care recognizes death as a natural process and attempts to cure the illness are terminated. Palliative care aims to maximize comfort and acknowledges that keeping patients comfortable helps them to live fully during the time that they have remaining. Palliative care measures do not hasten or postpone death (Hospice & Palliative Nurses Association & ANA, 2014).

Hospice and palliative care nursing occurs in homes, residential hospices, extended-care facilities, and hospitals. This special area of practice offers employment opportunities for nurse generalists, clinical nurse specialists (CNSs), and NPs. RNs can take the certification examination offered by the Hospice and Palliative Nurses Association. Some university nursing education programs offer graduate degrees while others offer postgraduate certificates in palliative care. Nursing roles in hospice and palliative care also include case managers, first-line and middle nurse administrative opportunities, and executive positions (Hospice and Palliative Nurses Association & ANA, 2014).

Business Opportunities

Nurses can also find employment opportunities in the business sector. Business career opportunities enable nurses to make an impact on client care by bringing the care ethic to corporations that supply products and reimbursement for health care.

Insurance and Managed Care Companies

Insurance and managed care companies use nurses to evaluate care delivered to customers. Third-party payers frequently use nurses as gatekeepers to verify that company resources have been used effectively to provide services. Responsibilities of nurses employed by these companies include reviewing medical records and activities to evaluate the need for care, ensuring that the appropriate level of care was received, and determining whether quality care was delivered in a timely fashion.

Along with quality management, third-party payers use nurses to staff telephones to certify insurance coverage before service delivery. Nurses who fill certification positions need a strong clinical background and an ability to grasp the global picture of the issues surrounding care delivery. However, nurses employed in this position frequently encounter many ethical dilemmas when working with complex clinical issues and deciding when to certify care. If a wrong decision is made, the nurse may be solely accountable for it, especially if the nurse is a company manager.

Telephone Triage and Health Care Advice Lines

Managed care companies, physician offices, clinics, and hospitals frequently use professional nurses to staff call centers devoted to determining the urgency of care needed, providing health information, referring clients to appropriate health care providers, scheduling appointments with health care providers, and offering health advice. Although triage and health care advice lines started out as a marketing strategy, they quickly

demonstrated the ability to streamline the use of health care services, thereby reducing health care costs. Some managed care companies require that subscribers call the triage nurse to certify trips to emergency departments.

Nurses use assessment and therapeutic communication skills to determine the extent of the health problems of callers. Because some clients become frequent callers, telephone triage nurses may develop long-term relationships with them. Some nurses report that they schedule the time to call clients to follow-up on the decisions they made.

Marketing and Sales

Companies that sell products such as pharmaceuticals, equipment, and monitors often hire professional nurses as sales representatives. Nurses provide credibility for product promotion, especially when they have used the product in clinical practice. Nurses also provide insight into product improvements and future products that may be useful in client care delivery. When complex equipment is purchased, the company often provides staff education in the use of the equipment.

Nurses can be effective sales representatives because they know how to approach other nurses and anticipate questions and problems that nurses may experience. Sales representatives must be energetic and self-motivated. Because most sales representatives work from their homes and travel a lot, they work in flexible hours. Much time is spent meeting with prospective customers. Nurses entering the corporate sales world require knowledge related to the business world and principles of operating a home office. Some companies provide a base salary that does not meet the salary earned in clinical practice. However, significant bonuses can be earned on commissions from successful sales.

Occupational Health and Worker's Compensation Programs

Many businesses have occupational health departments or contract with businesses that offer occupational health services to offer employee health services. Occupation health services are designed to manage workplace injuries, prevent work-related illnesses, screen for environmental or occupational hazards, and provide employee health education services. Occupational health nurses may offer CPR training and health promotion education for company employees. However, more importantly, they also respond to work-related injuries or medical emergencies that occur. Some companies rely on the occupational health nurse to track the progress of workers recovering from work-related injuries. Other companies use nurses employed by the worker's compensation insurance plan to monitor worker progress. Nurses often develop light-duty work programs for employees who cannot perform all regular job duties but can provide some work for the company.

Take Note!
Through a career in the business sector, nurses can impact client care by bringing the care ethic to pharmaceutical and medical device companies and to organizations that provide reimbursement for health care.

Private Consulting

When a nurse identifies a problem, an area for consulting has surfaced. As companies outsource employee services, demands for consultants increase. Health care organizations use consulting firms to prepare for accreditation visits, apply for quality awards, meet employee educational needs, engage in work redesign, and look for ways to reduce operating costs. Some consultants have insider status, with which they provide special services within a system that employs them. Other consultants have outsider status; they work either as an independent contractor or for a company that provides services to organizations (Norwood, 1998). For example, a hospital may employ an enterostomal therapist specifically to provide ostomy care and education for clients and families. However, when the need arises for staff education related to ostomy care, the hospital uses the enterostomal therapist to provide a staff program. Extended-care facilities may use external nurse consultants for monthly client assessments or to provide client services such as foot or ostomy care. Health care consumers may use nurse consultants to assist in selecting an extended-care facility for a family member, paying medical bills, or learning relaxation techniques.

The success of nursing consultants depends on having proficiency in the area in which consultation is provided; strong theoretical, business, and clinical skills; the ability to solve problems quickly; and the ability to compete with other consultants. Consulting or working as an independent contractor can be done part-time until the business becomes established and profitable (Norwood, 1998).

Legal nurse consultants (LNCs) have been in existence for many years. As our society grows more litigious, the demand for LNCs is rising. Because of the nature of the work, the skills required for LNCs include an ability to quickly find relevant nursing and medical literature pertaining to a case, effective computer skills (internet-search proficiency), well-developed critical thinking skills, and detailed knowledge of legal issues surrounding nursing and health care delivery. LNCs assume the following roles and responsibilities: (1) clarify medical terminology; (2) review medical records to determine if harm was caused directly by a health provider's actions or inactions; (3) find and review current medical nursing and health care literature relevant to cases; (4) develop timelines and summaries to explain events of a case or claim; (5) locate or serve as an expert witness; (6) conduct interviews with clients, witnesses, or other parties; (7) assist in the development of case strategy; (8) educate attorneys and clients on medical issues; (9) identify and present relevant standards of current medical and nursing; (10) estimate the long-term costs of care associated with case injuries; (11) be present at independent medical examinations; (12) provide expert nurse testimony for cases; (13) evaluate elements of causation and damages sustained; and (14) provide support to clients during legal proceedings.

LNCs may be independent contractors or employees of a law firm. When working for a law firm, the LNC enjoys the benefits of working within an organization and does not need to assume the responsibility of running a business (American Association of Legal Nurse Consultants, 2016; Zorn, 2015). Community colleges, 4-year universities, and law schools have educational programs for nurses interested in becoming LNCs. The American Association of Legal Nurse Consultants offers certification examinations that assess the key knowledge and skills required for legal nurse consulting as well demonstrating a commitment to this specialized area of professional nursing.

In recent years, many nurse consultants have become entrepreneurs. Starting and running an independent business is a complex undertaking. Some nurses who have specialized education in complementary health care practices, such as massage, therapeutic touch, aromatherapy, or magnet therapy, may assume the role of nurse consultant when they use these practices or help others to incorporate them into client care.

ADVANCED NURSING PRACTICE CAREER OPTIONS

Most APRN careers require some education beyond the baccalaureate degree. Currently, APRN practice is recognized in the roles of NP, certified nurse-midwife (CNM), certified registered nurse anesthetist (CRNA), and CNS.

In the United States, the practice of nursing is determined at the state level. Some states recognize professional certification as a nurse-midwife or practitioner as the credential to obtain an advanced practice nursing license. However, because of the multiple entry paths into professional nursing, the NCSBN and professional nurses have pushed for APRNs to obtain a second nursing license to provide assurance that a minimum set of professional competencies is met. In addition, licensure as an APRN enables some nurses to prescribe medications and receive direct insurance (private and/or government policies) reimbursement for rendered services in most states. In most states, APRN licensure and statutes for advanced practice falls under the jurisdiction of State Board of Nursing (SBN). However, some states may have legal statutes and regulations for APRN practice with the Board of Healing Arts (BHA). There are some states (especially those who do not require collaborative practice agreements) that statutes and regulations for APRN practice are determined by both the SBN and BHA.

As APRNs move across state and national borders, credentialing becomes increasingly important. Credentialing provides documentation that an individual is recognized by a regulatory body and has met the standards to use a particular title. In health care, credentialing serves as a vehicle to protect the public against people who fail to meet the set standards and preparation to execute certain duties. Because of the variance among state nurse practice acts, some states require credentialing prior to attainment of the second advanced nursing practice license. Along with providing initial documentation of qualifications for advanced practice, most states require that the APRN fulfill continuing education and specific practice requirements (a certain number of clinical practice hours) to maintain certification (Jansen & Zwygart-Stauffacher, 2010).

Doctor of Nursing Practice

The American Association of Colleges of Nursing (AACN, 2006) passed a resolution recommending that all APRNs should be educated in a new program called the Doctor of Nursing Practice (DNP). In 2010, the NCBSN and the AACN adopted the Licensure, Accreditation, Certification, and Education model to regulate advanced practice nursing in the United States. This model is slated to be fully implemented by 2015. Although recommended, the DNP is not an educational requirement for nurses to take advanced practice nurse certification examinations. Nurses with master's degrees can also take these certification examinations.

Under the Licensure, Accreditation, Certification, and Education model, the nurse would be licensed according to role and population focus after passing a national certification examination. Licensure in an advanced practice role is a legal requirement before engaging in advanced nursing practice. The APRN would pass an examination in one of the six following population foci: family (across the lifespan), adult-gerontology, neonatal, pediatric, women's health/gender-related, or psychiatric/mental health. Certifying bodies include the American Nurses Credentialing Center; American Academy of Nurse Practitioners; American Association of Critical Care Nurses; American Psychiatric Nurses Association; Association for Women's Health, Obstetrics and Neonatal Nursing; National Board of Pediatric Nurse Practitioners and Associates; and the Oncology Nursing Society. The Council for the Advancement of Comprehensive Care has developed a certification examination for DNP graduates who have undertaken comprehensive care programs (Jansen & Zwygart-Stauffacher, 2010).

The DNP remains controversial for several reasons. Some states do not recognize the DNP for APRN practice, and others have statutory restrictions regarding the use of the title "Doctor," limiting its use in health care settings to medical or osteopathic physicians and surgeons, podiatrists, and dentists. Rhodes (2011) outlined facilitating factors and barriers to the DNP as entry level for APRNs. Adoption of the DNP by the National Council of State Boards of Nursing and individual states would provide APRNs with advanced competencies for the ever-increasing complexity of clinical, faculty, and leadership roles; enhance knowledge to improve nursing practice and client outcomes; improve the match between program requirements and earned degree; provide parity with other professional health team members; attract people to nursing from non-nursing backgrounds; increase the supply of clinical nursing faculty; and improve the image of the nursing profession. Currently, 264 universities have enrolled students into DNP programs, and 60 more DNP programs are planned (AACN, 2015a).

With the shortage of primary care physicians, the increased time required to prepare APRNs for preventive and primary care services to consumers could mean reduced access for the public to health care services, increased health care costs, and the rise of physician assistants as the cost-effective primary care provider (who have poorer outcomes than APRNs) (Newhouse, Bass, Steinwachs, et al., 2011). In addition, faculty with nursing doctorates would need to complete postgraduate education (in DNP programs), resulting in fewer qualified faculty to teach in undergraduate nursing programs and exacerbating the current and projected professional nursing shortage.

The DNP as entry level for APRN practice has been rejected by the ANA, American College of Nurse Midwives, American Organization of Nurse Executives, and the National Association of Nurse Practitioners in Women's Health. The American Association of Nurse Anesthetists has accepted DNP as the entry degree into practice provided that full implementation be delayed until 2025 (Rhodes, 2011).

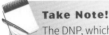

Take Note!

The DNP, which may become the entry level for APRN practice, remains controversial.

Additional Advanced Practice Opportunities

In addition to opportunities as an NP, CNS, CRNA, and CNM, other emerging advanced practice opportunities include parish nurses, case managers, clinical transplant coordinators, childbirth educators, advanced diabetes managers, genetic advanced practice nurses, and wound, ostomy, and continence nurses (Hamric & Hanson, 2013). However, many of these practice areas may not require graduate collegiate education. Instead, nurses who enter these specialized practice areas typically take specific continuing education courses and practice a specified number of hours within a given specialty to qualify to take certification exams (offered by a specialty nurse organization or the American Nurses Credentialing Center). Once they pass the certification exam, they become recognized nurse specialists.

Global APRN Practices

The APRN movement is not confined to the United States. Progress toward education, regulation, and utilization has occurred globally, especially in Australia, Africa, the Americas, and Europe. The United States remains the only nation with specified regulations for APRN practice in the NP, CNM, CNS, and CRNA roles. Canada has regulations for the CNS and NP roles. Less defined roles and regulations for NPs occur in Latin America, South Africa, and Botswana. In Mexico, Honduras, and Bolivia, there is no requirement for advanced nursing education. Japan and China have embraced the role of CNS, but there is no formalized regulation. South Korea started developing APRN practice roles in the 1950s starting with CNMs. In South Korea, 10 types of APRNs are recognized across multiple specialty

areas, each of which requires an advanced nursing degree and is regulated by the Ministry of Health. In Thailand, thousands of NPs provide care across a variety of specialties. Australian APRNs practice as CNSs and NPs and abide by the regulations similar to those in the United States. Advanced practice is common in Europe, with the CNS and NP roles dominating, and in all European countries with the exception of Nordic countries, which have formal regulations for APRN practice.

Effectiveness of APRNs

Multiple research studies suggest that NPs provide safe, efficient, cost-effective care to consumers (Sheer & Wong, 2008). Newhouse et al. (2011) conducted a comprehensive systematic review of studies addressing APRN outcomes, the results of which are presented in Focus on Research, "APRNs Versus Physicians: A Study of Outcomes." This study has been used as a basis for governmental agencies and health insurance companies to approve APRN care services.

FOCUS ON RESEARCH

APRNs Versus Physicians: A Study of Outcomes

The investigative team conducted a systematic review of studies addressing APRN outcomes. Research articles included in the study were found from a systematic database search using PubMed, the Cumulative Index to Nursing and Allied Health Literature, and Proquest. The inclusion criteria for study literature were randomized controlled trials (RCTs) or observational studies of at least two provider groups (APRNs working independently or in a team with physicians compared to physicians working alone or in teams without an APRN); and quantitative studies conducted in the United States regarding APRN outcomes published between 1990 and 2008. Each study was evaluated for quality by two team members for comparability of participants and practice settings, sample size, reported validity and reliability, ways to control bias, and at least one outcome that could be linked directly to APRNs.

Study data were analyzed and synthesized first by creating detailed tables for each APRN role. High evidence ranking was reserved for groups of studies that contained at least two RCTs or one RCT and two high-quality observational studies. Of the 107 reviewed studies, only 45 were ranked as high-evidence studies.

Thirty-seven studies addressed NP patient outcomes. When comparing NP care and physician care, the studies provided high levels of evidence that patients had equal levels of satisfaction with received care, perceived health status, functional abilities, glucose levels, blood pressure, use of inpatient care, emergency room visits, and mortality rates. There was a high level of evidence that NPs managed patient serum lipid levels better than physicians.

Twenty-one studies were aggregated for CNM outcomes. High levels of evidence were identified for equivalent outcomes for physicians and CNMs for Apgar scores, levels of labor augmentation, and low–birth-weight infants. High evidence levels were found for CNMs for lower rates of epidural use, labor induction, vaginal operative deliveries, labor analgesia, third- and fourth-degree lacerations, and lower rates of infant admissions to neonatal intensive care units. CNMs were found to have higher rates of breast feeding compared to physicians.

Eleven studies were analyzed for CNS outcomes. High levels of evidence were found for shorter hospital stays, lower care costs, and, and fewer complications.

Studies of CRNAs were focused on clinical interventions, and very few outcome studies could be found. Only single observational studies were found that suggested equivalent mortality and complications from anesthesia when comparing CRNA care and anesthesiologist care.

This systematic review revealed that NP and CRNA care outcomes are equivalent to those achieved by physicians. CNMs tend to have fewer invasive interventions than physicians that may result in reduced complication rates. CNMs also provide care primarily to women who have uncomplicated pregnancies and deliveries, which may account for the reduced number of interventions. CNMs and physicians appear to have similar outcomes of pregnancy and deliveries. With the Centers for Medicare and Medicaid Services reimbursement schedule of 85% of physician rate for APRN services, APRN care may provide a substantial reduction in costs to the government for delivery of health care in the United States.

Newhouse, R., Bass, E., Steinwachs, D., et al. (2011). Advanced practice nurse outcomes 1990–2008: A systematic review. *Nursing Economic, 29*(5), 230–250.

OPPORTUNITIES FOR APRNs

The following discussion presents information on the most common forms of advanced nursing practice. NPs, CNSs, and CNMs sometimes practice case management as a way to coordinate health care services across the continuum of care (Lundy & Huch, 2009). In acute care settings, NPs and CNSs assist patients and their significant others as they negotiate the complex maze of health care delivery, set realistic health outcomes, determine health care needs following facility dismissal, and develop strategies to improve health (education or supportive services). Home health agencies and community health centers use APRNs as case managers to coordinate needed health care services to keep people at home. Providing home care is more cost-effective than providing inpatient or residential care.

Nurse Practitioners

NPs provide primary health care services to consumers, including assessing client health using a holistic framework; identifying medical and nursing diagnoses; planning and prescribing treatments; managing health care regimens for individuals, families, and communities; promoting wellness; preventing illness and injury; and managing acute and chronic health conditions. The NP role surfaced during a physician shortage in the 1960s. The first NPs attended certification programs that lasted from a few weeks to as long as 2 years. NPs carved out a distinct difference in practice from the medical model by using a holistic approach to care based on nursing theory.

As the recognition of NPs grew (mostly related to the reduced cost of primary care and positive health outcomes for clients) NP programs in higher education settings proliferated. Education at the master's level dominates the education of NPs. Specialty practice areas for NPs include family care, adult care, pediatrics, geriatrics, acute care, and women's health. Primary care NPs typically practice in outpatient settings; provide health care services aimed at health promotion, disease prevention, and management of simple, acute, and chronic health conditions; and establish a partnership with their clients.

Acute care NPs provide health care services to clients who may be hospital inpatients or clients seeking care in emergency room, urgent care or clinic settings. They work in a variety of clinical specialties, including diabetes management, orthopedics, oncology, neurology, neurosurgery, and cardiovascular services. Acute care NPs frequently perform procedures that residents perform in teaching hospitals, such as lumbar punctures (neurologic acute NP), bone marrow aspirations (oncology acute NP), harvesting saphenous vein grafts during coronary bypass surgery (cardiovascular surgery acute NP), or serving as first assistants during surgery. They may work with physicians or they may have independent practice privileges at hospitals (Jansen & Zwygart-Stauffacher, 2010). NPs also provide health care services to the underprivileged and people living in underserved areas (Bureau of Labor Statistics, U.S. Department of Labor, 2016b).

In 2015, 136,060 NPs were employed and earned a mean salary of $101,260. NPs who are employed in surgical and acute care settings earn more than those employed in primary care. (Bureau of Labor Statistics, U.S. Department of Labor, 2016b). To qualify for direct third-party reimbursement, NPs must obtain certification. Most NPs are required to renew their certification every 5 years. This process requires documented practice and evidence of continuing education (Jansen & Zwygart-Stauffacher, 2010). NPs have earned the respect of clients and other health team members.

Certified Nurse-Midwives

Certified nurse-midwives independently manage women's health care with a special emphasis on pregnancy, childbirth, postpartum care, newborn care, family planning, and well-woman care (Fig. 20.2). Well-woman care focuses on family planning, screening for female-related cancer, and management of perimenopause and postmenopause. CNM care supports the natural processes of birth, growth, development, and aging; CNMs intervene only if absolutely indicated.

Of all the advanced practice roles, midwifery is the oldest. Records of midwifery practice are documented in the Bible. As the profession of medicine arose, midwifery declined. Mary Breckenridge, who received midwifery education in Scotland, became the first practicing

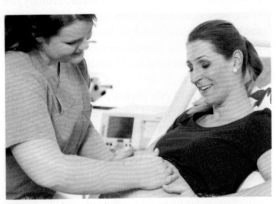

FIGURE 20.2 Certified nurse midwives provide material care before, during, and after delivery.

nurse-midwife in the United States when she established the Frontier Nursing Service in 1925. In 1932, the first American nurse-midwifery education program opened in the Maternity Center of the Lobenstein Clinic in New York City. Slow growth in nurse-midwifery occurred, and it was not until 1955 that the American College of Nurse-Midwives was established. The modern midwife emerged with a pilot project in Madera County, California, in the early 1960s. By the 1970s, nurse-midwifery was in demand by consumers seeking a more natural approach to childbirth. In 1971, a national certification examination became the standard for entry into practice by the American College of Nurse-Midwives. However, CNM practice is regulated by individual states, thereby creating variances in prescriptive authority, educational preparation, employment contracts, and practice arrangements. In 2015, the Bureau of Labor Statistics, U.S. Department of Labor (2016b) reported that there were 7,340 CNMs employed in the United States who earned a mean income of $93,610.

Although they started as certificate programs, nurse-midwifery programs progressed to graduate nursing education. By the 1990s, many CNMs were graduating from university-based programs (Hamric & Hanson, 2013). Forty-seven nurse-midwifery programs are housed in American universities, all but seven of which are incorporated into master of nursing programs. The AACN (2006) adopted the DNP as the desired degree for CNMs by 2015.

Research indicates that CNMs contribute substantially to the quality of maternal–child health care. The Bureau of Health Professions (BHPR) (2003) reported reduced cesarean section rates and fewer medical interventions for women at low risk cared for by CNMs when compared with women at low risk cared for by physicians. Studies report significantly lower neonatal mortality and infant mortality, as well as higher birth weights of infants when women were attended by CNMs. Along with improved outcomes, CNMs provide women with health care at reduced costs (BHPR, 2003; Gaudier, 2003; Rosseter, 2013).

Clinical Nurse Specialists

CNSs are highly skilled clinical experts in a specialized area of nursing practice and use all the steps of the nursing process to promote health, prevent complications, and manage health problems. CNSs work in many settings, including hospitals, schools, extended-care facilities, homes, and community agencies. In 2010, the BHPR estimated that close to 60,000 CNSs were in practice, earning an average annual salary of $74,918.

In 1954, Hildegard Peplau established the first graduate level CNS program at New Jersey's Rutgers University to prepare psychiatric CNSs. CNSs provide expert patient care, serve as professional role models, and act as client advocates. They also provide indirect care services when they act as consultants or resources to other health team members, supervise care delivery, act as liaisons between the client system and the care providers, initiate and direct change for client care, and engage in research and evidence-based nursing projects through clinical research. Some CNSs have prescriptive privileges. Second licensure as an APRN is not required for CNS practice in some states.

Hamric and Hanson (2013) noted that changing population demographics, health care cost containment issues, accessibility and affordability of care delivery, the ever-expanding knowledge base for specialty nursing practice arenas, and shortages of physicians and nurses have resulted in the role blending of CNS and NP. When CNSs have prescriptive privileges, typically most states require a second advanced practice nursing license. Nurses who have merged the roles of NP and CNS usually have had graduate educational preparation in both roles. The blended role offers nurses an opportunity to cross health care settings, provide comprehensive health care services to a narrowly defined clinical population, and serve as team members in primary, secondary, and tertiary care settings.

Early CNSs worked primarily in hospitals to provide support for patients and nursing staff. However, with the advent of managed care, many hospitals enlisted CNSs to serve as case managers. CNSs coordinate care of highly acute patients within the hospital and have been used as discharge planners. They practice in many subspecialty fields, including pulmonology, oncology, neuroscience, geriatrics, rehabilitation, diabetes, hospice, and palliative care. In the 1990s, CNSs assumed case management positions within their specialty area of practice. Case management by APRNs is expected to evolve and, perhaps, become more commonplace as the population ages and more elderly people with chronic illnesses have complex health care needs (Hamric & Handon, 2013). In 2006, the AACN proposed a new academic degree, the clinical nurse leader, which is a master's degree aimed at facilitating seamless health care delivery across the health care continuum.

Certified Registered Nurse Anesthetists

CRNAs provide anesthesia and anesthetic-related services to health care consumers (Fig. 20.3). Along with completing the 24-month program consisting of

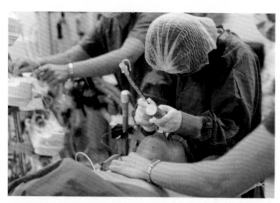

FIGURE 20.3 Certified registered nurse anesthetists deliver anesthesia including patient intubation as well as perform advanced procedures for pain relief.

advanced study in anatomy, physiology, chemistry, and pathophysiology, and 90 hours emphasizing the principles of anesthesia, an RN must administer at least 450 anesthetics before taking the certification examination (Hamric & Hanson, 2013).

All 50 states recognize CRNA practice. According to the American Association of Nurse Anesthetists (2013), CRNA practice includes preanesthetic assessment; anesthetic plan development and implementation; anesthesia induction; selection, application, and insertion of noninvasive and invasive monitoring devices; anesthetic selection, acquisition, and administration; fluid and ventilatory support; administration of medications and fluids to facilitate the emergence and recovery from anesthesia; patient discharge and follow-up care after anesthesia administration; airway support and management in medical emergencies; and implementation of various acute and chronic pain treatment modalities. Despite rigorous, standardized education requirements, approximately 80% of CRNAs practice anesthesia with a group of physician anesthesiologists. The other 20% practice independently to provide anesthesia services to outpatient clinics and rural hospitals (more than 70% of rural hospitals rely on CRNAs for anesthesia services). CRNAs receive payment for services directly from third-party payers and assume full legal responsibility for their own actions (Hamric & Hanson, 2013). The Bureau of Labor Statistics, U.S. Department of Labor (2016b) reported that in 2015, there were 39,410 employed CRNAs who earned a mean income of $160,250.

Registered Nurse First Assistant

Registered nurse first assistants (RNFAs) may be employed by hospitals and physicians or may work as independent contractors. Practice settings for RNFAs include hospitals, ambulatory surgical centers, and physician offices. RNFAs work collaboratively with surgeons during surgery; they may prepare the skin for incisions, hold retractors, assist with clamping vessels, perform suction, perform cautery, irrigate surgical wound beds, and close the incisions. Along with working in the operating room, RNFAs collect client histories, perform preoperative assessments, make client preoperative visits, educate clients about procedures, and conduct postoperative visits (Siefert, 2014). RNFAs are widely used in rural hospitals.

The scope of responsibility of RNFAs varies according to the employment setting. RNFAs working in surgeons' offices tend to have more autonomy and responsibilities than those employed by hospitals. The Association of Operating Room Nurses published the first official statement on RNFAs in 1984, then structured an educational and certificate program for RNFAs in 1985. Qualifications for certification as an RNFA include current licensure as an RN, certification from the Association of Operating Room Nurses as a certified operating room nurse, a bachelor's degree in nursing or a master's degree in nursing with a bachelor's degree in another field of study, and 2,000 documented hours of RNFA practice with the first 120 hours being completed under the guidance of a surgeon preceptor (Siefert, 2014).

RNFAs are reimbursed for their services at a lower rate than are assisting surgeons. Medicare does not reimburse RNFAs for their services. Many receive payment from the surgeons or hospitals for which they work (Siefert, 2014).

INDIRECT CLIENT CARE ADVANCED NURSING CAREER OPTIONS

Nursing Administration

Most health care organizations and systems employ nurses as administrators or managers. Positions in **nursing administration** range from departmental heads (head nurse or nurse manager) to chief nursing officers or chief nurse executives (director of nursing). In many hospitals, the traditional "head nurse" position has been replaced with a "nurse manager," who may have to manage more than one unit. Many hospitals require advanced degrees for management or administrative positions. Many colleges and universities offer graduate nursing education in nursing administration. Some nursing administrative personnel have opted to pursue graduate degrees in business or health administration to facilitate role performance. Complex

budgetary considerations, institutional accreditation requirements, legal issues, strategic planning, and staff management concerns (including having enough staff for effective care) are some of the key dimensions of the nurse administration career option (Caroselli, 2008).

Nursing Academia

Teaching the new generation of nurses provides great rewards for nursing faculty members. A career in **nursing academia** (nursing education) enables experienced nurses to share their knowledge and expertise with future professional nurses. As a faculty member, the nurse has opportunities to polish clinical skills, expand the knowledge of clinical nursing, engage in nursing research, and participate in community service. Although most nursing programs require a master's degree in nursing and recent clinical experience for faculty appointment, some associate degree and vocational nursing programs may hire baccalaureate-prepared nurses. Most programs preparing certified nursing assistants use baccalaureate-prepared nurses as faculty. Nursing programs offering baccalaureate degrees prefer to hire faculty with nursing or educational doctorates. The AACN (2015a) recognized that both the doctor of philosophy degree in nursing and DNP are terminal degrees in nursing. Both degrees enable nurses with these advanced degrees to teach in collegiate and university settings. However, the AACN recommends that additional optional coursework in education should be added to DNP programs that would prepare nurse educators (AACN, 2015b).

State- and privately sponsored research universities require faculty to develop a program of nursing research. In these settings, faculty members develop research proposals, write grants to fund projects, engage in research, disseminate research findings, and fulfill teaching responsibilities. Nursing programs in the community college setting emphasize technical aspects of nursing and faculty members concentrate on teaching the students clinical skills. Many faculty members practice nursing outside the academic setting to maintain their clinical competence (Penn, 2008).

Distance learning programs pose different challenges for faculty. In addition to being content and practice experts, nurse faculty in these programs must have the knowledge and expertise to run computer hardware, use software to engage learners, work with technology support staff, and establish online student relationships. As technology continues to evolve, faculty must remain more flexible with online instruction, especially if the required technology fails (Penn, 2008).

Nurse Researcher

As health care facilities strive to deliver the best quality care, many have hired nurse researchers to fill director of nursing research positions. Director of Nursing Research roles vary across institutions. The Institute of Medicine's (2011) recommendation to include the use of best practices to provide safe, effective, and efficient health care has created a climate that values the input of evidence-based practices and protocols. In many facilities, the director of nursing research educates staff about the research process and how to critique research studies effectively. The director of nursing research also guides, supports, and assists staff as they engage in evidence-based quality improvement and nursing research projects (Dumont, 2008).

Nurse Entrepreneurs

Because of the complex factors and education needed to establish and maintain an independent business, the career as **nurse entrepreneur** fits the description of advanced nursing practice. Many nurse entrepreneurs experience some life-defining event that serves as the reason for a career change. Life-defining events may be a singular event, such as reaching a personally significant age, changing marital status, or having a child or children, or they may be a compilation of factors, such as job boredom, frustration with administration, an unfulfilled need, or a general feeling that life is being wasted. Setting out to become an entrepreneur can be a challenging yet fulfilling move (see Box 20.1, Learning, Knowing, and Growing, "The Road to Entrepreneurship").

Not all nurses have the personality needed to embark on the entrepreneurial career path. Key personality characteristics shared by successful entrepreneurs include a willingness to take risks, self-confidence, internal locus of control, determination, perseverance, interpersonal communication skills, willingness to delay gratification, business awareness, desire for total control, ability to direct others, physical stamina, mental resilience, and a strong need for achievement. Running a personal business requires detailed knowledge of the corporate world and governmental policies that guide small businesses (Vogel & Doleysh, 1997; Waxman, 2005; Bennis, 2016).

Waxman (2005) and Bennis (2016) identify the advantages and disadvantages of being a nurse entrepreneur. Advantages include a high level of autonomy, flexible working hours, constant change, meeting new people, using previously untapped skills (creativity and interpersonal), and being paid high hourly rates.

20.1 Learning, Knowing, and Growing

The Road to Entrepreneurship

Making the move from nursing practice to entrepreneurship generally follows these steps (Vogel & Doleysh, 1997; Bennis, 2016).

1. The nurse entrepreneur discovers an idea for a viable business. Frequently, the idea for a business appears while practicing professional nursing in a traditional institution.

2. The nurse entrepreneur gathers more information about the idea to provide a solid foundation for the new business concept.

3. The nurse entrepreneur develops the business concept by verifying the idea through the gathering of more information.

4. The nurse entrepreneur performs an initial test of the business concept for success.

5. The nurse entrepreneur consults someone to navigate the complex legal aspects of developing, and running a business.

6. If needed, the nurse entrepreneur seeks out a business loan or financial partner for the business.

7. The nurse entrepreneur expands the number and types of offered products or services.

8. The nurse entrepreneur expands the business to include organizational structures, employees, policies, and procedures.

Vogel, G., & Doleysh, N. (1997). *Entrepreneuring: A nurses' guide to starting a business (NLN Publication No. 41–2201).* New York: National League for Nursing; Bennis, P. A. (2016). *Self- Employed RN: Earn respect, independence & a higher income.* San Bernardino, CA: P.A. Bennis.

Disadvantages include, loss of employee-based fringe benefits, having to secure accounts payable, taking risks, loss of daily contact with other nurses, no paid time off, and loss of job structure. However, many nurses, especially those who enjoy working independently, find being an entrepreneur satisfying and rewarding.

▌ QUESTIONS FOR REFLECTION

1. What career options sound like they might appeal to you in the short term? In 10 years?
2. What further information about the career options presented in this chapter would you like?
3. What additional education or skills would you need to obtain to pursue a specific career option in nursing?

Summary and Significance to Practice

Professional nursing offers many career options for committed, caring nurses. Nurses have opportunities not afforded to the other health professions to change their specialty and practice areas. Many expanded and most advanced nursing practice roles require additional education. Most APRN roles require certification and additional licensure in some states. In the future, the educational preparation for these roles might be a nursing doctorate. Although some nurses find that discovering one's personal niche in the profession can be a challenging and complex process, especially when they take the time to explore the various available career options, after determining their personal passion and professional goals, nurses can make their career decisions with confidence.

REAL-LIFE REFLECTIONS

Recall Laura from the beginning of the chapter. How would you respond to Laura if she asked you about your current nursing practice or your career plans? Why would you respond this way?

From Theory to Practice

1. Whom would you contact if you wanted to explore one of the nursing career options presented in this chapter? Why would you select this person? What other resources might you use?

Nurse as Author

Based on the information you learned in this chapter, write an essay about what career in professional nursing most interests you. In the opening paragraph, identify the career and explain why it appeals to you. In the next two to four paragraphs, outline the steps you will need to take to become a practicing nurse in this area; what current barriers do you face and what resources will you need to overcome them?

Your Digital Classroom

Online Explorations

All Nursing Schools: **www.allnursingschools.com**
American Association of Nurse Anesthetists:
  http://www.aana.com/Pages/default.aspx

American Association of Nurse Practitioners:
  www.aanp.org/
American Nurses Association: **www.nursingworld.org**
Health Resources and Services Administration:
  http://www.hrsa.gov/index.html
International Association of Forensic Nurses:
  http://www.forensicnurses.org/
Johnson & Johnson's Campaign for Nursing's Future:
  www.discovernursing.com
Sigma Theta Tau International Honor Society of
  Nursing: **www.nursingsociety.org**
TravelNursing.com: **www.travelnursing.com**
U.S. Department of Labor, Bureau of Labor Statistics
  Occupational Outlook Handbook:
  http://www.bls.gov/ooh/

Expanding Your Understanding

1. Visit the Sigma Theta Tau International website (**www.nursingsociety.org**). At the top of the page, hover on the words "Advance & Educate." Select Careers by clicking on the word "Careers:" Explore all the resources available related to career advice. Did you find the information helpful? Why or why not?
2. Visit the American Nurses Association website and look for information about specialty practice certification and advanced practice nursing. Was this information useful? Why or why not? Do you see yourself becoming an advanced practice nurse? Why or why not?

Beyond the Book

Visit the**Point**® **www.thePoint.lww.com** for activities and information to reinforce the concepts and content covered in this chapter.

REFERENCES

American Association of Colleges of Nursing. (2006). *DNP roadmap task force report.* Retrieved from www.aacn.nche.edu/DNP/roadmapreport.pdf. Accessed February 26, 2013.

American Association of Colleges of Nursing. (2015a). *DNP fact sheet.* Retrieved from http://www.aacn.nche.edu/media-relations/fact-sheets/dnp. Accessed June 18, 2016.

American Association of Colleges of Nursing. (2015b). The Doctor of Nursing Practice: Current Issues and Clarifying Recommendations Report from the Task Force on the Implementation of the DNP. Retrieved from http://www.aacn.nche.edu/aacn-publications/white-papers/DNP-Implementation-TF-Report-8–15.pdf. Accessed June 18, 2016.

American Association of Legal Nurse Consultants. (2016). What is an LNC? Retrieved from http://www.aalnc.org/page/what-is-an-lnc. Accessed June 18, 2016.

American Association of Nurse Anesthetists. (2013). *Certified registered nurse anesthetists at a glance.* Retrieved from www.

aana.com/ceandeducation/becomeacrna/Pages/Nurse-Anes-thetists-at-a-Glance.aspx. Accessed February 26, 2013.

American Nurses Association. (2015). *Scope and standards of nursing practice* (3rd ed.). Silver Spring, MD: Author.

American Nurses Credentialing Center. (2014). *Certification through portfolio requirements.* Retrieved from http://www.nursecredentialing.org/CertificationPortfolioRequirements. Accessed June 12, 2016.

Association for Nursing Professional Development. (2016). *About ANPD.* Retrieved from http://www.anpd.org/?page = about. Accessed June 12, 2016.

Bennis, P. A. (2016). *Self-Employed RN 101: Earn respect, independence & a higher income.* San Bernardino, CA: P. A. Bennis.

Bicki, A., Silva, A., Joseph, V., Handoko, R., Rico, S.V., Burns, J., et al. (2013). A nurse-run walk-in clinic: cost-effective alternative to non-urgent emergency department use by the uninsured. *Journal of Community Health, 38,* 1042–1049. doi: 10.1007/s10900–013–9712-y

Bureau of Health Professions. (2003). *A comparison of changes in the professional practice of nurse practitioners, physician assistants, and certified nurse midwives: 1992–2000.* Retrieved from http://bhpr.hrsa.gov/healthworkface/reports/scope/scope1–2./htm. Accessed July 1, 2005.

Bureau of Labor Statistics. (1992). *Occupational outlook handbook.* Washington, DC: Author.

Bureau of Labor Statistics, U.S. Department of Labor. (2016a). *Occupational outlook handbook, 2016–17 edition, registered nurses.* Retrieved from http://www.bls.gov/ooh/healthcare/registered-nurses.htm#tab-3. Accessed June 12, 2016.

Bureau of Labor Statistics, U.S. Department of Labor. (2016b). May 2015 National Occupational Employment and Wage Estimates. Retrieved from http://www.bls.gov/oes/current/oes_nat.htm#29–0000. Accessed June 18, 2016.

Caroselli, C. (2008). The system chief nurse executive: More than the sum of the parts. *Nursing Administration Quarterly, 32*(3), 247–252.

Coddington, J. A., & Sands, L. P. (2008). Cost of health care and quality outcomes of patients at nurse-managed clinics. *Nursing Economic$, 26*(2), 75–83.

Dumont, C. (2008). Nurse researcher: A career, not just a job. *American Nurse Today, 3*(5), 33–34.

Gaudier, F. (2003). *Health encyclopedia: Special topics—certified nurse midwife profession.* Retrieved from www.henryford-health.org/12893.cfm. Accessed July 18, 2005.

Hamric, A. B., & Hanosn, C. M. (Eds.) (2013). *Advanced nursing practice: An integrated approach.* (5th ed.). St. Louis, MO: Elsevier Saunders.

Hospice and Palliative Nurses Association & American Nurses Association. (2014). *Palliative nursing: Scope and standards of practice.* Silver Spring, MD: Nursesbooks.org.

International Association of Forensic Nurses. (2016). *Sexual Assault Nurse Examiner—Adult/Adolescent (SANE-A®) and Pediatric (SANE-P®) CERTIFICATION EXAMINATION HANDBOOK 2016.* Retrieved June 12, 2016 from http://c.ymcdn.com/sites/www.forensicnurses.org/resource/resmgr/Certification/2016_SANE_CERTIFICATION_EXAM.pdf

International Association of Forensic Nurses & American Nurses Association. (2009). *Forensic nursing: scope & standards of practice.* Silver Spring, MD: Nursesbooks.org.

Institute of Medicine. (2011). *The future of nursing, leading change, advancing health.* Washington, DC: The National Academies Press.

Jansen, M., & Zwygart-Stauffacher, M. (2010). *Advanced practice nursing core concepts for professional development.* (4th ed.). New York: Springer Publishing Co.

Lundy, K., & Huch, M. (2009). Advanced nursing practice in the community. In Lundy, K. & James, S. (Eds.). *Community health nursing, caring for the public's health,* (2nd ed.). Sudbury MA: Jones & Bartlett.

Mitty, E. (2003). Assisted living and the role of the nurse. *American Journal of Nursing, 103,* 32–44.

Morrison, D. (2014). Travel nursing anyone? *American Nurse Today, 9*(11), 41–42.

National Council of State Boards of Nursing. (2012). *Mutual recognition: Frequently asked questions.* Retrieved from www.ncsbn.org/2002.htm. Accessed September 2, 2012.

Newhouse, R., Bass, E., Steinwach, D., et al. (2011). Advanced practice nursing outcomes 1990–2008: A systematic review. *Nursing Economic$, 29* (5), 230–251.

Norwood, S. L. (1998). *Nurses as consultants: Essential concepts and processes.* Menlo Park, CA: Addison-Wesley.

Penn, B. (Ed.). (2008). *Mastering the teaching role: A guide for nurse educators.* Philadelphia, PA: F. A. Davis.

Rhodes, M. K. (2011). Using effect-based reasoning to examine the DNP as the single entry degree for advanced practice nursing. *OJIN: The Online Journal of Issues in Nursing, 16*(3), 8. doi: 10.3912/OJIN.Vol16No03PPT01.

Rosseter, R. (2013). *Nurse practitioners: The growing solution in health care delivery.* Retrieved from www.aacn.nche.edu/media-relations/fact-sheets/nurse-practitioners. Accessed February 25, 2013.

Ross-Kerr, J. (2011). Credentialing in nursing. In J. Ross-Kerr, & M. Wood (Eds.), *Canadian nursing issues & perspectives.* Toronto: Elsevier Canada.

Sheer, B., & Wong, F. (2008). The development of advanced nursing practice globally. *Journal of Nursing Scholarship, 40*(3), 204–201.

Siefert, P. C. (Ed.) (2014). *Core curriculum for the RN first assistant.* (5th ed.). Denver: AORN.

Stevens, S. (2004). Cracking the case: Your role in forensic nursing. *Nursing, 34,* 54–56.

Vogel, G., & Doleysh, N. (1997). *Entrepreneuring: A nurses' guide to starting a business (NLN Publication No. 41–2201).* New York: National League for Nursing.

Waxman, K. (2005). *Nurse entrepreneurship: Do you have what it takes? 2005 pathways to success.* Hoffman Estates, IL: Nursing Spectrum.

Yee-Litzenberg, L. (2011). *Universal job skills: Skills to highlight in your resume/cover letter/job interview.* Retrieved from www.rackham.umich.edu/downloads/examples/snre_universal_job_skills.pdf. Accessed April 27, 2013.

Zorn, E. (2015). In house law firm legal nurse role: 30 year perspective. *The Journal of Legal Nurse Consulting, 26*(1), 26–32.

Chapter 21

Development of a Professional Nursing Career

KEY TERMS AND CONCEPTS

Values
Career goals
Passions
Envisioning
Personal vision
Career vision
Vision statement
Mission statement
Networking
Mentoring
Linear career paths
Nonlinear career paths
Career mapping
Professional nursing
   résumé
Professional portfolios

LEARNING OUTCOMES

By the end of this chapter, the learner will be able to:

1. Discuss the relationship between values and career goals.
2. Use a process to discover a passion for a specific area of professional practice.
3. Compose personal vision and mission statements for professional nursing practice.
4. Prepare a professional cover letter and résumé.
5. Compile a professional nursing portfolio.
6. Specify strategies to develop a professional nursing network.
7. Explain how networking and mentoring enhance career opportunities.
8. Design a career map for your future professional career.

REAL-LIFE REFLECTIONS

Glen and Patricia work together on an inpatient oncology unit. They both started as new graduates a year ago. During a shift report, Glen mentions that he is thinking about changing jobs because he no longer enjoys his work. Patricia responds, "Oh, I'm sorry to hear that you don't love the work the way I do. I feel so satisfied if I can get patients to smile, even for a minute, or have them share how they are coping with cancer. I think that I want to spend my entire career specializing in oncology nursing. But if you no longer enjoy the work, it might be best for you to consider something else."

- *What steps do these nurses need to take to establish a career tailored to best meet their personal needs and desires?*
- *How can other nurses support these two novice nurses as they pursue their career goals?*

As the health care delivery system changes, new opportunities for professional nursing practice arise. Nurses live in an exciting time in which their specialized and complex skills can dramatically affect client care and outcomes. Developing required competence for effective professional nursing practice, especially in

specialty areas, takes many years. As a profession, nursing offers a wide array of career opportunities. Nurses decide what type of nursing they wish to pursue and where they want to practice. How a nursing career develops depends on the individual nurse. Some nurses create detailed written career plans with established timelines for implementation. Other nurses rely on seizing opportunities as they arise. This chapter outlines how to match career goals with personal values, discover ways to instill personal passion into practice, consider factors to envision a future career, develop strategies to create and implement a career map, and successfully apply and interview for a nursing position.

Take Note!

The responsibility for professional nursing career development lies within each nurse.

▌ QUESTIONS FOR REFLECTION

1. Do you have a particular nursing career goal in mind? If so, what is it? Are you flexible enough to consider other available nursing career options? Why or why not?

2. Why is it important for nurses to support each other as they pursue their career goals?

VALUES AND CAREER GOALS

Values denote what a person perceives as being important in life and provide guidance to people as they interact with each other and the environment. Examples of values include truth, integrity, justice, peace, health, education, conservation, possessions, money, security, safety, career, and family. Life has many important values, and selecting which ones are the most important can be a difficult task. A clue to defining a personal set of values may reside in what people enjoy doing. In early life, values are formed in families, but a person's values may change over time. Self-betrayal occurs when personal behaviors fail to match a personal set of values.

When people share values, communities are formed (Barrett, 1998). However, even within the profession of nursing (a community), no two nurses share an identical set of values.

Nurses learn professional values as part of socialization into the profession. Certain areas of nursing cater to different value sets. Nurses who value technologically complex skills tend to pursue critical care, emergency, or perioperative nursing. Nurses who value long-term relationships and the wisdom of the elderly find great rewards in working with a geriatric population in long-term care facilities. Hospice nursing provides rewards for nurses who value providing comfort and peace in the dying process, rather than preserving life at all costs. Nurses for whom the generation of knowledge is a cherished value may become nurse

21.1 Learning, Knowing, and Growing

Values Clarification Exercises

- **Step 1:** Find a quiet, peaceful place where you can spend some time alone and free from interruption.
- **Step 2:** Close your eyes and ask yourself: What things in life are important to me as a person? Record the list.
- **Step 3:** Close your eyes and ask yourself: What things in life are important to me as a professional nurse? Record the list.
- **Step 4:** Identify the entries that are common to both of your lists to identify similarities between your personal and professional values. Create a list for these results.
- **Step 5:** Generate a list of activities in which you engaged during the past week and include the approximate amount of time spent in each activity. Place each activity in a list according to how much time you spent on it, with the activity in which you spent the most time at the top of the list.
- **Step 6:** Compare this list with the lists generated in Steps 2, 3, and 4. This represents the congruence between how you spend your time and your set of personal and professional values.
- **Step 7:** Answer the following questions:
    1. Am I living in accordance with my personal values?
    2. Am I living in accordance with my professional values?
    3. Are there any things that I could do differently to live out my personal and professional values?

Chang, R. (2000). *The passion plan.* San Francisco, CA: Jossey-Bass.

researchers or theorists. Unlike some other professions, nursing offers many career paths that mesh with one's personal values. Most nurses use personal values when determining their **career goals** (specific professional nursing aspirations). Box 21.1, Learning, Knowing, and Growing, "Values Clarification Exercises," can help you determine your values.

DISCOVERING YOUR PASSION IN NURSING

Chang (2000) defined passion as a "personal intensity, an underlying force that fuels our strongest emotions," and distinguished this from **passions**, which are described as "activities, ideas, and topics that elicit these emotions" (p. 19). When people perform with passion, they perceive the world as being full of opportunities, rather than obstacles, and they focus on personal abilities, rather than limitations. People who live out their life's passions follow their hearts. Passions change as life evolves. A life without passion becomes a life of regrets (Chang, 2000). Nursing is a content-based and context-based passion (the personal, intense desire to help others) with multiple passions (activities and specialized knowledge to care for others). Client care involves activities that require specialized knowledge and skills (passions) centered on a theme of helping others (passion).

Take Note!
All people have the capacity to live passionate lives.

Chang (2000) outlined a seven-step process to develop a passion plan for living that requires feeling, thinking, and acting. These steps are outlined in Box 21.2, Learning, Knowing, and Growing, "Developing a Passion Plan for Living."

21.2 Learning, Knowing, and Growing

Developing a Passion Plan for Living

1. **Start from the heart:** Acknowledge all your emotions and desires and recognize their power. Engage in a gradual process that requires identifying things that inspire or elicit deep, strong emotions. (This may mean rediscovering things from childhood.)

2. **Discover all your passions:** Make a list of everything in life that is meaningful to you and all that you wish to accomplish during your life.

3. **Clarify the purpose of your passions:** Identify the results of living out your life's passions. The purpose of each passion helps to determine how it will be followed.

4. **Define the actions to achieve each passion:** Develop an action plan for each passion.

5. **Perform with passion:** Implement the action plan developed in Step 4, which may require some form of risk taking.

6. **Spread the passion:** Share the passion and how it excites you with others, and let it permeate all your interactions with others.

7. **Persist in the passion:** Stay the course, despite any unexpected circumstances or obstacles that may arise.

Chang, R. (2000). *The passion plan.* San Francisco, CA: Jossey-Bass.

Passionate nurses provide client care from the depths of their hearts and souls. They hold to high ideals and have no fear in confronting situations that compromise client care. Their nursing colleagues and other members of the health care team "catch" their enthusiasm. Passionate nurses demonstrate authentic caring, making clients and their significant others feel safe and important. Nurses and clients deeply connect with each other, and the fond memories of the nursing situation last a lifetime.

QUESTIONS FOR REFLECTION

1. What deep emotions surface when you engage in nursing practice or think about your future nursing career?
2. What activities in clinical practice result in extremely high levels of personal satisfaction for you?
3. What passions, other than nursing, do you have currently in life?
4. Why is it important to have passions or interests other than nursing?

ENVISIONING YOUR NURSING CAREER

Envisioning means picturing oneself in the future (Agnes, 2005). A **personal vision** specifies a future desired state for oneself. Developing a **career vision** statement assumes that change in one's career will occur. The ideal professional nursing career vision would include nursing-related passions.

Like all people, nurses progress through life transitions, so personal career vision statements may be revised to address changes in physical, mental, and spiritual health status. For example, a nurse may leave a position to stay home with his or her children. A nurse may re-enter clinical practice because of a change in marital status, spousal unemployment, or reduced child care responsibilities. Because physical stamina declines with age, a nurse may decide to pursue a nursing position that requires less physical exertion.

Reviewing personal values and strengths facilitates the development of a career vision. All visions start with dreams. When developing a personal vision, let ideas flow without inhibition. Visions may be articulated in the present or future tense. A **vision statement** is a written declaration of a desired future state and may incorporate ideas for future improvement (Barrett, 1998; Covey, 1992, 2004; Wesorick, Shiparski, Troseth, & Wyngarden, 1997).

21.3 Professional Prototypes

Sample Vision and Mission Statements

Sample Vision Statement

I envision myself to be a professional nurse who demonstrates authentic caring toward and appreciation of all living people and things.

Sample Mission Statement

As an authentic professional nurse, my personal mission is to take time to listen genuinely to clients, families, nursing colleagues, and other members of the interdisciplinary health team to provide them with the highest quality of service that is humanly possible.

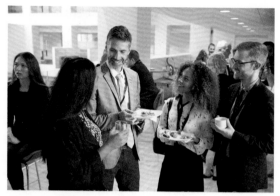

FIGURE 21.1 Networking enables nurses to learn about available professional nursing opportunities.

Vision statements relate closely to mission statements. A **mission statement** specifies how a vision may be actualized (Barrett, 1998) or the meaning and purpose behind work (Covey, 1992, 2004; Wesorick et al., 1997). Florence Nightingale (1929) viewed nursing as a spiritual calling. Barrett (1998) presented the concept of "soul work" as activities to be performed by the energy field occupying a living human body. For some, professional nursing may be one way to fulfill one's life purpose.

Mission statements clearly and concisely outline specific services using action verbs whose meaning comes from the heart (Wesorick et al., 1997; Meadows & Buckley, 2014). Mission statements related to a professional nursing career usually focus on client care. Box 21.3, Professional Prototypes, "Sample Vision and Mission Statements," provides a look at some commonly addressed areas.

When nurses create a career vision based on passions, they commit to living out a meaningful life as they engage in activities of the soul, rather than of the mind. Passionate nursing practice enables nurses to live out their life purpose of caring for others. Once personal visions and mission statements have been developed, nurses need to find a nursing position to fulfill them. Nurses use a variety of strategies to find and obtain a desired position.

NETWORKING

Networking consists of exchanging ideas and information among individuals, groups, or institutions (Agnes, 2005). Professional networks are interconnected groups of people who share similar work roles.

Professional networks may be interprofessional in nature or consist of people within a single profession. When nurses network, they become cognizant of career opportunities, learn about nursing care practice variances across settings, and support each other (Fig. 21.1). Strategies for developing effective professional networks include having the courage and willingness to reach out and connect with others as well as a genuine desire to help others, freely sharing information with others, distributing professional business cards, and actively participating in collaborative projects (Borgatti, 2008).

Opportunities for networking occur at work, school, professional organizational meetings, and community service activities. Networking beyond the boundaries of the nursing community enables nurses to expand their knowledge outside of nursing, share information about professional nursing with people who are not nurses, and explore other career options. Many nurse consultants and entrepreneurs rely on professional and community networking to generate business. Nurses who network effectively typically have a goal when interacting in professional or community groups (Borgatti, 2008; Waxman, 2005).

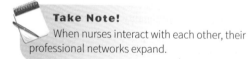

Take Note!

When nurses interact with each other, their professional networks expand.

QUESTIONS FOR REFLECTION

1. Why is it important to have strong collegial relationships?
2. What have you done during the past week to strengthen your relationships with your fellow students or nursing colleagues?

3. What networking opportunities are available to you as a nursing student?
4. Why is networking important in nursing education and practice?

MENTORING

For centuries, novices in various professions have sought the advice of experienced professionals. The term "mentor" has its roots in Greek mythology, when Odysseus entrusted the education of his son to his friend named Mentor (Agnes, 2005). Today, the word **mentoring** has come to denote the process of enlisting an experienced guide or trusted adviser who assumes responsibility for the professional growth and advancement of a less experienced person, called the protégé. Mentors open doors, create opportunities, and provide career role modeling for protégés while inspiring them. Mentors provide directions for nurses just entering the profession as well as those entering a specialized area of nursing practice. They also provide wisdom and help protégés develop professional networks. Mentors often actively sponsor protégés when career opportunities in the selected field arise (Falter, 1997). In addition, protégés help mentors by serving as trusted assistants who help clarify ideas (Malone, 1999).

Successful mentoring relationships require personal chemistry between the people involved. A novice nurse may not want to impose on a potential mentor's time, fear relationship failure, or have difficulty identifying the right person. Some mentoring relationships unfold naturally over the course of a career. People become mentors for various reasons, including the desire to help another, admiration for the novice's personal and professional goals and vision, recollection of a former younger self, and past experience as a protégé in a successful mentoring experience (Abrams, 2000; Malone, 1999). Successful mentoring requires mutual respect, complementary personalities, open attitudes, proper timing, and appropriate quality and quantity of guidance (Abrams, 2000).

To ease the burden of professional transition to clinical practice for new graduate nurses, some health care institutions offer mentoring, coaching, preceptor, or residency programs. These programs provide guidance for new nurses and those changing specialty practice areas. For nurses just entering the profession, coaching (or mentoring) typically eases the transition into independent, professional practice (Messmer, Jones, & Taylor, 2004; Sherman & Dyess, 2007).

Sometimes, these programs result in effective mentoring relationships. However, mentoring requires reciprocal investment in the relationship. Because most mentors have years of experience within a given field, they have much knowledge to impart to protégés (Sherman & Dyess, 2007). Mentoring provides mentors with the opportunity to fulfill developmental tasks related to older professional nurses. Sometimes, the mentor finds a protégé willing to continue the mentor's professional contributions as the mentor retires or loses interest in them as part of a natural career trajectory.

Residency programs differ from mentorship and other nursing orientation programs. Residency programs provide new graduate nurses entering the profession with expanded opportunities to understand and experience the transition arising from graduation from a nursing program to learning how to be a professional nurse in the clinical arena. In a nursing residency program, new graduate nurses receive detailed information of issues encountered during the first year (or two) of clinical practice. Along with understanding the transition process, new nurses are provided opportunities to refine their clinical skills, develop time management strategies, sharpen priority setting skills, and improve interprofessional and consumer communication skills. They also discuss transitions with each other. Residency programs assign each new nurse a seasoned nurse preceptor who guides them through agency (and unit) orientation and the professional transition processes (Institute of Medicine, 2011).

Nurses often experience a wide array of issues resulting in psychological distress during their first year of practice (see Box 21.4, Professional Building Blocks, "Issues Encountered by New Nurses That Lead to Psychological Distress") (Lavoie-Tremblay et al., 2008; Zimmerman & Ward-Smith, 2012). New graduate turnover has been reported to be 30% within the first year of licensure, and 57% of nurses leave their first nursing position by the second year (Candela & Bowles, 2005). Residency programs typically last 1 year and have been shown to facilitate transition to independent practice and reduce the turnover rates. The following Focus on Research brief "Transition to Practice Study in Hospital Settings" conducted by Spector and colleagues (2015) compares 6-, 9-, and 12-month outcomes of new nurses who were employed in acute care facilities with new transition into practice programs, established onboarding or nurse residency programs and no program other than new employee orientation.

FOCUS ON RESEARCH

Transition to Practice Study in Hospital Settings

The National Council of State Boards of Nursing (NCBSN) developed a transition into practice model program (TIPP) using the core competencies identified by Quality and Safety Education in Nursing. They wanted to know if the TIPP program provided a better transition for new graduate nurses in hospital settings. The TIPP contains basic facility orientation combined with five online modules addressing patient-centered care, communication and teamwork, evidence-based practice (EBP), quality improvement, and informatics. They wanted to examine the effects of TIPP on patient safety, overall nurse competence, specific QSEN competencies, job stress, job satisfaction, and retention of new graduate nurses.

Using a longitudinal, randomized comparative design, they looked at the study outcomes in 105 hospitals in the states of Illinois, Ohio, and North Carolina. Hospitals ranged in size of less than 100 to over 400 beds and were evenly distributed across urban, suburban, and rural locations. The hospitals were randomly assigned to TIPP and established program for onboarding new nurses ranging from basic facility orientation to well-established new graduate programs with preceptorships.

Data were collected on safety and negative safe practices, overall competence, work stress, job satisfaction at 6-, 9-, and 12-month intervals. Five hundred forty-four new nurses and 691 preceptors completed data collection at the 6-month interval; 518 new nurses and 675 preceptors provided data at the 9-month interval; and 281 new nurses and 336 preceptors complied with data collection at the 12-month interval. The following tools were used to collect data: the *NCSBN Practice Issues Index Revised* (self-report data on errors and positive and negative safety practices), *Overall Competency Tool* (perception of overall competence as a professional nurse), *Specific Competency Tool* (perception of competence in each of the QSEN competencies), *NCSBN 4 Questions on Job Stress* (self-reported levels of job stress), *Brayfield and Roth Index of Job Satisfaction,* and then retention rates reported at 12 months. The investigators reported elements of validity and reported reliabilities of 0.77 or higher for all tools used for data collection. They also reported minimum sample size required to achieve a power of 0.98 for the study.

Data were analyzed using Chi square for categorical data, analysis of variance for continuous data, and paired t-tests to compare measurements on tools used in the study. Initial data analysis comparing TIPP with control hospitals revealed control group hospitals had fewer errors, reported negative safety practice and reduced levels of job stress ($p < 0.05$). There were no statistical significant differences in overall competence and job satisfaction. TIPP participants reported statistically significant higher scores on patient-centered care, use of technology, and communication and teamwork ($p < 0.05$) and there were no statistically significant differences in quality improvement and EBP. Post hoc data analysis was done separating control groups with established preceptor orientation programs and those with only facility orientation. Established programs with preceptorships were found to have statistically significant lower job stress levels at the 6-month time frame. The only statistically significant difference reported was that TIPP had higher scores on the use of technology compared to all other programs. The study revealed no statistical significant differences in new graduate nurse retention.

This study provides solid support for preceptor use when onboarding new graduate nurses to acute care settings. Job stress peaks at 6 months into the role of professional nurse for all groups and then starts to decline. Job satisfaction showed steady declines until 9 months on the job and then it stabilizes or increases. Therefore, new graduate nurses need someone to help them during this difficult professional transition. More research is needed to address the effectiveness of the NCSBN TIP model and how it might be used in hospitals that provide only basic facility orientation for new graduate nurses and other interventions that might ease the stress of the transition to professional practice.

Spector, N., Blegen, M. A., Silvestre, J., Barnsteiner, J., Lynn, M. R., Ulrich, B., Fogg, L., & Alexander, M. (2015). Transition to practice study in hospital settings. *Journal of Nursing Regulation, 5*(4), 24–38. doi: 10.1016/S2155-8256(15)30031-4

21.4 Professional Building Blocks

Issues Encountered by New Nurses That Lead to Psychological Distress

- Lack of self-confidence
- Unrealistic expectations from clinical staff, supervisors, and other health team members
- Role ambiguity
- Lack of social support from nursing colleagues, unlicensed care providers, and/or supervisors
- Inadequate staffing
- High demands of the work of nursing
- Inability to use all capacities and qualifications to choose how to do one's work
- Job strain
- Imbalance between individual efforts and rewards from the work
- Unanticipated physical demands of the work of nursing
- Perceptions of being unprepared to work long hours
- Horizontal violence (bullying) by other nurses and health team members
- Feelings of being unprepared to manage patients or other staff members
- Perceptions of being unprepared to assume independent leadership roles
- Being unable to communicate effectively with physicians, residents, and/or interns
- Inability to organize all the tasks needed for effective delivery of nursing care
- Lack of confidence and ability to perform the complex skills required in practice
- Increasingly complex patient care requirements
- Difficulty in assertive communication resulting in the inability to advocate for oneself
- Lack of confidence in decision-making abilities
- Discomfort when working with dying patients and their significant others

Institute of Medicine. (2011). *The future of nursing: Leading change, advancing health.* Washington, DC: The National Academies Press; Lavoie-Tremblay, M., Wright, D., Desforges, N., Gélinas, C., Marchionni, C., & Drevniok, U. (2008). Creating a healthy workplace for new generation nurses. *Journal of Nursing Scholarship, 40*(3), 200–297; and Zimmerman, C., & Ward-Smith, P. (2012). Attrition of new graduate RN: Why nurses are leaving the profession. *The Missouri Nurse–Missouri Nurse Spring 2012,* 15–17.

▮ QUESTIONS FOR REFLECTION

1. What are the characteristics of an ideal mentor?
2. Why are these characteristics important?
3. If you were to select a professional nursing mentor today, whom would you choose?

CAREER DEVELOPMENT STRATEGIES

Once nurses identify a career direction on which to focus, they can use a variety of strategies to make their ideal career happen. Most authors addressing career development suggest beginning the process with a self-assessment of personal values followed by a period of dreaming about what a future career may look like (ANA Career Center Staff, 2015; Chang, 2000; Donner & Wheeler, 2001; Malone, 1999; McGillis Hall, Waddell, Donner, & Wheeler, 2004). A career in nursing equips nurses with many life skills that can transfer to other professions, while basic nursing knowledge transfers to a variety of professional nursing specialty areas.

Career Paths

No one career-planning process has proven to be superior to others. The process may be linear or nonlinear, and nurses select which path to follow based on their ability to tolerate uncertainty and ambiguity (Bongard, 1997a).

Linear career paths require nurses to follow a sequential series of steps. For example, staff nurses who enjoy working with students may decide they will pursue a career in nursing academia. They usually earn a master's degree in nursing before assuming nursing faculty positions. Once employed by a nursing program, they closely follow a tenure track system with specific criteria for advancement from instructor to full professor. Nurses who like structure and meeting designated deadlines prefer this approach to career development (Bongard, 1997b).

Nonlinear career paths rely on life circumstances and critical incidents that result in career changes. Nurses who follow nonlinear career paths frequently create careers by using their interests, outside experiences, and nursing skills. They seize opportunities as they arise. Nurses using a nonlinear approach to career development frequently create new nursing positions within a health care organization or become entrepreneurs. Today, nurses following nonlinear career paths have a better chance of professional survival, especially during times when health care organizations eliminate nursing positions (Bongard, 1997b).

Take Note!

No two nurses follow identical paths for career development.

Career Development Model

Donner and Wheeler (2001, p. 2) viewed career development as "an iterative and continuous" process and combine linear and nonlinear approaches to career development. They developed a five-phase career planning and development model, which starts with scanning the environment to understand current realities and future trends in society that have implications for nursing and create possibilities for new areas of clinical practice. Their model emphasizes the importance of periodic self-assessments and reality checks related to self-identity and how others view the individual nurse. If nurses find that their current employment situations do not fit with attributes discovered from their self-appraisals, Donner and Wheeler suggest that it may be time to pursue an alternative career path. They also advocate for the creation of a career vision to link current status with future possibilities. Nurses may then use the career vision as a motivating source for remaining in a current practice setting or making a change. Donner and Wheeler suggest that designing a strategic career plan around the career vision facilitates attainment of career goals. Finally, once a career plan has been established, efforts should be channeled into marketing professional skills by forming an expansive professional network, developing a mentoring relationship, and further refining verbal and written communication skills.

Career Mapping

Malone (1999) used the term **career mapping** to denote a continuous process of nursing career development in which career moves unfold as a person engages in professional practice and lifelong learning. This process starts with identifying values, determining the importance of each value, and envisioning a future. The following questions can facilitate the career mapping process:

- Why did I select a nursing career?
- Why do I have a specific job?
- What can I do now to impact my career?
- What strengths have I brought to clinical practice settings while serving the clients under my care?
- What is my 5-year career goal? (ANA Career Center Staff, 2015)

The future vision creates a blueprint for personal action to make that envisioned future become a reality.

To facilitate the preferred career vision, nurses can use a variety of resources that outline career trends. Resources for learning about current and future needs for professional nursing include the U.S. Department of Labor, the Bureau of Health Professions, the Bureau of Labor Statistics, the American Association of Colleges of Nursing, the National League for Nursing, and the American Nurses Association.

Once nurses determine their preferred career, specialty certification serves as an important step in the career-mapping process. Professional certification provides public acknowledgment of professional competence, enhances career opportunities, demonstrates the ability of the profession for self-regulation, and increases personal power (Malone, 1999). The American Nurses Credentialing Center offers 27 certification examinations across a variety of nursing practice areas. Nurses also can earn certification from a variety of nurse specialty organizations. Nurse specialty certification have found to be a contributing factor to better patient outcomes (Kendall-Gallagher, Aiken, Sloane, & Cimiotti, 2011).

For developing successful career maps, Malone (1999) identified networking and finding a mentor as key strategies. Nurses frequently overlook the importance of networking with professionals from other disciplines. Networking with other members of the health care team and with other professionals within the community enables nurses to gain a more global perspective on the meaning of health and the needs for future health care delivery. Malone specified that personal and professional mentors serve vital roles in the career-mapping process because mentors help shape professional values and instill confidence in young professionals to pursue their dreams.

MAKING A NURSING CAREER CHANGE

Nurses make career changes for a variety of reasons. Some pursue part-time employment to spend more time with families or pursue outside interests. Some nurses experience intense value conflicts with employers that result in an employment change. Some nurses follow partners when their employment situations change. Others lose their jobs during periods of economic downturn (Kelly, 2008). Nurses who earn advanced degrees frequently change jobs. Finally, when nurses get bored or burned out with their current position, they embark on a journey to either change jobs or pursue a different area of nursing practice.

Several strategies prove useful for nurses who wish to remain viable in today's employment market (Cardillo, 2001).

- Keeping a current résumé enables immediate action when an opportunity for employment surfaces.
- Refining personal interview skills provides confidence when interacting with future employers.
- Networking with other nurses at professional organizational meetings, career fairs, conventions, and

community service activities enables acquisition of key information about employment opportunities.

- Making lists of personal assets, strengths, and preferred professional activities helps identify the type of position best suited to the individual nurse.
- Exposing oneself to motivational information (print, audio, video, or online) arms the nurse considering change with a "can do" attitude.
- After accepting a new position, easing out of the old one gracefully makes it easier to return if the new job fails to meet expectations.

▌ QUESTIONS FOR REFLECTION

1. What is your ideal picture of your future nursing career?
2. How can you make this picture a reality?
3. What are the consequences of not envisioning an ideal future nursing career?

Finding Available Nursing Opportunities

Nurses can use a variety of resources to locate employment opportunities. Most hospitals and integrated health systems post internal job openings in areas accessible to employees and in human resource departments. Many organizations also list employment opportunities on their company websites (Enelow & Kursmark, 2010; Kelly, 2008; VGM Career Horizons, 2008). The internet also offers many commercial online job search sites. Nursing journals and periodicals contain classified advertisements with available nursing opportunities. Nurses can learn about career opportunities from networking with colleagues during professional nursing organizational events (Borgatti, 2008; VGM Career Horizons, 2008). In times of nursing shortages, some health care agencies turn to radio and television advertising to recruit nurses. Local newspapers publish classified advertisements related to employment opportunities in nursing. Social networking websites (e.g., Facebook, LinkedIn, and others) and other online applications also serve as useful tools for nurses to find employment and market themselves.

Marketing Your Skills

Employers need to verify that applicants have the necessary skills to meet the demands of the position. Tailoring cover letters and résumés to address specific skills outlined for a particular position may prove to be more successful in securing a new job than using generic cover letters and résumés. Documents showcasing professional skills should be saved as computer files and edited to fit the requested skills and previous professional experience delineated by the posted job. Special care must be taken to verify that all information sent to prospective employers and clients has no spelling or punctuation errors, and if being sent through the mail, is visually appealing. Poorly constructed documents readily find their way into the trash (Bongard, 1997b; Enelow & Kursmark, 2010; VGM Career Horizons, 2008).

Writing a Cover Letter

Cover letters provide a general introduction to prospective employers and offer an opportunity for the applicant to shed light on his or her personality. If the organization specifies a person to contact in its advertisement for the position, the cover letter should be addressed to the designated person.

Two forms of cover letter provide information to prospective employers. The traditional cover letter gives reasons for contact, expands on the rationale for applying for the position, and details how to contact the writer to set up an interview. The second form, a skill-matched cover letter, not only provides the same information as the traditional cover letter, but also outlines how the applicant's acquired credentials and skills match the job requirements. The skill-matched cover letter format saves time for people who screen applicants for interview invitations because they can easily read specific applicant qualifications. For an example of each type, see Box 21.5, Professional Prototypes, "Sample Cover Letters."

When using the postal system to submit your application, typewritten or printed addresses on all materials sent to prospective employers or clients create a better impression than handwritten ones. If sending the cover letter on paper, the signature may be the last item the human resource department reads, so applicants should ensure that is neat and legible.

The general rules for cover letter rules apply regardless of whether the applicant is communicating through the postal service or via email, personally delivering the cover letter, or communicating through a company's website.

Preparing a Résumé

The résumé originated as a solution for employers who wanted to interview only qualified job applicants. Human resource personnel find most résumés dull and boring. A good **professional nursing résumé** presents individual strengths while showcasing special skills and professional accomplishments (Enelow & Kursmark,

21.5 Professional Prototypes

Sample Cover Letters

Jane Doe, RN, BSN
111 E. Lilac Avenue
Springfield, MO 65106

November 1, 2017

Mary Ashcraft, RN
Nurse Recruiter
Human Resources Department
Springfield Medical Center
803 North Maple Street
Springfield, MO 65107

Dear Ms. Ashcraft:

As I was reading the Springfield Daily News, I spotted your advertisement for a nursing position on your oncology unit. I have recently moved to Springfield, Missouri and would like to work for Springfield Medical Center, the premier hospital in the area. My professional nursing background includes previous oncology nursing experience.

I am enclosing a copy of my résumé so that you may review my credentials. I would appreciate the opportunity to discuss my qualifications in person. Please call me at my home, 417-555-6464, at any time to schedule an interview. If I am not available to take your call, please leave a message and telephone number so I can contact you.

Thank you for reviewing my credentials. I look forward to meeting you soon.

Sincerely,

Jane Doe, RN, BSN

Jane Doe, RN, BSN

FIGURE 21.2 Traditional cover letter.

(continued on page 560)

21.5 Professional Prototypes (continued)

Sample Cover Letters (continued)

Jane Doe, RN, BSN
111 E. Lilac Avenue
Springfield, MO 65106

November 1, 2017

Mary Ashcraft, RN
Nurse Recruiter
Human Resources Department
Springfield Medical Center
803 North Maple Street
Springfield, MO 65107

Dear Ms. Ashcraft:

As I was reading the Springfield Daily News, I spotted your advertisement for a nursing position on your oncology unit. I have recently moved to Springfield, Missouri and would like to work for Springfield Medical Center, the premier hospital in the area. I have also read the exciting news about the current expansion of the oncology services at Springfield Medical Center.

My professional nursing background includes previous oncology nursing experience and the following summary outlines how my qualifications fit your nursing position requirements:

Your requirements	My qualifications
* Professional nursing licensure in Missouri	* Missouri nursing license for 6 years
* One year's experience in oncology nursing	* Five years' experience in oncology nursing at St. Luke's Hospital, Omaha, NE
* OCN certification	* Current OCN certification

I am enclosing a copy of my résumé so that you may review my credentials. I would appreciate the opportunity to discuss my qualifications in person. Please call me at my home, 417-555-6464, at any time to schedule an interview. If I am not available to take your call, please leave a message and telephone number so I can contact you.

Thank you for reviewing my credentials. I look forward to meeting you soon.

Sincerely,

Jane Doe, RN, BSN

Jane Doe, RN, BSN

FIGURE 21.3 Skill-matched cover letter.

TABLE 21.1 Comparison of the Chronologic and Functional Résumé Formats

	Chronologic Résumé	Functional Résumé
Description	Lists job titles and responsibilities in reverse chronologic order	Highlights professional skills (also called skill-based résumé)
Components	Contact information Job and career objectives Career summary that highlights dates of each position Education Special awards or honors Community service	Contact information Job and career objective List of skills specific for job Dates of previous positions, usually listed at the end or in smaller type Education and skills acquired from employment or community service activities
Situations for best use	Documentation of personal career growth Continued employment in a field without too many job changes	Professional career established Beginning of a career Career change with the goal to focus on relevant skills Stagnant or declining career Returning to the workforce after a prolonged absence
When best not to use	Frequent job changes (every 1–2 years) Just finishing school Seeking a career change	No situations
Advantages	Showcases detailed employment history Outlines specific job responsibilities and previous employers	Highlights skills, rather than employment history Makes it easier for human resource personnel to determine if skills match posted job description Can include skills gained from outside areas of past employment

Enelow, W., & Kursmark, L. (2010). *Expert resumes for health care careers* (2nd ed.). Indianapolis, IN: JIST Works; Yate, M. (2012). *Knock 'em dead resumes: How to write a killer resume that gets you job interviews* (10th ed.). Avon, MA: Adams Media; and VGM Career Horizons. (2008). *Resumes for nursing careers* (2nd ed.). Lincolnwood, IL: Author.

2010; Poulin, 2015; VGM Career Horizons, 2008). A good résumé will get the candidate an interview, and preparation of the résumé assists in interview preparation, especially for the common request during interviews for applicants to "tell me about yourself." Résumé preparation also provides time for reflection about one's career. All résumés strive to showcase professional achievements, attributes, and experience while minimizing any potential weaknesses and stimulating enough interest in the applicant to ensure an invitation for an interview (Enelow & Kursmark, 2010; Poulin, 2015). Many companies today use automated programs to screen résumés for key terms, and résumés should be modified as needed to ensure that the specific skill terminology mentioned in a job posting is included in the document.

The majority of job applicants use either a chronologic or a functional résumé format. Of the two, the chronologic format is the most common. Some people opt to combine the two formats when developing a résumé (Poulin, 2015; Yate, 2012). Table 21.1 outlines the chronologic and functional résumé formats and highlights the strengths of each. The selection of format depends on where a person is within his or her career trajectory, employment experiences, and the type of opportunity being considered. For an example

of each type, see Box 21.6, Professional Prototypes, "Sample Résumés." Résumé experts disagree on many aspects of résumé preparation. However, they do agree on several preparation principles.

Human resource personnel spend little time reading individual résumés. Résumé containing more than one to two pages will most likely not be read. Some potential employers use automated programs to screen résumés; résumés not containing critical key terms will be automatically rejected. Many experts on résumé preparation suggest inclusion of a job/career objective. However, when a job/career objective is present, some human resource department employees assume that if the objective fails to match the open position, the applicant will reject an offer if made. Therefore, it is imperative to verify that a job/career objective matches the desired position and editing the résumé to match each job application may be advisable. Résumés that incorporate the following suggestions are more likely to be efficiently processed.

1. Organize résumé categories in a logical manner.
2. For paper-based résumés:
   - use a font size of 11 to 14 pt from an easily readable font (e.g., Arial, Bookman, Times New Roman, Verdana), and keep the font style

21.6 Professional Prototypes

Sample Résumés

Jane Doe, RN, BSN
111 E. Lilac Avenue
Springfield, MO   65106
(417) 888-6464

Objective	Obtain a professional nursing position on an oncology client care unit

Experience	St. Luke's Hospital, Omaha NE Oncology Unit Evening Charge Nurse	**July 2017 to present**
	University of Nebraska Medical Center, Omaha NE Post Anesthesia Care Unit Staff Nurse	**June 2015 to July 2017**
	University of Nebraska Medical Center, Omaha NE East Seven (Surgical Nursing Unit) Staff Nurse	**June 2013 to May 2015**
	Longview Extended Care Licensed Practical Nurse	**May 2011 to June 2013**
Education	BSN, University of Nebraska LPN, Clarkson Technical School, Omaha, NE	**May 2013** **May 2009**
Professional Credentials	Missouri Professional Nursing License ACLS Certification Oncology Nursing Society Certification Oncology Nursing Society American Nurses' Association	

Professional and Personal References Available Upon Request

FIGURE 21.4 Sample chronologic résumé.

Jane Doe, RN, BSN
111 E. Lilac Avenue
Springfield, MO 65106
(417) 888-6464

Objective: Full-time professional nurse position on an adult oncology unit

Skills

- Certification in oncology nursing since June, 2017
- 5 years' experience in oncology nursing
- Experienced in insertion and removal of percutaneous intravenous central catheters
- Taught Oncology Certification Review courses on chemotherapy administration and radiation therapy for oncology staff
- Published newsletter for the local chapter of the Oncology Nursing Society
- Supervised staff of two RNs and three patient care technicians as evening charge nurse

Education

- BSN, University of Nebraska Medical Center, May 2013
- Oncology Certification Course, Omaha Chapter of the Oncology Nursing Society, May 2014
- 30 hours of continuing education in Oncology Nursing, May 2013 to July 2015
- LPN, Clarkson Technical School, May 2009

Professional Credentials

- Certification in oncology nursing by the Oncology Nursing Society
- Missouri Professional Nursing License #556087352
- Nebraska Professional Nursing License #N6670889
- Current certification in ACLS and BCLS

Professional Organizations

- Oncology Nursing Society (past secretary of the Omaha, Nebraska Chapter)
- American Nurses Association

Employment History

St. Luke's Hospital, Omaha NE
Oncology Unit
Evening charge nurse   July 2017 to present

University of Nebraska Medical Center, Omaha NE
Post Anesthesia Care Unit
Staff nurse   June 2015 to July 2017

University of Nebraska Medical Center, Omaha NE
East Seven (Surgical Nursing Unit)
Staff nurse   June 2013 to May 2015

Longview Extended Care
Licensed practical nurse   May 2011 to June 2013

Professional and Personal References Available on Request

FIGURE 21.5 Sample functional (skill-based) résumé.

consistent throughout the résumé (a larger size can be used effectively to present headings).

- use 8½″ by 11″ paper (standard letter size) because employers may photocopy the résumé for distribution to department managers and human resource files.
- select high-quality, white, cream, or pastel (avoid pink) paper of 16- to 25-lb weight.
- maintain strict alignment of margins within sections.
- keep a free-flowing appearance without any noticeable breaks.

3. Limit résumé blocks to five to seven lines (two to three sentences).
4. Use action verbs to describe all job skills and responsibilities. If key job skills are mentioned in an advertisement for a position, make sure those terms are used in your résumé
5. Have a friend or family member proofread the résumé before sending it.

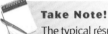

Take Note!

The typical résumés receive about a 30-second review.

Nurses may develop a résumé independently, seek the advice of career counselors, or have their résumé generated by a résumé specialist. Résumé preparation software can also be used. The internet is a great source of information for creating a professional résumé and for résumé templates. State employment agencies also may offer online assistance with résumé generation. Today, many organizations prefer electronic submission of job application materials over paper copies, either through a special portal on their websites or via email.

The résumé should include the applicant's name without any titles (unless it is a gender-neutral name that may create confusion), physical mailing address, telephone number, and email address. Applicants should refrain from using their current employer's email address or telephone number unless they have informed the current employer of their search for another job (Bongard, 1997b; VGM Career Horizons, 2008; Yate, 2012). If the applicant does not have an email address that sounds professional, he or she should create one. Google, Yahoo, and others offer free email accounts.

Finally, résumés lose power if they contain mistakes or possess certain characteristics. Yate (2012) offered the following suggestions for what *not* to do on a résumé.

1. Never give the document a title, such as "résumé" or "fact sheet."
2. Never state availability for employment.
3. Never specify reasons for leaving a previous or current job.
4. Never outline references (employers are legally obligated to obtain written consent from prospective employees before they check references).

The résumé provides applicants with a systematic format to showcase their professional skills and written communication abilities to prospective clients and employees. Usually, no verbal interaction occurs between the person screening the résumé and the applicant (and some are screened by computers!). Thus, utmost care should be taken when preparing a résumé to create the best impression.

References

As stated earlier, personal and professional references should not be listed on a résumé (VGM Career Horizons, 2008; Yate, 2012). The type and number of references required vary across organizations (typically three to six are required). Applicants usually find out how many references are required when they complete an employment application. When specifying references, common courtesy suggests that applicants inform the people whose names appear on the reference list. In addition, if people have used more than one surname during their employment, this information should be included somewhere because verifying references can become difficult if a married name is given to a reference when he or she knows the person only by her maiden name (Yate, 2012; Moore & Pierce, 2016).

Moore and Peirce (2016) offer suggestions for selecting and contacting persons for use as professional references. Human resource personnel typically ask professional references about job applicant knowledge, skills, attitudes, and work ethic. Because professional nurses may change positions throughout a career, some nurses keep a record of significant contacts with whom they have worked. Suggested professional references include past and present employers and professional colleagues. If the nurse has not informed persons in his or her current work setting, then he or she would use past employers and colleagues. For new graduate nurses, Moore and Pierce suggest using professors, clinical instructors, preceptors, and professional mentors. Classroom professors can address applicant work ethic and knowledge; whereas, clinical instructors can address applicant clinical skills more effectively. When making decision about who to include in a reference list, the job applicant should determine if the person being considered would share positive information about his or her abilities to fulfill the desired job responsibilities. Before finalizing a professional reference, nurses should considerer how much time has lapsed since having a working relationship. For example, a favorite professor from a nursing program would be an excellent choice as a reference especially for graduate nurses pursuing their first nursing position. However, if several years have lapsed and the nurse has had no contact with the professor, the professor would not be able to provide recent information about the nurse's professional abilities.

After professional references are identified, common courtesy specifies that applicants contact them, inform them about the nursing position and its requirements, and request how the identified reference might address job requirements. Professional references appreciate receiving a current résumé especially if the applicants are applying for positions if time has lapsed since working with them. Because employers and graduate nursing programs use a variety of ways to secure information from professional references, job applicants should inform each reference of the expectations (phone call, online survey, formal letter) and if there is a specific deadline for completing required materials (Moore & Pierce, 2016).

Professional references appreciate learning about career accomplishments for persons for whom they have provided information. Moore and Pierce (2016) suggest sending each reference a brief note expressing thanks to them for providing information to prospective employers and notifying them whether or not that they got the position. Additional ways of contacting references can also be email or through social media.

Professional Portfolios

Some nurses have developed **professional portfolios** to showcase their skills and accomplishments (Fig. 21.6). Some nursing programs have students generate nursing portfolios as part of the curriculum (Peddle, Jokwiro, Carter, & Young, 2016). In clinical practice, the professional nursing portfolio is used by some health care organizations as evidence that the employee deserves a promotion. In many Magnet facilities, a career ladder serves as a means for keeping experienced nurses at the bedside while offering them financial rewards for providing requisite nursing care and participating in shared governance activities. Nurses who have a professional portfolio may elect to take it to interviews to display evidence of professional accomplishments. Some nurses leave the portfolio with a prospective employer for review after all interviews have been completed

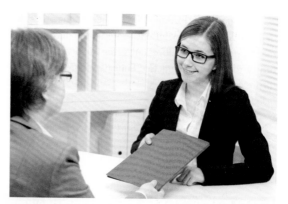

FIGURE 21.6 Presenting oneself as a polished professional is the first step in attaining a desired professional nursing position.

along with a specific time for the nurse to retrieve it (Bell, 2001). Box 21.7, Learning, Knowing, and Growing, "Building Your Portfolio," outlines the most common components you should consider including.

 21.7 Learning, Knowing, and Growing

Building Your Portfolio

Whether you are new to nursing or have many years of experience, it is never too soon to start building your portfolio. Your portfolio components may vary according to its intended use and the stage of your career. Williams and Jordon (2007) offered the following suggestions for things that may be included in a professional portfolio.

- Résumé
- Nursing philosophy statement
- Letter(s) of recommendation or appreciation
- Professional license
- Professional certifications
- Diplomas and continuing education certificates
- Special recognition such as honors or awards
- List of professional organizational memberships
- Copies of publications
- Photographs of podium or poster presentations
- Evidence of organizational service (e.g., shared governance committee participation) and community service
- List of inventions
- Written documentation of professional behaviors to facilitate client outcome attainment

Williams, M., & Jordon, K. (2007). The nursing professional portfolio: A pathway to career development. *Journal for Nurses in Staff Development, 3,* 125–131; Peddle, M., Jokwiro, Y., Carter, M., & Young, T. (2016). A professional portfolio of learning for undergraduate nursing students. *Australian Nursing & Midwifery Journal, 24*(4), 40.

Williams and Jordon (2007) specify that, besides being a vehicle to document professional accomplishments, portfolio development gives nurses the opportunity to reflect on practice endeavors and determine future career goals.

Take Note!
Professional portfolios provide documented evidence for meeting criteria for promotion.

Interview Skills

A face-to-face or phone interview enables potential employers or clients to assess applicants on a personal level and determine how they may fit with the organization. When an interview invitation is extended, applicants are one step closer to getting the desired position. Successful interview performance relies on adequate preparation. Table 21.2 outlines tips for effective performance during an employment interview. Although

TABLE 21.2 Tips for Effective Interviewing

Tips	Rationale
Learn as much as possible about the organization.	Knowledge of the organization's mission and philosophy enables the applicant to anticipate questions related to his or her personal fit with the organization.
Be prepared to answer questions related to your personal strengths, problem-solving skills, teamwork experiences, assessment for safe practice, organizational skills, priority setting, your expectations, areas for future professional growth and future career plans	Employers want to hire someone who has the capability to perform the roles and responsibilities of professional nursing safely and effectively. They also want nurses who have realistic appraisals of themselves and determine if the candidate may have potential to stay with the organization for an extended timeframe.
Dress conservatively in a business suit or well-tailored dress, not a uniform or scrubs.	Present a professional appearance. The employment interview rule is to dress one level above the position being considered.
Avoid wearing fragrances, smoking, or filling your car's gas tank right before the interview.	Fragrances create impressions. Heavy perfumes may trigger allergies, and the smell of smoke emphasizes the habit.
Groom the face and head impeccably with clean, neat hair and conservative make-up; avoid touching your face and hair during the interview.	Facial appearance and hair create an initial impression when interacting with others.
Groom the feet and lower legs impeccably with well-polished, clean shoes with no signs of wear and stockings or socks that blend with clothing.	A neat, clean appearance signifies attention to detail.
Rehearse the employment interview with a friend or family member.	This can allay nervousness and anxiety.
Bring nursing license and certification requirements with you.	Prospective employers may want to copy these for your file.
Prepare a set of questions related to the agency and position.	Asking questions may generate information to continue or stop pursuing the position. Questions also reveal interest.
Be armed with information related to the local market salary, bonus, and job expectations.	Verify that the position is aligned with others in the current market.
Arrive 5–10 minutes before the scheduled interview time.	Extra time allows you to relax immediately before the interview, allays potential anxiety related to tardiness, and demonstrates punctuality. However, arriving too early may make the interviewer feel rushed with a previous appointment.
Look busy while waiting: read a magazine, look over a list of questions, or review your résumé.	The interviewer may accompany his or her previous appointment to the waiting area, and making use of waiting time creates a positive first impression.
Do not bring friends or relatives to the interview site.	Concern for them may keep you from focusing on the interview and may give the impression that you lack self-confidence.
Greet the interviewer with direct eye contact and a firm handshake.	Business etiquette dictates use of a firm handshake when first meeting someone, and eye contact denotes assertiveness in Western culture.
Do not chew gum.	Chewing gum disrupts articulation of words, and the chewing motion creates an unprofessional appearance.

Tips	Rationale
Always ask a question if asked whether you have any questions.	Asking questions denotes interest in the organization and shows that you are focused on the interview.
Be honest and forthcoming with all answers.	Dishonesty or perceptions of covert information provide reasons for the interviewer not to continue the job application process.
If asked why you left previous places of employment, describe the situation specifically using positive terms.	Employers will assume that if an applicant speaks negatively about previous employment experiences, the applicant will do the same when he or she leaves this organization.
Wait for the interviewer to address salary, hours, and working conditions.	These topics are usually not covered in the first interview. However, they must be discussed before accepting a position.
Limit answers to each question to three statements, and share something about yourself related to the question.	Brief, targeted answers facilitate the interview process.
Come prepared to address professional experiences and include information related to teamwork.	Applicants are expected to share specific examples of how they executed various aspects of professional nursing and evidence of working in teams.
Carry a briefcase to store a portfolio or evidence of accomplishments, extra résumés, reference letters, and reference list.	Briefcases keep materials neat and project an air of professionalism.
Conclude the interview with a question related to the next step of the interview process.	This communicates continued interest in pursuing the position.
Send a thank-you note to the interviewer as soon as possible after the interview.	A follow-up note shows appreciation and highlights courtesy as a personal strength; it also provides one last opportunity to highlight a personal strength.

Bongard, B. (1997b). Managing your career. In B. Case (Ed.), *Career planning for nurses.* Albany, NY: Delmar Publishers; Pagana, K. (2012). Presenting yourself professionally. *American Nurse Today, 7*(7), 16–17; and Ulrich, D. L., & Stalter, A. M. (2015). Securing your first clinical nursing position. *Nursing 2015, 45*(8), 60–63. doi: 10.1097/01NURSE.0000466447,19807.6b

some nurses find the interview process stressful, it is important to remember that interview skills improve with practice. Rehearsing with someone who assumes the role of interviewer can be an effective strategy for interview preparation.

Prospective employers have legal limitations regarding the questions they may ask during an employment interview. Some organizations have prospective employees interview with a member of the human resource department, the nursing department manager, and staff members before an employment offer is extended. Nurses who inquire about the hiring process during the initial interview can better prepare themselves for any future interviews.

In times of nursing shortages, some employers offer large sign-on bonuses and other amenities to attract qualified nurses. When applying for positions with attractive bonuses and incentives, nurses should be aware of the risks associated with such enticements. Some incentives require nurses to sign contracts agreeing to a specified time commitment for employment. If nurses do not abide by conditions for the incentives, they usually must reimburse the employer for all or a portion of funds received.

Follow-Up Communication

Applicants should send a thank-you note within 24 hours after the interview, either by postal service or by email. Manners mean a lot to organizations that value customer service and teamwork. A thank-you note also gives applicants a chance to summarize interview highlights and make a final positive impression.

Summary and Significance to Practice

Developing a meaningful nursing career requires an open attitude, periodic self-assessment, lifelong learning, creativity, courage, and confidence. Along with personal characteristics, nurses rely on others for effective career development. Networking and mentoring are effective strategies for career development. Both require commitment, caring, and effective communication skills. To live out a preferred career vision, professional nurses must develop a plan and market their personal and professional skills to make the vision become a reality.

From Theory to Practice

1. What are the positive and negative consequences of staying in a particular nursing position for a long time?
2. Develop a professional nursing résumé and compile a portfolio. Analyze both projects. Are you on target to meeting your desired career goals? Why or why not?
3. Determine a nursing career goal. Design a career map to meet your desired career goal. You might find the four-step career planning process designed by the New Zealand Health Workforce website listed below useful as it contains a downloadable template. Share your plan with another nurse or your nurse manager (if you are already practicing nursing) or with a clinical nurse preceptor or nursing faculty (if you are a nursing student who has not engaged in professional clinical nursing practice). What are the advantages and disadvantages of having a career map?

Nurse as Author

1. Write a cover letter to accompany your résumé that could also be used as an email message to introduce yourself when applying for a nursing position. It is your choice whether to write a traditional or a skill-matched cover letter.
2. Create your own professional nursing résumé using either a chronologic or functional format.

Your Digital Classroom

Online Exploration

American Nurses Association:
www.nursingworld.org
Bureau of Labor Statistics *Occupational Outlook Handbook:* **www.bls.gov/ooh**
Career Mosaic: **www.careermosaic.org**

Monster: **www.monster.com**
New Zealand Health Workforce: Nurses: Four Step Career Planning Process
http://www.health.govt.nz/our-work/ health-workforce/career-planning
Nurse.com job listings: **www.nurse.com/jobs**
PONGO: **https://www.pongoresume.com/**
Résumé Writers: **www.resumewriters.com**
Sigma Theta Tau International: **www.nursingsociety.org**

Expanding Your Understanding

1. Develop two brief professional nursing résumés, one using PONGO and the other using a computer software program or website. Print the résumés and compare them. Would you use one of these while applying for a nursing position? Why or why not?
2. Visit the Résumé Writers website, and determine if it would be worth it for you to pay for a professionally generated résumé and cover letter. Why or why not?
3. Visit Nurse.com, and click on "Find a Nursing Job." Read about current job openings, including travel nursing positions and prospective employers. Do any of these positions appeal to you? Why or why not?

Beyond the Book

Visit the**Point®** **www.thePoint.lww.com** for activities and information to reinforce the concepts and content covered in this chapter.

REFERENCES

Abrams, S. L. (2000). *The new success rules for women.* Roseville, CA: Prima.

Agnes, M. (Ed.). (2005). *Webster's new world college dictionary* (4th ed.). Cleveland, OH: Wiley.

ANA Career Center Staff. (2015). 2015 Career resolutions for nurses. Retrieved from http://nursingworld.org/Content/Resources/2015-Career-Resolutions-for-Nurses.html. Accessed November 12, 2016.

Barrett, R. (1998). *Liberating the corporate soul, building a visionary organization.* Boston, MA: Butterworth-Heinemann.

Bell, S. K. (2001). Professional nurse's portfolio. *Nursing Administration Quarterly, 25,* 69–73.

Bongard, B. (1997a). Creating your own job: Using nonlinear strategies to reach your career goals. In B. Case (Ed.), *Career planning for nurses.* Albany, NY: Delmar.

Bongard, B. (1997b). Managing your career. In B. Case (Ed.), *Career planning for nurses.* Albany, NY: Delmar.

Borgatti, J. (2008). Networking for nurses. *American Nurse Today, 3*(4), 40–42.

Candela, L., & Bowles, C. (2005). Recent RN graduates perceptions of educational preparation. *Nursing Education Perspectives, 29*(5), 266–271.

Cardillo, D. (2001). Knowing when it's time to move on. *Nursing Spectrum, 2*, 20.

Chang, R. (2000). *The passion plan.* San Francisco, CA: Jossey-Bass.

Covey, S. (1992). *Principle-centered leadership.* New York: Simon & Schuster.

Covey, S. (2004). *The 8th habit: From effectiveness to greatness.* New York: Free Press.

Donner, G. J., & Wheeler, M. M. (2001). Taking control of your career and your future. *Excellence in Clinical Practice, 2*, 2.

Enelow, W., & Kursmark, L. (2010). *Expert resumes for health care career* (2nd ed.). Indianapolis, IN: JIST Works.

Falter, E. J. (1997). The nurse-manager-to-executive track. In B. Case (Ed.), *Career planning for nurses.* Albany, NY: Delmar Publishers.

Institute of Medicine. (2011). *The future of nursing: Leading change, advancing health.* Washington, DC: The National Academies Press.

Kelly, K. (2008). Coping with unexpected job loss. *American Nurse Today, 3*(7), 24–25.

Kendall-Gallagher, D., Aiken, L., Sloane, D., & Cimiotti, P. (2011). Nurse specialty certification, inpatient mortality and failure to rescue. *Journal of Nursing Scholarship, 43*(2), 188–194. doi: 10.1111/j.1547-5069.2011.01391.x

Lavoie-Tremblay, M., Wright, D., Desforges, N., Gélinas, C., Marchionni, C., & Drevniok, U. (2008). Creating a healthy workplace for new generation nurses. *Journal of Nursing Scholarship, 40*(3), 200–297.

Malone, B. L. (1999). Career mapping: Visioning your future. In C. A. F. Anderson (Ed.), *Nursing student to nursing leader: The critical path to leadership development.* Albany, NY: Delmar.

McGillis Hall, L., Waddell, J., Donner, G., & Wheeler, M. (2004). Outcomes of a career planning and development program for registered nurses. *Journal of Continuing Education, 21*(5), 231–238.

Meadows, K. L., & Buckley, J. J. (2014). You, Inc. *Journal of Healthcare Management, 59*(3), 173–176.

Messmer, P., Jones, S., & Taylor, B. (2004). Enhancing knowledge and self-confidence in novice nurses: The "shadow-a-nurse" ICU program. *Nursing Education Perspectives, 25*, 131–136.

Moore, G., & Pierce, Y. (2016). Selecting and preparing professional references. *American Nurse Today, 11*(1), 31–32.

Nightingale, F. (1929). *Notes on nursing.* New York: D. Appleton & Co.

Peddle, M., Jokwiro, Y., Carter, M., & Young, T. (2016). A professional portfolio of learning for undergraduate nursing students. *Australian Nursing & Midwifery Journal, 24*(4), 40.

Poulin, R. (2015). *Nurse résumé hacking: Shortcuts to outshining your peers & getting interviews.* Montreal, Canada: Richard Poulin.

Sherman, R., & Dyess, S. (2007). Be a coach for a novice nurse. *American Nurse Today, 2*(5), 54–55.

Spector, N., Blegen, M. A., Silvestre, J., Barnsteiner, J., Lynn, M. R., Ulrich, B., Fogg, L., & Alexander, M. (2015). Transition to practice study in hospital settings. *Journal of Nursing Regulation, 5* (4), 24–38. doi: 10.1016/S2155-8256(15)30031-4

VGM Career Horizons. (2008). *Resumes for nursing careers* (2nd ed.). Lincolnwood, IL: VGM Career Horizons.

Waxman, K. (2005). *Nurse entrepreneurship: Do you have what it takes? 2005 pathways to success.* Hoffman Estates, IL: Nursing Spectrum.

Wesorick, B., Shiparski, L., Troseth, M., & Wyngarden, K. (1997). *Partnership council field book.* Grand Rapids, MI: Practice Field.

Williams, M., & Jordon, K. (2007). The nursing professional portfolio: A pathway to career development. *Journal for Nurses in Staff Development, 3*, 125–131.

Yate, M. (2012). *Knock 'em dead resumes: How to write a killer resume that gets you job interviews* (10th ed.). Avon, MA: Adams Media.

Zimmerman, C., & Ward-Smith, P. (2012). Attrition of new graduate RN: Why nurses are leaving the profession. *The Missouri Nurse—Missouri Nurse Spring, 2012*, 15–17.

Chapter 22

Shaping the Future of Nursing

Future

Vision

Possible future

Plausible future

Probable future

Preferable future

Scenarios

Evidence-based nursing
  practice

Nurse licensure compact

By the end of this chapter, the learner will be able to:

1. Compare and contrast the terms possible future, plausible future, probable future, and preferable future.
2. Explain the implications of current trends on the nursing profession for each presented future scenario.
3. Outline strategies nurses can use to plan for the future.
4. Specify ways nurses can create a preferable future.
5. Outline how nursing education might better prepare nurses to meet the challenges of future health care delivery.
6. Discuss the role of nursing scholarship in the future of the nursing profession and health care.

Jing is a registered nurse (RN) who learned that the hospital where she has worked for 15 years is closing. Reasons for closing the hospital include the declining economy, fewer service demands, increased competition for clients among local health care providers, high unemployment, reduced government reimbursement for rendered care, inability to meet financial demands, and difficulty with nursing staff recruitment and retention. Jing is upset and wonders why she did not foresee the hospital closure. Because Jing has worked for the past 10 years on the day shift in the postpartum unit, she knows that her work hours and special area of practice most likely will change.

QUESTIONS FOR REFLECTION

1. How can you prepare yourself so that you maximize your knowledge, skills, and talents as a professional nurse?
2. Where would you like to be in the nursing profession 10 years from now?
3. What steps do you need to take to accomplish your future career vision?
4. What are the consequences for you as a professional nurse if you fail to consider what changes may occur within health care and the nursing profession in the next decade?

Humans have attempted to predict the future for centuries. Egyptian pyramids, for example, contain hieroglyphics that predict the future of the human race. Today, computer software programs and advanced statistical techniques have led to the development of sophisticated forecasting models. The random nature of the universe, however, prevents even the best forecasting methods from definitively predicting the future. Humans have come to realize that the only thing they can rely on is change.

Dramatic environmental and societal changes have influenced human health, health care delivery, professional nursing practice, nursing education, and nursing scholarship. Many of the forces influencing change have been detailed in earlier chapters in this text. Because the forces influencing professional nursing are intertwined with these changes in the world, an effort has been made to avoid redundancy. This chapter focuses on the future as a concept and outlines potential future scenarios so that the nursing profession and individual nurses can plan to meet the challenges of the 21st century and beyond. An entire book could be written about the myriad issues that impact the future of the nursing profession. To keep the subject manageable, this chapter provides a conceptual approach to the future and then uses it to address three critical societal issues: an aging American population, disasters, and increased rates of obesity.

A CONCEPTUAL APPROACH TO THE FUTURE

Depending on the context in which it is used, the word **future** means "that is to be or to come; of days, months, or years ahead . . . the time that has yet to come . . . what will happen; what is going to be" (Agnes, 2005, p. 576). In the plural form, "futures" refer to contracts made for goods or commodities that will be delivered at a date to come—for example, the rising price of crude oil in response to increased demand. In English (and many other languages), verbs have a future tense to communicate proposed actions. Whatever the definition, unless time ceases, the future will arrive soon.

Futurists use a variety of forecasting methods. Minkin (1995) proposed using a format that identifies and analyzes trends and determines their implications before making predictions. Other futurists use similar approaches to forecasting, with varying degrees of success (Aburdene & Naisbitt, 1992; Canton, 2015; Johnson & White, 2000; Naisbitt, 1996; Naisbitt & Aburdene, 1990; Sachs, 2008; Toffler, 1970, 1990; Toffler & Toffler, 2006). Some futurists, such as Thomas

Alva Edison, started with a vision (the concept of electric lighting) and then took steps to make the vision a reality. In terms of the future, the meaning of **vision** expands to include forecasting or prophecy.

There is much scholarly debate about the ability of mankind to shape the future. Minkin (1995) said the future is the only part of life that people can change based on their actions or inactions. Sullivan (1999, p. 5) identified two relevant assumptions about the future: "First, the future is uncertain. . . . Second, we choose and create major aspects of the future by what we do or fail to do." In contrast, many religions hold the belief that the future unfolds as part of a grand plan by a higher power.

Henchley (1978) specified four ways of looking at the future: possible, plausible, probable, and preferable. Henchley's approach considers the future from standpoints ranging from the wildest possible ideas to probable concepts based on human history and trends. This chapter presents definitions and scenarios for Henchley's four ways to approach the future, followed by selected key issues confronting the nursing profession and health care delivery.

The **possible future** considers all potential things that may occur, including the wildest ideas, even if they violate the laws of science (Henchley, 1978). Examples include unpredicted catastrophes, such as the catastrophic earthquake and tsunami affecting the Japanese northwestern coastline in 2011; potential, coordinated, multiple worldwide terrorists attacks; or a large meteor hitting and destroying the planet. Science fiction media and doomsday prediction exercises serve as sources for the possible future.

The **plausible future** focuses on what may occur based on current trends that may be combined to describe a range of potential futures (Henchley, 1978). Examples include increasing tensions between the United States and other nations, developing clean alternative energy sources, technologic advances, increasing disparity of income between the rich and poor, and increasing global warming and pollution.

The **probable future** presents a picture of what most likely will happen, with the future being primarily a mirror to the present with little or no actual change. Examples include continued financial strain on health care providers and businesses, a complex system of health care delivery, continued scientific and technologic advances, and the multifaceted dimensions of making life decisions.

The **preferable future** proposes the desired state for the future. Development of a preferred vision requires evolvement of common visions, shared values, and strategic plans among many groups of people. The preferable future starts by identifying a vision and taking steps to make that vision a reality. Indeed, this future results from deliberate actions or inactions. Examples include the unification of the government (federal, state, and local levels), insurance companies, and all health care providers to develop and implement a realistic health care system without resulting in national bankruptcy; the elimination of culturally biased health care service delivery by actively recruiting the best and the brightest of all cultural groups into the health care professions; and the development of strategies to integrate holistic health care practices into traditional scientific-based medical care methods.

Scenarios are forecasts, "an outline for any proposed or planned series of events, real or imagined" (Agnes, 2005, p. 1281). They raise awareness of the wide range of possible implications of external forces, sensitize people to potential threats and opportunities, and allow examination of alternative options for action. The scenarios presented in this chapter barely skim the issues that affect the future of professional nursing. Some of the presented scenarios are controversial. The scenarios without reference citations represent the author's predictions of what could happen.

FUTURE SCENARIOS FOR SOCIETY AND HEALTH CARE

Many of the forces that shape the future are beyond human control. Humans have yet to find ways to control acts of nature, such as weather patterns, earthquakes, certain epidemics, and famines. However, people do control governments, laws, and policies. Unfortunately, professional nurses lack the societal status and resources to become highly influential in the determination of laws, policies, and regulations. Nurses, thus, must build coalitions with more influential members of society to create a solid united front to create change. The following scenarios contain factors that cannot be controlled by the nursing profession alone. Nevertheless, nurses play a key role in being prepared to either confront these challenges or work collaboratively with others to steer action in a desired direction.

The Aging American Population

In 2014, 46.2 million Americans were over age 65 years (14.5% of the population). By 2040, 21.7% of the American population is expected to be over the age of 65 years (U.S. Department of Health and Human

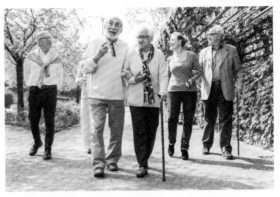

FIGURE 22.1 A major challenge in the future is promoting the health of the ever-expanding aging population.

Services, Administration on Aging, 2016). The doubling of the aging American population results in the need for more registered nurses in order to meet their needs for health care services (Fig. 22.1). The Institute of Medicine (IOM) (2008) proposed a three-step approach to prepare for this increase that includes improving the way health care is delivered, increasing the number of care providers specializing in geriatrics, and enhancing the geriatric competence of the health care workforce.

Demonstration of essential knowledge and competence in the care of older adults may become part of licensure and has been incorporated into some advanced practice nursing certification examinations (e.g., geriatric and family nurse practitioner examinations). More home health care nurses will be needed because increasing numbers of the elderly living at home will need help with activities of daily living and management of complex drug regimens. Elderly clients (if they have the cognitive ability to make sound, reasonable decisions) and their informal caregivers (family members and friends) will need to become active members of the health care team. New technologic devices such as computer-chipped bracelets, home alarms (for doors and stoves), and pressure sensor devices enable the elderly to stay at home safely under the care of family members, friends or hired help. Nurse geriatric consultants will help caregivers cope with the declining health of the elderly. When the elder persons can no longer manage their own personal and health care needs independently and become homebound, a primary or acute care geriatric nurse practitioner will make home visits aimed at keeping the person stable and safe at home. Finally, nursing research will be needed to determine needs and trends of the aging population along with ways to attract nurses to the field of geriatrics.

An aging nurse workforce compounds the issue of increased numbers of the elderly. In 2013, 34.96% of the nursing workforce was over 50 years of age and 38.3% of working registered nurses were 40 years of age or younger. One million registered nurses are expected to retire by 2025 (U.S. Bureau of Health Professions, Health Resources and Services Administration, 2013). Many of the older nurses reported reducing their working hours because of the physical demands of the job. According to a report published by the Robert Woods Johnson Foundation (2014), 74% of registered nurses over the age of 62 years and 24% of registered nurses over the age of 69 years have remained in the workforce. Several experts estimate that the United States will need to replace 900,000 to 1.2 million retiring nurses by 2025 (American Association of Colleges of Nursing [AACN], 2014; IOM, 2011; U.S. Bureau of Health Professions, Health Resources and Services Administration, 2013). Nursing programs have increased production of new professional nurse grades from 2001 to 2013 that has the potential to create an excess of registered nurses in 2025 if current trends continue (U.S. Bureau of Health Professions, Health Resources and Services Administration, 2013). However, if this trend reverses, the health care system will need to look for ways to entice retiring nurses to remain employed and retired nurses to return to work or volunteer their services (Neal-Boylan, Coccoa, & Carnoali, 2009).

Aging nurses might have an increased understanding of the needs of elderly clients as they experience caring for elderly relatives and recognize their own age-associated decline in physical abilities. Clinical issues projected to arise from the aging of the population include prevention of infectious diseases (especially human immunodeficiency virus, as sexually active seniors may refrain from condom use as pregnancy is not a potential outcome of intercourse), health promotion strategies for the elderly, supporting older persons with physical and cognitive limitations, and finding ways to support caregivers who care for loved ones in their homes.

Strategies for reversing the aging process may appear. Biotechnology also may create spare body parts, tissue transplants, and implanted computer chips for disabled people. Gene therapy, herbal therapies, and more drugs will be used to cease or reverse the aging process (Canton, 2015; Kaku, 2011; Toffler & Toffler, 2006). Kaku (2011) presents startling information on the use of nanotechnology to detect and treat life-threatening diseases, including breath analysis for health status in private home bathroom mirrors and the use of nanotechnology to detect and treat many forms of cancer, diabetes, and cardiovascular disease.

Healthy lifestyle choices, including proper exercise, diet, and stress management, will continue to be essential because of their positive effects on physical and mental fitness. With reduced costs of DNA testing at birth, everyone born may be genetically tested to obtain a DNA profile that might effectively predict lifespan, specific dietary recommendations and exercise prescriptions to enhance health and prolong life (Canton, 2015).

Possible Future

Often, elderly people with resources exhaust them to pay for health care services. As people age, they consume more health care services (IOM, 2008, 2011). By 2030, 20% of the American population will be over the age of 65 years and less than 20% will have defined pension plans (U.S. Department of Health and Human Services, Administration on Aging, 2012). Economic downturns and uncertainty have resulted in employers providing a fixed benefit pension plan to matched employee contribution plans. Today, some employees do not work for companies that provide pension plans, especially if they work part time jobs. Some large corporations (such as General Motor) have discontinued health care benefits for retirees. Retirees too young for Medicare benefits find themselves scrambling to secure health care coverage and may have to pay much more for coverage than they did in the past. Because most retirees cannot afford to be without supplemental health care coverage, many of them purchase supplemental insurance. Decisions retirees face will affect their health, well-being, and quality of life. For example, some elderly people must decide whether to buy food or prescription medications, move in with children, buy less nutritious food to reduce their grocery bill, or set thermostats to potentially dangerous settings (e.g., not using air conditioners during a heat wave) to stretch the resources they need to survive.

Forecasters predict that a possible intergenerational conflict may arise worldwide as Japan and several European nations have a similar problem with increasing elderly populations. Younger workers may revolt against paying high social security taxes to support the elderly (Canton, 2015; Kaku, 2011; Toffler & Toffler, 2006).

In the author's version of a worst-case and possible scenario, American society perceives the elderly as valueless people who do nothing but drain limited resources. Therefore, the elderly have an obligation to die in order to preserve precious commodities for younger, more productive world citizens. Governments enact laws to make euthanasia and assisted suicide legal, and the elderly who no longer want to burden their families or society willingly end their lives.

Plausible Future

A plausible scenario (especially for nations that have a democratic form of government and a large senior population) is that older people with cognitive capability exert energy on political activism, resulting in massive reformation in available senior services sponsored by government, businesses, and nonprofit agencies. For the financially solvent, elderly, specialized residences and extended-care facilities will be built to provide desired, individualized, and culturally relevant services. Older people without vast resources will find themselves living with children who gladly offer their homes to them, thereby creating multigenerational family units. As working adults serve as primary caregivers for the aged, geriatric day care programs will increase in number and some may even be employer sponsored. Caregiver programs will be developed to provide social and emotional support for exhausted and depressed family members caring for a debilitated aging adult. Legislation to provide funding for aging services, caregiver programs, medical care, and tax credits for home caregiving will be enacted. In this possible scenario, basic needs of the elderly are met and younger members of society value the elderly.

Probable Future

The probable scenario would be that the elderly might enjoy improved health from advances in medical science, remain a strong lobbying group, and demand increased governmental support for life and health care needs. Societal and governmental support for the health care of the elderly remains similar to what they are today.

Preferable Future

In the preferred scenario, the aging population makes health-promoting lifestyle choices (starting in middle adulthood) and develops strong ties with younger people. People of all ages, governmental agencies, businesses, and nonprofit foundations and organizations work together to develop policies related to health care delivery which provide equal access to services for all. The physically able elderly engage in volunteerism that results in a meaningful societal contribution. The elderly who have resources willingly assume financial responsibility for their health care services and residential care requirements. Public funding is reserved exclusively for the elderly and other societal members who cannot pay for basic life needs, including health care.

■ QUESTIONS FOR REFLECTION

1. How can the nursing profession prepare for the increased numbers of elderly who will need future nursing services?
2. What are the possible consequences for the nursing profession if it fails to address the aging population issue?
3. What are the possible consequences for the nursing profession if it fails to address the aging of the nursing workforce?

Man-Made Disasters

Any event resulting in great harm or damage can be considered a disaster. Man-made disasters occur because of human action. The very powerful or people who are disadvantaged and disenfranchised act in violent ways that result in human and environmental catastrophes (government corruption, rebellions, wars, and terrorism).

Before September 11, 2001, the United States considered itself immune to multiple terrorist attacks or acts of war. However, some people forewarned of a coordinated terrorist attack plan (National Institute of Medicine and National Research Council, 1999). Terrorist acts occur in many nations, and countless acts have been averted. The ease of securing plans for building bombs (some with nuclear, disease-producing, or noxious chemical capability) increases the likelihood of a large-scale terrorist attack. Technologic advances such as nanotechnology, biotechnology, and robotics offer the possibility of destroying the human race while leaving buildings and infrastructures intact. Sources of energy production become prime targets of terrorists because of the current reliance on these power sources for health, safety, and business (Kaku, 2011). Balancing societal needs for safety while preserving individual rights challenge those entrusted to provide public safety.

The terrorist attacks in the United States sparked a worldwide war on terrorism, with most of the actual combat occurring in Iraq and Afghanistan. Uprisings against oppressive governments trigger civil wars or government attacks against rebels. Recent terrorist attacks across the globe create fear and uncertainty for persons as they live their lives. As in all wars and

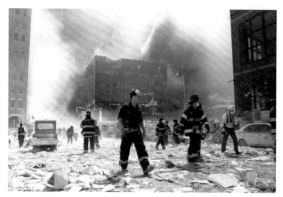

FIGURE 22.2 Nurses, other health care providers, and first responders must be ready to respond to an act of terror. Nurses may care for persons dealing with long term consequences of terrorism.

terrorist attacks, much environmental destruction has occurred and many people have died (including many innocent civilians) or sustained physical and/or psychological injury (Fig. 22.2).

Possible Future

A possible (and bleak) scenario is that terrorists obtain access to nuclear and biologic weaponry. Within a short time frame (perhaps weeks), terrorists execute a well-coordinated series of attacks on American soil resulting in many civilian casualties and widespread destruction. The United States launches a unilateral attack against terrorist cells with total disregard for national borders. The American action fuels international opinion that the United States will conquer the world to force democratic and capitalistic values on all people.

Plausible Future

A more plausible scenario results in the strengthening of the coalition of countries engaging in the war on terrorism because of attacks happening in many countries. In this scenario, the United Nations becomes the place where strategic plans are made to rid the world of terrorist acts initiated by well-organized groups with global networks. The United Nations also develops a global response plan to chemical and biologic attacks. However, acts of terrorism performed by individuals remain unpredictable, and the people responsible for such acts remain elusive.

Probable Future

Unfortunately, the probable scenario results in a future not much different from today. The United States and certain allies develop stronger ties, and the war on terrorism lasts for many years. In response to identified potential biologic attacks, the United States stockpiles medications and vaccines for future use, if needed.

Most Americans refuse to be intimidated by terrorist threats and continue with their usual life practices—working, shopping, and attending sporting and other recreational events as if the world is still a safe place. Some anxious citizens stockpile supplies in anticipation of a terrorist attack using nuclear devices. The government tries to stimulate the economy while spending vast amounts of money to preserve homeland security. Less money becomes available to provide services to the poor (food subsidies, health care) and to repair infrastructure (roads, sewage systems, power plants). American citizens live with minor inconveniences, such as having to arrive earlier and wait longer in lines when traveling by air. Health care workers voluntarily register to become members of federal, state, or local medical response teams (Veenema, 2013).

Preferable Future

The preferable future is one in which people have no need for violent acts because diverse values and approaches to life are valued. Rich nations foster the economic development of poorer countries. Agreement occurs on defining basic human rights and values across cultures while allowing for diversity when appropriate. All people are valued. People with more resources than what they can use support those who cannot meet basic human needs (food, water, shelter, and safety). Because all people feel valued and respected, there is no need for violence.

■ QUESTIONS FOR REFLECTION

1. How can the nursing profession prepare to confront the effects of terrorist acts?
2. Why is being prepared for terrorism important to the nursing profession?

Natural Disasters

Natural disasters occur as the result of climate or geologic events. In recent years, some climatic changes have been linked to the actions of humans (see Chapter 13, "Environmental and Global Health") (Canton, 2015; Kaku, 2011; Sachs, 2008; Veenema, 2013). Natural disasters can occur quickly and without warning (earthquakes, volcanic eruptions, some tornadoes, and flash floods), quickly and with warning (storms, tsunamis), or slowly and with warning (downstream flooding, environmental contamination, famines from prolonged drought). Hurricane Katrina revealed what can happen when a well-coordinated disaster response plan at the federal, state, and local state governmental levels is lacking.

Predicted effects of global climate change include more intense storms, rising sea levels, and geographical climate shifts (tropical forests become deserts, temperate zones become tropical, tundra becomes fertile farmland). Infectious diseases would follow climate changes and become prevalent in more temperate climate zones (Canton, 2015; Kaku, 2011; Sachs, 2008).

Possible Future

The possible future is one in which humans show an increasing disregard for the Earth. The need for human survival and desire for extravagant lifestyles dominate all human activities. Humans ravage the planet and expand their residential areas with total disregard for wildlife and plant life. Environmental impacts consolidate and results in catastrophic climate effects, such as those depicted in the film *The Day After Tomorrow* (Emmerich, 2004), in which climate change produces rapidly rising sea levels and a series of massive storms that culminate with rapidly falling temperatures affecting Europe, North America, and the northern half of Asia. Falling temperatures result in deep freezes that cannot support human existence. Not even the most powerful government can intervene to prevent the catastrophe.

Plausible/Preferable Future

A plausible (and perhaps preferable) scenario encompasses increased human awareness of our impact on the environment. The United Nations spearheads a binding global environmental treaty for all nations (even developing countries with fewer resources). The world works cohesively and collaboratively to reduce greenhouse gas emissions and air, soil, and water pollution, and facilitates action by offering incentives. Nature flourishes and counteracts the damage done by humans.

Probable Future

The probable future involves the continuation of existing international, national, and local environmental policies. Economic considerations supersede required actions for energy conservation and environmental preservation, with most people abiding by them and other people looking for ways around them because of increased personal expenditures. If (or when) sea levels begin to rise enough to threaten human life, storms become highly destructive, and plants and wildlife disappear (Canton, 2015; Kaku, 2011), then the human race might develop and implement stronger, environmentally friendly global policies.

Obesity

In 2015, the Centers for Disease Control National Center for Health Statistics reported that close to 70% of Americans were overweight (body mass index greater than 25 m²). The CDC also reported that 78.6 million American adults (34.9%) suffered from obesity (body mass index greater than 30 m²). Obesity is linked to many chronic illnesses, including type 2 diabetes, heart disease, stroke, and some cancers. In 2015, health care costs related to obesity were $147 billion and an obese person had $1,429 higher health care costs when compared to persons with healthy weights (CDC, 2015a). The CDC (2015b) projects that one in three Americans adults will develop diabetes (if current trends persist) by 2050.

Ancient humans survived as hunter-gatherers, and efficient storage of energy promoted the survival of the human race. In modern times, however, Americans (and citizens of other developed nations) engage in a sedentary lifestyle and have unrestricted access to high-calorie foods (Centers for Disease Control and Prevention [CDC], 2008, 2010; IOM, 2012). Obesity results from consuming more calories than are expended. Today's American lifestyle, communities, and individuals share the blame (see Box 22.1, Professional Building Blocks, "Factors Contributing to Obesity").

The epidemic of overweight and obese Americans has erased many of the achievements made in health and medicine over the past few decades. The economic costs for obesity-related health care are estimated to be close to $200 million, with childhood obesity costs exceeding $14 million. Being overweight and obese also contributes to the development of degenerative arthritis, hypertension, heart disease, stroke, gallbladder disease, sleep apnea, respiratory difficulties, and certain forms of cancer (CDC, 2008; IOM, 2012).

Some people indeed have genetic or biologic factors and for them obesity cannot be avoided. A population focus on obesity education and prevention does not deny the importance of specific biologic or genetic factors that cannot be ameliorated (IOM, 2012).

The IOM (2012) compiled a report and recommendations to combat and prevent obesity in the United States. In its 2012 report, the IOM recommended that individuals, families, community, and society need to be aware of and engage themselves in actions to actualize the following five goals.

1. Make physical activity an integral and routine part of life (p. 10).
2. Create food and beverage environments that ensure that healthy food and beverage options are the routine, easy choice (p. 11).

22.1 Professional Building Blocks

Factors Contributing to Obesity

- Cultural norms that specify that being overweight or obese is not an individual's fault, but rather the result of an illness, genetic defect, medication, or lack of resources for proper nutrition and exercise
- Poor food choices
- Lack of safe places outside to walk or play
- Retail stores and restaurants that sell only unhealthy foods
- Constant bombardment with advertisements for unhealthy foods and beverages
- Sedentary lifestyle
- Lack of education about healthy food choices and lifestyle
- Lack of time to exercise and prepare healthy meals
- Unclear nutritional standards for defining a healthy diet and nutritional labeling of all foods and beverages
- Inconsistent messaging about how much exercise is required to promote health and well-being
- Inconsistent standards for screening people of all ages for being overweight or obese
- Lack of access to routine obesity prevention, screening, diagnosis, and treatment
- Decreased time spent in physical education in schools
- Disparities in the amount of weight a woman should gain for a healthy pregnancy and while breastfeeding
- Inconsistent information and varying levels of commitment to maternal breastfeeding practices

Institute of Medicine. (2012). *Accelerating progress in obesity prevention: Solving the weight of the nation.* Washington, DC: The National Academies Press.

3. Transform messages about physical activity and nutrition (p. 13).
4. Expand the role of health care providers, insurers, and employers in obesity prevention (p. 14).
5. Make schools a national focal point for obesity prevention (p. 15).

As health care providers, nurses have the responsibility and opportunity to use evidence- or consensus-based guidelines to educate, screen, diagnose, and treat people of all ages for weight issues. Emphasis must be placed on helping others prevent obesity and maintain a healthy weight. Nurses can serve as role models by maintaining a healthy weight and if they become overweight, take action to lose weight. Some nursing interventions include providing education, emotional support, coaching, and periodic monitoring for clients as well as advocating them for improving resources to promote physical activity and health

dietary opportunities within their communities (IOM, 2012).

Possible Future

A possible scenario related to obesity is that science discovers ways to turn off the "thrifty gene" that makes humans conserve calories, block the chemicals responsible for hunger, and develop an effective weight loss pill that has few and insignificant adverse effects (Millett & Kopp, 1996). In addition, scientists realize that individual genetics determine how foods are metabolized and used by the body. Nutritional counseling based on individual genetic profiles becomes widespread (Canton, 2015; Underwood & Adler, 2005). Government support for weight reduction in obese and overweight citizens includes prescription drugs for weight loss, memberships to health clubs, and psychological counseling. In return, governments impose taxes on "junk" food and initiate tax surcharges on obese citizens to defray projected increased health care costs. Many people lose weight and adopt a healthy lifestyle (to avoid increased taxes), which results in reduced demand for secondary and tertiary health care services.

Plausible Future

In a plausible scenario, affluent citizens in developed nations continue to gain weight. They have unlimited access to food, engage in sedentary jobs, fail to exercise, and find comfort in passive entertainment (e.g., television, computer activities). Health problems once thought of as afflictions of aging, occur at younger and younger ages. Young, educated citizens find themselves incapable of performing any manual labor. They rely on housekeepers and gardeners to maintain a home or they live in condominiums or apartments where building and grounds maintenance is provided. Because of their size and health problems, young adults quickly find themselves unable to work, resulting in an increased incidence of worker disability. Some people become so large that they can no longer walk and rely on power chairs for mobility. They require assistive devices or robots for cleaning following elimination. The obese young and the elderly consume health care services to the point of exhaustion. Nurses caring for obese clients sustain more back injuries. Nursing becomes one of the most dangerous professions because of the high incidence of permanent disability related to work-related injuries.

Probable Future

A probable scenario related to increased obesity is that some obese and overweight people recognize the impact of weight on their overall health and daily lives. Corporate America recognizes ways to capitalize on the obesity epidemic. Employers reduce employee contributions to health care insurance for maintaining a healthy weight, provide incentives for employees to exercise more, and even provide them with free gym memberships. Many companies (including health care organizations) subsidize weight loss programs or offer employees incentives to lose weight. Companies develop weight reduction products and aggressively market them to consumers. Some persons blame others for their obesity, while others take steps to reduce their weight. Health insurance companies, employers, and highly futuristic, health-conscious people purchase time for virtual experiences during which they can watch an avatar of themselves age based on multiple lifestyle choices (Adler, Dunagan, Kreit, et al., 2009). There are legislative efforts to pass regulations and laws protecting consumers from poor eating habits, fraudulent weight reduction regimes, and to impose taxes on non-nutritious food and beverages (see Concepts in Practice, "Philadelphia Passes a Soda Tax"). People receive education on healthy lifestyles. Some people take advantage of psychological counseling or follow the advice of health care providers and lose weight, while others continue the cycle of temporary weight loss followed by weight gain. People (nurses and unlicensed care providers) caring for obese health care consumers have access to and use technologic and other assistive devices to prevent work-related injuries. Laws are enacted to require health care providers to use lifting devices and health care organizations establish hardline policies requiring their use.

Preferable Future

In the preferred future, more (ideally all) people adopt a healthy lifestyle. Health care professionals provide accessible education programs that address the health hazards of being obese and overweight, with consideration given to the current literacy levels of the targeted learners. The message is successful, and people lose their excess weight. They consume only the number of calories needed to maintain a healthy body weight and follow the recommendation for getting 60 minutes of vigorous exercise daily (IOM, 2012). Health care dollars are spent on health promotion, resulting in increased savings because of reduced consumption of secondary and tertiary health care services.

▌ QUESTIONS FOR REFLECTION

1. How does obesity affect the health of clients? Of nurses?

2. What are the potential adverse effects of obese clients on the nursing profession? On society?

3. What are the possible ways to minimize health hazards for nurses working with obese clients?

4. What safety devices are present in your current clinical practice setting for nurses to use when caring for obese clients?

5. Do you use the safety devices available to you? Why or why not?

Concepts in Practice `IDEA ──▶ PLAN ─▶ ACTION`

Philadelphia Passes a Soda Tax

On June 14, 2016 the Philadelphia City Council passed a tax of 18 cents on a can of soda, $1.08 on a 6-pack and $1.02 2-L bottle of soda. They included all forms of soda (diet and regular). The tax is in addition to the current 8% sales tax because in the state of Pennsylvania, soda is not classified as food.

The tax is estimated to raise $91 million annually. The city plans to use the generated revenue to expand pre-kindergarten education program, fund community school, improve parks, renovate add recreational centers. Unspent revenue will be placed into the city's general revenue fund where it can be used for other projects.

1. What do you think the tax assessment on sodas?

2. Would you support such a tax? Why or why not?

3. What action would you take as a professional nurse to support or not support such a tax?

Sahdi, J., & Smith, A. (2016). Philadelphia passes a soda tax. *CNNMoney. com* June 16, 2016. Retrieved from http://money.cnn.com/2016/06/16/pf/taxes/philadelphia-passes-a-soda-tax/index.html. Accessed July 3, 2016.

Advances in Genetics

The findings from the Human Genome Project are having profound effects on society. Genes for various diseases have been discovered; eventually these discoveries will lead to new disease detection and treatment techniques. Genomics or proteomics (the reactions of genetics on body metabolism) also plays a key role in the development of health-related problems. Genetic testing may result in determining suitable marriage partners, safe insurance risks, individualized diets, disease treatment interventions (certain medications or lifestyle changes), and human evolution (Canton, 2015). People also may receive genetically designed medication to prevent or treat illnesses. In addition, people known to be at risk for a particular affliction may begin screening for a particular disease earlier in life than would be recommended for the general population. For example, an RNA blood test has been determined to have 75% accuracy and 85% specificity for predicting lung cancer diagnosis (Zander et al., 2008). Genetic testing for certain forms of breast cancer is now a reality as well (see Concepts in Practice, "Genetic Testing for Breast Cancer").

Concepts in Practice IDEA ⟶ PLAN ⟶ ACTION

Genetic Testing for Breast Cancer

Helena, an RN, has a mother, maternal aunt, and sister who have all been diagnosed with breast cancer. Her maternal grandmother died from ovarian cancer. Helena is aware that there is a genetic link for increased incidence of breast cancer in women who have a family history of breast cancer. When she goes for her scheduled mammogram at the breast center, staff offer her the option for genetic testing because of her family history.

1. For female students—what would you do if you were Helena? For male students—what would you want your wife, sister, or mother to do?

2. List the pros and cons of genetic testing for Helena.

3. If the genetic test came back positive (a positive result on a genetic test would indicate more than a 75% chance the woman would develop breast cancer), what type of treatment options would be available to Helena? What professional advice would you give Helena based on this information? What would you do if she refused any treatments and just decided to continue routine screening?

4. Outline key ethical issues related to genetic testing for breast cancer.

Possible Future

A possible scenario comes from the movie *Gattaca* (Niccol, 1997), in which individuals receive genetic testing at birth to determine their future lives. The state selects the profession, education, and genetic composition for all citizens. Marriage is no longer needed because new human life is created using artificial insemination in women genetically designed to thrive during pregnancy and childbirth. Individuals lose the freedom to choose their destiny.

Plausible Future

A plausible scenario is one in which people undergo genetic testing at birth to determine potential health risks. For those with a genetic predisposition to cancer, screenings begin earlier in life than would be recommended for the general population. Drug companies use genetic research to design effective medications against previously incurable illnesses. In addition, genetically designed medications for individuals enhance disease prevention and treatment efforts (Adler et al., 2009; Canton, 2015; Institute for Alternative Futures, 2012). The cost of health care escalates as individually designed drugs increase costs for production and create more medications. Only the affluent have access to genetically designed medications. People requiring earlier and more frequent disease screenings receive them only if they can afford them.

Probable/Preferred Future

The probable scenario proposes that pharmaceutical companies and health care providers use information generated from human genetic research to find treatments for and ways to prevent illness. All people are offered genetic testing to determine optimal screening, prevention, and treatment modalities. Genetic testing is performed only with voluntary consent, costs only a few hundreds of dollars, and plays a key role in primary prevention. Persons become able to provide a bit of saliva and send it to a lab for a comprehensive report on their genome (Canton, 2015; Institute for Alternative Futures, 2012; Institute for the Future, 2016). Nurses assume the key role of helping people understand the results of genetic testing (Burke & Kirk, 2006; Tariman, 2008). Technology advances so much that a person can purchase inexpensive genetic testing, send in a sample of saliva, receive detailed interpretations of results with lifestyle recommendations for early disease detection and prevention, along with strategies for health promotion and enhancement. For this issue, the preferred scenario is also most likely the probable scenario.

▌ QUESTIONS FOR REFLECTION

1. What impact will advances in genetic research have on the nursing profession?
2. What additional knowledge and skills will nurses need in the future because of advances in genetic research and genetically based health care?
3. What are the potential hazards for consumers who undergo genetic testing?
4. What are the potential benefits of having a genetic health profile performed on all people?

FUTURE SCENARIOS FOR HEALTH CARE DELIVERY

Health care delivery has become increasingly complex. Recent safety and quality initiatives add to the complexity for all health care providers. Staying abreast of new discoveries about the human body (e.g., genetic, genomics, physiology, biochemistry, stem cells), healthy lifestyle strategies, and technology creates distress for some health care providers. Constant change seems to be the only thing on which providers and consumers can rely. In 1996, Bezold identified possible health care delivery scenarios for the 21st century. For this chapter section, Bezold's scenario titles are used, but updated information has been added based on current trends in health care delivery related to human physiology and disease etiology.

Hard Times Scenario (Possible Future)

This possible future assumes that times are tough for the economy as a whole and for health care. As unemployment increases, citizens pressure the federal government to create a universal health care plan. Because of consistent increases in government deficits, the plan offers a very frugal benefit package. The government refuses to pay providers for costs incurred from all preventable hospital-acquired conditions (Kurtzman & Buerhaus, 2008). Governmental health care plans cover only treatments based on comparative research. Governmental controls increase the amount of documentation health care providers must complete to justify reimbursement, and cost containment reduces the amount of federal funding for all forms of health care research. Health care innovations slow dramatically. Heroic measures once used to prolong life are limited to patients who are younger, have something to offer society, or can pay for them. A three-tiered health care system emerges, one for people relying exclusively on the government, another for those with resources for private insurance coverage, and another for people who have the ability to pay for health care costs independently. People who pay for their own health care travel abroad for nonemergent diagnostic tests and surgeries (reduced costs) and/or have a private physician who offers concierge services, including house calls on demand (Institute for Alternative Futures, 2012). For persons not able to afford health care services, they have to bear long lines to be seen by a health care professional.

Nursing care of acutely ill clients is important in this scenario, but nurses are poorly paid and have little prestige. Consequently, most nurses are from lower socioeconomic groups and from foreign countries. Some consumers of nursing services have less confidence in receiving care from a foreign-born nurse, especially when the consumer may not understand the nurse's instructions because of the nurse's accent or command of English. Clients who can pay are cared for in the home by private-duty nurses (Bezold, 1996).

To streamline the use of limited resources, Herzlinger (2004) suggested that government-financed and insurance-covered health treatments be limited to those with an established history of successful outcomes, based on reliable scientific evidence and documented emphasis on promoting client comfort (validated through comparative research).

Because of documented comparative research, advanced practice registered nurses (APRNs) are the main primary care providers. They rely on standardized protocols for preventing and treating specific health care problems. APRNs refer cases that require complex management to specialized physicians who would also use evidence-based practice treatment protocols shown to reduce costs but have optimal patient outcomes.

Paramedics start to fill the role of home health care nurses. They make routine visits to clients with whom they have received nonemergent call for situation such as helping them off the floor following a fall. APRNs and physicians make referrals for them to visit patients for glycemic control, dressing changes, and blood pressure monitoring. Consumers with knowledge and resources become empowered to act as equal partners with health care professionals. However, consumers without knowledge and/or resources are unable to access needed or direct their health care services.

Buyer's Market Scenario (Probable/Preferable Future)

In this probable future, Bezold (1996) and Herzlinger (2004) propose that the responsibility for health and health care expenditures is returned to the consumer. Insurance coverage includes a tax to help pay for the cost of care given to the poor. Health care providers are certified by the state on the basis of knowledge and competence. Health care providers, especially nurses, use evidence-based guidelines for practice. Competition for health care consumers becomes fierce, and health care organizations work hard to please consumers. People rely less on health care providers and have better tools for changing their lifestyles and preventing or managing illnesses. Consumers, rather than third-party payers, choose from various types of providers and treatments. Because health becomes a highly valued aspect of human life, consumers seek health care for illness prevention rather than disease treatment (Herzlinger, 2004).

This scenario offers real potential for nursing to achieve greater power and influence. Nursing practice based on scientific evidence elevates the level of professionalism for nurses. Nurses present solid evidence for optimal staffing patterns for positive client outcomes (Gordon, Buchanan, & Bretherton, 2008). Because nurses are seen by society as professionals who have altruistic concerns for clients and have reasonable workloads, more people choose to enter the profession. Nurses develop independent practices and demonstrate superiority in primary health care delivery. By accessing consumers directly, nurses have a major role in health promotion. Education emphasizes ways of teaching consumers how to promote individual, family, and community health. This scenario might be a preferable future for professional nursing because of its benefits for both nurses and consumers.

Business-As-Usual Scenario (Probable Future)

Another probable future, the business-as-usual scenario, assumes continued technologic ingenuity, proliferation of new pharmaceuticals, sophisticated communication, and high levels of consumption. Although most Americans are better off, the percentage of poor continues to rise. The Affordable Care Act remains in place, and the annual 2% cuts from direct Medicare funding result in substantial annual job losses in the health care industry—as many as 211,756 jobs lost in 2013 up to 330,127 jobs lost in 2021 (Tripp Umbach, 2012). However, advances in biomedical knowledge and technology make it possible to forecast, prevent, and manage illnesses earlier and more successfully. High-tech interventions such as performance-enhancing bionic implants and organoids (a new organ or organ part grown outside the body and then implanted) are widely available to those who can pay for them (Adler et al., 2009; Institute for Alternative Futures, 2012; Kaku, 2011). Small hospitals continue to close, patient acuity levels rise, early hospital dismissals become desired, and health care becomes more efficient. Wealthy for-profit and nonprofit hospitals develop integrated health systems and negotiate discounts with health insurance companies to obtain and maintain a stable patient base. Administrators rule and fewer hospitalists (but more acute care nurse practitioners) staff hospitals as employees. Insured consumers receive health care using inpatient, outpatient,

and home health care services. Health insurance plans cover emergency room—incurred costs only if the reason for the visit is determined to be a life-threatening or potential disability-producing event.

Because innovations continue, health care costs outpace inflation and eventually consume 20% of gross domestic product. Increased efficiency demands require providers to carry higher patient loads. The health professions become more devalued by society and fewer people enter professional nursing, thereby compounding the nursing shortage.

Healthy, Healing Communities Scenario (Preferred Future)

This preferred and probable scenario involves a focus on "healing the body, mind, and spirit of individuals and communities" (Bezold, 1996, p. 38). Neighbors look out for each other, and people work together to eliminate problems such as substance abuse, teenage pregnancy, and the effects of poverty. However, as information and technology increase worker productivity or replace workers altogether, unemployment grows to 25%. Community health centers serve as medical homes within neighborhoods. Health promotion efforts begin in early childhood. Older people find rewarding ways to contribute to the community, reducing disability, and the time spent in long-term care facilities. Advanced technologies lead to a comfortable life for most people, and bionics, robotics, smarter homes, and more caring neighborhoods allow disabled elderly individuals to remain in their homes.

Consumers become involved in decision making regarding their health as they learn how to access and evaluate health-related information through computer applications that track personal health information using semantic computing (i.e., looking at quantifiable personal health data and making clinical decisions). People become more comfortable sharing personal health data using electronic health records that connect to large databases that are used for research. Telehealth provides services for people who are homebound or live in remote rural areas (Adler et al., 2009; Institute for Alternative Futures, 2012; Kaku, 2011).

Technology becomes so advanced and inexpensive that consumers can swallow pills that safely collect comprehensive internal body information about their health that is automatically sent to their primary health care providers. Health care providers then send consumers advice for enhancing their health or treating identified health conditions. In addition, persons add sensors and cameras in their homes, to collect information about their health status and lifestyle measures that are automatically added to their health data cards. The health data cards consist of tiny microchips with wireless technology that are embedded into a piece of jewelry that can be worn attractively. Finally, physical environments of the home help humans to manage disease, enhance health, and facilitate healthy aging. Some of the physical environmental changes involve verbal reminders from computers or cell phone that respond to either the aforementioned pill consumed or in response to the home sensors or cameras (Institute for the Future, 2016). All persons, not just the affluent, have access to and can afford this technology for personal health management.

Nurses are full partners with consumers in this scenario, helping people with self-care and health promotion activities, interpreting the complex web of information received from computer applications, and providing information to support fully informed decision making. Consumers select a "medical home," a private outpatient office or community clinic that provides them with preventive and health promotion services in a coordinated care effort across the care continuum from primary care providers (including nurse practitioners). The medical home offers specialized services based on life span and specific health care needs (Institute for Alternative Futures, 2012; IOM, 2011; Vlasses & Smeltzer, 2007). Older people are valued and cared for at home whenever feasible. Nurses are recognized as highly educated professionals who make valuable contributions, such as providing psychosocial support to clients, engaging in surveillance activities to detect subtle changes in client health status, executing complex evidence-based clinical procedures and protocols confidently, and coordinating health care activities across the continuum of care (Formella & Rovin, 2004; Gordon et al., 2008; IOM, 2011).

EVOLVING HEALTH CARE NEEDS AND HEALTH CARE DELIVERY

Along with the aforementioned issues, Cetron and Davies (2008) of the World Future Society have identified additional trends that impact consumer health care needs and the delivery of health care services in the United States. Demographic trends reveal an ever-increasing population, with increased immigration to meet labor shortages. Immigration creates a diverse workforce and more culturally diverse clients seeking health care services. Issues on the economic

and occupational fronts include globalization, high unemployment (especially in the service sector), and younger people entering the workforce, a shrinking industrial workforce, and the continued expansion of information-based organizations. Rising education levels, altered gender roles, increased political participation by all citizens, increasing technologic sophistication and complexity, reliance on power, and knowledge dependency are societal trends that also impact health care needs and delivery.

Increased cultural diversity and immigration will force all health care providers to become more adept at delivering culturally sensitive and linguistically appropriate services. Health care providers must be attuned to signs of diseases never seen in the United States when working with people who have lived in different lands. Differences in genetic profiles and genomics also must be considered when caring for culturally diverse clients. In an ideal world, health care provider demographics should match the demographics of health care consumers. In 2013, the U.S. Bureau of Health Professions reported that 90.9% of nurses are female and have following ethnicity: 75.4% White, non-Hispanic, 9.9% African American, 4.8% Hispanic. Latino, 8.3% Asian, 0.4% American Indian/Alaskan Native, and 1.3% other (mixed—very different from the demographics of the American public) (IOM, 2011; Sullivan Commission, 2004).

Creating a culturally diverse workforce poses challenges to future health care delivery. Currently, the United States attracts internationally educated health care providers because the American health care system offers a higher income than what many health care providers can earn in their native homelands, and social status for nurses (especially from the Pacific Rim and Far East) is typically higher in the United States than in other countries (Kirk, 2007). Thus, salaries for physicians and nurses far exceed what they can make in their homelands.

Facilitating migration of nurses has been suggested as a remedy for the ever-growing nursing shortage. Currently, internationally educated nurses working in the United States come from the Philippines (50.2%), Canada (20.2%), the United Kingdom (8.4%), Nigeria (2.5%), Ireland (1.5%), India (1.3%), Hong Kong (1.2%), Jamaica (1.1%), and South Korea (1%). Clusters of internationally educated nurses work in California, Florida, New York, Texas, and New Jersey (Brush, 2008). Nurses from Canada, the United Kingdom, and Ireland typically do not have difficulty speaking English. Unfortunately, nurse migration to developed nations creates nursing shortages in the donor nations (Brush, 2008). In 2010, 7,189 foreign-educated nurses who passed the NCLEX-RN® on their first attempt came from the Philippines (72.3%), South Korea (10.5%), India (8.9%), Canada (5.9%), and Nigeria (2.4%) (U.S. Bureau of Health Professions, Health Resources and Services Administration, 2013). Kirk (2007) proposed that the global migration of professional nurses results in an international flow of skills and knowledgeable health care workers.

When working with a culturally diverse health care team, all members must demonstrate authenticity and encourage the full participation of everyone so that each person feels that he or she makes a valuable contribution to the team's efforts (see Chapter 11, "Multicultural Issues in Professional Practice"). Little things such as failure to include culturally diverse team members in informal conversations or outside-of-work activities may "have cumulative and profoundly negative effects" (Myers & Dreachslin, 2007, p. 294) on a team member's overall well-being and professional performance.

Take Note!
A large majority of RNs in the United States are white, non-Hispanic women—a demographic profile that in large part does not match that of the clients they serve.

Technologic advances in health care also pose challenges to health care delivery. All health team members need effective computer skills to access client health data; find current evidence-based best practice protocols; order client medications, interventions, and supplies; and document client plans, interventions, and outcomes (see Chapter 14, "Informatics and Technology in Nursing Practice"). In the future, people may carry computerized identification cards that include protected health information or will have online electronic personal health records (Adler et al., 2009; Canton, 2015; Institute for Alternative Futures, 2012; Institute for the Future, 2016; Kaku, 2011). Identification cards will be useful not only to verify client identity to prevent health insurance fraud but also, and more importantly, to provide a detailed, consistent health history, reducing the time spent conducting a detailed health history for each health care service encounter. Summaries for each time the person accesses and uses health care services will be recorded on the card, thereby fostering integration of health care services across the care continuum.

QUESTIONS FOR REFLECTION

1. What do you think the current health care system will look like in 10 years?
2. What knowledge and skills will be needed for effective nursing practice in 10 years?
3. How can nurses best prepare for the future health care delivery system?
4. What can the nursing profession do to help other nurses prepare for the challenges in the future health care delivery system?

THE FUTURE OF PROFESSIONAL NURSING PRACTICE

Many issues confront the nursing profession as it works to maintain sustainable numbers to meet the needs of society. Recent initiatives (including IOM recommendations to improve the quality and safety of American health care delivery from a series of IOM quality chasm series) (IOM, 2000, 2001, 2003, 2004, 2006) and Quality and Safety Education in Nursing (QSEN) (Sherwood & Barnsteiner, 2012) calling for improved quality and safety provide an opportunity for nurses to present evidence demonstrating the valuable contributions they make to health care. In addition, the profession needs to develop plans to accommodate a mobile society and increased geographical demands for nurses. If nurses fail to seize the current opportunities for leadership in health care delivery and fail to recruit new nurses, the profession may cease to exist. Nurses represent the largest percentage of all health team members.

Take Note!
Actions taken by the nursing profession today have profound implications for future clients, health care delivery, nurses, and society.

Evidence-Based Nursing Practice (Preferred/Probable Future)

Nursing research findings, quality improvement data results, and clinical experience provide the foundation for evidence-based nursing practice. **Evidence-based nursing practice** uses the best available sources of information to enable cost effective and clinically effective client care. Systematic nursing research and detailed evaluations of health care interventions provide strong evidence nurses can use as foundations for practice. Large databases such as those generated by the National Database of Nursing Quality Indicators (Dunton, 2008) and the Omaha System (Canham, Mao, Yoder, Connolly, & Dietz, 2008) facilitate the generation of solid evidence for use in quality management and clinical protocol development. In the past, nurses performed many tasks based on tradition and ritual. Evidence-based practice enables nurses to determine the effects of newly developed technology, alternative and complementary treatments, and the differences professional nurses make in client care outcomes. Nurses are doing a better job of producing and disseminating information about their impact on the delivery of high-quality care (Aiken, Clarke, & Sloane, 2000; Aiken, Smith, & Lake, 1994; Doran, 2003; Gordon et al., 2008; Havens & Aiken, 1999; Hinshaw, 2008; IOM, 2011; Porter-O'Grady & Malloch, 2015). However, more needs to be done to inform the public and policymakers of the substantial contributions professional nurses make to health care.

Evidence-based practice enables nurses to be taken more seriously by other health care providers and society. Scientific justification for nursing actions raises the level of professional practice. In addition, evidence-based practice may serve as the vehicle for the nursing profession to clearly define the term "nursing."

Multistate Compacts for Nursing Licensure in the United States (Probable Future)

Despite the recommendation by the Pew Health Professions Commission (1995) for health care professional regulation to remain controlled by individual states, the National Council of State Boards of Nursing (NCSBN) has initiated an effort for a mutual recognition model for professional nurse registration. The Multistate Compact started in 2000 and underwent a major revision in 2015 (NCSBN, 2015b). Under a mutual recognition model, RNs practicing nursing across state lines do not need a separate state nursing license provided that the states in which the practice participate in the **Nurse Licensure Compact**.

The interstate compact helps states with shortages of professional nurses by allowing nurses from bordering states to practice without needing to obtain an additional nursing license. Electronic- and telecommunication-based nursing practice frequently crosses state borders. The nurse would obtain licensure in the state of legal residence. To protect the integrity of individual state nurse practice acts, the nurse abides by the practice act of the state in which the client receives care (NCSBN, 2015b).

A single professional nursing license facilitates interstate practice, improves tracking of nurses with disciplinary problems, increases cost effectiveness, simplifies the nursing licensure process, eliminates duplicate listing of licensed nurses, and enhances interstate commerce. In addition, interstate licensure simplifies the licensing process for nurses who are employed by traveling nursing agencies (NCSBN, 2015b). Also, multistate compacts enable nurses to practice in diverse geographical locations, such as when many retired people follow desirable weather and establish residences in the northern United States in the summer and in southern states during the winter.

Although multistate professional licensure may seem appealing, several disadvantages accompany it. State boards of nursing may need to raise licensing fees for professional nurses to replace the revenue generated by nurses who formerly would have held more than one-state nursing license. Nurses with a disciplinary action record may not be able to obtain a fresh start in professional nursing after recovering from chemical addiction or after meeting the disciplinary requirements of a state board of nursing. Multistate licensure also would enable nursing agencies to provide replacement nurses for institutions experiencing shortages because their nurses decide to engage in collective bargaining or strikes to improve working conditions.

To maintain state control of professional nursing licensure, individual states must pass legislation to participate in the multistate licensure compact. As of May 2015, efforts to enact legislation have been successful in 25 states[1] (National Council of State Boards of Nursing, 2015a). Some failures in states attempting to participate in the Nurse Licensure Compact have been the result of failure of all nurses to support the idea. For example, some state nurses' associations oppose some elements contained in the language of the Compacts. In some states, participation in a multistate compact is prohibited by the state constitution, thereby creating another obstacle for multistate nursing licensure compact legislation.

The Demise of the Profession (Possible Future/Worst-Case Scenario)

The demise of the nursing profession is a possible future scenario. The nursing workforce continues to age and the proportion of associate degree nursing

---

[1]AK, Alaska; AZ, Arizona; CO, Colorado; DE, Delaware; IA, Iowa; ID, Idaho; KY, Kentucky; ME, Maine; MD, Maryland; MS, Mississippi; MO, Missouri; MT, Montana; NE, Nebraska; NH, New Hampshire; NM, New Mexico; NC, North Carolina; ND, North Dakota; RI, Rhode Island; SC, South Carolina; SD, South Dakota; TN, Tennessee; TX, Texas; UT, Utah; VA, Virginia; WI, Wisconsin.

graduates exceeds baccalaureate program nursing graduates. Nurses start to focus exclusively on the technical aspects of nursing practice resulting in increased patient mortality, morbidity, and adverse care events. The few BSN-prepared nurses enter the world of advanced practice nursing within a few years of graduation. Some states expand practice of emergency medical technicians to include providing services that currently fall within the scope of professional nursing practice in emergency departments and intensive care units.

Increased pressure for health care organizations to make profits or stay financially viable results in professional nurses assuming a subservient role to health care administrators. Creative ideas have surfaced to measure individual nurse productivity. For example, wireless communication devices enable administration to track every move made by every nurse. Although such devices reduce the time for nurses to meet client care requests (Kuruzovich, Angst, Faraj, & Agarwal, 2008), nurses receive negative performance evaluations for spending too much time providing education and emotional support to clients, completing required documentation, reporting to colleagues during shift changes, and taking breaks. Frustrated nurses dissuade others from entering the profession and the nursing workforce shrinks even more.

Efforts at private and federal funding for nursing students prove to be unsuccessful in attracting persons to enter the profession. Nursing ceases to be perceived by the public as the most ethical of all the professions because nurses must cater to the whims of employers. In response to the loss of professional power, nurses begin fighting with each other.

Because nurses fail to produce a united front for resolving practice and educational issues, they continue to lose power and autonomy. The lack of unity confuses policymakers and society. The marginalized status of nurses means they are denied participation in health care reform efforts, and a system is created that encourages increased workloads, multiple practice entries, and division within the profession (Allan, Tschudin, & Horton, 2008). Nurses are seen as the reason why errors occur in health care. Thus, nursing becomes the weakest link in acquiring and maintaining high-quality and safe health care delivery.

Nursing Gains Clout in Health Care (Preferred/Possible Future)

A more optimistic approach to and preferred scenario for the future of professional nursing would be that the profession becomes cohesive, provides solid evidence

for contributions made to health care, and is valued by society and other health professionals. Nurses have debated with each other for generations on issues such as entry-level education for professional practice, collective bargaining, defining professional nursing practice, and control of professional practice (e.g., American Nurses Association [ANA] vs. NCSBN, staff nurses vs. nurse administrators). Professional nurses work to safeguard the public against threats to health. Nurses have assumed the role of client advocate for many decades by protecting consumers from unscrupulous care providers and serious treatment errors. The movement toward a multidisciplinary health team approach to client care provides nurses with an opportunity to showcase their knowledge and expertise.

Research efforts demonstrate that outcomes are improved when clients receive care from professional nurses. Reductions in failure to rescue, nosocomial infections, and adverse effects of immobility also reduce hospital costs (Aiken et al., 1994, 2000; Buerhaus, Donelan, Ulrich, Norman, & Dittus, 2007; Doran, 2003; Gordon et al., 2008; Havens & Aiken, 1999; Unruh, 2008). However, executing studies does not mean changes in health care delivery happen automatically. Changes in public health care policy require an integrated and unified approach by the public, government, and nurses (Gordon et al., 2008; Milstead, 2008). Thus, professional nurses must determine a means to disseminate research findings to the public, inform the government of their needs and desires, and involve elected officials who draft legislation for policy changes (see Chapter 19, "The Professional Nurse's Role in Public Policy").

Take Note!

As nurses provide solid evidence for the contributions they make to health care, society, and other health team members will realize their value.

Along with improved societal status, professional nurses also become valued members of the health care team. Shared governance shifts from an exclusively nurse form of governance to an interdisciplinary form of governance (Porter-O'Grady & Malloch, 2015). Because of increased efforts of collaborative interdisciplinary teamwork, the health professions embark on providing interprofessional learning experiences that result in long-lasting effects. All team members understand their roles and gain increased respect for nursing's contributions to the interprofessional team efforts (Hylin, Nyholm, Mattiasson, & Ponzer, 2007; IOM, 2011).

When nurses demonstrate specialized knowledge and expertise that make differences in client care outcomes, society and other health team members will greatly value the profession. Nurses will enjoy greater autonomy and higher salaries. Then, the profession of nursing will have no difficulty attracting the best and brightest young people.

■ QUESTIONS FOR REFLECTION

1. What areas of nursing knowledge need further development?
2. How can nursing research affect the nursing profession and clinical practice?
3. What are the advantages and disadvantages of a multidisciplinary approach to health and health care research?
4. What might be some specific areas where a nursing approach to health and health care research might be beneficial to health care consumers and the delivery of health care services?

THE FUTURE OF NURSING EDUCATION

The knowledge base and technology used in providing nursing care will continue to increase, as will nurses' need for skill and ability in a number of areas.

1. Providing care to acutely ill clients
2. Monitoring for adverse effects of diagnostic tests, medications, radiation, and surgical interventions
3. Making critical clinical decisions
4. Using complex computer systems and technology effectively in clinical practice
5. Teaching clients, families, and caregivers how to manage health care needs effectively
6. Coordinating interprofessional health care teams
7. Delegating tasks to unlicensed assistive personnel
8. Collaborating with clients and health care professionals to improve the quality of health
9. Understanding and using research to provide a strong scientific base for nursing practice
10. Communicating to the public and health care providers the unique contributions nurses make to health care
11. Participating in political processes for shaping health care policies

In the future, more than ever, nurses will need a broad-based education, assertiveness skills, technical competence, and the ability to deal with rapid change. However, research and technology may provide the instruments nurses require for defining professional nursing, demonstrating that professional nursing care affects client care outcomes, and marketing professional nursing to the public.

Patterns of Nursing Education

Since the 1960s, there has been an intensive national effort to promote the Bachelor of Science in Nursing (BSN) degree as the entry level for professional nursing. In that time, although there has been an increase in the number of nurses prepared at the BSN level, there also has been a dramatic increase in the percentage of nurses prepared at the ADN level. More than 70% of currently practicing nurses are prepared at the technical level of nursing.

In the United States, education for entry into professional nursing can occur at one of four levels: the associate degree, the baccalaureate degree, the master's degree, or the doctoral degree. Thus, there are at least four different patterns of education that create nurses with different levels of knowledge and expertise. Importantly, having multiple entry levels into nursing creates confusion for health care consumers, who consider that all nurses are alike.

The current pattern of more professional nurses entering the profession at the ADN rather than the BSN level may continue. As a profession, nursing has been closely associated with upward mobility, especially for women. Most ADN programs are located in community colleges, making them financially and geographically accessible. Demand for an increased supply of licensed workers can readily be met in a short time. ADN-prepared nurses frequently work in the same positions as BSN-prepared nurses. However, some facilities require a minimum of a BSN for supervisory positions. As the complexity of professional nursing increases and nursing care moves to the community, where delivery settings have many uncontrolled variables, ADN-prepared nurses may lack the theoretical knowledge to deliver safe, effective nursing care. The Pew Task Force on Accreditation of Health Professions Education (1998) proposed an educational ladder for RNs with ADNs, and this practice was supported by the IOM (2011). Some nursing programs have developed creative approaches to advancing the level of nursing education. Examples of these programs include the RN to master's degree in nursing and the RN to nursing doctorate.

Before undertaking their baccalaureate studies, many students with an RN perceive nursing education at the BSN level as additional and partially redundant, rather than as different and enriching. Little incentive for professional education is provided by the delivery system, which lacks differential salary structures or clearly articulated differences in job expectations. Licensure as an RN after ADN education has reinforced this model.

However, in recognition of the improved patient outcomes noted in research studies, the IOM (2011) recommended to increase the proportion of nurses with BSN degrees from 50% to 80% by 2020. Many nursing organizations, including the ANA and the National League for Nursing, have endorsed this goal.

Take Note!

An increasing number of nurses are seeking baccalaureate education because of increased opportunities for promotion, perceived increased professional marketability, and improved job security.

Clinical Nurse Leader Program

In response to recommendations in reports generated by the IOM, the Joint Commission, and the Robert Wood Johnson Foundation for reducing fragmentation and increasing safety and quality of health care, AACN (2007) developed the Clinical Nurse Leader (CNL) program. The goal of this program is to provide a nurse generalist position with advanced education to offer leadership to clinical staff while coordinating client care across various health care settings. The CNL curriculum focuses on enhancing nursing leadership, managing clinical outcomes, understanding organizational and health care systems, facilitating change, and managing clinical environments using a complexity theory framework. Ideally, the graduate nursing program would develop partnerships with clinical facilities for clinical learning experiences while educating CNLs about needed services for a facility or health system (Begun, Hamilton, Tornabeni, & White, 2006; Gabuat, Hilton, Kinnaird, & Sherman, 2008; Magg, Buccheri, Capella, & Jennings, 2006; Rusch & Bakewell-Sachs, 2007).

Clinical Nurse Leaders concern themselves with microsystems (individual facilities or clinical units within a small geographical location). As the role has evolved, Rankin (2016) emphasizes how the CNL serves as a coach and mentor while providing professional role modeling for all health care team members. The CNL has a purpose to assess, intervene, and improve processes to optimize patient outcomes which is accomplished by assessing for patterns within the microsystem. The CNL serves as a provider of direct patient care, rapid response team member and

clinical resource for nursing staff members. When a patient becomes unstable, the CNL assists nursing staff by implementing interventions to stabilize the patient. The CNL directly monitors patient care and take prophylactic actions to avid potentially fatal care error. In addition, the CNL provides education to the interprofessional health care team when the need arises (Rankin, 2016).

The Nursing Doctorate

Currently, nurses basically have two paths to earn a nursing doctorate: the Philosophy (PhD) in nursing or the Doctor of Nursing Practice (DNP). Because of increasing confusion with the multiple doctoral nursing degrees and the high number of credit hours required for advanced practice nurse preparation, the AACN has determined that doctoral preparation in the form of the DNP will serve as the entry level to advanced nursing practice (AACN, 2015b; National Council State Board of Nursing [NCSBN], 2008). According to Advanced Practice Registered Nurse Consensus Model (NCSBN, 2008), the DNP degree is the preferred degree for advanced practice nursing roles (certified nurse midwife, nurse practitioner, clinical nurse specialist, and the certified registered nurse anesthetist). In 2015, 322 institutions of higher learning were conferring the DNP degree and another 60 DNP programs are in the planning phase (AACN, 2015a).

The DNP focuses attention on advanced practice nursing and the PhD aims to prepare nurse scientists who generate new nursing knowledge and develop a lifelong program of nursing research. The DNP degree also prepares nursing faculty, especially faculty who engage in clinical instruction of student (AACN, 2015b). However, some nursing faculty recognize the importance of education as a distinct discipline and have opted to earn PhDs in education, curriculum, and instruction or educational doctorates (EdD). The AACN (2015b) affirms that education is not an area of advanced nursing practice and that DNP programs should include education courses if the earned DNP is preparing future nurse educators.

Nursing Faculty Shortages

A barrier to increasing the number of nurses and their educational level is a shortage of nursing faculty (IOM, 2011). The current faculty shortage has prevented tens of thousands of people interested in pursuing a nursing career from gaining entry into nursing programs. According to the AACN (2015c), the average age of a doctoral-prepared professor was 61.6 years, associate professor 57.6 years, and assistant professor 51.4 years. The average age of an MSN-prepared assistant professor is 51.2 years.

Besides age, the following reasons have been identified for the growing nursing faculty shortage: (1) the profound gap in clinical and academic salaries for comparable or higher education, (2) the expense and time of pursuing a PhD in nursing, (3) the lack of effective educational preparation for assuming the full-time nurse faculty role (Fauteux, 2007), and (4) demands for nursing faculty to engage in research (sometimes, tenure decisions rely on the ability of faculty to secure extramural research grants), publication, service, and clinical practice. Like nurses in clinical practice, nursing faculty needs to engage in evidence-based teaching. For some faculty, keeping up with these multiple demands seems impossible, especially if they strive for an effective work–life balance.

Competition for Clinical Sites for Student Practice

Because nurse academia has increased the number of students accepted into nursing programs, educators sometimes have difficulty finding clinical placements for student clinical education. Hands-on, faculty supervised clinical placement has been required by state boards of nursing and the required number of clinical hours varies from state to state. With the introduction of high fidelity patient simulators, many educators have discovered that they can provide students with nearly identical clinical situations using case-based scenarios and high fidelity patient simulators. Nursing faculty can program the simulators to act in certain ways in order to assess student assessment and clinical decision-making skills. Clinical simulation provides students with a safe environment to practice skills and make clinical decisions in response to the simulator's condition (Curl, Smith, Chisholm, McGee, & Das, 2016; Forneris et al., 2015; Cazzell & Anderson, 2016). Educational outcomes for nursing students appear to be similar when clinical simulation replaces clinical setting practice hours according to the "National Council of State Boards of Nursing National Simulation Study" that is summarized in the following Focus on Research. Since the publication of the landmark National Simulation Study, more research has been published thereby adding to the credibility of its findings (Cummings, 2015; Curl et al., 2016; Forneris, et al., 2015; Cazzell & Anderson, 2016).

FOCUS ON RESEARCH

Comparing the Effects of Student Nurse Clinical Practice with High Fidelity Clinical Simulation in Prelicensure Nursing Education

The National Council of State Boards of Nursing National Simulation Study: A longitudinal, randomized, controlled study replacing clinical hours with simulation in prelicensure nursing education.

The National Council of State Boards of Nursing wanted to examine the effects of simulation (sim) on nursing student clinical competence, nursing knowledge, readiness for practice (student and nurse manager), and student perception of having learning needs met. They also wanted to determine how much simulation could replace student nurse direct clinical instruction hours.

The investigators of this study employed a longitudinal, randomized control study design using 10 American nursing traditional prelicensure education programs. Associate degree and bachelor of science degree programs were included in the study. Six hundred sixty-six students participated in the entire study that lasted 2 years. Three study groups were used. A control group with no more than 10% of clinical time spent in high fidelity simulation and two groups in which higher amounts of time during which high fidelity simulation substituted for actual student clinical practiced (25% and 50%).

Nursing knowledge was measured using the ATI Predictor®. Nursing competence was measured using the Creighton Competency Evaluation Instrument, New Graduate Performance Survey, Global Assessment of Clinical Competence, and Readiness for Practice tool. Critical thinking was measured using the Critical Thinking Diagnostic tool that measures problem recognition clinical decision making, prioritization, clinical implementation, and refection. Student perceptions of having learning needs met was assessed by the Clinical Learning Environment Comparison Survey. Minimal competence for safe clinical nursing practice was measured by the NCLEX-RN®. All instrument used in the study were reported to have effective validity and reliability.

Results of the study revealed that the control group had the lowest student program completion rate (79%). There were no statistically significant difference among the groups on the ATI Comprehensive Predictor® (control group—69.1%, 25% sim—88.4%, and 50% sim group—70.1%), NCLEX-RN® first-time pass rates (control group—96.4%, 25% sim—85.5, and 50% sim—87.1), nurse manager perceptions of clinical competence and readiness for practice, and student perception of having learning needs met (control group—96.4%, 25% sim—97.1%, and 50% sim—93.9%). There was a statistically significant attrition of minority students who participated in the study.

Findings of this study suggest that high fidelity simulation (up to 50% of clinical hours) can effectively replace nursing student clinical practice in professional nursing education programs. Nursing State Boards could relax the requirements for actual clinical setting practice hours for professional nursing students without compromising desired educational outcomes. Nursing faculty could increase the number of clinical simulation and decrease the number of direct clinical instruction hours knowing that student educational outcomes would be achieved. However, caution should be exercised if changes are made on the basis of the results of one well-designed research study.

Hayden, J. K., Smiley, R., Alexander, M., Kardong-Edgren, S., & Jeffires, P. (2014). The National Council of State Boards of Nursing National Simulation Study: A longitudinal, randomized, controlled study replacing clinical hours with simulation in prelicensure nursing education. *Journal of Nursing Regulation, 5*(2): July 2014 Supplement, S1–S66. doi: http://cmps-ezproxy.mnu.edu:2109/10.1016/j.ecns.2012.07.070

Future Scenarios for Nursing Education

Because of its newness, the outcomes of these radical changes in graduate and postgraduate nursing education have yet to be determined. A possible future (worst-case scenario) includes intense backlash against the revised model by current APRNs, a failure of higher learning institutions to provide required resources, a lack of available clinical facilities to develop service—education partnerships, increased nursing faculty shortages, and a failure of other health care professionals, along with general and specialty nursing organizations, to support the endeavor. There would be too few nursing faculty and clinical sites for students to learn the art and science of professional nursing at the associate, baccalaureate, graduate, and doctoral levels

of education. In the long term, there would be very few professional nurses available to meet the demands for nursing services.

The preferred future would be substantial improvements in client outcomes, heightened professional stature of the nursing profession, wide support for the revised nursing education plan by all health care stakeholders, and an increased supply of nursing faculty. The best and brightest persons would want to become nurses, and nursing academia would have ample faculty, well-stock nursing labs, high-tech simulation centers, and adequate clinical sites to teach the art and science of nursing effectively.

A more probable future scenario consists of mixed support and high criticism from other interprofessional health team and nurses (Silva & Ludwick, 2006). Nurses who want a career in research-oriented academic settings perceive the need to pursue a PhD, whereas nurses desiring a career in advanced nursing practice would pursue a DNP. DNP-prepared nurses would then be used as clinical faculty, leaving PhD-prepared nurses to assume classroom teaching and research activities (Loomis, Willard, & Cohen, 2007).

Adapting Nursing Education for the Future

The nursing profession needs to better articulate and publicize (both internally and to the public) the contributions of professionally educated practitioners to health promotion and restoration and illness prevention. This book has identified the knowledge base and values that characterize the professional nurse in the hope that this will be the first step toward acceptance of scholarship and demonstration of professional competence in practice.

All educational programs must continue to modify their curricula to include changes in the theoretical and technical database for professional nursing practice. For example, computer technology has had and will continue to have an enormous impact on discovery, communication, information storage, and instructional techniques. Clinical simulation learning experiences using high-tech manikins, software programs to simulate client responses, and well-designed case studies provide students with the opportunity to practice clinical decision making and skills in a safe environment (Fig. 22.3).

Many nursing programs provide online distance education as the primary means for instruction. Other programs offer hybrid nursing courses in which

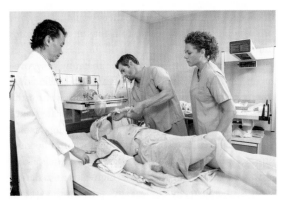

FIGURE 22.3 High fidelity simulation provides a mechanism for interprofessional education to train nurses to respond to clinical emergencies in health care facilities or in the community.

schools have included interdisciplinary educational learning activities with some success and long-term effects (Dinov, 2008; Hylin et al., 2007; IOM, 2011). In an ideal world, all members of the health care team should learn together, beginning with the first day of their professional education. Faculty from all respective disciplines also would learn and work collaboratively to prepare students to grasp individual discipline content while assessing interdisciplinary processes during carefully designed and conducted seminars.

Ironside and Valiga (2006) outlined a preferred future for nursing education (see Box 22.2, Professional Building Blocks, "Characteristics of an Ideal Nursing Education Program"). Unfortunately, their

content is provided using both online teaching strategies and face-to-face classroom instruction. Hybrid nursing courses typically use online methods for content acquisition (online lectures, podcasts) for student preparation. Students then apply content covered in preparatory activities in the classroom with faculty, solving clinical problems, completing a case study, or other contextual-based learning.

To create a nursing profession that meets the needs of a multicultural population, nurse educators must work to recruit students from a variety of cultural backgrounds. Professional nurses from various cultural backgrounds can help faculty in the recruitment and retention of a culturally diverse student population. More importantly, nurse educators must work to retain students from minority backgrounds once they are enrolled in nursing education programs. Special educational support systems may be required for remediation of reading and writing skills (especially for students for whom English is a second language). Curricular content and educational materials must include information regarding international cultural differences.

Culturally diverse students rely on faculty of similar backgrounds for an effective connection within nursing programs. However, until faculties become culturally diverse, current faculty members need to make special efforts to connect with minority students to help them succeed in nursing education, and perhaps, attract them to the world of nursing academia (IOM, 2011; Sullivan & Clinton, 1999; Sullivan Commission, 2004).

As the multidisciplinary health team approach to health care delivery grows, nurses will need education related to other health care providers and information on how to work as a team. Some health professional

22.2 Professional Building Blocks

Characteristics of an Ideal Nursing Education Program

An ideal nursing education program would

- include an open, flexible curriculum that responds to individualized student learning needs.
- provide a clinical practice focus in all nursing courses.
- include base course selection on student's individual interests (resulting in an individualized curriculum).
- include base faculty teaching assignments on areas of nursing in which they have great passion.
- include lively classroom discussions of significant issues.
- provide an atmosphere where students and faculty learn with each other.
- include course syllabi with suggested learning goals and activities.
- eliminate required textbooks with the understanding that students would discover effective learning materials.
- embrace and value diversity.
- include reciprocal challenges by students and faculty.
- employ faculty who work smarter, not harder.
- demonstrate visible thinking of faculty when interacting with students (including the admission of not knowing something).
- have supportive deans and directors who provide rewards and required resources for faculty to excel in teaching.

Ironside, P., & Valiga, T. (2006). Creating a vision for the future of nursing education: Moving toward excellence through innovation. *Nursing Education Perspectives, 27*(3), 120–121.

idea of nursing education would most likely not fulfill educational requirements outlined by most state boards of nursing. However, an egalitarian approach to learning the art and science of professional nursing would instill confidence in students as they master the cognitive, communication, and clinical skills required for effective professional nursing practice.

THE FUTURE OF NURSING SCHOLARSHIP

Within the past two decades, nursing research has received increased support from professional nurses and policymakers. In 2006, the National Institute of Nursing Research (NINR) celebrated its 20th anniversary as part of the National Institutes of Health. The NINR provides grant funding for nurse researchers, including studies that look at specific clinical care situations, ways to improve patient safety, and strategies to increase the professional nurse workforce. Results of funded nursing research are disseminated at annual NINR meetings.

Nursing research–based protocols have been developed for client care in the areas of skin management, cognitive impairment, culturally relevant care, pain control, and postoperative and chemotherapy-induced nausea and vomiting. Nursing research findings frequently cross health care disciplines. As interdisciplinary approaches to health care demonstrate improved client outcomes, nurses will be asked to participate in multidisciplinary research efforts. The National Institutes of Health's Roadmap to the Future offers opportunities for nurses to engage in multidisciplinary research projects.

Rapid development in nursing theory and research during the past quarter-century points to a promising outlook for the future. Nursing needs to develop and explicate theories to predict nursing outcomes. Increasingly, nursing research has validated models and theories for nursing care to provide foundations for care. As this trend continues, nursing will develop a unique knowledge base to fulfill the criteria defined for a profession.

Summary and Significance to Practice

Although the future cannot be predicted with great accuracy, nurses can accurately predict that health care delivery and the nursing profession will change. By visualizing several possible futures and identifying a preferred future, nurses can shape the future

of professional practice while planning for potential problems. The preferred future is one in which health care consumers, policymakers, and providers value the contributions nurses make to health care. To create the preferred future, nurses must use cognitive skills (to develop research projects demonstrating the value of professional nurses, make effective clinical decisions in practice, and find meaning in their careers), clinical skills (to effectively execute safe client care and promote client comfort and well-being), and communication skills (to collaborate with all health team members, including clients and families; promote public awareness of nursing's valuable contributions to society; shape health care policies; and recruit future nurses and sustain them once they enter the profession). The IOM (2011, p. 3) issued the following key messages for professional nursing and the health care delivery system.

1. Nurses should practice to the full extent of their education and training.
2. Nurses should achieve higher levels of education and training through an improved education system that promotes seamless academic progression.
3. Nurses should be full partners with physicians and other health care professionals in redesigning health care in the United States.
4. Effective workforce planning and policymaking require better data collection and an improved information infrastructure.

Table 22.1 outlines actions that individual nurses can take to facilitate implementation of the IOM's recommendations for nurses to lead change and advance the health of Americans in the future.

Take Note!
Competent nurses see opportunities to improve health care delivery and have the ability to work in today's increasingly complex health care environment while coping with constant change.

REAL-LIFE REFLECTIONS

Recall Jing from the beginning of the chapter. What assumptions did Jing make regarding her nursing career? How did these assumptions create a future problem for her? What advice would you give Jing to help her deal with her situation? How might Jing react to your advice? Specify reasons for each possible reaction that you identify.

TABLE 22.1 Individual Professional Nurse Action to Implement IOM Recommendations

IOM Recommendation	Nurse Action
Remove scope-of-practice barriers	Work with national, state, and local professional nursing organizations to develop a common strategic approach to contact governmental officials to pass legislation and revise current regulations to promote independent practice for APRNs and recognize contributions of nurse generalists in health care delivery.
Expand opportunities for nurses to lead and diffuse collaborative improvement efforts	Seek out opportunities to engage in workplace quality improvement processes such as performing concurrent or retrospective chart audits and auditing care in clinical settings to verify that best practices are being followed. Conduct quality improvement and evidence-based nursing research projects. Assist nurse researchers in the conduction of nursing research studies. Serve on nursing and organizational quality improvement committees. Document all care delivered to patients accurately so that efforts are forwarded to nursing national databases. Participate in quality improvement activities within professional nursing organizations.
Implement nurse residency programs	Serve on a planning committee that develops a nurse residency program in your facility. Offer to help staff educators with a local nurse residency program. Serve as a preceptor for a new graduate nurse. Enable new graduate nurses to participate in all nurse residency program activities. Support new graduate nurses as they experience the transition to independent practice.
Increase the proportion of nurses with a baccalaureate degree to 80% by 2020	Return to college to earn a BSN or higher degree. Encourage colleagues without a BSN to return to school. Talk positively about educational experience with colleagues after returning to school. Take advantage of employer-sponsored and available government programs that offer financial assistance to earn a BSN. Share with prospective nursing students' information about all educational opportunities for professional nursing, including how to start as an unlicensed care provider and how to earn a BSN (or even a nursing doctorate).
Double the number of nurses with a doctorate by 2020	Return to school to earn a graduate and postgraduate degree. Consider seriously a career in nursing academics. Utilize employer-sponsored and governmental programs that provide support to nurses earning nursing doctorates. Share with nursing colleagues and potential nursing students information about educational opportunities, especially how to start as an unlicensed assistive personnel and end with a nursing doctorate.
Ensure that nurses engage in lifelong learning.	Complete professional continuing education (CE) programs online or attend nursing CE programs. Take full advantage of any employer-sponsored CE education programs and educational funding opportunities. Subscribe to and read general nursing journals and those pertinent to the area of practice. Seek professional certification in the practice area. Subscribe to online resources that provide periodic updates on clinical practice, health policy, and scientific findings.
Prepare and enable nurses to lead change to advance health	Assume personal responsibility for professional growth. Speak up and advocate for change in clinical practice settings. Join and actively participate in professional nursing organizations. Request to and become involved with making budget requests and the budgeting process in the workplace. Serve on a board, executive management team, or other community-based committee (e.g., parent–teacher associations, faith-based groups, neighborhood associations). Run for a leadership position for any community association or organizational committee. Run for political office.
Build an infrastructure for the collection and analysis of interprofessional health care workforce data	Complete governmental surveys that collect data regarding professional nurses (e.g., National Sample of Registered Nurses Survey, State Board of Nursing Surveys). Register as a professional nurse to serve as a responder for a disaster at the local, state, or federal level.

Institute of Medicine. (2011). *The future of nursing: Leading change, advancing health* (pp. 3–7). Washington, DC: National Academies Press.

From Theory to Practice

1. Make a list of the scenarios in this chapter that seem implausible and those with which you do not agree. Conduct a literature search to substantiate your viewpoints on the list of identified scenarios. Develop a more realistic scenario.
2. What actions can you take to promote a preferred future for the nursing profession? Why are these actions important?

Nurse as Author

Pretend that you are a time traveler visiting the year 2050. Describe the condition of the nursing profession in the United States, taking into account the quality of nursing education and health care delivery. What challenges confront the profession? How might the profession as it exists today prepare to meet the future challenges you describe?

Your Digital Classroom

Online Exploration

American Association of Colleges of Nursing: **www.aacn.nche.edu**
American Nurses Association: **www.nursingworld.org**
Institute for Alternative Futures: **http://altfutures.com/**
Institute for the Future: **http://www.iftf.org/home/**
National League for Nursing: **www.nln.org**
Sigma Theta Tau International: **www.nursingsociety.org**
Stem Cell Information (National Institutes of Health): **http://stemcells.nih.gov/Pages/Default.aspx**
The Campaign for Nursing's Future: **www.discovernursing.com**

Expanding Your Understanding

1. Visit the home page of Sigma Theta Tau International www.nursingsociety.org, and click on "About STTI." You will see a heading "Position Papers," on the left side of the screen. Click on it. On the next screen you will see a heading "Position Statements and Resource Papers." Find the Resource Papers heading and underneath it you will see "ARISTA 3: Nurses and Health: A Global Future"; click on this title to read about the findings of the Sigma Theta

Tau Think Tank along with proposed initiative for the future of nursing. Do you think the preferred future outlined in this document is desirable? Why or why not? How can you contribute to the preferred future of the nursing profession outlined in this document?
2. Visit the AACN web site and read the position statement published by the TriCouncil on the Nursing Shortage. (American Association of Colleges of Nursing, American Nurses Association, American Organization of Nurse Executives & National League for Nursing) **http://www.aacn.nche.edu/publications/position/tri-council-shortage**. What can we do collectively as a profession to alleviate the nursing shortage? What can you do as an individual? What are the potential consequences of inaction in this future crisis for health care and the nursing profession?

Beyond the Book

Visit **thePoint®** **www.thePoint.lww.com** for activities and information to reinforce the concepts and content covered in this chapter.

REFERENCES

Aburdene, P., & Naisbitt, J. (1992). *Megatrends for women.* New York: Villard.

Adler, R., Dunagan, J., Kreit, B., et al. (2009). *HC2010 perspectives.* Palo Alto, CA: Institute for the Future.

Agnes, M. (2005). *Webster's new world college dictionary* (4th ed.). Cleveland, OH: Wiley.

Aiken, L., Clarke, S., & Sloane, D. (2000). Hospital restructuring: Does it adversely affect care and outcomes? *Journal of Nursing Administration, 30,* 457–465.

Aiken, L., Smith, H., & Lake, E. (1994). Lower Medicare mortality among a set of hospitals known for good nursing care. *Medical Care, 32,* 771–785.

Allan, H., Tschudin, V., & Horton, K. (2008). The devaluation of nursing: A position statement. *Nursing Ethics, 15*(4), 549–556.

American Association of Colleges of Nursing. (2007). *White paper on the role of the clinical nurse leader.* Retrieved from www.aacn.nche.edu/Publications/WhitePapers/ClinicalNurseLeader.htm. Accessed March 5, 2013.

American Association of Colleges of Nursing. (2014). *Nursing shortage.* Retrieved from http://www.aacn.nche.edu/media-relations/fact-sheets/nursing-shortage.Accessed July 3, 2016.

American Association of Colleges of Nursing. (2015a). *Fact sheet, The Doctor of Nursing Practice.* Retrieved from http://www.aacn.nche.edu/media-relations/fact-sheets/dnp. Accessed July 4, 2016.

American Association of Colleges of Nursing. (2015b). *The Doctor of Nursing Practice: Current Issues and Clarifying Recommendations.* Retrieved from http://www.aacn.nche.edu/aacn-publications/white-papers/DNP-Implementation-TF-Report-8–15.pdf

American Association of Colleges of Nursing. (2015c). *Nursing faculty shortage fact sheet.* Retrieved from http://www.aacn.nche.edu/media-relations/FacultyShortageFS.pdf. Accessed July 4, 2016.

Begun, J., Hamilton, J., Tornabeni, J., & White, K. (2006). Opportunities for improving patient care through lateral integration: The clinical nurse leader. *Journal of Healthcare Management, 51*(1), 19–25.

Bezold, C. (1996). Your health in 2010: Four scenarios. *The Futurist, 30,* 35–39.

Brush, B. (2008). Global nurse migration today. *Journal of Nursing Scholarship, 40*(1), 20–25.

Buerhaus, P., Donelan, K., Ulrich, B., Norman, L., & Dittus, R. (2007). State of the registered nurse workforce in the United States. *Nursing Economic$, 25*(1), 6–12.

Burke, S., & Kirk, M. (2006). Genetics education in the nursing profession: A literature review. *Journal of Advanced Nursing, 38,* 228–227.

Canham, D., Mao, C., Yoder, M., Connolly, P., & Dietz, E. (2008). The Omaha system and quality measurement in academic nurse-managed centers: Ten steps for implementation. *Journal of Nursing Education, 47*(3), 105–110.

Canton, J. (2015). *Future Smart: Managing the game-changing trends that will transform your world.* Philadelphia, PA: Da Capo Press.

Cazzell, M., & Anderson, M. (2016). The impact of critical thinking on clinical judgment during simulation with senior nursing students. *Nursing Education Perspectives, 37*(2), 83–90. doi: 2109/10.5480/15–1553

Centers for Disease Control and Prevention. (2008). *CDC behavioral risk factor surveillance system.* Retrieved from www.cdc.gov/brfss/. Accessed March 5, 2013.

Centers for Disease Control and Prevention. (2010). Number of Americans with diabetes projected to double or triple by 2050. Retrieved from http://www.cdc.gov/media/pressrel/2010/r101022.html. Accessed June 26, 2013.

Centers for Disease Control and Prevention. (2015a). Adult obesity facts. Retrieved from http://www.cdc.gov/obesity/data/adult.html. Accessed July 3, 2016.

Centers for Disease Control and Prevention. (2015b). Diabetes 2014 Report Card. Retrieved from http://www.cdc.gov/diabetes/pdfs/library/diabetesreportcard2014.pdf. Accessed July 3, 2016.

Centers for Disease Control and Prevention, National Center for Health Statistics. (2015). Health, United States-2015 Health and risk factors. Retrieved from http://www.cdc.gov/nchs/data/hus/2015/058.pdf. Accessed July 3, 2016.

Cetron, M., & Davies, O. (2008). *Trends shaping tomorrow's world forecasts and implications for business, government and consumers.* Bethesda, MD: World Future Society.

Cummings, C. (2015). Evaluating clinical simulation. *Nursing Forum, 50*(2), 109–115. doi: 2109/10.1111/nuf.12075

Curl, D., Smith, S., Chisholm, L. A., McGee, L. A., & Das, K. (2016). Effectiveness of integrated simulation and clinical experiences compared to traditional clinical experiences for nursing students. *Nursing Education Perspectives, 37*(2), 72–77. doi:2109/10.5480/15–1647

Dinov, I. (2008). Integrated, multidisciplinary and technology-enhanced science education: The next frontier. *MERLOT Journal of Online Learning and Teaching, 4*(1), 84–93.

Doran, D. (Ed.). (2003). *Nursing-sensitive outcomes: State of the science.* Sudbury, MA: Jones & Bartlett.

Dunton, N. (2008). Take a cue from the NDNQI. *Nursing Management, 39*(4), 20, 22, 23.

Emmerich, R. (2004). *The day after tomorrow [motion picture].* Los Angeles, CA: 20th Century Fox.

Fauteux, N. (2007). The nursing faculty shortage: Public and private partnerships address a growing need. In *Charting nursing's future.* Princeton, NJ: Robert Wood Johnson Foundation.

Formella, N., & Rovin, S. (2004). Creating a desirable future for nursing. Part 2: The issue. *Journal of Nursing Administration, 34,* 264–267.

Forneris, S. G., Neal, D. O., Jone, T., Keihn, M. B., Meyer, H. M., Blazovich, L. M., et al. (2015). Enhancing clinical reasoning through simulation debriefing: A multisite study. *Nursing Education Perspectives, 36*(5), 304–310. doi: 10.5480/15–1672

Gabuat, J., Hilton, N., Kinnaird, L., & Sherman, R. (2008). Implementing the clinical nurse leader role in a for-profit environment: A case study. *Journal of Nursing Administration, 38*(6), 302–307.

Gordon, S., Buchanan, J., & Bretherton, T. (2008). *Safety in numbers: Nurse-to-patient ratios and the future of health care.* Ithaca, NY: Cornell University Press.

Havens, D., & Aiken, L. (1999). Shaping systems to promote desired outcomes. *Journal of Nursing Administration, 29,* 14–20.

Henchley, N. (1978). Making sense of the future. *Alternatives, 7,* 24–26.

Herzlinger, R. (2004). *Consumer-driven health care.* San Francisco, CA: Jossey-Bass.

Hinshaw, A. (2008). Navigating the perfect storm: Balancing a culture of safety with workforce changes. *Nursing Research, 57*(1, Suppl 1), S4–S10.

Hylin, U., Nyholm, H., Mattiasson, C., & Ponzer, S. (2007). Interprofessional training in clinical practice on a training ward for healthcare students: A two-year follow-up. *Journal of Interprofessional Care, 21*(3), 277–288.

Institute for Alternative Futures. (2012). *Primary care 2025: A scenario exploration.* Alexandria, VA: Author. Retrieved from www.altfutures.com/pubs/pc2025/IAF-PrimaryCare2025Scenarios.pdf. Accessed March 5, 2013.

Institute for the Future. (2016). Health Aware World Map. Retrieved from http://www.iftf.org/our-work/health-self/health-horizons/healthaware/. Accessed July 3, 2016.

Institute of Medicine. (2000). *To err is human: Building a safer health system.* Washington, DC: National Academies Press.

Institute of Medicine. (2001). *Crossing the quality chasm: A new health system for the 21st century.* Washington, DC: National Academies Press.

Institute of Medicine. (2003). *Health professions education: A bridge to quality.* Washington, DC: National Academies Press.

Institute of Medicine. (2004). *Keeping patients safe: Transforming the work environment of nurses.* Washington, DC: National Academies Press.

Institute of Medicine. (2006). *Identifying and preventing medication errors.* Washington, DC: National Academies Press.

Institute of Medicine. (2008). *Retooling for an aging America.* Washington, DC: National Academies Press.

Institute of Medicine. (2011). *The future of nursing: Leading change, advancing health.* Washington, DC: The National Academies Press.

Institute of Medicine. (2012). *Accelerating progress in obesity prevention: Solving the weight of the nation.* Washington, DC: The National Academies Press.

Ironside, P., & Valiga, T. (2006). Creating a vision for the future of nursing education: Moving toward excellence through innovation. *Nursing Education Perspectives, 27*(3), 120–121.

Johnson, T., & White, A. (2000). Six business principles for the 21st century. *Civilization, 61*(2), 57.

Kaku, M. (2011). *The physics of the future.* New York: First Anchor Books.

Kirk, H. (2007). Towards a global nursing workforce: The "brain circulation." *Nursing Management, 12*(10), 26–30.

Kurtzman, E., & Buerhaus, P. (2008). New Medicare payment rules: Danger or opportunity for nursing? *American Journal of Nursing, 108*(6), 30–35.

Kuruzovich, J., Angst, C., Faraj, S., & Agarwal, R. (2008). Wireless communication in patient response time. *CIN Computers, Informatics Nursing, 26*(3), 159–166.

Loomis, J., Willard, B., & Cohen, J. (2007). Difficult professional choices: Deciding between the PhD and the DNP in nursing. *Online Journal of Issues in Nursing, 12*(1), 6. Retrieved from http://www.nursingworld.org/MainMenuCategories/ANAMarketplace/ANAPeriodicals/OJIN/TableofContents/Volume122007/No1Jan07/ArticlePreviousTopics/tpc28_816033.html. Accessed June 24, 2013.

Magg, M., Buccheri, R., Capella, E., & Jennings, D. (2006). A conceptual framework for a clinical nurse leader program. *Journal of Professional Nursing, 22*(6), 367–372.

Millett, S., & Kopp, W. (1996). The top 10 innovative products for 2006: Technology with a human touch. *The Futurist, 30,* 16–20.

Milstead, J. A. (2008). *Health policy and politics: A nurse's guide* (3rd ed.). Sudbury, MA: Jones & Bartlett.

Minkin, B. H. (1995). *Future in sight.* New York: Macmillan.

Myers, V., & Dreachslin, J. (2007). Recruitment and retention of a diverse workforce: Challenges and opportunities. *Journal of Healthcare Management, 52*(5), 290–298.

Naisbitt, J. (1996). *Megatrends Asia.* New York: Simon & Schuster.

Naisbitt, J., & Aburdene, P. (1990). *Megatrends 2000.* New York: Penguin.

National Council of State Boards of Nursing. (2008). *Consensus Model for APRN Regulation: Licensure, Accreditation, Certification & Education.* Retrieved from https://ncsbn.org/Consensus_Model_for_APRN_Regulation_July_2008.pdf. Accessed July 4, 2016.

National Council of State Boards of Nursing. (2015a). 25 Nurse Licensure Compact (NLC). States. Retrieved from https://www.ncsbn.org/NLC_Implementation_2015.pdf. Accessed July 3, 2016.

National Council of State Boards of Nursing. (2015b). Nursing Licensure Compact. Retrieved from https://www.ncsbn.org/NLC_Final_050415.pdf. Accessed July 3, 2016.

National Institute of Medicine and the National Research Council. (1999). *Chemical and biological terrorism.* Washington, DC: National Academies Press.

Neal-Boylan, L., Coccoa, K., & Carnoali, B. (2009). The benefits to working for retired RNs. *Geriatric Nursing, 30*(6), 378–383.

Niccol, A. (1997). *Gattaca [motion picture].* Los Angeles, CA: Columbia Pictures.

Pew Health Professions Commission. (1995). *Critical challenges: Revitalizing the health professions for the twenty-first century.* San Francisco, CA: University of California, San Francisco Center for the Health Professions.

Pew Task Force on Accreditation of Health Professions Education. (1998). *Recreating health professional practice for a new century.* San Francisco, CA: University of California, San Francisco Center for the Health Professions.

Porter-O'Grady, T., & Malloch, K. (2015). *Quantum leadership: Building better partnerships for sustainable health* (4th ed.) Burlington, MA: Jones & Bartlett. Learning.

Rankin, V. (2016). Clinical nurse leader: A role for the 21st century. *MedSurg Nursing, 24*(3), 199–201.

Robert Woods Johnson Foundation. (2014). Older nurses push retirement envelope. Retrieved from http://www.rwjf.org/en/library/articles-and-news/2014/12/older-nurses-push-retirement-envelope.html. Accessed July 3, 2016.

Rusch, L., & Bakewell-Sachs, S. (2007). The CNL: A gateway to better care? *Nursing Management, 38*(4), 32, 34, 36, 37.

Sachs, J. (2008). *Common wealth: Economics for a crowded planet.* New York: Penguin.

Sherwood, G., & Barnsteiner, J. (2012). *Quality and safety in nursing.* Chichester, UK: John Wiley & sons.

Silva, M., & Ludwick, R. (2006). Is the doctor of nursing practice ethical? *Online Journal of Issues in Nursing, 11*(2). Retrieved from http://www.medscape.com/viewarticle/536482. Accessed June 24, 2013.

Sullivan, E. J. (Ed.). (1999). *Creating nursing's future.* St. Louis, MO: Mosby.

Sullivan, E. J., & Clinton, J. F. (1999). Achieving a multicultural nursing profession. In E. J. Sullivan (Ed.), *Creating nursing's future: Issues, opportunities, and challenges.* St. Louis, MO: Mosby.

Sullivan Commission. (2004). *Missing persons: Minorities in the health professions: A report of the Sullivan Commission on diversity in the healthcare workforce.* Retrieved from www.aacn.nche.edu/media-relations/sullivanreport.pdf. Accessed March 5, 2013.

Tariman, J. (2008). Technologic advancements in cancer care. *ONS Connect, 22*(7), 8–12.

Toffler, A. (1970). Future shock. New York: Random House.

Toffler, A. (1990). *Powershift: Knowledge, wealth, and violence at the edge of the 21st century.* New York: Bantam.

Toffler, A., & Toffler, H. (2006). *Revolutionary wealth: How it will be created and how it will change our lives.* New York: Currency Doubleday.

Tripp Umbach. (2012). *The negative employment impacts of the Medicare cuts in the Budget Control Act of 2011.* Retrieved from www.aha.org/content/12/12sep-bcaeconimpact.pdf. Accessed March 5, 2013.

Underwood, A., & Adler, J. (2005). Diet and genes. *Newsweek, 145,* 39–48.

Unruh, L. (2008). Nurse staffing and patient, nurse and financial outcomes. *American Journal of Nursing, 108*(1), 62–71.

U.S. Department of Health and Human Services, Administration on Aging. (2012). *Older Americans 2012 Key Indicators or Well-being.* Retrieved from http://www.agingstats.gov/agingstatsdotnet/Main_Site/Data/2012_Documents/Docs/EntireChartbook.pdf. Accessed July 3, 2016.

U.S. Department of Health and Human Services, Administration on Aging. (2016). Aging statistics. Retrieved from http://www.aoa.gov/Aging_Statistics/. Accessed July 3, 2016.

U.S. Bureau of Health Professions, Health Resources and Services Administration. (2013). The U.S. Nursing Workforce: Trends in supply and education. Retrieved from http://bhpr.hrsa.gov/healthworkforce/reports/nursingworkforce/nursingworkforcefullreport.pdf. Accessed July 3, 2016.

Veenema, T. (Ed.). (2013). *Disaster nursing and emergency preparedness for chemical, biological and radiological terrorism and other hazards* (3rd ed.). New York: Springer.

Vlasses, F., & Smeltzer, C. (2007). Toward a new future for healthcare and nursing practice. *Journal of Nursing Administration, 37*(9), 375–380.

Zander, T., Debey-Pascher, S., Eggle, D., Staratschek-Jox, A., Stoelben, E., Linseisen, J., et al. (2008, May). *Predictive value of transcriptional changes in peripheral blood for future clinical onset of lung cancer in asymptomatic smokers [Abstract 1509].* Paper presented at the annual meeting of the American Society of Clinical Oncology, Chicago.

American Nurses Association Standards of Professional Nursing Practice*

STANDARDS OF PRACTICE

Standard 1. Assessment
The registered nurse collects pertinent data and information relative to the health care consumer's health or the situation.

Standard 2. Diagnosis
The registered nurse analyzes the assessment data to determine actual or potential diagnoses, problems, and issues.

Standard 3. Outcomes Identification
The registered nurse identifies expected outcomes for a plan individualized to the health care consumer or the situation.

Standard 4. Planning
The registered nurse develops a plan that prescribes strategies to attain expected, measurable outcomes.

Standard 5. Implementation
The registered nurse implements the identifed plan.

Standard 5A. Coordination of Care
The registered nurse coordinates care delivery.

Standard 5B. Health Teaching and Health Promotion
The registered nurse employs strategies to promote health and a safe environment.

Standard 6. Evaluation
The registered nurse evaluates progress toward attainment of goals and outcomes.

STANDARDS OF PROFESSIONAL PERFORMANCE

Standard 7. Ethics
The registered nurse practices ethically.

Standard 8. Culturally Congruent Practice
The registered nurse practices in a manner that is congruent with cultural diversity and inclusion principles.

Standard 9. Communication
The registered nurse communicates effectively in all areas of practice.

Standard 10. Collaboration
The registered nurse collaborates with health care consumer and other key stakeholders in the conduct of nursing practice.

Standard 11. Leadership
The registered nurse leads within the professional practice setting and the profession.

Standard 12. Education
The registered nurse seeks knowledge and competence that reflects current nursing practice and promotes futuristic thinking.

Standard 13. Evidence-Based Practice and Research
The registered nurse integrates evidence and research findings into practice.

Standard 14. Quality of Practice
The registered nurse contributes to quality nursing practice.

Standard 15. Professional Practice Evaluation
The registered nurse evaluates one's own and others' nursing practice.

Standard 16. Resource Utilization
The registered nurse utilizes appropriate resources to plan, provide, and sustain evidence-based nursing services that are safe, effective, and financially responsible.

Standard 17. Environmental Health
The registered nurse practices in an environmentally safe and healthy manner.

Note: Page number followed by b, f, and t indicates text in box, figure, and table, respectively.